Principles and Practice of Clinical Cardiovascular Genetics

Principles and Practice of Clinical Cardiovascular Genetics

EDITED BY

Dhavendra Kumar, MD, FRCP, FRCPCH, FACMG

Consultant Clinical Geneticist, Institute of Medical Genetics,
University Hospital of Wales, Cardiff, UK

Perry Elliott, MD, FRCP

Reader in Inherited Heart Disease and Hon. Consultant Cardiologist,
The Heart Hospital, University College Hospital, London, UK

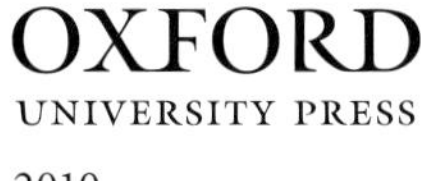

2010

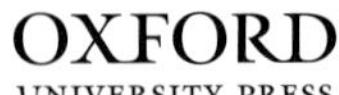

Oxford University Press, Inc., publishes works that further
Oxford University's objective of excellence
in research, scholarship, and education.

Oxford New York
Auckland Cape Town Dar es Salaam Hong Kong Karachi
Kuala Lumpur Madrid Melbourne Mexico City Nairobi
New Delhi Shanghai Taipei Toronto

With offices in
Argentina Austria Brazil Chile Czech Republic France Greece
Guatemala Hungary Italy Japan Poland Portugal Singapore
South Korea Switzerland Thailand Turkey Ukraine Vietnam

Published by Oxford University Press, Inc.
198 Madison Avenue, New York, New York 10016
www.oup.com

Library of Congress Cataloging-in-Publication Data
Principles and practice of clinical cardiovascular genetics / edited by Dhavendra Kumar, Perry Elliott.
p. ; cm.
Includes bibliographical references and index.
ISBN 978-0-19-536895-6
1. Cardiovascular system—Diseases—Genetic aspects. I. Kumar, Dhavendra. II. Elliott, Perry.
[DNLM: 1. Cardiovascular Diseases—genetics. 2. Cardiovascular Diseases—diagnosis.
3. Cardiovascular Diseases—therapy. 4. Genetic Predisposition to Disease. WG 120 C641 2009]
RC669.P673 2009
616.1'.04—dc22
2009066873

9 8 7 6 5 4 3 2 1

Printed in China
on acid-free paper

If there were no individual variability, medicine would have been science not an art.

Sir William Osler (1849–1919)

Chief Physician,
Johns Hopkins Hospital,
Baltimore, Maryland (1888)
Regius Professor of Medicine, 1905
Oxford University

Foreword

At the end of 2007, Science recognized human genetic variation as the "Breakthrough of the Year." After nearly 7 years from the announcement of the draft human genome in 2000, there has been quite a remarkable avalanche of discoveries of genes and pathways that represent the underpinnings of complex traits. This unprecedented discovery work has been an outgrowth of three major concurrent fronts of progress. First, the Human Genome Project itself laid the groundwork of sequencing the 3.1 million haploid base pairs. Second, it took the International HapMap and related projects to breakdown the billions of base pairs to heritable linkage disequilibrium blocks that could be tagged with one or more single nucleotide polymorphisms (SNPs). And third, advances in ultrahigh-throughput genotyping set up the potential to assay up to 1 million SNPs per individual, paving the way for contemporary whole genome association studies. In the past year alone, more than 40 common diseases have undergone such study, which has identified new genes and pathways that were never conceived of relating to the disease or trait of interest. In a short time of a year or two, the knowledge base of the molecular underpinnings of diseases has exploded and transcended decades of prior biomedical research effort. The textbooks of medicine need to be rewritten, as our insights about so many common diseases have been greatly enhanced.

A new textbook on the subject of cardiovascular genetics is particularly welcome in the midst of the ongoing revolution. With cardiovascular diseases still the number one cause of death and disability in the world, progress in genomics and genetics is especially vital. Two cardiovascular genetic experts, Drs. Dhavendra Kumar and Perry Elliott, have carefully edited a comprehensive textbook that presents beyond state-of-the-art reviews of virtually every pertinent topic in this field. The first section provides a superb foundation in classification, epidemiology, and even delves into imaging. This is followed in the second section by 25 chapters, each of which zooms on particular conditions from arrhythmias, structural disorders, systemic diseases, and the most important condition from the standpoint of public health—coronary artery disease. The third and final section gets into the management and practical issues, providing critical context of how the findings in cardiovascular genetics should influence day-to-day clinical care. The authors are internationally recognized authorities in the topics that are reviewed.

This effort will surely be seen as a tour de force in the cardiovascular arena. At just a time when there has been such exceptional progress through intensive research, the editors and authors have managed to cull together such a valuable resource. This also comes at a time when genetic testing, once only a research tool in cardiovascular medicine, is coming out and starting to be part of mainstream medicine. This is the new era when individuals can order their own genome-wide scan of 1 million SNPs that tag most of the heritable linkage disequilibrium bins, providing association data to many common complex cardiovascular diseases such as myocardial infarction, abdominal aortic aneurysm, intracranial aneurysm, peripheral arterial disease, the variety of lipoprotein abnormalities, and atrial fibrillation. When patients are armed with this genomic information and approach their cardiologists, it will become increasingly important for the medical community to keep up with the remarkable pace of discovery in this discipline. This goes well beyond the longstanding debates about rare Mendelian traits such as long QT syndrome and hypertrophic cardiomyopathy as to whether genotyping should be part of the routine work up. And before the second edition of this textbook is ready, whole genome sequencing will become a reality and further catapult the definition of cardiovascular diseases at the molecular level.

Clinical Cardiovascular Genetics is a superb textbook that will prove as a valuable resource to cardiovascular practitioners and researchers, and the health care team of cardiovascular nurses and genetic counselors. The timing of this comprehensive and practically minded monograph could not possibly have been better!

Eric J Topol, MD, FACC, FESC, FAHA, FACP
Dean, Scripps School of Medicine
Director, Scripps Translational Science Institute
Professor of Translational Genomics,
The Scripps Research Institute
Senior Consultant of Cardiovascular Diseases,
Scripps Clinic
La Jolla, California

Acknowledgments

Any major undertaking such as developing the idea of a new book and bringing this to real existence requires concerted efforts of several people with varying skills and dedication. This new book, probably first of its kind, was conceived out of sheer imagination when both of us argued on a number of issues related to inherited cardiovascular diseases. It became evidently clear that there was a huge gap in the available medical literature to offer a balanced and up-to-date account to the busy clinician and some one with a special interest in genetic conditions of heart and blood vessels. We both appreciated this need and embarked on this project. Most of our colleagues welcomed the idea and encouraged us to develop this further.

Several colleagues from Cardiff and London offered support and advice in early stages of planning, notably Prof. Peter Harper, Prof. Julian Sampson, Prof. Angus Clarke, Dr. Annie Procter, Mrs. Mary Nicol, and Prof. Bill McKenna. We are grateful to both Peter Harper and Bill McKenna for agreeing to mentor us as advisory editors. The mammoth task of planning and selecting the expert authors for individual chapters was facilitated by several experts from Cardiology and Medical Genetics including Teri Manolio (NIH/NHBRI, USA), Mark Rees (Swansea, Wales), Paul Brennon (New Castle upon Tyne, England), Sally Davies (Cardiff, Wales), Pier Lambiase (London, England), Zaheer Yousef (Cardiff, Wales), Michael Patton (London, England), and Silvia Priori (Pavia, Italy).

We are fortunate to have the privilege of editing several well-written and masterly presented manuscripts covering the vast field of clinical cardiovascular genetics. We are convinced that each chapter is a detailed and comprehensive account of the specific condition or subject. We have taken into consideration that the whole field is rapidly evolving and fast developing, and therefore a reader might find few gaps in the literature cited. However, all authors and contributors have worked extremely hard to offer the readership the core and factual information on a broad range of inherited cardiovascular conditions. As editors we will always remain indebted to them for this huge undertaking on their part. This is also acknowledged and appreciated by Prof. Eric Topol (San Diego, USA) in his excellent foreword.

Compiling and editing a book of this size is impossible without the secretarial/editorial support. Ms. Cetra Hastings (Oxford, England) deserves special thanks for providing this support. Finally, we are grateful to Bill Lamsback and Tracy O'Hara from Oxford University Press (New York) for their enthusiastic support and patience in bringing our dream to reality. We humbly present this book to our readers and hope that this fulfills its obligations. Any controversial opinion or statement would reflect individual author's view and should be referred to the respective author(s). All errors and omissions are entirely ours.

Dhavendra Kumar
Perry Elliott

Contents

Contributors

Ibrar Ahmed, MRCP
Department of Cardiovascular Medicine
The Medical School University of Birmingham
Edgbaston
Birmingham, UK

Robert H Anderson, MD, FRCPath
Professorial Fellow
Institute of Child Health
University College
London, UK

Elijah R Behr, MD
Cardiac and Vascular Division
St George's University of London
London
SW17 0RE, UK

Jamie Bentham
Department of Paediatric Cardiology
Oxford Children's Hospital
Oxford, OX3 9DU

Shoumo Bhattacharya, MD, FRCP
Professor of Cardiology
Department of Cardiovascular Medicine
Wellcome Trust Centre for Human Genetics
University of Oxford
Roosevelt Drive
Oxford, UK

Elena Biagini
Institute of Cardiology
University of Bologna
S.Orsola-Malpighi Hospital
Bologna, Italy

John P Bourke, MD, FRCP
Department of Cardiology
Freeman Hospital
Institute of Human Genetics
University of Newcastle upon Tyne
England, UK

Paul Brennan, FRCP
Northern Genetics Service
Institute of Human Genetics
Newcastle upon Tyne, UK

Ulrich Broeckel, MD
Departments, Human and Molecular Genetics, Physiology and Medicine
Medical College of Wisconsin
Milwaukee, WI, USA
and Department of Pediatrics
Children's Hospital of Wisconsin
Milwaukee, WI, USA

Nigel A Brown, BSc, PhD
Professor/Dean, Faculty of Medicine and Biomedical Sciences
Head, Division of Basic Medical Sciences
St. George's, University of London
Cranmer Terracew
London, UK

Kate Bushby, MD FRCP
Act. Res. Chair of Neuro-muscular Genetics
Institute of Human Genetics, International Centre for Life
Newcastle University
Newcastle upon Tyne, UK

John Camm, MD, FRCP
Professor of Cardiology
Department of Cardiovascular Medicine
St. George's Hospital Medical School
Tooting
London, UK

Mark Caulfield, FRCP
Professor of Cardiovascular Medicine
William Harvey Research Institute
Barts and The London, Queen Mary's School of Medicine and Dentistry
John Vane Building
Charterhouse Square
London, UK

Mike Champion, MRCP, FRCPCH
Department of Paediatrics
Evelina Children's Hospital
St. Thomas's Hospital and Medical School
London, SE1, UK

Patrick F Chinnery, PhD, FRCPath, FRCP. FMedSci
Professsor of Neurogenetics, Newcastle University
Honorary Consultant Neurologist, Newcastle upon Tyne Hospitals NHS Foundation Trust
Newcastle upon Tyne, UK

Seo-Kyung Chung
Institute of Life Science, School of Medicine
Swansea University
Singleton Park
Swansea SA2 8PP, UK

Paolo Ciliberti
Institute of Cardiology
University of Bologna and S.Orsola-Malpighi Hospital
Bologna, Italy

Angus Clarke, DM, FRCP
Professor of Clinical Genetics
Institute of Medical Genetics
School of Medicine Cardiff University, UK

Maureen Cleary, MRCP, MRCPCH, MD
Department of Metabolic Medicine
Great Ormond Street Hospital NHS Trust
Institute of Child Health
London, WC1, UK

Helen Cox, MD, FRCP
West Midlands Regional Genetics Service
Birmingham Women's Hospital
Birmingham, UK

Mark D Davies, MRCP
Institute of Medial Genetics
School of Medicine, Cardiff University
Cardiff, UK

Sally J Davies, FRCP
Institute of Medical Genetics
University Hospital of Wales
Cardiff, UK

John CS Dean, MD, FRCP
Department of Clinical Genetics
Aberdeen
Scotland, UK

Susan L Drinkwater, MD
Department of Vascular Surgery
St. Mary's Hospital
University of London
London, UK

Girish Dwivedi, MRCP
Department of Cardiovascular Medicine
The Medical School University of Birmingham
Edgbaston
Birmingham, UK

Perry Elliott, MD, FRCP
The Heart Hospital
16-18 Westmoreland Street
University College Hospital
London, UK

Siv Fokstuen
Department of Medical Genetics
University Hospital
Geneva, Switzerland

Ian Frayling, MB, BChir, PhD, FRCPath
All-Wales Medical Genetics Service
Institute of Medical Genetics
University Hospital of Wales
Cardiff, UK

Michael Frenneaux, MD, FRCP
BHF Professor of Cardiovascular Medicine
The Medical School University of Birmingham
Edgbaston
Birmingham, UK

Keiichi Fukuda, MD, PhD
Professor and Chair
Department of Regenerative Medicine and Advanced Cardiac Therapeutics
Keio University School of Medicine
35 Shinanomachi
Shinjukuku
Tokyo 160-8582, Japan

Judith Goodship, MD, FRCP
Professor of Clinical Genetics
Institute of Human Genetics
Newcastle University
Newcastle upon Tyne
England UK

Grainne Gorman, MD, FRCPI
Biomedical Research Centre
Newcastle upon Tyne Hospitals NHS Foundation Trust & Newcastle University
Newcastle upon Tyne, UK

S Gaye Hadfield
Centre for Cardiovascular Genetics
Department of Medicine
University College London
5 University Street
London, UK

Michael Harrison, BA
Department of Physiology
Medical College of Wisconsin
Milwaukee, WI, USA

Steve E Humphries, PhD
Centre for Cardiovascular Genetics
Department of Medicine
University College London
5 University Street
London, UK

Sahoko Ichihara
Department of Human Functional Genomics
Life Science Research Center
Mie University
Tsu, Mie, Japan

Diala Khraiche
Department of Radiology
The Heart Hospital
UCL, University of London
Westmoreland Street
London, UK

Dhavendra Kumar, MD, FRCP, FRCPCH, FACMG
All-Wales Medical Genetics Service
Institute of Medical Genetics
University Hospital of Wales
Cardiff, UK

Pier D Lambiase, PhD, MRCP
The Heart Hospital, UCL
Westmoreland Street
London, UK

Stephen Leadbeatter, FRCPath
Department of Forensic Medicine
Cardiff University
Cardiff, UK

Bart Loeys, MD, PhD
Professor of Clinical Genetics
Center for Medical Genetics
University of Ghent
Ghent, Belgium

Simone Longhi
Institute of Cardiology
University of Bologna and S.Orsola-Malpighi Hospital
Bologna, Italy

Ivan Macciocca
Genetic Counselor
Genetic Health Services Victoria
Murdoch Children's Research Institute
Parkville
Victoria, Australia

Calum A MacRae
Cardiovascular Division
Brigham and Women's Hospital
Thorn 11, 20 Shattuck Street
Boston, MA 02115

Teri A Manolio, MD, PhD
Director, Office of Population Genomics
National Human Genome Research Institute
National Institutes of Health
Bethesda, MD

Karen Maresso, MPH
Human & Molecular Genetics Center
Medical College of Wisconsin
Milwaukee
WI, USA

Ian FW McDowell, MD, FRCP, FRCPath
Department of Medical Biochemistry and Immunology
University Hospital of Wales
Cardiff, UK

William J McKenna, MD, DSc, FRCP
Professor of Cardiology
The Heart Hospital
UCL/UCLH (University College London Hospitals Trust)
16-18 Westmoreland Street
London, W1G 8PH
UK

Martin C Michel
Professor of Pharmacology Department Pharmacology Pharmacotherapy
Academic Medical Center
University of Amsterdam
Meibergdreef 15
Amsterdam, The Netherlands

James Moon
Department of Radiology
Lead-Cardiac Magnetic Resonance
The Heart Hospital
UCL, University of London
Westmoreland Street
London, UK

Antoon FM Moorman, PhD
Professor of Embryology and Molecular Biology of Cardiovascular Diseases
Heart Failure Research Center
Academic Medical Center
University of Amsterdam
Amsterdam, The Netherlands

Patricia B Munroe, PhD
Clinical Pharmacology and Barts and The London Genome Centre
William Harvey Research Institute
Barts and The London School of Medicine
Charterhouse Square
London, UK

Elizabeth Nabel, MD, PhD
Director, National Heart, Lung and Blood Institute
National Institutes of Health
Bethesda, MD

Carlo Napolitano, MD, PhD
Molecular Cardiology
IRCCS Fondazione Maugeri
Department of Cardiology
University of Pavia
Pavia, Italy

Ruth Newbury-Ecob, MD, FRCP
Department of Clinical Genetics
Institute of Child Health
Bristol Children's Hospital
St. Michael's Hill
Bristol, UK

Stephen J Newhouse, PhD
Clinical Pharmacology and Barts and the London Genome Centre
William Harvey Research Institute
Barts and the London School of Medicine
Charterhouse Square
London, UK

Tamotsu Nishida
Department of Human Functional Genomics
Life Science Research Center
Mie University
Tsu, Mie, Japan

Constantinos O'Mahony
The Heart Hospital
University College London Hospitals NHS trust
London, UK

Juan Pablo-Kaski
The Heart Hospital
16-18 Westmoreland Street
University College
London, UK

Michael A Patton, MB, MSc, FRCP
Professor of Clinical Genetics
Department of Medical Genetics
St. George's University of London Cranmer Terrace
London, UK

Denis Pellerin, PhD
Department of Radiology
Lead-Cardiac Ultrasound
The Heart Hospital
UCL, University of London
Westmoreland Street
London, UK

Enrica Perugini
Institute of Cardiology
University of Bologna
S.Orsola-Malpighi Hospital
Bologna, Italy

Michael F Pope, MD, FRCP
Professor of Clinical Genetics and Dermatology
Ehlers Danlos National Diagnostic Service
Kennedy Galton Centre
Northwick Park Hospital, Watford Rd
Harrow Middlesex, HA1 3UJ and Department of Dermatology
West Middlesex University Hospital
Twickenham Rd, Isleworth
TW7 6AS, London England

Pieter G Postema, MD
Department of Cardiology
Academic Medical Center
University of Amsterdam
Amsterdam, The Netherlands

Silvia G Priori, MD, PhD
Professor of Cardiology
Molecular Cardiology
Maugeri Foundation
University of Pavia
Via Maugeri 10/10A
Pavia, Italy

Candida Cristina Quarta
Institute of Cardiology
University of Bologna and S.Orsola-Malpighi Hospital
Bologna, Italy

Claudio Rapezzi
Institute of Cardiology
University of Bologna
S.Orsola-Malpighi Hospital
Bologna, Italy

Mark I Rees
Institute of Life Science, School of Medicine
Swansea University
Singleton Park
Swansea SA2 8PP, UK

Cardiac Inherited Disease Group
Auckland Hospital
Grafton, Auckland
New Zealand

Institute of Medical Genetics
School of Medicine
Cardiff University
Heath Park
Cardiff CF14 4XN, UK

Letizia Riva
Institute of Cardiology
University of Bologna and S.Orsola-Malpighi Hospital
Bologna, Italy

Tom Rossenbacker, MD, PhD
Molecular Cardiology
IRCCS Fondazione Maugeri
Department of Cardiology
University of Pavia
Pavia, Italy

Dieter Rosskopf
Professor of Pharmacology
Department Pharmacology
Center for Pharmacology and Experimental Therapeutics
Ernst-Moritz-Arndt University
Friedrich Loeffler Str. 23
Greifswald, Germany

Fabrizio Salvi
Department of Neurology
Bellaria Hospital
Bologna, Italy

Jonathan R Skinner
Cardiac Inherited Disease Group
Auckland Hospital
Grafton, Auckland
New Zealand

Department of Paediatric Cardiology
Starship Hospital
Grafton, Auckland
New Zealand

Petros Syrris, PhD
The Heart Hospital
Department of Medicine
University College London
16-18 Westmoreland Street
London, W1G 8PH
UK

Peter Taylor, FRCS
Professor of Surgery
Department of Vascular Surgery
St.Thomas's/Guy's/King's
University of London
London, UK

Jennifer Thomson, MD, MRCP
Yorkshire Regional Clinical Genetics Service
Chapel Allerton Hospital
Leeds, UK

Eric J Topol, MD, FACC, FESC, FAHA, FACP
Dean, Scripps School of Medicine
Director, Scripps Translational Science Institute
Professor of Translational Genomics
The Scripps Research Institute
Senior Consultant of Cardiovascular Diseases
Scripps Clinic
La Jolla
California, USA

Richard C Trembath, FRCP, F Med Sci
Professor of Medical Genetics
Division of Genetics and Molecular Medicine
Guy's Hospital Medical School
King's College
University of London
London, UK

Pascal FHM van Dessel, MD, PhD
Department of Cardiology
Academic Medical Center
University of Amsterdam
Amsterdam, The Netherlands

Malcolm J Walker, MD, FRCP
Hatter Cardiovascular Institute
University College Hospital
University of London
London, NW1, UK

Arthur AM Wilde, MD, PhD
Professor of Cardiology
Department of Cardiology
Academic Medical Center
University of Amsterdam
Amsterdam, The Netherlands

Christopher Wren, MBChB, FRCP, FRCPCH
Department of Paediatric Cardiology
Freeman Hospital
Newcastle upon Tyne
England, UK

Yoshiji Yamada, MD, PhD
Department of Human Functional Genomics
Life Science Research Center, Mie University
1577 Kurima-machiya, Tsu
Mie, Japan

Shinsuke Yuasa, MD, PhD
Center for Integrated Medical Research
Department of Regenerative Medicine and Advanced Cardiac Therapeutics
Cardiology division, Department of Medicine
Keio University school of Medicine, 35-Shinanomachi Shinjuku-ku Tokyo, 160-8582 JAPAN

Zaheer Yousef, MD, MRCP
Department of Cardiovascular Medicine
University Hospital of Wales
Cardiff
CF14 4XW, UK

Introduction: The Challenges of Inherited Cardiovascular Conditions

Dhavendra Kumar and Perry Elliott

Diseases of the heart and blood vessels are a major contributor to human morbidity and mortality. A substantial proportion of cardiovascular disease is caused by genetic mechanisms including major chromosomal structural aberrations, submicroscopic chromosomal microdeletions and microduplications, mutations in single genes, and the interaction of low-penetrance genes or polymorphisms with environmental factors. It is estimated that the total burden of inherited cardiovascular disorders is greater than cancer, some forms of which are also caused by genetic mechanisms.

Clinicians regularly encounter patients and family members with known or presumed inherited conditions affecting the heart and blood vessels. Some of these disorders manifest for the first time with sudden unexplained death in a young person, whereas others present with progressive symptoms or may simply be detected incidentally. Over the past two decades, substantial progress has been made in unraveling the genetic basis of many cardiac disorders, but it is only recently that this knowledge has started to percolate into everyday clinical practice. In Europe, Australasia, and North America, specialist multidisciplinary services are being created in order to improve diagnosis and treatment of a wide range of diseases. This book is designed to support the development of such services by providing health care professionals of all backgrounds with a comprehensive resource on the principles and practice of cardiovascular genetics.

One of the challenges that we faced when designing this book was the range of healthcare professionals that can be involved in the diagnosis and care of patients with inherited cardiovascular disease. We were aware that a number of excellent textbooks (see *Related titles*) dealing with one or more aspects of cardiovascular genetics and genomics already existed. However, many of these titles were research oriented and predominantly focused on basic molecular biology. Few if any of the existing textbooks addressed cardiovascular genetic conditions primarily from a clinical perspective. This textbook consists of commissioned contributions from experts in cardiovascular genetics and applied clinical cardiology. Chapters on specific conditions provide a detailed and comprehensive account of the molecular genetics and clinical practice related to the disorder or group of disorders. In most chapters, key points are presented in a box for quick reference. Relevant references to the literature are listed at the end of each chapter. The text in each chapter is supported by illustrations and tables.

The book is arranged in three sections. The first deals with general topics, relevant to cardiac development, disease classification, and diagnosis of inherited cardiovascular disease; the second is dedicated to specific genetic diseases that affect the cardiovascular system; and the third reviews generic issues relevant to service development and the management of patients with genetic cardiovascular diseases.

Part I

Chapters 1 (*Development of the Heart*) and 2 (*The Molecular Basis of Cardiac Development*) review the complex molecular and genetic aspects of the developmental anatomy and physiology of cardiovascular system. Chapter 3 (*The Classification of Inherited Cardiovascular Conditions*) describes the classification and pattern of inheritance of the commonest cardiovascular diseases including chromosomal abnormalities, classical Mendelian (autosomal dominant, autosomal recessive, X-linked recessive, and X-linked dominant), mitochondrial, and polygenic. Chapter 4 (*Genetic Epidemiology of Cardiovascular Diseases*) reviews the epidemiology of genetic cardiovascular disease in the context of population incidence and prevalence, genetic variability, interaction with dietary and other environmental factors, and the role of lifestyle in causation and clinical outcomes. Chapters 5 (*Cytogenetic Testing in Clinical Cardiovascular Genetics*) and 6 (*Molecular Diagnosis in Clinical Cardiovascular Genetics*) present overviews of the techniques of cytogenetic and molecular genetic testing relevant to cardiovascular disease. Chapters 7 (*Cardiac Magnetic Resonance Imaging in Cardiovascular Genetics*) and 8 (*Ultrasound Imaging in Cardiovascular Genetics*) provide an introduction to the techniques of cardiac magnetic resonance imaging and echocardiography, respectively, considering their role in the diagnosis of structural heart diseases. These general overviews are complemented by additional information in later chapters dealing with specific disorders.

Part II

This section is dedicated to individual disorders or groups of conditions. A number of major structural and functional cardiac abnormalities are associated with chromosome aberrations. These include aneuploidies (e.g., Down's syndrome), X-chromosome abnormalities (as seen in Turner syndrome), chromosome rearrangements, and chromosome microdeletions (e.g., 22qdel syndrome), and duplications. In Chapter 9 (*Congenital Cardiovascular Malformations*) the underlying molecular pathology, clinical phenotype, and clinical management of some of the more common genetic cardiovascular disorders associated with chromosome abnormalities are reviewed. Empirically all pregnancies are at risk of being associated with a major or minor congenital cardiovascular malformation. These may include a small nonspecific vascular malformation (e.g., a strawberry nevus), an aneurysm, a major structural cardiac anomaly (such as Fallot's tetralogy), a septal defect (such as an ASD or VSD), a major blood vessel anomaly (e.g., coarctation of aorta or anomalous venous drainage), and isomerism (e.g., dextrocardia). Chapter 10 (*Malformation Syndromes with Heart Disease*) reviews the genetic basis of various malformation syndromes and discusses issues in clinical and genetic management.

Chapter 11 (*Marfan Syndrome and Related Disorders*) deals with the natural history, clinical manifestations, molecular genetics, management, and related medical and ethical issues of Marfan syndrome. Individuals with Marfan's syndrome live with a major risk of sudden death due to ruptured aneurysm in the ascending aorta. Diagnosis and identification of new patients is essential to ensure long-term medical care. Inherited in autosomal dominant manner, the disorder is characterized by high penetrance and marked phenotypic variation. At least three genes are implicated in Marfan syndrome, the most common of which are mutations in microfibrillin-1 (*FBN1*). Mutations in the same gene are also associated with other clinically distinct genetic diseases, collectively called "microfibrillinopathies."

Familial aortic aneurysm without other phenotypic manifestations is a distinct familial disorder with autosomal dominant inheritance. Some families do not meet the criteria for a monogenic disorder, but a genetic causation is inferred by the observation of multiple affected family members. Genetic association studies suggest molecular heterogeneity reflecting different pathophysiological mechanisms in the descending thoracic and infrarenal abdominal aortic segments. It is also possible that such genetic differences are population specific. Major clinical, molecular, and management aspects of thoracic and abdominal aortic aneurysms are reviewed in detail in Chapter 12 (*Thoracic and Abdominal Aortic Aneurysms*).

Chapters 13 and 14 are dedicated to the more common forms of inherited heart muscle disease (cardiomyopathies): specifically hypertrophic (HCM), dilated (DCM), restrictive cardiomyopathy (RCM), and arrhythmogenic right ventricular cardiomyopathy (ARVC). These are usually inherited in a Mendelian, autosomal dominant manner with marked clinical and genetic heterogeneity. Hundreds of mutations in genes encoding various structural and functional myocardial proteins have been identified. Together with the variable and age-related phenotype this makes genetic counseling complex and challenging in most families. However, clinical and molecular diagnoses offer the opportunity for presymptomatic diagnosis and targeting of health care resources. Chapter 15 (*Ventricular Noncompaction*) reviews the clinical and molecular aspects of a rarer and more recently recognized heart muscle disorder, left ventricular noncompaction (LVNC). Cardiomyopathies associated with dysmorphic syndromes and metabolic diseases are reviewed in Chapters 10 and 26.

Disorders of cardiac rhythm are common in the general population where they cause considerable morbidity and mortality, particularly in middle age and beyond. In a number of patients, arrhythmias arise as the result of monogenetic disorders that affect cardiac ion channels, most notably long QT syndrome, short QT syndrome, Brugada syndrome, and catecholaminergic polymorphic ventricular tachycardia. Arrhythmia may also be the presenting feature of genetic diseases that affect structural proteins or cardiac metabolism. The basic molecular biology of cardiac arrhythmia is reviewed in Chapter 16 (*Molecular Genetics of Arrhythmias*). More detailed accounts of specific disorders are presented in Chapters 17 (*The Long QT Syndrome and Catecholaminergic Polymorphic Ventricular Tachycardia*), 18 (*Acquired Repolarization Disorders*), 19 (*Brugada Syndrome*), and 20 (*Inherited Conduction Disease and Familial Atrial Fibrillation*).

Inherited disorders of lipid metabolism and related biochemical disorders are among the commonest genetic diseases. Routine testing for hyperlipidemias is an essential component of any clinical service dealing with complex cardiovascular disease, but a discussion on all forms of inherited hyperlipidemias is beyond the scope of this book. Instead, we focus on the most frequent disease, familial hypercholesterolemia, which has a population prevalence of 1 in 500 individuals and is a major risk determinant for coronary heart disease (Chapter 21—*Familial Hypercholesterolemia*).

Complex cardiovascular diseases comprise a large group of disorders of the heart and blood vessels with multifactorial genetic etiology. Key diseases in this group include congenital malformations, coronary artery disease, myocardial infarction, systemic hypertension, peripheral vascular disease, and stroke. These disorders are discussed in detail in separate chapters. Coronary artery disease (CAD) is a major cause of death and long-term morbidity leading to enormous social, economic, and psychological burden in developed countries and increasingly in the developing world. Chapter 21 (*Genetics of Coronary Artery Disease*) deals with the most important biological factor underlying CAD, atherosclerosis, and reviews the impact of genome-based science and technology, particularly in high-throughput population screening.

A small number of monogenic disorders, including familial renal disorders such as autosomal dominant adult onset polycystic kidney disease (ADPKD) can cause systemic hypertension but these are rare. Chapter 23 (*Genetics of Essential Hypertension*) describes the genetic epidemiology and molecular genetics of essential hypertension, a disorder that affects hundreds of thousands of people in developed and developing countries. Several epidemiologic studies indicate higher prevalence among males, and those of African and Hispanic origin. However, lifestyle factors such as high salt intake and obesity are also important.

Chapter 24 is dedicated to the issue of stroke, a major cause for long-term morbidity and mortality in people over the age of 60 years. There are two distinct forms, hemorrhagic and ischemic, the latter being the most frequent. A family history is encountered in approximately 10% of stroke victims and genome-wide genetic association studies have suggested several potential loci. Genetic linkage studies in selected multiplex families provide support for genetic causation following autosomal dominant inheritance related to low-penetrance pathogenic mutations. One of the best characterized examples of Mendelian stroke are mutations of the notch, drosophila, homolog of 3 gene (*NOTCH3*) in cerebral arteriopathy, autosomal dominant, with subcortical infarcts and leukoencephalopathy (CADASIL), a condition that leads to lacunar infarcts and vascular dementia.

Primary pulmonary hypertension is an uncommon autosomal dominant disorder characterized by incomplete penetrance and variable clinical manifestations. Affected individuals experience long-term morbidity caused by poor effort-tolerance, breathlessness, congestive cardiac failure, and face early death. Chapter 25 (*Pulmonary Arterial Hypertension*) discusses the clinical pathologic aspects of the disease and reviews data on disease-causing mutations in *BMPR2* gene at 2q33.

Inherited metabolic and neuromuscular diseases are individually rare, but collectively they comprise a significant medical burden often manifesting with cardiac involvement, usually cardiomyopathy. Chapter 26 (*Heart and Metabolic Disease*) summarizes the more metabolic common disorders that affect the heart including glycogen storage disease (Pompe disease), disorders of glycosylation, mucopolysaccharidoses (Hurler; Hurler-Sheie), and lysosomal storage disease (Fabry disease).

In Chapter 27 (*Heart and Neuromuscular Disease*), the more important neuromuscular diseases that affect the heart are reviewed. The most common are the X-linked recessive muscular dystrophies (Duchenne and Becker type) that typically cause dilated cardiomyopathy, even in female carriers. Cardiomyopathy and disturbance of cardiac rhythm also occur in autosomal Emery-Dreiffus muscular dystrophy caused by mutations in lamin A/C mutation and in autosomal dominant myotonic dystrophy.

Inherited disorders of collagen are a relatively common case of cardiovascular disease. Chapter 28 (*Cardiovascular Complications in Ehlers-Danlos Syndromes)* focuses on the Ehlers-Danlos syndrome (EDS). Structural abnormality of mitral and aortic valves is common in several forms of EDS. Patients with type EDS IV, perhaps the only lethal form, are prone to rupture of middle-sized arteries. In addition, the cardiovascular involvement is an important feature in the phenotype of some forms of genetic skeletal dysplasia. Understanding the molecular genetics is of major importance in genotype–phenotype correlations in genetic collagen diseases.

Cardiac manifestations are an important complication of a number of inherited hematological diseases, in particular those associated with excessive tissue iron storage whether as a primary component (hemochromatosis) or secondary resulting from multiple blood transfusions (hemoglobinopathies). The pathogenesis and molecular basis of cardiac involvement in selected inherited blood disorders are reviewed in detail in Chapter 29 (*The Heart and Inherited Diseases of Hemoglobin*). Hematologic diseases are also important in the amyloidoses, a group of disorders caused by extracellular deposition in various tissues of proteinaceous material with a characteristic cross-ß-sheet quaternary structure (Chapter 30—*Familial Amyloidoses and the Heart*). Hematological disorders associated with excessive light chain (AL) immunoglobulin production are the commonest cause of cardiac amyloid. Familial forms caused by the accumulation of mutant proteins (transthyretin or A-apolipoprotein) have variable cardiac involvement.

Mitochondrial diseases are a clinically heterogeneous group of disorders resulting from dysfunction of the mitochondrial respiratory chain. They can be caused by mutations of nuclear or mitochondrial DNA (mtDNA). Some mitochondrial disorders may only affect one organ (e.g., eye in Leber hereditary optic neuropathy) but multisystem involvement is more common presenting with a combination of features such as muscle weakness, deafness, stroke like episodes, seizures, and dementia. Chapter 31 (*Cardiac Involvement in Mitochondrial Disease*) reviews the cardiovascular manifestations of mitochondrial diseases.

Tumors of the heart are uncommon and usually benign, but a small number, for example, cardiac myxoma, can be inherited in autosomal dominant manner. Some cardiac tumors occur as part of the multisystem pleiotropic manifestations of cancer predisposing Mendelian disorders such as tuberous sclerosis. The clinical features and genetics of familial cardiac neoplasia are reviewed in Chapter 32 (*Inherited Cardiac Tumors*).

Part III

Sudden cardiac death in a young person (under 40 years of age) is a tragic consequence of some genetic cardiovascular diseases. Such deaths have profound psychological, legal, and social implications for affected families and society at large. Examples of diseases that cause sudden cardiac death include hypertrophic cardiomyopathy, long QT syndrome, and familial thoracic and abdominal aortic aneurysm. Chapter 33 (*The Sudden Arrhythmic Death Syndrome*) reviews the genetic epidemiology of sudden cardiac deaths associated with an apparently normal postmortem and outlines approach that should be taken to the evaluation of other family members who may themselves be at risk. Applications of the new genomic technology in population/family screening for selecting and targeting the high-risk individuals are also discussed.

The outlook for patients with a range of genetic and acquired cardiovascular disease has been substantially improved over the past two decades by the systematic use of modern pharmacotherapy. It is clear, however, that individual patient responses to drug treatment vary. This variation is at least in part explained by genetic factors that affect drug action (*pharmacodynamics*) and the fate of the drug in the organism (*pharmacokinetics*). Chapter 34 (*Cardiovascular Pharmacogenomics*) discusses the relevance of both these factors to the action of the most commonly used cardioactive drugs.

Examples of successful therapeutic applications of germline and/or somatic gene therapy in clinical cardiology are few, but tremendous progress has been made in understanding the basic biology of stem cells. Chapter 35 (*Stem Cell Therapy in Cardiovascular Medicine*) reviews the current state-of-the-art technology[for cardiovascular regenerative medicine with a particular focus on the potential sources for stem cells.

The process of genetic counseling in cardiovascular genetics can be complex and challenging as different approaches are necessary in individual conditions. The process also has to take into account the emotional and psychological state of counselees particularly in the context of a sudden cardiac death in a relative. The basic principles of genetic counseling are reviewed in Chapter 36 (*Genetic Counseling in Cardiovascular Genetics*). The general ethical, legal, and social issues (ELSI) that accompany the diagnosis of a genetic disease are reviewed in Chapter 37 (*Social and Ethical Issues Arising in Cardiovascular Genetics*). The complex legal issues that can arise as a consequence of an autopsy are illustrated in Chapter 38 (*The Forensic Pathologist and Genetic Cardiovascular Disease: A U.K. Perspective*), which focuses on the specific duties and responsibilities of the coroners' service pathologist in the United Kingdom.

Clinical genetic services are an integral part of specialist medical services. Increasingly, clinical genetics itself has become subspecialized, for example, prenatal genetics, dysmorphology, metabolic diseases, and cancer genetics. Chapter 39 describes the emerging subspecialism of clinical cardiovascular genetics, emphasizing its multidisciplinary structure and dependence on key competences.

We are aware that some of the material included in this book are relatively new and have not had sufficient professional scrutiny to justify a place in established clinical practice of cardiology and clinical genetic communities. However, we hope that the contents, interpretations, views, and speculations for the future contained within this book will be helpful to the broad range of clinicians and health professionals for whom this book was originally conceived and developed. All errors and emissions are entirely the responsibility of contributors and editors.

Related Book Titles

1. Cardiovascular diseases—Genetics, Epidemiology and Prevention, Oxford Monographs on Medical Genetics, OUP, 1991.
2. *Molecular Genetics and Gene Therapy of Cardiovascular Disease*, Mercel Dekker, New York, 1996
3. *Cardiovascular Genetics for Clinicians*, Kluwer/ Springer, 2001
4. *Genetics of Cerebrovascular Disease*, Blackwell Publishing, New York, 1999.
5. *Genetics and Genomics for the Cardiologist*, Kluwer Academic, 2002.
6. *Cardiovascular Pharmacogenetics*, Springer-Verlag, Heidelberg, 2004
7. *Molecular Genetics of Cardiac Electrophysiology*, Kluwer Academic, 2000.
8. Cardiovascular Genetics and Genomics for the Cardiologists, Blackwell, 2007.

Part I

General Aspects of Cardiovascular Genetics

1

Development of the Heart

Robert H Anderson, Nigel A Brown, and Antoon FM Moorman

Introduction

Over the past decade, much has been learnt concerning the development of the heart. Much of this knowledge, in turn, mandates the need for marked changes in our approach to the morphogenesis of cardiac malformations. The heart is no more than a specialized component of the vascular system. Perhaps the greatest change to have occurred over that past decade in understanding its development relates to the origin of its so-called segments. Cardiac embryologists and pediatric cardiologists, over the years, have used the term segment in a fashion that is foreign to those trained in biology. To biologists, segments are parts of an organism that have uniform structure. To those dealing with the heart, both during its development and in postnatal life, segment has been used to describe the atrial, ventricular, and arterial parts of the organ. These parts are markedly different in their morphological makeup. For better or worse, those concerned primarily with congenital cardiac malformations will continue to use the word in the latter sense. Hence, that is the way we will use it in this chapter. Until recently, it was believed that the linear heart tube, when first seen during development of the organ, contained the precursors of all these segments. We now know that this is not the case. Instead, material is added continually to the tube as it grows and loops (Kelly et al. 2001; Mjaatdvedt et al. 2001; Waldo et al. 2001). The part of the tube first seen during development eventually forms little more than the definitive left ventricle. Only as the new material is added at the venous and arterial poles does the tube loop, with the larger parts of the walls of the atrial and ventricular chambers then ballooning from the cavity of the primary tube (Moorman and Christoffels 2003). The concept of expansion of the chambers from a linear tube is itself far from original, having been well described by Davis (1927). It is an appreciation of the changes to the molecular phenotype of the myocardium making up the walls that has advanced our knowledge of development (Anderson et al. 2006). Such studies of molecular phenotype have also served to resolve ongoing controversies. We will discuss the formation of the heart tube, and the initial appearance of the cardiac components, in the opening sections of our chapter. Thereafter, we will provide an account of the maturation of the various segments. In this way, we hope to provide the necessary background to understand the anomalous development leading to deficient septation, and why some congenitally malformed hearts have abnormal connections between the segments as their major feature. To appreciate our descriptions, the reader should also note discrepancies in the use of adjectives to describe the relationship of cardiac components between biologists and clinicians. When biologists and embryologists have used the term *anterior*, they describe structures that are toward the head, using *posterior* to describe structures toward the feet. For the clinician, of course, these terms means structures adjacent to the sternum as opposed to the spine. We circumvent these problems by describing cranial and caudal, and ventral and dorsal structures. Fortunately, there are no problems with the use of right and left.

Formation of the Heart Tube

It had long been suggested (Patten and Kramer 1933; Viragh and Challice 1973; Arguello et al. 1975) that cells were continuously added during development to both the venous and arterial poles of the newly formed linear heart tube. Those producing the evidence to substantiate these notions initially described the source of this new material as the anterior heart field (Mjaatvedt et al. 2001), pointing out that the cellular populations formed the right ventricle and the outflow tract of the developing heart. It is now realized that this anterior field is part of a more extensive second heart field, which also contributes to the developing venous pole (Cai et al. 2003). With ongoing investigations, however, it can be questioned whether it is justifiable to identify two specific developmental fields rather than one, or even three or more. We do not know, as yet, whether the cells derived from the alleged first and second fields are irreversibly committed to distinct anatomic compartments within the definitive heart. Recent advances made concerning the mechanics of formation of the linear tube itself throw some light on these ongoing conundrums (Moorman et al. 2007).

The heart tube is formed relatively early in the developmental sequence, occurring subsequent to gastrulation, the embryo having acquired its three germ layers during the latter process. These layers are the ectoderm, endoderm, and an intermediate mesodermal layer. At the stage of formation of the germ layers, the embryo itself is disc shaped, the layers of the disc merging at its margins with the extra-embryonic tissues formed by the amnion and yolk sac. It is during the stage at which the embryo is a disc that the cells eventually forming the heart migrate from the cranial part of the midline of the disc, this region known as the primitive streak (Figure 1–1). The migrating cells move between the ectodermal and endodermal layers, giving rise to two heart-forming regions on either side of the midline in the middle mesodermal layer (Rosenquist 1970; Garcia-Martinez and Schoenwolf 1993). Further migrations from these heart-forming areas then form the cardiac crescent toward the cranial end of the disc. With subsequent remoulding, the cells initially derived from the crescent form a trough, which closes by a process of zipping in cranial and caudal directions from the middle to form the initial linear heart tube. During this folding and zipping, it is the part of the crescent initially positioned peripherally, or the primary heart field, that becomes the linear tube. The part of the cardiac crescent that was initially positioned centrally is the so-called secondary heart field (Figure 1–1). This central location permits this part of the crescent to contribute new material, albeit with a temporal delay, to the initial linear tube. With ongoing development, further new material, known as mediastinal myocardium (Soufan et al. 2004) is added at the venous pole. The part of the heart formed by this mediastinal myocardium, as we will explain, provides not only the site of entry for the pulmonary veins, but also the roof of the developing atrium, the latter then providing the site of growth of the primary atrial septum. At the arterial pole, it is the tissues that will form the right ventricle and outflow tract that are added from the anterior component of the second heart field, with further ingrowth at this pole providing the nonmyocardial components of the intrapericardial arterial trunks along with their valves and sinuses.

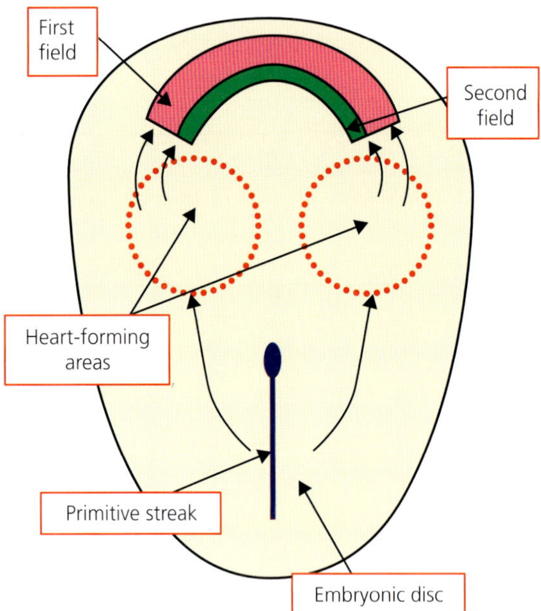

Figure 1–1 Embryonic disc. The cartoon shows the structure of the embryonic disc and the migrations of cells from the primitive streak that form, first, the heart-forming areas within the middle mesodermal layer, and subsequently the cardiac crescent. We now know that the cells from the periphery of the cardiac crescent, shown in purple, form the initial linear heart tube, with subsequent addition of material from the central part of the cresenct, shown in green, forming most of the atrial part of the heart along with the right ventricle and the outflow tract. The cartoon does not show the important overlapping of the first and second fields, with the differences between the parts being temporal as much as morphologic.

In essence, therefore, the second heart field provides the basis for the formation of the components of the pulmonary circulation (Moorman et al. 2007). The evidence confirming that new myocardium is added to the already functioning myocardial heart tube has come primarily from studies of molecular lineages (Cai et al. 2003; Zaffran et al. 2004). It is likely that differences of opinion with regard to the structures formed from the so-called second field are more apparent than real, since the initial boundaries seen between different areas do not necessarily retain their location within the maturing organ. The cells contained within the initial heart-forming fields have the capacity to form all parts of the heart, depending on their position in the field and the time at which they migrate into the definitive heart tube (Rana et al. 2007). It is probably differences in the concentration of diffusing morphogens that create the different fates for a given cell, promoting diversity within a field that was initially homogeneous.

Looping of the Heart Tube

Soon after the formation of the straight heart tube it becomes S-shaped by a process known as looping (Figure 1–2). Looping is an intrinsic feature of the developing heart (Orts Llorca and Roana Gil 1967; Manasek and Monroe 1972), although the exact cause has still to be determined. With normal development, the tube loops to the right (Figure 2–2, lower panel). Such rightward turning is independent of the overall left–right asymmetry of the developing embryo, and gives no indication of the subsequent lateralization of the cardiac components.

The Cardiac Components

It is only subsequent to looping that it is possible to recognize the primordiums of the developing cardiac segments. The outlet component becomes evident at this time, which gives rise to the right ventricle, as well as the intrapericardial arterial trunks. The distal end of the outlet is continuous with the aortic sac, which in turn supports the arteries extending through the pharyngeal arches. At the same time, there is expansion of the atrial component, which receives on each side the terminations of the venous tributaries. Looping also sets the scene for expansion of the cavities of the definitive atrial and ventricular chambers by a process now known as ballooning. As the walls of the chambers balloon from the linear tube, so do the myocytes within them develop a markedly different molecular phenotype than those forming the walls of the initial tube. The myocytes within the initial tube are negative for connexin 40 and atrial natriuretic peptide, these features permitting their identification as primary myocardium (Moorman and Christoffels 2003). Subsequent to looping, and growth of the outlet component, the outlet of the tube achieves a position directly ventral to the developing atrium. The cavities of the right and left atrial appendages then balloon in parallel to either side of the outlet component (Figure 1–3, left panel). Within the ventricular part of the loop, in contrast, the cavities of the developing ventricles balloon in series, with the apical part of the left ventricle developing from the inlet, and the right ventricle from the outlet parts of the loop (Figure 1–3, right panel). This ballooning of the ventricles takes place from the outer curvature of the loop, and the primordium of the ventricular septum becomes evident as the apical parts extend outward. The myocytes making up the ballooning components

A

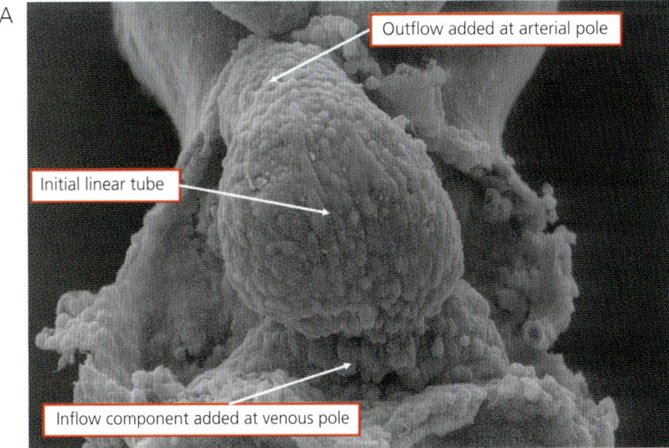

B

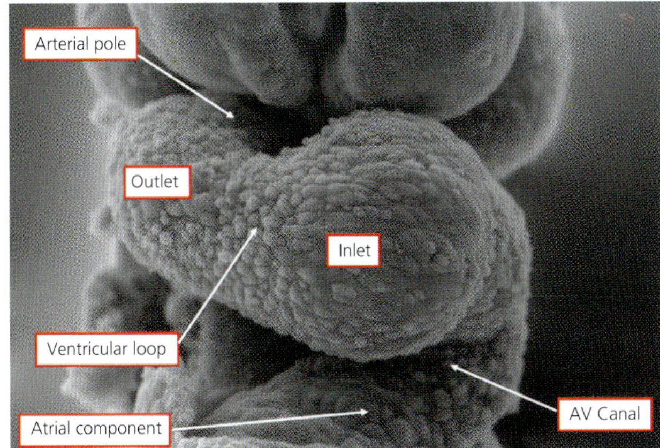

Figures 1–2a and 1–2b Scanning electron micrographs. These scanning electron micrographs of the developing mouse heart show the morphology of the heart tube after having removed the pericardium. The upper panel shows the linear heart tube subsequent to the initial addition of material at the venous and arterial poles. With still further addition of material from the second heart field, the tube loops, as shown in the lower panel. Note that the atrial component of the tube will be common to both the developing right and left atrial chambers, whereas the inlet and outlet of the ventricular part of the loop are formed in series, and will give rise to the developing left and right ventricles, respectively.

A

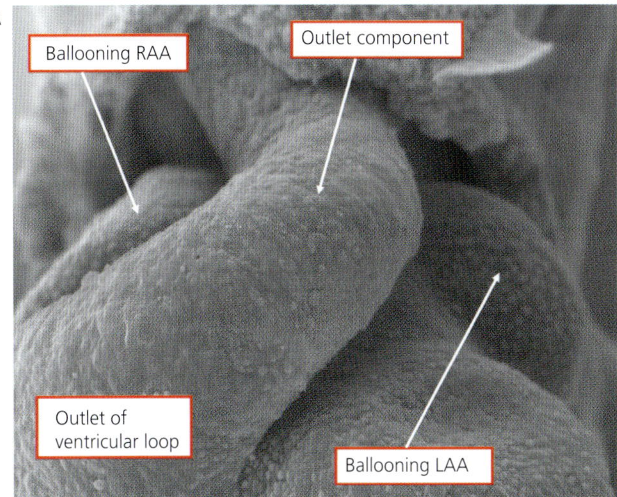

B

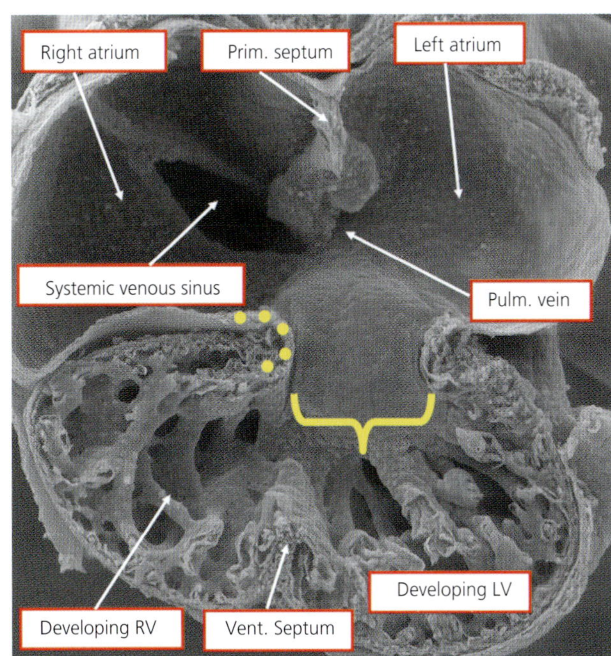

Figures 1–3a and 1–3b Scanning electron micrographs. These scanning electron micrographs, again of the mouse heart, show in the upper panel the cranial part of the developing heart of an embryo with 42 somites, and in the lower panel a "four-chamber" dissection across the atrioventricular canal (yellow bracket) of another embryo at the same stage. The upper panel shows how the atrial appendages (RAA, LAA) have ballooned to either side of the outflow tract, while the lower panel shows the ballooning of the apical parts of the ventricles (RV, LV) from the inlet and outlet parts of the ventricular component of the primary heart tube. Note that the walls of the developing right atrium and ventricle are already in continuity through the inner curvature (yellow dotted line) despite the fact that most of the circumference of the atrioventricular canal is supported by the inlet component of the tube. Note also that the systemic venous sinus is now committed to the developing right atrium, while the pulmonary (pulm.) vein opens to the left atrium, with the primary (prim) atrial septum beginning to grow between them.

are positive for both connexin 40 and atrial natriuretic peptide (Moorman and Christoffels 2003), distinguishing them from the primary myocardium, and permitting their designation as chamber myocardium. Significantly, it is these components formed from chamber myocardium that serve to distinguish the chambers postnatally when the heart is congenitally malformed. Equally significantly, the atrial appendages ballooning in symmetrical and parallel fashion from the atrial component of the primary tube, the pouches formed extending to either side of the outflow tract from a common atrial lumen (Figure 1–3, upper panel). By this stage, nonetheless, the atrial component itself has received a third population of molecularly distinct cells. These are the mediastinal myocytes, which are positive for connexin 40 but negative for atrial natriuretic peptide (Soufan et al. 2004). It is the mediastinal myocytes that form the pulmonary venous component of the left atrium, along with a small part of the dorsal wall of the right atrium and the area in the atrial roof that gives rise to the primary atrial septum (Mommersteeg et al. 2006).

In contrast to the atrial ballooning, however, the pouches that balloon from the ventricular part of the loop do so in series, rather than in parallel (Figure 1–3, lower panel). Thus, the apical part of the developing left ventricle grows from the inlet part of the ventricular loop, while the apical part of the right ventricle taking its origin from the outlet part.

The formation of chamber myocardium enlarges the cavities of the developing atriums and ventricles and sets the scene for subsequent septation. Septation also requires significant remodeling of the initial cavity of the heart tube itself. The cavity of the initial tube can be considered to represent the inner heart curvature. After looping, and the initial phases of ballooning, the greater part of the circumference of the atrioventricular canal, by now evident between the common atrial chamber and the ventricular loop, is supported by the ventricular inlet. Already, nonetheless, the rightward margin of the canal provides a direct connection between the walls of the developing right atrium and right ventricle (Figure 1-3, lower panel). At the same stage, the greater part of the circumference of the developing outlet component is supported by the outlet of the ventricular loop. The stream of blood from the developing left ventricle, nonetheless, is able to pass directly through the initial linear tube and reach the developing aortic pathway. It is remodeling within the initial primary heart tube, therefore, which eventually separates the pulmonary and systemic circuits.

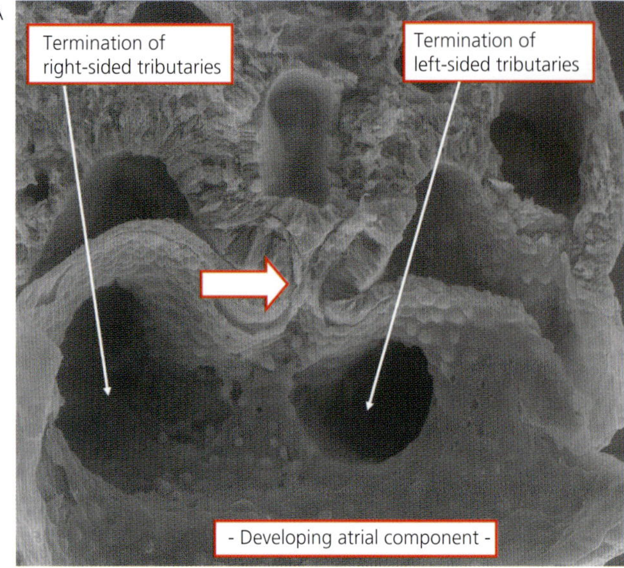

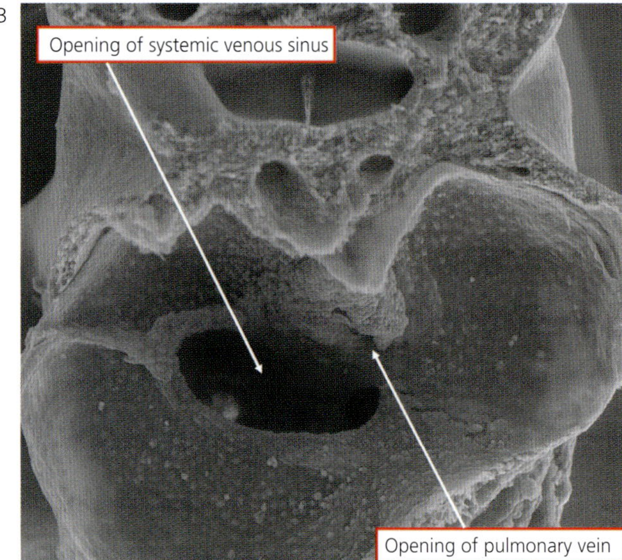

Figures 1–4a and 1–4b Scanning electron micrographs. These scanning electron micrographs, once more of developing mouse embryos, show the reorientation of the systemic venous tributaries. At an early stage (upper panel) the tributaries from both sides of the embryo drain to the common atrial chamber, although already the mouth of the right-sided tributaries is larger than the left. It is only after the opening of the tributaries has shifted to the right (lower panel) that the valves forming the boundary between the systemic venous sinus and the atrium become evident. The upper panel shows how initially the back of the atrial chamber is connected to the pharyngeal mesenchyme through the dorsal mesocardium (arrow). In the bottom panel, this area has provided the site of entry for the developing pulmonary vein.

1. Development of the Venous Components

At the stage of the beginning of ballooning of the atrial appendages, the systemic venous tributaries are relatively symmetrical. At this early stage, venous channels drain into the developing atrial component from both sides of the embryo, and also bilaterally from the yolk sac and from the placenta. Many accounts of cardiac development have described these tributaries as forming a "sinus venosus," with the right and left sides described as sinus horns. At the early stages, there are no anatomic landmarks permitting recognition of the venous tributaries as a discrete cardiac segment. Instead, the tributaries simply drain to the developing atrial component, albeit that even from the earliest stages the mouth of the right-sided channel is broader than its left-sided counterpart (Figure 1–4, upper panel). Only after remoulding of the systemic venous tributaries, such that they drain asymmetrically to the right side of the common atrial component, are structures seen demarcating their borders, namely the valves of the systemic venous sinus, or the so-called venous valves (Figure 1–4, lower panel). The remoulding of the systemic venous tributaries involves formation of anastomoses between the venous systems on the right and left of the embryo such that left-sided venous return is shunted to the right. The anastomoses formed result in all the return from the placenta, reaching the heart through the umbilical veins, being diverted to the cardinal venous system, with the anastomotic channel persisting as the venous duct. The veins draining the yolk sac, or the vitelline veins, become incorporated for the larger part into the venous system of the liver, which develops adjacent to the heart in the transverse septum. Within the embryo itself, the formation of the left brachiocephalic vein serves to divert the venous return from the left side to the right side of the embryo, the blood returning to the heart through the superior caval vein. Concomitant with this change, and increasing diminution of the venous return through the left-sided channels, the left superior caval vein, retaining its walls becomes incorporated into the left half of the developing atrioventricular junction (Figure 1–5, lower panel). This vein, along with the cranial and caudal right-sided tributaries, then opens into the newly formed right atrium within the confines of the systemic venous sinus (Figures 1–4, 1–5 lower panels).

Concomitant with this remodeling of the systemic venous tributaries, there has been formation of the lungs and pulmonary veins. The lungs themselves develop as buds from the tracheobronchial tube in the ventral part of the mediastinal mesenchyme. Prior to formation of these buds, the developing atrium itself retains its initial connection to the mediastinum through the dorsal mesocardium (Figure 1–4, upper panel). Then, as veins canalize within the forming lung buds, they use this connection

A

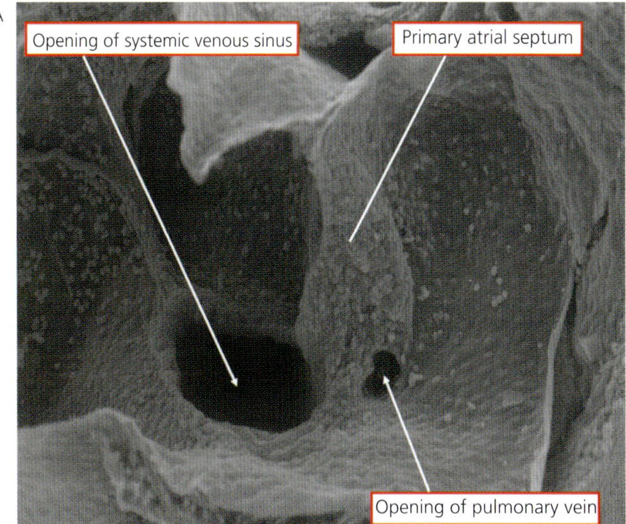

B

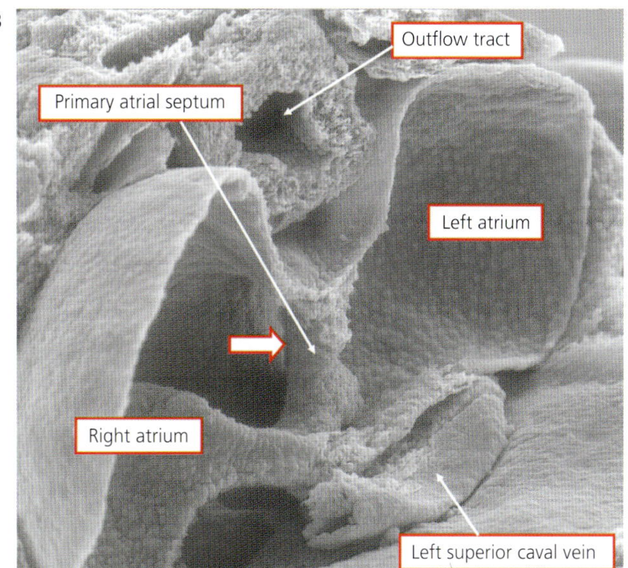

Figures 1–5a and 1–5b Scanning electron micrographs. The upper panel, similar to the preparation shown in the lower panel of Figure 1–4, but from a different animal, is orientated to show the mouth of the pulmonary vein and the beginning of growth of the primary atrial septum from the roof of the common atrial chamber. The lower panel shows the situation after the primary atrial septum has grown toward the atrioventricular endocardial cushion, but has not yet fused with them, but the upper part of the septum has broken down to form the secondary interatrial foramen (arrow). By this stage, the channel draining the systemic tributaries from the left side of the embryo has become incorporated into the left atrioventricular junction, retaining its own walls, and becoming the left superior caval vein. The vein opens to the developing right atrium within the confines of the systemic venous sinus.

through the mesocardium to gain entrance to the atrium (Figure 1–5, upper panel). Controversy has raged over the relationship of the newly formed pulmonary vein and the systemic venous sinus for over a century. The morphologic findings (Webb et al. 1998, 2000, 2001), coupled with the lineage of the cells forming the pulmonary vein (Soufan et al. 2004; Mommersteeg et al. 2006, 2007a) show that the developing pulmonary vein has no connections with the systemic venous tributaries. From the outset it is positioned to the left of the primary atrial septum, which like the vein itself is derived from mediastinal myocardium. The lineage of the systemic venous tributaries can be traced on the basis of their expression of the transcription factor Tbx18. The developing pulmonary veins do not contain this protein (Christoffels et al. 2006). When first seen, the pulmonary vein drains into the heart directly adjacent to the developing atrioventricular junction. In the mouse, the vein persists as a solitary vessel opening to the dorsal wall of the left atrium (Figure 1–5, upper panel). In the human heart, in contrast, the vein, initially opening also to the atrium adjacent to the atrioventricular junction, becomes cannabalized by the left atrium, so that eventually four pulmonary veins open to the corners of the newly formed atrial roof (Webb et al. 2001). This is not completed until after growth of the primary atrial septum and its fusion with the atrioventricular endocardial cushions (see below). And only at this stage is there formation of the superior interatrial groove, or the so-called septum secundum.

2. Septation of the Atrial Chambers

As we have described, it is the rightward shift of the tributaries of the systemic venous sinus that sets the scene for atrial septation. It is concomitant with reorientation of the systemic venous tributaries that the mediastinal myocardium has been added to the common atrial component of the primary tube to form the larger part of the body of the developing left atrium, and provide the site of formation of the primary atrial septum. The atrioventricular canal, of course, was present from the outset and is composed of primary myocardium. The walls of the initial common atrial component of the heart tube are also composed of primary myocardium. The two appendages budding dorsocranially in symmetrical and lateral fashion from this lumen, passing to either side of the developing outflow tract, are made up of chamber myocardium, while the forming pulmonary venous component of the left atrium, the atrial roof, and a small part of the developing right atrium are all made up of mediastinal myocardium. With the rightward shift of the systemic venous tributaries, and the appearance of the mediastinal myocardium, there is also a rightward shift of the corridor of primary myocardium that continues to form the floor of the systemic venous sinus. It is at this stage that we first see the appearance of the primary atrial septum, or *septum primum*, which grows as an interatrial shelf from the atrial roof (Figure 1–5, upper panel). Already by the time of appearance of the primary atrial septum, mounds of endocardial tissue, the atrioventricular endocardial cushions, have appeared on the dorsal and ventral walls of the atrioventricular canal. With ongoing development, these cushions grow toward each other and fuse, separating the canal itself into right-sided and left-sided channels (Figure 1–6). As the cushions grow toward each other to divide the canal, so the primary septum grows toward the cushions, carrying on its leading edge a further collection of endocardial tissue, the so-called mesenchymal cap. By the time the primary septum and mesenchymal cap approach the cushions, the cranial part of the septum, at its origin from the atrial roof, has broken down, creating the secondary interatrial foramen (Figure 1–5, lower panel). The primary atrial foramen is the space between the mesenchymal cap and the fusing atrioventricular endocardial cushions (Figure 1–7). It is then fusion of the mesenchymal cap with the endocardial cushions that obliterates the primary atrial foramen. This process occurs to the right side of the initial opening of the pulmonary vein into the common atrial chamber through the site of the dorsal mesocardium. By the time

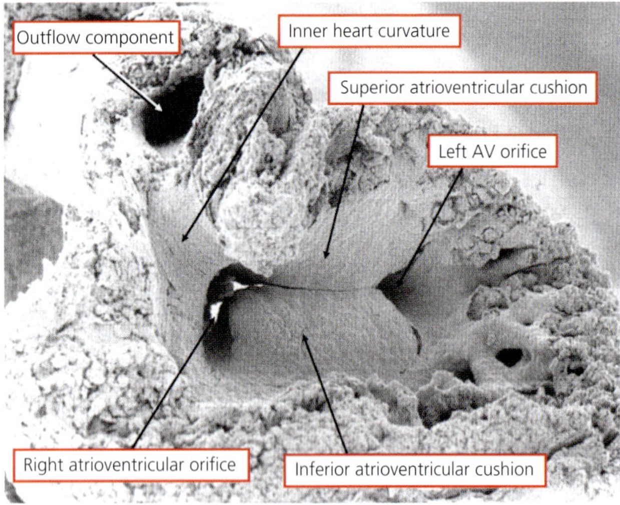

Figure 1–6 Scanning electron micrograph. Dissection of a human embryo. The scanning electron micrograph shows a dissection of a human embryo at the stage of fusion of the atrioventricular (AV) endocardial cushions. The ventricular mass has been cut away, and the developing atrioventricular junctions are viewed from the ventricular aspect. The cushions have been formed by a process of endothelial to mesenchymal transformation along the ventral and dorsal aspects of the canal, but are now positioned cranially, or superiorly, and caudally, or inferiorly, when considered relative to the landmarks of the body.

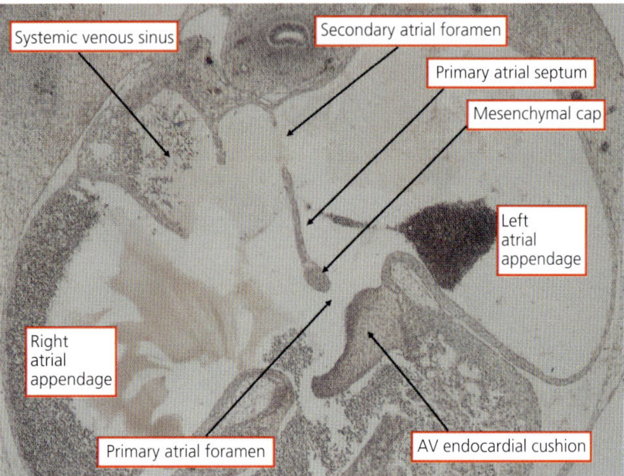

Figure 1–7 Human embryo sectioned in "four chamber" plane. This section from a human embryo is sectioned in the "four chamber" plane. It shows the stage at which the primary atrial septum, carrying a mesenchymal cap on its leading edge, is growing toward the atrioventricular cushions. Already the cranial part of the septum has broken down to form the secondary atrial foramen. The primary foramen is the space between the mesenchymal cap and the endocardial cushion. Note the venous valves delimiting the extent of the systemic venous sinus within the right atrium.

the primary septum has fused with the cushions, the right side of the pulmonary venous orifice itself has enlarged due to ingrowth of tissue from the pharyngeal mesenchyme through the so-called dorsal mesocardial protrusion (Snarr et al. 2007), or the vestibular spine (Webb et al. 1997; Anderson et al. 1998). The mesenchymal tissue of the spine, together with the mesenchymal cap on the primary septum, then muscularizes to form a buttress at the base of the newly formed atrial septum. In the definitive right atrium, the conjoined caudal end of the valves of the systemic venous sinus extend through this muscularized buttress, forming one of the landmarks of the triangle of Koch, thus marking the location of the atrioventricular node (see below). The processes complete the formation of the basal part of the atrial septum, with the muscularized vestibular spine forming the ventrocaudal margin of the oval foramen, the primary septum itself forming the flap valve of the foramen. The foramen itself is the hole formed by the breakdown of the cranial part of the primary septum. This hole is an essential part of the fetal circulation, permitting the richly oxygenated placental return to reach the left side of the developing heart so as to pass to the developing brain. Although many texts describing cardiac development describe formation of a secondary septum in the atrial roof, there is no such structure to be found in the human heart. The upper margin of the oval foramen is no more than a cranial interatrial fold. This does not appear until after the pulmonary veins have achieved their definitive positions at the corners of the atrial roof (Webb et al. 2001).

To summarize the development of the atrial components (Figure 1–8), each atrium possesses a part of the body derived from mediastinal myocardium, with the larger part committed to the morphologically left atrium. Each atrium also possesses an appendage, with walls formed from chamber myocardium, and derived by ballooning from the primary myocardium of the heart tube. Each atrium also possesses a vestibule, formed from the primary myocardium of the atrioventricular canal. The venous components, however, have disparate origins. The systemic venous myocardial component is formed by differentiation of Tbx18-positive tissues into myocardium. The pulmonary venous myocardial component, in contrast, is derived, along with the atrial septum, from Islet1-positive mediastinal mesenchyme, itself developing from the secondary heart field (Soufan et al. 2004; Zaffran et al. 2004; Mommersteeg et al. 2007a). The knowledge concerning the mechanisms of septal formation also permits distinction to be made between the various types of interatrial communication. Not all holes between the atrial chambers are due to deficient atrial septation (Anderson et al. 1999). On the contrary, the morphology of some of the defects shows that they cannot be formed until after the completion of atrial septation, whereas as we will discuss below, the essence of the so-called *primum* defect is failure of formation of the atrioventricular, rather than the atrial, septum. The true septal defects are those found within the confines of the oval fossa. These defects are found when the flap valve of the oval foramen, derived from the primary atrial septum, is fenestrated, or is of insufficient area to overlap the rims formed caudoventrally by muscularization of the vestibular spine, and cranially by the infolded atrial walls. It is also possible for defects to be found within the buttress formed by muscularization of the vestibular spine, but these are very rare (Sharratt et al. 2003). The more frequent sinus venosus defects, along with the rarer coronary sinus defect, are positioned outside the confines of the oval fossa. Indeed, their distinction is dependent on the finding of intact rims of the oval fossa, although the floor of the fossa can be deficient. The sinus venosus defect exists because of anomalous connections of the right pulmonary veins, which create an extraseptal conduit between the cavities of the right and left atriums (Al Zaghal et al. 1997), while the coronary sinus defect exists because of fenestration of the walls that usually divide the sinus from the left atrium (Knauth et al. 2002).

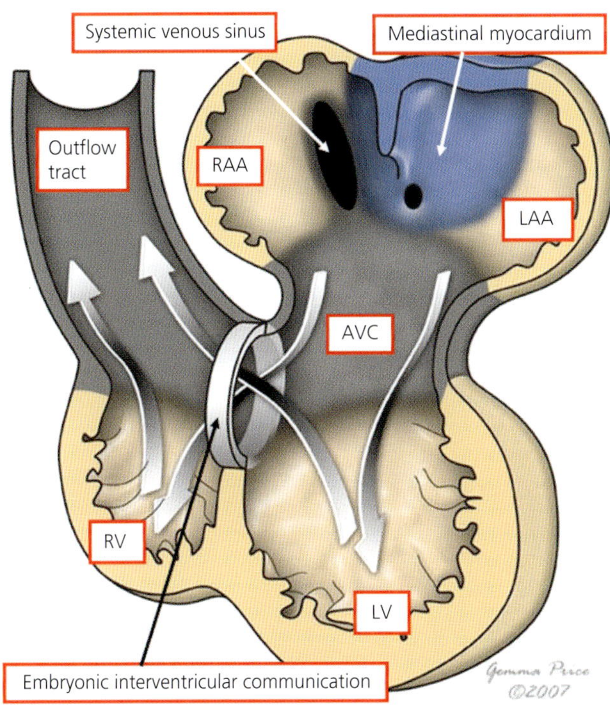

Figure 1–8 Postlooping of the heart tube. The cartoon shows the situation subsequent to looping of the heart tube, ballooning of the apical components of the ventricles, and formation of the atrial chambers. The gray area is the primary tube, while the chamber myocardium is shown in yellow-orange, and the mediastinal myocardium in blue. Note the orifice of the pulmonary vein within the area of mediastinal myocardium, and the growth of the primary atrial septum from within this area. The cartoon also shows how, from the outset, there is streaming of right-sided and left-sided pathways through the embryonic interventricular communication, even though at the stage illustrated the larger part of the atrioventricular canal is supported by the developing left ventricle, and the outlet segment arises almost exclusively from the developing right ventricle. See also Figure 1–3, lower panel.

3. The Atrioventricular Canal

The atrioventricular canal is the part of the primary heart tube positioned between the common atrial component and the inlet of the ventricular loop. As we have described, the canal is septated by fusion of the superior and inferior atrioventricular endocardial cushions (Figure 1–6). Having fused together, the cushions provide an intermediate septal structure, buttressed on the atrial side by the ingrowth and muscularization of the vestibular spine. On the ventricular side, subsequent to closure of the embryonic interventricular communication, to be described below, the tissue derived from the cushions becomes the atrioventricular component of the membranous septum (Allwork and Anderson 1979). The cushions themselves, as we will also describe, provide the foundations for formation of the aortic leaflet of the mitral valve, and the septal leaflet of the tricuspid valve. The initial formation of the cushions within the atrioventricular canal depends on the process of endothelial to mesenchymal transformation (Markwald et al. 1990). In the past, it was usually thought that failure of fusion of the cushions underscored the development of hearts with a common atrioventricular junction, these lesions often being labelled as *endocardial cushion defects* (Van Mierop et al. 1962). Recent studies, nonetheless, have identified inadequate formation of the vestibular spine as the mechanism underscoring persistence of the common atrioventricular junction (Webb et al. 1997, 1998; Snarr et al. 2007). If development proceeds normally, the cushions fuse with each other, thus dividing the atrioventricular canal into right-sided and left-sided channels (Figure 1–6). With ongoing development, the musculature of the atrioventricular canal itself becomes sequestrated as the atrial vestibules (Lamers et al. 1992). If the cushions fuse appropriately, aided by ingrowth of the vestibular spine on the atrial aspect, they pin together the central part of the atrioventricular canal, then permitting expansion of the forming tricuspid and mitral valvar orifices in figure of eight fashion. Should these processes not occur, then there is persistence of a common atrioventricular junction, and almost always a hole in the middle of the heart permitting communication between all four cardiac chambers. It is the common atrioventricular junction that is the essence of so-called atrioventricular septal defects. The *ostium primum* defect is an example of such a lesion, albeit with shunting through the atrioventricular septal defect confined at atrial level because the leaflets derived from the atrioventricular cushions are fused to the crest of the ventricular septum. More frequently, however, patients with an atrioventricular septal defect have a common atrioventricular valvar orifice, with shunting at both atrial and ventricular levels, although in some cases shunting may be confined at ventricular level, or there may even be spontaneous closure of the septal defect (Mahle et al. 2006).

4. Further Development of the Ventricular Loop

Functional separation of the left-sided and right-sided bloodstreams takes place long before the completion of ventricular septation, with two parallel bloodstreams, rather than a single one, traversing the segments as they develop in serial fashion (Figure 1–8). Further development requires partitioning of these blood streams so that the right-sided channel through the atrioventricular canal becomes connected to the pulmonary trunk, whilst the one traversing the left side of the atrioventricular canal is committed eventually to the aorta. This requires remodeling of the part of the heart initially derived from the primary tube, along with appropriate septation of the outlet component.

It is expansion of the right side of the atrioventricular junction that places the cavity of the right atrium in more direct communication with the apical component of the right ventricle ballooned from the outlet of the ventricular loop. It was the fate of a ring of cells marked by the antibody to the nodose ganglion of the chick that clarified this process (Lamers et al. 1992). The ring identified in this fashion initially encircles the communication between the inlet and outlet components of the ventricular loop (Figure 1–9, left panel). With ongoing development, the cells become sequestrated in the vestibule of the tricuspid valve and form a ring around the aortic outflow from the left ventricle. The differences in location of the cells show that the entirety of the right ventricle is derived from the outlet part of the ventricular loop, whilst the subaortic component of the outflow segment is reorientated to become the left ventricular outlet (Figure 1–9, right panel). As this reorientation of the cavity of the initial primary tune has been taking place, so has the outflow tract itself been septated by formation and fusion of a further set of endocardial cushions or ridges, formed as with the atrioventricular cushions by a process of endothelial to mesenchymal transformation (Markwald et al. 1990). We will describe this process in our section devoted to the outlet. It is the remodeling of the cavity of the primary heart tube, nonetheless, providing the inlet to the apical part of the right ventricle, and the

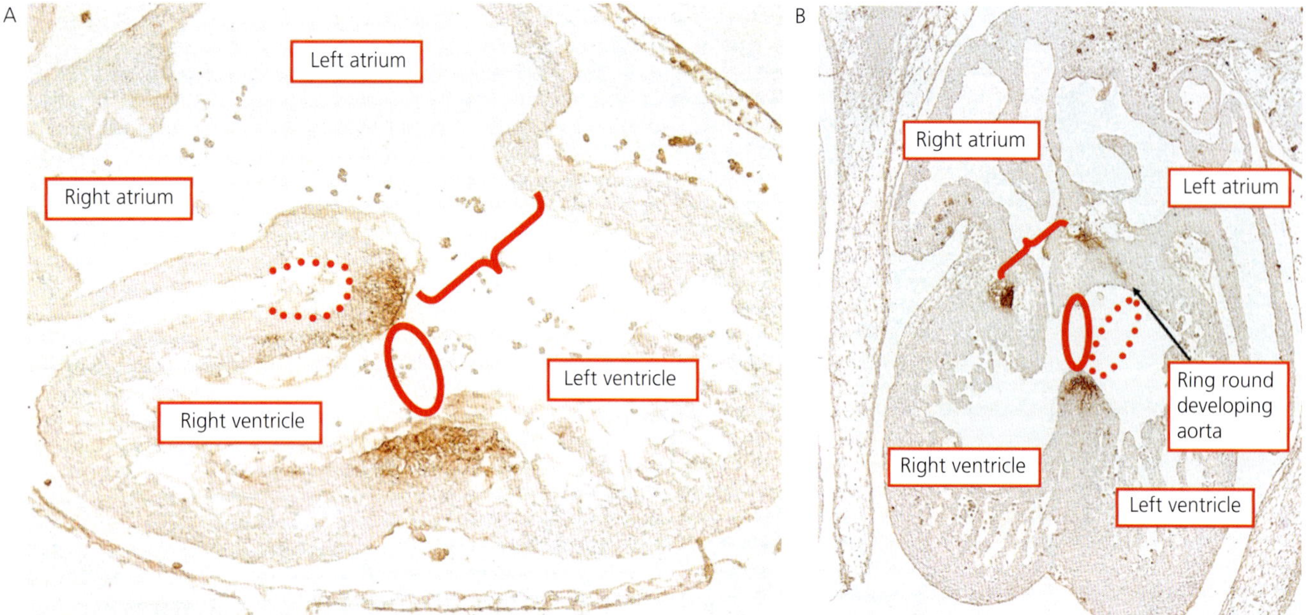

Figures 1–9a and 1–9b Reorientation of the initial embryonic interventricular communication. The figures show the reorientation of the initial embryonic interventricular communication as shown by use of the antibody to the nodose ganglion of the chick. The antibody has stained in brown a ring of cells in these human embryos. At the early stage (left (a) panel) the ring surrounds the embryonic interventricular communication (red oval). Note that most of the circumference of the atrioventricular canal (red bracket) is supported by the developing left ventricle, but that already the wall of the right atrium is directly continuous with that of the right ventricle in the inner heart curvature (red dotted line). As shown in Figure 1–8, there is already separation of right-sided and left-sided streams at this stage. Subsequent to ongoing septation (right panel), the ring of cells, still stained brown, has encircled the newly formed tricuspid valvar vestibule (red bracket), and is passing round the aortic outflow tract as the subaortic component of the outlet is committed to the left ventricle (red dotted oval). Note the plane of the initial interventricular communication (solid red oval).

outlet for the apical part of the left ventricle, which permits the plane of the initial interventricular communication to be closed by apposition of the atrioventricular and outlet endocardial cushions (Odgers 1937–1938; McBride et al. 1981).

5. The Outlet Segment

It is the knowledge regarding mechanics of formation, septation, and separation of the pulmonary and aortic channels of the outlet segment that has benefited most from the recent studies of cardiac development. We now know that this part of the developing heart is derived from a secondary source, different at least in terms of the timing of its commitment to the heart from that producing the initial linear tube (Kelly et al. 2001; Mjaatvedt et al. 2001; Waldo et al. 2001). We have also learnt that, although most of the walls of the definitive intrapericardial outflow tracts have an arterial phenotype, when first formed the entirety of the outlet segment possesses walls made of myocardium (Ya et al. 1998; Anderson et al. 2003). Studies using the scanning electron microscope have shown that the aortic sac is no more than a manifold supporting the arteries that extend through the arches of the pharyngeal mesenchyme (Figure 1–10). It has previously been presumed that this sac, and the outlet segment itself, are septated by growth of an aortopulmonary septum. The recent studies show that the process is much more complicated than growth of a septum in the fashion analogous to division of the atriums by growth of the primary atrial septum. At the same time, it has been shown that migration of cells from the neural crest (Waldo et al. 1998) is crucial for normal separation of the outlet into its pulmonary and aortic channels, but that the population of cells from the neural crest is but one of the new lineages populating the outflow tract (Soufan et al. 2004).

Understanding of these processes is helped by taking note of anatomic boundaries, although there is no certainty that these boundaries themselves are static during the process of development. The developing outlet segment extends to the margins of the pericardial cavity, beyond which it becomes confluent with the aortic sac (Figure 1–10, lower). When first formed, the outlet is a tube with a solitary lumen, taking its origin from the outlet of the ventricular loop. At this early stage, the walls of the tube are exclusively myocardial. When viewed externally, the tube has an obvious bend, permitting the distinction of proximal and distal parts (Figure 1–10, upper). The arteries taking origin from the aortic sac (Figure 1–10, lower) extend through the pharyngeal mesenchyme, encircling the gut and the developing tracheobronchial groove, and uniting dorsally to form the descending aorta. Cartoons representing this stage usually show five pairs of arteries, but in reality there are never more than two or three pairs of arches, along with their arteries, to be seen at any one time. By the time that the arteries of the fourth, or systemic and sixth, or pulmonary arches are seen, the arteries of the third arches have already become moulded into the presumptive carotid vessels, and the arteries of the initial two arches are no longer seen as encircling structures. By this time, the cavity of the aortic sac is little more than the continuation of the lumen of the outlet segment beyond the pericardial boundaries (Figure 1–10, lower). Within the lumen of the outlet segment, nonetheless, the endocardial tissue formed by endothelial to mesenchymal transformation thickens to form opposing and spiraling cushions. When traced from proximally to distally, the parietal

A

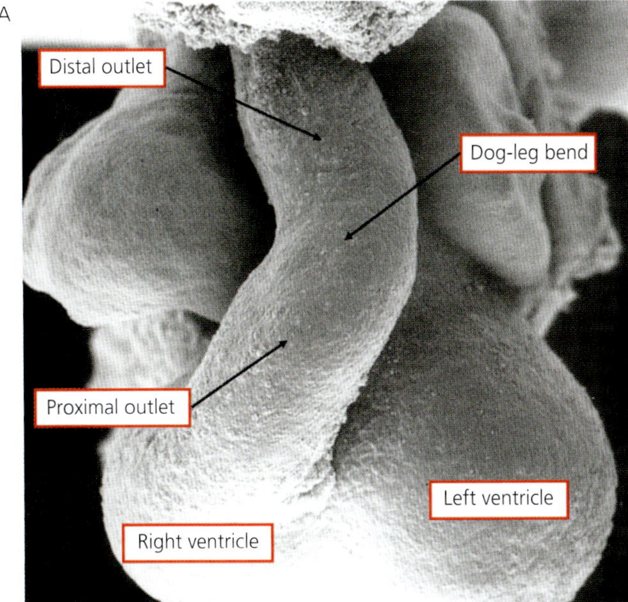

B

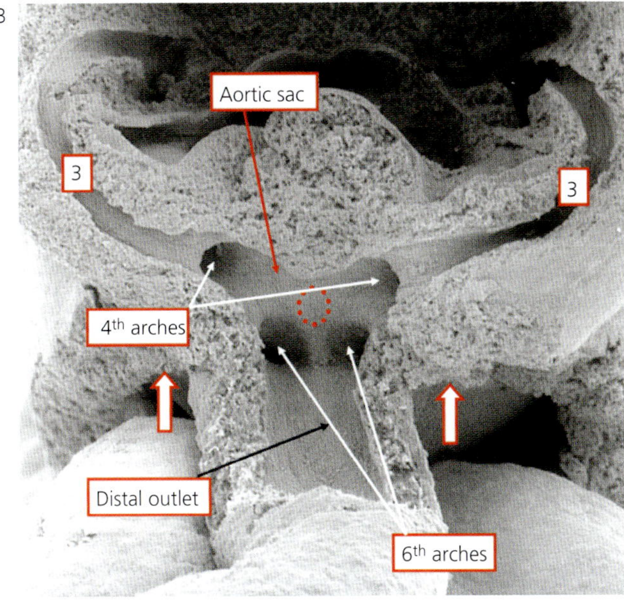

Figures 1–10a and 1–10b Scanning electron micrographs of human embryos. These scanning electron micrographs of human embryos show the structure of the developing outflow tract and aortic sac. The upper (a) panel shows the dogleg configuration of the intrapericardial outflow tract, which is supported at this stage almost exclusively above the right ventricle. During this phase of development, the bend permits recognition of proximal and distal components of the outflow tract. The lower panel shows a dissection of the distal segment, which becomes confluent with the aortic sac at the margins of the pericardial cavity (arrows). The aortic sac is no more than a manifold giving rise to the arteries running through the pharyngeal arches. At this stage, it is possible to recognize the symmetrical arteries of the third, fourth, and sixth arches. The dorsal wall of the sac (dotted red area) represents the putative aortopulmonary septum.

ridge turns at the bend beneath the cushion initially located septally, achieving a caudal location within the distal outflow tract. Subsequent fusion of the cushions along their facing surfaces, therefore, septates the proximal outflow tract into ventral and dorsal channels, but produces right-sided and left-sided channels distally. The fusion commences distally and zips up the outflow tract in proximal direction. Concomitant with development of the cushions, important changes take place within the aortic sac.

There is marked diminution in size, and eventual obliteration, of the right-sided arteries running from the sac to join the descending aorta. As these right-sided arteries begin to involute, so it becomes possible to recognize the developing pulmonary arteries, which descend caudally within the pharyngeal mesenchyme to supply the developing lungs (Figure 1–11, left). After these changes, only two arterial orifices, located cranially and caudally, arise from the aortic sac. Ingrowth of the dorsal wall of the pharyngeal mesenchyme between the origins of arteries running to the fourth and sixth arches, creating an arterial spine that functions as an aortopulmonary septum, then permits fusion with the distal ends of the outlet cushions so that the right-sided aortic channel becomes connected to the fourth arch, and the left-sided pulmonary channel to the sixth arch (Figure 1–11, right). By this time, cells have also begun to invade the parietal walls of the distal outlet from the pharyngeal mesenchyme, replacing the initially myocardial walls between the ends of the cushions. The ingrowth of this tissue, which rapidly arterializes, gives a fish mouth appearance to the myocardial border of the distal outlet (Bartelings and Gittenberger de Groot 1989). By the time that the arterial spine, corresponding to the aortopulmonary septum, has fused with the distal edges of the middle parts of the endocardial cushions, the myocardial border of the outlet is seen at the junction of its distal and proximal parts, the distal parts themselves having become the intrapericardial parts of the aorta and pulmonary trunk (Figure 1–12).

At this stage of development, with the distal part of the initially muscular outflow tract now replaced by the intrapericardial parts of the aorta and pulmonary trunk, the cushions within the proximal outlet are fused distally, but remain unfused more proximally. The cushions within this proximal part of the outlet are still encased within a turret of myocardium. At the margins of the more distal part of this turret, now separated into aortic and pulmonary components, additional intercalated cushions have formed, again by a process of endothelial to mesenchymal transformation. The cushion in the pulmonary component is positioned appreciably more cranially than the aortic cushion. Cavitation now occurs within the distal ends of these cushions, along with either ends of the fused outflow cushions, to produce the primordiums of the aortic and pulmonary valves. With cavitation of the cushions, the part of the cushion adjacent to the myocardial turret arterializes and becomes the arterial valvar sinus. At the same time, the part of each cushion, adjacent to the arterial lumen, becomes converted into the valvar leaflets. The edges of the outlet cushions at their margins do not fuse so that the combination with the intercalated cushions is able to produce the trifoliate configuration of the aortic and pulmonary valves. The middle part of the cushions, in contrast, breaks down along a line at right angles to their plane of fusion, thus separating the newly formed arterial roots. This middle part of the fused cushions was initially occupied by the cells derived from the neural crest (Waldo et al. 1998). It is these cells that then die by apoptosis (Sharma et al. 2004) so as to produce the plane of cleavage between the arterial roots. Should there be excessive fusion along the line of union between the cushions, this would result in formation of an arterial valve with only two leaflets, the so-called bicuspid valve.

At the commencement of cavitation of the distal margins of the cushions, the proximal parts of the cushions remain unfused.

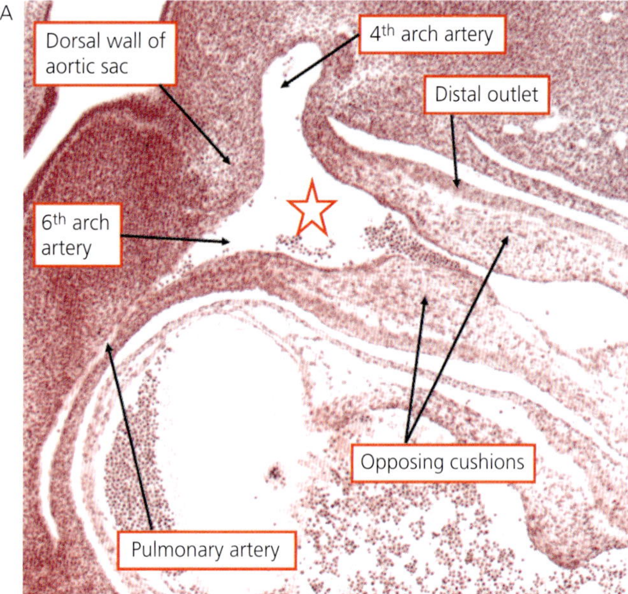

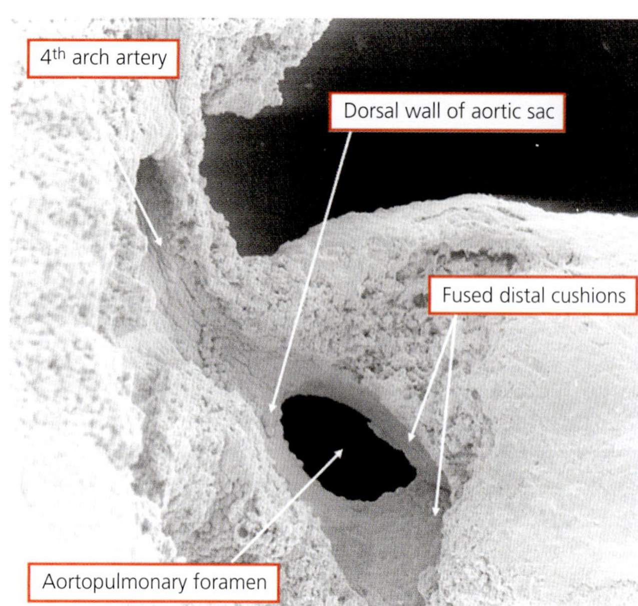

Figures 1–11a and 1–11b Location of the aortopulmonary foramen. The left (a) hand panel is a sagittal section through the distal outflow tract of a human embryo just prior to fusion of the distal outflow cushions, while the right panel is a comparable dissection revealed with the scanning electron microscope to show the fused cushions and the right-sided channel arising from the aortic sac to feed the systemic aortic arch. Closure of the aortopulmonary foramen (star in left panel) will connect the aortic channel in the distal outlet segment with the fourth arch, and pulmonary channel with the left sixth arch and the pulmonary arteries, which now arise from the caudal part of the aortic sac.

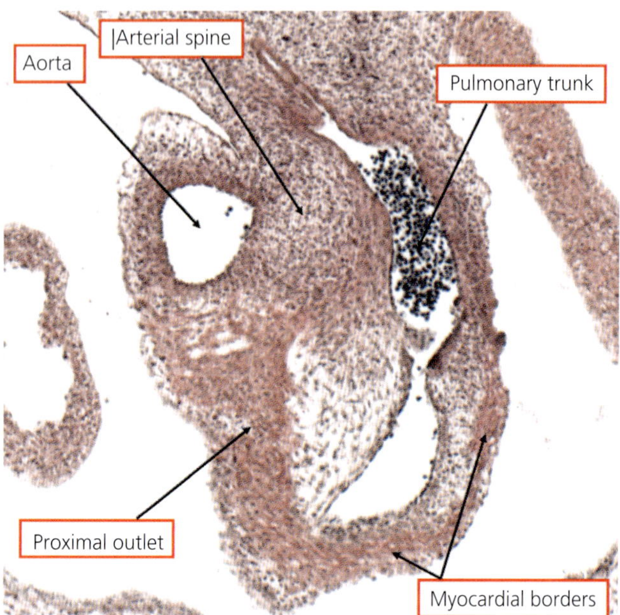

Figure 1–12 Frontal section of developing human outflow tracts. This cross-section through the outlets of a human embryo shows how the distal part has arterialized, with ingrowth of an arterial spine separating the aorta from the pulmonary trunk, while the more proximal part remains encased within a myocardial turret, and has yet to progress to form the arterial valves and the subpulmonary infundibulum.

It is the fusion of these proximal cushions with each other, and also with the crest of the muscular ventricular septum formed concomitant with the ballooning of the apical ventricular components, which walls the aorta into the left ventricle. As they fuse, the most proximal parts of the cushions also muscularize, while the central part of the cushion mass, again initially occupied by the cells taking their origin from the neural crest, disappears by the process of apoptosis (Sharma et al. 2004). In this way, the cranial part of the proximal outlet becomes the subpulmonary infundibulum, the disappearance of the cells migrating from the neural crest creating the tissue plane between it and the aortic root. The fusion of the muscularized cushions with the crest of the muscular ventricular septum sets the scene for final closure of the embryonic interventricular foramen by formation of the membranous septum (Odgers 1937–1938), with ongoing delamination of the septal leaflet of the tricuspid valve serving to divide the septum into its interventricular and atrioventricular components (Allwork and Anderson 1979). The musculature of the inner heart curvature initially continues to separate the developing leaflets of the aortic valve, by now committed to the left ventricle, from the aortic leaflet of the mitral valve. This muscle does not disappear until a much later stage, giving the aortic-to-mitral valvar continuity characteristic of the postnatal heart. It is also at much later stages that the muscular cuff surrounding the developing arterial roots is removed, once more by a process of apoptosis (Sharma et al. 2004).

Formation of Valves

There are valves formed at several positions within the developing heart. The valve-like structures formed at the sinuatrial junction are most conspicuous during the early stages of development (Figure 1–13). They do remain recognizable to various extents postnatally. The ventral portion guards the orifice of the coronary sinus, the Thebesian valve, while the dorsal part persists as the Eustachian valve, guarding the orifice of the inferior caval vein.

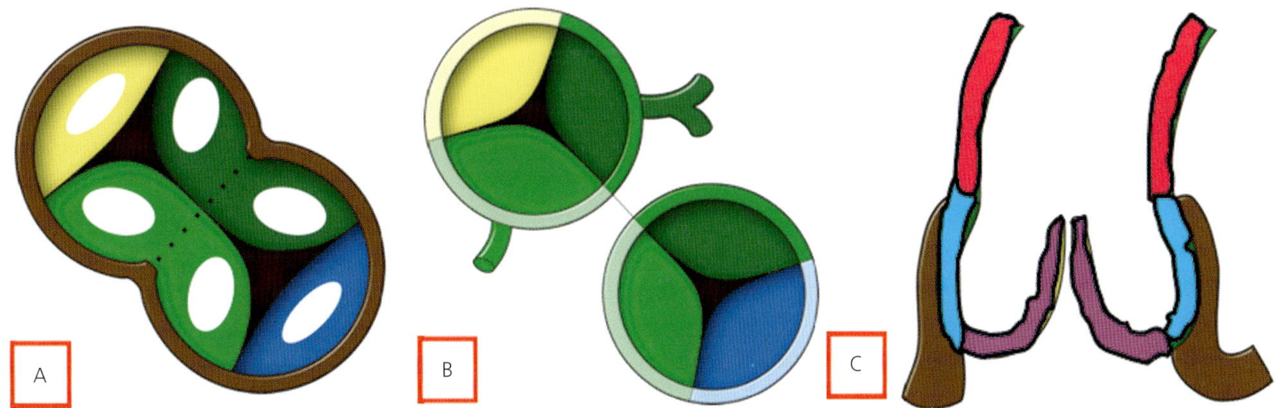

Figure 1–13 Development of the arterial valves. The cartoons show the steps involved in formation of the arterial valves and their supporting sinuses from the excavating distal ends of the outflow cushions. Panel A shows the arrangement at the beginning of cavitation of the cushions, as seen in plan form, with the cavitation shown in longitudinal section in panel C. Panel B shows the formation of the separate aortic and pulmonary roots. In panel C, the myocardial turret is shown in brown, with the walls of the arterial trunk in red, the sinus in pale blue, and the leaflets in purple.

As we have already described, the atrioventricular canal is initially lined by a continuous mass of cardiac jelly, from which develop gradually, by the process of mesenchymal to endothelial transformation, the superior and inferior atrioventricular endocardial cushions. These cushions themselves function as valves during early development. They then provide the scaffold for formation of the definitive valvar leaflets. The left ventricular components fuse to form the aortic leaflet of the mitral valve, while the right ventricular parts give rise to the septal leaflet of the tricuspid valve (de Lange et al. 2004; Kanani et al. 2005). Formation of new cushions in the lateral parts of the atrioventricular canal provides the primordiums of the other valvar leaflets. In addition, there is delamination of superficial ventricular myocardium at the sites of the cushions, but the definitive leaflets have been shown to lack any myocardial heritage (de Lange et al. 2004), so the delaminating myocardium must subsequently disappear. The points of attachment of the delaminated myocardium, nonetheless, compact and persist as the papillary muscles. Formation of the septal leaflet of the tricuspid valve is an extremely late event, and undermining of this leaflet is the mechanism responsible for formation of the atrioventricular and interventricular parts of the membranous septum (Allwork and Anderson 1979).

We have already described at length the processes involved in formation of the arterial valves. We will not repeat this information, other than to state that, as yet, it remains to be determined how the cushions give rise, on the one hand the valvar leaflets, and on the other hand the supporting valvar sinuses.

The Conduction System

The genetic and molecular advances of the past decade have also served to elucidate our knowledge of the development of the conduction tissues. During early development of the heart, it is not possible to recognize areas of myocardium that are distinguished in the fashion of the postnatal nodes and ventricular conduction pathways. Even at these early stages, however, it is possible to record an electrocardiogram from the developing embryo, this feature becoming evident as soon as the heart tube is differentiated to give areas permitting fast as opposed to slow conduction, this coinciding with the ballooning of the chamber myocardium from the primary myocardium of the linear heart tube (Moorman et al. 2005). The feature of chamber myocardium is that it conducts rapidly, while the primary myocardium conducts slowly. After ballooning of the atrial appendages, the primary myocardium of the atrial component forms a dorsal corridor extending from the atrioventricular canal to the orifices of the systemic venous tributaries. In the developing murine heart, this myocardium can be recognized by its content of the *Tbx3* gene. This gene also marks the entirety of the atrioventricular canal at an early stage, and shows the location of the ring of cells demarcated by the Gln1 antibody in the human heart (Figure 1–9). Eventually, only the atrioventricular node and the sinus node remain *Tbx3* positive, although the location of the tissues initially positive for *Tbx3* within the atrial vestibules, around the mouth of the coronary sinus, and along the terminal crest offers some explanation for the origins of arrhythmic activity in patients with atrial arrhythmias (Mommersteeg et al. 2007b).

Myocardial Vascularization

In the early stage of development, there is no requirement for any specific vascularization of the myocardial walls, since the myocardium itself is no more than a mass of individual trabeculations lined by endocardium. The first indication of the epicardial trunks that feed the mural vessels is seen with the appearance of a subepicardial endothelial plexus. This network, continuous with endothelial sprouts that encircle the developing proximal outlet, forms a ring around the developing arterial valves. Sprouts from the ring then invade the aortic wall from the outside (Bogers et al. 1989). Only two of these multiple sprouts eventually develop a lumen, thus producing the orifices of the definitive right and left coronary arteries.

Myocardial Maturation

The maturation of the myocardium forming the ventricular walls is intimately connected to the development of the mural coronary arterial supply. It is these processes which underscore the compaction of the ventricular walls. As yet, our knowledge of the precise steps involved in removal of the initially extensive trabecular myocardial network, and the thickening of the compact layer, remains rudimentary (Freedom et al. 2005; Lurie 2008). In the sixth and seventh weeks of development, immediately prior to closure of the embryonic interventricular foramen, there is an extensive trabecular meshwork filling the larger part of the ventricular lumens. The compact layer of the myocardium is very thin at this stage in relation to the thickness of the trabeculated layer. It is subsequent to closure of the embryonic interventricular communication that a marked reduction becomes evident in the extent of the trabeculations, along with a thickening of the compact layer. It does not seem that the trabeculations themselves coalesce to produce the compact layer, but persistence of the embryonic trabecular layer is almost certainly the substrate for ventricular noncompaction. Signaling from the developing epicardium, nonetheless, has been shown to play a key role in thickening of the developing compact layer (Lavine et al. 2005).

References

Allwork SP, Anderson RH. Developmental anatomy of the membranous part of the ventricular septum in the human heart. *Br Heart J.* 1979;41:275–280.

Al Zaghal AM, Li J, Anderson RH, Lincoln C, Shore D, Rigby ML. Anatomical criteria for the diagnosis of sinus venosus defects. *Heart.* 1997;78:298–304.

Anderson RH, Brown NA, Moorman AFM. Development and structures of the venous pole of the heart. *Dev Dyn.* 2006;235, 2–9.

Anderson RH, Webb S, Brown NA. The mouse with trisomy 16 as a model of human hearts with common atrioventricular junction. *Cardiovasc Res.* 1998;39:155–164.

Anderson RH, Webb S, Brown NA. Clinical anatomy of the atrial septum with reference to its developmental components. *Clin Anat.* 1999;12:362–374.

Anderson RH, Webb S, Brown NA, Lmers W, Moorman A. Development of the heart: (3) Formation of the ventricular outflow tracts, arterial valves, and intrapericardial arterial trunks. *Heart.* 2003;89:1110–1118.

Arguello C, De la Cruz MV, Gomez CS. Experimental study of the formation of the heart tube in the chick embryo. *J Embryol Exp Morphol.* 1975;33:1–11.

Bartelings MM, Gittenberger-de Groot AC. The outflow tract of the heart—embryologic and morphologic correlations. *Int J Cardiol.* 1989;22:289–300.

Bogers AJJC, Gittenberger-de Groot AC, Poelmann RE, Peault BM, Huysmans HA. Development of the origin of the coronary arteries, a matter of ingrowth or outgrowth. *Anat Embryol.* 1989;180:437–441.

Cai CL, Liang X, Shi Y, et al. Isl1 identifies a cardiac progenitor population that proliferates prior to differentiation and contributes a majority of cells to the heart. *Dev Cell.* 2003;5:877–889.

Christoffels VM, Mommersteeg MTM, Trowe MO, et al. Formation of the venous pole of the heart from an Nkx 2.5 negative precursor population requires Tbx 18. *Circ Res.* 2006;98:1555–1563.

Davis CL. Development of the human heart from its first appearance to the stage found in embryos of 20 paired somites. *Contrib Embryol.* 1927;19:247–293.

de Lange de Lange FJ, Moorman AFM, Anderson RH, et al. Lineage and morphogenetic analysis of the cardiac valves. *Circ Res.* 2004;95:645–654.

Freedom RM, Yoo SJ, Perrin D, Taylor G, Petersen S, Anderson RH. The morphological spectrum of ventricular noncompaction. *Cardiol Young.* 2005;15:345–364.

Garcia-Martinez V, Schoenwolf GC. Primitive streak origin of the cardiovascular system in avian embryos. *Dev Biol.* 1993;159:706–719.

Kanani M, Moorman AFM, Cook AC, et al. Development of the atrioventricular valves: clinicomorphologic correlations. *Ann Thorac Surg.* 2005;79:1797–1804.

Kelly RG, Brown NA, Buckingham ME. The arterial pole of the mouse heart forms from Fgf10-expressing cells in pharyngeal mesoderm. *Dev Cell.* 2001;1:435–440.

Knauth A, McCarthy KP, Webb S, et al. Interatrial communication through the mouth of the coronary sinus. *Cardiol Young.* 2002;12:364–372.

Lamers WH, Wessels A, Verbeek FJ, et al. New findings concerning ventricular septation in the human heart. Implications for maldevelopment. *Circulation.* 1992;86:1194–1205.

Lavine KJ, Yu K, White AC, et al. Endocardial and epicardial derived FGF signals regulate myocardial proliferation and differentiation in vivo. *Dev Cell.* 2005;8:85–95.

Lurie P. Ventricular non-compaction. A nonogenarian's perspective. *Cardiol Young.* 2008;18:243–249.

Mahle WT, Shirali GD, Anderson RH. Echo-morphological correlates in patients with atrioventricular septal defect and common atrioventricular junction. *Cardiol Young.* 2006;16(suppl 3):43–51.

Manasek FJ, Monroe RG. Early cardiac morphogenesis is independent of function. *Dev Biol.* 1972;27:584–588.

Markwald RR, Mjaatvedt CH, Krug EL, Sinning AR. Inductive interactions in heart development: role of cardiac adherons in cushion tissue formation. In: Bockman DE, Kirby ML, eds. *Embryonic Origins of Defective Heart Development. Ann N Y Acad Sci.* 1990;588:13–25.

McBride RE, Moore GW, Hutchins GM. Development of the outflow tract and closure of the interventricular septum in the normal human heart. *Am J Anat.* 1981;100:309–331.

Mjaatvedt CH, Nakaoka T, Moreno-Rodriguez R, et al. The outflow tract of the heart is recruited from a novel heart-forming field. *Dev Biol.* 2001;238:97–109.

Mommersteeg MTM, Brown NA, Prall OWG, et al. Pitx2c and Nkx2.5 are required for the differentiation and identity of the pulmonary myocardium. *Circ Res.* 2007a;101:902–909.

Mommersteeg MTM, Hoogars WMH, Prall OWJ, et al. Molecular pathway for the localized formation of the sinoatrial node. *Circ Res.* 2007b;100:354–362.

Mommersteeg MTM, Soufan AT, de Lange F, et al. Two distinct pools of mesenchyme contribute to the development of the atrial septum. *Circ Res.* 2006;99:351–353.

Moorman AFM, Christoffels VM. Cardiac Chamber Formation: Development, Genes and Evolution. *Physiol Rev.* 2003;83:1223–1267.

Moorman AFM, Christoffels VM, Anderson RH. Anatomic substrates for cardiac conduction. *Heart Rhythm.* 2005;2:875–886.

Moorman AFM, Christoffels VM, Anderson RH, van den Hoff MJB. The heart-forming fields--one or multiple? *Phil Trans R Soc B.* 2007;362:1257–1265.

Odgers PNB. The development of the pars membranacea septi in the human heart. *J Anat.* 1937–1938;72:247–259.

Orts Llorca F, Ruano Gil D. A causal analysis of the heart curvatures in the chicken embryo. *Roux Archiv für Entwicklungsmechanik der Organismen.* 1967;158:52–63.

Patten BM, Kramer TC. The initiation of contractions in the embryonic chicken heart. *Am J Anat.* 1933;53:349–375.

Rana MS, Horsten NCA, Tesink-Taekema S, Lamers WH, Moorman AFM, van den Hoff MJB. Trabeculated right ventricular free wall in the chicken heart forms by ventricularization of the myocardium initially forming the outflow tract. *Circ Res.* 2007;100:1000–1007.

Rosenquist GC. Location and movements of cardiogenic cells in the chick embryo: the heart forming portion of the primitive streak. *Dev Biol.* 1970;22:461–475.

Sharma PR, Anderson RH, Copp AJ, Henderson DJ. Spatiotemporal analysis of programmed cell death during mouse cardiac septation. *Anat Rec A Discov Mol Cell Evol Biol.* 2004;277(2)A:355–369.

Sharratt GP, Webb S, Anderson RH. The vestibular defect: an interatrial communication due to a deficiency in the atrial septal component derived from the vestibular spine. *Cardiol Young.* 2003;13:184–190.

Snarr BS, O'Neal JL, Chintalapudi MR, et al. Isl1 expression at the venous pole identifies a novel role for the second heart field in cardiac development. *Circ Res.* 2007;101:971–974.

Soufan AT, van den Hoff MJB, Ruijter JM, et al. Reconstruction of the patterns of gene expression in the developing mouse heart reveals an architectural arrangement that facilitates the understanding of atrial malformations and arrhythmias. *Circ Res.* 2004;95:1207–1215.

Van Mierop LHS, Alley RD, Kausel HW, Stranahan A. The anatomy and embryology of endocardial cushion defects. *J Thor Cardiovasc Surg.* 1962;43:71–82.

Viragh S, Challice CE. Origin and differentiation of cardiac muscle cells in the mouse. *J Ultrastruct Res.* 1973;42:1–24.

Waldo K, Miyagawa-Tomita S, Kumiski D, Kirby ML. Cardiac neural crest cells provide new insight into septation of the cardiac outflow tract: aortic sac to ventricular septal closure. *Dev Biol.* 1998;196:129–144.

Waldo KL, Kumiski DH, Wallis KT, et al. Conotruncal myocardium arises from a secondary heart field. *Development.* 2001;128:3179–3188.

Webb S, Brown NA, Anderson RH. Cardiac morphology at late fetal stages in the mouse with trisomy 16: consequences for different formation of the atrioventricular junction when compared to humans with trisomy 21. *Cardiovasc Res.* 1997;34:515–524.

Webb S, Brown NA, Anderson RH, Richardson MK. Relationship in the chick of the developing pulmonary vein to the embryonic systemic venous sinus. *Anat Rec.* 2000;259:67–75.

Webb S, Brown NA, Wessels A, Anderson RH. Development of the murine pulmonary vein and its relationship to the embryonic venous sinus. *Anat Rec.* 1998;250:325–334.

Webb S, Kanani M, Anderson RH, Richardson MK, Brown NA. Development of the human pulmonary vein and its incorporation in the morphologically left atrium. *Cardiol Young.* 2001;11:632–642.

Ya J, van den Hoff MJB, de Boer PAJ, et al. The normal development of the outflow tract in the rat. *Circ Res.* 1998;82:464–472.

Zaffran S, Kelly RG, Meilhac SM, Buckingham ME, Brown NA. Right ventricular myocardium derives from the anterior heart field. *Circ Res.* 2004;95:261–268.

2

The Molecular Basis of Cardiovascular Development

Jamie Bentham and Shoumo Bhattacharya

Introduction

Congenital heart disease (CHD) is the commonest birth defect and a major cause of childhood morbidity and mortality. In live-born infants the incidence ranges from 0.4% to 1.2% (Burn and Goodship 2002; Hoffman 2002). CHD is typically characterized by lesions such as atrial, ventricular, and atrioventricular septal defects (ASD, VSD, and AVSD), outflow tract malformations [e.g., tetralogy of Fallot (TOF), common arterial trunk (CAT), transposition of great arteries (TGA), and double outlet right ventricle (DORV)], and aortic arch malformations [e.g., patent ductus arteriosus (PDA), aortic coarctation or interruption (Clark 2001)].

Surgical and medical advances over the past three decades have had a tremendous impact on mortality. A major translational goal is the prevention of CHD. The paradigm here is the use of folate as prophylaxis against neural tube defects, which has led to the prevention of 50% to 75% of cases (Blom et al. 2006; De Wals et al. 2007). A major aim of genetic studies is to identify pathways that could be manipulated to prevent CHD or modify the course of disease. Another major goal is to understand the genetic architecture of CHD and the underlying biological mechanisms. This will allow us to better predict the likelihood of CHD based on a particular genetic background. It will also enable us to understand how disease causing mutations on many occasions do not result in a phenotype—that is, are buffered by gene–gene and gene–environment interactions. Our understanding of CHD is critically dependent on using animal models that will allow identification of the key genetic and environmental mechanisms likely to cause disease in man (Box 2–1).

Box 2–1

- The mouse is a good model for understanding cardiac development and congenital heart disease (CHD).
- Genes necessary for mouse heart development will be CHD candidate genes in man.
- Identifying the components of cardiac genetic networks will be crucial for evaluating the roles genes play in causing CHD.
- Identification of cardiac developmental genes and their regulatory sequences will be crucial in developing new therapeutic and preventive strategies for CHD.

Genetic Architecture of CHD

Heritable syndromes account for approximately 7.4% of CHD, and studies of such families have identified several genes that control cardiac development (Ferencz et al. 1989; Ferencz and Boughman 1993; Burn and Goodship 2002). The genetic mechanisms underlying "sporadic" CHD are in general poorly understood. Approximately 11.9% arises from chromosomal abnormalities such as Down or DiGeorge (22q11 deletion) syndrome, which affect cardiac developmental gene copy number (Ferencz and Boughman 1993; Burn and Goodship 2002). In addition, some patients with nonsyndromic "sporadic" CHD also have 22q11 deletion (Pierpont et al. 2007). Moreover, analysis of the human gene variation database (http://projects.tcag.ca/variation/ November 29, 2007) shows that in apparently normal individuals 70 of 284 cardiac developmental genes have some form of copy number variation (CNV), suggesting a potential role for this mechanism in CHD, for instance, by random assortment leading to multiple cardiac gene CNV in a single individual. Point mutations in cardiac developmental genes have also been identified in CHD (e.g., Goldmuntz et al. 2002; McElhinney et al. 2003) but currently account for only a small proportion (a few percent) of "sporadic" CHD, for example, 0.77% for CITED2 (Sperling et al. 2005) and 2% for NKX2–5 (McElhinney et al. 2003). However, these studies of human genetic architecture do not provide a mechanistic understanding of gene function in cardiac development, and analyses of gene–gene and gene–environment interactions in humans remain a challenge.

Rationale for Using the Mouse as a Model for CHD

Mouse models are powerful experimental tools for understanding human disease and those genes that have a major role in mouse heart development are likely candidate genes for CHD in man. Like the human, the mouse has a four-chambered heart with a septated outflow tract, left-sided great arteries, and parallel pulmonary and systemic circulations (Kent and Carr 2001). Thus it is a good anatomical model for common cardiac malformations [e.g., ASD, VSD, TOF, TGA, CAT, PDA, interrupted aortic arch, and isomerism (Figure 2–1)]. These cannot be identified in other genetically tractable model organisms such as the fruit fly or zebra fish that lack parallel pulmonary and systemic circulations. Extensive chromosomal synteny, phylogenetic closeness, and the availability of complete mouse and human genomic sequence make the identification of orthologous human genes considerably easier. Of 239 human genes associated with CHD, 150 have been knocked out or mutated in the mouse. Of these genes, the large majority (133) have either a lethal or a cardiac developmental phenotype that recapitulates the human malformation. These observations support the use of the mouse as a model for human CHD.

Molecular Mechanisms in Cardiac Development

We can consider molecular mechanisms in terms of the interrelated processes of heart tube development, left-right patterning, atrioventricular septation, outflow tract development, valvulogenesis, pharyngeal arch artery patterning, and myocardial development. These developmental processes have been recently reviewed (Hamada et al. 2002; Harvey 2002), but it is useful to outline the principal embryological events required to form a four-chambered mammalian heart as background for discussing the molecular basis of CHD.

Cardiac Precursors and Specialization

Cardiac malformations can broadly be considered to arise from defects in progenitor cell specialization, or abnormal patterning during development. The heart, although induced by endodermal signals, is essentially mesodermal in origin, with a minor contribution from the ectodermal neural crest (Moorman and Christoffels 2003). These three embryonic lineages arise from the epiblast (Tam and Gad 2004). Following gastrulation, mesodermal progenitors migrate anteriorly to form two closely appositioned primary and secondary heart fields (embryonic day E7–7.5) (Harvey 2002; Kelly and Buckingham 2002; Cai et al. 2003; Solloway and Harvey 2003). These cells specialize into cardiomyocyte, endothelial, and

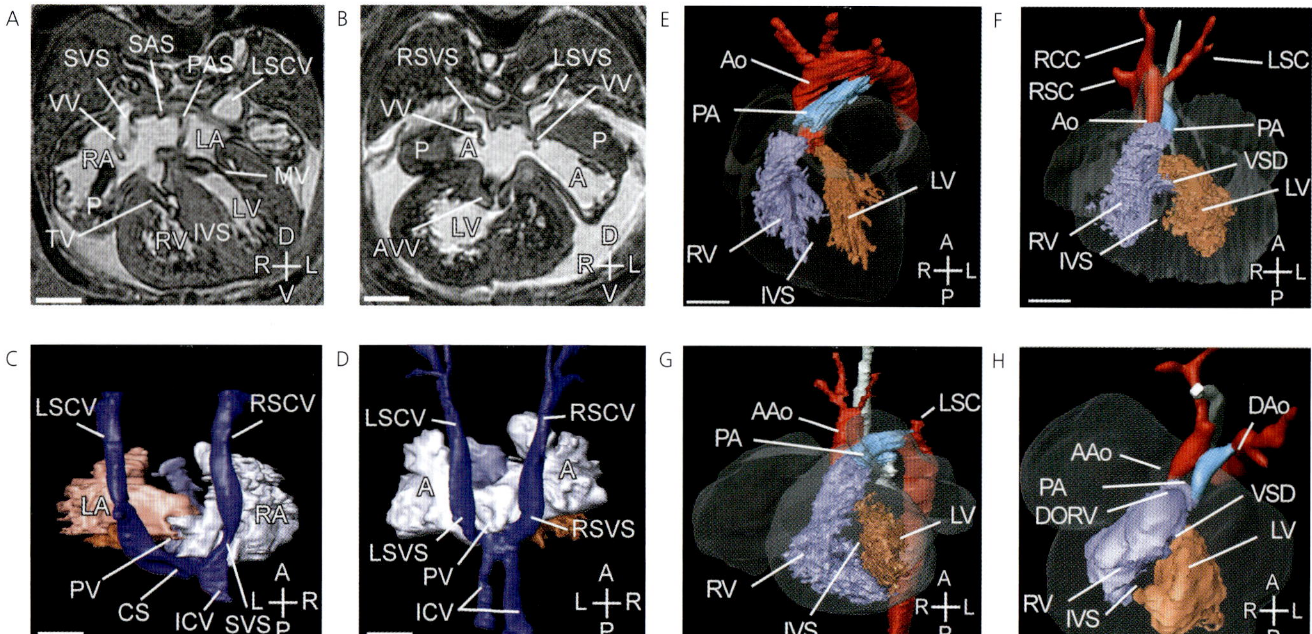

Figure 2–1 Cardiac malformations in 15.5dpc embryos. (a–d) Magnetic resonance images of wild-type and littermate transgenic knockout mice. Reprinted by permission from Macmillan Publishers Ltd. (*Nat Genet*) (Bamforth SD, Braganca J, Farthing CR, et al. Cited2 controls left-right patterning and heart development through a Nodal-Pitx2c pathway. *Nat Genet.* 2004;36:1189–1196), copyright (2004). (a) Transverse section of a wild-type embryo. The interventricular septum (IVS) separates the right and left ventricles (RV, LV), the cardiac apex is to the left and there are separate atrioventricular valves (MV, TV); the pectinated (P) right atrium (RA), the primary and secondary atrial septa (PAS, SAS), and superior venous sinus (SVS) are shown. The cardiac anatomy is normal. (b) Transverse section of a left-right patterning gene transgenic embryo [littermate of (a)]. The apex is to the right; there is right atrial isomerism [characterized by a common atrial chamber, loss of the primary atrial septum, pectination of the left atrium as well as the right (P), and loss of the coronary sinus (CS) with the superior caval vein (SCV) entering to the left of the common chamber directly). There is an atrioventricular septal defect (common atrioventricular valve (AVV)]. (c,d) The 3D reconstruction of the same hearts as in (a,b) enables the entry of the left superior vena cava into the right atrium through the coronary sinus (CS) in the normal heart (c) to be viewed. (e–h) 3D magnetic resonance image cardiac reconstructions of wild-type and littermate transgenic knockout mice. (e) Wild-type mouse with a normal heart. The ascending aorta (Ao) and pulmonary artery (PA) are shown. (f) 3D reconstruction of a transgenic mouse heart. The aorta arises anterior in parallel and to the right of the pulmonary artery (transposition of the great arteries) and arises from the right ventricle (DORV). The aortic arch descends to the right of the trachea. There is a large VSD. (g,h) 3D reconstructions of transgenic mouse hearts demonstrating interruption of the aortic arch. In (g) the arch is interrupted after the left common carotid (LCC), in (h) the arch is interrupted before the left common carotid. Both great arteries arise from the right ventricle (DORV). Right subclavian artery (RSC), left subclavian artery (LSC), right common carotid artery (RCC), ascending aorta (AAo), descending aorta (DAo), and pulmonary veins (PV). Scale bars = 500 μm; axes: D—dorsal; V—ventral; R—right; L—left; A—anterior; P—posterior.

epicardial lineages that form the heart. Neural crest cells differentiate into the mesenchyme of the great arteries and transiently contribute to the outflow tract (conotruncal) and aorticopulmonary septa (Jiang et al. 2000; de Lange et al. 2004).

1. Heart Tube Formation

Cardiac crescent in anterior lateral mesoderm forms the heart tube as the initial event in heart morphogenesis (primary or posterior heart field) (Harvey 2002). Cells in the caudal region of the cardiac crescent (the venous pole) give rise to myocardium of the atrioventricular canal, atria, and inflow tract. At the arterial pole of the heart extracardiac cells from the pharyngeal mesoderm elongate the heart tube further to form the myocardial wall of the outflow tract (secondary or anterior heart field) (Kelly et al. 2001; Mjaatvedt et al. 2001; Waldo et al. 2001). Cardiac neural crest cells, which populate the heart during the last stages of arterial pole elongation, drives septation of the outflow tract to generate systemic and pulmonary ventriculoarterial connections and contribute to the semilunar and atrioventricular valves (Kirby and Waldo 1995; Sugishita et al. 2004).

2. Left-Right and Pharyngeal Arch Arterial Patterning

Left-right patterning also plays a key role in creating a four-chambered heart (Harvey 2002; Moorman and Christoffels 2003). The heart tube is initially linear (E7.5–8), with venous tributaries draining into the developing atria at the posterior or inflow end, and connecting to the ventral aorta at its anterior or outflow end. The initially symmetrical atria subsequently develop distinct left-right identities. The heart tube undergoes dextral looping beginning E8.25 and remodeling between E10.5 and E12.5, processes that are necessary to position the developing atria cranial to the ventricles and to connect the left and right atria to the respective ventricles (Harvey 2002). The aorta and carotid and pulmonary arteries arise by remodeling of the initially bilateral pharyngeal arterial arch system, beginning at E11.5 (Hiruma et al. 2002). Cardiovascular left-right patterning is created, in part, by *Nodal* activated transcription of target genes such as *Nodal*, *Pitx2c*, and *Lefty2* in left-lateral plate mesoderm, and *Lefty1* in the prospective floor plate (Hamada et al. 2002; Ramsdell 2005). Mutation affecting genes in the *Nodal* signaling pathway results in abnormal topology of atria, lungs, ventricles, and pharyngeal arch arteries (Figure 2–1) (Oh and Li 1997; Gaio et al. 1999; Kitamura et al. 1999; Lin et al. 1999; Lu et al. 1999; Yan et al. 1999; Liu et al. 2001; Yamamoto et al. 2001; Brennan et al. 2002; Saijoh et al. 2003).

3. Myocardial and Coronary Vessel Development

Myocardial cell proliferation plays a key role in cardiac growth during embryogenesis (reviewed in Sucov 1998; Chen et al. 2002; Pasumarthi and Field 2002). The mouse embryonic ventricle is a thin-walled chamber at E9.5. By E10.5, projections of trabecular myocardium into the ventricular cavity can be identified. By E11.5 the epicardial myocardium begins to thicken giving rise to the compact zone (reviewed in Sedmera et al. 2000). Lineage tracing experiments have shown that embryonic cardiomyocytes divide to give rise to clonal cell populations of new cardiomyocytes (Reese et al. 2002; Meilhac et al. 2003). The compact and trabecular zones are clonally related, with wedge-shaped clones, wider at the epicardial surface, extending to the endocardial surface (Meilhac et al. 2003). The epicardium, coronary vasculature, and interstitial cardiac fibroblasts arise from an outgrowth of the septum transversum called the proepicardial organ (reviewed in Reese et al. 2002; Luttun and Carmeliet 2003). In the mouse epithelial cells from this structure envelop the heart between E9.5 and E10.5 to form the epicardium (Moore et al. 1999; Merki et al. 2005). Some of this epithelium turns into mesenchymal cells by E11.5–12.5. These cells migrate into the underlying subepicardial space and the myocardium, and give rise to the smooth muscle cells of the coronary vasculature and a subset of intermyocardial fibroblasts (Merki et al. 2005). The coronary endothelium in the mouse does not appear to be derived from the proepicardial organ and originates by invagination from the endocardium (Viragh and Challice 1981; Mikawa and Gourdie 1996; Merki et al. 2005). The coronary arteries finally connect to the aorta by E13, joining the systemic circulation (Viragh and Challice 1981). The development of the coronary system is initiated at the time the compact zone begins to thicken, suggesting that the two processes are biologically coupled.

Genetic and Molecular Interaction Networks

Identifying Cardiac Developmental Genes

The roles of individual genes in these processes can be identified using mutagenesis approaches such as knockouts, ENU mutagenesis, and gene trapping. A key question for CHD is the number of genes that control cardiovascular development. Examination of the Mouse Genome Informatics (MGI) database reveals that of 4,373 genes that have been knocked out, there are 246 with abnormal cardiac morphology or development resembling CHD. If this is extrapolated to 28,000 genes (the estimated number of genes in the mouse genome; Waterston et al. 2002), we expect that there will be approximately ~1,500 genes that are necessary for heart development. We have systematically examined the MGI database to identify 311 mouse mutations with a cardiovascular phenotype that resembles CHD (Table 2–1), and classified the phenotypes in terms of the processes described above. We also classified the genes in terms of their best-established molecular function (with the caveat that many genes have a number of different molecular functions). This analysis shows that diverse genes have shared phenotypes—indicating that they probably act within the same developmental process.

Genetic Interaction Networks

A major limitation of our current understanding of molecular mechanisms is how these genes interact in these developmental processes. Genetic interaction networks can be systematically mapped by identifying synthetic phenotypes created by compound mutations (Hartman et al. 2001), and have provided powerful insights into yeast and worm biology (Tong et al. 2004; Lehner et al. 2006). Such complex networks can maintain overall function despite removal or malfunction of one or more nodes (Newman 2003), that is, they provide a mechanism for *buffering* of genetic variation (Hartman et al. 2001). Mechanisms include compensation by a normally functioning second allele or a duplicated gene that maintains residual function, distributed network robustness (e.g., from negative feedback mechanisms that regulate flux in metabolic networks, and cooperative regulatory mechanisms observed in gene regulatory networks), and from epigenetic mechanisms such as molecular chaperones (Hartman et al. 2001). Cardiac genetic interaction networks studied in the mouse include those in the left-right patterning module (e.g., between *iv* and *Actr2b*; *Nodal*, and *Actr2b*; *Nodal* and *Zic3*; *Nodal* and *Smad2;* and *Nodal* and *Foxa2*) (Collignon et al. 1996; Nomura and Li 1998; Oh and Li 2002; Ware et al. 2006), the secondary heart field module

Table 2–1 Human Orthologs of Mouse Genes with Mutant Phenotypes Resembling Human Congenital Heart Disease Divided by Cardiac Developmental Process

Cardiac Developmental Process	Receptor Binding Molecule	Receptor	Intracellular Signaling Molecule	Transcription Factor	Cell Cycle and Apoptosis	Structural Protein	Energy Metabolism	Membrane Transporter	Miscellaneous
LR patterning	CFC1, *CHRD, DLL1*, FGF10, GDF1, *IFT88*, LEFTY1, LEFTY2, NODAL, NOG	ACVR2B, DISP1, NOTCH2, NOTCH1, SMO	SMAD1, *SMAD5*, SUFU	CITED2, FOXA2, FOXJ1, HIRA, MEOX2, PITX2, RFX3, SMAD2, SNAI1, ZIC3	RPGRIP1L	DNAH11, *DYNC2H1*, DYNC2LI1, INVS, KIF3A, *KIF3B*, OFD1, *RTTN*			DAND5, IFT172, IFT57, MGAT1, MGRN1, PCSK6, *PKD2*
Heart tube development	BMP2, CDH2, CFC1, *CHRD, DLL1*, ENG, *EPHB4*, FGF8, *IFT88*, NODAL, NOG, TGFB2	APC, ACVR2B, CXADR, DISP1, FGFR1, NOTCH1, NOTCH2, PTPRB, SMO	ADRBK1, HGS, MAPK7, *PDPK1, PKD2*, PRKAR1A, PTEN, SHH, SMAD1, *SMAD5*, SUFU,	CITED2, *CTBP2*, FOXA2, *FOXH1*, FOXO1, FOXP4, GATA4, GSC, HAND1, HAND2, HIF1A, HIRA, ISL1, MEF2C, MESP1, MIXL1, NKX2-5, NR2F2, OVOL2, RBL2, *RERE*, RFX3, SMAD2, SMAD3, SNAI1, T, TAL1, TBX20, TBX5, ZIC3	GAS1	*AXIN1, DYNC2H1*, DYNC2LI1, INVS, KIF3A, *KIF3B, MYL7, NCKAP1*, OFD1, *RTTN*, TMOD1, WASF2	ALDH1A2,	CACNB2, GJC1	CHMP5, CYP26A1, DAND5, EVI1, FURIN, IFT172, IFT57, MEOX2, *MGAT1*, MIBI, *PCSK6*, PSEN1, PSEN2
Outflow tract	BMP4, CFC1, *CHRD, DVL1*, DVL2, ENG, *FGF19*, FGF8, LEFTY1, NTF3, SEMA3C, TGFB2, VEGFA	ACVR2B, ACVR1, *BMPR1A*, EDNRA, FGFR2, NRP1, NRP2, *NTRK3*, PDGFRA, PDGFRB, PLXND1, SMO, TGFBR2	KRAS, MAP2K5, PTPN11, SMAD6,	CITED2, FOXC2, FOXG1, *FOXH1*, FOXJ1, FOXP1, GATA4, GATA6, HAND1, HAND2, HHEX, HIF1A, HOXA3, ISL1, JUN, MESP1, MKL1, MKL2, *NFATC1*, NKX2-5, *PAX3*, PITX2, RARA, RARB, RARG, *RXRA*, SNAI1, *SOX11*, TBX1, TBX2, TFAP2A, ZFPM2		FLNA, *FN1*, HAS2, *HSPG2*, INVS, *LTBP1*, MYH10, *MYL7, PDLIM3*	ALDH1A2, *POR*	GJA1	*ADAM19*, ATE1, ECE1, *ECE2*, MEOX2, *NF1, PCSK6*, SSR1
Valvulogenesis	BMP10, BMP2, BMP4, BTC, *EPHA3*, FGF8, HBEGF, LEFTY1, SEMA3C, LEFTY2, *NRG1*, NTF3, TGFB2	ACVR1, ACVRL1, *BMPR1A, BMPR2*, CXADR, CXCR7, EFNB2, EGFR, ERBB2, ERBB3, *ERBB4, FBN1*, FGFR2, *HTR1B*, KDR, *NTRK3*	KL, KRAS, MAP2K5, NOS3, *PKD1*, PLCE1, PTPN11, SHC1, SMAD6,	CITED2, CREBBP, FOXC1, FOXC2, *FOXM1*, FOXP1, GATA4, HAND1, HEY1, HEY2, HHEX, HOXA3, IGHMBP2, MESP1, *NFATC1*, NKX2–5, NKX2–6, *PAX3*, PITX2, RARA, RARB, RARG, *RXRA*, SALL4, SIRT1, SMAD4, SOX4, *SOX9*, TBX1, TBX2, TBX5, *ZFPM1*, ZFPM2	CDK2, CDK4, WRN	COL2A1, FLNA, *FN1*, FREM2, HAS2, *HSPG2*, INVS, JUP, LOX, MYH10, *MYL7*, POSTN, RBP4, CAN, VCL	ALDH1A2	GJA1, GJA5, GJC1, SLC6A4, *SLC8A1*	*ADAM12*, ADAM17, *ADAM19*, ARSB, ECE1, *ECE2*, IDUA, MEOX2, *NF1, SGSH*, SSR1

Aortic arch	BMP2, BMP4, CFC1, *CHRD*, *FGF19*, TGFB2, VEGFA	ACVR1, ACVRL1, EDNRA, NRP1, PDGFRA, PLXND1, SMO, TGFBR2	CRKL, EDN1, FGF8, MAP3K7,	CITED2, FOXA2, FOXC1, FOXC2, FOXG1, *FOXH1*, FOXO1, GATA4, GATA6, GBX2, GSC, HAND2, HDAC7A, HIF1A, HOXA3, ISL1, JUN, MEF2C, MESP1, MKL2, NKX2–5, *PAX3*, PITX2, PRRX1, PRRX2, RARA, RARB, TBX1, TBX2, TFAP2A, VEZF1, ZIC3	CCNE1, CCNE2,	KRIT1, *LTBP1*	ALDH1A2,	GJA5, SEMA3C	APOE, CST3, ECE1, MYST3
AV Septation	*BMP1*, BMP10, BMP2, BMP4, CDH2, CFC1, *CHRD*, *DLL1*, DLL4, DVL2, ENG, *EPHA3*, *EPHB4*, FGF10, *FGF19*, FGF2, FGF8, *FGF9*, FKBP1A, *IFT88*, JAG1, LEFTY1, LEFTY2, NODAL, NOG, NTF3, PDGFA, PDGFC, SEMA3C, SMO, TGFB2, VEGFA	ACVR1, ACVR2B, ACVRL1, AGTR1, APC, *BMPR2*, CXADR, CXCR4, CXCR7, DISP1, EDNRA, ERBB2, F2R, *FBN1*, FGFR1, FGFR2, JMJD6, LY6E, NOTCH1, NOTCH2, NRP1, NRP2, *NTRK3*, PDGFRA, PDGFRB, PTPRB, ROR1, *ROR2*, TGFBR2, TGFBR3, VCAM1	ADRBK1, CRKL, CXCL12, EDN1, *GAB1*, GAB2, GDF1, *GNA11*, GNAQ, HGS, KRAS, MAPK7, NOS3, *PDPK1*, *PKD1*, *PKD2*, PRKAR1A, PTEN, PTPN11, SHH, SMAD1, *SMAD5*, SUFU,	ATF2, ATF7, CITED2, CREBBP, *CTBP2*, EGLN1, EP300, FOXA2, FOXC1, FOXC2, FOXG1, *FOXH1*, FOXJ1, *FOXM1*, FOXO1, FOXP1, FOXP4, GATA4, GATA6, GBX2, GSC, HAND1, HAND2, HDAC2, *HDAC5*, *HDAC9*, HEY1, HEY2, HHEX, HIF1A, HIRA, *HOXB4*, ISL1, JARID2, JUN, MEF2C, MED24, *MEN1*, MESP1, MIXL1, MKL2, MYCN, NCOA6, NKX2–5, NR2F2, OSR1, OVOL2, PITX2, PPARG, RARA, RARB, RARG, RBL2, *RERE*, RFX3, *RXRA*, SALL1, SALL4, SIRT1, SMAD2, SMAD3, SMYD1, SNAI1, *SOX11*, SOX4, *SOX9*, SRF, T, TAL1, TBX1, TBX2, TBX20, TBX5, TCEB3, *ZFPM1*, ZFPM2, ZIC3	*CCND1*, *CCND2*, CCND3, CCNE1, CCNE2, CDK2, CDK4, GAS1, LATS2, PDS5B, RPGRIPIL	*AXIN1*, CAV1, CA3, *DES*, DNAH11, *DYNC2H1*, DYNC2LI1, FLNA, HAS2, INVS, KIF3A, *KIF3B*, *KRT19*, MYH10, MYL2, *MYL7*, *NCKAP1*, OFD1, *PDLIM3*, *RTTN*, THBS1, TMOD1, *TTN*, WASF2	ALDH1A2, ATP2A2, *FXN*, *GYS1*, *PNPLA2*, *TXNRD2*	CACNB2, GJA1, GJA5, GJC1, *RYR2*, *SLC39A4*	*ADAM12*, ADAM17, *ADAM19*, ADAM9, ATE1, *CALR*, CHD7, CHMP5, CYP26A1, DAND5, DNMT3B, ECE1, EVI1, FKBP1B, FURIN, IDUA, IFT172, IFT57, MAP3K7IP1, MED1, MEOX2, *MGAT1*, MGRN1, MIB1, *MOSPD3*, *NF1*, PBRM1, *PCSK6*, PSEN1, PSEN2, SSR1, TH, *TLL1*, UBR1, UBR2

Data are based on searches of the MGI database for the following keywords: Left-right patterning: MP:0000644; MP:0004133; MP:0000542; MP0004252; MP:0003178; MP0001706; MP0006061; MP:0000531; MP:0002767; MP:0002766. Heart tube: MP:0000270; MP:0004187. Outflow tract. MP:0002633; MP:0004110; MP:0006127; MP:0005674; MP:0006126. Valvulogenesis: MP:0000285; MP:0000287; MP:0003958; MP:0006049; MP:0002746; MP:0006115; MP:0006117; MP:0006047; MP:0002747; MP:0002748; MP:0006128; MP:0006048; MP:0006130; MP:0006122; MP:0006045; MP:0006119; MP:000286; MP:0006124; MP:0006044; MP:0006123; MP:0002745. Aortic arch: MP:0004113; MP:0006356; MP:0006355; MP:0006354; MP:0002977; MP:0002672. AV Septation: MP:0004225; MP:0000279; MP0000301; MP0003808; MP:0000299; MP:0000300; MP:0000298; MP:0000297.

For each category, genes are listed by their predominant molecular function. Genes are underlined if variations have been identified in human subjects. Genes are in italics if CNV has been identified in normal individuals. This table was compiled by interrogating the following databases: MGI database (http://www.informatics.jax.org/), the database of human genetic variation (http://projects.tcag.ca/variation/data/variation.hg18.txt), and Ensembl release 45 via Biomart (http://www.ensembl.org/biomart/martview/).

(e.g., *Pitx2* and *Tbx1*) (Nowotschin et al. 2006), or in septation (e.g., *Tbx20* and *Nkx2-5*) (Stennard et al. 2005), and chamber development modules (e.g., *Nkx2-5* and *Hand2*; *Gata4* and *Gata6*) (Yamagishi et al. 2001; Xin et al. 2006). It also becomes clear that to identify the links between the network nodes will potentially require the analysis of 1,500×1,499 / 2 (i.e., over a million) pair-wise genetic crosses and analysis of compound mutant embryos.

Phenotypic Heterogeneity in Mouse and Man

This analysis also shows that single genes often act in distinct cardiac developmental processes, resulting in phenotypic heterogeneity. Of 311 mouse gene mutations with cardiac phenotypes, 122 have malformations that affect more than one cardiac structure, that is, atria, ventricles, valves, outflow tract, or aortic arches (see Table 2–1). Variability in phenotype resulting from different mutations in the same gene may result from involvement of the gene in multiple developmental processes such as left-right patterning, atrioventricular septation, outflow tract, and aortic arch development. Alternatively, a primary requirement in an early process such as left-right patterning may have knockon effects on later processes such as atrioventricular septation. Variability in phenotype resulting from the same single gene mutation can partly be explained by variation in genetic background, as seen in mice lacking *Cited2* (Bamforth et al. 2001; Bamforth et al. 2004), as well as by environmental and/or epigenetic mechanisms.

Phenotypic heterogeneity is also observed in humans, with important implications. Mutation in certain genes [e.g., *CFC1* (Bamford et al. 2000; Goldmuntz et al. 2002), *CITED2* (Sperling et al. 2005), *CREBBP/EP300* (Stevens and Bhakta 1995; Petrij et al. 1995; Roelfsema et al. 2005), *CRELD1* (Robinson et al. 2003), *CHD7* (Vissers et al. 2004; Bosman et al. 2005; Jongmans et al. 2006), *GATA4* (Garg et al. 2003; Hirayama-Yamada et al. 2005), *NKX2-5* (Benson et al. 1999; Goldmuntz et al. 2001; McElhinney et al. 2003), *NOTCH1* (Krebs et al. 2000; Garg et al. 2005; Mohamed et al. 2006), and *ZIC3* (Gebbia et al. 1997; Megarbane et al. 2000; Ware et al. 2004)] results in diverse cardiovascular malformations that affect septation, outflow tract, or aortic arch development in mouse and man (Tables 2–2 and 2–3). Such pleiotropy, (i.e., "many turnings"), is of clinical importance: malformations such as TGA or TOF have substantially poorer outcomes than, for instance, an ASD (Hoffman et al. 2004). NKX2.5, the most commonly mutated gene identified in human CHD, is a good example resulting most frequently in ASD and conduction defects but also in DORV, aortic stenosis, TOF, and Ebstein's anomaly (see Table 2–3 for examples; Goldmuntz et al. 2001; McElhinney et al. 2003).

Role of Copy Number Variation

Large-scale structural variation has a clear role in many classic chromosomal syndromes that have CHD as a major component. These include Alagille, Down, DiGeorge, Williams-Beuren, and Trisomy 18 (Pollex and Hegele 2007; Thienpont et al. 2007). The importance of intermediate-scale CNV (1kb–3Mb) in non-Mendelian/nonchromosomal CHD is not known. However, analysis of the human gene variation database indicates that 80 of 311 genes, which when mutated in the mouse result in a CHD-like phenotype, have a CNV overlapping with the gene (Table 2–1: genes where CNV has been identified are in italics). The locus-specific mutation rate for CNV is approximately 2–4 orders of magnitude greater than nucleotide-specific rates for base substitution, suggesting that de novo CNV in cardiac developmental genes could be a mechanism for CHD (Table 1–3 in Lupski 2007). From these observations we may expect that patients with CHD could have high mutational loads (e.g., from commonly occurring CNVs or from de novo CNVs) in genetic networks that are necessary for cardiac development.

Table 2–2 Mouse Genes with Mutant Phenotypes Resembling Human Congenital Heart Disease

Phenotypic Heterogeneity Score[a]	Mouse Genes
0–1	*Adrbk1, Agtr1b, Apc, Apoe, Axin1, Bmp1, Btc, Calr, Cav1, Cav3, Ccnd1, Ccnd2, Ccnd3, Cdh2, Chd7, Chmp5, Col2a1, Cst3, Ctbp2, Cxcl12, Cxcr4, Cyp26a1, Disp1, Dll1, Dll4, Dnahc11, Dnmt3b, Dvl1, Dync2h1, Dync2li1, Efnb2, Egfr, Egln1, Ep300, Ephb4, Erbb3, Erbb4, Evi1, F2r, Fgf10, Fgf2, Fgf9, Fgfr1, Fkbp1a, Fkbp1b, Foxp4, Frem2, Furin, Fxn, Gab1, Gas1, Gna11, Gnaq, Gys1, Hbegf, Hdac5, Hdac7a, Hdac9, Hgs, Htr1b, Ift172, Ift57, Ift88, Jarid2, Jmjd6, Jup, Kdr, Kif3a, Kif3b, Kl, Krit1, Krt19, Lats2, Lox, Ly6e, Map3k7, Map3k7ip1, Mapk7, Men1, Mgat1, Mib1, Mixl1, Mkl1, Mospd3, Mycn, Myl2, Myst3, Nckap1, Ncoa6, Nkx2–6, Nog, Notch1, Nr2f2, Nrg1, Ofd1, Ovol2, Pbrm1, Pdgfa, Pdgfc, Pdpk1, Plce1, Pnpla2, Por, Postn, Pparbp, Pparg, Prkar1a, Prrx1, Prrx2, Psen1, Psen2, Pten, Rbl2, Rbp4, Rere, Rfx3, Ror1, Ror2, Rttn, Sall1, Sgsh, Shc1, Shh, Slc6a4, Slc8a1, Smad1, Smad2, Smad4, Smad5, Smyd1, Sufu, T, Tal1, Tceb3, Tgfbr3, Th, Thbs1, Thrap4, Tll1, Txnrd2, Vcam1, Vcan, Vcl, Vezf1, Wasf2, Wrn*
1–2	*Adam12, Adam17, Adam9, Atp2a2, Bmp10, Bmpr1a, Bmpr2, Cdk2, Cdk4, Dand5, Dvl2, Ece2, Edn1, Eng, Erbb2, Fbn1, Foxj1, Foxm1, Foxo1, Gbx2, Gdf1, Gja7, Hey1, Hspg2, Jag1, Map2k5, Mgrn1, Nfatc1, Nodal, Nos3, Notch2, Nrp2, Osr1, Pcsk6, Pdlim3, Pkd2, Plxnd1, Smad6, Sox11, Sox4, Srf, Tbx20, Tcfap2a, Tmod1, Ubr1, Ubr2*
2–3	*Acvr2b, Acvrl1, Ate1, Ccne1, Ccne2, Chrd, Crebbp, Crkl, Cxadr, Ednra, Fgfr2, Foxc1, Foxg1, Foxp1, Gata6, Hand1, Has2, Hey2, Hhex, Hif1a, Hoxa3, Invs, Jun, Mef2c, Mkl2, Myh10, Myl7, Nrp1, Pax3, Pdgfra, Pkd1, Rarg, Sall4, Sirt1, Sox9, Ssr1, Tbx5, Tgfbr2, Vegfa, Zfpm1, Zic3,*
3–4	*Acvr1, Adam19, Bmp2, Cfc1, Ece1, Fgf15, Flna, Foxc2, Foxh1, Gja1, Gja5, Hand2, Isl1, Nf1, Ntf3, Ntrk3, Ptpn11, Rara, Rarb, Rxra, Sema3c, Smo, Tbx2, Zfpm2*
4–5	*Aldh1a2, Bmp4, Cited2, Fgf8, Gata4, Mesp1, Nkx2–5, Pitx2, Tbx1, Tgfb2*

[a]For each gene, aortic arch, outflow tract, valve/endocardial cushion, ventricle/heart tube, and atrial abnormalities were scored as 0 or 1 if absent or present. These scores were summed to create a phenotypic heterogeneity score for each gene. Of the 311 genes identified, 122 had a phenotypic heterogeneity score > 1, that is, mutation in these genes affected more than one cardiac structure.

Table 2–3 Phenotypic Heterogeneity in Patients with Congenital Heart Disease Resulting from Nonsynonymous Mutations in Single Genes and Certain Chromosomal Disorders

Gene	Cardiac phenotypes
CFC1	TGA, ASD, AVSD, VSD, PDA, L-atrial isomerism, DORV, heterotaxy
CITED2	TOF, ASD, VSD, TAPVR, TGA
CRELD1	AVSD, heterotaxy
GATA4	TOF, AVSD, AS, PS, dextrocardia
LEFTY A	HLHS, AVSD, dextrocardia, heterotaxy
TBX5	ASD, VSD, AVSD, HLHS, TOF, CAT, TA, DORV, TAPVR
TBX20	ASD, VSD, valve defects
JAG1	ASD, AVSD, VSD, TOF, PA, PDA, PS, right aortic arch, coarctation of aorta, CAT
NKX2–5	ASD, VSD, TOF, DORV, L-TGA, IAA, coarctation of aorta, HLHS, PAVSD
NOTCH1	AS, TOF, VSD, bicuspid aortic valve
PROSIT240	TGA, VSD, coarctation of aorta
PTPN11	PS, hypertrophic cardiomyopathy, PDA, ASD, peripheral pulmonary artery stenosis
ZIC3	Situs inversus, TAPVR, HLHS, VSD, TGA, DORV, PS, right aortic arch
22q11del	IAA, VSD, CAT, PAVSD, TOF, absent pulmonary valve syndrome
Trisomy 21	AVSD, VSD, TOF

Notes: TAPVR (total anomalous pulmonary venous return), HLHS (hypoplastic left heart syndrome), IVC (inferior vena cava) IAA (interrupted aortic arch), PAVSD (pulmonary atresia ventricular septal defect with aortopulmonary collaterals), CAT (common arterial trunk), DORV (double outlet right ventricle), L-TGA (congenitally corrected transposition of great arteries), PA (pulmonary atresia), TA (tricuspid atresia).

Sources: Information compiled from Basson et al. 1994, 1999; Petrij et al. 1995; Stevens and Bhakta 1995; Newbury-Ecob et al. 1996; Gebbia et al. 1997; Schott et al. 1998; Bruneau et al. 1999; Kosaki et al. 1999; Satoda et al. 1999; Bamford et al. 2000; Satoda et al. 2000; Megarbane et al. 2000; Tartaglia et al. 2001; McElhinney et al. 2002; Garg et al. 2003; McElhinney et al. 2003; Ware et al. 2004; Garg et al. 2005; Muncke et al. 2005; Hirayama-Yamada et al. 2005; Sperling et al. 2005; Kirk et al. 2007; Pierpont et al. 2007; Schluterman et al. 2007; Sznajer et al. 2007.

Conclusions

An understanding of the genetic basis of CHD can be greatly facilitated by using mouse models. Candidate genes can be efficiently isolated using mouse genetic techniques and applied to human disease. The key future challenges, however, involve understanding the mechanisms that create and disrupt genetic buffering of developmental networks. High-throughput techniques such as magnetic resonance imaging of mouse embryos (Schneider et al. 2003; Schneider and Bhattacharya 2004; Schneider et al. 2004) will enable investigation of gene–gene and gene–environment interactions and the effects on cardiac developmental networks. A long-term goal in CHD is to manipulate these networks to enhance buffering and prevent or modify disease.

References

Bamford RN, Roessler E, Burdine RD, et al. Loss-of-function mutations in the EGF-CFC gene CFC1 are associated with human left-right laterality defects. *Nat Genet.* 2000;26:365–369.

Bamforth SD, Braganca J, Eloranta JJ, et al. Cardiac malformations, adrenal agenesis, neural crest defects and exencephaly in mice lacking Cited2, a new Tfap2 co-activator. *Nat Genet.* 2001;29:469–474.

Bamforth SD, Braganca J, Farthing CR, et al. Cited2 controls left-right patterning and heart development through a Nodal-Pitx2c pathway. *Nat Genet.* 2004;36:1189–1196.

Basson CT, Cowley GS, Solomon SD, et al. The clinical and genetic spectrum of the Holt-Oram syndrome (heart-hand syndrome). *N Engl J Med.* 1994;330:885–891.

Basson CT, Huang T, Lin RC, et al. Different TBX5 interactions in heart and limb defined by Holt-Oram syndrome mutations. *Proc Natl Acad Sci U S A.* 1999;96:2919–2924.

Benson DW, Silberbach GM, Kavanaugh-McHugh A, et al. Mutations in the cardiac transcription factor NKX2.5 affect diverse cardiac developmental pathways. *J Clin Invest.* 1999;104:1567–1573.

Blom HJ, Shaw GM, den Heijer M, Finnell RH. Neural tube defects and folate: case far from closed. *Nat Rev Neurosci.* 2006;7:724–731.

Bosman EA, Penn AC, Ambrose JC, Kettleborough R, Stemple DL, Steel KP. Multiple mutations in mouse Chd7 provide models for CHARGE syndrome. *Hum Mol Genet.* 2005;14:3463–3476.

Brennan J, Norris DP, Robertson EJ. Nodal activity in the node governs left-right asymmetry. *Genes Dev.* 2002;16:2339–2344.

Bruneau BG, Logan M, Davis N, et al. Chamber-specific cardiac expression of Tbx5 and heart defects in Holt-Oram syndrome. *Dev Biol.* 1999;211:100–108.

Burn J, Goodship J. Congenital heart disease. In: Rimoin DL, Connor JM, Pyeritz RE, Korf BR, eds. *Principles and Practice of Medical Genetics.* London: Churchill Livingstone; 2002.

Cai CL, Liang X, Shi Y, et al. Isl1 identifies a cardiac progenitor population that proliferates prior to differentiation and contributes a majority of cells to the heart. *Dev Cell.* 2003;5:877–889.

Chen TH, Chang TC, Kang JO, et al. Epicardial induction of fetal cardiomyocyte proliferation via a retinoic acid-inducible trophic factor. *Dev Biol.* 2002;250:198–207.

Clark EB. Etiology of congenital cardiac malformations: epidemiology and genetics. In: Allen HD, Gutgessell HP, Clark EB, Driscoll DJ, eds. *Moss and Adams' Heart Disease in Infants, Children, and Adolescents.* Philadelphia: Lipincott Williams & Wilkins; 2001.

Collignon J, Varlet I, Robertson EJ. Relationship between asymmetric nodal expression and the direction of embryonic turning. *Nature.* 1996;381:155–158.

de Lange FJ, Moorman AF, Anderson RH, et al. Lineage and morphogenetic analysis of the cardiac valves. *Circ Res.* 2004;95:645–654.

De Wals P, Tairou F, Van Allen MI, et al. Reduction in neural-tube defects after folic acid fortification in Canada. *N Engl J Med.* 2007;357:135–142.

Ferencz C, Boughman JA. Congenital heart disease in adolescents and adults. Teratology, genetics, and recurrence risks. *Cardiol Clin.* 1993;11:557–567.

Ferencz C, Boughman JA, Neill CA, Brenner JI, Perry LW. Congenital cardiovascular malformations: questions on inheritance. Baltimore-Washington Infant Study Group. *J Am Coll Cardiol.* 1989;14:756–763.

Gaio U, Schweickert A, Fischer A, et al. A role of the cryptic gene in the correct establishment of the left-right axis. *Curr Biol.* 1999;9:1339–1342.

Garg V, Kathiriya IS, Barnes R, et al. GATA4 mutations cause human congenital heart defects and reveal an interaction with TBX5. *Nature.* 2003;424:443–447.

Garg V, Muth AN, Ransom JF, et al. Mutations in NOTCH1 cause aortic valve disease. *Nature.* 2005;437:270–274.

Gebbia M, Ferrero GB, Pilia G, et al. X-linked situs abnormalities result from mutations in ZIC3. *Nat Genet.* 1997;17:305–308.

Goldmuntz E, Bamford R, Karkera JD, dela Cruz J, Roessler E, Muenke M. CFC1 mutations in patients with transposition of the great arteries and double-outlet right ventricle. *Am J Hum Genet.* 2002;70:776–780.

Goldmuntz E, Geiger E, Benson DW. NKX2.5 mutations in patients with tetralogy of fallot. *Circulation.* 2001;104:2565–2568.

Hamada H, Meno C, Watanabe D, Saijoh Y. Establishment of vertebrate left-right asymmetry. *Nat Rev Genet.* 2002;3:103–113.

Hartman JLT, Garvik B, Hartwell L. Principles for the buffering of genetic variation. *Science.* 2001;291:1001–1004.

Harvey RP. Patterning the vertebrate heart. *Nat Rev Genet.* 2002; 3:544–556.

Hirayama-Yamada K, Kamisago M, Akimoto K, et al. Phenotypes with GATA4 or NKX2.5 mutations in familial atrial septal defect. *Am J Med Genet A.* 2005;135:47–52.

Hiruma T, Nakajima Y, Nakamura H. Development of pharyngeal arch arteries in early mouse embryo. *J Anat.* 2002;201:15–29.

Hoffman JI, Kaplan S, Liberthson RR. Prevalence of congenital heart disease. *Am Heart J.* 2004;147:425–439.

Hoffman JIE. Incidence, mortality and natural history. In: Anderson RH, Baker EJ, Macartney FJ, Rigby ML, Shinebourne EA, Tynan M, eds. *Paediatric Cardiology.* London: Churchill Livingstone; 2002:111–139.

http://projects.tcag.ca/variation/. November 29, 2007. *Database of Genomic Variants.*

Jiang X, Rowitch DH, Soriano P, McMahon AP, Sucov HM. Fate of the mammalian cardiac neural crest. *Development.* 2000;127:1607–1616.

Jongmans MC, Admiraal RJ, van der Donk KP, et al. CHARGE syndrome: the phenotypic spectrum of mutations in the CHD7 gene. *J Med Genet.* 2006;43:306–314.

Kelly RG, Brown NA, Buckingham ME. The arterial pole of the mouse heart forms from Fgf10-expressing cells in pharyngeal mesoderm. *Dev Cell.* 2001;1:435–440.

Kelly RG, Buckingham ME. The anterior heart-forming field: voyage to the arterial pole of the heart. *Trends Genet.* 2002;18:210–216.

Kent GC, Carr RK. *Comparative Anatomy of the Vertebrates.* Boston: McGraw Hill. 2001.

Kirby ML, Waldo KL. Neural crest and cardiovascular patterning. *Circ Res.* 1995;77:211–215.

Kirk EP, Sunde M, Costa MW, et al. Mutations in cardiac T-box factor gene TBX20 are associated with diverse cardiac pathologies, including defects of septation and valvulogenesis and cardiomyopathy. *Am J Hum Genet.* 2007;81:280–291.

Kitamura K, Miura H, Miyagawa-Tomita S, et al. Mouse Pitx2 deficiency leads to anomalies of the ventral body wall, heart, extra- and periocular mesoderm and right pulmonary isomerism. *Development.* 1999;126:5749–5758.

Kosaki K, Bassi MT, Kosaki R, et al. Characterization and mutation analysis of human LEFTY A and LEFTY B, homologues of murine genes implicated in left-right axis development. *Am J Hum Genet.* 1999;64:712–721.

Krebs LT, Xue Y, Norton CR, et al. Notch signaling is essential for vascular morphogenesis in mice. *Genes Dev.* 2000;14:1343–1352.

Lehner B, Crombie C, Tischler J, Fortunato A, Fraser AG. Systematic mapping of genetic interactions in *Caenorhabditis elegans* identifies common modifiers of diverse signaling pathways. *Nat Genet.* 2006;38:896–903.

Lin CR, Kioussi C, O'Connell S, et al. Pitx2 regulates lung asymmetry, cardiac positioning and pituitary and tooth morphogenesis. *Nature.* 1999;401:279–282.

Liu C, Liu W, Lu MF, Brown NA, Martin JF. Regulation of left-right asymmetry by thresholds of Pitx2c activity. *Development.* 2001;128:2039–2048.

Lu MF, Pressman C, Dyer R, Johnson RL, Martin JF. Function of Rieger syndrome gene in left-right asymmetry and craniofacial development. *Nature.* 1999;401:276–278.

Lupski JR. Genomic rearrangements and sporadic disease. *Nat Genet.* 2007;39:S43–S47.

Luttun A, Carmeliet P. De novo vasculogenesis in the heart. *Cardiovasc Res.* 58:378–389.

McElhinney DB, Geiger E, Blinder J, Benson DW, Goldmuntz E. NKX2.5 mutations in patients with congenital heart disease. *J Am Coll Cardiol.* 2003;42:1650–1655.

McElhinney DB, Krantz ID, Bason L, et al. Analysis of cardiovascular phenotype and genotype-phenotype correlation in individuals with a JAG1 mutation and/or Alagille syndrome. *Circulation.* 2002;106:2567–2574.

Megarbane A, Salem N, Stephan E, et al. X-linked transposition of the great arteries and incomplete penetrance among males with a nonsense mutation in ZIC3. *Eur J Hum Genet.* 2000;8:704–708.

Meilhac SM, Kelly RG, Rocancourt D, Eloy-Trinquet S, Nicolas JF, Buckingham ME. A retrospective clonal analysis of the myocardium reveals two phases of clonal growth in the developing mouse heart. *Development.* 2003;130:3877–3889.

Merki E, Zamora M, Raya A, et al. Epicardial retinoid X receptor α is required for myocardial growth and coronary artery formation. *Proc Natl Acad Sci U S A.* 2005;102:18455–18460.

Mikawa T, Gourdie RG. Pericardial mesoderm generates a population of coronary smooth muscle cells migrating into the heart along with ingrowth of the epicardial organ. *Dev Biol.* 1996;174:221–232.

Mjaatvedt CH, Nakaoka T, Moreno-Rodriguez R, et al. The outflow tract of the heart is recruited from a novel heart-forming field. *Dev Biol.* 2001;238:97–109.

Mohamed SA, Aherrahrou Z, Liptau H, et al. Novel missense mutations (p.T596M and p.P1797H) in NOTCH1 in patients with bicuspid aortic valve. *Biochem Biophys Res Commun.* 2006;345:1460–1465.

Moore AW, McInnes L, Kreidberg J, Hastie ND, Schedl A. YAC complementation shows a requirement for Wt1 in the development of epicardium, adrenal gland and throughout nephrogenesis. *Development.* 1999;126:1845–1857.

Moorman AF, Christoffels VM. Cardiac chamber formation: development, genes, and evolution. *Physiol Rev.* 2003;83:1223–1267.

Muncke N, Niesler B, Roeth R, et al. Mutational analysis of the PITX2 coding region revealed no common cause for transposition of the great arteries (dTGA). *BMC Med Genet.* 2005;6:20.

Newbury-Ecob RA, Leanage R, Raeburn JA, Young ID. Holt-Oram syndrome: a clinical genetic study. *J Med Genet.* 1996;33:300–307.

Newman MEJ. The structure and function of complex networks. *SIAM Review.* 2003;45:167–256.

Nomura M, Li E. Smad2 role in mesoderm formation, left-right patterning and craniofacial development. *Nature.* 1998;393:786–790.

Nowotschin S, Liao J, Gage PJ, Epstein JA, Campione M, Morrow BE. Tbx1 affects asymmetric cardiac morphogenesis by regulating Pitx2 in the secondary heart field. *Development.* 2006;133:1565–1573.

Oh SP, Li E. The signaling pathway mediated by the type IIB activin receptor controls axial patterning and lateral asymmetry in the mouse. *Genes Dev.* 1997;11:1812–1826.

Oh SP, Li E. Gene-dosage-sensitive genetic interactions between inversus viscerum (iv), nodal, and activin type IIB receptor (ActRIIB) genes in asymmetrical patterning of the visceral organs along the left-right axis. *Dev Dyn.* 2002;224:279–290.

Pasumarthi KB, Field LJ. Cardiomyocyte cell cycle regulation. *Circ Res.* 2002;90:1044–1054.

Petrij F, Giles RH, Dauwerse HG, et al. Rubinstein-Taybi syndrome caused by mutations in the transcriptional co-activator CBP. *Nature.* 1995;376:348–351.

Pierpont ME, Basson CT, Benson DW Jr, et al. Genetic basis for congenital heart defects: current knowledge: a scientific statement from the

American Heart Association Congenital Cardiac Defects Committee, Council on Cardiovascular Disease in the Young: endorsed by the American Academy of Pediatrics. *Circulation.* 2007;115:3015–3038.

Pollex RL, Hegele RA. Copy number variation in the human genome and its implications for cardiovascular disease. *Circulation.* 2007;115:3130–138.

Ramsdell AF. Left-right asymmetry and congenital cardiac defects: getting to the heart of the matter in vertebrate left-right axis determination. *Dev Biol.* 2005;288:1–20.

Reese DE, Mikawa T, Bader DM. Development of the coronary vessel system. *Circ Res.* 2002;91:761–768.

Robinson SW, Morris CD, Goldmuntz E, et al. Missense mutations in CRELD1 are associated with cardiac atrioventricular septal defects. *Am J Hum Genet.* 2003;72:1047–1052.

Roelfsema JH, White SJ, Ariyurek Y, et al. Genetic heterogeneity in Rubinstein-Taybi syndrome: mutations in both the CBP and EP300 genes cause disease. *Am J Hum Genet.* 2005;76:572–580.

Saijoh Y, Oki S, Ohishi S, Hamada H. Left-right patterning of the mouse lateral plate requires nodal produced in the node. *Dev Biol.* 2003;256:160–172.

Satoda M, Pierpont ME, Diaz GA, Bornemeier RA, Gelb BD. Char syndrome, an inherited disorder with patent ductus arteriosus, maps to chromosome 6p12-p21. *Circulation.* 1999;99:3036–3042.

Satoda M, Zhao F, Diaz GA, et al. Mutations in TFAP2B cause Char syndrome, a familial form of patent ductus arteriosus. *Nat Genet.* 2000;25:42–46.

Schluterman MK, Krysiak AE, Kathiriya IS, et al. Screening and biochemical analysis of GATA4 sequence variations identified in patients with congenital heart disease. *Am J Med Genet A.* 2007;143:817–823.

Schneider JE, Bamforth SD, Farthing CR, Clarke K, Neubauer S, Bhattacharya S. Rapid identification and 3D reconstruction of complex cardiac malformations in transgenic mouse embryos using fast gradient echo sequence magnetic resonance imaging. *J Mol Cell Cardiol.* 2003;35:217–222.

Schneider JE, Bhattacharya S. Making the mouse embryo transparent: identifying developmental malformations using magnetic resonance imaging. *Birth Defects Res C Embryo Today.* 2004;72:241–249.

Schneider JE, Bose J, Bamforth SD, et al. Identification of cardiac malformations in mice lacking Ptdsr using a novel high-throughput magnetic resonance imaging technique. *BMC Dev Biol.* 2004;4:16.

Schott JJ, Benson DW, Basson CT, et al. Congenital heart disease caused by mutations in the transcription factor NKX2-5. *Science.* 1998;281:108–111.

Sedmera D, Pexieder T, Vuillemin M, Thompson RP, Anderson RH. Developmental patterning of the myocardium. *Anat Rec.* 2000;258:319–337.

Solloway MJ, Harvey RP. Molecular pathways in myocardial development: a stem cell perspective. *Cardiovasc Res.* 2003;58:264–277.

Sperling S, Grimm CH, Dunkel I, et al. Identification and functional analysis of CITED2 mutations in patients with congenital heart defects. *Hum Mutat.* 2005;26:575–582.

Stennard FA, Costa MW, Lai D, et al. Murine T-box transcription factor Tbx20 acts as a repressor during heart development, and is essential for adult heart integrity, function and adaptation. *Development.* 2005;132:2451–2462.

Stevens CA, Bhakta MG. Cardiac abnormalities in the Rubinstein-Taybi syndrome. *Am J Med Genet.* 1995;59:346–348.

Sucov HM. Molecular insights into cardiac development. *Annu Rev Physiol.* 1998;60:287–308.

Sugishita Y, Watanabe M, Fisher SA. The development of the embryonic outflow tract provides novel insights into cardiac differentiation and remodeling. *Trends Cardiovasc Med.* 2004;14:235–241.

Sznajer Y, Keren B, Baumann C, et al. The spectrum of cardiac anomalies in Noonan syndrome as a result of mutations in the PTPN11 gene. *Pediatrics.* 2007;119:e1325–e1331.

Tam PP, Gad JM. Gastrulation in the mouse embryo. In: Stern CD, ed. *Gastrulation: From Cells to Embryo.* Cold Spring Harbor: Cold Spring Harbor Press; 2004:233–262.

Tartaglia M, Mehler EL, Goldberg R, et al. Mutations in PTPN11, encoding the protein tyrosine phosphatase SHP-2, cause Noonan syndrome. *Nat Genet.* 2001;29:465–468.

Thienpont B, Mertens L, de Ravel T, et al. Submicroscopic chromosomal imbalances detected by array-CGH are a frequent cause of congenital heart defects in selected patients. *Eur Heart J.* 2007;28:2778–2784.

Tong AH, Lesage G, Bader GD, et al. Global mapping of the yeast genetic interaction network. *Science.* 2004;303:808–813.

Viragh S, Challice CE. The origin of the epicardium and the embryonic myocardial circulation in the mouse. *Anat Rec.* 1981;201:157–168.

Vissers LE, van Ravenswaaij CM, Admiraal R, et al. Mutations in a new member of the chromodomain gene family cause CHARGE syndrome. *Nat Genet.* 2004;36:955–957.

Waldo KL, Kumiski DH, Wallis KT, et al. Conotruncal myocardium arises from a secondary heart field. *Development.* 2001;128:3179–3188.

Ware SM, Harutyunyan KG, Belmont JW. Heart defects in X-linked heterotaxy: evidence for a genetic interaction of Zic3 with the nodal signaling pathway. *Dev Dyn.* 2006;235:1631–1637.

Ware SM, Peng J, Zhu L, et al. Identification and functional analysis of ZIC3 mutations in heterotaxy and related congenital heart defects. *Am J Hum Genet.* 2004;74:93–105.

Waterston RH, Lindblad-Toh K, Birney E, et al. Initial sequencing and comparative analysis of the mouse genome. *Nature.* 2002;420:520–562.

Xin M, Davis CA, Molkentin JD, et al. A threshold of GATA4 and GATA6 expression is required for cardiovascular development. *Proc Natl Acad Sci U S A.* 2006;103:11189–11194.

Yamagishi H, Yamagishi C, Nakagawa O, Harvey RP, Olson EN, Srivastava D. The combinatorial activities of Nkx2.5 and dHAND are essential for cardiac ventricle formation. *Dev Biol.* 2001;239:190–203.

Yamamoto M, Meno C, Sakai Y, et al. The transcription factor FoxH1 (FAST) mediates Nodal signaling during anterior-posterior patterning and node formation in the mouse. *Genes Dev.* 2001;15:1242–1256.

Yan YT, Gritsman K, Ding J, et al. Conserved requirement for EGF-CFC genes in vertebrate left-right axis formation. *Genes Dev.* 1999;13:2527–2537.

3

The Classification of Inherited Cardiovascular Conditions

Dhavendra Kumar and Ruth Newbury-Ecob

All major body systems have a complex anatomical and physiological arrangement to ensure smooth functioning throughout the life span. This requires a complex and coordinated functional arrangement of several hundred genes that code for or modify several protein families. Some of these are evolutionarily conserved as would be expected in the taxonomical context. In humans this is evident when compared to other primates and nonprimate mammals. Some of these are relevant for very basic biological functions, for example, mitosis, meiosis, cell structure, and cell function. An interested reader may find a detailed account on this subject in any of the text books on molecular biology or molecular genetics (see *Further reading*).

The anatomy and physiology of the cardiovascular system (CVS) is complex. Almost all body organs, regions and systems are intricately linked with CVS, and it is involved directly or indirectly in several hundred genetic diseases. These could be primary CVS diseases or diseases of other body systems with secondary CVS involvement. However, several disorders simultaneously or sequentially affect multiple organs or body systems including CVS. For example, inherited metabolic diseases often present with symptoms and signs referable to CVS. It is difficult to categorize these as primary or secondary CVS diseases with a genetic etiology. In simple phenotypic terms, inherited disorders of the heart and the vascular system can be discussed under three broad headings—primary, secondary, and multisystem disorders.

In the genetic context, it is important that the reader has a basic understanding of genes, molecular cell biology, and patterns of inheritance. It is recommended that the interested reader refer to any of the text books listed in *Further reading*. Several of the genetic terms that appear in this chapter and other chapters are defined in the *Glossary*. It is beyond the scope of this chapter to provide a detailed account of the basic principles of human genetics and genomics. However, a brief description of patterns of inheritance and related information is provided to assist the reader in understanding the complexity and diversity of the inherited disorders of the CVS. Major disorders are addressed in detail in the second section of the book. Inevitably, the reader will find that a few disorders are discussed in more than one chapter.

All inherited diseases are classified as chromosomal (numerical or structural), single gene, or Mendelian; multifactorial/polygenic complex diseases; congenital anomalies or diseases associated with specific mitochondrial gene mutations (Table 3–1). Apart from chromosomal disorders, essentially all genetic disorders result from some form of alteration or mutation occurring in a specific gene (single gene diseases) or involving multiple loci spread across the human genome (polygenic disorders). The major impact of chromosomal disorders occurs before birth and carries a serious health burden throughout childhood and during the early years of life (Figure 3–1). Single gene diseases can pose a real medical and health burden from the perinatal period to adult age with a peak around mid-childhood. In contrast, the polygenic/multifactorial diseases tend to present late, except for developmental anomalies that require active multidisciplinary care during early life.

Traditional Patterns of Inheritance

Traditionally, the genetic conditions (Table 3–1) include chromosomal abnormalities (aneuploidies, structural aberrations, and mosaicism), Mendelian diseases or single gene disorders (autosomal dominant, autosomal recessive, X-linked recessive, and X-linked dominant), polygenic/multifactorial, and mitochondrial diseases. This conventional approach may not be applicable in explaining the underlying genetic mechanisms in certain conditions. Newer, nontraditional approaches and concepts, for example, genomic rearrangement, genomic imprinting, and copy number variations, are now being applied in dissecting the underlying genetic etiology

Table 3–1 The Classification of Genetic Disorders

Chromosomal	Numerical-aneuploidy; structural-deletion; duplication; inversion; isochromosome; ring chromosome; reciprocal or Robertsonian translocation
Mendelian	Autosomal recessive
	Autosomal dominant
	X-linked recessive
	X-linked dominant
Multifactorial/ polygenic	Gene–environment interaction; genetic/genomic polymorphisms
Mitochondrial	Deletion; point mutations; mtDNA polymorphisms

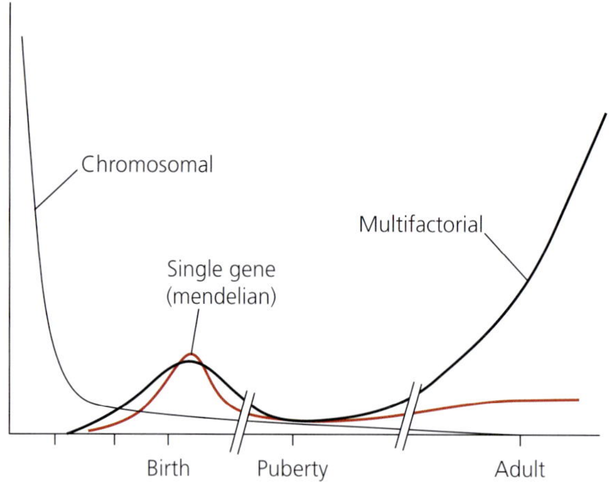

Figure 3–1 Distribution of different genetic disorders in various age groups. Adopted with permission from *Principles of Medical Genetics* by Thomas D Gelehrter, Francis S Collins, and David Ginsburg, Williams and Wilkins, Baltimore, USA, Second edition, 1998.

and pathogenesis. Several well-defined and recognizable CVS disorders exist, which follow one of these inheritance patterns. It is now possible to carry out online database searches to obtain information on any of these diseases or syndromes. Currently, clinicians and researchers alike regularly use databases, such as Victor McKusick's "On-line Mendelian Inheritance of Man" (www.ncbi.nlm.nih.gov/omim), Albert Schizel's catalog of phenotypes associated with chromosome abnormalities (Human cytogenetics database, Oxford Medical Databases), and DECIPHER (https://decipher.sanger.ac.uk/). There are other databases that document mutations and polymorphic variants in relation to human disease phenotypes that are also useful in clinical medicine, for example, ENSEMBL genome browser (www.ensembl.org/) and Cardiff Human Mutation Database (www.hgmd.cf.ac.uk).

1. Chromosomal Disorders

The entire human genome is spread over 23 pairs of chromosomes including one pair specifically assigned to male (XY) and female (XX) gender, designated the sex-chromosome pair. The chromosomal constitution of man is complex and comprises variable amounts of euchromatin and heterochromatin that exhibit with a characteristic "banding pattern" and is essential for the physical and distinct appearance of a particular chromosome. Typically, a chromosome pair includes two homologs each comprising a short arm (p) and a long arm (q) separated by the central heterochromatin-G-C rich region designated the centromere. A detailed account of chromosome structure and fundamental changes that occur during meiosis and mitosis can be found in any leading textbook on basic genetics (see *Further reading*).

Chromosomal disorders are essentially disorders of the genome resulting from either loss or addition of a whole chromosome (aneuploidy) or parts of chromosomes (structural). A chromosome abnormality results in major disturbance in the genomic arrangement since each chromosome or part thereof consists of thousands of genes and several noncoding polymorphic DNA sequences. The physical manifestations of chromosome disorders are often quite striking, characterized by growth retardation, developmental delay, and a variety of somatic abnormalities. A number of chromosomal syndromes are now recognizable. The diagnosis and genetic management of these disorders fall within the scope of the subspecialty "clinical cytogenetics." Chapter 5 deals with this subject in detail.

The management of chromosomal disorders requires a coordinated and dedicated team approach involving a wide range of clinicians and health professionals. A typical example is Down syndrome resulting from either three copies of chromosome 21 (trisomy) or an addition to the long arm of chromosome 21 usually resulting from an unbalanced meiotic rearrangement of a parental chromosomal translocation between chromosomes 21 and one of the other acrocentric (centromere located at the end) chromosomes (Robertsonian translocation). Down syndrome occurs in about 1 in 800 live births and increases in frequency with advancing maternal age. It is characterized by growth and developmental delay, often with severe mental retardation, and the characteristic facial appearance recognized with upward slanting eyes. A major cause of death in these individuals is associated congenital heart defects that can complicate the clinical management in a significant proportion of Down syndrome cases. Prenatal diagnosis and antenatal assessment of the maternal risk for Down syndrome employing a variety of imaging and biochemical markers is now established clinical and public health practice in most countries.

Clinically significant chromosome abnormalities occur in nearly 1% of live-born births and account for about 1% of pediatric hospital admissions and 2.5% of childhood mortality (Hall et al. 1978). The loss or gain of whole chromosomes is often incompatible with survival, and such abnormalities are a major cause of spontaneous abortions or miscarriages. Almost half of the spontaneous abortuses are associated with a major chromosomal abnormality. It is estimated that about a quarter of all conceptions may suffer from major chromosome problems because approximately 50% of all conceptions may not be recognized as established pregnancies, and 15% of these end in a miscarriage. Essentially, the major impact of chromosomal disorders occurs before birth or during early life (Figure 3–1).

The delineation of rare and uncommon chromosomal disorders has been crucial in the gene mapping of several Mendelian (single gene) disorders such as X-linked Duchenne muscular dystrophy (*dystrophin*), type 1 neurofibromatosis (*neurofibromin*), and Williams syndrome/familial supraventricular aortic stenosis (SVAS) (*elastin*). The chromosomal regions involved in deletion, duplication, inversion, and breakpoints involved in a complex chromosomal rearrangement provide an important clue and assist the keen researcher in focusing on genes located within the chromosomal segment.

2. Single Gene (Mendelian) Disorders

About 4,000 human diseases are caused by mutations in single genes and constitute a major health burden. Single gene disorders account for approximately 5%–10% of pediatric hospital admissions and childhood mortality. The major impact of these disorders occurs in the newborn period and early childhood. However, these also constitute a significant proportion of adulthood diseases, notably late onset neurodegenerative diseases and various forms of familial cancer. Although the majority of single gene diseases are rare, some are relatively common and pose a major health problem. For example, familial hypercholesterolemia, a major predisposing factor in premature coronary artery disease, occurs in about 1 in 500 people. Other good examples would be familial breast and colorectal cancers, which affect approximately 1 in 300. Some single gene disorders are specific for certain populations, for example, Tay-Sachs disease among Ashkenazi Jews, cystic fibrosis in white Caucasians, thalassemias among people from southeast Asia and the Mediterranean countries, and sickle cell disease in people of western African origin. Techniques in molecular biology have enabled characterization of a number of mutated genes. Sickle cell disease was the first single gene disorder to be defined at the molecular level. This has revolutionized the diagnosis and management of these disorders. The single gene disorders are inherited in a simple Mendelian manner, and hence justifiably called *Mendelian disorders*. The genetic transmission of altered genes or traits follow principles as set out by the Austrian monk Gregor Mendel in 1865, based on his seminal work on garden pea plants. Mendel inferred that "those characteristics that are transmitted entire, or almost unchanged by hybridization, and therefore constitute the characters of the hybrid, are termed dominant, and those that become latent in the process, recessive."

The nomenclature of these disorders reflects the gender-specific transmission and is supported by localization of an altered gene on either an autosome (1–22) or the X chromosome. Mendelian disorders are described as autosomal dominant, autosomal recessive, and X-linked recessive (Figure 3–2) or X-linked dominant (Figure 3–3). The latter pattern differs from the X-linked recessive by having an excess of affected females in a family because the heterozygous mutation on the X chromosome can be transmitted to the daughter from an affected mother as well as the affected father. Sporadic X-linked dominant diseases are encountered in a female as these are lethal in the male. A detailed family history and careful interpretation of the pedigree are essential prerequisites in the diagnosis of a Mendelian disease. Accurate risk estimates, for use in genetic counseling, are not possible in the absence of a reliable and comprehensive pedigree. The major features of the individual inheritance manner are described in leading genetics text books (see *Further Reading*). All human disorders and traits that follow the Mendelian principles are listed in a major resource—McKusick's catalog of "Mendelian Inheritance of Man." An online version (OMIM) is available and regularly updated.

3. Multifactorial/Polygenic Disorders

This group of disorders includes the most common and least understood human genetic diseases. These diseases result from interaction of certain environmental factors with multiple genes, some of

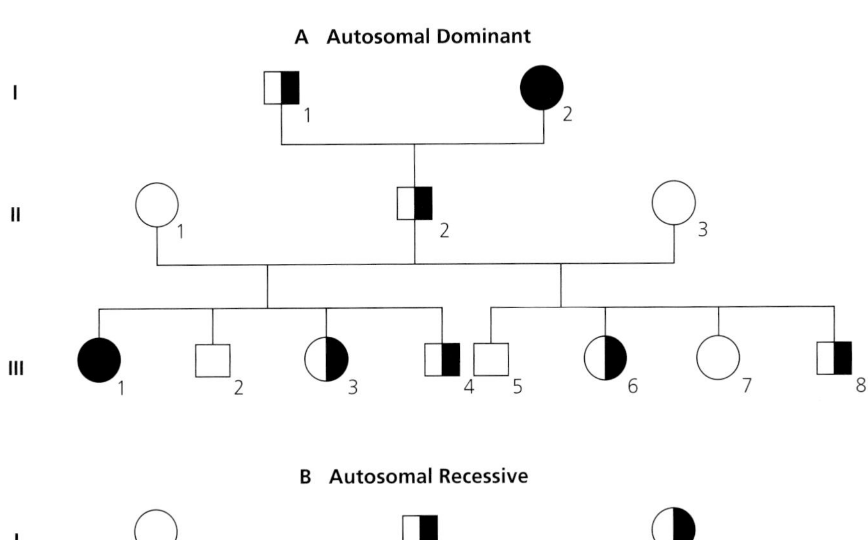

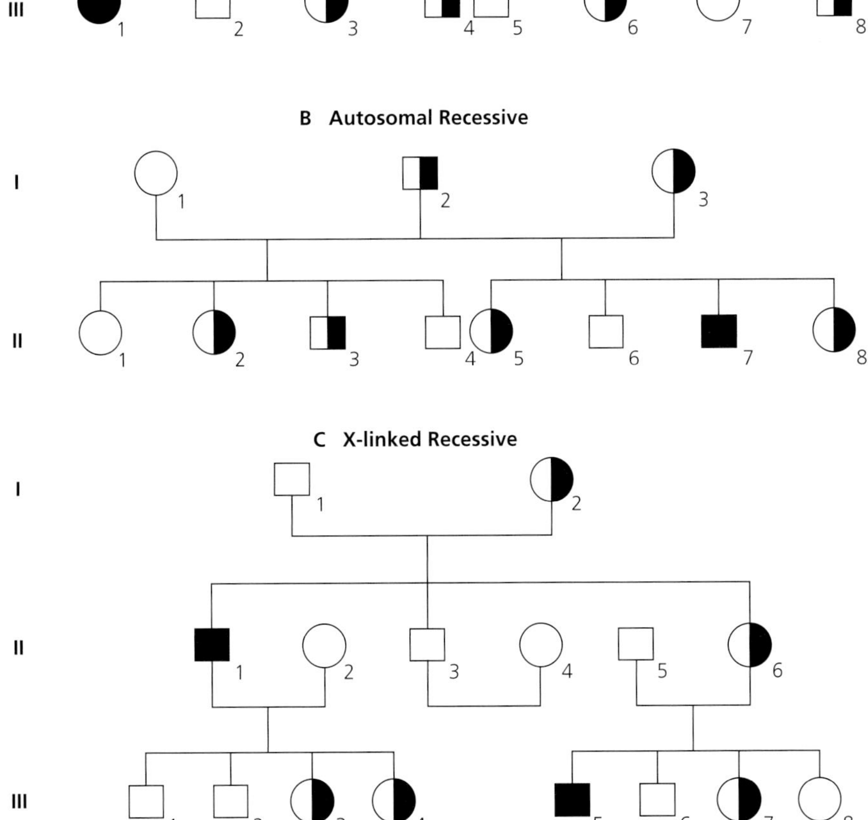

Figure 3–2 Typical pedigrees in Mendelian inheritance. Key to symbols: blank square - unaffected male; open circle - unaffected female; black filled - affected (homozygous); half black filled - carrier (heterozygous).

Figure 3–3 A pedigree with an X-linked dominant disorder: note absence of "male-male" transmission; all daughters of an affected male would be heterozygous and thus could be symptomatic. Adopted with permission from *Principles of Medical Genetics* by Thomas D Gelehrter, Francis S Collins, and David Ginsburg, Williams and Wilkins, Baltimore, USA, Second edition, 1998.

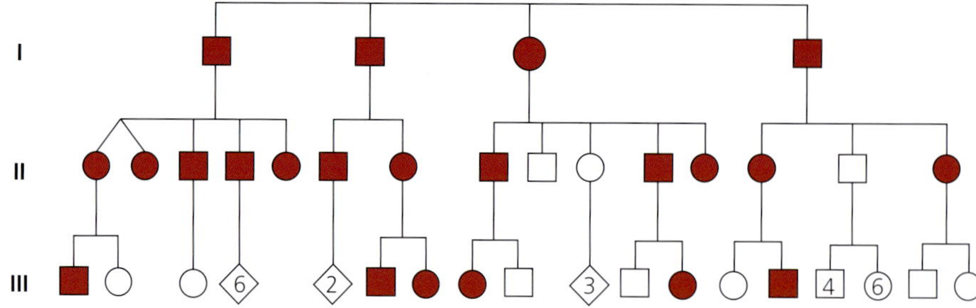

which may have a major effect, but the majority carry only a relatively minor effect. The minor additive effect of these multiple loci lowers the *threshold* of an organ or a body system to withstand environmental pressures resulting in either a developmental anomaly or an abnormal disease state. Examples include common congenital anomalies such as cleft lip, cleft palate, neural tube defects, and most congenital heart diseases. The common chronic medical diseases fall within this category of genetic disorders including diabetes mellitus, coronary heart disease, hypertension, arthritis, and schizophrenia. Understanding the genetic basis of common diseases remains the major challenge facing modern genetics and genomics.

The clinical impact of multifactorial diseases is significant in both the neonatal period and in adult life. It is estimated that about 25%–50% pediatric hospital admissions are related to these groups of disorders and associated with 25%–35% of childhood mortality. There is an even greater medical and health burden of these disorders during adult life due to a chronic natural history of resulting medical diseases. For instance, diabetes mellitus and obesity account for about 40% of the adult medical problem in the developed and developing world.

Identification of any such disorder or condition is important in assessing risks to close relatives. A comparison of general population and multiple cases in a family would indicate a shift of the bell-shaped Gaussian curve to the right reflecting a lowered threshold with an increased incidence (Figure 3–4). The precise additional risk would be dependent upon the degree of relationship with the index case in the family. In addition, the gender of the index case

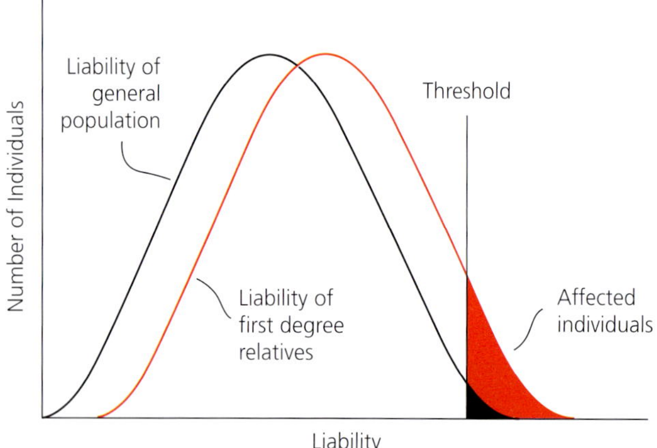

Figure 3–4 The "Gaussian" bell shaped curve to illustrate *genetic threshold,* indicated by liability in the general population (shown in black). A shift to the right (in gray) indicates increased liability in first-degree relatives with an increased risk of recurrence. Reprinted with permission, Weatherall, 1991, Oxford University Press, UK.

is also important in assessing the liability. The genetic liability is estimated to be greater if the index case is of the gender with lowest incidence. For example, in the case of pyloric stenosis, greater risk would be applicable if the index case were a female, which carries the lowest birth prevalence. Finally, recurrence risks for a given population group is estimated to equal the square root of the birth incidence. For instance, the birth incidence of ventricular septal defect is approximately 3 per 1,000, the recurrence risk to first-degree relative, such as the next child, would be the square root of 0.003 or 3%. These figures are useful in genetic counseling of a family following the birth of a child with a congenital anomaly.

This group of diseases poses the challenge of working out the mechanisms that determine the additive or interactive effects of many genes creating predisposition to diseases, which in turn manifest only in the presence of certain environmental factors. It is hoped that a combination of molecular genetic approaches, gene mapping, and functional genomics will allow a clearer definition of these genetic diseases. Several sections in this book will address this issue at length and focus on specific disease groups and systems.

4. Mitochondrial Disorders

Apart from the nuclear DNA (nDNA), a small proportion of DNA is also found in mitochondria in the cytoplasm of cells (mtDNA). Each cell contains 2–100 mitochondria, each of which contains 5–10 circular chromosomes. The 16.5 kb mtDNA molecule is free from any noncoding intronic regions and encodes two ribosomal RNA (rRNA) genes, 22 transfer RNAs (tRNA), and 13 polypeptides that are parts of multisubunit enzymes involved in oxidative phosphorylation. In comparison to nuclear DNA, mtDNA is 20 times more prone to recurrent mutations resulting in generation of mutagenic oxygen radicals in the mitochondria. The inheritance of mtDNA is exclusively maternal due to its cytoplasmic location. The mature sperm cytoplasm contains very little mitochondria as it is almost completely lost during the fertilization process, apparently at the loss of the tail that carries the bulk of the cytoplasm. Owing to the wholly maternal cytoplasmic location, only females can transmit mitochondrial diseases to their offspring of either gender (Figure 3–5).

Since mtDNA replicates separately from nDNA, and mitochondria segregate in daughter cells independently of the nuclear chromosomes (replicative segregation), the proportion of mitochondria carrying an mtDNA mutation can differ among somatic cells. This mitochondrial heterogeneity is also called heteroplasmy and plays an important part in the variable and tissue-specific phenotype of mitochondrial disease. Since different tissues have varying degrees of dependence on oxidative phosphorylation, with heart, muscle, and central nervous system being the most dependent, the common manifestations of mitochondrial disease include cardiomyopathy, myopathy, and encephalopathy. Furthermore, oxidative phosphorylation declines with age, probably related to the accumulation of successive mtDNA mutations. Thus the clinical

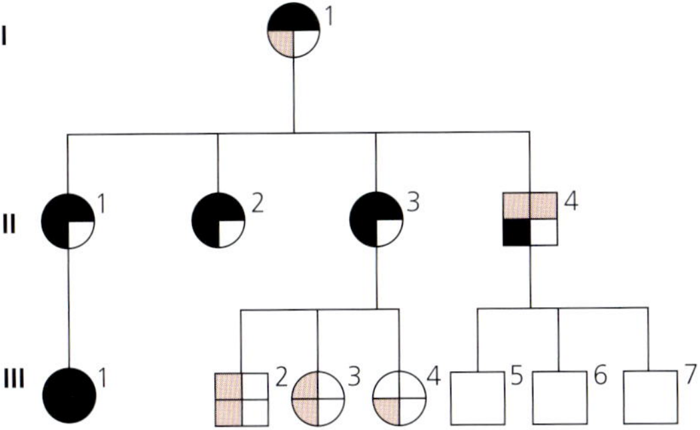

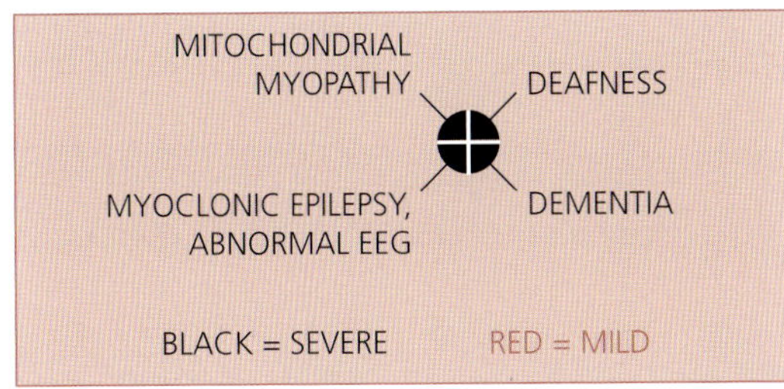

Figure 3–5 Pedigree of a family with mitochondrial encephalopathy with ragged-red muscle fibers (MERRF)–note segregation of different features with variable severity in the affected family members. Adopted with permission from *Principles of Medical Genetics* 2nd ed. by Thomas D Gelehrter, Francis S Collins, and David Ginsburg, Williams and Wilkins, Baltimore, USA, 1998.

phenotype in a mitochondrial disease is not simply or directly related to mtDNA genotype, but it reflects several factors, including the overall capacity for oxidative phosphorylation determined by both mtDNA and nDNA genes, the accumulation of somatic mtDNA mutations and the degree of heteroplasmy, tissue-specific requirements of oxidative phosphorylation, and age.

Several mitochondrial diseases have now been characterized (see also Chapter 31). One of the best characterized is Leber's hereditary optic neuropathy (LHON), which exclusively affects males. There is loss of central vision secondary to optic nerve degeneration. The vision loss usually occurs in the twenties and can progress rapidly in some men. Eleven different missense mtDNA mutations in three different mitochondrial genes encoding respiratory chain enzyme subunits have been described. The phenotype in other mitochondrial diseases tends to include a combination of heart, muscle, and central nervous system manifestations with considerable intra/interfamilial variability for the same mtDNA mutation. In addition, mitochondrial dysfunction can be part of the phenotype in some Mendelian diseases where the mutant gene product presumably has pathogenic influence on the mitochondrial-mediated metabolic pathway. Examples include Barth syndrome and autosomal recessive respiratory enzyme disorders. Genetic counseling and decision for prenatal diagnosis can be difficult in mitochondrial disorders due to the difficulty in predicting the phenotype in the affected pregnancy.

Finally, a high degree of sequence variation (polymorphism) is known to occur in the noncoding region of the mitochondrial chromosome (the D-loop). This polymorphism has been used in anthropologic and evolutionary studies to trace back the origins and links of human populations. In addition, this information has been applied in forensic analysis to match maternal grandparent mtDNA with an orphaned child whose parents have "disappeared" during war, a natural disaster, or in mysterious circumstances.

Nontraditional Patterns of Inheritance

Recent advances in molecular genetics have enabled us to identify specific groups of disorders that result from characteristic mechanisms involving specific areas of the human genome. Often these do not conform to the standard basic principles of genetics. A broad term "genomic disorders" has been coined to describe these conditions (Table 3–2).

A number of hereditary disorders present with complex genetic pathology that do not follow the conventional principles of inheritance as outlined in the previous sections. There is now overwhelming evidence within these disorders that indicates unusual mechanisms suggesting *nontraditional inheritance*. The mechanisms involve certain genomic regions that directly or indirectly influence regulation and expression of one or more genes manifesting in complex phenotypes. Currently, some of these disorders are listed as either chromosomal or single gene disorders.

1. Disorders of Genomic Imprinting: Epigenetic Diseases

The term "epigenetics" refers to heritable factors that affect gene expression without any change in the gene coding sequence. These factors could be operational either during meiosis or mitosis and are often selective and preferential on the basis of *parent of origin*. The term "imprinting" is commonly used to describe this important biological mechanism, which is recognized to influence wide-ranging physical and molecular phenotypes. A number of human diseases have now been confirmed to result from epigenetic changes in various parts of the genome. The term "epigenetic diseases" or "genomic imprinting disorders" refers to this group of diseases. Basic mechanisms related to the phenomenon of epigenetics or epigenomics are reviewed elsewhere (Wolffe and Matzke 1999) (Table 3–3).

Epigenetic initiation and silencing is regulated by the complex interaction of three systems, including DNA methylation, RNA-associated silencing, and histone modification (Egger et al. 2004). The relationship between these three components is vital for expression or silencing of genes (Figure 3–6). Disruption of one or other of these interacting systems can lead to inappropriate expression or silencing of genes resulting in epigenetic diseases. Methylation of the C^5 position of cytosine residues in DNA has long been recognized as an epigenetic silencing mechanism of fundamental importance (Holliday and Pugh 1975). The methylation of CpG sites within the human genome is maintained by a number of DNA methyltransferases (DNMTs) and has multifaceted roles for silencing transportable elements, for defense against viral sequences and for transcriptional repression of certain genes. A strong suppression of the CpG methyl-acceptor site in human DNA results from mutagenic changes in 5-methylcytosine, causing C:G to T:A transitions. Normally CpG islands, which are GC rich evolutionary conserved regions of more than 500 bp, are kept free of methylation. These stretches of DNA are located within the promoter region of about 40% of mammalian genes and, when methylated, cause stable heritable transcriptional silencing. Aberrant de

Table 3–2 Classification of Genomic Disorders

Disorders of genomic imprinting (epigenetic diseases)
Disorders of genome architecture
Trinucleotide repeats disorders
Complex genomic diseases

Table 3–3 Recognizable Epigenetic Dysmorphic Syndromes (Egger et al. 2004)

Disease	Main Features	Epigenetic Mechanism
ATR-X syndrome	α-Thalassemia, facial dysmorphic features, neurodevelopmental disabilities	Mutations in *ATRX* gene; hypomethylation of repeat and satellite sequences
Fragile X syndrome	Chromosome instability, physical and learning/ behavioral difficulties	Expansion and methylation of CGG repeat in *FMR1* 5' UTR, promoter methylation
ICF syndrome	Chromosome instability, immunodeficiency	*DNMT3* mutations; DNA hypomethylation
Angelman syndrome	Seizures and intellectual disabilities	Deregulation of one or more imprinted genes at 15q11–13 (maternal)
Prader-Willi syndrome	Obesity, intellectual disabilities	Deregulation of one or more imprinted genes at 15q11–13 (paternal)
Beckwith-Wiedemann syndrome (BWS)	Organ overgrowth, childhood tumors	Deregulation of one or more imprinted genes at 11p15.5 (*IGF2, CDKN1C, KvDMR1* etc.)
Russel-Silver syndrome	Growth delay, body asymmetry	Deregulation of one or more imprinted genes at 7p (maternal)
Rett syndrome	Seizures, intellectual disabilities	*MeCP2* mutations
Rubinstein-Taybi Syndrome	Facial dysmorphism, intellectual disabilities	Mutation in CREB-binding protein (histone acetylation)
Coffin-Lowry syndrome	Facial dysmorphism, developmental delay	Mutation in *RSk-2* (histone phosphorylation)

Abbreviations: ATR-X, α-thalassemia, X-linked mental retardation; UT, untranslated region; ICF, immunodeficiency, chromosome instability, facial anomalies; CREB, cAMP-response-element-binding protein.

novo methylation of CpG islands is a hallmark of human cancers and is found early during carcinogenesis (Jones and Baylin 2002).

In addition to DNA methylation, histone modifications have also been found to have epigenetic effects. Acetylation and methylation of conserved lysine residues of the amino terminal tail domains are the key elements in histone modification. Generally, the acetylation of histones marks active, transcriptionally competent regions, whereas hypoacetylation histones are found in transcriptionally inactive euchromatic and heterochromatic regions. On the other hand, histone methylation can be a marker for both active and inactive regions of chromatin. Methylation of lysine residue 9 on the N terminus of histone 3 (H3-K9) is a hallmark of silent DNA and is evenly distributed throughout the heterochromatic regions such as centromeres and telomeres, including the inactive X chromosome. In contrast, methylation of lysine 4 of histone 3 (H3-K4) denotes activity and is predominantly found at promoter regions of active genes (Lachner and Jenuwein 2002). This constitutes a "histone code," which can be read and interpreted by different cellular factors. There is evidence that DNA methylation depends on methylation of H3-K9, and can also trigger its methylation. Recently, evidence has accumulated on the role of RNA in posttranscriptional silencing. In addition, RNA in the form of antisense transcripts (Xist or RNAi) can also lead to mitotically heritable transcriptional silencing by the formation of heterochromatin. For example, transcription of antisense RNA led to gene silencing and to the methylation of the structurally normal α-globin gene in patients with α-thalassemia. This is possibly one of the many human diseases resulting from epigenetic silencing due to antisense RNA transcripts (Tufarelli et al. 2003).

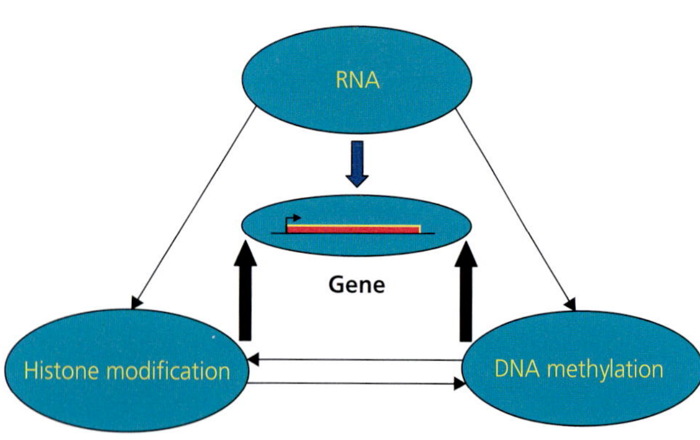

Figure 3–6 Interaction between RNA, histone modification, and DNA methylation in gene expression and silencing. Reprinted from Egger G, Liang G, Aparicio A, Jones P. Epigenetics in human disease and prospects of epigenetic therapy. *Nature*. 2004;429:457–463, with permission.

Mutations in genes that affect genomic epigenetic profiles can give rise to human diseases that can be inherited or somatically acquired (Table 3–4). These epigenetic mutations can be either due to hypermethylation (silencing) of a regulating gene or loss of methylation (LOM) (activation) of another gene that has a positively modifying effect on the phenotype. The parental imprinting effect can be inferred by demonstrating the parental origin of the mutant allele. Similarly, either loss or gain of a chromosomal segment can result in the same situation. Confirmation of a specific chromosomal deletion or duplication is usually possible by using the fluorescence in situ hybridization (FISH) method. The paternal imprinting in this situation is commonly demonstrated by genotyping a set of polymorphic markers located within the chromosomal segment. Inheritance of the whole chromosomal homolog from one parent effectively confirms the imprinting phenomenon since the regulatory gene sequences for the pathogenic gene would be missing from the other parent. This characteristic abnormality is commonly referred to as "uniparental disomy" or UPD, and could be isodisomy (similar parental homologs) or heterodisomy (parental and grandparental homologs) (Figure 3–7). The origin of UPD is believed to be the loss of the additional chromosomal

Table 3–4 Contiguous Gene Syndromes as Genomic Disorders

Disorder (OMIM)	Inheritance	Locus	Gene	Rearrangement	Recombination (Kb) (normal range)
Williams-Beuren syndrome (194050)	AD	7q11.23	*ELN*	del;inv	1600 (> 320)
Prader-Willi syndrome (176270)	AD	15q11.2q13	?	del	3500 (> 500)
Angelman syndrome (105830)	AD	15q11.2q13	*UBE3A*	del	3500 (> 500)
Dup(15)(q11.2q13)	?AD	15q11.2q13	?	dup	3500 (> 500)
Triplication 15q11.2q13	?	15q11.2q13	?	trip	? (> 500)
Smith-Magenis syndrome (18290)		17p11.2	*RA13*	del	4000 (~ 250)
Dup(17(p11.2p11.2)	AD	17p11.2	*PMP22*	dup	4000 (~ 250)
DiGeorge/VCFS (188400)	AD	22q11.2	*TBX1*	del	3000/1500 (~ 225–400)
Male infertility (415000)	YL	Yq11.2	*DBY,*	del	800 (~ 10)
AZFa microdeletion			*USP9Y*		
AZFc microdeletion (400024)	YL	Yq11.2	*RBMY*	del	3,500 (~ 220)
			DAZ	?	

Abbreviations: del, deletion; dup, duplication; inv, inversion; D, direct; C, complex.

homolog, failing which the conceptus would be trisomic. This mechanism is also called *trisomic rescue*.

For a maternally imprinted disorder, paternal UPD would be confirmatory, and maternal UPD would be diagnostic for the paternally imprinted condition. For example, maternal UPD is diagnostic for Prader-Willi syndrome, and paternal UPD for Angelman syndrome, both conditions being associated with a microdeletion of 15q11 region. The parental origin of the 15q microdeletion follows the expected epigenetic pattern and is in keeping with the clinical diagnosis. Recurrence risk estimates vary dependent on the specific epigenetic pattern. This information is crucial in offering accurate genetic counseling in any genomic imprinting disorder.

Many epigenetic diseases are associated with chromosomal alterations and manifest with physical and learning difficulties. For example, mutations in X-linked mental retardation with the α-thalassemia phenotype (*ATRX*) result in consistent changes in the methylation pattern of ribosomal DNA, Y-specific repeats,

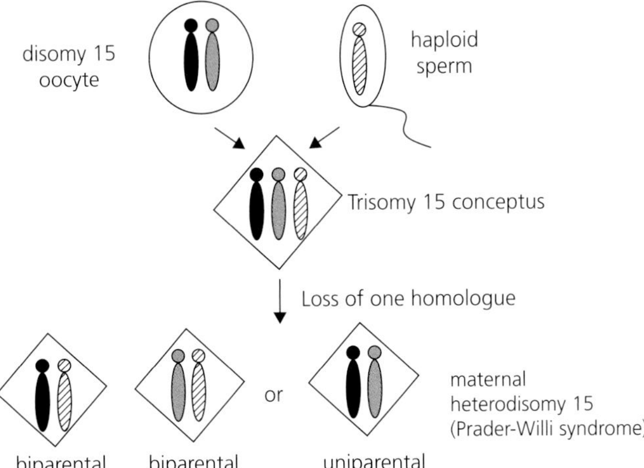

Figure 3–7 The origin of uniparental disomy 15 in Prader-Willi syndrome through trisomic rescue during early embryogenesis—note different homologs (maternal heterodisomy).

and subtelomeric repeats. Another X-linked recessive mental retardation syndrome, associated with a visible "fragile site" on the terminal part of the long arm of the X chromosome (fragile X syndrome), results from de novo silencing of the pathogenic gene *FMR1*. This syndrome is characteristically associated with an abnormal expansion of CGG triplet repeats in the *FMR1* 5' untranslated terminal region. Methylation of the expansion leads to silencing of the *FMR1* gene and under certain cultural conditions creates the visible *fragile site* on the X chromosome.

Epigenetic silencing is probably also significant in other neurodevelopmental disorders. For example, in Rett syndrome, a common cause of intellectual disability in young girls, mutations of the *MeCP2* gene are seen in about 80% of cases. The MeCP protein binds to methylcytosine residues and causes derepression of genes normally suppressed by DNA methylation. Despite lack of firm evidence, it is likely that *MeCP2* might have a key role in the control of neuronal gene activity resulting in the pathology of Rett syndrome (Chen et al. 2003). Interaction with another pathogenic gene (*CTKL5* or *STK9*) in Rett syndrome is likely to be important in the pathogenesis of this neurodevelopmental disorder (Slager et al. 2003). On a wider genomic level, mutations in the *DNMT3b* gene, causing the ICF (immunodeficiency, centromeric region instability, and facial anomalies) syndrome, result in deregulation of DNA methylation patterns. A notable example is that of Beckwith-Wiedemann syndrome, an overgrowth syndrome predisposing to Wilms' tumor and other childhood tumors, which is associated with duplications and rearrangements of a small chromosomal region on the short arm of chromosome (11p15.5). This region contains a cluster of genes, which is susceptible to a number of epigenetic alterations, manifesting with the BWS phenotype and tumorigenesis, particularly, Wilms' tumor and other childhood embryonal tumors. Loss of methylation in imprinting control regions (such as *KvDMR1*) can cause deregulation of imprinting and either biallelic expression (*IGF2* and *H19*) or silencing (such as *CDKN1C*) of imprinted genes, which is seen in most sporadic cases.

The epigenetic phenomenon is probably significant for the phenotypic manifestations in some cardiovascular disorders. More importantly the epigenetic changes are probably important in a number of other complex cardiovascular phenotypes, such as coronary artery disease (Chapter 22), essential hypertension (Chapter 23), and stroke (Chapter 24).

2. Disorders of Genome Architecture

Recent completion of the human genome project and sequencing of the total genomes of yeast and other bacterial species have enabled investigators to view genetic information in the context of the entire genome. As a result, it is now possible to recognize mechanisms of some genetic diseases at the genomic level. The evolution of the mammalian genome has resulted in the duplication of genes, gene segments, and repeat gene clusters (Lupski 1998). This aspect of genome architecture provides recombination hot spots between nonsyntenic regions of chromosomes distributed across the whole genome. These genomic regions become susceptible to further DNA rearrangements that may be associated with an abnormal phenotype. Such disorders are collectively grouped under the broad category of *genome architecture disorders* (Figure 3–8).

The term "genome architecture disorder" refers to a disease that is caused by an alteration of the genome that results in complete loss, gain, or disruption of the structural integrity of a dosage sensitive gene(s) (Shaw and Lupski 2004; Lupski and Stankiewicz 2005). Notable examples include a number of chromosome deletion/duplication syndromes (Table 3–5). In these conditions, there is a critical rearranged genomic segment flanked by large (usually >10 kb), highly homologous low-copy repeat (LCR) structures that can act as recombination substrates. Meiotic recombination between nonallelic LCR copies, also known as nonallelic homologous recombination (NAHR), can result in deletion or duplication of the intervening segment.

Similarly, other chromosomal rearrangements (Table 3–5), including reciprocal, Robertsonian and jumping translocations, inversions, isochromosomes, and small marker chromosomes, may also involve susceptibility to rearrangement related to genome structure or architecture. In several cases, LCRs, A-T rich palindromes and pericentromeric repeats are located at such rearrangement breakpoints. This susceptibility to genomic rearrangements is not only implicated in disease etiology, but also in primate genome evolution (Shaw and Lupski 2004).

An increasing number of Mendelian diseases (Table 3–6) are recognized to result from recurrent inter- and intrachromosomal rearrangements involving unstable genomic regions facilitated by LCRs. These genomic regions are predisposed to NAHR between paralogous genomic segments. LCRs usually span approximately 10–400 kb of genomic DNA, share ≥97% sequence identity, and provide the substrates for NAHR, thus predisposing to rearrangements. LCRs have been shown to facilitate meiotic DNA rearrangements associated with several multiple malformation syndromes and some disease traits (Table 3–5). Seminal examples include microdeletion syndromes [Williams-Beuren syndrome (7q11del), DiGeorge syndrome (22q11del)], autosomal dominant Charcot-Marie-Tooth disease type 1A (PMP22 gene duplication), Hereditary Neuropathy of Pressure Palsy (HNPP: PMP22 gene deletion) mapped to 17p11.2, and Smith-Magenis, a contiguous gene syndrome (CGS) with del (17)(p11.2p11.2). Dominantly inherited male infertility related to AZF gene deletion follows a similar mechanism. In addition, this LCR-based complex genome architecture appears to play a major role in primate karyotype evolution, pathogenesis of complex traits, and human carcinogenesis.

Similar observations were also made in relation to Smith-Magenis syndrome (SMS), a contiguous gene syndrome associated with a microdeletion of 17p11.2 segment (Greenberg et al. 1991). Affected children present with facial dysmorphic features, severe

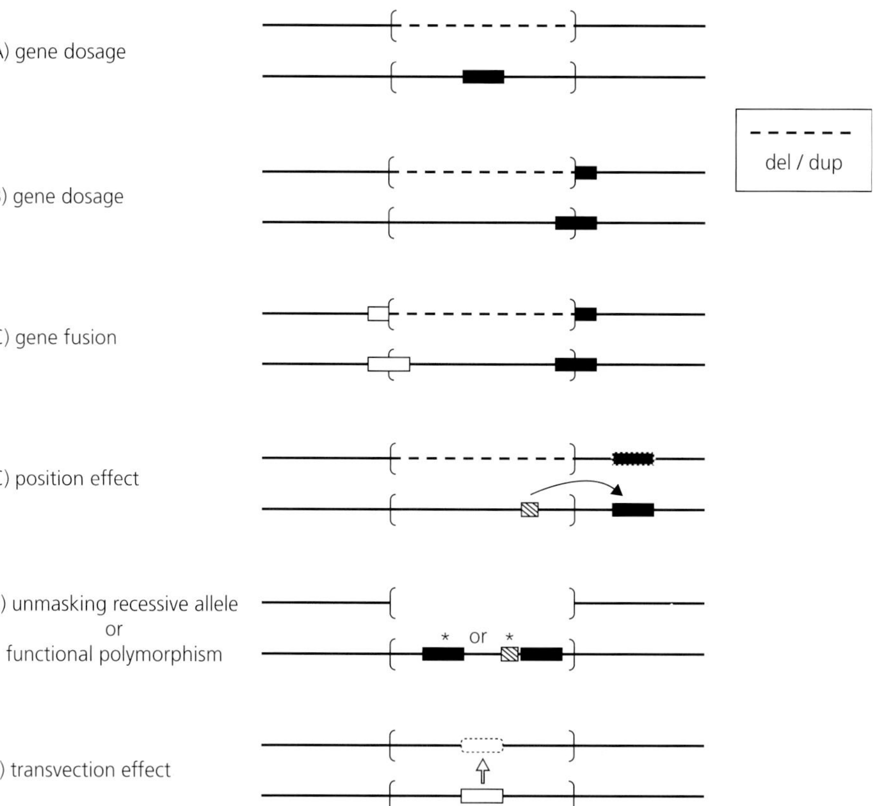

Figure 3–8 Molecular mechanisms for genomic disorders. Dashed lines indicate either deleted or duplicated region; the rearranged genomic interval is shown in brackets; gene is depicted by filled horizontal rectangle; regulatory gene is shown as horizontal hatch-marked rectangle; asterisks denote point mutations. Reprinted from Lupski JR, Stankiewicz P. Genomic disorders: molecular mechanisms for rearrangements and conveyed phenotypes. *PlOS Genetics* 2005;1(6):e49, with permission.

Table 3–5 Genomic Diseases Resulting from Recurrent Chromosomal Rearrangements

		Recombination Substrates		
Rearrangement	Type	Repeat Size	% Identity	Orientation Type
Inv dup(15)(q11q13)	Inverted dup	>500		C
Inv dup(22)(q11.2)	Inverted dup	~225–400	97–98	C
Idic(X)(p11.2)	Isodicentric			I?
Inv dup(8)(pterp23.1::p23.2pter); Olfactory	inv/dup/del	~400	95–97	I
Del(8)(p23.1p23.2)				Receptor gene cluster
dup(15)(q24q26)	Dup	~13–60		?

Abbreviations: del, deletion; dup, duplication; inv, inversion; D, direct; C, complex; I, inverted.

speech delay, and behavioral problems with signs of self-harm. A specific junction fragment was detected by PFGE (SMS-REP) that was involved in recurrent rearrangement resulting in either SMS or reciprocal 17p11.2 duplication. Pathogenic mutations in *RAI1* gene, mapped to the 17p11.2 chromosomal region, are now shown to be etiologically linked with SMS (Slager et al. 2003). It is also possible to have both duplication and deletion at the same time, resulting from DNA rearrangements on both homologs of chromosome 17. This was demonstrated in a patient with mild delay and a family history of autosomal dominant carpal tunnel syndrome (Potocki et al. 1999). The occurrence of both the 17p11.2 duplication and HNPP deletion in this patient reflects the relatively high frequency at which these abnormalities arise and the underlying molecular characteristics of the genome in this region.

It is perfectly reasonable to accept the argument that similar molecular mechanisms apply in causing disorders with diverse phenotypes. The human genome has evolved an architecture that may make us as a species more susceptible to rearrangements causing genomic disorders (Lupski 2003).

3. Disorders with Trinucleotide (Triplet) Repeats

Several disorders are recognized to have a phenomenon of earlier age at onset of disease in successive generations. This is known as *anticipation*. This observation failed to secure a valid biological explanation and had been put aside simply on the basis of biased ascertainment of probands or random variations in the age of onset. With the identification of unstable DNA repeats distributed across the genome, a molecular basis has been found for the phenomenon of anticipation. These unstable DNA repeats tend to increase in size during meiosis over successive generations. The abnormal expansion is correlated with reducing age of onset and increasing severity with further expansion of DNA repeats. The characteristic pattern of the DNA repeat involving a set of three nucleotides is commonly referred to as *tri-nucleotide* or *triplet* repeats. This soon became established as a novel class of mutation and offered a plausible explanation for the phenomenon of anticipation and variable clinical severity in a number of neurodegenerative diseases (Table 3–6).

The X-linked recessive spinal bulbar atrophy (SBA) was one of the first hereditary neurological disorders recognized to be associated with CAG triplet repeats (Warren 1996).

The expanded region can occur anywhere in the gene and thus can disrupt the expression of the gene. In the case of X-linked fragile X syndrome (FRAXA), the CGG repeats are found in the 5'-untranslated region of the first exon of *FMR1*, the pathogenic gene for FRAXA. However, in the case of Friedreich's ataxia (FA), an autosomal recessive form of spinocerebellar ataxia (SCA), the expanded triplet repeat allele (GAA) occurs in the first intron of *X25*, the gene encoding frataxin. In Huntington disease (HD) and other inherited neurodegenerative disorders, the CAG triplet repeats occur within exons and encode an elongated polyglutamine tract.). However, the expanded CTG triplet repeats of myotonic dystrophy (DM) are found in the 3'-untranslated region of the last exon of the DM protein kinase (myotonin) gene (*DMPK*).

Each class of trinucleotide repeats exists in normal individuals. A pathogenic expansion is the one that is seen in clinically symptomatic individuals. Carriers for an X-linked disease also have an expanded allele (premutation), which does not usually result in abnormal phenotype. However, it is likely that some carrier females might exhibit some manifestations as in fragile X syndrome. An expanded allele in the premutation range in a male would not be associated with any clinical manifestations (normal transmitting male, NTM), but this could further expand resulting in all daughters being carriers. However, recent studies have provided data on the existence of late onset gait ataxia in NTMs (Greco et al. 2006). On the other hand, a normal size CGG repeat in a normal male could undergo further expansion during meiosis leading to a carrier daughter. This usually comes to light when a symptomatic grandson is confirmed to have pathogenic FRAXA expansion. Prior to availability of molecular testing in FRAXA, this kind of unusual pedigree pattern in fragile X syndrome was called the *Sherman paradox*. Detailed molecular studies in the family are often necessary to offer accurate genetic counseling to *at-risk* carrier females. Carrier females are at an additional risk for developing premature ovarian failure, usually diagnosed when investigated for secondary infertility (Ennis et al. 2006).

4. Complex Genomic Diseases

All inherited disorders have a genetic abnormality present in the DNA of all cells in the body including germ cells (sperm and egg) and can be transmitted to subsequent generations. In contrast, a genetic abnormality present only in specific somatic cells can not be transmitted. The genetic abnormality in a somatic cell can occur at any time from the postconception stage to late adult life. The paradigm of somatic cell genetic disorder is cancer, where the development of malignancy is often the consequence of mutations in genes that control cellular growth. There are several such genes and these are designated oncogenes. It is now accepted that all human cancer results from mutations in the nDNA of a specific somatic cell, making it the most common genetic disease.

The clinical course and outcome of treatment in a number of acute and chronic medical conditions depend upon various factors. For instance, there is overwhelming evidence that highly polymorphic cytokine, interferon, and interleukin families of complex

Table 3–6 Disorders with Trinucleotide (Triplet) Repeat Expansion

Disorder	Triplet	Location	Normal	Mutation
Fragile X syndrome	CGG	5'UTR	10–50	200–2,000
Friedreich's ataxia	GAA	Intronic	17–22	200–900
Kennedy disease (SBMA)	CAG	Coding	17–24	40–55
Spinocerebellar ataxia 1(SCA1)	CAG	Coding	19–36	43–81
Huntington disease	CAG	Coding	9–35	37–100
Dentatorubral-Pallidoluysian Atrophy (DRPLA)	CAG	Coding	7–23	49->75
Machado-Joseph disease (SCA3)CAG	Coding	12–36	67->79	
Spinocerebellar ataxia 2(SCA2)	CAG	Coding	15–24	35–39
Spinocerebellar ataxia 6(SCA6) CAG	Coding	4–16	21–27	
Spinocerebellar ataxia 7(SCA7) CAG	Coding	7–35	37–200	
Spinocerebellar ataxia 8(SCA8) TG	UTR	16–37	100->500	
Myotonic dystrophy	CTG	3'UTR	5–35	50–4,000
Fragile site E (FRAXE)	CCG	Promoter	6–25	>200
Fragile site F (FRAXF)	GCC	?	6–29	>500
Fragile site 16 A (FRA16A)	CCG	?	16–49	1,000–2,000

Abbreviation: UTR, untranslated region.

proteins influence the host response to acute infection and physical injury. All these proteins are encoded by several genes. Similarly, association of human leucocyte antigens (HLA) in the pathogenesis of a number of acute and chronic medical disorders is well known. In addition, interaction of mutations within these genes and with several other genomic polymorphisms, such as single nucleotide polymorphisms (SNPs) is probably important in several acute medical conditions including trauma. This will have a major impact in critical care and acute medicine. The role of SNPs in modulating complex medical disorders, such as diabetes mellitus, coronary heart disease, hypertension, and various forms of cancer is unclear. However, the complexity of interaction of SNPs with other genetic traits and loci is probably important in the prognosis of these disorders, in particular the outcome of therapeutic interventions. This argument probably justifies separating some of these disorders under the title of "complex genomic diseases."

Various cancers and degenerative diseases occur with increasing frequency in old age. However, these may also present at a younger age, such as childhood leukemias. The molecular mechanisms in these diseases are not entirely clear, but probably include defects in DNA repair mechanisms, accelerated apoptosis, deregulation of imprinted genomic regions, and de novo chromosome rearrangements involving specific genomic regions. Although these disorders can arguably be included under the broad category of multifactorial/polygenic diseases, the pattern of distribution and recurrence does not follow the agreed principles of multifactorial/polygenic inheritance as discussed elsewhere in this chapter.

As described in the previous section on *epigenetics*, epigenetic changes play a major role in the development of human cancer (Egger et al. 2004). A high percentage of patients with sporadic colorectal cancer (CRC) possess microsatellite instability and show methylation and silencing of the gene encoding *MLH1* (Kane et al. 1997). It is thus likely that epigenetic changes also predispose to genetic instability. In some cases, promoter-associated methylation of *MLH1* is found not only in the tumor but also in normal somatic tissues, including spermatozoa. These germline "epimutations" predispose individuals carrying abnormal methylation patterns to multiple cancers. Indeed, disruption of pathways that lead to cancer is often caused by the de novo methylation of the relevant gene's promoters (Jones and Baylin 2002). Epigenetic silencing has been recognized as a third pathway satisfying Knudson's "two-hit" hypothesis for the silencing of tumor suppressor genes (Jones and Laird 1999).

Chromosomal rearrangements have long been associated with human leukemias. These result in formation of fusion proteins including histone acetyltransferases and histone methyltransferases that influence upregulation of target genes. In acute promyelocytic leukemia, the oncogenic fusion protein PML-RARα (promyelocytic leukemia-retinoic acid receptor-α) causes repression of genes that are essential for differentiation of hematopoietic cells. Similarly in acute myeloid leukemia, AML-ETO fusions recruit the repressive N-COR-Sin3-HDAC1 complex and inhibit myeloid development (Jones and Saha 2002). There are further examples of complex genomic arrangements that result in other cancers, and which can modify the therapeutic response. For example, mutations in genes for ATPase complex are associated with poorer prognosis in patients with nonsmall-cell lung cancer (Roberts and Orkin 2004).

Genetic Heterogeneity and Pleiotropy

The genetic evaluation of any disorder, phenotype, or trait requires an understanding of the fundamental principles of medical genetics. Genetic heterogeneity and pleiotropy are the two basic concepts that need to be addressed in any human genetic disorder.

Genetic heterogeneity refers to different genetic etiologies assigned to a given phenotype or a combination of phenotypes recognized as a disorder or syndrome. For example hypertrophic cardiomyopathy (HCM) and dilated cardiomyopathy (DCM) are related to mutations in several different genes (Table 3–7a and Table 3–7b). The term pleiotropy on the other hand refers to variable expressivity of a single genetic etiology, for example, a chromosomal abnormality or mutation in a single gene. However, it

Table 3–7a Genetic Heterogeneity in Hypertrophic Cardiomyopathy (Marion 2007)

Gene/Protein	Gene Symbol	Locus	Mutations%
β-myosin heavy chain	*MYH7*	14q112	35–40
Myosin binding protein C	*MYBPC3*	11p11.2	15–20
Cardiac troponin T	*TNNT2*	1q32	5–10
Cardiac troponin I	*TNNTI*	19p13.2	~5
α-Tropomyosin	*TPM1*	15q22.1	<5
Cardiac alpha actin	*ACTA*	11q	<5
Essential myosin light chain	*MYL3*	3p21.3-p21.2	<5
Regulatory myosin light chain	*MYL2*	12q23-q24.3	<5
Titin	*TTN*	2q24.3	<5
Cardiac troponin C	*TNNCI*	3p21	Rare
Telethonin (Titin cap)	*TCAP*	17q12	Rare
Cardiac myosin light peptide			
Kinase	*MYLK2*	20q13.3	Rare
α-myosin light chain	*MYH6*	14q12	Rare
Caveolin 3	CAV3	3p25	Rare
Phospholamban	*PLN*	6p22.1	Rare

Table 3–7b Genetic Heterogeneity in Dilated Cardiomyopathy (Esfandiarei et al. 2007)

Gene/Protein	Locus	Phenotype	Inheritance
Dystrophin	Xp21	Duchenne/Becker myopathy	XLR X-linked DCM
Emerin	Xq28	Emerin-Dreifuss myopathy	XLR
Tafazin	Xq28	Barth syndrome	XLR/Mt
Desmins	Various	DCM	AD
Lamins A/C	1q11-q23	Emerin-Dreifuss myopathy	AD
Lamins A/C	1p1-q21	DCM/conduction system disease	AD
Sarcoglycans			
(α,β,γ,δ)	Various	DCM/ LGMD	AD
Actin	1q11-q21	DCM/ LGMD	AD
Actin	Various	DCM/conduction system disease	AD

Abbreviations: XLR, X-linked recessive; Mt, Mitochondrial; AD, autosomal dominant; DCM, dilated cardiomyopathy; LGMD, limb girdle muscular dystrophy.

may be argued that pleiotropy would only apply to variable phenotypic manifestation associated with a specific mutation. This concept holds true when dealing with the contentious issue of genotype–phenotype correlation of a specific mutation or polymorphism. Often the term clinical heterogeneity is used to discuss variable or complex phenotypes to support the argument of different etiologies. Clinical heterogeneity is helpful in the clinical context whilst the term pleiotropy is preferable in the genetic context referring to diverse phenotypes related to a single genetic etiology, for example, firbrillin-1 gene related several clinical phenotypes (Table 3–8). Nevertheless, both the above two basic principles apply to the practice of clinical cardiovascular genetics.

Genetic heterogeneity may refer to different alleles within a gene (allelic heterogeneity) or different loci (locus heterogeneity). Mutations in the respiratory complex genes or mitochondrial regulatory genes in the nuclear DNA (nDNA) and within the mitochondrial DNA (mtDNA) would be acceptable as an example of genetic heterogeneity. It is essential that the recognition of the phenotype or clinical syndrome should be based on accepted criteria before one considers the question of genetic heterogeneity. For example, familial cardiomyopathy in itself would not be a single disorder, and thus the question of genetic heterogeneity would not have any basis. On the other hand, one could provide evidence for both locus heterogeneity and allelic heterogeneity in hypertrophic cardiomyopathy (HCM).

Locus heterogeneity is indicated by the presence of several genes at different loci coding for a number of sarcomere proteins that form the cardiac myofibril. On the other hand, several different mutations within a single gene account for the clinical phenotype of HCM (Table 3–8) (see also Chapter 13). This is also applicable for ion channelopathies manifesting with a number of different types of familial arrhythmias (see Chapter 15).

There are several examples where the principle of pleiotropy could be applied. Most of these disorders or syndromes have complex phenotypes (clinical, biochemical, electrophysiological, and radiological) involving multiple body systems. For example, disorders associated with genes encoding microfibrillin and matrix metalloproteins manifest with complex variable phenotypes. Marfan syndrome and other microfibrillopathies are good examples of pleiotropy. A number of disorders or phenotypes are associated with mutations in the *FBN1* gene (Table 3–8) (see also Chapter 11). The reader will find similar examples in other sections of this book.

Table 3–8 Spectrum of Diverse Phenotypes with FBN1 Gene Mutations (OMIM)

Clinical Phenotype	MIM	*FBN1* Mutation(s)
Marfan classic	154700	GLY1013ARG; CYS1129TYR; TYR754CYS; IVS46 + 5G-A; 33-BP INS, IVS46, G-A, + 1; IVS2DS, G-A, + 1; ARG529TER; CYS1265ARG; CYS2307SER; 366-BP DEL; TRP2756TER; CYS1249SER; CYS1663ARG; CYS2221SER; TYR2113TER, EX51DEL; TYR2113TER, EX51DEL; ASN548ILE; ASP723ALA
Severe classic		ARG1137PRO
Mild variable		GLY1127SER
Atypical neonatal		ARG122CYS; GLY985GLU CYS1074ARG; IVS31AS, A-T, -2; IVS32DS, G-A, + 1; LYS1043ARG; CYS1221TYR;
Marfanoid skeletal		ARG2726TRP
Subclinical variant		ARG1170HIS
Ectopia lentis	129600	GLU2447LYS; ARG240CYS
MASS	604308	4-BP INS, NT5138
Shprintzen-Goldberg	182212	CYS1223TYR; CYS1221TYR
Weill-Marchesani	608328	24-BP DEL

The Classification of Inherited Cardiovascular Conditions

It is not possible to accurately document all genetic cardiovascular conditions in the context of inheritance patterns. The complexity of the whole field is evident from the broad and variable phenotypic spectrum associated with chromosomal abnormalities. Similarly, the extent of etiological contribution of mutations in several genes scattered across the nuclear and the mitochondrial genomes is not currently possible. However, it is possible to estimate the prevalence of a broad range of cardiovascular disorders that are directly or indirectly associated with recognizable Mendelian diseases, traits, or loci. Some of these are relevant in the context of abnormal chromosomal phenotypes and have indirect influence on the functioning of the mitochondrial genome.

An online search of OMIM using *heart, cardiac, cardiovascular,* and *vascular* prompts brings up almost all known disorders, genes/mutations, and polymorphisms directly or indirectly linked with a cardiovascular disorder (Table 3–9). The enormity of the genetic cardiovascular disease burden can be judged by the huge numbers that amount to about half of the known human Mendelian phenotypes! Not surprisingly there is considerable overlap and repetition in these searches, as one condition may have several of the search prompts, which could give erroneous prevalence figures and an overestimate of Mendelian disorders and traits. Entries in OMIM do not cover the chromosomal disorders and some of the polygenic/multifactorial traits and disorders.

All inherited disorders of the CVS can be divided on the basis of the major anatomic or physiological components involved (Table 3–10). This should be the first step in delineating whether the condition refers to anatomic structure, an abnormality of the large or medium-sized blood vessels, structural or functional disturbance of the cardiac musculature, or an abnormality of the conduction system. The next logical approach could be to consider the possible molecular mechanism (Table 3–11a). This approach, although attractive and scientifically plausible, is less likely to be useful to the practicing clinician as it is rapidly evolving and

Table 3–9 Cardiovascular Genetic Related Entries in Victor McKusick's Mendelian Inheritance in Man (OMIM)* http://ncbi.nlm.nih.gov/sites/enterez/OMIM (Accessed July 22, 2007)

Search Prompt	Number of Entries
Heart	3,293
Cardiac	1,244
Cardiovascular	681
Vascular	950

Table 3–10 Major Clinical Categories of Inherited Cardiovascular Condition

Anatomic	Congenital heart defects - single/multiple malformation syndromes
Vascular	Congenital anomalies Functional abnormalities
Muscular	Primary cardiomyopathies Secondary cardiomyopathies
Conduction	Congenital conduction blocks Familial arrhythmias

Table 3–11a The Molecular Classification of Inherited Cardiovascular Conditions*

Genes/ Protein Family	Disorder(s) (OMIM#)
T-box genes-related	
T-Box1	Conotruncal anomaly face syndrome (217095); Velo-cardio-facial syndrome (192430); DiGeorge syndrome (188400)
T-Box3	Ulnar-mammary syndrome (181450)
T-Box5	Holt-Oram syndrome (142900)
RAS/MAPK pathway	Noonan syndrome (163950, NS1); Cardiofaciocutaneous syndrome, CFC (115150); Costello syndrome (218040); LEOPOLD syndrome (151100)
Ion channelopathies	
Sodium	Brugada syndrome, BS1, SCN5A (601144); Long QT syndrome type3, LQT3, SCN5A (603830); LQT10, SCN4B (608256)
Potassium	Long QT syndrome-1, LQT1, KCNQ1 (192500); Jervell and Lange-Nileson syndrome, KCNQ1 (220400); LQT2, KCNH2(152427); LQT5, KCNE1(176261); LQT6, KCNE2 (603796); LQT7, Anderson cardiodysrhythmic periodic paralysis, KCNJ2 (170390);
Calcium	LQT8, Timothy syndrome, CACNA1C (601005); Brugada syndrome-3, BS3, CACNA1C (611875); Brugada syndrome-4, BS4, CACNB2 (611876)
Sarcomere genes-related	Familial hypertrophic cardiomyopathy:CMH1(160760); CMH2 (115195); CMH3 (11596); CMH4 (115197); CMH6 (600858); CMH7 (191044), CMH8 (160790); CMH9 (188840); CMH10 (160781). Familial dilated cardiomyopathy: CMD1D (601494); CMD1S (160760); CMD1Y (611878);
Actin genes-related	Familial dilated cardiomyopathy, CMD: CMD1R (102540); familial atrial septal defect (160710); arterial tortuosity syndrome (208050)
Microfibrillins	
FBN1	Marfan syndrome, MF1 (154700); Ectopia lentis (129600); Shprintzen-Goldberg syndrome (182212); Weill-Marchesani syndrome (608328); MASS syndrome (604308)
FBN2	Congenital contractural arachnodacytly(121050)
Transforming growth factors-related	
TGFBR1(190181)	Loeys-Dietz syndrome, LDS1A (609192); LDS2A (608967)
TGFBR2(190182)	Loeys-Dietz syndrome, LDS1B (610168); LDS2B (610380)
Mitochondrial	Barth syndrome (302060); cataract and cardiomyopathy (212350)
Lamins-related	Familial dilated cardiomyopathy, CMD, CMD1A (115200); limb girdle muscular dystrophy, LGMD1B (159001); Emery-Dreifuss muscular dystrophy, autosomal dominant, ADEMD (181350); quadriceps myopathy with dilated cardiomyopathy (607920); lipoatrophic diabetes with hypertrophic cardiomyopathy (608056)
Dystrophin-related	Familial dilated cardiomyopathy, CMD1A (115200); CMD3B (302045); CMD1L (606685); Duchenne/Becker muscular dystrophy (310200 and 300376); nemaline type cardioneuromyopathy (606842); Bethlem myopathy (158810); limb girdle muscular dystrophy, LGMD2E(604286);
Desmin-related	Familial restrictive cardiomyopathy (609578); arrhythmogenic right ventricular cardiomyopathy/dysplasia, ARVC/ARVD, type 7 (609160); type 8 (607450);
Collagen genes-related	Ehler-Danlos syndrome type 4, EDSIV (130050)

*Based on entries in OMIM accessed on May 31, 2008.

numerous additions and deletions are made with fast turnover of research outcomes. A pragmatic approach would be to attempt categorizing as either primary or secondary dependent upon the pathogenesis (Table 3–12). In addition, several inherited metabolic conditions manifest with recognizable cardiac phenotypes, notably cardiomyopathy (Table 3–11b; see also Chapters 26 and 31.). However, this approach may be problematic as there are several multisystem inherited conditions with a significant CVS manifestation. This approach to categorizing inherited disorders of the CVS is probably a convenient method that might be acceptable to clinicians across all disciplines. The majority of the genetic (or possibly genetic) cardiovascular conditions are listed in OMIM with an assigned number. In this chapter, OMIM numbers are used (Table 3–12) to enable the reader to refer to this indispensable database. Nevertheless there is clearly a need for a dedicated database with classified information on all inherited cardiovascular conditions listing cardiovascular phenotypes, proteins, genes, loci, traits, and polymorphic variants.

Table 3–11b Inherited Metabolic Diseases Presenting with Cardiomyopathy (Clarke 2002)

Metabolic Disease	OMIM#	Major Clinical Features
Glycogen metabolism disorders		
Pompe disease (GSD II)	232300	Profound skeletal myopathy, early death
GSD IV (debrancher enzyme deficiency)	232500	Hepatomegaly and variable hypoglycemia
GSD VI (brancher enzyme deficiency)	232700	Mild hepatic involvement
Phosphorylase b kinase deficiency	261750	Predominantly cardiomyopathy
Triosephosphate isomerase deficiency	190450	Chronic hemolytic anemia, progressive dystonia, and spasticity; early death
Disorders of fatty acid metabolism		
Systemic carnitine deficiency	212140	Skeletal myopathy, Reye-like acute encephalopathy
LCAD deficiency	609016	Skeletal myopathy, exercise induced myoglobinuria, and Reye-like acute encephalopathy
Carnitine-acylcarnitine translocase deficiency	212138	Hepatomegaly, hepatocellular dysfunction, hyperammonemia, hypotonia, and early onset encephalopathy
Organic acidopathies		
Propionic academia	606054	Metabolic acidosis, ketosis, hyperammonemia, neutropenia
Methylmalonic academia	251000	-As above-
HMG-CoA lyase deficiency	246450	-As above-
B-ketothiolase deficiency	203750	Intermittent metabolic acidosis
(α-Methylacetoacetic aciduria)	203750 607809	Metabolic acidosis and ketosis Clinically 'ketotic hyperglycinemia syndrome'
Glutaric aciduria type II (multiple acyl-CoA dehydrogenase deficiency)	231680	Facial dysmorphism, multiple malformations, hepatomegaly, nonketotic hypoglycemia, metabolic acidosis, and hyperammoneima
Amino acidopathies		
Hepatorenal tyrosinemia	276700	Acute hepatocellular dysfunction, hypoglycemia, renal tubular acidosis, pophyria
Alkaptonuria	203500	Dark urine, calcification of cartilage, arthritis
Homocystinuria	236200	Marfanoid habitus, psychomotor retardation, lens dislocation, thromboembolic episodes
Mitochondrial cardiomyopathies		
Kearns-Sayre syndrome	530000	PEO, retinal degeneration, cerebellar ataxia, growth failure, sensorineural hearing loss
Lethal infantile encephalopathy	232500- Glycogen storage disease IV (Hepatic form) 24510 - Fatal infantile lactic acidosis 252010 Mitochondrial complex deficiency (see OMIM for more conditions with similar clinical phenotype)]	WPW and other cardiac dysrhythmias; early death
Leigh disease	256000 (AutRec)	
Subacute necrotizing encephalomyelopathy	308930 (X-linked)	Psychomotor retardation, seizures, failure to thrive, lactic acidosis, and oculomotor dysfunction
Hypertrophic cardiomyopathy and myopathy	611705	Skeletal myopathy, diabetes mellitus, cataracts, cardiac dysrhythmias

(Continued)

Table 3–11b (Continued)

Metabolic Disease	OMIM#	Major Clinical Features
Barth syndrome	302060	Skeletal myopathy, chronic neutropenia and 3-methylglutonic academia
Benign infantile mitochondrial myopathy and cardiomyopathy	500000	Hypotonia, respiratory failure, severe lactic acidosis, variable course cardiomyopathy
MELAS	540000	Psychomotor retardation, growth failure, seizures, stroke-like episodes with lactic acidosis
MERRF	545000	Cerebellar ataxia, skeletal myopathy, psychomotor retardation, myoclonus, and seizures
Lysosomal storage disorders		
Fabry disease	301500	Recurrent neuritic pain (hands and feet), angiokerotomas, corneal opacities, progressive renal failure, left ventricular hypertrophy, cardiac dysrhythmias, and early cerebrovascular disease
Hurler disease (MPS IH)	607014	Facial dysmorphism, hepatosplenomegaly, dysostosis multiplex, progressive psychomotor retardation, corneal clouding, and urinary glycosylaminoglycans (GAGs)
Hunter disease (MPS II)	309900	Facial dysmorphism, hepatosplenomegaly, dysostosis multiplex, progressive psychomotor retardation, and urinary glycosylaminoglycans (GAGs)
Maroteaux-Lamy disease (MPS VI)	253200	Short stature, dysostosis multiplex, corneal clouding, normal intelligence, and urinary GAGs
GM1 gangliosidosis		Facial dysmorphism, hepatosplenomegaly, variable dysostosis multiplex, oligoacchariduria
Type1	230500	
Type2	230600	
GM2 gangliosidosis	230700	Chronic progressive encephalopathy, seizures, cherry-red retinal spots, and blindness
Gaucher disease (type 1)	230800	Hepatosplenomegaly, anemia, thrombocytopenia, and bone crises
Niemann-Pick disease (type A)	257200	Hepatosplenomegaly and chronic progressive encephalopathy
I-cell disease (Leroy disease) (neuraminidase deficiency)	256550	Hurler-like appearance, hepatosplenomegaly, and dysostosis multiplex
Juvenile neuronal ceroid lipofuscinosis	204200	Psychomotor retardation, seizures, progressive visual impairment

Table 3–12 The Clinical Classification of Inherited Cardiovascular Conditions

1. Primary	Familial congenital heart defects
	Atrioventricular septal defect 2, AVSD2 (606217)
	Atrioventricular septal defect, AVSD; atrioventricular canal defect, AVCD (600309)
	Coarctation of aorta (120000)
	Conotruncal heart malformations, CTHM (217095)
	Endocardial fibroelastosis, autosomal recessive (226000)
	Endocardial fibroelastosis, X-linked (305300)
	Epstein anomaly (224700)
	Familial anomalous origin of right pulmonary artery and other anatomic cardiac anomalies (610338)
	Familial aortic valve disease (109730)
	Familial atrial septal defect (108800)
	Familial heart malformation (234750)
	Familial mitral valve prolapse, MVP (157700)
	Familial patent ductus arteriosus (169100)
	Familial pulmonary stenosis (265500)
	Familial supravalvular aortic stenosis (185500)
	Hypoplastic left heart syndrome (241550)
	Isolated situs inversus (270100)
	Marfanoid habitus with situs inversus (609008)
	Noncompaction of left ventricular myocardium with congenital heart defects (606617)
	Pulmonary atresia with intact interventricular septum (265150)
	Pulmonic stenosis, atrial septal defect, and unique electrocardiographic abnormalities (178650)
	Secondum atrial septal defects with other cardiac and noncardiac defects (603642)

Supravalvular aortic stenosis (185500)
Tricuspid atresia (605067)
X-linked Cardiac valvular dysplasia, CVD1 (314400)

Familial cardiomyopathies

Hypertrophic cardiomyopathy, familial, CMH, (192600)
type 8, CMH8 (608751)
type 10, CMH10 (608758)
with Wolff-Parkinson-White syndrome (600858)

Dilated cardiomyopathy, DCM,
type 1A, CMD1A (115200)
type IB, CMD1B (600884)
type 1D, CMD1D (601494)
type1F, CMD1F (602067)
type 1G, CMD1G (604145)
type 1J, CMD1J (605362)
type 1M, CMD1M (607482)
type 1O, CMD1O (608569)
type IP, CMD1P (609909)
autosomal recessive type (212110)

Arrhythmogenic right ventricular cardiomyopathy, ARVC (107970)

Arrhythmogenic right ventricular dysplasia, Familial, ARVD
type I, ARVD1 (107970)
type II, ARVD2 (600996)
type III, ARVD3 (602086)
type IV, ARVD4 (602087)
type VI, ARVD6 (604401)
type VIII, ARVD8 (607450)
type IX, ARVD9 (609040)
type X, ARVD10 (610193)
type XI, ARVD11 (610476)

Naxos disease (601214)
Left ventricular noncompaction type (605906)
Restrictive cardiomyopathy, RCM (115210)
Cardiomyopathy with cataract (212350)

Familial arrhythmias

Anderson cardiodysrhythmic periodic paralysis (170390)
Atrial septal defect with atrioventricular conduction defects (108900)
Atrial tachyarrhythmia with short PR interval (108950)
Brugada syndrome (601144)
Cardiac conduction defect, SCD (115080)
Catecholaminergic polymorphic ventricular tachycardia, CPVT (604772)
Congenital heart block (234700)
Familial atrial fibrillation (163800)
Familial atrial fibrillation, ATFB1 (607554); ATFB2 (608583)
Familial heart block type 1 (113900)
Familial heart block type 2 (140400)
Familial ventricular tachycardia (192605)
Familial Wolff-Parkinson-White, WPW (194200)
Jervell and Lange-Nielson syndrome, JLNS1 (220400)
Long QT syndrome LQT (192500)
Long QT syndrome 3, LQT3 (603830)
Progressive familial heart block type I, PFHBI (113900)
Progressive familial heart block type II, PFHBII (140400)
Short QT syndrome (609620)
Sick sinus syndrome with bradycardia, LQT4 (600919)
Sick sinus syndrome, autosomal dominant (163800)
Sick sinus syndrome, autosomal recessive (608567)

Familial vascular disorders

Arterial tortuosity syndrome (208050)
Cerebral autosomal dominant arteriopathy with subcortical infarcts and leukoencephalopathy, CADASIL (125310)
Cerebral autosomal recessive arteriopathy with subcortical infarcts and leukoencephalopathy, CARASIL, Maeda syndrome (600142)
Cerebral hemorrhage with amyloidosis, hereditary, Dutch type, HCHWAD (609065)
Aortic aneurysm, abdominal, dissection (100070)

(Continued)

Table 3–12 (Continued)

	Aortic aneurysm, familial thoracic 1 (607086)
	Aortic aneurysm, familial thoracic 4 (132900)
	Ischemic stroke (601367)
	Total anomalous pulmonary venous return 1, TAPVR1 (106700)
	Transposition of great arteries, dextro-looped, DLGA (608808)
	X-linked visceral heterotaxy; X-linked transposition of great arteries (306955)
	Familial cardiac tumors
	Familial myxoma syndrome (see Carney complex)
	Carney complex, CNC1 (160980)
	Familial myxoma, intracardiac (255960)
	Paraganglionoma, PGL1 (168000)
	Primary systemic hypertension
	Glucocorticoid-remediable aldosteronism (GRA, 103900)
	Apparent mineralocorticoid excess (AME, 207765)
	Primary aldosteronism (Liddle's, 177200)
	Familial pheochromocytoma (171300)
	Essential hypertension (145500)
	Early onset hypertension, autosomal dominant with severe exacerbation in pregnancy (605115)
	Pulmonary arterial hypertension
	Primary pulmonary hypertension, PPH1 (178600)
	Secondary pulmonary hypertension
	Hereditary hemorrhagic teleangiectasia, HHT, Osler-Rendu-Weber disease (187300; 600376)
	Familial coronary artery disease
	Familial coronary artery disease, ADCAD1 (608320)
	Familial hypercholesterolemia, FH (143890)
	Familial combined hyperlipidemia, FCHL (144250)
	Familial defective apolipoprotein B100 (FDB, 107730)
	Coronary heart disease, susceptibility to (300464, 608316,608901, 607339, 608318, 610938)
	Apolipoprotein (a), LPA (152200)
	Apolipoprotein B, ApoB (107730)
	Apolipoprotein E, ApoE (107741)
	Familial hyperhomocystinemia (603174, 607093)
	Homocystinemia (603174)
	Earlobe disease (128950)
	Cerebrotendinous xanthomatosis (213700)
	Metabolic syndrome (605552)
	Familial hypertriglyceridemia (145750)
	Autosomal recessive hypercholesterolemia, ARH (603813)
	Primary cardiac metabolic disorders
	Familial cardiac lipidosis (212080)
	Danon disease (300257)
2. Secondary	Familial connective tissue disorders
	Marfan syndrome I, MFSI (154700)
	Marfan syndrome II, MFSII (154705)
	Marfanoid hypermobility syndrome (154750)
	Ehlers-Danlos syndrome
	type I, EDSI (130000)
	type II, EDSII (130010)
	type III, EDS (130020)
	type IV, EDSIV, vascular form (130050)
	type VI, EDSVI (225400)
	autosomal recessive cardiac valvular form (225320)
	with platelet dysfunction from fibronectin abnormality (225310)
	Beals congenital contractural arachnodactyly (121050)
	Loeys-Dietz syndrome, LDS (609192)
	Pseudoxanthoma elasticum (PXE) (264800)
	Aplasia cutis congenital (107600)
	X-linked dilated cardiomyopathy
	Duchenne/Becker myopathy, DMD/BMD (310200, 302045)
	Emery-Dreiffus muscular dystrophy, X-linked EDMD (310300)
	Barth syndrome (302060)
	Dilated cardiomyopathy with Triplet Repeat syndromes
	Dentato-Rubro-Pallidoluysian atrophy, DRPLA (125370)
	Fragile X syndrome; FRAXA (300624; 309550)

Fragile XE syndrome, FRAXE (309548)
Friedreich's ataxia, FRDA (229300, 601992)
Huntington disease (143100)
Kennedy's disease (313200)
Myotonic dystrophy (160900)
Spinocerebellar ataxia type 1, SCA1 (164400)

Cardiomyopathy in other primary myopathies
Bethlem myopathy (158810)
Cardiomyopathy with hyaline masses and nemaline rods (606842)
Cardiomyopathy with quadriceps myopathy (607904)
Cardiomyopathy with woolly hair and keratoderma (606676)
Central core disease
Centronuclear myopathy, autosomal recessive (255200)
Congenital fiber type disproportion, CFTD
type 1, CFTD1, autosomal recessive (255310)
type 2, CFTD2, X-linked (300580)
Congenital muscular dystrophy IC, MDC1C (606612)
Distal myopathy 1, MPD1 (160500)
Emery-Dreifuss muscular dystrophy, autosomal dominant type, EDMD2 (181350)
Facioscapulohumeral muscular dystrophy 1A, FSHMD1A (158900)
Fukuyama congenital muscular dystrophy, FCMD (253800)
Inclusion body myopathy with early onset Paget disease and frontotemporal dementia (167320)
Infantile autophagic vacuolar myopathy (609500)
Limb girdle muscular dystrophy, LGMD
type 1B, LGMD1B (159001)
type 2C, LGMD2C (253700)
type 2B, LGMD2B (253601)
type 2D, LGMD2D (608099)
type 2E, LGMD2E (604286)
type 2G, LGMD2G (601954)
type 2I, LGMD2I (607155)
type 2J, LGMD2J (608807)
Muscular dystrophy, cardiac type, X-linked (309930)
Myofibrillar myopathy, desmin related (601419)
Myofibrillar myopathy, ZASP related (609452)
Myopathy with excessive autophagy, X-linked, MEAX (310440)
Myopathy, mysosin storage (608358)
Myotilinopathy (609200)
Progressive pecto-dorsal muscular dystrophy (310095)

Cardiac manifestation in other genetic neurological disorders
Alpha-thalassemia/mental retardation syndrome, ATR-X, X-linked (301040)
Charcot-Marie-Tooth disease with ptosis and Parkinsonism (118301)
Charcot-Marie-Tooth disease, demyelinating type 1B, CMT1B (118200)
Charcot-Marie-Tooth disease, Guadalajara neuronal type (118230)
Charcot-Marie-Tooth peroneal muscular atrophy and Friedreich ataxia combined, X-linked (302900)
Dystrophia myotonica DM2 (602668)
Dystrophia myotonica, DM1 (160900)
Fragile X mental retardation syndrome, FRAXA, X-linked (300624)
Friedreich ataxia with congenital glaucoma (229310)
Hereditary sensory and autonomic neuropathy III (223900)
Malignant hyperthermia, MHS1, King-Denborough syndrome (145600)
Mental retardation, febrile seizures, keratoconus and sinoatrial block (609438)
Mental retardation, X-linked with Marfanoid habitus, Lujan-Fryns syndrome (309520)
Myoclonic epilepsy of Lafora, EPM2B (24780)
Periventricular heterotopia, X-linked (300049)
Progressive external ophthalmoplegia with mitochondrial DNA deletions, autosomal recessive (258450)
Progressive external ophthalmoplegia with mitochondrial DNA deletions, autosomal dominant (609283)
Sensory ataxic neuropathy, dysarthria, and ophthalmoparesis (607459)
Spinal muscular atrophy type 1, SMA1 (253300)
Stiff-person syndrome, SPS including progressive encephalomyelitis with rigidity (PERM) (184850)

Cardiac manifestations in phakomatoses
Neurofibromatosis type 1 (162200)
Tuberous sclerosis, TS (191100)

Chronic pulmonary diseases
Cystic fibrosis, CF (219700)
Primary ciliary dyskinesis (??)

(Continued)

Table 3–12 (Continued)

	Chronic renal disease
	Adult onset polycystic kidney disease 1, APKD, PKD1 (173900)
	Autosomal recessive polycystic kidney disease, ARPKD (263200)
	Barter syndrome (601678)
	Denys-Drash syndrome (194080)
	Nephrogenic syndrome of inappropriate diuresis, NSIAD (300539)
	Nephronopthisis 2, NPHP2 (602088)
	Polycystic kidney disease 2, PKD2 (173910)
	Hematological disorders
	Asplenia with cardiovascular anomalies (208530)
	Benign familial thrombocytosis (601977)
	Diamond-Blackfan anemia, DBA (105650)
	Familial atransferrinemia/hypotransferrinemia (209300)
	Fanconi anemia, FA (227650)
	Glucose-6-phosphate dehydrogenase deficiency, G6PD (305900)
	Hemochromatosis, HFE (235200)
	Hemophilia A (306700)
	Hermansky-Pudlak syndrome (203300)
	Idiopathic hypereosinophilic syndrome, HES (607685)
	Juvenile hemochromatosis, JH (602390)
	Multiple coagulation factor deficiency, pseudoxanthoma elasticum like (610842)
	Neonatal hemochromatosis (231100)
	Primary amyloidosis
	Primary polycythaemia vera (263300)
	Sideroblastic anemia, X-linked (301300)
	Thalassemias
	Thiamine responsive megaloblastic anemia (249270)
	Thrombocytosis, X-linked (300331)
	Thrombocytopenia-absent radius syndrome, TAR (274000)
3. Multisystem	Chromosomal syndromes
	Aneuploidies
	Cat eye syndrome, CES (115470)
	Down/trisomy 21 (190685; 602917)
	Edward/trisomy 18/trisomy 18 like syndrome (601161)
	Patau/trisomy 13, pseudotrisomy 13 syndrome (264480)
	Turner syndrome (45X, IsoXq, Xpring, Xpdel etc.)
	Microdeletions/microduplications
	18q deletion syndrome (601808)
	Di George/ 22 q deletion syndrome (188400; 601279)
	Miller-Dieker lissenchephaly, MDLS (247200)
	Monosomy 1p36 syndrome (607872)
	Smith-Magenis syndrome, SMS (182290)
	Williams-Beuren syndrome (194050)
	9q subtelomeric deletion syndrome (610253)
	10q microdeletion syndrome (609625)
	Other chromosomal disorders
	Emanuel syndrome, supernumerary der (22) syndrome
	Pallister-Killian syndrome, tetrasomy 12p (601803)
	Multiple malformation syndromes
	Acrocallosal syndrome 1, ACLS1 (200990)
	Acrofacial dysostosis 1, Nager type, AFD1 (154400)
	Adams-Oliver syndrome (100300)
	Agenesis of corpus callosum with facial anomalies and Robin sequence (217980)
	Alagille syndrome (118450; 610205)
	Alstrom syndrome, ALMS (203800)
	Ankyloblepharon-ectrodactyly-cleft lip/palate (106260)
	Antley-Bixler syndrome, ABS (207410)
	Apert type acrocephalosyndactyly (101200)
	Aplasia cutis congenital with coarctation of aorta, ACCCA (107601)
	Arthrogryposis multiplex congenita, neurogenic type, AMCN (208100)
	Atrioventricular septal defect with Dandy-Walker malformation (220210)
	Atrioventricular septal defect with blepharophimosis and anal and radial defects (600123)
	Aurocephalosyndactyly (109050)
	Baller-Gerold syndrome, BGS (218600)
	Bardet-Biedl syndrome, BBS (209900)

Basal cell nevus syndrome, BCNS, Gorlin syndrome (109400)
Beckwith-Wiedemann syndrome, BWS (130650)
Borrone dermatocardioskeletal syndrome (211170)
Bowen multiple malformation syndrome (211200)
Burn-McKeown syndrome (608572)
C syndrome (211750)
Camptomelic dysplasia (114290)
Cardiac defect, cleft palate, genital anomalies, and ectrodactyly (600460)
Cardiac malformation, cleft lip/palate, microcephaly, and digital anomalies (600987)
Cardiofaciocutaneous syndrome, CFC (115150)
Cardiogenital syndrome (212120)
Cardiomyopathy, hypogonadism, and collagenoma syndrome (115250)
Cardioskeletal syndrome, Kuwaiti type (212135)
Carpenter syndrome (201000)
Catel-Manzke syndrome (302380)
Cayler cardiofacial syndrome (125520)
Cerebrocostomandibular syndrome (117650)
Cerebrofaciothoracic dysplasia (213980)
Char syndrome (169100)
CHARGE syndrome (214800)
Chondrodysplasia punctata syndrome (215015)
Cleft-Limb-Heart malformation syndrome (215850)
Cleidocranial dysplasia with micrognathia, absent thumbs and distal aphlanagia, and congenital heart defects (216340)
Cockayne syndrome, type A, CSA (216400)
Coffin-Lowry syndrome (303600)
Coffin-Siris syndrome (135900)
Cohen syndrome, COH1 (216550)
Congenital anomalies of the heart and peripheral vasculature with distichiasis (126320)
Congenital dislocation of hip, congenital heart defects, hyperextensibility of fingers, facial dysmorphism (601450)
Congenital heart defect, ectrodactyly of lower limbs and micrognathia (601348)
Congenital heart defects, hamartomas of tongue and polysyndactyly (217085)
Congenital heart defects, Hirschprung disease, laryngeal
anomalies and preaxial syndactyly (604211)
Congenital heart defects, hypertelorism, microtia and facial clefting syndrome (239800)
Congenital heart defects, thumb agenesis, short stature, and immune deficiency (274190)
Congenital heart disease, blepharophimosis, blepharoptosis, hypoplastic teeth, and mental retardation (249620)
Congenital heart disease, congenital pancreatic hypoplasia with diabetes mellitus (600001)
Congenital heart disease, craniofacial anomalies, cataracts, sacral neural tube defect, and growth and developmental retardation (608227)
Congenital heart disease, microcephaly, unilateral renal agenesis, and hyposegmented lungs (249620)
Congenital heart disease, sagittal craniostenosis, mandibular ankylsos, and mental deficiency (218450)
Congenital hemidysplasia with icthyosiform erythroderma and limb defects, X-linked (308050)
Cornelia de Lange syndrome, CDLS1 (122470)
Costello syndrome (218040)
Cranioectodermal dysplasia (218330)
Craniofacial dysmorphism with ocular coloboma, absent corpus callosum, and aortic dilatation (218340)
Dandy-Walker syndrome, DWS (220200)
Diastrophic dysplasia (222600)
Donnai-Barrow syndrome (222448)
Duane-Radial ray syndrome, DRRS (607323)
Ellis-van Creveld syndrome, EVC (225500)
Faciocardiomelic dysplasia, lethal (227270)
Faciocardiorenal syndrome (227280)
Faciogenital dysplasia (305400)
Fallot's complex with severe growth and mental retardation (601127)
FATCO (fibular aplasia, tibial camptomelia, congenital heart defect, oligosyndactyly) syndrome (246570)
Fibrochondrogenesis (228520)
Frank-Ter Haar syndrome, Melnick-Needles (249420)
Frontometaphyseal dysplasia, FMD, X-linked (305620)
Frontonasal dysplasia (136760)
Fronto-ocular syndrome (605321)
Fryns syndrome (229850)
Geleophysic dysplasia (231050)

(Continued)

Table 3–12 (Continued)

	Genito-patellar syndrome (606170)
	GOMBO (growth retardation, ocular abnormalities, microcephaly, brachydactyly, and oligophrenia) syndrome (233270)
	Gorlin syndrome
	Hallermann-Streiff syndrome (234100)
	Heart-Hand syndrome, Slovenian type (610140); Spanish type (140450)
	Hemifacial microsomia, HFM (164210)
	Hennekam lymphangiestasia-lymphedema syndrome (235510)
	Holt-Oram syndrome (142900)
	Holtzgreve syndrome (236110)
	Humerospinal dysostosis (143095)
	Hutchinson-Gilford progeria syndrome, HGPS (176670)
	Hydrolethalus syndrome 1 (236680)
	Hypergonadotrophic hypogonadism with congestive cardiomyopathy (212112)
	Hypertrichotic osteochondrodysplasia (239850)
	Hypogonadism, alopecia, diabetes mellitus, mental retardation, and extrapyramidal syndrome (241080)
	Immunodeficiency with cleft lip/palate, hypopigmentation, and absent corpus callosum (242840)
	Incontinentia pigmenti, IP (308300)
	Iris coloboma with ptosis, hypertelorism, and mental retardation (243310)
	Isoretinoin embryopathy-like syndrome (243440)
	Jacobsen syndrome, JBS (147791)
	Johanson-Blizzard syndrome (243800)
	Johnson neuroectodermal syndrome (147770)
	Kabuki syndrome (147920)
	Kallmann syndrome, X-linked, KAL1 (308700); autosomal dominant, KAL2 (147950)
	Kapur-Toriello syndrome (244300)
	Kartagener syndrome (24400)
	Keutel syndrome (245150)
	Klippel-Feil syndrome, autosomal recessive (214300)
	Klippel-Trenaunay-Weber syndrome (149000)
	Knobloch syndrome, type II (608454)
	Larsen syndrome, autosomal dominant (150250)
	Larsen syndrome, autosomal recessive (245600)
	LEOPARD syndrome (151100)
	Lethal congenital heart disease, cleft lip/palate with characteristic facies, and intestinal malrotation (601165)
	Lowry-Maclean syndrome (600252)
	Lymphedema-Distichiasis syndrome (153400)
	Lymphedema-hypoparathyroidism syndrome (247410)
	Marden-Walker syndrome (248700)
	Marshall-Smith syndrome (602535)
	Marstolf syndrome (212720)
	McDonough syndrome (248950)
	McKusick-Kaufman syndrome, MKKS (236700)
	Meckel syndrome type 1, MKS1 (249100)
	Melnick-Needles syndrome, MNS (309350)
	Mesoaxial hexadactyly with cardiac malformation (249670)
	Microgastrial-limb reduction defects, MLRD (156810)
	MOHR syndrome (252100)
	Mowat-Wilson syndrome (235730)
	Mulberry nanism (253250)
	Multiple pterygium syndrome, Escobar variant (265000)
	Multiple pterygium syndrome, lethal type (253290)
	Multiple pterygium syndrome, X-linked (312150)
	Nasodigitoacoustic syndrome (255980)
	Neonatal progeroid syndrome (264090)
	Neu-Laxova syndrome, NLS (256520)
	Neurofaciodigitorenal syndrome (256690)
	Noonan syndrome (163950)
	Oculocerebral syndrome with hypopigmentation (257800)
	Opitz syndrome (300000)
	Oro-facial-digital syndrome 1, OFD1 (311200)
	Osteodysplastic primordial dwarfism, type 1 (210710)
	Osteogenesis imperfecta, type IIA (166210)
	Osteopathia strata with cranial sclerosis, OSCS (300373)

Oto-palato-digital syndrome II, OPDII (304120)
Pallister-Hall syndrome, PHS (146510)
Patent ductus arteriosus and bicuspid aortic valve with hand anomalies (604381)
Persistence of Mullerian derivatives with postaxial polydactyly and lymphangiectasia (235255)
Peters-plus syndrome (261540)
PHACES syndrome—posterior fossa brain malformations, hemangiomas of the face (large or complex), arterial anomalies, cardiac anomalies, eye abnormalities, sternal clefting, and supraumbilical raphe (606519)
Phocomelia-ectrodactyly-earmalformation-deafness-sinus arrhythmia (171480)
Poland syndrome (172800)
Postaxial polydactyly with dental and vertebral anomalies (263540)
Potter-type polycystic kidney disease with microbrachycephaly, hypertelorism, and brachymelia (263210)
Pottocki-Lupski syndrome (610883)
Progeria with hand and cardiac anomalies (602249)
Progressive occlusive disease with hypertension, heart defects, bone fragility, and brachysyndactyly (602531)
Proteus syndrome (176920)
Renal hamartomas, neuroblastomatosis, and fetal gigantism (267000)
Rett syndrome (312750)
Rieger syndrome type 2, RIEG2 (601499)
Roberts syndrome, RBS (268300)
Robinow syndrome, autosomal dominant (180700)
Robinow syndrome, autosomal recessive (268310)
Roifman syndrome- spondyloepiphyseal dysplasia, retinal dystrophy, and antibody deficiency (300258)
Runinstein-Taybi syndrome, RSTS (180849)
Saethre-Chotzen syndrome, SCS (101400)
SC Phocomelia syndrome (269000)
Schinzel-Giedion midface-retraction syndrome (269150)
Scimitar anomaly-multiple cardiac malformations, craniofacial and central nervous system abnormalities (608281)
Short rib-polydactyly syndrome type III (263510)
Shprintzen-Goldberg craniosynostosis syndrome (182212)
Shwachman-Diamond syndrome, SDS (260400)
Silver-Russel syndrome, SRS (180860)
Simpson-Golabi-Behmel syndrome type 1, SGBS1 (312870)
Situs inversus viscerum (270100)
Skeletal dysplasia with progressive central nervous system degeneration, lethal (602613)
Skin fragility-Wooly hair syndrome (607655)
Smith-Lemli-Optiz syndrome, SLOS (270400)
Sonoda syndrome (270460)
Sotos syndrome (117550)
Spondylocostal dysostosis with anal atresia and urogenital anomalies (271520)
Spondylocostal dysostosis, autosomal recessive, SCOD1 (277300)
Spondyloepimetaphyseal dysplasia with joint laxity, SEMDJL (271640)
Spondylometaphyseal dysplasia, Sedaghatian type (250220)
Steinfeld syndrome (184705)
Stickler syndrome (108300)
Subaortic stenosis- short stature syndrome (271960)
Sudden infant death with dysgenesis of testis, SIDDT (608800)
Tetra-amelia, autosomal recessive (273395)
Thoracoabdominal syndrome, THAS, X-linked (313850)
Thoracopelvic dysostosis (187770)
Townes-Brock syndrome, TBS (107480)
Trigonocephaly with short stature and developmental delay (314320)
Ulnar/fibular ray defect, brachydactyly, and cardiac anomalies (608571)
Uruguay faciocardiomusculoskeletal syndrome (300280)
VACTERL association with hydrocephalus (276950)
Valvular heart lesions, ptosis, and disproportionate short stature (126190)
Varadi-Papp syndrome (277170)
VATER/VACTERL association (192350)
Velo-cardio-facial syndrome (192430) (see DiGeorge/ 22q deletion syndrome, 188400)
Watson syndrome (193520)
Weill-Marchesani syndrome, autosomal dominant (608328)
Weil-Marchesani syndrome, autosomal recessive (277600)

(*Continued*)

- Werner syndrome, WRN (277700)
- Wolf-Hirschhorn syndrome, WHS (194190)
- Wolfram syndrome (222300)
- Xeroderma pigementosum (278760)
- Young-Simpson syndrome (60736)
- Zimmermann-Laband syndrome, ZLS (135500)
- Zunich neuroectodermal syndrome (280000)

Mitochondrial genetic disorders
- Cyclic vomiting syndrome, CVS (500007)
- Leber hereditary optic neuropathy (535000)
- Mitochondrial myopathy, lethal infantile, LIMM (551000)
- Myoclonic epilepsy with lactic acidosis and stroke, MELAS (540000)
- Kearn-Sayers syndrome, KSS (530000)
- Mitochondrial complex deficiency (124000)

Metabolic diseases
- 3-αhydroxyacyl-CoA dehydrogenase deficiency (231530)
- Acyl-CoA dehydrogenase deficiency, medium chain, MCAD (201450)
- Acyl-CoA dehydrogenase deficiency, short chain, SCAD (201470)
- Acyl-CoA dehydrogenase deficiency, very long chain (201475, 201460)
- Alkaptonuria (203500)
- Aminoadipic aciduria (204750)
- Aromatic L-aminoacid decarboxylase deficiency (608643)
- Aspartylglucosaminuria, aspartylglucodaminidase, AGA (208400)
- Cardiac lipidosis, familial (212080)
- Carnitine palmitoyl transferase I deficiency (255120)
- Carnitine palmitoyl transferase II deficiency, lethal neonatal (608836); Infantile (600649)
- Cerebrohepatorenal syndrome, variant types (214110)
- Combined oxidative phosphorylation deficiency (610505; 610498)
- Congenital adrenal hyperplasia, CAH, 21-hydroxylase deficiency (201910)
- Congenital disorder of glycosylation, CDG
  - type 1K, CDG1K (608540)
  - type2F, CDG2F (603585)
- Congenital generalized lipodystrophy type2, CGL2 (269700)
- Dopamine hydroxylase deficiency, congenital (223360)
- Fabry disease (301500)
- Fatal infantile cardioencephalopathy due to cytochrome c oxidase deficiency (604517)
- Fucosidosis, alpha-L fucosidase 1 (230000)
- Gaucher disease type IIIC (231005)
- Gaucher disease, lethal perinatal (608013)
- Glycogen storage disease, GSD
  - GSD I (232200)
  - GSD IB (232220)
  - GSDII, Pompe's disease (232300)
  - GSD III/ GSD IIIa (232400)
  - GSD IV, classic hepatic type (232500)
  - GSD VI (232700)
- Hartnup disorder (234500)
- Homocystinuria (236200)
- Homocystinuria due to deficiency of MTHFR (236250)
- Infantile sialic storage disorder (269920)
- Lethal congenital glycogen storage disease of heart (261740)
- Lipodystrophy, partial familial (608600)
- Malonyl-CoA decarboxylase deficiency (248360)
- Mannosidosis, alpha B, Lysosomal (248500)
- Menkes disease (309400)
- Methylmalonic aciduria due to methylmalonic-CoA mutase deficiency (251000)
- Mitochondrial complex I deficiency (252010)
- Mitochondrial complex II deficiency (252011)
- Mitochondrial complex III deficiency (124000)
- Mitochondrial complex IV deficiency (220110)
- Mucopolysaccharidoses, MPS
- MPS I, Hurler syndrome (607014)
  - MPS I, Hurler-Sheie syndrome (607015)
  - MPSII, Hunter syndrome (309900)
  - MPS IIIA (252900)
  - MPS IIIB (252920)

MPS IIIC (252930)
MPS IIID (252940)
MPS IVA, galactosamine-6-sulfate sulfatase, GALNS (253000)
MPS IVB (253010)
MPSVI, arylsulfatase B, ARSB (253200)
MPSVII, beta-glucuronidase, GUSB (253220)
Mucolipidosis II (252500)
Mucolipidosis IIIA (252600)
Mucolipidosis type IIIA (252600)
Multiple acyl-CoA dehydrogenase deficiency, MADD (231680)
Multiple sulfatase deficiency (272200)
Ornithine transcarbamylase deficiency, OCT (311250)
Peroxisomal disorders
Phenylketonuria (261600)
Phosphoribosylpyrophosphate synthetase, PRPSI (311850);PRPS II (311860)
Porphyrias
Coproporphyria (121300)
Porphyria variegata (176200)
Porphyria, acute intermittent type (176000)
Primary carnitine deficiency, systemic (212140)
Primary hyperoxaluria type 1 (259900)
Propionic academia (606054)
Pyruvate decarobxylase deficiency (312170)
Refsum disease (266500)
Sandhoff disease, adult type (268800)
Tangier disease (205400)
type 1a, CDGIa (212065)
type 1M, CDG1M (610768)
type IIa, CDG2A (212066)
type IIf, CDH2F (603585)
type Ik, CDG1K (608540)
Tyrosinemia type 1 (276700)
Unclassified MPS types (252700)
Wilson disease (277900)
Zellweger syndrome, ZS (214100)

Summary

This chapter introduces fundamental aspects of inheritance patterns. A busy clinician without genetic knowledge may find this helpful in understanding the likely genetic mechanism and/or inheritance pattern. This is supported by several examples and illustrations that are in general generic, although some examples are unrelated to CVS. The reader will find introduction to both molecular and clinical approaches to classifying inherited cardiovascular conditions. Both approaches are valid but with practical limitations. A busy clinical cardiologist may prefer to rely on the clinical approach whilst a molecular cardiologist, clinical geneticist, and molecular geneticist would likely go along the molecular route. Several other medical specialist practices have slowly adopted the molecular approach as this helps in avoiding the clinical bias and ambiguity. The molecular approach provides the scientific basis to the practice of clinical cardiovascular genetics. It is important that all clinicians engaged in the care of patients and families affected with an inherited cardiovascular condition should be equipped with the molecular understanding essential in planning and interpreting the genetic laboratory investigations and applying results in the clinical practice.

References

Chen WG, Chang Q, Lin Y, et al. Derepression of BDNF transcription involves calcium-dependent phosphorylation of MeCP2. *Science.* 2003;302:885–889.

Egger G, Liang G, Aparicio A, Jones P. Epigenetics in human disease and prospects of epigenetic therapy. *Nature.* 2004;429:457–463.

Ennis S, Ward D, Murray A. Nonlinear association between CGG repeat number and age of menopause in FMR1 premutation carriers. *Eur J Hum Genet.* 2006;14(2):253–255.

Esfandiarei M, Yanagawa R, McMannus BM. Dilated cardiomyopathy and other cardiomyopathies. In: Dzau VJ, Liew C-C, eds. *Cardiovascular Genetics and Genomics for the Cardiologist'.* Blackwell Futura, Oxford, UK; 2007:55–82.

Greco CM, Berman RF, Martin RM, et al. Neuropathology of fragile X-associated tremor/ataxia syndrome (FXTAS). *Brain.* 2006;129 (Pt 1):243–255.

Greenberg F, Guzzetta V, de Oca-Luna RM, et al. Molecular analysis of the Smith-Magenis syndrome: a possible contiguous-gene syndrome associated with del(17)(p11.2). *Am J Hum Genet.* 49:1207–1218.

Hall JG, Powers EK, Mcllvaine, Ean VH. The frequency and financial burden of genetic disease in a pediatric hospital. *Am J Med Genet.* 1978;1:417–436.

Holliday R, Pugh JE. DNA modification mechanisms and gene activity during development. *Science.* 1975;187:226–232.

Jones LK, Saha V. Chromatin modification, leukaemia and implications for therapy. *Br J Haematol.* 2002;118:714–727.

Jones P, Baylin SB. The fundamental role of epigenetic events in cancer. *Nat Rev Genet.* 2002;3:415–428.

Jones PA, Laird PW. Cancer epigenetics comes of age. *Nat Gen.* 1999;21:163–167.

Kane MF, Loda M, Gaida GM, et al. Methylation of hMLH1 promoter correlates with lack of expression in sporadic colon tumours and mismatch repair defective human cancer cell lines. *Can Res.* 1997;57:808–811.

Lachner M, Jenuwin T. The many facets of histone lysine methylation. *Curr Opin Cell Biol.* 2002;14:286–298.

Lupski JR. Genomic disorders: structural features of the genome can lead to DNA rearrangements and human disease traits. *Trends Genet.* 1998;14:417–420.

Lupski JR. Genomic disorders: recombination-based disease resulting from genome architecture. *Am J Hum Genet.* 2003;72:246–252.

Lupski JR, Stankiewicz P. Genomic disorders: molecular mechanisms for rearrangements and conveyed phenotypes. *PlOS Genetics.* 2005;1(6):e49.

Marion AJ. Hypertrophic cardiomyopathy. In: Dzau VJ, Liew C-C, eds. *Cardiovascular Genetics and Genomics for the Cardiologist.* Blackwell Futura, Oxford, UK; 2007:30–54.

Potocki L, Chen K-S, Koeuth T, et al. DNA rearrangements on both homologues of chromosome 17 in a mildly delayed individual with a family history of autosomal dominant carpal tunnel syndrome. *Am J Hum Genet.* 1999;64:471–478.

Roberts CW, Orkin SH. The SW1/SNF complex-chromatin and cancer. *Nat Rev Cancer.* 2004;4:133–142.

Shaw CJ, Lupski JR. Implications of human genome architecture for rearrangement-based disorders: the genomic basis of disease. *Hum Mol Genet.* 2004;13(1):R57–R64.

Slager RE, Newton TL, Vlangos CN, Finucane B, Elsea SH. Mutations in *RAII* associated with Smith-Magenis syndrome. *Nat Gen.* 2003;33:466–468.

Tufarelli C, Stanley JA, Garrick D, et al. Transcription of antisense RNA leading to gene silencing and methylation as a novel cause of human genetic disease. *Nat Gen.* 2003;203:157–165.

Warren ST. The expanding world of trinucleotide repeats. *Science.* 1996;271:1374–1375.

Wolffe AP, Matzke MA. Epigenetics: regulation through repression. *Science.* 1999;286(5439):481–486. DOI: 10.1126/science.286.5439.481.

Further Reading

1. On-line Mendelian Inheritance in Man (OMIM) accessed at -http://www.ncbi.nlm.nih.gov/sites/entrez?db=omim
2. Oxford Desk Reference-Clinical Genetics (eds. Firth and Hurst), Oxford University Press, Oxford, 2005.
3. Principles of Medical Genetics (eds. Gelehrter, Collins and Ginsburg), 2nd ed. Williams and Wilkins, Baltimore, 1998.
4. Textbook of Cardiovascular Medicine (ed. Topol), Lippincot, Williams and Wilkins, 3rd ed. Philadelphia, 2007."

4

Genetic Epidemiology of Cardiovascular Diseases

Teri A Manolio and Elizabeth Nabel

Introduction

Genetic epidemiology has been defined as the study of "the role of genetic factors and their interaction with environmental factors in the occurrence of disease in human populations" (Khoury et al. 1993). It involves a variety of study designs, including classic etiologic epidemiologic designs such as case-control and cohort studies examining the risk of disease associated with a positive family history, as well as family study designs such as twin, sibling, and parent–offspring studies examining familial resemblance in disease occurrence. In addition, pedigree studies have facilitated the investigation of inheritance patterns, such as dominant or recessive inheritance, which are needed for modeling of genetic transmission through segregation analysis (Khoury et al. 1993). Pedigree studies have also been the critical substrate for genetic linkage analysis, especially with the advent of techniques for effective amplification of very small amounts of DNA and for assay of highly polymorphic, anonymous microsatellite markers (Mullis et al. 1987; Weber and May 1989). Indeed, identification of genetic linkage, or alleles at a marker locus that cosegregate with alleles at a putative trait locus, has been described as the strongest statistical evidence for an underlying genetic mechanism (Elston 1981).

Investigations of heritability, segregation, and linkage have tended to be most useful in studies of Mendelian or single gene disorders, though extensions have been developed to assess polygenic inheritance (Weeks and Lange 1992; Blangero and Almasy 1997). While much has been and remains to be learned from the relatively rare cardiovascular disorders influenced by a single major gene (Nabel 2003) such as familial hypercholesterolemia (Williams et al. 1999), Hutchinson-Gilford progeria (Capell et al. 2007), and familial long QT syndromes (Roden and Spooner 1999), the vast majority of cardiovascular disease is likely due to the interplay of multiple genetic and environmental factors, and is thus an excellent and challenging example of a complex genetic disease (Lander and Schork 1994; Risch 2000). Here we examine methodologic issues related to phenotypic, genetic, and environmental complexity of cardiovascular disease, as well as evidence from major genetic epidemiologic study designs of the role of genetic factors in the development and progression of cardiovascular disease.

Cardiovascular Disease as a Paradigm of a Complex Disease

Phenotypic Complexity

Cardiovascular disease provides an outstanding illustration not only of genetic but of phenotypic complexity, since cardiovascular disorders represent a vast and diverse array of conditions (Table 4–1). Phenotypic complexity is often cited as a reason for failing to find potentially causative genetic variants in genetic studies, particularly if the trait under study is believed to represent several heterogeneous disorders with differing underlying genetic influences. This situation is similar to genetic heterogeneity, discussed below, in which each of several different loci and mutations produce very similar phenotypes (Shaw et al. 2002).

Table 4–1 Conditions Included under the Rubric of "Diseases of the Circulatory System," International Classification of Diseases, 10th Version (ICD-10)

ICD-10 Code	Condition
I00–I02	Acute rheumatic fever
I05–I09	Chronic rheumatic heart diseases
I10–I15	Hypertensive diseases
I20–I25	Ischemic heart diseases
I26–I28	Pulmonary heart disease and diseases of pulmonary circulation
I30–I52	Other forms of heart disease
I60–I69	Cerebrovascular diseases
I70–I79	Diseases of arteries, arterioles, and capillaries
I80–I89	Diseases of veins, lymphatic vessels, and lymph nodes, not elsewhere classified
I95–I99	Other and unspecified disorders of the circulatory system

Adapted from ICD-10 online 2007, accessed at http://www.who.int/classifications/apps/icd/icd10online/.

Table 4–2 Gene Mutations that Cause Unexplained Left Ventricular Hypertrophy

Gene (Designation)	Chromosome	Frequency	Number of Mutations	Phenotype
HCM-sarcomere proteins				
ß-Myosin heavy chain (*ß-MHC*)	14q1	30%–40%	>80	Typically obvious disease with significant LVH; several severe phenotypes
α-Myosin heavy chain (*α-MHC*)	14q1	Rare	<5	
Cardiac myosin binding protein C (*cMYBPC*)	11q1	30%–40%	>50	Typically more mild disease, but severe phenotypes have been described; associated with elderly-onset HCM
Cardiac troponin T (*cTnT*)	1q3	15%–20%	>20	Typically mild LVH but increased association with sudden death
Cardiac troponin I (*cTnI*)	19p1	<5%	>10	
Cardiac troponin C (*CTnC*)	3p	Rare	1	
α-Tropomyosin (*α-TM*)	15q2	<5%	8	
Myosin essential light chain (*MLC-1*)	3p	Rare	2	Skeletal myopathy
Myosin regulatory light chain (*MLC-2*)	12q	Rare	8	Skeletal myopathy
Actin	11q	Rare	5	
Titin	2q3	Rare	1	
Metabolic cardiomyopathies				
γ-Subunit AMP kinase (*PRKAG2*)	7q3	?	4	Ventricular preexcitation and conduction disease
Linked lysosome-associated membrane protein (*LAMP2*)	X	?	6	Ventricular preexcitation, elevated liver transaminases, cognitive impairment

Adapted from Ho CY, Seidman CE. A contemporary approach to hypertrophic cardiomyopathy. *Circulation*. 2006;113(24):e858–862.

Few investigators would attempt to investigate the genetics of conditions as different as acute rheumatic fever and pulmonary hypertension together, but even a seemingly specific phenotype such as hypertrophic cardiomyopathy, which involves only two ICD-10 codes (I42.1, "Obstructive hypertrophic cardiomyopathy," and I42.2, "Other hypertrophic cardiomyopathy") can be quite complex phenotypically (Arad et al. 2002). The cardiac phenotype, for example, may differ in age of onset, clinical course, penetrance, and severity and pattern of hypertrophy. While some of these differences are partly explained by differences in the proteins that are mutated in different patients, a reflection of genetic heterogeneity, diverse phenotypes may also be accompanied by other cardiac manifestations such as preexcitation and progressive conduction system delays, or by extracardiac evidence of metabolic, infiltrative, or storage diseases such as Fabry's disease (Arad et al. 2002). Unexplained left ventricular hypertrophy (LVH) might be considered to be a very specific phenotype that can be measured with reasonable reliability, but the presence of other clinical manifestations may be a clue to phenotypic diversity reflecting substantial underlying genetic heterogeneity (Table 4–2; Ho and Seidman 2006). Differing genetic influences have been identified for severe versus mild LVH, for example, as well as for LVH associated with sudden death or skeletal myopathy (Ho and Seidman 2006). Knowledge of the specific causal variant in hypertrophic cardiomyopathy patients may thus provide important prognostic information (Niimura et al. 1998).

Phenotypic diversity may not necessarily indicate genetic heterogeneity, however, since many factors influence the manifestation of underlying genetic variants, such as genetic background, gender, medication use, and acquired conditions (Arad et al. 2002; Roden 2002). Studies of the extraordinarily comprehensive genealogical information available in Icelanders, for example, have suggested a shared genetic linkage in such diverse forms of stroke as hemorrhagic, large vessel ischemic, small vessel ischemic, and cardioembolic subtypes (Gretarsdottir et al. 2002), as well as a shared linkage for stroke and myocardial infarction (Helgadottir et al. 2004). Conversely, phenotypic diversity may not necessarily be the result of genetic heterogeneity, but rather of variable manifestations or associations with a single gene.

Many genes have multiple, or pleiotropic, effects and can be associated with a variety of seemingly disparate conditions, depending possibly on the genetic background or environmental milieu in which they occur. This is exemplified by the recent demonstration that variants near the cell cycle genes *CDKN2A* and *CDKN2B* are associated with both diabetes and, independently, with myocardial infarction (McPherson et al. 2007; Scott et al. 2007), and that *PTPN22* variants are associated with both type I diabetes and rheumatoid arthritis (Wellcome Trust Case Control Consortium 2007).

These and similar observations have led some to propose a final common pathway hypothesis, in which multiple genetic variants in a physiologic pathway, such as inflammation or coagulation, produce very similar phenotypic manifestations (Bowles et al. 2000). In long QT syndromes, for example, mutations in ion channel proteins such as *KVLQT1*, *KCNE1*, *HERG*, *SCN5A*, and *KCNE2* have all been associated with hereditary syndromes of ventricular arrhythmias, suggesting that ion channelopathies may be a final common pathway leading to potentially fatal ventricular arrhythmias. Similarly, mutations in sarcomeric proteins, as described in Table 4–2, appear to be a common pathway to familial hypertrophic cardiomyopathy, while mutations in genes encoding cytoskeletal proteins may be a common pathway to inherited and acquired forms of dilated cardiomyopathy (Bowles et al. 2000). Alterations in renal sodium handling have been suggested as a common final pathway for regulation of blood pressure, for example, based on single gene mutations affecting sodium reabsorption such as mutations in genes encoding the mineralocorticoid receptor or enzymes that activate it, subunits of the renal epithelial sodium channel, and the *WNK* kinases (Turner and Boerwinkle 2003). That these rare syndromes converge on a similar metabolic pathway suggests that common genetic variations affecting blood pressure regulation on a population basis may act in the same pathways, with similar phenotypic expression; considerable evidence is available to support this hypothesis (Turner and Boerwinkle 2003).

The potential importance of metabolic pathways in dissecting the genetics of complex diseases has led to the suggestion that phenotypic measures used for gene discovery be as close to the gene or gene product as possible, including assays for cellular phenotypes such as gene expression (Stranger et al. 2005) or cell surface markers (Grimaldi et al. 2007). In complex disease genetics, this has led to the examination of intermediate phenotypes, sometimes called endophenotypes. These are phenotypes presumed to be more proximal in the chain of pathophysiologic events leading from a specific gene to a distant clinical manifestation and thus less likely to be influenced by environmental variation (Williams et al. 1990; Timberlake et al. 2001). Intermediate phenotypes in hypertension, for example, might include non-modulation of renal blood flow in response to angiotensin II or increased urinary free cortisol (Timberlake et al. 2001). Because it is difficult without knowing the causative gene to know where in the pathway from gene to disease manifestation a particular phenotype may lie, and because identifying the causative gene is the goal of many genetic epidemiology studies, choice of intermediate phenotypes can be difficult. Characteristics of such phenotypes that might make them particularly valuable for gene discovery have been described, and include strong association with the trait of interest and ease of measurement (Table 4–3; Timberlake et al. 2001). Perhaps the key requirement for a phenotype suitable for genetic studies is that it be documented to have a high heritability, and thus likely to be influenced by genetic factors (Newton-Cheh and Hirschhorn 2005).

A final critical consideration in selection of phenotypes in genetic epidemiology studies is the reliability of the measurement—that is, a low potential for misclassification error in assigning the phenotype. Misclassification of case status can have disastrous effects on study power in case-control association studies, particularly when the specificity of a disease measure is low so that a large number of unaffected individuals are misclassified as affected (Burton et al. 2009). This is because, regardless of sensitivity, if specificity is high, all of the subjects classified as cases truly have the disease, and the great majority of controls (if the disease is not common) will be selected from the large group of truly unaffected persons rather than the few affected persons incorrectly classified as disease free. In contrast, if specificity is not high, the number of unaffected persons incorrectly classified as affected (false positives) will greatly outnumber those who truly have the disease (true positives) and power to detect any differences between them will rapidly decay. For example, sampling cases of a disease with 10% prevalence from a population of 500,000 using a measure with 100% sensitivity and 90% specificity (a fairly respectable level of specificity, in fact) will produce 50,000 true cases of disease and 45,000 subjects incorrectly classified as diseased, so that nearly half the cases will truly be unaffected. For a condition with prevalence of 1% using a measure with the same 100% sensitivity and 90% specificity, the pool of potential cases will include 5,000 subjects correctly classified as having the disease, and 49,500 healthy subjects incorrectly classified as diseased, so that less than 10% of the cases will actually have the disease (Burton et al. 2009).

Table 4–3 Characteristics of Intermediate Phenotypes Making Them Particularly Valuable for Gene Discovery (Timberlake et al. 2001)

- Strong association with trait of interest
- Easy to assess and relatively noninvasive, to make its measurement suitable in relatives of affected probands
- High heritability
- High penetrance
- Early expression in offspring of affected parents, to facilitate estimates of heritability
- Bimodal distribution
- Causality in the pathogenesis of the trait
- Suggestive of testable candidate genes

Population-based measures of clinical cardiovascular events, such as patient- or physician-reported stroke or heart failure, can have substantial misclassification rates that greatly diminish the power of a study to identify genetic factors conferring relatively small (relative risks of 1.3–1.5) degrees of increased risk. For this reason, more objective measures with less potential for misclassification and other biases have been suggested for genetic studies, such as ultrasonographically defined carotid atherosclerosis (Manolio et al. 2004) and cerebral white matter hyperintensities (Turner et al. 2003). A major additional advantage of such measures is the potential for examination of a continuous rather than a dichotomous outcome, which tends to provide greater power for identification of risk factors (O'Leary et al. 1999).

Genetic Complexity

"Genetic heterogeneity," a form of genetic complexity, is a concept arising from linkage studies in that "in some families a disease is caused by a gene located in the vicinity of a marker locus, while in other families the same disease phenotype is due to a disease gene located elsewhere, or the disease is not due to a single gene" (Ott 1991). The concept has primarily been applied to single gene disorders caused by numerous individual genetic variants, each of large effect and each often limited to a given family, sometimes called *private mutations* (Reitsma and Rosendaal 2007). Good examples of this are the many mutations that can produce long QT syndrome or hypertrophic cardiomyopathy (as above), giving rise to variable phenotypic effects and substantial clinical variability (Botstein and Risch 2003). Although some of the variability in phenotypic expression in Mendelian disorders has been ascribed to "variable penetrance," or unexplained variation in the probability that an individual with the causative gene will be affected (Khoury et al. 1993), recognition is growing that modifier genes and environmental factors influence the expression of even "simple" Mendelian disorders (Botstein and Risch, 2003). Such influences are likely to be the rule rather than the exception in understanding the genetics of non-Mendelian, complex disorders, in which many genetic variants, each of small effect, may act together in a single individual to increase disease risk. In such a case, all loci contributing to a complex disease could be considered to be modifiers since there is no single locus of large effect (Botstein and Risch 2003).

Genetic complexity has been conceptualized in terms of two extreme models of an allelic spectrum of common diseases, or number and population frequency of disease-predisposing alleles at a given locus (Reich and Lander 2001). One extreme is that common alleles at multiple loci interact to cause disease, and the other is that rare alleles at many loci, either acting alone or with other genetic or environmental influences, cause disease. The distinction is important, because common alleles (generally defined as allele frequency of 5% or greater, International HapMap Consortium 2003) are easier to discover and more practical to test clinically (Reich and Lander 2001). The pursuit of rare alleles in common diseases is beyond the scope of this chapter, other than noting that sequencing studies of persons with extreme phenotypes such as very low or high cholesterol levels or blood pressure levels has led to identification of rare genetic variants of great value in understanding disease pathogenesis and potential pathways to treatment (Halushka et al. 1999; Cohen et al. 2004; Kotowski et al. 2006). In contrast, the pursuit of common alleles through genome-wide association studies, greatly facilitated by the recent cataloguing of the vast majority of *common* human variation (International HapMap Consortium 2005) and the development of high-throughput, dense genotyping platforms, has gained preeminence in the approach to gene discovery for common diseases (see below). Such studies have demonstrated conclusively that genetic variants of relatively modest effect (genotype relative risks of 1.2–1.5) exist for common diseases and can be detected in samples of adequate size and phenotypic characterization (Hunter and Kraft 2007).

Environmental Complexity

Cardiovascular disease could also be considered to be an "environmentally complex" disease, since a wide variety of environmental and lifestyle exposures and other nongenetic factors are known to be related to disease development (Table 4–4). These exposures are complex not only because they may interact with each other to produce disease, as demonstrated by the increased risk of coronary disease associated with cigarette smoking in men with elevated cholesterol levels in the Honolulu Heart Program (Robertson et al. 1977), but also because they often vary within an individual over time and space. Particulate air pollution levels, for example, are highly variable geographically and temporally (Dockery 2001), and dietary intakes and smoking exposure vary substantially both day to day and throughout a lifetime. Environmental exposures are also complex because they are very challenging to measure—many current measures rely on self-report, which can involve substantial biases, especially after the onset of disease (Neugebauer and Ng 1990).

Efforts to improve assessment of environmental exposures and lifestyle factors are underway, particularly through the U.S. National Institutes of Health's Genes, Environment, and Health Initiative (GEI, http://www.gei.nih.gov/). Traditional methods of assessing potentially toxic environmental exposures include measuring the potential toxin in environmental samples or in biospecimens such as blood or urine, or through estimates of frequency, duration, and severity of exposure reported in questionnaires (Schwartz and Collins 2007). Even the reliable and cost-effective assays developed for human biospecimens, however, do not permit assessment of extent of exposure, individual biological response, or temporal relationship between exposure and biologic response. While technologies appear to be at hand to provide precise measures of potentially toxic exposures at the point of contact or to characterize the biological fingerprint of, or physiologic response to, environmental stressors, much work is needed to bring these to the point of widespread application in population-based studies, particularly for examination of their influence on associations of genetic variants with disease (Schwartz and Collins 2007).

Table 4–4 Environmental and Lifestyle Exposures and Nongenetic Factors Implicated in Etiology of Atherosclerotic Cardiovascular Disease

- Tobacco use
- High dietary saturated fat and cholesterol intake
- High dietary salt intake
- Physical inactivity
- Particulate air pollution
- Psychological stress
- Social isolation
- Low socioeconomic status
- Periodontal disease
- Elevated homocysteine levels
- Elevated C-reactive protein levels
- Infections
- Age

Gene–Environment Interactions in Cardiovascular Disease

Gene–environment interactions, or differing associations of genes with disease in the presence or absence of an environmental factor (or vice versa), have been suggested to be at the root of most recent epidemics of common diseases. This is because the human genome has not changed substantially in the timespan of these epidemics, yet substantial familial aggregation independent of shared environment can be demonstrated for many of them (Manolio et al. 2006). Interactions can be qualitative, in which a specific allele might be associated with reduced risk in the absence of an environmental factor but increased risk in the presence of that factor, or quantitative, in which the *magnitude* of an allelic association is greater in the presence than in the absence of the environmental factor but the *direction* of association is the same (Szklo and Nieto 2004).

Examples of qualitative interactions are relatively rare, but an interesting one has been suggested in the modification of the relationship of hepatic lipase (*LIPC*) to HDL-cholesterol (HDL-C) levels by dietary fat intake in the Framingham Heart Study (Ordovas et al. 2002). Predicted levels of HDL-C were shown in that study to be highest among TT homozygotes and lowest among CC homozygotes in persons with low dietary fat intake (Figure 4–1, panel A), but this relationship was reversed in persons with high fat intake (Figure 4–1, panel C). Quantitative interactions are more common and are exemplified by the stronger protective association against myocardial infarction of moderate alcohol intake reported in men homozygous for the gamma2 allele of the *ADH3* gene (relative risk of MI compared to light drinkers = 0.14) compared to men homozygous for the gamma1 allele (relative risk of MI compared to light drinkers = 0.62, p for interaction = 0.01; Hines et al. 2001).

Gene–environment interactions are critical to identify in studies of cardiovascular genetics because they can mask the

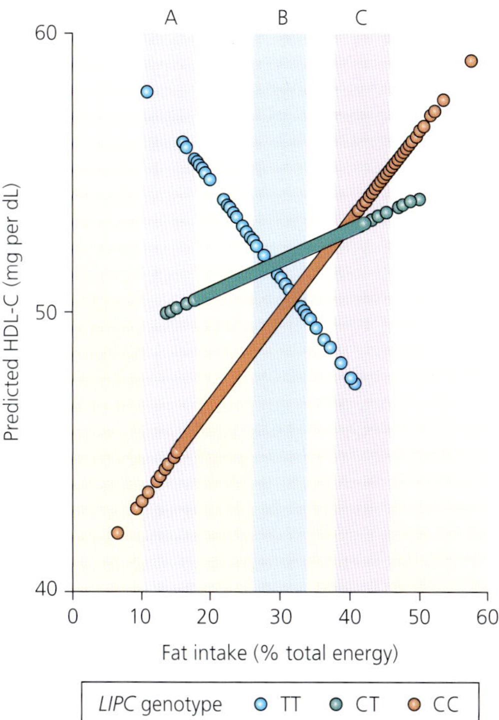

Figure 4–1 The importance of gene–environment interactions—an example. Predicted values of high-density lipoprotein cholesterol (HDL-C) are shown for different hepatic lipase (LIPC) genotypes at different total levels of dietary fat intake (data from Ordovas et al. 2002). Low fat intake (band A) combined with the TT genotype results in the highest HDL-C level. For a moderate fat intake (band B), there is no relationship between genotype and HDL-C level. For a high fat intake (band C), the TT genotype has the lowest HDL-C level. Gene–environment interactions are therefore important in identifying genetic and environmental determinants of medically relevant phenotypes such as HDL-C levels; depending on the dietary fat intake, one could conclude that the TT genotype produces high (band A) or low (band C) HDL-C levels, or that it is not associated with HDL-C levels at all (band B). Reprinted from Manolio TA, Bailey-Wilson JE, Collins FS. Genes, environment and the value of prospective cohort studies. *Nat Rev Genet.* 2006;7(10):812–820, with permission from Nature Publishing Group.

detection of a genetic (or an environmental) effect, as in the *LIPC* example above, where, in persons with moderate dietary fat intake (Figure 4–1, band B), one would conclude there is no relationship between genotype and HDL-C levels at all (Ordovas et al. 2002). They are also important because they can lead to inconsistencies in gene–disease associations, as in panels A and C of the *LIPC* example. Most importantly, however, they may suggest approaches for modifying deleterious gene effects, by avoiding a deleterious exposure (such as dietary phenylalanine in persons with phenylketonuria) or by promoting a beneficial exposure. Examples of beneficial environmental exposures are harder to come by but have been suggested by the apparent alleviation of elevated homocysteine levels, and possibly risk of colon cancer, in persons homozygous for the thermolabile methylenetetrahydrofolate reductase variant who also have high dietary folate intake (Jacques et al. 1996; Le Marchand et al. 2005). The search for additional such beneficial exposures may be a fertile area for future epidemiologic research.

A major challenge in identifying gene–environment interactions lies in the sample sizes needed to detect them, which can be enormous. This is because, for low frequency minor alleles and infrequent exposures, persons with both the risk allele and the environmental exposure (and thus providing the most information on interaction of the two) will usually make up the smallest proportion of the study subjects. A rough estimate is that the sample size needed to detect an interaction of two factors is at least four times the sample size needed to detect the main effect of each factor (Smith and Day 1984; Hunter 2005). This was recently demonstrated in estimates of the smallest detectable odds ratios for cohorts of a fixed size and disease incidence (Manolio et al. 2006). Although a cohort of 200,000 persons, for example, could detect an odds ratio of about 2.5 for a disease of 0.05% incidence and an environmental exposure of 10% prevalence in that analysis, and could detect an odds ratio of about 2 for an allele of 10% frequency, the smallest detectable odds ratio for their interaction was about 7 (Figure 4–2).

Evidence for Genetic Influences on Cardiovascular Disease Risk

The potential role of genetic factors in the occurrence and course of cardiovascular disease can be examined epidemiologically through studies of familial clustering, genetic linkage, and genetic association. Evidence for genetic influences on CVD provided by each of these approaches is briefly reviewed below.

Familial Clustering of Cardiovascular Disease

Cardiovascular diseases have long been known to cluster in families, a strong but not infallible indicator of genetic factors at work. Reports of familial occurrence of coronary disease date back at least to the mid-1950s, and most often were assessed by comparing the presence of a positive family history of disease, usually among parents, in coronary disease cases and controls (Thomas and Cohen 1955; Russek and Zohman 1958). Early studies typically showed a three- to fourfold greater reported family history of coronary disease among coronary disease cases, even after accounting for reporting and selection bias (Rose 1964; Slack and Evans 1966). These findings have been replicated in prospective assessments of the risk of incident disease in persons with and without positive family histories (Barrett-Connor and Khaw 1984, Colditz et al. 1986). Considerable debate has ensued as to whether this clustering was due primarily to known clustering of cardiovascular disease risk factors, such as hypertension and hyperlipidemia (Deutscher et al. 1969; Perkins 1986), but studies adjusting for these factors have clearly demonstrated the independence of the associated risk (Friedlander et al. 1985; Myers et al. 1990).

A positive family history has generally been associated with a 1.5- to 2-fold increased risk of coronary disease among first-degree relatives after adjustment for other risk factors, with risk consistently stronger for early onset cases (Deutscher et al. 1970; Higgins 2000). Not only is this true of early disease onset in the person at risk—that is, younger persons with coronary disease are more likely to have had family members with coronary disease at any age than are older persons with coronary disease, who are in turn more likely to have had family members with coronary disease than are persons without coronary disease—but also of early disease onset in the relatives conferring the risk. In this latter case, persons at any age with relatives developing coronary disease at younger ages are more likely to develop coronary disease

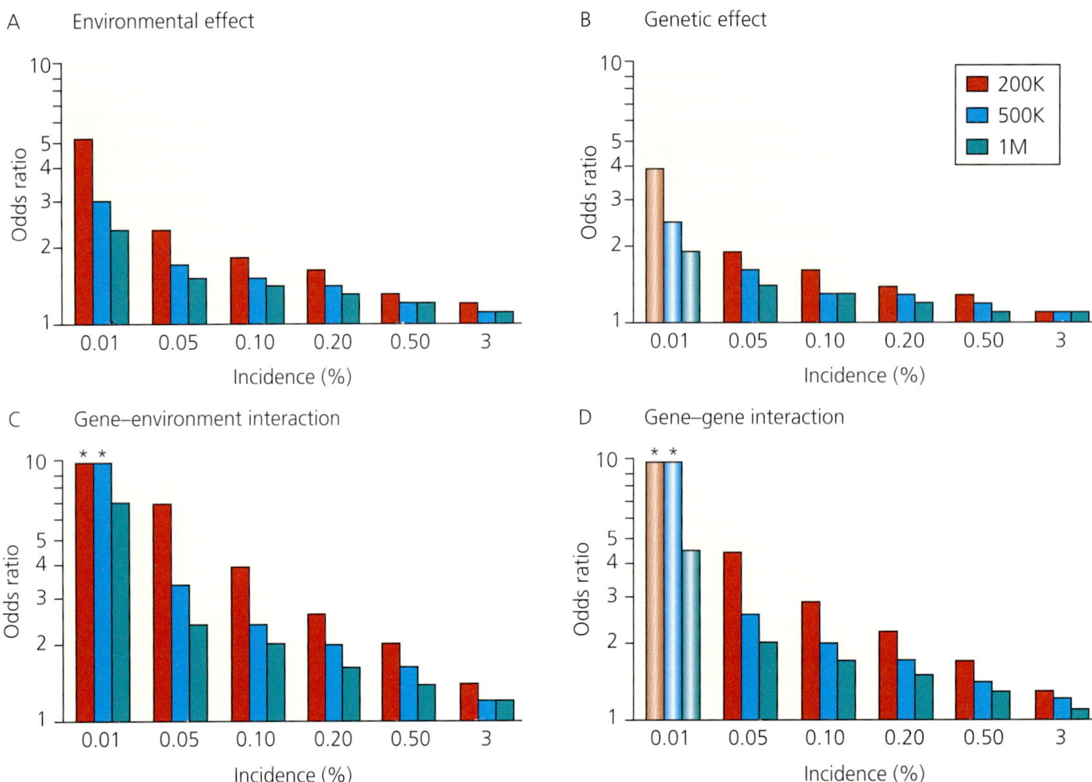

Figure 4–2 Sample size requirements for detecting interactions. Reprinted from Manolio TA, Bailey-Wilson JE, Collins FS. Genes, environment and the value of prospective cohort studies. *Nat Rev Genet.* 2006;7(10):812–820, with permission from Nature Publishing Group.

themselves than are persons with relatives who developed coronary disease at older ages (Hopkins and Williams 1989). The age dependence of familial risk of cardiovascular disease, the variability in family sizes, and the high incidence of coronary disease in general have led to the development of family risk scores (Higgins 2000). These scores compare the observed number of coronary disease cases in a given family to that expected based on the number, age, sex, and in some cases other risk factors of each family member (Hunt et al. 1986). Such scores can be quite useful in categorizing persons as to level of familial risk for screening and risk reduction purposes (Williams et al. 2001).

The genetics literature often reports familial risks in terms of recurrence risk ratio, λ_R, or the ratio of prevalences of disease in relatives of type R of affected cases divided by the prevalence in the general population (Risch 1990). Relative risk among siblings of affected cases is thus often referred to as λ_s, though strictly speaking λ was defined as a prevalence ratio; other studies may report familial relative risk of disease incidence instead of λ (Burton et al. 2005). For diseases with a prominent genetic component, recurrence risk ratios should be higher among more closely related relatives, and highest of all among identical twins. Decline in familial risk by degree of relatedness is nicely demonstrated in data from the extensive Icelandic genealogical database, demonstrating a nearly stepwise decline in risk of atrial fibrillation from 1.77 (95% confidence interval, 1.67–1.88) in first-degree relatives to 1.05 (95% confidence interval, 1.02–1.07) in fifth-degree relatives (Arnar et al. 2006).

Familial clustering can also be assessed by analyses of mixtures of distributions, familial correlations, and heritability. Analysis of mixtures of distributions, or commingling analysis, is infrequently used at present, but was a common approach in the past as a prelude to formal segregation analysis (Khoury et al. 1993). The first step in these analyses is to search for evidence of major gene effects on a trait, whether the trait is quantitative, such as lipid or blood pressure levels, or qualitative, such as presence or absence of disease, though this tends to be easier to conceptualize and display for quantitative traits. For example, if a single gene with two alleles determines a quantitative trait such as LDL-cholesterol levels, one would anticipate a population sample to consist of three underlying distributions of the trait if alleles are codominant or two distributions if alleles are recessive or dominant (Boerwinkle et al. 1986). Friedlander et al. nicely demonstrated two underlying distributions for LDL-cholesterol peak particle diameter in Israeli families, as shown in Figure 4–3 (Friedlander et al. 1999). Multiple distributions in both related and unrelated individuals have been shown for other cardiovascular traits such as left ventricular mass (Chien et al. 2006) and angiotensinogen levels (Guo et al. 1999).

Phenotypic resemblance among relatives can also be estimated either by regressing one relative's value (such as the offspring's) on that of another (such as the parent's) or by using the correlation between the pairs' phenotypic values. Twice the parent–offspring correlation estimates the proportion of additive genetic variance in the trait and can be used to estimate heritability (Fisher 1918). If the trait is under genetic control, one would expect trait correlations among closer relatives to be greater than those among more distant relatives, under the critical assumption that environmental similarity does not differ with degree of relatedness (Cavalli-Sforza and Bodmer 1971). Spouse correlations are often used to gauge the effects of shared environment, though they may be increased by assortative mating (persons tending to

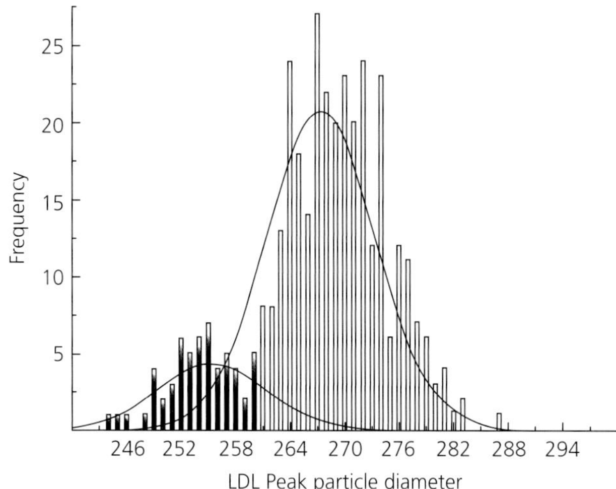

Figure 4–3 Distribution of adjusted LDL-cholesterol peak particle diameter for 373 family members with LDL subclass phenotypes B (solid bars), I (striped bars), and A (open bars) with the two-component distributions as predicted from commingling analysis. Reprinted from Friedlander Y, Kark JD, Sinnreich R, Edwards KL, Austin MA. Inheritance of LDL peak particle diameter: results from a segregation analysis in Israeli families. *Genet Epidemiol.* 1999;16(4):382–396, with permission.

choose mates who resemble them in demographics, physical characteristics, or behaviors) or shared lifestyles, or decreased by sex differences.

Data from the Busselton Population Health Studies demonstrated consistently stronger correlations among first-degree relatives than between spouses in a variety of cardiovascular disease risk factors (Table 4–5; Knuiman 1996). In that study and many others, most spouse correlations were small but were not zero, with spouses tending to resemble each other most for height and body mass index (Ellison et al. 1999; Harrap et al. 2000). Perhaps not surprisingly, spouse correlations may actually exceed those for first-degree relatives for lifestyle factors such as smoking, alcohol, exercise, and diet, as demonstrated in the National Heart, Lung, and Blood Institute (NHLBI) Family Heart Study (Higgins 2000). The contributions to these correlations of assortative mating and shared family environment can be assessed by comparing repeated examinations over time, or among relative pairs of different ages. One would expect that correlations due to assortative mating would decline or remain constant with time or age, while those due to shared environment would increase; none of the spouse correlations in the Busselton Study increased with time (Knuiman et al. 1996). In contrast, correlations among parents and offspring that are due to shared environment would be expected to decrease with time, as also demonstrated in Busselton, where all correlations declined with increasing age of the offspring.

A more general measure of familial clustering is heritability (h^2), defined as the proportion of total phenotypic variance attributable to the average effects of genes, and estimated as the ratio of genetic variance to total phenotypic variance (Khoury et al. 1993). Heritability can be calculated as twice the correlation coefficient between parents and offspring, as noted above, but information from other types of relatives is often included in variance components models of heritability (Burton et al. 2005). Heritability for most cardiovascular disease risk factors other than obesity is generally estimated in the 20%–40% range (i.e., 20%–40% of the total population variability in these traits appears due to genetic factors), with obesity having somewhat higher heritability, at least prior to the recent epidemic of obesity (Table 4–5, Knuiman et al. 1996). Measures of heritability depend importantly on the degree of variation in both the genetic and the environmental factors contributing to the trait, since population variation in a setting with little environmental variation (e.g., folate levels in a population with uniformly high dietary intakes of folate) will be disproportionately due to genetic factors, thus inflating estimates of heritability, and vice versa (Falconer and MacKay 1996).

Twin studies provide a special model for estimating heritability that has been widely used in cardiovascular disease (Berg 1987; Austin 1993; Evans et al. 2003). This method relies upon comparison of correlations between monozygotic (MZ) and dizygotic (DZ) twin pairs, recognizing that MZ pairs are genetically identical while DZ twins share on average only half their genes. The difference between MZ and DZ correlations for a given trait can be used to estimate heritability, as greater concordance between MZ than between DZ pairs suggests a role for genetic factors, while any discordance within MZ pairs suggests a role for environment (Khoury et al. 1993). The twin design relies heavily, however, on several key assumptions, the most questionable of which is that the degree to which environmental factors are shared is the same for MZ as for DZ twins (Eaves et al. 2003; Richardson and Norgate 2005). Heritability estimates from twin studies tend to be higher than those from other study designs, a difference that has been ascribed to the potential weakness of its underlying assumptions, but this does not diminish the value of the design for other investigations of genetic and environmental influences on disease (Evans et al. 2003).

Almost regardless of the manner in which it is assessed, so long as biases are minimized, estimation of heritability is a critical first step in identifying phenotypic measures likely to have demonstrable genetic influences, as noted above. In general, the higher the heritability of a trait, the more likely one is to find a genetic influence on it, though most cardiovascular disease traits cluster in the modest (< 40%) range of heritability. Identification of phenotypes that can be shown repeatedly, in diverse settings relatively free of bias, to have high heritability is a promising area for research in the genetic epidemiology of cardiovascular disease.

Linkage Analysis

The identification of alleles at a genetic marker locus that cosegregate with alleles at a putative trait locus, or "linkage," has been described as the strongest statistical evidence for an underlying genetic mechanism (Elston 1981). Linkage, generally assessed by a "LOD" (log-odds) score exceeding 3.0, can be sought with "known," or "candidate" loci, or with polymorphic loci with no known functional significance but having known locations throughout the genome ("anonymous markers"). Both approaches have been used to identify genes for cardiovascular disease (the use of ABO blood group markers, for example, to implicate catechol-O-methyl-transferase in essential hypertension) (Wilson et al. 1984); but use of anonymous markers increased dramatically in the last decade with the advent of extensive marker maps and efficient technologies for assaying highly polymorphic microsatellite markers (Weber and May 1989). Such maps were widely applied to large-scale family studies of heart disease through NIH-supported efforts such as the Mammalian Genotyping Service at the Marshfield Clinic and the Centers for Inherited

Table 4–5 Familial Correlations (95% confidence intervals) for Selected Cardiovascular Risk Factors in 1,319 Nuclear Families Involving 4,178 Adults from the Busselton Population Health Studies (Knuiman et al. 1996)

Risk Factor	Spouse	Parent-Offspring	Siblings	Overall Heritability
Systolic blood pressure	0.06 (0.01, 0.12)	0.09 (0.05, 0.14)	0.34 (0.27, 0.42)	27%
Diastolic blood pressure	0.05 (−0.02, 0.11)	0.12 (0.08, 0.16)	0.19 (0.12, 0.26)	27%
Cholesterol	0.12 (0.05, 0.19)	0.20 (0.15, 0.24)	0.14 (0.07, 0.21)	37%
Body mass index	0.10 (0.04, 0.17)	0.25 (0.21, 0.29)	0.29 (0.22, 0.36)	52%
Triceps skinfold	0.06 (−0.03, 0.15)	0.10 (0.06, 0.14)	0.14 (0.09, 0.20)	23%

Disease Research at Johns Hopkins University, as well as international efforts such as the Icelandic genealogy database studied by deCODE Genetics Inc (Gulcher et al. 2001) and the British Heart Foundation Family Heart Study (Samani et al. 2005).

This approach initially looked quite promising, particularly for single gene disorders, and early successes in cardiovascular disease included identification of the ATP-binding cassette transporter as the causative gene for Tangier disease (Brooks-Wilson et al. 1999) as well as genes for several uncommon monogenic forms of hypertension (Lifton 2004–2005). Progress in complex cardiovascular disorders has been more limited, but is perhaps best exemplified by the identification of arachidonate 5-lipoxygenase-activating protein (*ALOX5AP*) as a potential causative gene for myocardial infarction and stroke among Icelandic families (Helgadottir et al. 2004). Several of the challenges of this approach are clearly demonstrated in that analysis: the initial linkage peak failed to reach conventional definitions of genome-wide significance (LOD score of 2.86); the peak spanned a 7.6-Mb-region containing 40 known genes; extensive fine mapping and haplotype analyses were needed to localize the association (Figure 4–4); and replication in an independent sample produced inconsistent results (Helgadottir et al. 2004).

Other challenges in using linkage analysis for the study of complex disorders include its inherently low power in the presence of genetic heterogeneity, which tends to flatten and widen linkage peaks (Pollex and Hegele 2005) and requires large numbers of large families for success (Khoury et al. 1993). Other confounding factors such as variable penetrance, effects of genetic background and parental allelic origin, and environmental influences all tend to reduce the ability of linkage analysis to identify candidate loci or regions (Pollex and Hegele 2005). In addition, the extended length of linkage disequilibrium (LD) blocks shared among relatives, despite the current availability of dense marker maps, means that fine mapping of additional markers within linkage peaks often fails to show enough differences between relatives with and without disease to narrow the linkage signal sufficiently to identify a causative gene or variant. This has led to a number of promising linkage findings that could never be resolved into a causative gene, as exemplified by the report of strong linkage of familial combined hyperlipidemia to the *APOA1/C3/C4* gene cluster (Wojciechowski et al. 1991), which 13 years later had still not yielded a causative gene (Pollex and Hegele 2005). For these reasons, emphasis on linkage studies in the genetic epidemiology of cardiovascular disease has tended to decline in favor of genetic association studies.

Genetic Association Studies

Genetic association studies, like association studies of any type, are designed to identify genetic variants that are present among persons with (or who develop) a disease more frequently than in those without disease. Most often carried out in case-control or prospective cohort designs, association studies can be conducted in unrelated individuals, and are often more powerful in this setting than in groups of relatives because the genomes of relatives are not independent, making the effective sample size smaller. Conversely, because they are conducted in unrelated individuals one cannot take advantage of inheritance patterns and LD that are fundamental to linkage studies.

Association studies are of two primary types: candidate gene studies, in which variants are selected for study based on their presence within a gene known or suspected to be related to the phenotype of interest; and genome-wide studies, in which the entire genome is surveyed in an unbiased manner for regions that might harbor causative variants, whether these occur within genes or not. Candidate genes can be selected on a variety of evidence, such as the encoded protein being implicated in the biology of the disease or in the mechanism of action of a disease-modifying drug, or the gene being shown in animal studies, monogenic diseases, linkage scans, or prior association studies to be related to the disease or trait (Hattersley and McCarthy 2005). A recent review identified several candidate genes related to lipid metabolism, vascular homeostasis, hemostasis, inflammation, and other factors that are under intense investigation as possible genes for coronary disease (Table 4–6; Nordlie et al. 2005).

A major shortcoming of initial candidate gene association reports, however, has been their failure to replicate in other studies—indeed, it sometimes seems that nearly as much has been written about failure to replicate candidate gene associations as about the initial associations themselves (Hattersley and McCarthy 2005). Potential reasons for failure to replicate are legion but include differences between study populations in the allele frequency of interest, in genetic background or environmental exposures, or in a host of potential biases that can afflict both case-control and cohort studies (Manolio et al. 2006). Many initial reports, especially in small studies prone to sampling bias, may simply have been spurious (i.e., due to chance alone). A comprehensive review of 600 candidate genes for common diseases reported that only six of those studied three or more times had been consistently replicated (Hirschhorn et al. 2002); one of these six, Factor V Leiden, is a risk factor for venous thromboembolism. Similar comprehensive reviews (Lohmueller et al. 2003;

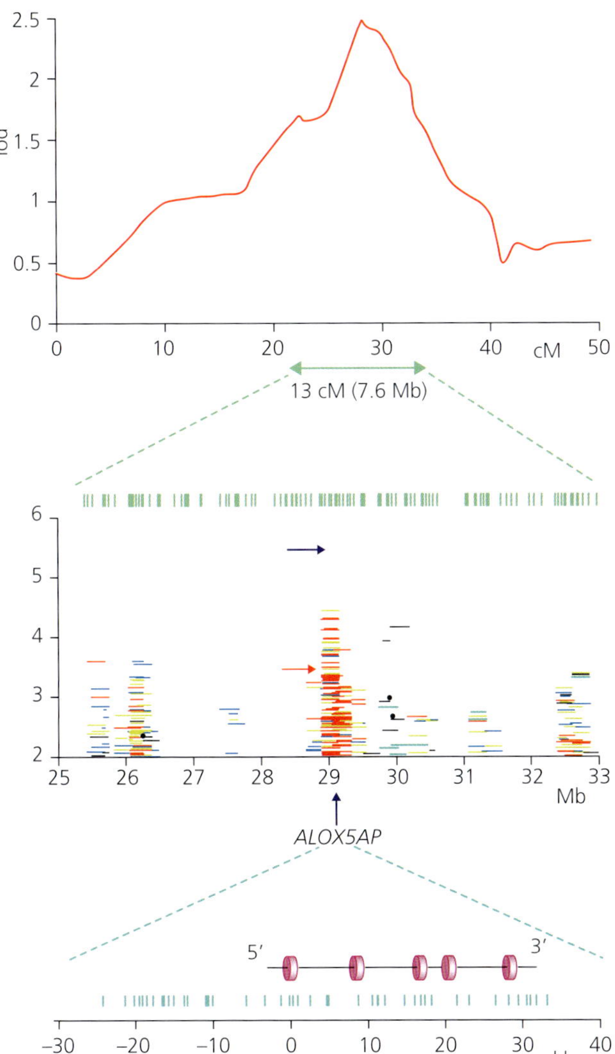

Figure 4–4 Identification and pursuit of the linkage signal for *ALOX5AP* in myocardial infarction. (a) The linkage scan for females with myocardial infarction and the one-log drop region that includes *ALOX5AP*. (**b**) Microsatellite association for all individuals with myocardial infarction: single-marker association (black dots) and two-, three-, four- and five-marker haplotype association (black, blue, green, and red horizontal lines, respectively). The blue and red arrows indicate the location of the most significant haplotype association across *ALOX5AP* in males and females, respectively. (**c**) *ALOX5AP* gene structure, with exons shown as colored cylinders, and the locations of all SNPs typed in the region. The green vertical lines indicate the position of the microsatellites (**b**) and SNPs (**c**) used in the analysis. Reprinted from Helgadottir A et al. The gene encoding 5-lipoxygenase activating protein confers risk of myocardial infarction and stroke. *Nat Genet*. March 2004;36(3):233–239, with permission.

Trikalinos et al. 2004), including one specific to carotid atherosclerosis (Manolio et al. 2004), have produced similar outcomes, and have generated a lively debate on what constitutes sufficient evidence for association (Neale and Sham 2004; Patterson and Cardon 2005; Todd 2006).

The advent of genome-wide association studies, building on the completion of the human genome sequence and human haplotype maps of the most common form of genetic variation, the single nucleotide polymorphism (SNP), may be changing

Table 4–6 Selected Candidate Genes Reported or Suggested to be Related to Coronary Disease (Nordlie et al. 2005)

Lipid metabolism
Apolipoprotein E (*APOE*)
Lipoprotein lipase (*LPL*)
Apolipoprotein B (*APOB*)
Vascular Hemostasis
Endothelial cell nitric oxide synthase (*ecNOS*)
Angiotensin convertin enzyme (*ACE*)
Angiotensin II type 1 receptor (*AT1R*)
Angiotensinogen (*AGT*)
Aldosterone synthase (*CYP11B2*)
Hemostasis
Glycoprotein Ia/IIa complex (*ITGA2*)
Glycoprotein IIb/IIa (*ITGB3*)
Thrombospondin II and IV (*THBS2, THBS4*)
Factor V Leiden
Prothrombin variant G20210A
Plasminogen activator inhibitor-1 (*PAI-1*)
Other
Methylenetetrahydrofolate reductase (*MTHFR*)
Interleukin 6 (*IL-6*)
Alcohol dehydrogenase (*ADH*)

this discouraging picture (International HapMap Project 2003; International Human Genome Sequencing Consortium 2004). Genome-wide association studies assay hundreds of thousands of SNPs designed to capture the great majority of human genomic variation in a cost-efficient and reliable manner. They identify SNPs associated with a disease or trait in much the same way analytically that candidate gene studies do, but without the reliance on prior knowledge, imperfect as it is, of genes likely to be related to the trait of interest. Instead, they survey the entire genome in a systematic, even agnostic, manner, relaxing the dependence on strong prior hypotheses (Chanock et al. 2007).

The stunning success of this approach has been evident across a wide variety of common diseases, as described by Hunter and Kraft, who note there have been few, if any, similar bursts of discovery in the history of medical research (Hunter and Kraft 2007). This technique has its weaknesses as well, chief among which is distinguishing the small number of true positive SNP-disease associations from the hundreds or even thousands of false positive, spurious ones. Although statistical techniques, including setting very stringent p-values for significance (10^{-7} or less) and comparing observed to expected associations after random permutation (Wacholder et al. 2004; Dudbridge et al. 2006), are under development to address this problem, the best solution is replication in independent samples (Todd 2006; Chanock et al. 2007). Adequate replication of the generally small odds ratios (1.2–1.5) detected in these studies has required many tens of thousands of subjects.

Despite the arduous nature of genome-wide association studies, the benefits to date have been substantial, as evidenced by the large number of hitherto unsuspected associations identified. For noncardiovascular diseases, these include complement factor H in age-related macular degeneration (Klein et al. 2005) or the HLA locus in control of human immunodeficiency virus infection (Fellay et al. 2007). In the cardiovascular field, Ozaki and colleagues conducted what was probably the first true genome-wide association study ever, of over 90,000 gene-centric SNPs in 94 cases of myocardial infarction and 658 controls in Japan (Ozaki et al. 2002). They identified two SNPs in the lymphotoxin A gene, each associated with a 1.7-fold increased risk of myocardial infarction in the homozygous state, that unfortunately failed to replicate in large-scale follow-up studies (Clarke et al. 2006). This early work opened the door, however, to a new generation of genome-wide findings that have been replicated and are now widely accepted as real.

Several such studies have identified robust, replicated, potentially causative genetic variants for cardiovascular diseases and traits, including associations of coronary disease with variants in the chromosome 9q21 region near the cell cycle variants *CDKN2A* and *CDKN2B* (Helgadottir et al. 2007; McPherson et al. 2007; Wellcome Trust Case Control Consortium 2007); with variants on chromosome 6q25.1, in the gene for methylenetetrahydrofolate dehydrogenase (NADP$^+$-dependent) 1-like protein (*MTHFD1L*); and with variants in chromosome 6p21.2, in a region currently known to harbor only a pseudogene (Samani et al. 2007). Evidence for four other potential loci with weaker associations was also uncovered in that study, suggesting that other variants remain to be found. Other genome-wide association studies have uncovered associations with atrial fibrillation in a region with no known genes (Gudbjartsson et al. 2007) and QT interval prolongation in the gene for nitric oxide synthase 1 (neuronal) adaptor protein, *NOS1AP* (Arking et al. 2006). In nearly all of these cases, the identified genetic variant has conferred only a modest relative risk, in the range of 1.2–1.5 for the heterozygote, and evidence for additional variants has been suggested. Genome-wide association would thus seem to be a powerful technique for gene discovery, despite the substantial sample sizes required. Several such studies are currently in progress, as described in the National Heart, Lung, and Blood Institute Strategic Plan (available at http://apps.nhlbi.nih.gov/strategicplan/).

As valuable as genome-wide association studies are for gene discovery, they are only a first step in identifying a disease gene. As noted above, initial findings must be replicated, preferably in a variety of population samples with differing genetic background and environmental exposures, so that the impact of these differences on the observed associations can be assessed. Fine-mapping, or typing of variants near or between the SNPs associated in initial genome scans, can help narrow the region of interest or select the potential causative gene from a number of possibilities in the region. If evidence of additional genetic influence on a trait remains after accounting for known variants, additional variants may need to be identified through sequencing studies of persons with extreme phenotypes, as noted above (Cohen et al. 2004; Lifton 2004–2005). Investigation then often shifts to the laboratory for determination of a gene's function, through in vitro studies or animal models, but epidemiologic approaches can provide important clues here as well. Typing potentially causative variants in well-characterized cohorts with a host of other phenotypic and exposure measures may provide important epidemiologic clues to gene function by demonstrating physiologic pathways in which they appear to be important or environmental factors that may modulate their effects. These findings then need to be translated into diagnostic or therapeutic strategies, much as sarcomere protein and ion channel variants are used in the diagnosis of familial cardiomyopathies and arrhythmia syndromes, or as the discovery of the LDL-receptor led to the new generation of lipid-lowering agents, the hydroxymethylglutaryl-CoA reductase inhibitors. These steps will take enormous additional effort, and will require collaboration across the numerous disciplines of genetics, epidemiology, clinical medicine, policy, and public health. They are critical to pursue, however, if the recent explosion of fascinating information about genomic structure and function is to be translated to improved human health.

Key Points

1. Genetic epidemiology is the study of the role of genetic factors and their interaction with environmental factors in the occurrence of disease in human populations.
2. Much of the current knowledge about genes related to cardiovascular diseases comes from studies of monogenic conditions that tend to be rare.
3. The majority of cardiovascular disease is likely due to the interplay of multiple genetic and environmental factors, and should thus be considered a "complex" genetic disease.
4. Genetic complexity may be a result of convergence of gene effects on a single common pathway, as for renal sodium handling and hypertension.
5. Key considerations in selecting intermediate phenotypes for investigation in genetic studies include strong association with the disease of interest, accurate measurement methods, and high heritability.
6. Genetic heterogeneity is defined as different single loci influencing a trait in different families, or as a trait not due to a single gene.
7. Developing better methods of measuring environmental exposures is critical to accurate identification of gene–environment interactions.
8. Methods for assessing familial clustering include estimates of familial relative risk, mixtures of distributions, familial correlations, and heritability.
9. Linkage analysis is a valuable tool for identifying large, potentially causative chromosomal regions, typically of 5–10 MB in size, in related individuals and families.
10. Candidate gene association studies are prone to false positive results but can be useful in assessing the contribution of a variant to disease on a population basis.
11. Genome-wide association studies are a valuable and highly productive method of interrogating the vast majority of genomic variation, in a relatively "agnostic" way, to identify genetic variants related to complex diseases.

Conclusion

Cardiovascular diseases present significant challenges to the identification of genetic factors related to human health and disease, primarily because the vast majority of cardiovascular disease is likely due to the interplay of multiple genetic and environmental factors. Like many other fields, much of the early success in gene discovery in cardiovascular disease has been in single gene, "Mendelian" disorders such as familial cardiomyopathy and arrhythmia syndromes (Robin et al. 2007). The relevance of traditional genetic epidemiologic approaches such as family linkage studies to complex disorders is less clear, and more recent successes such as genome-wide association studies have arisen from research in unrelated individuals. Newer technologies are on the horizon for assaying rarer genetic variants than are currently captured by genome-wide studies, and for assaying epigenetic modifications such as DNA methylation and histone modification that may regulate the expression of genes (Shendure et al. 2004; Bernstein et al. 2007).

Much epidemiologic research remains to be done before a large number of genetic variants will be ready for clinical use on a large scale, though here again single gene disorders will likely lead the way (Robin et al. 2007). In the interim, however, identification of persons with strong family histories of cardiovascular disease is an outstanding approach for selecting those at high risk for targeted interventions, even if those interventions are limited to more aggressive application of proven risk reduction strategies for other risk factors (Guttmacher et al. 2004). Fruitful areas of research in genetic epidemiology to facilitate the discovery and application of genetic risk information are likely to include improved methods for measuring environmental exposures, identification of intermediate phenotypic traits with high heritability, investigation of beneficial environmental exposures to reduce the adverse impact of deleterious variants, and examination of phenotypic and environmental correlates of potentially causative variants in well-characterized cohort studies. The future of genetic epidemiology has never been brighter.

References

Arad M, Seidman JG, Seidman CE. Phenotypic diversity in hypertrophic cardiomyopathy. *Hum Mol Genet.* 2002;11(20):2499–2506.

Arking DE, Pfeufer A, Post W, et al. A common genetic variant in the NOS1 regulator NOS1AP modulates cardiac repolarization. *Nat Genet.* 2006;38(6):644–651.

Arnar DO, Thorvaldsson S, Manolio TA, et al. Familial aggregation of atrial fibrillation in Iceland. *Eur Heart J.* 2006;27(6):708–712.

Austin MA. The Kaiser-Permanente Women Twins Study data set. *Genet Epidemiol.* 1993;10(6):519–522.

Barrett-Connor E, Khaw K. Family history of heart attack as an independent predictor of death due to cardiovascular disease. *Circulation.* 1984;69(6):1065–1069.

Berg K. Twin studies of coronary heart disease and its risk factors. *Acta Genet Med Gemellol (Roma).* 1987;36(4):439–453.

Bernstein BE, Meissner A, Lander ES. The mammalian epigenome. *Cell.* 2007;128(4):669–681.

Blangero J, Almasy L. Multipoint oligogenic linkage analysis of quantitative traits. *Genet Epidemiol.* 1997;14(6):959–964.

Boerwinkle E, Chakraborty R, Sing CF. The use of measured genotype information in the analysis of quantitative phenotypes in man. I. Models and analytical methods. *Ann Hum Genet.* 1986;50(Pt 2):181–194.

Botstein D, Risch N. Discovering genotypes underlying human phenotypes: past successes for mendelian disease, future approaches for complex disease. *Nat Genet.* 2003;33(suppl):228–237.

Bowles NE, Bowles KR, Towbin JA. The "final common pathway" hypothesis and inherited cardiovascular disease. The role of cytoskeletal proteins in dilated cardiomyopathy. *Herz.* 2000;25(3):168–175.

Brooks-Wilson A, Marcil M, Clee SM, et al. Mutations in ABC1 in Tangier disease and familial high-density lipoprotein deficiency. *Nat Genet.* 1999;22(4):336–345.

Burton PR, Hansell AL, Fortier I, et al. Size matters: realistic power calculations for genetic association studies in the genomics age. *Int J Epidemiol.* 2009;38(1):263–273.

Burton PR, Tobin MD, Hopper JL. Key concepts in genetic epidemiology. *Lancet.* 2005;366(9489):941–951.

Capell BC, Collins FS, Nabel EG. Mechanisms of cardiovascular disease in accelerated aging syndromes. *Circ Res.* 2007;101(1):13–26.

Cavalli-Sforza LL, Bodmer WF. *The Genetics of Human Populations.* San Francisco: W.H. Freeman and Company; 1971.

Chanock SJ, Manolio T, Boehnke M, et al. Replicating genotype-phenotype associations. *Nature.* 2007;447(7145):655–660.

Chien KL, Hsu HC, Su TC, Chen MF, Lee YT. Heritability and major gene effects on left ventricular mass in the Chinese population: a family study. *BMC Cardiovasc Disord.* 2006;6:37.

Clarke R, Xu P, Bennett D, Lewington S, et al. Lymphotoxin-alpha gene and risk of myocardial infarction in 6,928 cases and 2,712 controls in the ISIS case-control study. *PLoS Genet.* 2006;2(7):e107.

Cohen JC, Kiss RS, Pertsemlidis A, Marcel YL, McPherson R, Hobbs HH. Multiple rare alleles contribute to low plasma levels of HDL cholesterol. *Science.* 2004;305(5685):869–872.

Colditz GA, Stampfer MJ, Willett WC, Rosner B, Speizer FE, Hennekens CH. A prospective study of parental history of myocardial infarction and coronary heart disease in women. *Am J Epidemiol.* 1986;123(1):48–58.

Deutscher S, Epstein FH, Keller JB. Relationships between familial aggregation of coronary heart disease and risk factors in the general population. *Am J Epidemiol.* 1969;89(5):510–520.

Deutscher S, Ostrander LD, Epstein FH. Familial factors in premature coronary heart disease—a preliminary report from the Tecumseh Community Health Study. *Am J Epidemiol.* 1970;91(3):233–237.

Dockery DW. Epidemiologic evidence of cardiovascular effects of particulate air pollution. *Environ Health Perspect.* 2001;109(suppl 4):483–486.

Dudbridge F, Gusnanto A, Koeleman BP. Detecting multiple associations in genome-wide studies. *Hum Genomics.* 2006;2(5):310–317.

Eaves L, Foley D, Silberg J. Has the "Equal Environments" assumption been tested in twin studies? *Twin Res.* 2003;6(6):486–489.

Ellison RC, Myers RH, Zhang Y, et al. Effects of similarities in lifestyle habits on familial aggregation of high density lipoprotein and low density lipoprotein cholesterol: the NHLBI Family Heart Study. *Am J Epidemiol.* 1999;150(9):910–918.

Elston RC. Segregation analysis. *Adv Hum Genet.* 1981;11:63–120.

Evans A, Van Baal GC, McCarron P, et al. The genetics of coronary heart disease: the contribution of twin studies. *Twin Res.* 2003;6(5):432–441.

Falconer DS, Mackay TFC. *Introduction to Quantitative Genetics.* 4th ed. Harlow, Essex: Addison Wesley Longman Limited; 1996.

Fellay J, Shianna KV, Ge D, et al. A whole-genome association study of major determinants for host control of HIV-1. *Science.* 2007;317(5840): 944–947.

Fisher RA. The correlation between relatives on the supposition of Mendelian inheritance. *Trans Roy Soc Edinburgh.* 1918;52:399–433.

Friedlander Y, Kark JD, Sinnreich R, Edwards KL, Austin MA. Inheritance of LDL peak particle diameter: results from a segregation analysis in Israeli families. *Genet Epidemiol.* 1999;16(4):382–396.

Friedlander Y, Kark JD, Stein Y. Family history of myocardial infarction as an independent risk factor for coronary heart disease. *Br Heart J.* 1985;53(4):382–387.

Gretarsdottir S, Sveinbjornsdottir S, Jonsson HH, et al. Localization of a susceptibility gene for common forms of stroke to 5q12. *Am J Hum Genet.* 2002;70(3):593–603.

Grimaldi MP, Vasto S, Balistreri CR, et al. Genetics of inflammation in age-related atherosclerosis: its relevance to pharmacogenomics. *Ann N Y Acad Sci.* 2007;1100:123–131.

Gudbjartsson DF, Arnar DO, Helgadottir A, et al. Variants conferring risk of atrial fibrillation on chromosome 4q25. *Nature.* 2007;448(7151): 353–357.

Gulcher J, Kong A, Stefansson K. The genealogic approach to human genetics of disease. *Cancer J.* 2001;7(1):61–68.

Guo X, Rotimi C, Cooper R, et al. Evidence of a major gene effect for angiotensinogen among Nigerians. *Ann Hum Genet.* 1999;63(Pt 4):293–300.

Guttmacher AE, Collins FS, Carmona RH. The family history—more important than ever. *N Engl J Med.* 2004;351(22):2333–2336.

Halushka MK, Fan JB, Bentley K, et al. Patterns of single-nucleotide polymorphisms in candidate genes for blood-pressure homeostasis. *Nat Genet.* 1999;22(3):239–247.

Harrap SB, Stebbing M, Hopper JL, Hoang HN, Giles GG. Familial patterns of covariation for cardiovascular risk factors in adults: The Victorian Family Heart Study. *Am J Epidemiol.* 2000;152(8):704–715.

Hattersley AT, McCarthy MI. What makes a good genetic association study? *Lancet.* 2005;366(9493):1315–1323.

Helgadottir A, Manolescu A, Thorleifsson G, et al. The gene encoding 5-lipoxygenase activating protein confers risk of myocardial infarction and stroke. *Nat Genet.* 2004;36(3):233–239.

Helgadottir A, Thorleifsson G, Manolescu A, et al. A common variant on chromosome 9p21 affects the risk of myocardial infarction. *Science.* 2007;316(5830):1491–1493.

Higgins M. Epidemiology and prevention of coronary heart disease in families. *Am J Med.* 2000;108(5):387–395.

Hines LM, Stampfer MJ, Ma J, et al. Genetic variation in alcohol dehydrogenase and the beneficial effect of moderate alcohol consumption on myocardial infarction. *N Engl J Med.* 2001;344(8):549–555.

Hirschhorn JN, Lohmueller K, Byrne E, Hirschhorn K. A comprehensive review of genetic association studies. *Genet Med.* 2002;4(2):45–61.

Ho CY, Seidman CE. A contemporary approach to hypertrophic cardiomyopathy. *Circulation.* 2006;113(24):e858–e862.

Hopkins PN, Williams RR. Human genetics and coronary heart disease: a public health perspective. *Annu Rev Nutr.* 1989;9:303–345.

Hunt SC, Williams RR, Barlow GK. A comparison of positive family history definitions for defining risk of future disease. *J Chronic Dis.* 1986;39(10):809–821.

Hunter DJ. Gene-environment interactions in human diseases. *Nat Rev Genet.* 2005;6(4):287–298.

Hunter DJ, Kraft P. Drinking from the fire hose--statistical issues in genomewide association studies. *N Engl J Med.* 2007;357(5):436–439.

International HapMap Consortium. The International HapMap Project. *Nature.* 2003;426(6968):789–796.

International HapMap Consortium. A haplotype map of the human genome. *Nature.* 2005;437(7063):1299–1320.

International Human Genome Sequencing Consortium. Finishing the euchromatic sequence of the human genome. *Nature.* 2004;431(7011): 931–945.

Jacques PF, Bostom AG, Williams RR, et al. Relation between folate status, a common mutation in methylenetetrahydrofolate reductase, and plasma homocysteine concentrations. *Circulation.* 1996;93(1):7–9.

Khoury MJ, Beaty TH, Cohen BH, eds. *Fundamentals of Genetic Epidemiology.* New York: Oxford University Press; 1993.

Klein RJ, Zeiss C, Chew EY, et al. Complement factor H polymorphism in age-related macular degeneration. *Science.* 2005;308(5720):385–389.

Knuiman MW, Divitini ML, Welborn TA, Bartholomew HC. Familial correlations, cohabitation effects, and heritability for cardiovascular risk factors. *Ann Epidemiol.* 1996;6(3):188–194.

Kotowski IK, Pertsemlidis A, Luke A, et al. A spectrum of PCSK9 alleles contributes to plasma levels of low-density lipoprotein cholesterol. *Am J Hum Genet.* 2006;78(3):410–422.

Lander ES, Schork NJ. Genetic dissection of complex traits. *Science.* 1994;265:2037–2048.

Le Marchand L, Wilkens LR, Kolonel LN, Henderson BE. The MTHFR C677T polymorphism and colorectal cancer: the multiethnic cohort study. *Cancer Epidemiol Biomarkers Prev.* 2005;14(5):1198–1203.

Lifton RP. Genetic dissection of human blood pressure variation: common pathways from rare phenotypes. *Harvey Lect.* 2004–2005;100:71–101.

Lohmueller KE, Pearce CL, Pike M, Lander ES, Hirschhorn JN. Meta-analysis of genetic association studies supports a contribution of common variants to susceptibility to common disease. *Nat Genet.* 2003;33(2):177–182.

Manolio TA, Bailey-Wilson JE, Collins FS. Genes, environment and the value of prospective cohort studies. *Nat Rev Genet.* 2006;7(10):812–820.

Manolio TA, Boerwinkle E, O'Donnell CJ, Wilson AF. Genetics of ultrasonographic carotid atherosclerosis. *Arterioscler Thromb Vasc Biol.* 2004;24(9):1567–1577.

McPherson R, Pertsemlidis A, Kavaslar N, et al. A common allele on chromosome 9 associated with coronary heart disease. *Science.* 2007;316(5830):1488–1491.

Mullis KB, Faloona EA. Specific synthesis of DNA in vitro via a polymerase-catalyzed chain reaction. *Methods Enzymol.* 1987;155:335–350.

Myers RH, Kiely DK, Cupples LA, Kannel WB. Parental history is an independent risk factor for coronary artery disease: the Framingham Study. *Am Heart J.* 1990;120(4):963–969.

Nabel EG. Cardiovascular disease. *N Engl J Med.* 2003;349(1):60–72.

Neale BM, Sham PC. The future of association studies: gene-based analysis and replication. *Am J Hum Genet.* 2004;75(3):353–362.

Neugebauer R, Ng S. Differential recall as a source of bias in epidemiologic research. *J Clin Epidemiol.* 43(1990):1337–1341.

Newton-Cheh C, Hirschhorn JN. Genetic association studies of complex traits: design and analysis issues. *Mutat Res.* 2005;573(1–2):54–69.

Niimura H, Bachinski LL, Sangwatanaroj S, et al. Mutations in the gene for cardiac myosin-binding protein C and late-onset familial hypertrophic cardiomyopathy. *N Engl J Med.* 1998;338(18):1248–1257.

Nordlie MA, Wold LE, Kloner RA. Genetic contributors toward increased risk for ischemic heart disease. *J Mol Cell Cardiol.* 2005;39(4):667–679.

O'Leary DH, Polak JF, Kronmal RA, Manolio TA, Burke GL, Wolfson SK Jr. Carotid-artery intima and media thickness as a risk factor for myocardial infarction and stroke in older adults. Cardiovascular Health Study Collaborative Research Group. *N Engl J Med.* 1999;340(1):14–22.

Ordovas JM, Corella D, Demissie S, et al. Dietary fat intake determines the effect of a common polymorphism in the hepatic lipase gene promoter on high-density lipoprotein metabolism: evidence of a strong dose effect in this gene-nutrient interaction in the Framingham Study. *Circulation.* 2002;106(18):2315–2321.

Ott J. *Analysis of Human Genetic Linkage* (revised edition). Johns Hopkins University Press, Baltimore; 1991:203–204.

Ozaki K, Ohnishi Y, Iida A, et al. Functional SNPs in the lymphotoxin-alpha gene that are associated with susceptibility to myocardial infarction. *Nat Genet.* 2002;32(4):650–654.

Patterson M, Cardon L. Replication publication. *PLoS Biol.* 2005;3(9):e327.

Perkins KA. Family history of coronary heart disease: is it an independent risk factor? *Am J Epidemiol.* 1986;124(2):182–194.

Pollex RL, Hegele RA. Complex trait locus linkage mapping in atherosclerosis: time to take a step back before moving forward? *Arterioscler Thromb Vasc Biol.* 2005;25(8):1541–1544.

Reich DE, Lander ES. On the allelic spectrum of human disease. *Trends Genet.* 2001;17(9):502–510.

Reitsma PH, Rosendaal FR. Past and future of genetic research in thrombosis. *J Thromb Haemost.* 2007;5(suppl 1):264–269.

Richardson K, Norgate S. The equal environments assumption of classical twin studies may not hold. *Br J Educ Psychol.* 2005;75(Pt 3):339–350.

Risch N. Linkage strategies for genetically complex traits. I. Multilocus models. *Am J Hum Genet.* 1990;46(2):222–228.

Risch NJ. Searching for genetic determinants in the new millennium. *Nature.* 2000;405(6788):847–856.

Robertson TL, Kato H, Gordon T, et al. Epidemiologic studies of coronary heart disease and stroke in Japanese men living in Japan, Hawaii and California. Coronary heart disease risk factors in Japan and Hawaii. *Am J Cardiol.* 1977;39:244–249.

Robin NH, Tabereaux PB, Benza R, Korf BR. Genetic testing in cardiovascular disease. *J Am Coll Cardiol.* 2007;50(8):727–737.

Roden DM. The problem, challenge and opportunity of genetic heterogeneity in monogenic diseases predisposing to sudden death. *J Am Coll Cardiol.* 2002;40(2):357–359.

Roden DM, Spooner PM. Inherited long QT syndromes: a paradigm for understanding arrhythmogenesis. *J Cardiovasc Electrophysiol.* 1999;10(12):1664–1683.

Rose G. Familial patterns in ischaemic heart disease. *Brit J Prev Soc Med.* 1964;18:75–80.

Russek HI, Zohman BL. Relative significance of heredity, diet and occupational stress in coronary heart disease of young adults; based on an analysis of 100 patients between the ages of 25 and 40 years and a similar group of 100 normal control subjects. *Am J Med Sci.* 1958;235(3):266–277.

Samani NJ, Burton P, Mangino M, et al. A genomewide linkage study of 1,933 families affected by premature coronary artery disease: the British Heart Foundation (BHF) Family Heart Study. *Am J Hum Genet.* 2005;77(6):1011–1020.

Samani NJ, Erdmann J, Hall AS, et al. Genomewide association analysis of coronary artery disease. *N Engl J Med.* 2007;357(5):443–453.

Schwartz D, Collins F. Medicine. Environmental biology and human disease. *Science.* 2007;316(5825):695–696.

Scott LJ, Mohlke KL, Bonnycastle LL, et al. A genome-wide association study of type 2 diabetes in Finns detects multiple susceptibility variants. *Science.* 2007;316(5829):1341–1345.

Shaw T, Elliott P, McKenna WJ. Dilated cardiomyopathy: a genetically heterogeneous disease. *Lancet.* 2002;360(9334):654–655.

Shendure J, Mitra RD, Varma C, Church GM. Advanced sequencing technologies: methods and goals. *Nat Rev Genet.* 2004;5(5):335–344.

Slack J, Evans KA. The increased risk of death from ischaemic heart disease in first degree relatives of 121 men and 96 women with ischaemic heart disease. *J Med Genet.* 1966;3(4):239–257.

Smith PG, Day NE. The design of case-control studies: the influence of confounding and interaction effects. *Int J Epidemiol.* 1984;13(3):356–365.

Stranger BE, Forrest MS, Clark AG, et al. Genome-wide associations of gene expression variation in humans. *PLoS Genet.* 2005;1(6):e78.

Szklo M, Nieto FN. *Epidemiology: Beyond the Basics.* Jones and Bartlett Publishers, Sudbury, MA; 2004:238–240.

Thomas CB, Cohen BH. The familial occurrence of hypertension and coronary artery disease, with observations concerning obesity and diabetes. *Ann Intern Med.* 1955;42(1):90–127.

Timberlake DS, O'Connor DT, Parmer RJ. Molecular genetics of essential hypertension: recent results and emerging strategies. *Curr Opin Nephrol Hypertens.* 2001;10(1):71–79.

Todd JA. Statistical false positive or true disease pathway? *Nat Genet.* 2006;38(7):731–733.

Trikalinos TA, Ntzani EE, Contopoulos-Ioannidis DG, Ioannidis JP. Establishment of genetic associations for complex diseases is independent of early study findings. *Eur J Hum Genet.* 2004;12(9):762–769.

Turner ST, Boerwinkle E. Genetics of blood pressure, hypertensive complications, and antihypertensive drug responses. *Pharmacogenomics.* 2003;4(1):53–65.

Wacholder S, Chanock S, Garcia-Closas M, El Ghormli L, Rothman N. Assessing the probability that a positive report is false: an approach for molecular epidemiology studies. *J Natl Cancer Inst.* 2004;96: 434–442.

Weber JL, May PE. Abundant class of human DNA polymorphisms which can be typed using the polymerase chain reaction. *Am J Hum Genet.* 1989;44(3):388–396.

Weeks DE, Lange K. A multilocus extension of the affected-pedigree-member method of linkage analysis. *Am J Hum Genet.* 1992;50(4): 859–868.

Wellcome Trust Case Control Consortium. Genome-wide association study of 14,000 cases of seven common diseases and 3,000 shared controls. *Nature.* 2007;447(7145):661–678.

Williams RR, Hopkins PN, Stephenson S, Wu L, Hunt SC. Primordial prevention of cardiovascular disease through applied genetics. *Prev Med.* 1999;29(6 Pt 2):S41–S49.

Williams RR, Hunt SC, Hasstedt SJ, et al. Multigenic human hypertension: evidence for subtypes and hope for haplotypes. *J Hypertens Suppl.* 1990;8(7):S39–S46.

Williams RR, Hunt SC, Heiss G, et al. Usefulness of cardiovascular family history data for population-based preventive medicine and medical research (the Health Family Tree Study and the NHLBI Family Heart Study). *Am J Cardiol.* 2001;87(2):129–135.

Wilson AF, Elston RC, Siervogel RM, Weinshilboum R, Ward LJ. Linkage relationships between a major gene for catechol-O-methyltransferase activity and 25 polymorphic marker systems. *Am J Med Genet.* 1984;19(3):525–532.

Wojciechowski AP, Farrall M, Cullen P, et al. Familial combined hyperlipidaemia linked to the apolipoprotein AI-CII-AIV gene cluster on chromosome 11q23-q24. *Nature.* 1991;349(6305):161–164.

5

Cytogenetic Testing in Cardiovascular Genetics

Helen Cox

Introduction

Congenital heart disease (CHD) occurs in association with aneuploidies (altered chromosomal number, e.g., trisomy 21), mosaic chromosomal abnormalities (e.g., Cat Eye syndrome), segmental deletions (of which the commonest is chromosome 22q11 deletion), and translocations. Whilst translocations are a rare cause of CHD they can lead to identification of genes with a role in cardiogenesis, which may be implicated in the etiology of other cases of isolated CHD [e.g., the elastin gene in supravalvar aortic stenosis (SVAS)]. Summaries of the well-defined clinical phenotypes associated with chromosomal imbalance are included in this chapter but it is important to be aware that CHD is common in individuals with previously unreported de novo chromosome abnormalities.

Cytogenetic Techniques—Past, Present, and Future

Human chromosomes have been studied by examining lymphocytes treated by G-banding using light microscopy since the 1960s (Seabright 1971). Figure 5–1 shows the normal complement of 46 chromosomes—22 pairs of autosomes and the sex chromosomes. The characteristic banding pattern of each chromosome allows it to be identified and facilitates the detection of gains or losses of over approximately 5 Mb (megabases) at the highest possible resolution. Modifications in cell culture conditions have improved resolution; however, gain or loss of up to 5 Mb may not be visible on high-resolution (850 bands per haploid genome) chromosome analysis. This is equivalent to gain or loss of in the order of tens of genes.

The introduction of new molecular cytogenetic techniques, particularly array-based comparative genomic hybridization (aCGH) is bringing higher resolution chromosome analysis into the diagnostic laboratory. Gains or losses of 500 kb (kilobases) or less can be detected, which may contain as few as one gene. The human genome project has clarified the sequence of the human genome, and microarray results have the potential to clarify the human disease phenotypes caused by gains or losses of specific genes.

Cytogenetic Methods Used to Diagnose Chromosome Abnormalities

About 1% of newborns have abnormal chromosomes when tested using conventional cytogenetics (Jacobs et al. 1992). The clinical features found in individuals with common chromosome abnormalities have been studied extensively (see below for descriptions of abnormalities commonly causing CHD).

Sometimes, the phenotype of a specific chromosome imbalance is found when the karyotype is normal using conventional cytogenetic methods. For example, chromosome 22 rearrangements were found by conventional cytogenetics in an infant with DiGeorge syndrome before it was recognized that submicroscopic deletions of chromosome 22q11 were responsible for over 95% of cases of DiGeorge syndrome. Submicroscopic deletions have been identified using fluorescence in situ hybridization (FISH) since the 1990s. FISH tests are requested when a specific microdeletion is suspected based on the clinical picture. Figure 5–2 shows images obtained from a patient with deletion of chromosome 22q11.2.

When to Check Chromosomes in the Patient with Congenital Heart Disease

The standard G-banded karyotype is abnormal in 12.9% of patients with CHD (Ferencz et al. 1989). A number of syndromes are now known to be associated with chromosomal deletions that are not reliably detected by standard karyotyping. These account for an additional unknown percentage of all cases of CHD.

Suggested indications for requesting a karyotype for a patient with CHD include

- If there are multiple congenital malformations, dysmorphic features, pre- and postnatal retardation of growth, unexplained developmental delay, or any combination of these features in association with CHD, but the features do not fit with a recognizable pattern (syndrome), chromosome analysis should be requested.
- Chromosome analysis should also be undertaken when there is a family history of congenital malformations as the index case and other affected individuals might have inherited an

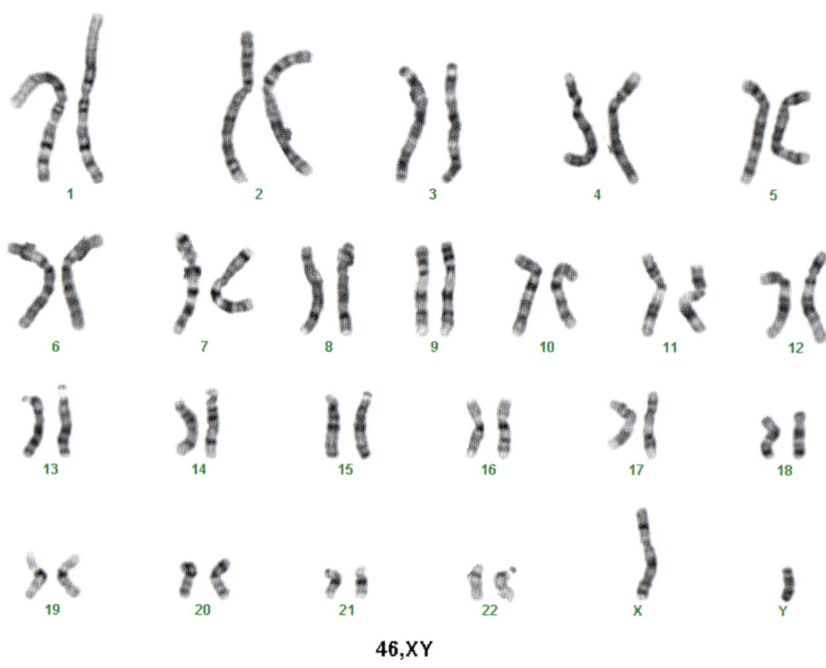

Figure 5–1 The normal male chromosome complement, 46,XY. G-banding has been used to stain the chromosomes. The recognizable pattern of dark and light bands also facilitates identification of small gains or losses of chromosome material.

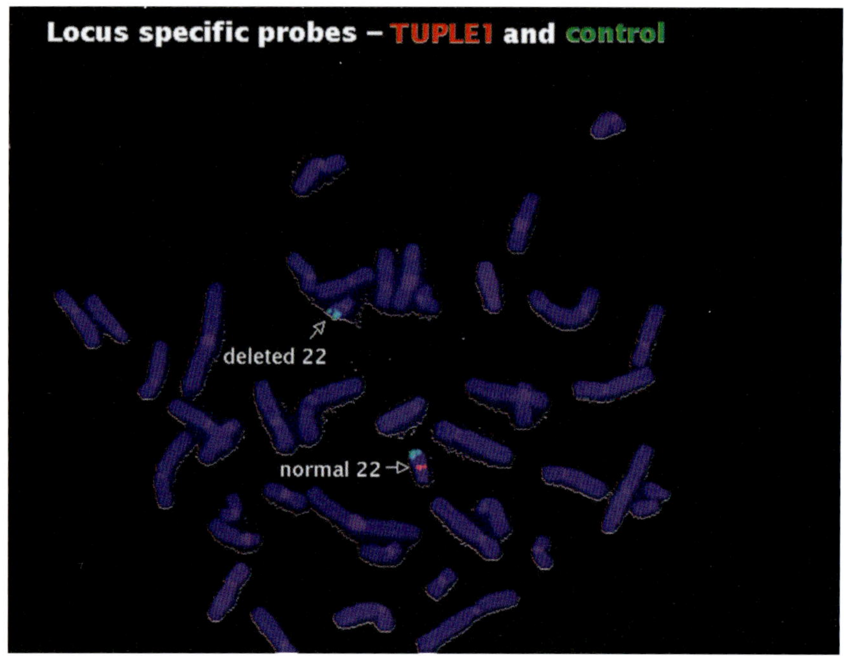

Figure 5–2 FISH in a patient with 22q11 deletion. The green control probe hybridizes to the end of the long arm, identifying both copies of chromosome 22. The red TUPLE1 probe hybridizes to 22q11.2, which is deleted from one chromosome 22.

unbalanced (meaning chromosome material has been gained and/or lost) chromosome rearrangement from an unaffected parent carrying a balanced (no apparent gain or loss of chromosome) or unbalanced translocation.

There is evidence that certain types of CHD are more or less likely to be associated with a chromosome abnormality (Harris et al. 2003). For example, at one end of the spectrum 0.9% of children with transposition of the great arteries (d-TGV) have a chromosome abnormality, compared to 68.4% with endocardial cushion defects. In postnatal life, this knowledge is less useful in deciding which children's chromosomes to check and which not to than careful clinical assessment and following the guidelines laid out above. However, when there is a statistically significant association between a cardiac defect and a *specific* chromosome imbalance, it may tell us about genomic regions that contain genes important for specific aspects of cardiac development and, as such, is useful to the study of developmental genetics of the heart.

If a child is found to have a chromosomal translocation (balanced or unbalanced) parental chromosomes should also be analyzed. For straightforward trisomies it is not necessary to analyze parental chromosomes. Chromosome deletions (or duplications) associated with severe developmental delay are usually de novo but it is important to check parental karyotypes if the phenotypic spectrum associated with a deletion is variable as finding that the deletion is inherited has implications for recurrence risks.

How Karyotyping Has Changed Our Clinical Practice

The ability to study chromosomes has made it possible to confirm clinical diagnoses, to anticipate the natural history of a child's condition and to provide appropriate management. It has also led to identification of new syndromes.

- The association between Down syndrome and CHD was recognized many years before the cause of Down syndrome, namely having three copies of chromosome 21, was known (Lejeune et al. 1959). By checking chromosomes, clinical diagnoses such as Down syndrome can be confirmed.
- The clinician can use the karyotype to identify those individuals whose CHD is caused by chromosome imbalance and manage them accordingly. For example, the child with 22q11 deletion and CHD is at risk of hypocalcemia predisposing to seizures, immunodeficiency, and congenital renal anomalies, all of which should be screened for (Greenhalgh et al. 2003).
- Clinicians have been able to identify and define new syndromes caused by chromosome imbalance. For example, deletion of chromosome 1p36 is associated with CHD in 71% and noncompaction cardiomyopathy in 23% (Battaglia et al. 2008). The distinctive dysmorphic features and the developmental profile of individuals with this deletion are described below. This knowledge can be used by clinicians to diagnose the deletion and by clinicians and families to guide management.
- Families have been able to make use of the results of chromosome analysis to understand the cause of their child's developmental abnormalities and to help them to make reproductive decisions. Knowing that a specific chromosome abnormality is responsible for CHD allows them to get accurate advice on the chances of recurrence and, if desired, prenatal testing in future pregnancies. As outcomes for children born with CHD improve and growing numbers have children of their own, a cytogenetic diagnosis informs advice offered about recurrence risk. For example, the patient with 22q11 deletion can receive genetic counseling to understand the 50% offspring risk and the types of clinical problem that can occur with this chromosome abnormality. The option of pre- or postnatal testing is available to plan management.

The following brief summaries are not intended to be comprehensive accounts of the phenotypes seen in chromosome abnormalities. For such descriptions, the reader is referred to reference works including Smith's *Recognizable Patterns of Human Malformations* (Jones 2006), *Malformations of the Head and Neck* (Gorlin et al. 2001), and *Catalogue of Unbalanced Chromosome Aberrations in Man* (Schinzel 2001). Each account aims to highlight interesting aspects of the CHD associated with the chromosome abnormality. The genetics of cardiovascular development is complex—different children with the same chromosome abnormality have different cardiovascular malformations (CVMs), so knowledge of a child's karyotype is a poor predictor of cardiovascular anatomy. However, knowing that a child has a chromosome abnormality associated with a high incidence of CHD will make the clinician more likely to undertake a detailed cardiovascular assessment. Similarly, although some CVMs are strongly associated with a specific chromosome abnormality (e.g., atrioventricular septal defect [AVSD] and Down syndrome, conotruncal malformations, and 22q11 deletion), the majority of children with CHD (particularly those who are nondysmorphic and have no other congenital malformations) have normal chromosomes.

Chromosome Aneuploidies Associated with CHD

Down Syndrome (Trisomy 21)

The birth prevalence of Down syndrome is approximately 1/700. Babies with Down syndrome are hypotonic and have a flat facial profile with upslanting palpebral fissures, brachycephaly, and small round ears. In some infants there is redundant nuchal skin. Single palmar creases are present in just under half of affected children and the most frequent extracardiac congenital malformation is duodenal atresia. Atlantoaxial instability affects 12%–20%. Short stature and developmental delay are seen during childhood. Approximately, a quarter of individuals with Down syndrome have seizures, often of adult onset. Provision of medical services for ongoing surveillance for hypothyroidism and celiac disease and assessment of mental state for signs of depression as much as for Alzheimer's disease is important for adults with Down syndrome. In a study of 481 children with Down syndrome undertaken by Digilio and colleagues, 381 (80%) had CHD. These comprised 229 AVSD cases (47%), 121 ventricular septal defect (VSD) (25%), 25 tetralogy of fallot (TOF), 3 atrial septal defect (ASD), and 3 with an isolated mitral cleft (Marino 1996). In addition to the congenital malformations, mitral valve prolapse and aortic regurgitation in adult life are more common in Down syndrome than in the general population, mitral valve prolapse occurring in 44%–57% of adults with Down syndrome and aortic regurgitation in approximately 11%–14% (Hamada et al. 1998).

The majority of cases of Down syndrome are caused by straightforward free trisomy 21 and in these cases there is no need to karyotype parents. In 5% of cases the additional chromosome 21 is due to an unbalanced translocation, classically though not in all cases a Robertsonian translocation, in which two acrocentric chromosomes have fused at the centromere or within the short arm. In these cases parental karyotyping should be arranged because a parent carrying a balanced Robertsonian translocation involving chromosome 21 is at risk of future recurrence of Down syndrome.

Edwards Syndrome (Trisomy 18)

Trisomy 18 or Edwards syndrome is the second most common autosomal aneuploidy after Down syndrome. In a review of trisomy 18 over a 6-year period in Northern England 66 babies and fetuses were identified in 282,583 births giving a prevalence at 18 weeks gestation of 1 in 4,274 and a birth prevalence of 1 in 8,333 (Embleton et al. 1996).

This is an important bedside diagnosis, because the poor prognosis influences medical management. Median survival of those born alive was 3 days with no babies living longer than a year though the cardiac problem was rarely implicated as the cause of death (Embleton et al. 1996).

The typical finger clenching with second and fifth overlapping third and fourth is a useful diagnostic clue. Babies are small for gestational age, have a prominent occiput, low-set ears, micrognathia, small palpebral fissures, and a short sternum. Extracardiac malformations can affect most systems, but commonly the gastrointestinal (e.g., umbilical hernia, omphalocele) and urogenital systems (horseshoe kidney, hydronephrosis, polycystic kidneys) are involved.

Echocardiograms or autopsy findings were available for 25 cases and CHD was found in 21 of these (87% of those for whom there was data). These twenty-one cases comprised seven VSD, five AVSD, three hypoplastic left heart (HLH), two double outlet right ventricle (DORV), one TOF, one subvalvar pulmonary stenosis, one transposition of the great arteries (TGA), and one coarctation of the aorta (COA) (Embleton et al. 1996).

Patau Syndrome (Trisomy 13)

In a review of trisomy 13 over an 8-year period in Northern England, 36 cases were reviewed, 16 of which were born alive giving a birth prevalence of 1 in 20,258 (0.049/1000 live births) (Wyllie et al. 1994).

Cleft lip and/or palate (often bilateral), postaxial polydactyly, structural brain abnormalities (commonly holoprosencephaly), scalp defects, and other congenital malformations are frequent features of trisomy 13. As for trisomy 18, early diagnosis is important because the poor prognosis influences medical management. The median survival in this series was 4 days and the longest survival 3.5 months (Wyllie et al. 1994).

Echocardiography or postmortem findings were available for 14 of the 16 cases, only 2 of which had a normal heart. The twelve CVMs comprised five VSD, two ASD and VSD, one AVSD, one TOF, one DORV, one VSD with pulmonary stenosis (PS), and one case of left isomerism (Wyllie et al. 1994).

Most cases of Patau syndrome have straightforward trisomy 13. In these cases there is no need to karyotype parents. In others the additional chromosome 13 is due to an unbalanced translocation, classically though not in all cases a Robertsonian translocation. In these cases parental karyotyping should be arranged because a parent carrying a balanced Robertsonian translocation involving chromosome 13 is at risk of future recurrence of Patau syndrome.

Turner Syndrome

The birth incidence of Turner syndrome is approximately 1/2,000 girls (Gøtzsche et al. 1994).

Redundant nuchal skin or neck webbing, a low posterior hairline, edema of the dorsum of hands and feet in the perinatal period that resolves later, and deep-set, hyperconvex nails may lead the clinician to suspect Turner syndrome. The chest can be broad, the nipples widespaced. CHD affects less than 50% (estimates vary between series), and up to 60% have structural renal malformations (e.g., horseshoe kidney). Growth retardation, failure to develop secondary sexual characteristics, and infertility all occur in girls with a 45,X karyotype. Intelligence is in the normal range in most cases.

Regarding the CVM found among girls with Turner syndrome, those with a 45,X karyotype had aortic coarctation and/or aortic valve malformations in 38% in one population-based series (Gøtzsche et al. 1994).

A karyotype of 45,X is seen in approximately 50% of cases (Birkebaek et al. 2002) but others have structural abnormalities of the X chromosome, of which there are many variations including isochromosomes comprising two copies of Xq(iXq), deletions, and mosaicism. Phenotype, including the risk of CVM, can vary with the specific karyotype. All clinical features can be milder or even absent if there is mosaicism with a normal cell line. Girls with mosaicism can have normal secondary sexual development and fertility followed by premature ovarian failure.

Mosaic Chromosome Abnormalities Associated with CHD

Cat Eye Syndrome

Cat eye syndrome is the name given to the phenotype caused by tetrasomy for 22q11.2. The name derives from the coloboma of the iris seen in around 60% (Rosias et al. 2001). Colobomata can be unilateral or bilateral and can extend to involve the choroid and retina. Preauricular pits and tags are found in around 87% of cases (Rosias et al. 2001). In addition, the pinna can be malformed or even absent, with or without associated atresia of the external auditory meatus. Unlike other chromosome abnormalities, cat eye syndrome can be associated with normal growth in at least 50% of affected children and development can be normal, with 50% showing developmental delay of mild to moderate severity (Rosias et al. 2001). Urogenital abnormalities (such as horseshoe kidneys, unilateral renal hypoplasia, imperforate anus with a fistula, and cryptorchidism in males) and CHD both affect at least one-third of patients.

Cardiac abnormalities include anomalous pulmonary venous drainage in 19% (Rosias et al. 2001).

The additional piece of chromosome, made up of two copies of material from chromosome 22, is identifiable on a standard karyotype as an extra piece of chromosome (a marker extra structurally abnormal or ESAC chromosome). As the marker chromosome is unstable, it is often lost from some cells, leading to the mosaic karyotype (see Chapter 9).

Chromosome Deletions and Microdeletions Associated with CHD

Cri du Chat Syndrome

The incidence of this microdeletion syndrome is 1/50,000 in newborn infants. Cri du Chat syndrome should be suspected in a child with pre- and postnatal growth retardation, microcephaly, a "catlike" cry in infancy (from which the syndrome takes its name), and developmental delay. It is important to look for the characteristic round face, hypertelorism, high nasal bridge, micrognathia, as, as with other microdeletion syndromes, many cases are only diagnosed after a specific FISH test is requested. Talipes, congenital hip dislocation, and inguinal herniae are described. Tone improves beyond infancy and the facial characteristics described above change (Van Buggenhout et al. 2000). Premature graying of the hair is seen in adulthood. CHD is estimated to affect between 15% and 20% of patients, as summarized by Hills et al. (2006).

A review of published cases found that around 40% of children with CHD had a septal defect (mostly VSD, some ASD). A further 40% had patent ductus arteriosus (PDA) and up to 10% had either TOF or pulmonary stenosis (Hills et al. 2006). Although percentages vary between series, septal defects and PDA are consistently most common.

The cause of Cri du Chat syndrome is a microdeletion of chromosome 5p. Some larger deletions are detected on a standard karyotype; however, if the diagnosis is strongly suspected and the karyotype appears normal, FISH testing should be requested. In 85% of cases there is a de novo deletion of 5p and 15% of cases are the unbalanced product of a parental balanced translocation. The latter will have a risk of recurrence in future pregnancies, so genetic counseling—and karyotyping—for parents is important.

Chromosome 1p36 Deletion

Deletion of chromosome 1p36 is among those microdeletion syndromes that have been more recently identified. Its incidence has been estimated to be as high as 1 in 5,000 (Heilstedt et al. 2003). Developmental delay, hypotonia, and seizures are associated with a characteristic facial appearance, with deep-set eyes, straight eyebrows, and a broad nasal bridge.

In addition to structural heart defects, cardiomyopathy also occurs. For example, in one series deletion of chromosome 1p36 was associated with CHD in 71% and noncompaction cardiomyopathy in 23% (Battaglia et al. 2008). Septal defects (VSD, ASD) are most frequent, but a significant proportion of children are also born with PDA, TOF, and valve abnormalities (Battaglia et al. 2008). Chromosome 1p36 deletion is particularly interesting because of its association with Ebstein anomaly and other tricuspid valve defects.

Deletions vary in size—some are cytogenetically visible but the majority are only identified with a specific FISH test. For example, in one series around 25% of deletions were cytogenetically visible (Battaglia et al. 2008).

Chromosome 11q23-qter Deletion (Jacobsen Syndrome)

Terminal deletion of the long arm of chromosome 11 is an uncommon chromosome abnormality affecting fewer than 1 in 100,000 children (Penny et al. 1995). CHD is common in affected individuals, with an excess of HLH.

Jacobsen syndrome is the eponymous name given to terminal 11q deletions. There is a distinctive clinical phenotype that includes congenital malformations affecting the CVS, thrombocytopenia and abnormal leukocyte function, craniosynostosis, renal tract, CNS and eye malformations, and facial dysmorphism. Reviews have described and compared the physical characteristics of over 100 individuals with partial monosomy for 11q (Grossfeld et al. 2004). Some clinical problems associated with 11q deletions are distinctive; for example, metopic synostosis causing trigonocephaly accounts for less than 20% of craniosynostosis overall but affects over half of Jacobsen syndrome patients (Grossfeld et al. 2004). An unusual type of thrombocytopenia (Paris-Trousseau thrombocytopenia; Breton-Gorius et al. 1995) affects up to 94% of patients in some series (Grossfeld et al. 2004). Between 50% and 60% of patients have CHD.

The CHD seen in Jacobsen syndrome is also distinctive. HLH accounts for around 1.5% of all cases of CHD overall, yet 13% of individuals with 11q23-qter deletion have HLH and an additional 11% have mitral stenosis. These probably reflect the same developmental abnormality as severe mitral stenosis or mitral atresia forms part of HLH (Grossfeld 1999).

In most cases of Jacobsen syndrome a cytogenetically visible 11q deletion is identified. This can be de novo or it can be the unbalanced product of a balanced parental translocation.

Chromosome 22q11 Deletion

The phenotype associated with chromosome 22q11 deletion is highly variable. CHD, cleft palate or velopharyngeal insufficiency, hypocalcemia, and immunodeficiency are all well recognized features. Growth retardation, developmental delay, particularly speech and language delay, structural renal tract anomalies, and an increased risk of psychiatric disorder in adult life occur. Although the association between the deletion and a phenotype was first detected through investigation of children with DiGeorge syndrome it rapidly became apparent that the same deletion was present in children with velocardiofacial syndrome (VCFS) and conotruncal anomaly face syndrome (Burn et al. 1993). The term "22q11 deletion syndrome" is more useful than the eponyms "DiGeorge" and "VCFS" because there is such marked phenotypic variation. Within a single family one can find individuals who have never presented to medical attention, individuals with velopharyngeal insufficiency and learning difficulties and also individuals with hypocalcemia, low T cell counts, and CHD (DiGeorge syndrome) all resulting from the same deletion.

Congenital heart disease affects 75% (Ryan et al. 1997). Of these 14% have VSDs, 14% have interruption of the aortic arch, 10% have pulmonary atresia (with or without VSD), and 17% have TOF (Ryan et al. 1997). A further 9% have truncus arteriosus—overall, a high proportion of all children with 22q11 deletion have serious CHD that is likely to require surgical correction or palliation.

The deletion is rarely visible on routine karyotype hence a specific test should be requested when the diagnosis is considered, either FISH on chromosome spreads or a DNA-based test depending on your diagnostic laboratory. Around 90% of deletions are de novo, 10% are familial, so genetic counseling is recommended. Clinical presentation in an affected parent or sibling can be mild. Parental karyotyping should always be performed.

The principle of investigating the relatively small genomic region shared in common by CHD patients with microdeletion syndromes to find a gene or genes that are involved in cardiogenesis is well illustrated by research that identified *TBX1*. There are two lines of evidence that *TBX1*, a cardiac transcription factor within the 22q11 deleted region is a major player in the cardiac phenotype.

In 2001, Lindsay et al. found that mice heterozygous for a deletion that included *TBX1* had aortic arch abnormalities (Lindsay et al. 2001). A second group went on to show that the cardiac phenotype was partially rescued by a BAC containing the human *TBX1* gene (Merscher et al. 2001). Jerome and Papaioannou produced a *TBX1* null mutation in the mouse (Jerome and Papaioannou 2001). Mice heterozygous for this mutation had a high incidence of cardiac outflow tract anomalies. Homozygous mice had additional congenital malformations, including thymic and parathyroid hypoplasia, cleft palate, abnormal facial structures, and vertebral anomalies (Jerome and Papaioannou 2001). This phenotype closely resembles that seen across the spectrum of 22q11.2 deletions. Since *TBX1* was first proposed as the gene responsible for the cardiac phenotype in 22q11.2 deletion, point mutations in this gene have been found in human subjects with conotruncal heart lesions (Yagi et al. 2003). However, *TBX1* mutations do not seem to be a common cause of isolated conotruncal CVM.

Williams Syndrome

Williams syndrome is a condition causing developmental delay, short stature, hypercalcemia, and characteristic facies with stellate irides, periorbital fullness, and prominent lips.

Supravalvar aortic stenosis and peripheral pulmonary artery stenosis are typical cardiac malformations. Arterial stenosis can affect other organs (e.g., kidneys).

Similarly, in one study, of the 53% of children with Williams syndrome and CHD, 73% have SVAS and 41% have pulmonary arterial stenosis (Eronen et al. 2002).

Ninety-six percent of Williams syndrome cases have a deletion of chromosome 7q11.23 that is identified on a standard FISH test (Lowery et al. 1995).

Supravalvar aortic stenosis accounts for <1% of all CHD, but a high proportion of the cardiac defects found in patients with Williams syndrome. The explanation for this became clear as a result of the work of several research groups. The genetic basis of SVAS was elucidated through investigation of a family in which nonsyndromic SVAS segregated with a balanced chromosome translocation. One breakpoint of this reciprocal translocation disrupted the elastin gene at chromosome 7q11.23 (Curran et al. 1993), a locus that had already shown to be linked to SVAS in two unrelated families with autosomal dominant SVAS (Ewart et al. 1993). Point mutations in *ELN* have since been found in autosomal dominant SVAS (Li et al. 1997; Metcalfe et al. 2000) and *ELN* maps to the Williams syndrome critical region, confirming that this is the gene responsible for CHD in Williams syndrome. Patients who lack one functional copy of *ELN* typically have stenotic lesions of the outflow tract but the range of cardiac phenotypes includes a normal cardiovascular system to a persistent truncus arteriosus. Metcalfe et al. found point mutations in *ELN* in 35/100 SVAS patients (Metcalfe et al. 2000).

Wolf Hirschorn Syndrome

Prevalence is 1 in 50,000.

The characteristic facies, microcephaly, and pre- and postnatal growth retardation lead the clinician to suspect this diagnosis. The nasal bridge is prominent and broad, giving rise to comparison with the appearance of a "Greek Helmet." This and the arched eyebrows, sometimes associated with ptosis, make up the characteristic facial appearance. Forty-five percent have CHD, 50% have seizures, and development is delayed in the majority. Cleft palate, talipes, and hypospadias are all common.

Congenital heart defects are most often ASDs and VSDs.

The cause is a deletion of terminal 4p and, although visible on a standard karyotype in 58% of cases, specific FISH testing should be requested if this diagnosis is suspected and chromosomes are normal. Submicroscopic deletions account for the remaining 42% of cases.

About 85% of cases occur de novo. Parental karyotypes should be checked to ensure that balanced translocations involving 4p16.3 are not missed as a cause.

The Future: How Advances in Cytogenetics Could Increase Our Understanding of the Genetics of Cardiac Development

Chromosome Abnormalities and Congenital Heart Defects: Study of Unbalanced Chromosome Rearrangements

Overall around 30% of all children with a chromosome abnormality have CHD (Pierpont and Moller 1987). Some chromosome abnormalities (e.g., trisomy 18) are associated with a very high rate of CHD, whereas, in others CHD is much less common. Some chromosome deletions or duplications also have a strong association with a *specific* congenital heart defect (e.g., duplication of chromosome 21 in Down syndrome and AVSD). Researchers have used this knowledge to look for chromosome regions that may be associated with specific CVMs. Brewer et al. (1998, 1989) constructed a chromosomal map of autosomal deletions and duplications associated with 47 different congenital malformations based on clinical and cytogenetic data from 1,753 nonmosaic single autosomal deletions and 1,621 duplications. Positive associations between defined, deleted, and duplicated chromosome regions and specific malformations were found. In total, 29 chromosome regions for which deletion or duplication showed a statistically significant association with congenital heart defects were identified (Brewer et al. 1998, 1989). Those for which the association is

Table 5–1 Chromosome Regions for Which Deletion or Duplication Showed a Statistically Significant Association with Congenital Heart Defects Are Tabulated against Specific CVM for Which the Association Is Highly Statistically Significant ($p<0.001$)

Congenital Heart Defect	Deleted Chromosome Region
VSD	22q11, 4q31
Pulmonary stenosis	22q11, 20p11–13
Aortic stenosis	11q23–24
HLH	11q23–25
Truncus arteriosus	22q11, 2q22
Congenital heart defect	**Duplicated chromosome region**
PDA	16q22
VSD	8q24
Pulmonary Stenosis	8q22–24
Tetralogy of Fallot	8q22–24
HLH	16q22–24

Sources: From Brewer et al. (1998, 1989).

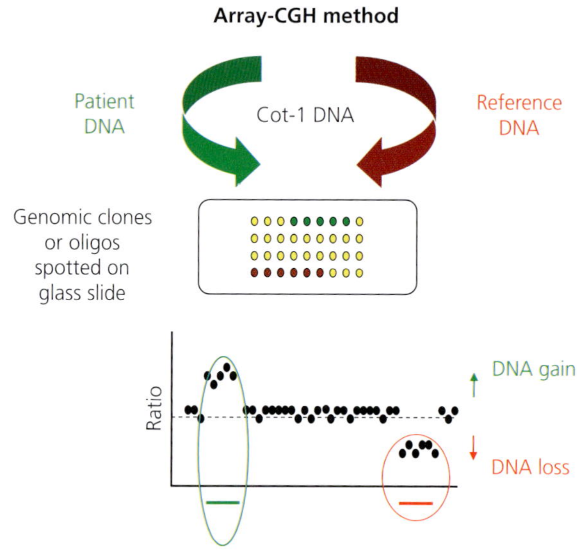

Figure 5–3 To illustrate the principles of aCGH. This molecular cytogenetic technique can identify deletions and duplications the size of which is measured in kilobases (compared with megabase imbalances detected by light microscopy, illustrated in Figure 5–1). Information on the position of the imbalance and thus the genes that lie within it is also more precise. Adapted from Fiegler H, Redon R, Carter NP. Construction and use of spotted large-insert clone DNA microarrays for the detection of genomic copy number changes. *Nature protocols.* 2007;2:(3)577, with permission.

highly statistically significant ($p<0.001$) are tabulated in Table 5–1. This included chromosome 11q23 deletion and HLH—this region has been studied in detail and a candidate gene, JAM3 has been identified (Phillips et al. 2002). The critical genes in many of these chromosome bands have yet to be found; however, each band contains a large number of genes from which candidates need to be identified.

The introduction of new molecular cytogenetic techniques, particularly array based comparative genomic hybridization (aCGH), is bringing higher resolution analysis into the diagnostic laboratory and gains or losses of as little as 500 kb can be detected. The term "genomic disorders" is used for these small deletions and duplications. Figure 5–3 is a diagram illustrating the principles of aCGH. Although this work is in its infancy it is possible that it may define new syndromes and identify much smaller critical regions containing genes that cause CHD. The genetic basis for some of the syndromes described in Chapter 10 is currently unknown and it is possible that at least some are genomic disorders.

Conclusions

Examining chromosomes using conventional cytogenetics finds an underlying diagnosis to explain the occurrence of CHD in a significant proportion of children. Using the combined skills of the cardiologist and clinical geneticist, children and families who are most likely to benefit from cytogenetic (or molecular genetic) investigation can be selected.

New ways of looking at chromosomes, especially FISH and array-based CGH, have improved on the resolution of the standard karyotype and identified the cause of CHD in more children. These advances have helped clinicians in the management of children with specific syndromes and their families who wish to understand both the cause and familial implications of their child's CHD. They offer new tools with which to investigate the genetics of cardiac development.

Acknowledgments

Thanks to the West Midlands Regional Genetics Unit for Figures 5–1 and 5–2 and to Professor Judith Goodship for her advice and collaboration.

References

Battaglia A, Hoyme HE, Dallapiccola B, et al. Further delineation of 1p36 syndrome in 60 patients: a recognizable phenotype and common cause of developmental delay and mental retardation. *Pediatrics.* 2008;121:404–410.

Birkebaek NH, Cruger D, Hansen J, Nielsen J, Buun-Petersen G. Fertility and pregnancy outcome in Danish women with Turner syndrome. *Clin Genet.* 2002;61:35–39.

Breton-Gorius J, Favier R, Guichard J, et al. A new congenital dysmegakaryopoetic thrombocytopenia (Paris-Trousseau) associated with giant platelet α-granules and chromosome 11 deletion at 11q23. *Blood.* 1995;85:1085–1814.

Brewer C, Holloway S, Zawalnyski P, Schinzel A, Fitzpatrick D. A chromosomal deletion map of human malformations. *Am J Hum Genet.* 1998;63:1153–1159.

Brewer C, Holloway S, Zawalnyski P, Schinzel A, Fitzpatrick D. A chromosomal duplication map of malformations: regions of suspected haplo- and triplolethality and tolerance of segmental aneuploidy in humans. *Am J Hum Genet.* 1999;64:1702–1708.

Burn J, Takao A, Wilson D, et al. Conotruncal face syndrome is associated with a deletion within chromosome 22q11. *J Med Genet.* 1993;30:822–824.

Curran ME, Atkinson DL, Ewart AK, Morris CA, Leppert MF, Keating MT. The elastin gene is disrupted by a translocation associated with supravalvular aortic stenosis. *Cell.* 1993;73:159–168.

Embleton ND, Wyllie JP, Wright MJ, Burn J, Hunter S. Natural history of trisomy 18. *Arch Dis Child Fetal Neonatal Ed.* 1996;75:F38–F41.

Eronen M, Peippo M, Hiippala A, et al. Cardiovascular manifestations in 75 patients with Williams Syndrome. *J Med Genet.* 2002;39:554–558.

Ewart AK, Morris CA, Ensing GJ, et al. A human vascular disorder, supravalvar aortic stenosis, maps to chromosome 7. *Proc Nat Acad Sci.* 1993;90:3226–3230.

Ferencz C, Neill CA, Boughman JA, Rubin JD, Brenner JI, Perry LW. Congenital cardiovascular malformations associated with chromosome abnormalities: an epidemiological study. *J Pediatr.* 1989;114:79–86.

Fiegler H, Redon R, Carter NP. Construction and use of spotted large-insert clone DNA microarrays for the detection of genomic copy number changes. *Nat protoc.* 2007;2:(3)577.

Gorlin RJ, Cohen MM, Hennekam RCM. *Syndromes of the Head and Neck*, 4th ed. Oxford University Press; 2001.

Gøtzsche C-O, Krag-Olsen B, Nielsen J, Sørensen KE, Kristensen BØ. Prevalence of cardiovascular malformations and association with karyotypes in Turner's syndrome. *Arch dis Child.* 1994;71:433–436.

Greenhalgh KL, Aligianis I, Bromilow G, et al. 22q11 deletion: a multisystem disorder requiring multidisciplinary input. *Arch Dis Child.* 2003;88:523–524.

Grossfeld PD. The genetics of hypoplastic left heart syndrome. *Cardiol Young.* 1999;9(6):627–632.

Grossfeld PD, Mattina T, Lai Z, et al. 11q Consortium The 11q terminal deletion disorder: a prospective study of 110 cases. *Am J Med Genet.* 2004;129A:51–61.

Hamada T, Gejyo F, Koshino Y, et al. Echocardiographic evaluation of cardiac valvular abnormalities in adults with Down's syndrome. *Tokohu J Exp Med.* 1998;185:31–35.

Harris JA, Fracannet C, Pradat P, Robert E. The epidemiology of cardiovascular defects, part 2: a study based on data from three large registries of congenital malformations. *Pediatr Cardiol.* 2003;24:222–235.

Heilstedt HA, Ballif BC, Howard LA, Kashorf CD, Schaffer LG. Population data suggest that deletions of 1p36 are a relatively common chromosome abnormality. *Clin Genet.* 2003;64:310–316.

Hills C, Moller JH, Finkelstein M, Lohr J, Schimmenti L. Cri du Chat syndrome and congenital heart disease: A review of previously reported cases and presentation of an additional 21 cases from the Paediatric Cardiac Care Consortium. *Pediatrics.* 2006;117:e924–e927.

Jacobs PA, Browne C, Gregson N, Joyce C, White H. Estimates of the frequency of chromosome abnormalities detectable in unselected newborns using moderate levels of banding. *J Med Genet.* 1992;29: 103–108.

Jerome LA, Pappaioannou VE. DiGeorge syndrome phenotype in mice mutant for the T-box gene Tbx1. *Nat Gen.* 2001;27:286–291.

Jones KL. *Smiths Recognizable Pattern of Human Malformations.* 6th ed. Harcourt Brace Jovanovitch Inc., W.B. Saunders Company; 2006.

Lejeune J, Gautier M, Turpin R. Etudes des chromosomes somatiques de neufs enfant mongoliens. *Comp Rend Acad Sci.* 1959;248:1721–1722.

Li DY, Toland, AE, Boak BB, et al. Elastin point mutations cause an obstructive vascular disease, supravalvar aortic stenosis. *Hum Molec Genet.* 1997;6:1021–1028.

Lindsay EA, Vitelli F, Su H, et al. Tbx1 haploinsufficiency in the DiGeorge syndrome region causes aortic arch defects in mice. *Nature.* 2001;410: 97–101.

Lowery MC, Morris CA, Ewart A, et al. Strong correlation of elastin deletions, detected by FISH, with Williams Syndrome: evaluation of 235 patients. *Am J Hum Genet.* 1995;57:49–53.

Marino B. Patterns of congenital heart disease and associated anomalies in children with Down Syndrome. In: Marino B, Peuschel SM, (eds) *Heart disease in Persons with Down Syndrome.* Paul H Brookes Publishing Co. Baltimore; 1996:134.

Merscher S, Funke B, Epstein JA, et al. TBX1 is responsible for cardiovascular defects in velo-cardio-facial/DiGeorge syndrome. *Cell.* 2001; 104:619–629.

Metcalfe K, Rucka AK, Smoot L, et al. Elastin: mutational spectrum in supravalvar aortic stenosis. *Eur J Hum Genet.* 2000;8:955–963.

Penny L, Dell'Aquila M, Jones MC, et al. Clinical and molecular characterisation of patients with distal 11q deletions. *Am J Hum Genet.* 1995;56:676–683.

Phillips H, Renforth GL, Spalluto C, et al. Narrowing the critical region within 11q24-qter for hypoplastic left heart and identification of a candidate gene JAM3, expressed during cardiogenesis. *Genomics.* 2002;79:475–478.

Pierpont MEM, Moller JH. Chromosome abnormalities. In: Moller JH, Pierpoont MEM, eds. *The Genetics of Cardiovascular Disease.* Boston, MA: Nijhoff; 1987:13–24.

Rosias PPR, Sijstermans JMJ, Theunissen PMVM, et al. Phenotypic variability of the Cat Eye syndrome. Case report and review of the literature. *Genet Counsel.* 2001;12:273–282.

Ryan AK, Goodship JA, Wilson DI, et al. Spectrum of clinical features associated with interstitial chromosome 22q11 deletions: a European collaborative study. *J Med Genet.* 1997;34:798–804.

Schinzel A. *Catalogue of Unbalanced Chromosome Aberrations in Man.* 2nd ed. Berlin: Walter de Gruyter & Co.; 2001.

Seabright M. A rapid banding technique for human chromosomes. *Lancet.* 1971;297:971–972.

Van Buggenhout GJ, Pijkels E, Holvoet M, Schaap C, Hamel BC, Fryns JP. Cri du chat syndrome: changing phenotype in older patients. *Am J Med Genet.* 2000;90:203–215.

Wyllie JP, Wright MJ, Burn J, Hunter S. Natural history of trisomy 13. *Arch Dis Child.* 1994;71(4):343–345.

Yagi H, Furutani Y, Hamada H, et al. Role of TBX1 in human del 22q11.2 syndrome. *Lancet.* 2003;362:1342–1343.

6

Molecular Diagnosis in Cardiovascular Genetics

Karen Maresso, Michael Harrison, Ian Frayling, and Ulrich Broeckel

Introduction

As new technological developments lead to fundamental changes in our understanding of disease mechanisms, the ways in which we diagnose and treat patients are ultimately changed. In the past two decades, basic science breakthroughs have enabled advances in the field of cardiovascular genetics. These advances have contributed to a better molecular understanding of both Mendelian cardiovascular conditions, such as the cardiomyopathies and long QT syndrome (LQTS), as well as atherosclerotic cardiovascular disease. Beginning in the 1990s, the identification of the first gene for hypertrophic cardiomyopathy (HCM), cardiac-β myosin heavy chain (Solomon et al. 1990), and the identification of the first two genes for LQTS in 1995, *KCNH2* (Curran et al. 1995) and *SCN5A* (Wang et al. 1995), revolutionized the field of clinical cardiovascular genetics. With the discovery of these genes and the subsequent identification of their causative mutations for two of the most common cardiovascular disorders, the field witnessed the earliest possibilities of personalized medicine, where patients could be managed according to their own molecular signatures.

Since then, the completion of the Human Genome Project (HGP) in 2003 has moved the field even closer to the ultimate goal of individualized medicine. The HGP, along with technological advancements in mass-throughput genotyping, have allowed the field to transition from focusing primarily on the genetics of the more common cardiovascular Mendelian conditions to more complex cardiovascular outcomes, such as coronary artery disease (CAD) and myocardial infarction (MI). In recent years, genome-wide association (GWA) studies have allowed for the discovery of novel genes and variants for both CAD and MI, as well as other related cardiovascular traits. Innovations in genotyping technology now allow millions of single nucleotide polymorphisms (SNPs) to be affordably assayed in an individual in a matter of days. This high-throughput genomic technology has been behind the success of GWA studies, where a vast majority of the genome can now be tested for statistical associations with CAD/MI and other complex diseases (The Wellcome Case Control Study Consortium 2007). In addition, both genome-wide expression arrays and proteomic tools are also quickly becoming commonly used tools to help identify CAD/MI disease genes and protein biomarkers. The combined use of high-throughput DNA, mRNA, and protein level analyses in order to understand disease processes better can be termed "functional genomics." Such studies are capable of finding truly novel genes and proteins that will ultimately improve the field's molecular understanding of CAD/MI and may even directly impact the diagnosis and treatment of patients with these very common conditions.

Even as challenges remain in translating research findings on the Mendelian cardiovascular disorders into the clinic, a challenge in coming years will also be translating the results and technology of functional genomic studies into clinical practice. This chapter discusses the molecular diagnostic techniques commonly used in any modern diagnostic genetic laboratory. These are not specific to a particular system or group of disorders. We have included the methods that are commonly used in the molecular diagnosis of the common Mendelian inherited cardiovascular conditions and their application to clinical practice. In addition, molecular cytogenetic techniques used in investigating congenital cardiac anomalies and associated malformation syndromes are also described (see also Chapters 7 and 8). We also include a discussion on the newer genomic approaches, such as high-throughput SNP arrays and genome expression profiling that are currently being developed for diagnosing the more complex, polygenic conditions of CAD and MI. A final section on the feasibility of population/community level screening in cardiovascular genetics is also included.

Molecular Cytogenetic Techniques

Classical cytogenetics is the standard method of rapidly and relatively cheaply carrying out a whole genome scan. At the simplest level it allows enumeration of chromosomes, but a number of different techniques for revealing structure within chromosomes, otherwise known as banding techniques, have been developed (reviewed in Craig and Bickmore 1993). Giemsa banding (G-banding) is the most widely used method for routine analysis of human chromosomes. Metaphase spreads of chromosomes are subjected to treatment with a protease, such as trypsin, after first

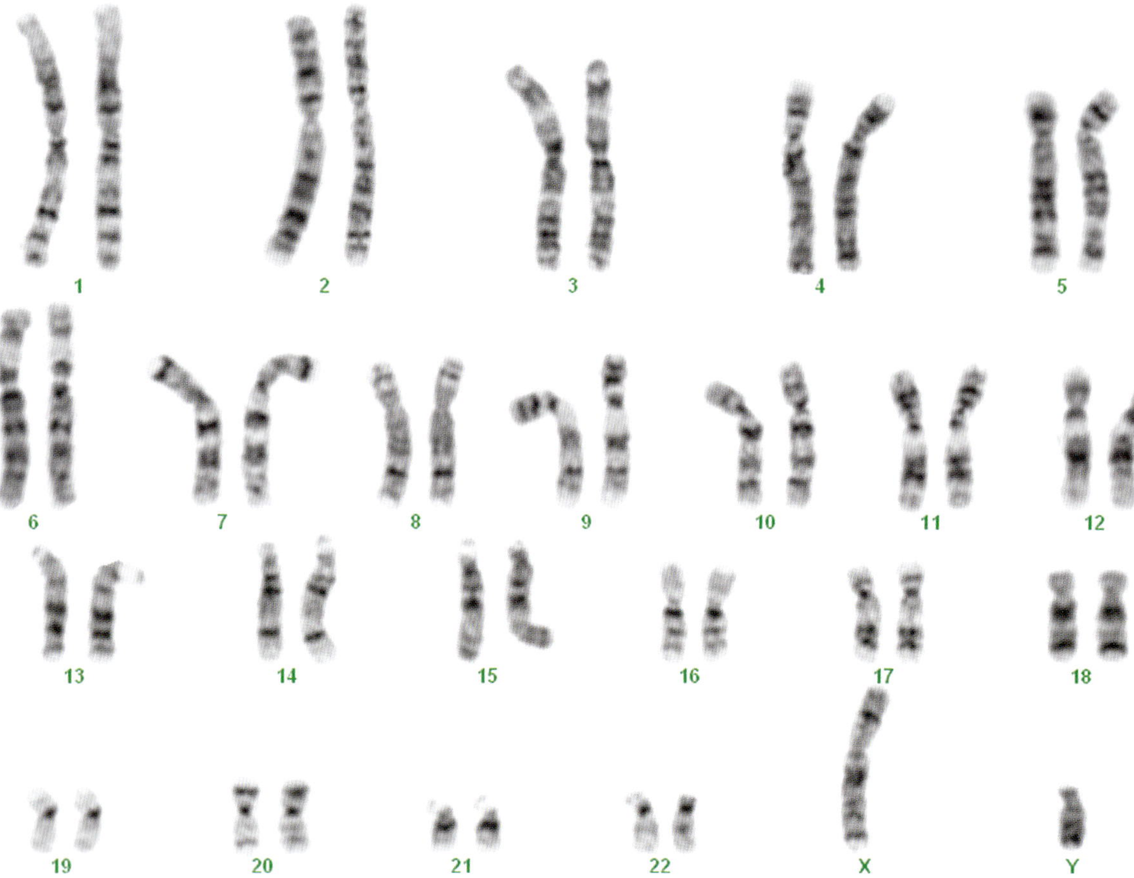

Figure 6–1 A G-banded karyotype from a normal human male (46, XY) Courtesy of Dr Peter Thompson, Cytogenetics Laboratory, Institute of Medical Genetics, Cardiff, UK.

some sort of aging, for example, 3–5 days at room temperature, or ca. 56°C overnight (Seabright 1972). Giemsa stain contains eosin and a mixture of thiazine dyes, and the latter bind to DNA, resulting in differential staining. Late-replicating, transcriptionally quiet A/T-rich DNA stains darkly (G-positive), while early-replicating, transcriptionally active relatively G/C-rich DNA stains light (G-negative). The highest quality G-banded preparations are able to give 850 bands/points of comparison across the genome, to which if one adds the total number of different chromosomes, totals nearly 1,000 [International System for human Cytogenetic Nomenclature (ISCN) 2005; Figure 6–1]. Thus, a G-banded chromosome preparation can be thought of as a 1 K whole genome array, arranged in a linear anatomical fashion. Such analysis can reveal loss or gain of material down to only a few Mb in size, though exactly how small depends on the location of the defect. It can also reveal balanced events such as translocations and inversions, where no net gain or loss of material has occurred. Thus, chromosomal analysis is capable of giving not just dosage but also data on location and orientation.

Other banding methods include Q-banding, where a fluorescent dye such as quinacrine, DAPI, or Hoechst 33258, binds preferentially to A/T-rich sequences; R-banding, which is the reverse of G-banding, uses high-molar low pH phosphate buffer heat denaturation of chromosomes and/or acridine orange staining, to produce a banding pattern complementary to that produced by G-banding; T-banding, which is directed at R-bands toward the telomeres by especially strong heat treatment prior to Giemsa staining; and C-banding, where denaturation with, for example, barium hydroxide, before Giemsa staining, brings out the so-called constitutive heterochromatin at centromeres. All these techniques can reveal complementary information about the structure and organization of the genome at the chromosomal level. Q-banding is commonly used in combination with FISH to precisely locate hybridization signals.

Fluorescence In Situ Hybridization

In situ hybridization techniques, in particular *fluorescence in situ hybridization* (FISH), have allowed study of the structure of the genome at a level of detail greater than that seen by conventional banding techniques (Pinkel et al. 1986; Trask et al. 1988; Trask 1991; van Ommen et al. 1995). The method depends on the specific hybridization of a probe DNA sequence to its complementary sequence in the genome, and an early description shows how it was used to study satellite DNA location within cells(Jones 1970). Labeling of the probe with a fluorescent dye allows its location to be revealed by laser excitation microscopy, usually in combination with some form of Q-banding (Figure 6–2). Cot-1 DNA competitive hybridization suppresses unwanted signals. The probes used in FISH experiments are typically derived from cloning human sequences into bacterial artificial chromosomes (BACs), with sizes of around 100 kb. For a practical consideration see Mundle and Koska (Mundle and Koska 2005).

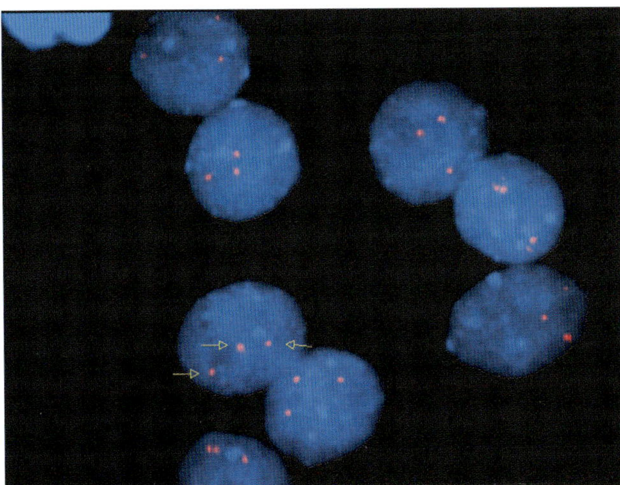

Figure 6–2 Interphase FISH. For the rapid prenatal diagnosis of common aneuploidies, FISH can be performed on cells in interphase obtained at amniocentesis, rather than having to spend time culturing them with arrest at metaphase. A probe to the chromosome of interest is hybridized to interphase nuclei, together with a counterstain, blue in this instance. In this example, the probe is to chromosome 21, and all the nuclei contain three red signals, establishing a diagnosis of trisomy 21 (Down syndrome). It is necessary to count a sufficient number of nuclei to make the analysis statistically valid. Unlike conventional cytogenetic analysis this technique only indicates the number of copies of the probe region, which does not necessarily equate to the number of copies of whole chromosomes. Courtesy of Dr Peter Thompson, Cytogenetics Laboratory, Institute of Medical Genetics, Cardiff, UK.

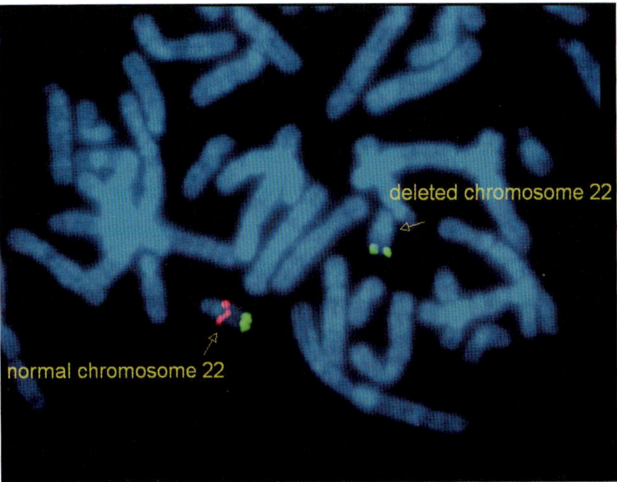

Figure 6–3 Fluorescence in situ hybridization (FISH). Specific target sequences in the genome can be analyzed by the use of DNA probes (typically 100–150 kb in size) labeled with a fluorescent dye. These can be hybridized to a metaphase chromosome spread, together with a contrasting dye that stains all chromosomes, to give information on both position within the genome and copy number.

The figure shows an experiment to test a patient for the common chromosomal microdeletion on the long arm of chromosome 22 associated with DiGeorge syndrome: del22q11.2. A blue counter stain is used to show the chromosomes, while a control FISH probe to the end of the long arm (22q) is labeled green and is present on both copies of chromosome 22. However, only one copy of chromosome 22 is labeled (red) by the test probe to the DiGeorge region on 22q11.2, showing clearly that the patient has a deletion and thus confirming a diagnosis of DiGeorge syndrome. Courtesy of Dr Peter Thompson, Cytogenetics Laboratory, Institute of Medical Genetics, Cardiff, UK.

The HGP has resulted in an almost complete tiling path consisting of approximately 32,000 BACs, and hence there are only very few regions of the genome not amenable to FISH experiments. The HGP required individual FISH experiments to ensure that any given BAC clone's sequence was defined and unique, and not subject to duplication or rearrangement. FISH can be performed on both metaphase spreads and interphase nuclei. Simple and rapid enumeration of chromosomes can be achieved on interphase nuclei, given that no culturing of cells is necessarily required (Figure 6–3). On metaphase spreads with contrasting Q-banding highly specific positional and dosage information can be obtained, and FISH is an excellent tool in gene mapping and diagnosis (Figure 6–4).

One application of FISH technology that gives highly specific and accurate positional and dosage information is fiber-FISH. In this, individual strands of DNA are stretched out on a glass slide and the FISH probes hybridized. The probes can be as small as individual exons, that is, only a few hundred bp, far smaller than conventional FISH probes. Fiber-FISH can thus reveal deletion, duplication, or rearrangement of exons in specific genes, for example, DMD (Florijn et al. 1995). Developments in FISH have recently been reviewed (Murthy and Demetrick 2006).

Comparative Genome Hybridization, M-FISH, and Chromosome Painting

If the probe DNA used in a FISH experiment is derived from a whole chromosome, rather than a smaller specific sequence cloned in a vector, then it will reveal a whole chromosome. The ability to flow sort chromosomes and then carry out some form of in vitro amplification before labeling with a mixture of dyes to

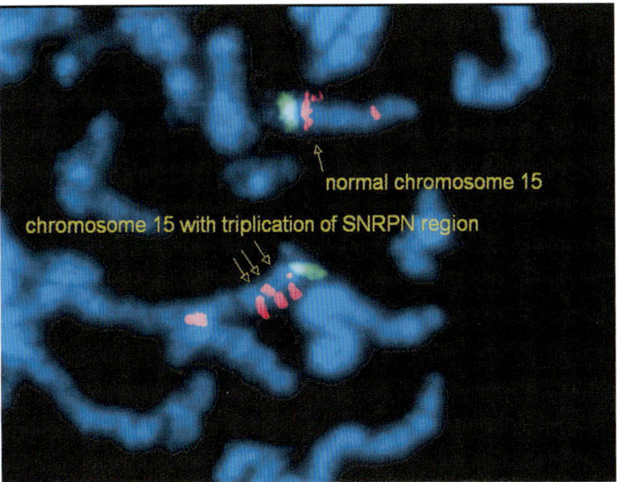

Figure 6–4 Fluorescence in situ hybridization (FISH). The figure shows the results of an experiment to investigate a patient with features including learning difficulties, autism and seizures, suggestive of Prader-Willi Syndrome (PWS), which is frequently due to deletion of the *SNRPN* region on chromosome 15. The FISH experiment, however, reveals three copies of the *SNRPN* region, enabling the conclusion that the patient in fact has 15q11-q14 triplication syndrome, a condition with overlapping clinical phenotype with PWS (Ungaro et al. 2001).

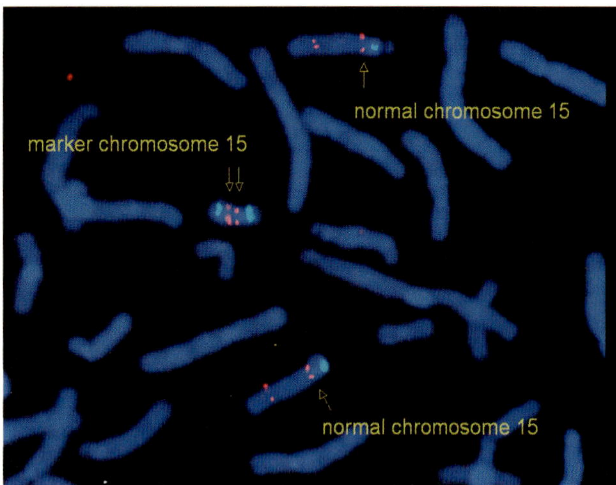

Figure 6–5 Identification of extra genetic material. A marker chromosome is a small supernumerary chromosome. Its origin in this case is revealed in a FISH experiment. Specific FISH probes indicate that it is derived from chromosome 15 material, and hence is likely to be pathogenic.

give a specific color signal has enabled probes to be produced for all 24 human chromosomes. If the desired experiment is simply to investigate one or two different chromosomes, that is, chromosome painting, then conventional FISH image analysis will suffice. This is good for detecting abnormal arrangements of chromosomes, such as translocations, and identification of the origin of material in, for example, marker chromosomes, which may otherwise have no identifying features. If all 24 different chromosome paints are applied the technique becomes even more sophisticated and is known by the term multicolor FISH (M-FISH), further developed as spectral karyotyping (SKY) (Schröck et al. 1996, 1997). This is especially good at determining the many and complicated rearrangements that occur in cancer cells (Figure 6–5). By means of specialized image analysis dosage across the genome can be measured in an M-FISH/SKY experiment, chromosome by chromosome, and this is the technique of choice.

Array Comparative Genomic Hybridization

While FISH experiments using individual probes can give useful information about the dosage and location of a particular sequence in the genome, it is simply unfeasible to carry out 32,000 different FISH experiments to cover the whole of the human genome in cases where this might be appropriate. However, a number of technological developments have made it possible to put small and uniform amounts of many different DNA probes onto a suitable substrate, for example, a 1" x 3" glass microscope slide, in the form of an array, often referred to by the colloquial name of DNA or gene "chip." If then DNA from a test subject or patient is labeled with one fluorochrome (e.g., red), and DNA from a pool of control individuals is labeled with another color (e.g., green), and equal amounts are mixed and then hybridized to the probes on the glass slide, the relative amounts of red versus green signal from each probe will indicate relative dosage, that is, loss or gain of that probe sequence in the test subject. This is array comparative genomic hybridization (CGH) (Pinkel et al. 1998; Pollack et al. 1999; Veltman et al. 2002; Mantripragada et al. 2004a; Figures 6–6 and 6–7).

To begin with, a few thousand probes have been used in array CGH. Choosing every tenth BAC clone covering the genome, such that every 1 Mb or so a region of ca. 100 kb is probed requires a set of around 3,000 BACs, that is, a 3K CGH array. More recently, it has become possible to produce arrays of 32,000 clones almost completely covering the whole genome (32K arrays). While these clearly have the ability to detect smaller changes, it remains to be seen whether this is, in fact, useful in the clinical setting. Having obtained a result from an array CGH experiment that suggests gain or loss of a particular probe region, it is then necessary to carry out further experiments to determine if this is the case and whether there has been some other complication, such as a rearrangement. These extra confirmatory experiments can take a number of forms, from, for example, one or more FISH experiments on metaphase spreads to a Southern blot (see subsequent text), or some other molecular dosage technique. Indeed, array CGH is revealing that some apparently balanced translocations do harbor gain or loss of material.

In the clinical setting, array CGH is useful in those circumstances where significant abnormalities are present in the patient, such as learning difficulties and dysmorphic features, but no one feature, or combination of features, is diagnostic of a particular syndrome. Thus, the clinician cannot suggest that the laboratory carry out a specific FISH test for a particular microdeletion syndrome, and the laboratory can do no more specific test than a karyotype analysis by G-banding, plus perhaps a screen of subtelomeric regions for deletions. However, armed with an array of 3,000 or even 32,000 FISH probes in one array it does become feasible to carry out in effect a genome-wide FISH experiment (Shaw-Smith et al. 2004). Many of those working in the field are pooling their data in the Database of Chromosomal Imbalance and Phenotype in Humans using Ensemble Resources (DECIPHER; at http://www.sanger.ac.uk/PostGenomics/decipher/). There are two main reasons for this: array CGH studies are revealing the complexity of variation within the normal human genome, and the subtleties and complexity of clinical features constituting the phenotype of individual patients necessitates the most careful data collection if comparisons are to be meaningful (Buckley et al. 2005; de Bustos et al. 2006). There are understandable concerns about interpreting possible abnormality in the face of so much normal variation, but in principle the problem is no different from the interpretation of point mutations in genes, something which molecular geneticists don't underestimate, but have been getting to grips with for some time. At least, it is encouraging that a problem involving a similar large amount of data processing resulted, over 60 years ago, in the development of the machine that is being used to produce this book, the electronic digital computer (Copeland 2006). It seems unlikely to be beyond the wit of man to solve the problem of array CGH data interpretation.

Powerful approaches using a combination of techniques, such as DNA microarrays and chromosome sorting, are showing that positional data can be obtained about aberrant chromosomes, as well as dosage (Gribble et al. 2004). Cross species experiments are revealing details of primate genome evolution (Locke et al. 2003). Given the delays inherent in producing a karyotype analysis because of the cell culturing required, prenatal testing has always been problematic; however, array CGH opens up the possibility that rapid testing, currently carried out by FISH or PCR for only the most common of defects, may soon be carried out by array

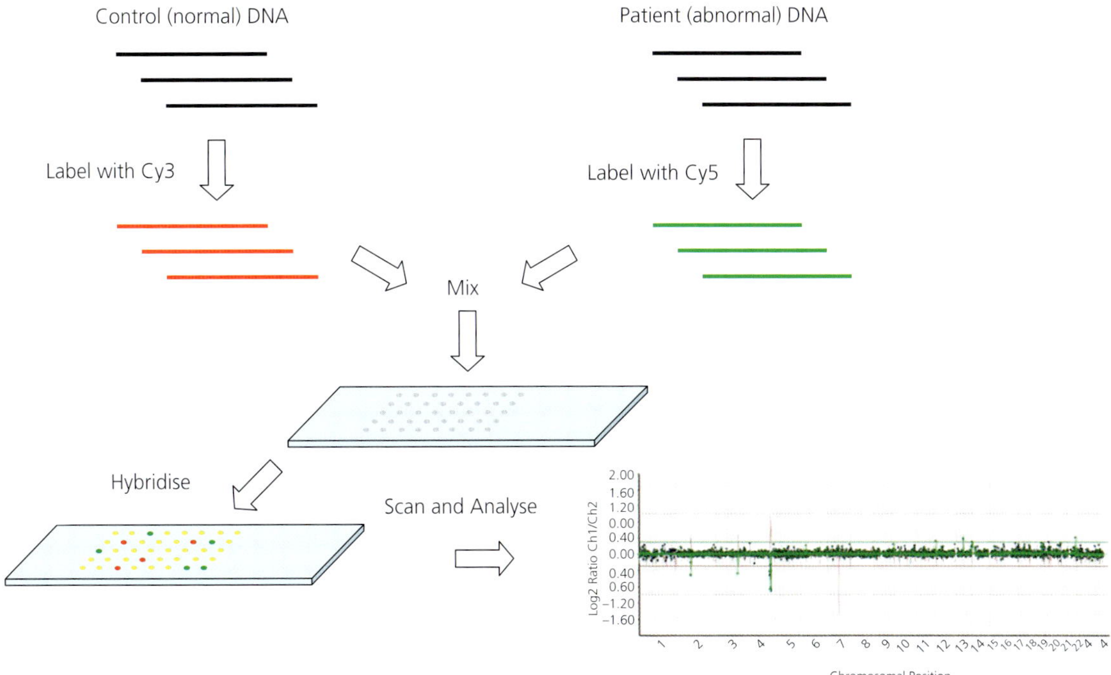

Figure 6–6 Simplified Schematic of an array CGH Experiment. Test and control DNAs are labelled with fluorescent dyes of contrasting colours, and mixed together. The mixture is denatured and then hybridised with an array of genomic DNA probes which are adherent to the surface of a solid substrate (typically a 1" × 3" glass slide). The relative copy number of the probe sequences in the control versus test DNAs determines the relative fluorescence of the colours. This is measured by a high resolution photometric scanner. The position of any one probe on the array is known to the analysis software, hence the relative copy number of that probe's region in the test genome can be determined. This is presented by the software to show relative copy number across the whole genome.

CGH, which would have the additional benefit of the comprehensive detection of microdeletions (Le Caignec et al. 2005; reviewed by Rickman et al. 2005). One of the drawbacks of array CGH up to now has been that it requires large amounts of DNA; however, in an exciting recent advance it has been shown that robust results can be obtained from single cells, with the use of whole genome amplification by PCR using degenerate oligonucleotide primers (Le Caignec et al. 2006).

Targeted Arrays

There are a number of forms of targeted arrays. One is simply an array of BAC clone probes, of the type used in whole genome arrays, but restricted to a particular region of interest in the genome (Bruder et al. 2001; Buckley et al. 2002; Locke et al. 2004; Sharp et al. 2005). To achieve higher density coverage in more detail cosmid probes have been used (Mantripragada et al. 2003). One potential clinical application of this principle is in an array designed for the purposes of prenatal diagnosis of common chromosomal abnormalities, from trisomy 21 to various microdeletion syndromes, and requiring only 600 BAC clones, rather than 3,000 or more (Rickman et al. 2006). This would have the effects of reducing cost not only because fewer clones are required but also because several replicates of the array can be printed on one slide.

Another form of targeted array involves the use of smaller probes of either PCR product size (ca. 200–2,000 bp), or even oligonucleotide arrays, allowing resolution down to the level of individual exons (Mantripragada et al. 2004b, 2006; Ren et al. 2005; Selzer et al. 2005; Urban et al. 2006; Figure 6–8). Care has to be taken that the PCR probes used in such arrays are derived from nonrepetitive regions of the genome, but the resolution offered by such arrays is impressive (Figure 6–8).

Oligonucleotide arrays for the determination of SNPs can be used to determine copy number changes in the genome in, for example, cancer cells. Where a series of contiguous SNPs become apparently homozygous, that is, there is loss of heterozygosity, then it can be assumed that a deletion of one allele has occurred, and if no signal should be obtained then a homozygous deletion can be assumed (Lindblad-Toh et al. 2000; Wang et al. 2006; reviewed by Zhou et al. 2005). Advances in the technology of oligonucleotide-based array production are enabling ever higher densities of probes: 500K SNP arrays are now commonplace, and arrays with one million or more features are becoming available.

Southern Analysis

The gel transfer method known the world over as "Southern analysis," or more colloquially "Southern blotting," is with PCR one of the best-known techniques in molecular biology. It has the unique ability to give data simultaneously on position, orientation, dosage, and even methylation of sections of the genome from ca. 100 bp up to several Mb (Southern 1975, 2000, 2005).

The method depends on the combination of a number of techniques. First, DNA is fragmented in a controlled fashion using a restriction endonuclease, which will cut the DNA at defined sites. Next, the digested DNA fragments are separated by size using gel electrophoresis, and the DNA then transferred to membrane capable of binding the DNA and immobilizing it, usually nitrocellulose or nylon, to produce a "blot." The size fractionated DNA on

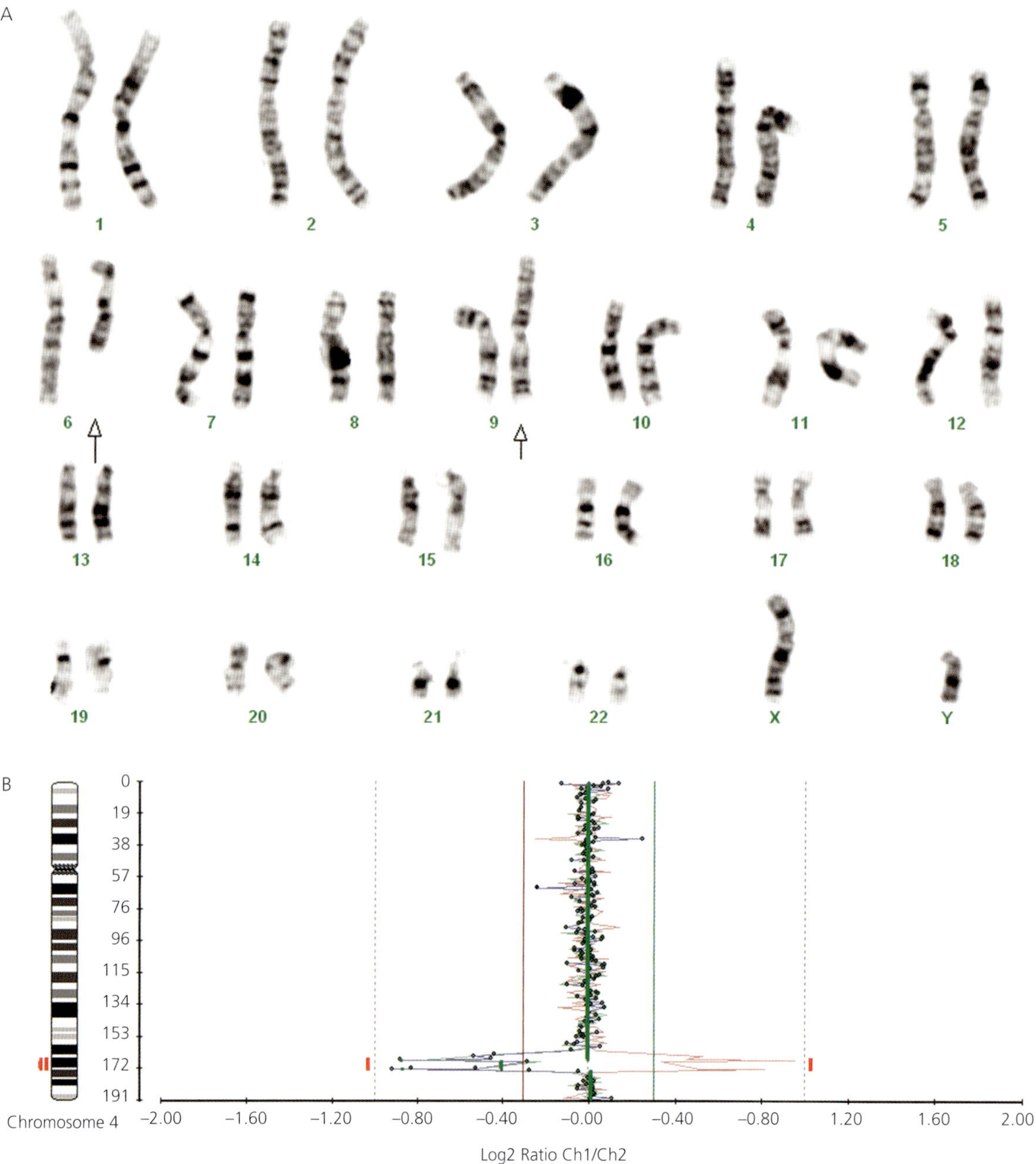

C

4

Figure 6–7 Use and value of array CGH in clinical diagnosis. A 3-year old male presented to a Clinical Geneticist, with developmental delay, poor speech, positional talipes, a left squint, atrial septal defect, and short stature (2nd percentile), but head circumference on the 50th percentile. He was found by conventional cytogenetic analysis (G-banding) to have an apparently balanced translocation between chromosomes 6 and 9 [46, XY, t(6;9)(q16.2;p22–24) de novo], as shown by the arrows (Figure 6–7a).

Subsequent array CGH analysis, using a whole genome array of 0.1 Mb BAC clones spaced ~1 Mb apart, showed that there is no loss of DNA in the regions of the breakpoints on chromosomes 6 and 9. However, it revealed that there had been loss of ~8.7 Mb of DNA from chromosome 4 (region shown by vertical red bar in Figure 6–7b), which in retrospect is just visible on the karyotype (Figure6–7a and 6–7c). The deletion was determined to be between 4q32.2 and 4q34.2, and hence the patient's karyotype is properly described as 46, XY, del(4)(q32.2q34.2)de novo, t(6;9)(q16.2;p22–24)de novo. The loss of ~8.7 Mb of DNA from chromosome 4 is highly likely to be the cause of the patient's phenotype, and the 6;9 translocation is therefore merely an incidental finding.

(Courtesy of Sian Morgan, Clinical Cytogeneticist, Cytogenetics Laboratory, and Dr Daniela Pilz, Consultant in Clinical Genetics, Institute of Medical Genetics, Cardiff, UK.)

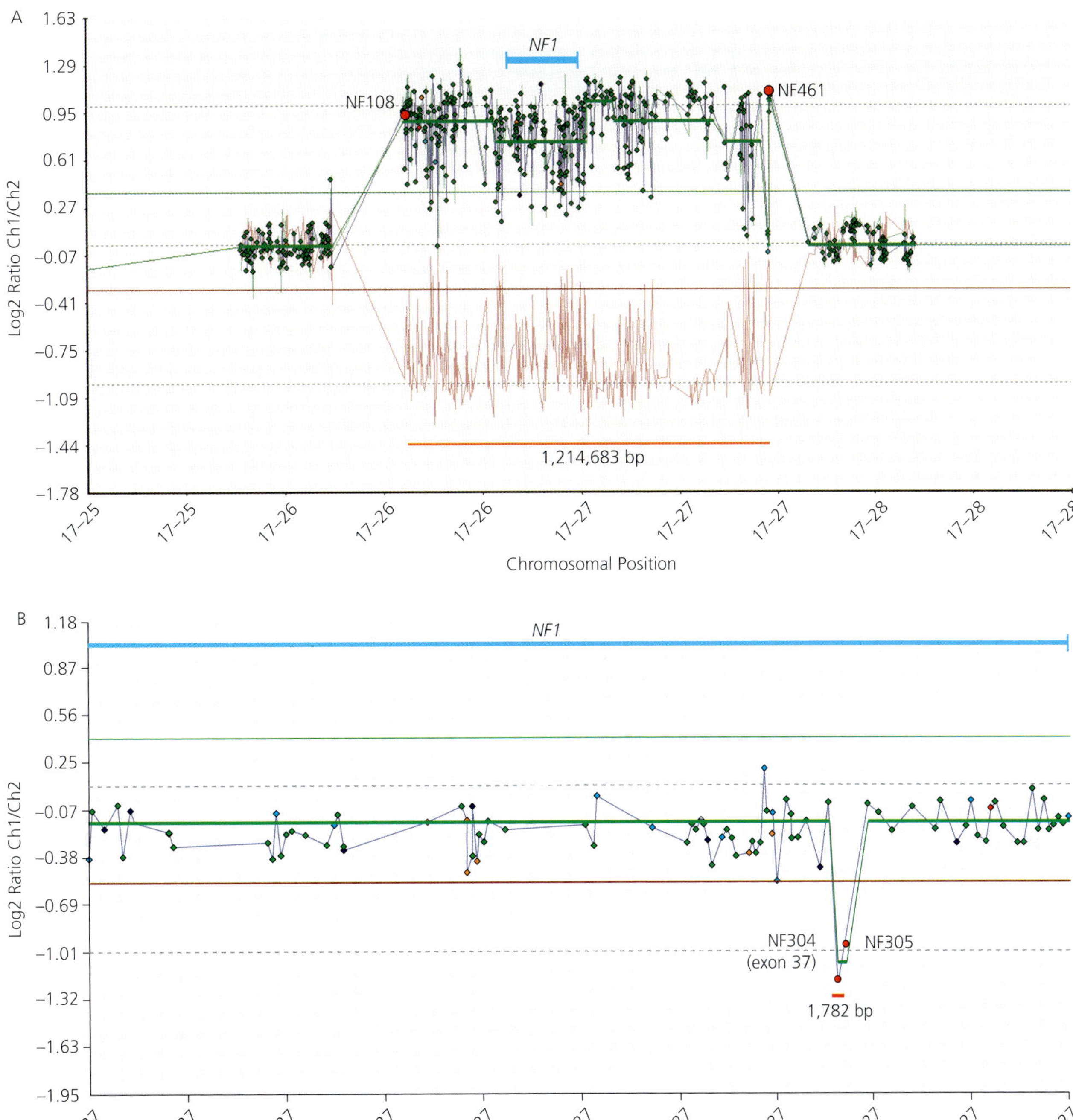

Figure 6–8 (Continued)

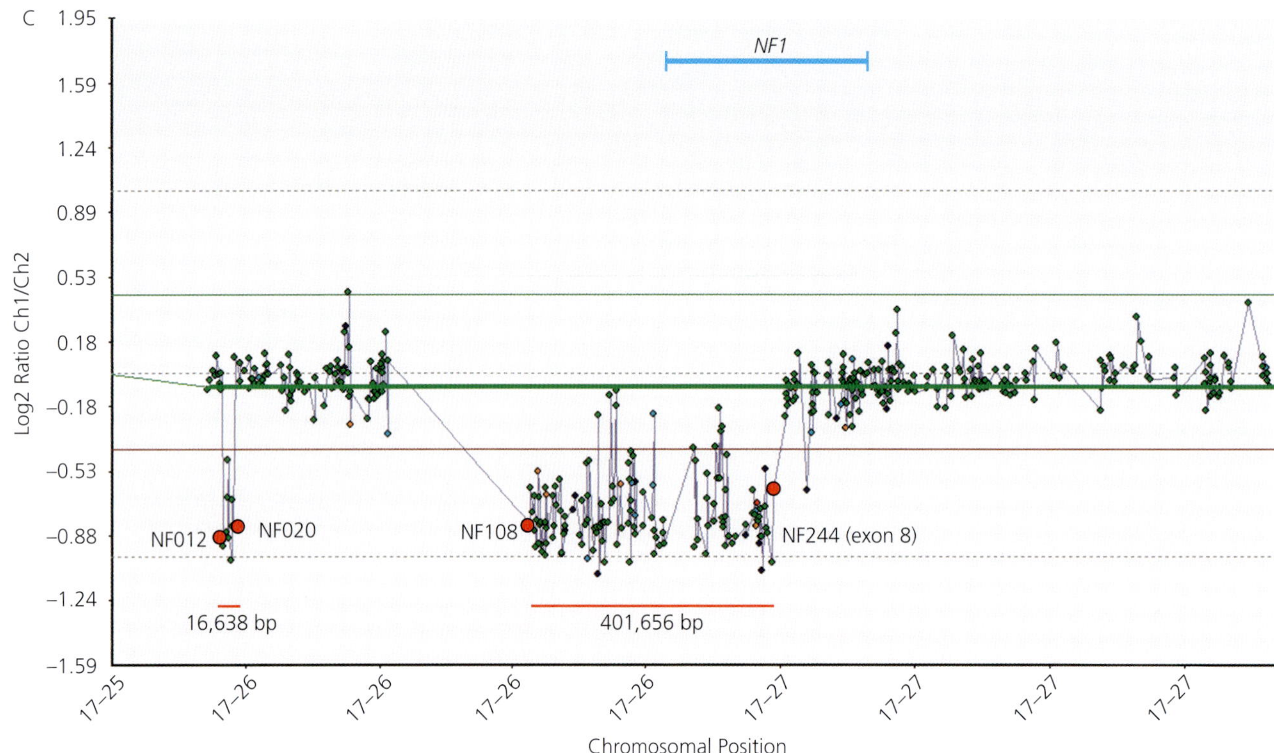

Figure 6–8 Use of an array targetted to a specific locus. Targeted arrays can be used to analyse specific regions of the genome in great detail. Mutations in the *NF1* gene on chromosome 17 can lead to neurofibromatosis type 1. These mutations can take many forms and range in size from a single bp (point mutations) up to 1–2 Mb, or larger. Detecting and defining the larger mutations can be difficult as the *NF1* gene lies in a region of the genome containing many repeated and repetitive sequences. By constructing a targeted array of 515 probes, between 200 and 999 bp in size and generated by PCR, the whole 2 Mb region around *NF1* can be studied.

Test (patient) DNA and normal DNA are labelled with different fluorescent dyes, mixed together and then hybridised to the PCR probes immobilised as spots on the array. The positions of the probes along the chromosome are shown on the X axis, with the position of the coding region of the *NF1* gene itself shown by the light blue bar (probes 209–328). The relative amounts of fluorescence at each probe are measured and hence the relative copy number of the probes determined in the test sample (Y axis).

In Case 1 (Fig. 6–8a), probes 108 and 461 (shown by large red dots), and all those in between, have been deleted, encompassing a region of at least 1,214,683 bp (shown by the thick red line). The green line shows the results when test DNA is labelled green and normal DNA red, the thin red line shows the results of a "dye swop experiment" when the test and normal DNAs are labelled the other way round: this provides extra confidence in the result.

In Case 2 (Fig. 6–8b) only two probes have been deleted, 304 (in exon 37) and 305, representing a mere 1,782 bp.

In Case 3 (Fig.6–8c) a more complicated picture is revealed. The patient has two regions deleted, between probes 12 to 20, and 108 to 244 (in exon 8). What an array can't determine is the relative orientation of the remaining parts of the genome, it may well be that the retained region between probes 20 and 108 has become inverted.

(Courtesy of Dr Ming Hong Shen, NHS R&D Laboratory, Institute of Medical Genetics, Cardiff, UK)

the membrane is then hybridized with a labeled probe DNA (usually radiolabeled), which is then put up against radiosensitive photographic film, revealing where on the membrane there are target sequences that match the probe sequence. Hence, the actual and relative sizes of the fragments can be determined. The principle is sound and robust, but the beauty lies in the variations that can be used to address specific questions.

As there are hundreds of different restriction endonucleases ("restriction enzymes") recognizing distinct, typically 6–8 bp sequence motifs, so information can be gleaned about hundreds of different sites in the DNA. Combinations of restriction endonucleases can be used, and the information on fragment sizes can be used to construct a genomic map of a region. Restriction endonucleases that cut at commonly occurring sites will tend to produce small fragments, while "rare cutters" will produce large fragments useful for longer-range mapping. As Southern found in his original studies, if a restriction endonuclease cutting within a repetitive sequence should be used then information about such regions, such as the size of repeats, would be gleaned (Southern 2005). Some restriction endonucleases are specific for methylated or unmethylated motifs, so the methylation status of a stretch of DNA can be determined, potentially down to the level of individual restriction sites (Marcaud et al. 1981; Wolf and Migeon 1982; Gronostajski et al. 1985). Use of a combination of methylation sensitive and insensitive restriction endonucleases is employed in the diagnosis of Fragile X(A) syndrome, where the presence is sought of an expansion at the FMR1 locus that is also methylated (reviewed by Tsongalis and Silverman 1993; Oostra and Willemsen 2001); the Southern analysis also gives dosage information (one allele in males, two in females), and often shows somatic heterogeneity/mosaicism in the sizes of pathological expansions, which is manifest as a smear on the blot (Figure 6–9).

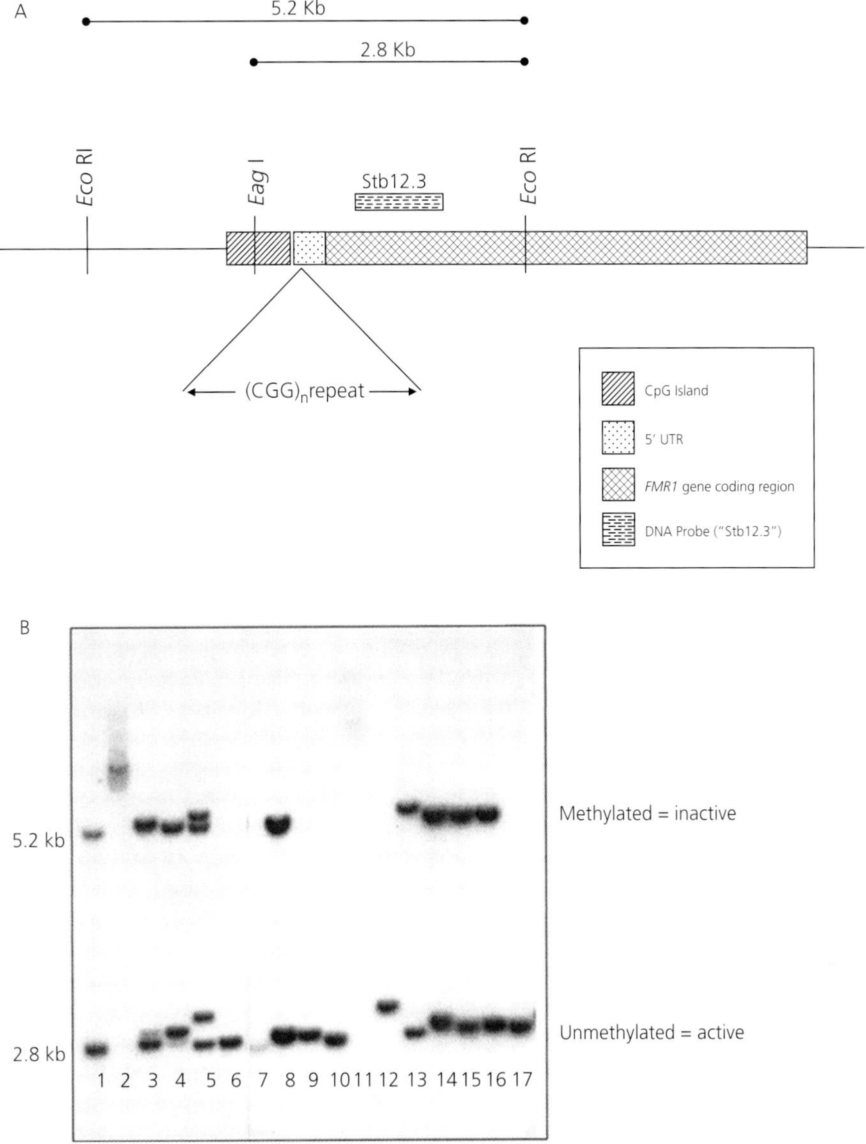

Figure 6–9 Testing for Fragile X Syndrome (FraX). FraX syndrome is caused by pathogenic expansions of a CGG repeat in the 5′ untranslated region (5′ UTR) of the *FMR1* gene, located on the X chromosome. It is so named because such expansions are liable to cause chromosome breakage at the resultant fragile site in cultured cells used for karyotype determination. Large expansions of the CGG repeat lead to methylation of it and the *FMR1* gene's promoter in the adjoining CpG island, causing down-regulation of the gene. Small expansions which do not cause methylation, but which may expand in subsequent generations are known as premutations. Methylation, and hence inactivation of the single copy of *FMR1* in males causes the syndrome, which includes mental retardation. In normal females one copy of the X chromosome in each cell is anyway randomly and naturally inactivated by being methylated, so the condition is typically less manifest in them. Southern analysis is very useful in molecular diagnosis of the condition.

A map of the region surrounding the *FMR1* locus is shown in Figure 6–9a. Sites which can be cut by the restriction enzymes *Eco* RI and *Eag* I are shown, and it should be noted that the *Eag* I site lies within the CpG island. Because *Eag* I does not cut DNA that is methylated, then it is able to discriminate between methylated (inactive) and unmethylated (active) alleles, in both males and females. The approximate distances between the restriction sites is shown, as is the region of DNA which corresponds to the probe sequence, called Stb12.3. DNA digested by a combination of *Eco* RI and *Eag* I is separated by electrophoresis and then transferred to a suitable membrane that binds the DNA fragments which have been sorted by size by the gel. The probe is then radioactively labelled and hybridised with the membrane, in the process binding to unmethylated fragments (2.8 kb; *Eag* I – *Eco* RI), or methylated fragments (5.2 kb: *Eco* RI – *Eco* RI) and exposed to X-ray film.

Figure 6–9b shows the results obtained with a variety of controls and test samples. Lanes 1 and 14–16 show normal females, 50% of whose X chromosomes are randomly inactivated by methylation, hence two bands are seen, one of 2.8 kb plus another of 5.2 kb. Lanes 6, 9, 10 and 17 show normal males: a single unmethylated allele of 2.8 kb in size. Lane 2 shows a male with a pathological methylated expansion of >5.2 kb (somatic mosaicism of the unstable expanded region causes the smeared indistinct band). Lane 12 shows a male with an unmethylated, but expanded, allele, i.e. a premutation. Lane 5 shows a female with a premutation: as the natural X chromosome inactivation methylates both the normal and premutation-carrying chromosomes there are two bands seen at 2.8 and 5.2 kb, the slightly larger one in each case being derived from the premutation chromosome.

(Courtesy of Dr Moira MacDonald, Molecular Genetics Laboratory, Institute of Medical Genetics, Cardiff.)

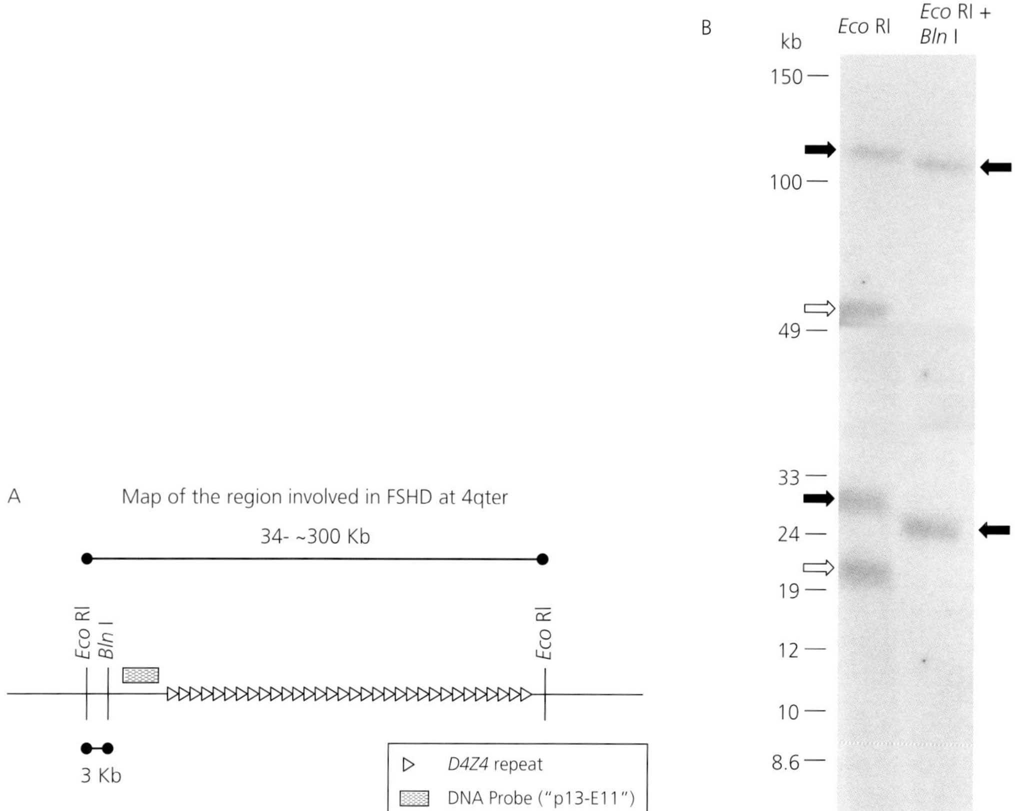

Figure 6–10 Testing for facio-scapulo-humeral muscular dystrophy (FSHD). FSHD is a form of muscular dystrophy that affects muscles of the face and upper limb girdle. The precise underlying genetic cause remains obscure, but most cases are associated with the presence of a shortened array of repetitive DNA sequences, called *D4Z4*, towards the end of the long arm of chromosome 4. Because of the large sizes of the regions of DNA involved, sometimes over 100 kb, a special technique called pulsed-field gel electrophoresis (PFGE) is necessary to give good separation of the fragments. A complication is that similar repeats are found on chromosome 10, but have nothing to do with FSHD.

A map of the FSHD-associated region of chromosome 4 is shown in Figure 6–10a, showing the probe region (p13-E11) between two *Eco* RI sites and near to the region of *D4Z4* repeats. Each *D4Z4* repeat is 3.3 kb in size. Normal individuals usually have at least 11 and sometimes up to approximately 90 *D4Z4* repeats on each chromosome 4, so the distance between the two *Eco* RI sites can vary between 34 and ~300 kb. Individuals with FSHD commonly have less than 11 repeats, thus having an *Eco* RI fragment <34 kb. Although there is a similar region on chromosome 10, fortunately type 10 repeats contain within them a site for the restriction enzyme *Bln* I, which distinguishes them from the true D4Z4 repeats on chromosome 4: thus digestion with *Bln* I reduces the probe binding fragment to such a small size it does not appear. Note, however, that there is a *Bln* I site 3 kb inside the left hand of the chromosome 4 *Eco* RI fragment.

Hence, in Figure 6–10b in the left hand lane, which is genomic DNA digested with *Eco* RI, there are four bands at 120, 50, 29 and 20 kb, while in the right hand lane (DNA digested with both *Eco* RI and *Bln* I) there are only two bands at approximately 115 kb and 26 kb, the difference in size being the distance between the *Eco* RI and *Bln* I sites of about 3 kb. Thus, *D4Z4*-containing fragments can be identified (solid arrows), distinct from the chromosome 10-derived ones (hollow arrows). The presence in this individual of an *Eco* RI fragment derived from chromosome 4 and of <34 kb is consistent with their clinical diagnosis of FSHD.

(Courtesy of Dr Gill Spurlock and Prof. Meena Upadhyaya, NHS R&D Laboratory, Institute of Medical Genetics, Cardiff, UK.)

If a particular restriction site should be polymorphic, then Southern analysis can be used to determine the frequency of the polymorphism, but perhaps more importantly these restriction fragment length polymorphisms (RFLPs) can be used in linkage experiments to locate genes (Solomon et al. 1976; Jeffreys 1979). Loss of heterozygosity for an RFLP can be and has been used to locate tumor suppressor genes (Solomon et al. 1987; Ward et al. 1993).

It is possible to use different probes, and this can even be done on the same blot as probes can be stripped off under appropriate conditions that denature the target DNA/probe hybrid. This will give information, for example, on probe sites being located together, or not, on the same restricted fragment of DNA. Cross species hybridization experiments can also be carried out, to find homologous or related genes.

Densitometric measurement of band intensities on the X-ray film, or actual counting of radioactivity on the membrane itself using, for example, a phosphorimager can give dosage information: useful in studies of gene amplification, for instance (Cowan et al. 1982; reviewed by Stark and Wahl 1984). Given the wealth of information obtainable from a Southern blot, at one and the same time, data can be obtained on copy number and rearrangements (Sabbir et al. 2006).

For a long time one of the limitations of Southern analysis was that it could not be used to study DNA fragments any larger than about 50 kb in size, because that was the maximum size resolvable on conventional agarose gel electrophoresis. However, this has been overcome by an understanding of the physics of DNA migration within gels leading to the development of pulsed-field gel electrophoresis, able to resolve DNA fragments of up to several Mb in size (Schwartz and Cantor 1984; Southern et al. 1987). An ability to analyze such large fragments has been critical in helping to understand a number of conditions, for example, facioscapulohumeral muscular dystrophy, by first mapping the region of interest and then facilitating laboratory diagnosis, and also fusion genes in malignancy (Min et al. 1990; Wijmenga et al. 1993; Galluzzi et al. 1999; Figure 6–10).

Other Techniques: MLPA, MAPH, Long-Range PCR

As well as the techniques described above, there are a number of methods that can give genomic data. Advances in PCR now enable amplicons of up to 20 kb to be routinely generated, and with care even up to 30 kb. This has facilitated the study and identification of, for example, chromosomal breakpoints and fusion genes, as well as haplotype mapping (Waggott et al. 1995; Klockars et al. 1996; Michalatos-Beloin et al. 1996; Wu et al. 2005; reviewed by Eisenstein 2006).

Notwithstanding the power of Southern blotting to detect deletions, duplications, and rearrangements, diagnostic laboratories have long sought a simpler and easier alternative to such mutations affecting exons. Quantitative PCR is one approach, but the technique of multiplex ligation-dependent probe amplification (MLPA) has really taken off as a robust and now increasingly routine option. It relies on the ligation of oligonucleotides that hybridize specifically to the region/exon of interest: ligation is only possible if there are no mismatches at the adjoining ends of the primers. The primers have generic sequences at their opposing ends, which then enable a PCR amplification to produce an amplicon corresponding to the ligation product, and most importantly quantitatively. By varying the length of intervening sequences between the specific and generic parts of the primers, a whole series of reactions can be amplified in the same tube, thus allowing quantitative analysis of all exons in the *BRCA1* gene (Schouten et al. 2002; Hogervorst et al. 2003). While MLPA can confidently give information on exon dosage, it does not give data on how these exons are arranged. Another technique that gives similar data to MLPA is multiplex amplifiable probe hybridization (MAPH) (Akrami et al. 2005; Patsalis et al. 2005).

Molecular Genetic Techniques

A modern molecular genetic laboratory employs several laboratory techniques in diagnosing a broad range of Mendelian disorders. Essentially the laboratory methods, the structure of the laboratory result reports, and interpretation of results follow a pattern that is in keeping with universally agreed protocols. Apart from the laboratory scientific staff, the ultimate responsibility is with the clinician whether a cardiologist or a clinical geneticist. All individuals involved are expected to follow guidelines as laid down by the respective professional statutory body or organization. A detailed technical description of each technique used is beyond the scope of this chapter. A brief outline for each method is given here to assist the reader in understanding issues and limitations in carrying out molecular analysis whether for confirmation of the diagnosis or in genetic risk assessment of a close family member seeking advice for own risks and long-term implications.

In a clinical setting, commonly the following situations arise:

- a previously known disease-causing mutation in the family
- a known mutation or intragenic polymorphism in the family with uncertain pathogenic significance
- a newly detected mutation with known pathogenic significance reported in the literature or in another family
- a newly diagnosed sequence variation in the promoter or an intronic region of one of the genes associated with the disease but not yet confirmed to have any pathogenic significance
- another genetic mechanism indirectly influencing the function of the gene, for example, methylation or parental imprinting
- involvement of more than one gene, for example, a mitochondrial gene and related nuclear gene

In view of the above situations, it is important that the clinician involved prepares the patient or the family member seeking genetic or clinical advice. Genetic counseling and discussion needs to be nonjudgmental and nondirective so that the decision is made in a clearly informed manner.

Direct Mutation Detection Using Polymerase Chain Reaction

Direct testing involves the analysis of a patient's DNA sample to determine if a particular genotype is present, usually a pathogenic mutation within a specific gene. To perform direct testing, we must not only know the particular gene(s) to test, but we must also have knowledge of the normal or wild-type sequence. Almost all direct testing methods, as described below, rely on polymerase chain reaction (PCR). Southern blotting is one technique that does not require PCR; however, applications of this method are generally limited to testing for gene deletions or other major gene disruptions. Owing to its sensitivity, PCR can be applied to a broad spectrum of samples; while a blood sample is the most common source of patient DNA, PCR can also be applied to mouthwash or buccal swab samples, hair, semen, or archived pathological samples (Strachan and Read 1999).

With direct testing methods, it is important to distinguish between cases in which a known, specified mutation is being analyzed, and cases in which a gene is being scanned for the identification of *any* mutation present. Testing a sample for a specific sequence change is a much simpler task than screening an entire gene for any mutation. Consequently, the techniques differ between the two instances. Common methodologies used to test for the presence or absence of a specific mutation include dot blot hybridization using allele-specific oligonucleotide (ASO) probes, the amplification refractory mutation system (ARMS) test, and the oligonucleotide ligation assay (OLA). However, as most cardiovascular disorders are the result of extensive allelic heterogeneity, there is often the need to scan a gene(s) for the presence of *any* mutation, rather than simply testing for one specific change. Therefore, the techniques described below are those commonly used in the diagnostic laboratory for mutation scanning.

Denaturing High-Performance Liquid Chromatography

Denaturing high-performance liquid chromatography (dHPLC) offers a sensitive, gel-free method of mutation scanning, and it is a form of HPLC, where either fully denaturing or partially denaturing conditions, as opposed to nondenaturing conditions, are used to achieve separation of nucleic acids bound to a column by increasing the concentration of an organic solvent. For mutation scanning, partially denaturing conditions are employed. After the initial step of hetero- and homoduplex formation, samples are run over a hydrophobic column and are bound to it by a pairing ion, such as triethylammonium acetate (TEAA). TEAA binds to DNA through its positively charged ammonium group and binds to the column via its hydrophobic ethyl groups. Separation of the nucleic acids bound to the column is achieved at an optimized temperature by increasing the concentration of an organic solvent, such as acetonitrile. This solvent competes with the hydrophobic interactions between the column and TEAA, resulting in the elution of the DNA. Under partially denaturing conditions, the optimal temperature for separation is between 52°C and 75°C (Frueh and Noyer-Weidener 2003). In this optimal temperature range, any disruption of the helix caused by incorrect base pairing due to a potential mutation is most pronounced. This allows for discrete separation of hetero- and homoduplexes. Heteroduplexed DNA will elute before homoduplex DNA at a lower concentration of the organic solvent, as it makes fewer ion-pairing bonds due to its lower helicity. UV or fluorescence can be used for signal detection and samples can be retained for downstream analysis, such as sequencing.

This particular method was first applied to the analysis of genetic variation in 1996 (Underhill et al. 1996, 1997; Ophoff et al. 1996). A number of reports have documented the accuracy and specificity of this method for detecting genetic variation (Orita et al. 1989; Choy et al. 1999; Gross et al. 1999; Bunn et al. 2002). However, it has a potential limitation in that a sample that is homozygous for a mutation will not generate heteroduplexes, unless reference DNA is added. Thus, its sensitivity is not necessarily as high as sequencing. Although it has been used extensively in research settings to study the mutations associated with LQTS and the cardiomyopathies, there is concern in diagnostic laboratories at the technique's potentially reduced sensitivity, especially as families are found to harbor more than one mutation at the same locus. These diseases and their associated mutations are discussed in detail in other chapters in this book (see Table of Contents).

DNA Sequencing

DNA sequencing is considered the gold standard of molecular methods in the identification of genetic mutations. High-throughput automated fluorescent sequencers based on capillary gel electrophoresis have considerably reduced costs and speeded up analysis, providing the ability to sequence numerous samples and/or genes simultaneously. Allied with data analysis softwares, and robotics to set up PCR and sequencing reactions, sequencing is thus now increasingly performed as the method of choice for both detecting and defining mutations in the diagnostic laboratory. Advantages of sequencing include its ability to identify all sequence changes within the DNA fragment submitted for sequencing, as well as revealing the exact position and nature of the change(s). It can equally well reveal mutations in the homo- or heterozygous state. In conditions such as LQTS where dominant, codominant, and recessive patterns of inheritance may operate, it is possible for a patient to have mutations in both alleles of the same gene, and thus direct sequencing becomes a distinct advantage, particularly in the case where a patient may be homozygous for a mutation, which would not necessarily be detected by a method such as dHPLC, which relies on conformational differences between DNA strands.

The chemistry for automated sequencing is based on a double-stranded template and cycle sequencing, where the actual sequencing reactions are performed in a thermal cycler. In order for there to be automated reading of the DNA sequence ladder, the sequence fragments must be labeled with a fluorescent dye. Four distinct colors are used to distinguish the four different bases. Dye-terminator chemistry is the most commonly used method to label the DNA fragments with fluorescent dyes. Fragments are labeled with the dye corresponding to their last dideoxynucleotide (ddNTP). Dideoxynucleotides lacking the 3' hydroxyl group in order to terminate the chain after the incorporation of the labeled nucleotide are used in the sequencing reactions, just as in the manual version of the Sanger sequencing method. Fragments ending in ddATP will be labeled with "green" dye and read as "A" in the sequence, fragments ending in ddTTP will be labeled with "red" dye and read as "T" in the sequence, and so on. Incorporation of the four distinct dyes allows all four sequencing reactions to be performed in the same tube or plate well, rather than four separate tubes. Once the sequencing reaction is complete, the sample must be purified in order to remove excess ddNTPs. Purification can be done by ethanol precipitation or by various column or bead methods, the latter of which can be easily automated and performed by robotics. Samples are then denatured, as separation during electrophoresis occurs strictly by size. Each sample is loaded into one lane of the capillary gel and fragments migrate by size, or samples in 96- or 384-well plates can be loaded onto machines with 16, 48, or even 96 capillaries, circumventing the need for potentially error-prone manual loading and the preparation of gels. Each fragment in turn passes by a laser beam that excites the fluorescent dye, causing it to emit its color, which is then captured by a detector. The detector converts the fluorescence to an electrical signal that is read by a computer software program as a peak of color. The readout from this software, called an electropherogram, displays the sequence as peaks of colors and assigns a text letter to each peak corresponding to the appropriate base. A number of publicly and commercially available software programs currently exist, which can then interpret and apply the sequencing data. Collectively, these programs call the bases and assign a quality score to each base (Phred), assemble contigs (Phrap), determine single nucleotide changes (Polyphred), and allow for viewing and editing of the sequence (consed). In this way, large amounts of data can be filtered so that interpretational effort can be directed to putative mutations. Sequencing is quantitative, if reference is made to the original fluorescence intensity data, rather than the possibly manipulated data displayed in the sequence traces. Thus, it is capable of detecting mosaicism or heteroplasmy when the proportion of the minor allele is more than 5%–10%.

A number of parameters are capable of affecting the quality of the sequence read, including the PCR reaction, the amount, quality and size of the template, as well as the sequence content. PCR reactions must be cleaned before using the amplicons as sequencing templates, as leftover components of the PCR reaction can interfere with the sequencing reaction. In addition, low-quality DNA that has been degraded, or a low starting amount of template, will result in poor sequencing reads. The length of the template to be sequenced can also affect final sequence quality. Most sequencing chemistries are capable of accurately reading 400 to 500 bases (Buckingham and Flaws 2007), although, sequences with a high GC content are often difficult to read due to intrastrand hybridization within the template. Using special dGTPs such as 7-deaza-dGTP in place of standard dGTP can improve sequencing reads around GC bands (Buckingham and Flaws 2007).

In addition to the above-described automated Sanger sequencing method, pyrosequencing is a relatively new method that also allows for the determination of the order of nucleotides in a DNA sample. Pyrosequencing does not require the generation of a DNA ladder, as in the Sanger method, and it does not require fluorescent dyes or gels. This method is based on the generation of light when a nucleotide is added to a growing DNA strand. One advantage of this method is that it is quantitative, allowing for the measurement of the relative amounts of alleles. However, read lengths are generally limited to less than 100 bases. It is therefore most appropriate for short to moderate sequence analysis. This may be useful when determining the presence or absence of a specific mutation, but may not be ideal when scanning a whole gene or large parts of a gene for the presence of any mutation.

Molecular Testing for Cardiovascular Genetic Disorders

Genetic mechanisms and classification of cardiovascular genetic disorders are discussed elsewhere in this book (Chapter 3). The classification of inherited cardiovascular disorders includes several disorders that exhibit Mendelian inheritance patterns. In addition, mitochondrial inheritance pattern is also seen in some conditions with similar phenotype inherited in the Mendelian manner (see also Chapter 31). It is beyond the scope of this chapter to discuss all Mendelian disorders as these are discussed elsewhere in this book (see Table of Contents). Tables 6–1 and 6–2 list cardiomyopathic and arrhythmic syndromes for which molecular diagnosis is available for clinical purposes; however, because new tests are being introduced all the time, it is recommended that web sites that list diagnostic genetic tests be consulted for up-to-date information, for example, the U.K. National Health Service Genetic Testing Network (NHS UKGTN: http://www.ukgtn.nhs.uk/gtn/Home), Orphanet (www.orpha.net/), Eurogentest (www.eurogentest.org/), and GeneTests (www.genetests.org/). Request for molecular testing is now frequently received from clinical cardiologists or clinical geneticists. Specialist clinics are now operational dealing with a specific disorder or for a single group of Mendelian inherited cardiovascular disorder. This chapter will only discuss molecular testing in reference to cardiomyopathies and LQTS, which are the two most common Mendelian cardiovascular disorders encountered in the clinical setting.

Table 6–1 Molecular Genetic Diagnosis in Mendelian Cardiovascular Disorders

Disease	Laboratory Method
Hypertrophic cardiomyopathy	Direct mutation detection and sequencing
Dilated cardiomyopathy	Direct mutation detection and sequencing
Arrhythmogenic right	
Ventricular hypertrophy	Direct mutation detection and sequencing
Duchenne/Becker MD	Exon dosage and sequencing
Left ventricular noncompaction	Direct mutation detection and sequencing
Long QT syndrome	Direct mutation detection and sequencing
Brugada syndrome	Direct mutation detection and sequencing
Metabolic heart disease	Cardiac and skeletal muscle histology; biochemical
Pompe, Danon disease, Mitochondrial	Assay; direct mutation analysis

Cardiomyopathies define any disease of the heart that arises from a primary abnormality present in the myocardium (Richardson et al. 1996). These diseases can lead to significant morbidity and mortality (Karkkainen and Peuhkurinen 2007) and while most cases are considered idiopathic, there is mounting evidence that shows that a significant amount of the cases are influenced by genetic factors. Understanding these genetic factors and risks could lead to early detection and better therapies to cardiomyopathy patients. Cardiomyopathies are heterogeneous and are generally classified into two broad categories—dilated cardiomyopathy (Box 6–1) and HCM (Box 6–2). Mendelian disorders of cardiac rhythm and conduction are equally heterogeneous. The LQTS is the most common condition within this group. This is defined by the prolongation of the recovery period [the T interval on electrocardiograms (ECGs)] of the cardiac ventricles following their depolarization (the Q interval). Owing to fatal ventricular arrhythmias caused by LQTS, it is perhaps the most common genetic cause of sudden unexplained death (SUD) of cardiac origin with a structurally normal heart (Ackerman 2005). Much like the cardiomyopathies, it is characterized by substantial genotypic and phenotypic heterogeneity.

The Molecular Genetics of Cardiomyopathies

DCM was once considered to have a genetic origin in only rare cases, but in the past 15 years, researchers have described many mutations and genes thought to play a role in the etiology of DCM. Estimates vary and between 30% and 50% of the cases of DCM are genetic in origin with autosomal dominant being the most reported form of inheritance (Keeling et al. 1995; Baig et al. 1998; Grunig et al. 1998; Gregori et al. 2001), although autosomal recessive, X-linked, and mitochondrial inheritance does occur in rare cases (Suomalainen et al. 1992; Remes et al. 1994; Silvestri et al. 1994; Marin-Garcia et al. 1996; Li et al. 1997; Arbustini et al. 1998; Baig et al. 1998; Grunig et al. 1998; Mestroni et al. 1999; Seliem et al. 2000; Murphy et al. 2004). Many genes have been identified as causal candidates for DCM and several mutations within these genes have been found to be associated with the disease (Table 6–2).

HCM is a familial disease in which most of the cases are inherited in an autosomal dominant pattern. Much is known about the genetics underlying HCM. Most HCM cases are thought to have a genetic origin with the majority following an autosomal dominant inheritance pattern (Marian et al. 2001; Wigle 2001; Maron 2002) and the rest either being sporadic mutations or rare autosomal recessive mutations (Poetter et al. 1996; Richard et al. 2003). Despite this relatively simple mode of inheritance, the genetics of this disease is quite complex. The presentation of HCM is extremely variable, which has historically made the disease very difficult to diagnose. This variability of disease is a direct reflection of the underlying genetic heterogeneity.

Treatment for HCM based on the identification of one of the known mutations remains a goal of HCM research. Some genotype–phenotype correlations have been made, though they have not been observed consistently. Family studies initially identified gene-specific phenotypes, with clear "malignant" and "benign" mutations emerging. For example, various mutations in the β-myosin heavy chain gene were associated with a mild or benign clinical course of HCM, while others in this same gene were associated with early disease presentation, rapid progression, and increased risk of sudden death (Watkins et al. 1992; Anan et al. 1994). However, subsequent studies in a number of different populations of unrelated individuals have not seen these types of clear-cut correlations (Ackerman et al. 2002; Jääskeläinen et al. 2002;

Table 6–2 Genes and Proteins Mutated in Dilated and Hypertrophic Cardiomyopathy

Cardiomyopathy	Locus	Gene	Protein	References
DCM				
	12p12.1	*ABCC9*	Sulfonylurea receptor 2A	(Bienengraeber et al. 2004)
	1q43	*ACTN2*	A-Actinin	(Mohapatra et al. 2003)
	2q35	*DES*	Desmin	(Li et al. 1999)
	1q22	*LMNA*	Lamin A/C	(Fatkin et al. 1999; Becane et al. 2000; Brodsky et al. 2000; Hershberger et al. 2002; Arbustini et al. 2002; MacLeod et al. 2003; Verga et al. 2003; Sebillon et al. 2003; Taylor et al. 2003a; Genschel and Schmidt 2000; Karkkainen et al. 2004b, 2006; van Berlo et al. 2005)
	6q22.1	*PLN*	Phospholamban	(Haghighi et al. 2003; Schmitt et al. 2003)
	3p22–25	SCN5A	Sodium channel type 5α	(Olson and Keating 1996; McNair et al. 2004)
	5q33	SGCD	Δ-Sarcoglycan	(Tsubata et al. 2000)
	17q12	TCAP	Telethonin	(Knoll et al. 2002)
	12q22	TMPO	Thymopoietin	(Taylor et al. 2005)
	3p21	TNNC1	Cardiac troponin C	(Mogensen et al. 2004)
	2q31	TTN	Titin	(Siu et al. 1999; Gerull et al. 2002; Itoh-Satoh et al. 2002; Gerull et al. 2006)
	10q22.2	VCL	Metavinculin	(Olson et al. 2002)
	10q23.2	ZASP/LBD3	Cypher/LIM binding domain 3	(Vatta and Mohapatra 2003; Arimura et al. 2004)
X-linked DCM	Xp21.2	DMD	Dystrophin	(Muntoni et al. 1993; Towbin et al. 1993)
	Xq28	TAZ/G4.5	Tafazzin	(Bione et al. 1996; D'Adamo et al. 1997)
HCM				
	19q13.2–13.3	DMPK	Dystrophia myotonica protein kinase	(O'Cochlain et al. 2004)
	9q13	FXN	Frataxin	(Filla et al. 1996; Isnard et al. 1997)
	12q23–24.3	MYL2*	Ventricular myosin regulatory light chain	(Poetter et al. 1996)
	3p21.2–21.3	MYL3*	Ventricular myosin essential light chain	(Poetter et al. 1996)
	20q13.3	MYLK2	Myosin light polypeptide kinase	(Davis et al. 2001)
	7q36	PRKAG2	AMP-activated protein kinase γ2 regulatory subunit	(Blair et al. 2001; Gollob et al. 2001; Arad et al. 2002, 2003)
X-linked HCM	Xq22	GLA	α-Galactosidase A	(Matsuzawa et al. 2005; Garman and Garboczi 2004)
Mitochondrial inheritance	mtDNA	MTTG	Mitochondrial transfer RNA-glycine	(Taylor ct al. 2003b)
	mtDNA	MTTI	Mitochondrial transfer RNA-isoleucine	(Taylor et al. 2003b)
DCM and HCM				
	15q14	ACTC*	Cardiac actin	(Olson et al. 1998)
	11p15.1	MLP/CSRP3	Cardiac LIM protein	(Knoll et al. 2002; Mohapatra et al. 2003)
	11p11.2	MYBPC*	Myosin-binding protein C	(Daehmlow et al. 2002)
	14q12	MYH6	A-myosin heavy chain	(Niimura et al. 2002)
	14q12	MYH7*	β-myosin heavy chain	(Kamisago et al. 2000; Daehmlow et al. 2002; Karkkainen et al. 2004; Villard et al. 2005)
	19q13.4	TNN13*	Cardiac troponin I	(Murphy et al. 2004)
	1q32	TNNT2*	Cardiac troponin T	(Durand et al. 1995; Kamisago et al. 2000; Li et al. 2001; Hanson et al. 2002; Stefanelli et al. 2004)
	15q22.1	TPM1*	α-Tropomyosin	(Olson et al. 2001)

*Indicates those genes for which a commercially available test is now offered.
Abbreviations: DCM, dilated cardiomyopathy, HCM, hypertrophic cardiomyopathy.

Box 6–1 Key Points about Dilated Cardiomyopathy

- DCM occurs in approximately 1 out of every 2,500 individuals and accounts for the majority of cardiomyopathies.
- It is associated with substantial mortality due to heart failure, arrhythmias, and thromboembolic events.
- Diagnosis relies on an echocardiogram but symptoms are often vague in the early stages of disease and there is great variability in clinical presentation.
- Of idiopathic DCM, 25%–30% has been shown to be the result of inherited gene mutations.
- The genetics of DCM are complex, with hundreds of mutations spanning numerous genes related to sodium and potassium channels, the sarcomere, and cytoskeleton.
- Mutation screening and genetic testing are not yet available for routine use, in part due to its extensive genetic heterogeneity.
- Advances in genetics and genomics are critically needed to allow for earlier detection and more tailored therapy.

Box 6–2 Key Points about Hypertrophic Cardiomyopathy

- The prevalence of HCM is estimated to be 1 in 500 young adults and symptoms most commonly present in the 10–25-year age group.
- Unlike DCM, it is characterized by myocyte hypertrophy and disarray, as well as interstitial fibrosis.
- Over 50% of those with unexplained left ventricular hypertrophy harbor one of the known causal HCM mutations, making it the most commonly inherited cardiovascular disease.
- The variability of HCM is in part due to its underlying genetic heterogeneity, with over 100 different mutations in at least 11 different genes, many of which are related to the sarcomere.
- Diagnostic genetic testing is now available for the eight commonly mutated sarcomeric genes.
- Genetic and genomic advances can assist in earlier diagnosis and in establishing better genotype–phenotype correlations to guide treatment.

Erdmann et al. 2003; García-Castro 2003; Mörner et al. 2003; Van Driest et al. 2005b). Observations from these more recent studies suggest a much more nebulous picture of genotype–phenotype correlations, with a clear picture yet to emerge. More research in this area is needed in order to attach prognostic significance to any of the HCM mutations and to consequently allow for gene-based therapy in the management of this disease.

Genes Associated with Dilated and Hypertrophic Cardiomyopathies

Since cardiomyopathies are diseases classified by cardiac muscle dysfunction, it follows that most of the genes and mutations identified for this class of disease are involved in the mechanism of muscle contraction and the sarcomere. The sarcomere is the complex of proteins that is involved in generating the force necessary for contraction. The sarcomere is composed of a thick filament, a thin filament, and various structural and regulatory proteins. The thick filament consists of α- and β-myosin heavy chains, essential and regulatory myosin light chains, and myosin binding protein C. The heavy chains are involved in the hydrolysis of ATP to create the movement necessary to shorten the length of the sarcomere and cause contraction. The thin filament is made of actin, tropomyosin, and the troponin complex and is highly regulated. The heads of the myosin heavy chains bind the thin filament and the action of the power stroke causes the thin filaments to slide past and shorten the sarcomere. In addition to the structural roles of the previously mentioned proteins, titin, nebulin, and other proteins provide structure for the sarcomere.

As expected, mutations in the genes of the proteins that make up the sarcomere have been implicated in the pathogenesis of both DCM and HCM. Even though DCM and HCM follow different disease courses, the pathologic mechanisms behind them are remarkably similar because both involve improper performance of the sarcomere. Many other structural and regulatory genes have been identified as candidates for DCM and HCM, but genes and mutations referenced in this section represent the most common and well-known genes studied in the field of cardiomyopathy genetics. A majority of these genes have been found using the candidate gene approach due to their respective roles in muscle function. For a more complete listing of genes associated with cardiomyopathies, please refer to Table 6–2.

1. β-Myosin Heavy Chain

Myosin, the thick filament, is a large motor protein than is responsible for the actin-based motility of the cardiac myocyte. The heavy chain of myosin is responsible for hydrolysis of ATP and directly interacts with actin. This protein is essential for contraction. This gene was first identified through linkage analysis and later verified as the cause of HCM in a family study (Jarcho et al. 1989; Geisterfer-Lowrance et al. 1990). Most mutations occur at the head region of the protein and may interfere with myosin–actin binding (Kamisago et al. 2000). In DCM, mutations have been found in both familial (Kamisago et al. 2000) and sporadic cases (Daehmlow et al. 2002). In HCM, despite many cases of familial mutations, the discovery of identical mutations in patients with different haplotypic backgrounds points to the importance of sporadic mutations in this disease (Watkins et al. 1993). More mutations have been found in the *MYH7* gene than any other candidate gene for HCM and mutations within this gene are some of the most frequent mutations found in cardiomyopathies, appearing in roughly 25% of all HCM cases (Richard et al. 2003).

2. Myosin Binding Protein-C

MYBPC3 encodes the protein myosin binding protein C that binds to the myosin heavy chain and affects the binding of tropomysin. Mutations within this gene are frequent in families with HCM (Richard et al. 2003). In a study by Niimura and colleagues, 16 families were evaluated and found to have 12 different *MYBPC3* mutations that appeared to have a complex inheritance pattern and worse outcomes compared to patients without mutations (Niimura et al. 1998). Mutations in this gene appear to be mostly splice-site mutations that result in incomplete proteins that are unable to fully function in their roles of binding the myosin heavy chain (Okagaki et al. 1993; Bonne et al. 1995; Watkins et al. 1995a; Freiburg and Gautel 1996), but missense mutations have also been recorded (Moolman-Smook et al. 1998). There has also been a study that showed a *MYBPC3* mutation in association with human DCM (Daehmlow et al. 2002) and a study of homozygous mutant mice that showed DCM (McConnell et al. 1999).

3. Actin

Actin, a major component of the thin filament, is also an integral part of the contraction mechanism of the cardiac myocyte. The cardiac actin gene (*ACTC*) has been an area of research since the discovery of two missense mutations in DCM that are located near the dystrophin binding site (Olson et al. 1998; Komajda et al. 1999; Mogensen et al. 1999; Tsubata et al. 2000). These findings were quickly followed up by identification of a mutation in HCM, which is located in the myosin binding region (Mogensen et al. 1999). In either disease, these mutations are quite rare (Olson et al. 2000; Richard et al. 2003).

Troponin

The troponin complex consists of several troponins that bind to tropomyosin and form an integral regulatory portion of the thin filament. Troponin T (*TNNT2*) interacts with tropomyosin and other troponins, Troponin C (*TNNC1*) and Troponin I (*TNNI3*). TNNT2 mutations are frequent in cases of HCM (Watkins et al. 1995b) and typically result in poor prognosis and an increase in the possibility of sudden death. Mutations have also been found in DCM cases and one deletion, ΔLys210, is believed to reduce interaction between Troponin T and C and lead to a decrease in the power stroke (Kamisago et al. 2000; Hanson et al. 2002). Mutations have also been found in the *TNNI3* and *TNNC1* genes in both DCM and HCM patients (Kimura et al. 1997; Hoffmann et al. 2001; Mogensen et al. 2003, 2004; Murphy et al. 2004).

1. α-Tropomyosin

α-Tropomyosin (*TPM1*) is another important regulatory and structural protein on the thin filament. Mutations have been described in DCM in a region thought to control interactions between actin and α-tropomyosin and are possibly linked with a severe form of the disease (Olson et al. 2001). Several mutations have been identified in HCM patients and researchers have shown that some mutations change sarcomere force output and can lead to more severe disease processes such as early onset disease followed by heart failure or sudden death (Yamauchi-Takihara et al. 1996; Michele et al. 1999; Prabhakar et al. 2001).

2. Titin/Telethonin

Titin (*TTN*) is an extremely large protein (3,000 kDa) that is thought to support the myosin thick filament and provide a large component of the sarcomeric cytoskeleton. Mutations within this gene are rare, but have been described in both DCM (Gerull et al. 2002, 2006; Itoh-Satoh et al. 2002) and HCM (Satoh et al. 1999). Owing to the size of *TTN*, more mutations could easily be identified. DCM patients with *TTN* mutations tend to have accompanying arrhythmias and ECG abnormalities that often require implantation of a cardioverter-defibrillator. Mutations have also been found in rare occasions in DCM patients in the related telethonin gene (*TCAP*). TCAP is important in sarcomeric assembly and requires phosphorylation by TTN. Although this has only been found in a few patients, the disease appears to be severe in those with TCAP mutations (Knoll et al. 2002; Hayashi et al. 2004).

Mutation Detection and Genetic Testing in the Cardiomyopathies

Mutation detection in the cardiomyopathies has been conducted mainly in a research setting through the use of PCR and single-strand conformation polymorphism (SSCP) or denaturing high-performance liquid chromatography (dHPLC) analyses followed by direct sequencing (Ackerman et al. 2002; Blair et al. 2002; Van Driest et al. 2002a, 2002b; Yu et al. 2005). However, with the increased understanding of the relationship between phenotype and genotype and developments in analytical technology, diagnostic molecular genetic testing is now available for HCM. Genetic screening for cardiomyopathies, as with their diagnoses, is challenging due to the heterogeneous nature of this class of disease. Although cardiomyopathies tend to follow Mendelian inheritance patterns, variable penetrance complicates the interpretation and it is believed that additional modifying factors influence the actual disease expression and its course (Marian et al. 2001). With our currently limited understanding of all factors involved, clinical genetic testing is at this time limited to confirming a diagnosis in a proportion of cases, and when a causative mutation can be identified, to the identification of those at risk, or not at risk, in an affected family.

Clinical testing for HCM may be offered in two panels, the first of which screens for mutations within the five most common genes for HCM (*MYH7,MYBPC3, TNNT2, TNNI3*, and *TPM1*) and the second screens for mutations within three additional genes (*ACTC, MYL2*, and *MYL3*). The overall mutation detection rate of the first panel among patients with clinically evident HCM is estimated to be 50%–60% and the detection rate for the second panel is 5%–10%, yielding a combined detection rate of 55%–70% if both panels are tested (http://www.hpcgg.org/LMM/comment/print/HCM_info2007.pdf). Various cohort studies have suggested the yield to be in the range of 30%–60%, with an average of 42% (Van Driest et al. 2005a).

Since limited clinical diagnostic tests are being offered for DCM, a group in Finland has recently proposed screening for mutations within the Lamin A/C gene (*LMNA*) in patients that are believed to be at risk for familial DCM. Lamins play a role in connecting chromatin to the nuclear matrix and envelope. They propose that the mutations are frequent enough in this selected population to warrant genetic screening in first-degree relatives of clinically identified patients, especially considering that the phenotype is significantly more severe than average (Karkkainen and Peuhkurinen 2007). Knowing that a patient has a *LMNA* mutation would direct them to a more appropriate course of action, including more detailed follow-up.

One of the factors limiting the use of genetic testing results in the cardiomyopathies is the lack of data regarding genotype to phenotype correlation. There has historically been an emphasis on gathering this type of data, but more is needed before we can use a patient's sequence data to predict disease risk, progression, outcomes, and treatments. Additional studies with extensive patient follow-up are needed before we will be able to make more routine use of genetic screening data in the clinic.

Recent Genomic Advances in the Cardiomyopathies

There are many new techniques that are currently being developed that may aid in future genetic screening studies and clinical tests. Advances in technology are focusing on allowing clinicians to quickly, efficiently, and noninvasively identify genetic markers and mutations correlated to cardiomyopathies in a high-throughput manner at a low cost. Recently, Miller and colleagues have proposed taking advantage of new methods aimed at harvesting and preserving RNA to develop a new approach that is reported to allow sequence analysis of transcribed genes from <3 mL of peripheral blood (Miller et al. 2007b). They believe this technique is extremely valuable in the study of cardiovascular diseases such as DCM and HCM, because cardiac-restricted genes have proven difficult to acquire the necessary amounts of genetic testing material. By using inexpensive materials to isolate RNA directly from blood samples, they were able to quickly identify mutations by direct sequencing of *MYBPC3* mRNA at a greatly reduced cost when compared to similar studies. There are similar advances being made in the field of high-throughput mutational screening.

Zeller and colleagues recently completed a pilot study for large-scale mutation screening for both DCM and HCM using denaturing gradient gel electrophoresis (DGGE) (Zeller et al. 2006). They included 11 known and 14 putative candidate genes for cardiomyopathies and were able to screen 286 out of the total 312 exons for sequence variation that was detected by migration differences of homo- and heteroduplexes of PCR-generated amplicons. Once exons exhibiting migration differences on the gel were identified, they could then be sequenced to find mutations. Their method was able to identify known mutations, as well as several new variants that were associated with cardiomyopathies.

Another new platform being utilized to screen for mutations correlated to cardiomyopathies is the polony multiplex analysis of gene expression (PMAGE) method developed by Kim and colleagues (Kim et al. 2007). By clonally amplifying cDNA tags on a polony bead, this technique allows for the quantification of mRNA expression even in transcripts that are as rare as one transcript per three cells. PMAGE permits the analysis of as many as 5 million cDNA molecules per run, so the capability to run all the desired genes is in place. Kim and colleagues were able to identify many low-abundance transcripts in mice that they believe indicate transcriptional changes that occur long before clinical characteristics appear in a mouse model of HCM.

Genome-wide expression studies are quickly becoming a preferred method of determining the genetic profile of disease. In this way, Barth and colleagues have taken a major step in identifying a gene expression profile of DCM in their recent study of whole genome microarrays (Barth et al. 2006). They performed two genome-wide expression experiments in order to identify a genetic signature evident in patients with DCM when compared to nonfailing ventricular tissues. They subsequently found significant involvement of the immune response in end-stage DCM, as well as a robust profile of gene expression that allowed them to identify DCM patients with >90% accuracy.

With new tools such as whole genome sequencing and expression profiling, diseases such as DCM and HCM will be able to be better managed. Tests are now on the horizon that will allow physicians and researchers to easily determine a mutational or expression profile or simply sequence the ten most important genes in any patient suspected of having a cardiomyopathy. As testing costs decrease and high-throughput techniques continue to increase the amount of data output, the medical community comes closer to identifying patients at risk for cardiomyopathies before they have any symptoms. This is especially important for this class of disease as the first symptom could be sudden death. Ultimately, the goal will be that cardiomyopathies will no longer need to be classified into broad categories based on anatomical changes, but can be grouped into molecular mechanism of disease and be treated appropriately. If the current progress is any indication of the future, the field of cardiomyopathies, which is just now scratching the surface of genetic screening, may soon be leading the way into the genomics age.

In summary, dilated and hypertrophic cardiomyopathies are important diseases that are known to have a genetic component in many cases. With genetic factors playing an important role, the disease impacts not only the patient but also his family. Dozens of genes and hundreds of mutations have been identified that are associated with these diseases, but due to the heterogeneity and rarity of most of these mutations, genetic screening and characterization are not typical parts of most diagnostic and treatment procedures. As more mutations are identified and more studies are aimed at linking the mutations to disease and disease progression, our understanding of this class of disease will come into focus allowing us to better utilize the genetic tools available to not only identify patients, but treat them more effectively.

Molecular Diagnosis of Long QT Syndrome

Congenital LQTS is one of the most common Mendelian cardiovascular conditions, with an estimated prevalence of 1 in 5,000 (Ackerman 2005). The seriousness of this disorder is highlighted by its high risk of sudden death from ventricular arrhythmias. Its clinical presentation is heterogeneous in nature and often individuals are asymptomatic (Box 6–3). LQTS may result in death during infancy or those affected may remain asymptomatic throughout their lifetime. The genetics of this disease are equally heterogeneous as is the clinical presentation. Details of LQTS and related inherited arrhythmic disorders are discussed elsewhere in the book (see Table of Contents).

Molecular Genetics of LQTS

LQTS can be inherited in one of two ways, autosomal dominant or recessive. The recessive form is associated with deafness and is much rarer than the autosomal dominant type. There are also acquired forms of LQTS, which result from various drugs, including antidepressants and antiarrhythmics, as well as electrolyte imbalances. We will focus on the two inherited forms of LQTS. The first two genes identified for LQTS were the potassium channel gene *KCNH2* (formerly *HERG*) and the sodium channel gene *SCNA5* in 1995 (Curran et al. 1995; Wang et al. 1995). The identification of the third gene, *KCNQ1*, came in 1996 (Wang et al. 1996). Collectively, the hundreds of mutations scattered throughout these three genes account for 65%–75% of congenital LQTS cases and cause the three primary forms of the disorder (LQTS1–3) (Splawski et al. 2000; Ackerman 2005). Since then, seven other genes have been identified that are responsible for the less common subtypes of LQTS. All are either potassium, sodium, or calcium channel genes, with the exception of *ANK2* and *CAV3*, which are both scaffolding proteins (Table 6–3). The actual molecular defect behind LQTS is determined by the genotype; however, all result in a final common pathway of prolongation of the atrial action potential with decreased repolarization reserve (Roberts 2006). The effect of the potassium channel mutations is opposite that of the sodium channel mutations. Potassium channel mutations cause insufficient opening of the channels with consequent decreased outward current, while sodium channel mutations result

Box 6–3 Key Points about LQTS

- LQTS presents with considerable clinical heterogeneity and a high mortality rate if left untreated.
- Reliance on ECG findings to diagnose LQTS will miss cases of the disease, as many individuals do not show a clearly prolonged QT interval.
- The clinical heterogeneity of LQTS is matched by its genetic heterogeneity.
- There are three main types of LQTS caused by mutations in potassium and sodium channel-related genes.
- Strong genotype–phenotype correlations allow for gene-specific therapy.
- Genetic testing is now clinically available for the most common LQTS genes.

Table 6–3 Genes and Genotype-Phenotype Correlations in Long QT Syndrome (LQTS)

LQTS Subtype	Locus	Gene	Protein	Genotype–phenotype Correlations	References
LQTS1	11p15.5	*KCNQ1**	Voltage-gated potassium channel, KQT-like subfamily, member 1	Sympathetic activation can lead to events; low mortality; respond well to β-blockers Jervell and Lange-Nielsen syndrome.	(Wang et al. 1996)
LQTS2	7q35-q36	*KCNH2**	Voltage-gated potassium channel, subfamily H, member 2	Events triggered by sudden noises during periods of rest; ↑ risk of cardiac arrests during β-blocker therapy	(Curran et al. 1995)
LQTS3	3p21	*SCN5A**	Voltage-gated sodium channel, type 5, α subunit	↑ probability of death associated with first event; ↑ event rates during therapy; symptomatic after 10 years of age; ↑ use of ICDs	(Wang et al. 1995)
LQTS4	4q25-q27	*ANK2*	Ankyrin	Prolonged QT_c interval not a consistent feature; syncope; bradycardia; sinus arrhythmia; risk of sudden death. Suggested to be a distinct clinical entity	(Mohler et al. 2003; Mohler et al. 2004)
LQTS5	21q22.12	*KCNE1**	Voltage-gated potassium channel, Isk-related family, member 1	Rare; clinically managed as LQTS1	(Schulze-Bahr et al. 1997; Splawski et al. 1997)
LQTS6	21q22.12	*KCNE2**	Voltage-gated potassium channel, Isk-related family, member 2	Rare; clinically managed as LQTS2	(Abbott et al. 1999)
LQTS7	17q23.1-q24.2	*KCNJ2*	Potassium inwardly rectifying channel, subfamily J, member 2	LQTS occurs as part of Andersen-Tawil syndrome	(Plaster et al. 2001)
LQTS8	12p13.3	*CACNA1c*	Calcium channel, voltage-dependent, L type, α 1C subunit	LQTS occurs as part of Timothy syndrome	(Splawski et al. 2004)
LQTS9	3p25	*CAV3*	Caveolin-3	Nonexertional syncope; sinus bradycardia	(Vatta et al. 2006)
LQTS10	11q23.3	*SCN4B*	Voltage-gated sodium channel, type IV, β	Identified in Mexican family; similar to LQTS3	(Medeiros-Domingo et al. 2007)

* Indicates those genes for which a commercially available test is now offered.

in improper closing of the channels with consequent increased inward current. In the case of the calcium channel mutations (*CACNA1c* gene), reduced channel inactivation occurs, leading to maintained depolarizing L-type calcium currents (Splawski et al. 2004, 2005). The mechanism behind the *ANK2* mutation differs from either of the previous two mechanisms. The *ANK2* E1425G mutation leads to disruption of a number of ankyrin-binding proteins and is thought to possibly affect localization of sodium and calcium channel proteins (Mohler et al. 2003). The exact mechanism behind the *CAV3* mutation has yet to be defined, though it appears to affect the kinetics of the *SCN5A*-encoded voltage-gated sodium channel (Vatta et al. 2006).

As genetic testing has recently become available, and there are now some known limited genotype–phenotype correlations within LQTS, a form of gene-based therapy can be offered to patients. This will be discussed in more detail in the following section. While the ideal situation is one where the genotype is known before therapy is begun, genotype data is generally not immediately available. In addition, nearly 30%–35% of patients with LQTS do not carry one of the genotypes known to be associated with the disorder (Schwartz 2006). Consequently, given the high efficacy of β-blockers in LQTS, they are generally prescribed for all patients, with additional therapy, if needed, guided by a patient's genotype once it is known.

A number of genotype–phenotype studies have demonstrated clear differences between the three main forms of LQTS with regard to clinical presentation, event triggers, and the risk of cardiac arrest and sudden death (Moss et al. 1995; Zhang et al. 2000; Schwartz et al. 2001). These studies have allowed for gene-specific clinical management of the disease. The various forms of LQTS are discussed below along with their associated genes and known genotype–phenotype correlations.

1. LQTS1

This is the most common form of LQTS and is caused by heterozygous mutations within the *KCNQ1* gene, which encodes the potassium channel α subunit of I_{Ks}. Mutations in this gene are found in approximately 50% of affected individuals (Robin et al. 2007). Homozygosity or compound heterozygosity of mutations in this gene cause the recessive form of LQTS associated with hearing impairment (Jervell and Lange-Nielsen syndrome). Genotype–phenotype studies have shown that life-threatening events generally occur in this group during sympathetic activation, and hence, those with an LQTS1 genotype should not exercise or take part in competitive sports. Swimming is a particularly well-established trigger of events for this class (Ackerman et al. 1999; Schwartz et al. 2001). The rate of cardiac arrest and sudden death in this group is rather low, approximately 1% (Zareba et al. 2003; Priori et al. 2004), and the vast majority of these patients respond well to the use of β-blockers.

2. LQTS2

This is the second most common form of LQTS and involves mutations in the *KCNH2* gene (formerly *HERG*), encoding the I_{Kr} current. Mutations in this gene account for approximately 35%–40% of LQTS cases. Most events in this class are triggered by sudden noises during periods of rest (Wilde et al. 1999; Schwartz et al. 2001). Exercise and sports pose a very low risk to this group. However, they do not respond as well to β-blockers as those in LQTS1. Two studies demonstrated cardiac arrests in 4% and nearly 7% of LQTS2 study participants taking β-blockers (Schwartz et al.

2001; Priori et al. 2004), although neither report documented any sudden deaths among these patients. Those falling into this genotypic class of LQTS are typically managed with β-blockers, as with LQTS1; however, use of ICDs may be more prevalent in this class due to its rate of arrests during therapy.

3. LQTS3

The third most common type of LQTS is the result of mutations within the sodium channel α subunit gene *SCN5A* accounting for 10%–15% of cases. The management of patients within this group is more complicated than those in the previous two groups (Schwartz 2006). β-blockers appear to protect this group least effectively of the three main subtypes. Schwartz et al. and Priori et al. have shown event rates for the combined endpoint of cardiac arrests and sudden deaths to be 14%–17% in LQTS3 patients receiving therapy (Schwartz et al. 2001; Priori et al. 2004). An additional report suggests that there is a higher probability of death associated with the first event in those with this genotype (Zareba et al. 1998). Evidence also exists, which shows that many LQTS3 patients do not become symptomatic prior to the age of 10, particularly girls (Schwartz et al. 2001; Priori et al. 2003). Given this data, the course of treatment for these patients is less clear than for those in LQTS1 or LQTS2. As there is no evidence that β-blockers harm these patients, they are still recommended for use in this group. Additionally, these patients can be given mexiletine, a sodium channel blocker that has been shown to significantly shorten the QT interval in these patients (Schwartz et al. 1995). Finally, ICDs are commonly used in this group; however, given the fact that most in this class do not show symptoms before 10 years of age, the implantation of this device could be delayed (Schwartz 2006). Limited data suggest that LQTS3 patients may also derive benefit from LCSD for those who may not want an ICD (Schwartz et al. 2004).

4. LQTS4

The *ANK2* E1425G mutation has been shown to cause this subtype of LQTS (Mohler et al. 2003). This loss-of-function variant was identified in an extended French family. Since then, other unrelated individuals with cardiac dysfunction and sudden death have been shown to carry various loss-of-function mutations in *ANK2* (Mohler et al. 2004). Because these individuals displayed clinical features distinct from classic LQTS, it has been suggested that this form is actually a separate disorder (Mohler et al. 2004; Schwartz 2006).

5. LQTS5

This is a very rare form of LQTS and is caused by mutations in *KCNE1*, encoding the potassium channel β subunit of I_{Ks} (Schulze-Bahr et al. 1997; Splawski et al. 1997). Mutations in the gene account for nearly 2%–3% of LQTS. Owing to its rarity, LQTS5 is clinically managed as LQTS1 (Schwartz 2006).

6. LQTS6

Also a relatively uncommon form of LQTS, this type is the result of mutations in *KCNE2*, encoding the potassium channel β subunit of I_{Kr} (Abbott et al. 1999). Because of its rarity, this form is managed as LQTS2 (Schwartz 2006).

7. LQTS7

This form is caused by rare mutations within *KCNJ2*, which encodes the potassium channel α subunit I_{K1} (Plaster et al. 2001). This form is part of a larger syndrome (Andersen-Tawil syndrome) manifesting with skeletal deformities and periodic paralysis, in addition to prolonged QT intervals.

8. LQTS8–LQTS10

These three forms of LQTS are caused by mutations in *CACNA1c*, *CAV3*, and *SCN4B*, respectively. Mutations within each of these genes account for less than 1% of cases. In the case of LQTS8, LQTS generally occurs as part of a larger disorder known as Timothy syndrome. Mutations affect the cardiac L-type calcium channel $Ca_V1.2$ encoded by the *CACNA1c* gene (Splawski et al. 2004). Mutations in *Caveolin-3* result in LQTS9 (Vatta et al. 2006). The *CAV3* gene encodes a membrane structural protein, which forms microdomains on the cell membrane known as caveolae. The *SCN5A*-encoded voltage-gated sodium channel resides within these caveolae. The mechanisms behind CAV3 mutations appear to involve a gain-of-function increase in late sodium current (Vatta et al. 2006). Most recently, a novel susceptibility gene, *SCN4B*, which encodes a β subunit to $Na_V1.5$ (*SCN5A*), has been found in one patient from a Mexican family (Medeiros-Domingo et al. 2007). This has been termed LQTS10, but appears similar to LQTS3 both molecularly and electrophysiologically.

Mutation Detection and Genetic Testing in LQTS

Because of the strong genotype–phenotype correlations seen in LQTS, the role of genetic screening is more prominent in this disorder than in the cardiomyopathies. As with HCM, mutation detection has been performed in research labs for nearly a decade now (Tester et al. 2006). However, diagnostic testing is now increasingly available through accredited service laboratories (see e.g., http://www.ukgtn.nhs.uk/gtn/Home, www.genetests.org/, www.orpha.net/, and www.eurogentest.org/. It is critical to carry out genetic testing for an unknown mutation in an individual (or related individuals in the same family) with a precisely defined phenotype, because only in this way can the pathogenic significance of a mutation be determined. A mutation found at random in a healthy individual without a family history is likely of little consequence, whereas the same mutation found in an individual with physiologically proven LQTS and a family history of the same is most significant, and more so if the mutation segregates with disease in the kindred. Only then can predictive genetic testing be offered to relatives at risk of the same mutation. It is also necessary to bear in mind that the absence of a mutation indicates low but not zero risk: there may, for example, be more than one mutation in more than one locus that is segregating in a family, particularly a large kindred with a family history in more than one ancestral line. Also, depending on the technique/s used to detect mutations, there may be a greater or lesser chance of a mutation having escaped detection (finite sensitivity in mutation detection). Finding a pathogenic mutation in an individual with a clinical diagnosis of LQTS will help to confirm the diagnosis and to guide therapy, and enable first-degree relatives to be offered predictive genetic testing. Because of the high mortality and morbidity in untreated individuals, predictive genetic testing is of particular importance in asymptomatic, high-risk individuals. Another controversial strategy has been proposed for developing screening process to genotype suspected cases to expedite wide screening of those who might benefit from genetic testing (Napolitano et al. 2005). Genetic testing at the population level is currently not appropriate for numerous reasons, including but not limited to, the genetic heterogeneity of LQTS, the relatively high rates of nonpenetrance associated with some alleles and the lack of a rapid and cost-effective screening tool. Future molecular advances in the understanding of this disease and in sequencing and genotyping technologies may allow for genetic screening of specific at-risk subpopulations, such as young athletes.

Recent Genetic and Genomic Advances in LQTS

Recent advances in the genomics of LQTS have been greatly facilitated by the development of high-throughput genotyping methodologies. A number of recent large-scale linkage and association studies have identified genomic regions or particular SNPs that influence the heritability of the QTc interval among the general population. In a GWA report by Aarnoudse et al., two SNPs within the nitric oxide synthase 1 adaptor protein (NOS1AP) were highly significantly associated with QTc interval duration in a population-based, prospective cohort of over 6,000 individuals (Aarnoudse et al. 2007). A second study by Pfeufer et al. examining 270 SNPs in the *KCNQ1, KCNE1, KCNH2,* and *KCNE2* genes detected association of four variants with the QTc interval in the WHO KORA general population survey (Pfeufer et al. 2005). A third study detected suggestive evidence of linkage for the QT interval on a region on chromosome 3 harboring potassium and sodium channel genes, including *SCN5A*, in an unselected population (Newton-Cheh et al. 2005). These studies demonstrate the heritability of the QT interval and provide evidence as to some of the genes that may be influencing this complex trait within the general population. Such data should facilitate a better understanding of the molecular genetics of complex electrocardiographic traits, such as the duration of the QT interval, in both the healthy and diseased states.

An additional advance relates to the types of variants involved in LQTS. While most mutations are either single base pair alterations or small insertions and deletions occurring in exons or splice-site junctions, Koopmann et al. recently identified a large gene duplication in the *KCNH2* gene responsible for LQTS in a Dutch family (Koopmann et al. 2006). The authors state that these findings may be of particular relevance to those LQTS patients who are not found to harbor one of the previously identified point mutations by conventional genetic testing.

Finally, a few recent studies have cataloged the genetic variation existing within the LQTS genes in various ethnic populations, often demonstrating ethnicity-specific polymorphisms (Ackerman et al. 2004; Koo et al. 2006). These studies not only assist in the proper interpretation of genetic testing results but also provide a starting point for determining ethnicity-specific differences in susceptibility to LQTS.

Advances in genomics will assist in identifying novel genes and variants contributing to the pathological state of LQTS, as well as genes influencing complex electrocardiographic traits in the general population. As nearly 30% of LQTS patients are found not to carry one of the known point mutations, the identification of new genes and variants should allow for better diagnosis, management, and treatment of the disease. The cataloging of population-specific polymorphisms will facilitate research into ethnicity-specific differences in disease susceptibility and may elucidate previously unknown disease mechanisms.

Molecular Diagnosis in Complex Cardiovascular Disorders: Coronary Artery Disease and Myocardial Infarction

Disorders such as the cardiomyopathies and LQTS have a Mendelian mode of inheritance where one or a few genes contribute to the phenotype. Mendelian disorders, however, account for only a small percentage of the overall disease burden in patients seen by cardiologists. Consequently, with the help of recent advances in genomics, the focus has expanded toward improving our understanding of how genes and genetic factors contribute to the more complex forms of CVD, such as atherosclerosis and MI. It is generally accepted that complex CVD results from the interaction of several genetic and environmental factors, making it multifactorial (genes and environment) and polygenic (multiple genes required in each patient) in nature. This complex nature represents a substantial challenge to incorporating molecular genetic data on CAD and MI into the diagnosis, treatment, and care of cardiac patients. This section briefly discusses the current diagnostic methodologies for CAD and MI, as well as recent genetic and genomic discoveries in this area (Box 6–4).

Box 6–4 Key Points for CAD and MI

- CAD and MI are the leading causes of death in the world.
- Efforts to prevent CAD and MI have focused on lifestyle modifications with respect to the well-established risk factors.
- Family history remains the single strongest independent risk factor for development of the disease, indicating the importance of genetics in this complex disorder.
- Because CAD and MI result from the complex interplay of environmental and genetic factors, methods to identify CAD-related genes have not met with the same success as for some of the Mendelian cardiovascular disorders.
- There are currently no genetic tests commercially available for CAD or MI.
- GWA studies and the field of functional genomics offer the best possibilities for unraveling the genetics of this complex and deadly disease.

CAD and MI are the leading causes of death in the Western world. In 2004, an estimated 16 million adults had CAD and the estimated annual incidence of MI was 565,000 new attacks and 300,000 recurrent attacks (Association 2007). In terms of mortality, CAD was responsible for one in every five deaths in the United States in 2004 (Association 2007). Diagnosing CAD often requires the use of multiple tests, both noninvasive and invasive. Noninvasive tests include an exercise stress test along with an ECG, an echocardiogram, and a thallium study. If these tests are normal, usually no further work-up is required. However, if any of these tests are abnormal, a cardiac catheterization along with coronary angiography may be performed. This is considered the gold standard of CAD diagnosis, as it not only allows for its visual confirmation, but also allows for its extent and localization to be quantitatively determined.

While there are currently no laboratory assays that can diagnose CAD, intensive research efforts are focusing on the identification of genetic variants that will assist in the earlier detection and risk stratification of CAD. With both the human genome sequence and necessary high-throughput tools now available, recent advances in the area of functional genomics are enabling exceptional insights into the molecular basis of CAD, facilitating the search for new clinically relevant CAD genes and biomarkers. These data will be discussed in more detail in the section on *Functional Genomics of CAD and MI.*

Laboratory Tests for Myocardial Infarction

The definition and diagnosis of acute MI have been based on criteria set forth by the WHO. Patients are required to meet at least two of three criteria in order for an MI to be diagnosed: characteristic chest pain, diagnostic ECG changes, and elevation of the biochemical markers creatine kinase or troponin I in their blood samples. In 2000, these criteria were refined to give more prominence to the biochemical markers (Alpert et al. 2000). According to this new criterion, a rise in cardiac troponin accompanied by either typical symptoms, pathological Q waves, ST elevation or depression, or coronary intervention are diagnostic of MI.

The use of serum biomarkers in the diagnosis of MI first began in the 1950s with the use of the enzymes lactate dehydrogenase and aspartate aminotransferase to assess cardiac injury. However, these markers were not entirely cardiac specific and did not allow for the early detection of MI due to their time course in the blood and their labor-intensive methods of detection. Often with these markers, an MI could not be confirmed until days after the actual event. As early diagnosis of an MI has been shown to limit myocardial damage, markers were needed that could be detected relatively early in the blood after an MI. Throughout the 1960s and 1970s, much work focused on the use of creatine kinase (CK) and its more cardiac-specific isozyme, creatine kinase-MB (CK-MB). CK catalyzes the conversion of creatine to phosphocreatine and there are three different isozymes whose expression differs by tissue. CK-MB is predominantly expressed by cardiac muscle and was therefore more specific for cardiac injury than any of its predecessors; due to its time course in the blood, it allowed for a diagnosis within hours rather than days of an MI. In conjunction with technological advances that allowed for the rapid, automated, and high-throughput measurement of CK-MB, this biomarker became the gold standard of MI diagnosis throughout the 1980s. However, problems still remained with its specificity and sensitivity. With the subsequent ability to use monoclonal antibodies to select proteins specifically from myocardial cells, troponin T (cTnT) was identified as a marker of myocardial necrosis. cTnT is a cardio-specific myofibrillar protein and is one component of the larger troponin complex, which participates in cardiac calcium regulation. Eventually, attention was turned to another protein of this complex, cardiac troponin I (cTnI), the inhibitory subunit of this complex. One of the benefits of troponins over CK-MB is that they remain abnormally elevated for 4–10 days after an acute MI, allowing for diagnosis of infarctions with a delayed presentation. However, the true added value of troponins lies in the fact that they are a highly sensitive and highly specific marker for even minor myocardial injury and, therefore, allow for risk stratification in acute coronary syndromes, where an MI has been ruled out but some myocardial damage has nevertheless occurred. In addition, peak levels correlate nicely with infarct size (Licka et al. 2002; Panteghini et al. 2002). Because of this high sensitivity and specificity, and because troponins have been shown to have roles in prognostic risk assessment and even therapeutic choices (Heeschen et al. 1999; Newby et al. 2003; Babuin et al. 2005) they have become the new diagnostic standard for MI.

Despite the advances described above, the diagnosis of MI remains largely clinical. The measurements of any of the cardiac biomarkers must be interpreted within the context of the clinical findings. Because the early and rapid detection of MI can save lives and limit myocardial damage, markers are needed that allow the earliest possible detection and/or predict with high accuracy an impending MI. As the markers mentioned above are all indicative of myocardial necrosis, markers that precede necrosis and can detect myocardial ischemia before damage is induced are highly desirable. As with CAD, recent breakthroughs in functional genomics are greatly enhancing the search for new and improved markers of MI, including genetic variants that could determine an individual's susceptibility to MI (Box 6–5). This data is discussed in depth in the following section.

Box 6–5 Functional Genomics of CAD

- Functional genomics builds on DNA variation and takes into account what is occurring at the RNA and protein levels in order to characterize biological processes in the normal and abnormal states.
- Such a global view is now possible due to advances in high-throughput technologies that have been driven in part by the Human Genome Project.
- Owing to these advances, GWA studies incorporating nearly 1 million SNPs are now possible to assist in identifying CAD- and MI-related genes.
- Advances in expression profiling and proteomics are also enabling new discoveries into the processes behind atherosclerosis and MI.
- Future advances may focus on the identification of a biomarker(s) and/or gene expression signature, which can aid in risk stratification and treatment.
- A major challenge in the coming years in cardiovascular medicine will be integrating and interpreting the various types of data needed for a better molecular understanding of such a complex disease, as well as determining which data may have clinical utility.

Functional Genomics of CAD and MI

As a result of the Human Genome Project, we now know the building blocks that determine biological processes in humans (Lander et al. 2001). However, the knowledge about DNA sequence only provides a first glimpse into the molecular underpinnings of health and disease. Ultimately, RNA and proteins are responsible for carrying forward the information encoded in genes. Consequently, great emphasis is now placed on an integrated molecular view, linking all three components together to describe biological systems. Such a view is now possible in large part due to the development of technologies for genotyping, sequencing, expression analysis, and improved protein analyses. Such a global view is of particular importance to achieving a molecular understanding of highly complex, multifactorial diseases like CAD and MI.

The term *functional genomics* refers to the global view of integrative, systematic, and comprehensive analyses to identify and describe processes and pathways involved in normal and abnormal states. This type of analysis builds on the identification of DNA variation, mainly in the form of SNPs, and describes how this variation impacts diverse biological processes, particularly in the disease state. Ultimately, functional genomics will allow for a detailed molecular view of multifactorial, polygenic diseases, with resulting improvements in their molecular diagnostic tools and targets for improved treatment and drug development. In this section, we briefly review the individual components of functional genomics as applied to cardiovascular disease, with a specific focus on the analysis of DNA variation as the first step to identifying causal gene mutations that can be used for diagnostic tests in a clinical setting.

1. DNA Level

An intensive discussion regarding the methods to map and identify genes for common, polygenic diseases, such as CAD, has been ongoing for a number of years. In the past, there has been much success in mapping genes for Mendelian disease using linkage analysis, where several hundred microsatellites are typed within families to identify regions of the genome that are shared more often than expected by chance. However, this approach has proven more challenging for polygenic diseases. The genes typically identified with the linkage strategy have been those with low-frequency mutations causing a substantial effect on the phenotype, such as those for HCM and LQTS. Conversely, the gene variants believed to contribute to common disease are likely to have smaller effects. In such situations, it is well known that the linkage approach alone might not be sufficient to identify possible loci (Risch 1990). Consequently, there has been a need to develop further strategies to overcome these limitations. The greater power of association studies to identify the genes behind complex phenotypes was first demonstrated by Risch and Merikangas in 1996 (Risch et al. 1996). However, numerous challenges remained at that time before such studies could become a reality. Since then, candidate-gene association studies focusing on one or a few genes at a time have become commonplace. In relation to CAD and MI, numerous candidate-gene studies have examined genes known to be involved or related to atherosclerotic and/or ischemic disease processes. However, these studies have generally suffered from limited sample sizes and a lack of reproducibility. It is only within the past few years that large-scale GWA studies have become plausible. GWA studies offer a powerful, unbiased, comprehensive approach to identifying novel genes for common diseases. This paradigm shift has been enabled by the completion of the HGP, as well as advances in both high-throughput analysis techniques and bioinformatic data analysis methods. Nevertheless, there are still some unresolved issues related to association mapping in the context of complex phenotypes. This debate primarily concerns the nature of the allelic architecture of polygenic diseases. For example, it is still debated as to how many genes contribute to a particular disease risk, what is the likely frequency of mutations contributing to polygenic diseases (rare or common), and what is the effect of each mutation. The "common disease–common variant" hypothesis states that common diseases will result from common genetic variants, generally those variants with a frequency greater than 10% in the general population. Support for this theory builds the basis for the International HapMap project, which is currently developing a genome-wide haplotype map to be used for whole genome association scans. However, there is also support for models that favor the notion that rare alleles (< 10%) can contribute significantly to polygenic diseases as well (Pritchard et al. 2001). Despite these unresolved issues, the association study approach is now a widely accepted method of localizing genes for polygenic, multifactorial disease like CAD and MI.

The methodology of GWA scanning builds critically on technological platforms for high-throughput genotyping. This technology has recently matured to the point where several platforms are now commercially offered. Currently, two main platforms are available from Affymetrix (http://www.Affymetrix.com) and Illumina (http://www.Illumina.com) allowing for the simultaneous analysis of 500,000 or more SNPs (Figure 6–8a). The methodologies differ in the actual assay method. The Affymetrix chip incorporates oligonucleotides built onto an array, while the Illumina platforms uses oligonucleotides attached to micron-sized beads, which are then placed onto an array. The platforms also differ with respect to the markers that assayed. This is due in some part to technical constraints of the methods, but each platform is inherently based on a different strategy to ascertain full coverage of the genome. Illumina's arrays consist of maximally informative tagging SNPs (tSNPs), SNPs that are maximally correlated with other SNPs in the genome so as to allow the indirect capture of those other SNPs without actually assaying them. The Affymetrix arrays are based on a random panel of SNPs and do not rely on this correlation between SNPs. Although it is currently difficult to assess advantages of one platform over the other, a recent comparison between these two platforms concludes that both methods can be successfully used for GWA (Barrett et al. 2006; Pe'er et al. 2006).

With the availability of this new technology, the results of several GWA studies have been recently published, including the results of studies examining CAD and MI (The Wellcome Trust Case Control Consortium. Genome-wide association (2007)). Three independent groups have identified an interval on chromosome 9, which affects the risk of CAD and MI (Helgadottir et al. 2007; McPherson et al. 2007). The associated variant does not lie within any annotated genes but is near the tumor suppressor genes *CDKN2A* and *CDKN2B*. This region has not previously been associated with CAD, MI, or any of its established risk factors and represents an entirely novel finding with respect to this disease. Helgadottir et al. determined that carriers of the variant had nearly double the risk of MI when compared to noncarriers (Helgadottir et al. 2007). These findings are notable in that the same genomic region was identified in three independent studies, comprising numerous case-control samples of thousands of individuals. Further work is needed to determine the mechanism mediating this association. More GWA studies testing association with CAD and MI are currently underway. The identification of CAD and MI susceptibility genes and variants is, however, only a preliminary step in identifying markers that can facilitate our understanding of CAD and MI disease mechanisms, assist in its prevention and diagnosis, and impact therapeutic outcomes. Data such as that gleaned from GWA studies of genetic variants needs to be integrated with data from the RNA and protein levels in order to fully inform the molecular understanding, and hence prevention, diagnosis, and treatment of CAD and MI.

2. RNA Level

Because association studies do not provide any information with regards to SNP function, additional, complementary techniques must be used to follow-up a validated association signal. One such technique that can be used is the microarray analysis of gene expression levels; Figure 6–11 demonstrates the technique. As RNA is the downstream product of DNA, any disease processes influenced by DNA variation will be similarly reflected at the RNA level. Seminal work in cancer research has showed that changes in gene expression can be fundamental characteristics of pathogenesis, and that such changes correlate with prognosis and can therefore be used to molecularly classify patients, in addition to histologic criteria. It is hoped that a similar application will result from the growing use of high-throughput microarray technology and gene expression analyses in the cardiovascular field.

The application of microarray technology to study expression changes is rapidly increasing in the effort to gain a better molecular understanding of CAD and MI. Expression profiling has been performed across different CAD phenotypes and a variety of cells and tissues known to be involved in the CAD disease process. The basic design of such experiments consists of comparing gene expression patterns between those with and without the disease of interest. The end result of such experiments is generally a list of differentially expressed genes that can serve as a starting point for the identification of novel disease and/or therapeutic markers. However, there are a number of variations on this basic approach. While a healthy control group can be used, it is also worthwhile to compare expression differences between various disease phenotypes. This is particularly true for CAD, given the heterogeneity of this disease. For example, Healy et al. recently examined expression differences in

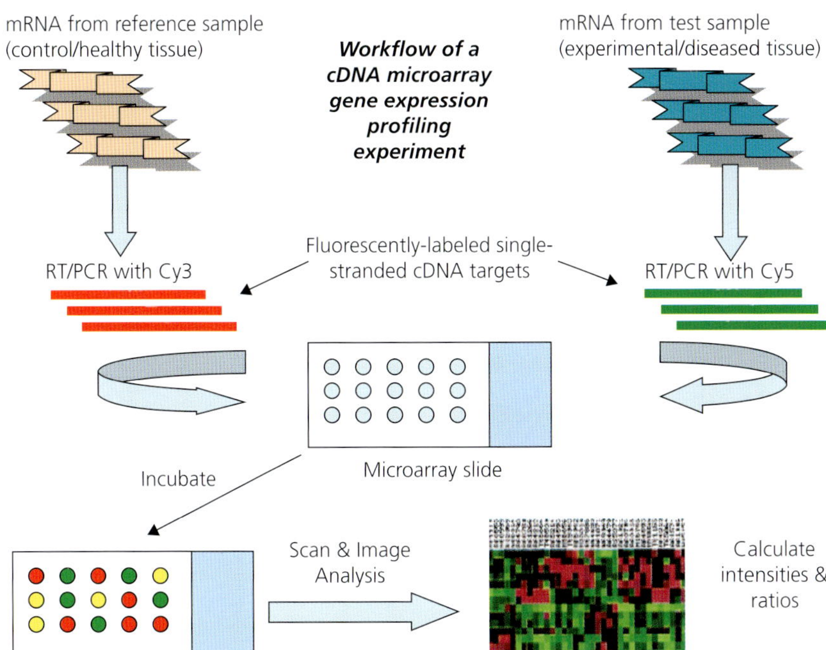

Figure 6–11 cDNA microarray gene expression profiling experiment.

the megakaryocyte-derived mRNAs of platelets in those with stable CAD and those with acute ST-segment elevation MI (STEMI) (Healy et al. 2006). Interestingly, they identified a gene that acted as a strong discriminator of STEMI and whose increasing plasma concentrations significantly predicted future coronary events in apparently healthy women. While circulating cells can be used to perform expression profiling, and they often are due to their accessibility, these cells do not necessarily represent the changes occurring in actual atherosclerotic lesions. Although this can be a more challenging approach, due to the heterogeneity of plaques, a number of studies have directly applied transcript profiling to coronary atheromata. Studies by Randi et al. and Faber et al. compared stable plaques to ruptured plaques, and a study by Archacki et al. compared severely diseased arteries to nondiseased arteries (Faber et al. 2001; Archacki et al. 2003; Randi et al. 2003). Each identified patterns of significantly altered gene expression between their respective groups. Additionally, expression profiling in CAD and MI can be used to determine the effect of various environmental stimuli on expression levels, as illustrated by a number of studies examining the effect of hemodynamic forces on gene expression in coronary endothelial cells and atherosclerotic plaques (Peters et al. 2002; Wasserman et al. 2002; Dai et al. 2004; Chiu et al. 2005).

While the above studies represent examples of the use of gene expression microarrays in the cardiovascular field, the challenges now happen to be the execution of such studies in conjunction with GWA studies, their convergent analysis, and the application of result to the clinic. While clinical tests based on such data are still in the future, the ability to use data from both the DNA and RNA levels to molecularly classify a disease state should allow placing a patient in a specific molecular subgroup with associated diagnostic and prognostic characteristics. This type of genetic- and genomic-derived classification can lead the prevention, diagnosis, and treatment of CAD and MI into the era of individualized medicine.

3. Protein Level

Proteomics is concerned with the high-throughput identification, characterization, and quantitative and functional analyses of proteins in cells. Systematically and comprehensively analyzing the proteome remains a daunting task, partly due to the significant complexity of proteins. However, recent developments in determining protein concentrations by mass spectrometry, and the development of protein arrays, have established the technological basis needed to increase the number of proteins that can be analyzed simultaneously. Figure 6–12 demonstrates the basic design of a proteomic experiment.

An important limitation of GWA and expression profiling studies is that they are unable to capture changes or processes occurring after transcription, such as alternative splicing or post-transcriptional modifications. In addition, assessing what is happening at the protein level is relevant because protein markers may more accurately reflect real-time pathological events occurring in the disease process (Miller et al. 2007a). The application of proteomics to cardiovascular disease has been more limited than either of the previous two technologies discussed and still faces significant challenges (Arab et al. 2006; Miller et al. 2007a). These challenges include, but are not limited to, the selection of appropriate tissue samples, the most appropriate technology platform(s) for analysis of the cardiovascular proteome, obtaining and processing usable samples, coordination of data among investigators, and its combination with genomic data (Arab et al. 2006; Miller et al. 2007a). Nevertheless, despite these issues, some progress has been made.

The Human Proteome Organisation (HUPO; www.hupo.org) was formed in 2001 in order to identify major proteomic challenges, foster collaborations around such issues, assist in the development of new proteomic technologies, and to provide education and training within the field. Under this organization, the Human Plasma Proteome Project was launched (www.hupo.org/research/hppp/). The pilot phase of this project included the analysis of plasma samples in 55 different laboratories worldwide using various proteomic approaches in an effort to accelerate the identification of disease biomarkers. Results from this pilot phase indicate that over 300 cardiovascular-related proteins can be identified in plasma and that they can be categorized into eight different groups, the largest of which is the markers of inflammation and CVD grouping (Berhane et al. 2005). These results provide a starting point from which to begin to identify novel cardiovascular biomarkers from human plasma. In contrast to using human plasma, an independent study examined the feasibility of identifying proteins directly

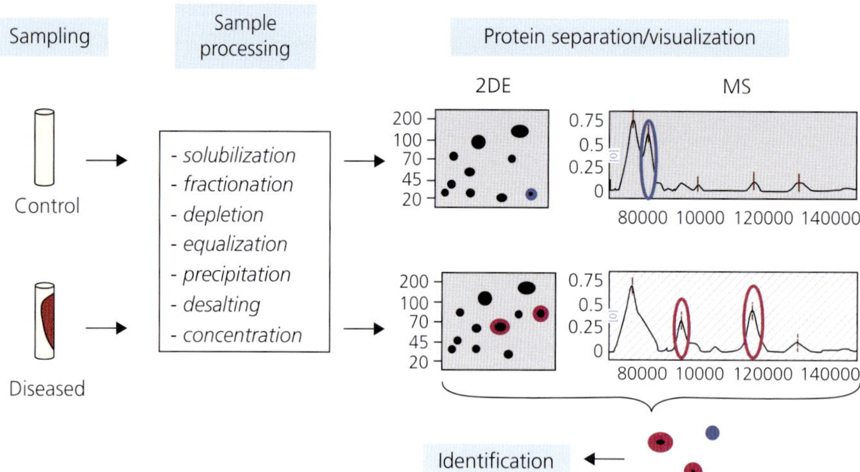

Figure 6–12 Basic Design of a Proteomic Experiment. Four distinct levels of sample preparation and analysis are required for a proteomic-based identification of differences in protein content from diseased tissues. First, tissue samples from diseased patients are attained. The corresponding control sample, same tissue type without disease, is used for comparison. Depending on the type of tissue and analysis required, samples are prepared for 2-dimensional electrophoresis (2DE) to separate proteins by molecular weight (Mw) and isoelectric point (pI). Following detection, differences in the protein content between the control and diseased samples are manifested in either the appearance (red) or disappearance (blue) of unique "spots." These differences (proteins) are subjected to mass spectrometry (MS) to identify either novel proteins or post-translational modifications present/absent in diseased tissues. Reprinted from Cardiovascular Research, Vol. 72(1), Blanco-Colio, et. al, Biology of Atherosclerotic Plaques: What We are Learning from Proteomic Analysis, pp. 18–29, Copyright (2006), with permission from Elsevier.

from archived frozen and paraffin-embedded human coronary arteries using a recently developed method termed *direct tissue proteomics* (DTP) (Bagnato et al. 2007). Results were promising, demonstrating the identification of over 800 proteins from atherosclerotic arteries. The authors state that these results provide the first large-scale human proteomic map of coronary plaques.

In the future, a comprehensive analysis of protein levels and activity will be an important component to understanding disease at the molecular level, particularly with diseases such as CAD and MI, given the heterogeneity of cell types involved in their underlying disease process. However, proteomic technologies are still maturing and their application to CVD carries its own set of challenges. The Human Plasma Proteome Project provides an initial blueprint to assist in establishing the basis of proteomics within the cardiovascular field and from which clinically relevant biomarkers can be identified.

4. In the Clinic

Currently, genetics does not play a prominent role in the evaluation of a patient in cardiology. The best approximation we have to account for the role of genetics in CAD and MI is the taking of a family history during a patient's initial evaluation. However, personalized medicine based on an individual's genetic make-up is now a vital goal of clinical medicine, as the contribution of genes to chronic disease becomes increasingly recognized. The diagnosis and treatment of patients based on their unique molecular signature will allow for more precise disease management and improved therapeutic outcomes. Perhaps of utmost importance with regard to the leading cause of morbidity and mortality across much of the globe, such knowledge can lead to enhanced primary prevention of atherosclerotic disease and its consequences, as those known to carry particular high-risk variants can be more aggressively monitored. While the full realization of individualized medicine is still in the future, we have come one step closer to this reality with the introduction of highly parallel, economical genome-wide arrays, like the SNP chips offered by Affymetrix and Illumina. As such technology is now in place, the challenges become how to interpret the massive amount of data such arrays provide and how to properly combine it with other patient data, whether genomic, proteomic, or otherwise. Large-scale genetic epidemiologic studies should assist with meeting these challenges. Nevertheless, a few limited applications of this type of technology being used in the clinic already exist.

One such example relates to optimizing therapeutic outcomes for a number of commonly prescribed drugs, including antiarrhythmics. While it is not a genome-wide test, it still displays the characteristics of functional genomics described previously and nicely represents the concept of individualized medicine and its benefits. The AmpliChip CYP450 test makes use of an Affymetrix array of more than 15,000 probes interrogating numerous SNPs in the *CYP2D6* and *CYP2C19* genes (www.amplichip.us). These genes are members of the cytochrome P450 family of genes that are responsible for metabolizing many drugs, including antidepressants and antipsychotics, as well as antiarrhythmics. On the basis of a patient's genotypes at SNPs within these two genes, patients can be classified into one of four metabolic phenotypes—ultrarapid, extensive, intermediate, or poor. Knowledge of this phenotype can assist physicians in prescribing the appropriate dosage. Currently, four labs within the United States perform the test. Results are received within days and the physician can then use that information to guide treatment. This test is novel in that it allows drug choice and dosing for an individual to be based on scientific data, prior to ever beginning treatment. This early example demonstrates how DNA-based arrays can be incorporated into the clinic and how such genomic data can directly contribute to personalized medicine. More such tests can be expected in the future as the field of functional genomics matures.

Conclusions

Technological development in genetics and genomics provides unprecedented opportunities to identify the underlying molecular basis of cardiovascular disease in all its forms, and increasingly in individuals at risk of inherited cardiac diseases through diagnostic molecular genetic testing, and their relatives. With the availability of the human genome sequence, including information on DNA variation, combined with new molecular analyses of the RNA and protein levels, cardiovascular disease might be more readily characterized at the molecular level in the future. Describing gene function and the specific role of DNA, RNA, and proteins in the disease processes behind CAD and MI will provide much-needed novel diagnostic tools and treatments. Ultimately, the goal is always to provide optimal therapy for each patient. Understanding how the unique genetic signature of an individual influences their risk and prognosis for cardiovascular disease will be the basis for individualized medicine in cardiology for years to come.

References

Aarnoudse AJ, Newton-Cheh C, de Bakker PI, et al. Common NOS1AP variants are associated with a prolonged QTc interval in the Rotterdam Study. *Circulation.* 2007;116(1):10–16.

Abbott GW, Sesti F, Splawski I, et al. MiRP1 forms IKr potassium channels with HERG and is associated with cardiac arrhythmia. *Cell.* 1999;97(2):175–187.

Ackerman MJ. Genetic testing for risk stratification in hypertrophic cardiomyopathy and long QT syndrome: fact or fiction? *Curr Opin Cardiol.* 2005;20:175–181.

Ackerman MJ, Splawski I, Makielski JC, et al. Spectrum and prevalence of cardiac sodium channel variants among black, white, Asian, and Hispanic individuals: implications for arrhythmogenic susceptibility and Brugada/long QT syndrome genetic testing. *Heart Rhythm.* 2004;1(5):600–607.

Ackerman MJ, Tester DJ, Porter CJ. Swimming, a gene-specific arrhythmogenic trigger for inherited long QT syndrome. *Mayo Clinic Proceedings.* 1999;74(11):1088–1094.

Ackerman MJ, VanDriest SL, Ommen SR, et al. Prevalence and age-dependence of malignant mutations in the beta-myosin heavy chain and troponin T genes in hypertrophic cardiomyopathy: a comprehensive outpatient perspective. *J Am Coll Cardiol.* 2002;39(12):2042–2048.

Akrami SM, Dunlop MG, Farrington SM, Frayling IM, MacDonald F, Harvey JF, Armour JA. Screening for exonic copy number mutations at *MSH2* and *MLH1* by MAPH. *Fam Cancer.* 2005;4:145–149.

Alpert JS, Thygesen K, Antman E, Bassand JP. Myocardial infarction redefined—a consensus document of The Joint European Society of Cardiology/American College of Cardiology Committee for the redefinition of myocardial infarction. *J Am Coll Cardiol.* 2000;36(3):959–969.

Anan R, Greve G, Thierfelder L, et al. Prognostic implications of novel beta cardiac myosin heavy chain gene mutations that cause familial hypertrophic cardiomyopathy. *J Clin Invest.* 1994;93(1):280–285.

Arab S, Gramolini AO, Ping P, et al. Cardiovascular proteomics: tools to develop novel biomarkers and potential applications. *J Am Coll Cardiol.* 2006;48(9):1733–1741.

Arad M, Benson DW, Perez-Atayde AR, et al. Constitutively active AMP kinase mutations cause glycogen storage disease mimicking hypertrophic cardiomyopathy. *J Clin Invest.* 2002;109(3):357–362.

Arad M, Moskowitz IP, Petel VV, et al. Transgenic mice overexpressing mutant PRKAG2 define the cause of Wolff-Parkinson-White syndrome in glycogen storage cardiomyopathy. *Circulation.* 2003;107(22):2850–2856.

Arbustini E, Diegoli M, Fasani R, et al. Mitochondrial DNA mutations and mitochondrial abnormalities in dilated cardiomyopathy. *Am J Pathol.* 1998;153(5):1501–1510.

Arbustini E, Pilotto A, Repetto A, et al. Autosomal dominant dilated cardiomyopathy with atrioventricular block: a lamin A/C defect-related disease. *J Am Coll Cardiol.* 2002;39(6):981–990.

Archacki SR, Angheloiu G, Tian XL, et al. Identification of new genes differentially expressed in coronary artery disease by expression profiling. *Physiol Genomics.* 2003;15(1):65–74.

Arimura T, Hayashi T, Terada H, et al. A Cypher/ZASP mutation associated with dilated cardiomyopathy alters the binding affinity to protein kinase C. *J Biol Chem.* 2004;279(8):6746–6752.

Association AH. Heart Disease and Stroke Statistics--2007 Update. Dallas, Texas, American Heart Association; 2007.

Babuin L, Jaffe AS. Troponin: the biomarker of choice for the detection of cardiac injury. *Can Med Assoc J.* 2005;173(10):1191–1202.

Bagnato C, Thumar J, Mayya V, et al. Proteomics analysis of human coronary atherosclerotic plaque: a feasibility study of direct tissue proteomics by liquid chromatography and tandem mass spectrometry. *Mol Cell Proteomics.* 2007;6(6):1088–1102.

Baig MK, Goldman JH, Caforio AL, Coonar AS, Keeling PJ, McKenna WJ. Familial dilated cardiomyopathy: cardiac abnormalities are common in asymptomatic relatives and may represent early disease. *J Am Coll Cardiol.* 1998;31(1):195–201.

Barrett JC, Cardon LR. Evaluating coverage of genome-wide association studies. *Nat Gen.* 2006;38(6):659–662.

Barth AS, Kuner R, Buness A, et al. Identification of a common gene expression signature in dilated cardiomyopathy across independent microarray studies. *J Am Coll Cardiol.* 2006;48(8):1610–1617.

Becane HM, Bonne G, Varnous S, et al. High incidence of sudden death with conduction system and myocardial disease due to lamins A and C gene mutation. *Pacing Clin Electrophysiol.* 2000;23(11 Pt 1): 1661–1666.

Berhane BT, Zong C, Liem DA, et al. Cardiovascular-related proteins identified in human plasma by the HUPO Plasma Proteome Project pilot phase. *Proteomics.* 2005;5(13):3520–3530.

Bienengraeber M, Olson TM, Selivanov VA, et al. ABCC9 mutations identified in human dilated cardiomyopathy disrupt catalytic KATP channel gating. *Nat Genet.* 2004;36(4):382–387.

Bione S, D'Adamo P, Maestrini E, Gedeon AK, Bolhuis PA, Toniolo D. A novel X-linked gene, G4.5 is responsible for Barth syndrome. *Nat Genet.* 1996;12(4):385–389.

Blair E, Redwood C, Ashrafian H, et al. Mutations in the gamma(2) subunit of AMP-activated protein kinase cause familial hypertrophic cardiomyopathy: evidence for the central role of energy compromise in disease pathogenesis. *Hum Mol Genet.* 2001;10(11):1215–1220.

Blair E, Redwood C, de Jesus Oliveira M, et al. Mutations of the light meromyosin domain of the beta-myosin heavy chain rod in hypertrophic cardiomyopathy. *Circ Res.* 2002;90(3):263–269.

Bonne G, Carrier L, Bercovici J, et al. Cardiac myosin binding protein-C gene splice acceptor site mutation is associated with familial hypertrophic cardiomyopathy. *Nat Genet.* 1995;11(4):438–440.

Brodsky GL, Muntoni F, Miocic S, Sinagra G, Sewry C, Mestroni L. Lamin A/C gene mutation associated with dilated cardiomyopathy with variable skeletal muscle involvement. *Circulation.* 2000;101(5):473–476.

Bruder CE, Hirvelä C, Tapia-Paez I, et al. High resolution deletion analysis of constitutional DNA from neurofibromatosis type 2 (NF2) patients using microarray-CGH. *Hum Mol Genet.* 2001;10(3):271–282.

Buckingham L, Flaws ML. *Molecular Diagnostics: Fundamentals, Methods, & Clinical Applications.* Philadelphia: F.A. Davis Company; 2007.

Buckley PG, Mantripragada KK, Benetkiewicz M, Tapia-Páez I, Diaz De Ståhl T, Rosenquist M, et al. A full-coverage, high-resolution human chromosome 22 genomic microarray for clinical and research applications. *Hum Mol Genet.* 2002;11(25):3221–3229.

Buckley PG, Mantripragada KK, Piotrowski A, Diaz de Ståhl T, Dumanski JP. Copy-number polymorphisms: mining the tip of an iceberg. *Trends Genet.* 2005;21(6):315–317.

Bunn CF, Lintott CJ, Scott RS, George PM. Comparison of SSCP and DHPLC for the detection of LDLR mutations in a New Zealand cohort. *Hum Mut.* 2002;19(3):311.

de Bustos C, Díaz de Ståhl T, Piotrowski A, et al. Analysis of copy number variation in the normal human population within a region containing complex segmental duplications on 22q11 using high-resolution array-CGH. *Genomics.* 2006;88(2):152–162.

Chiu JJ, Lee PL, Chang SF, et al. Shear stress regulates gene expression in vascular endothelial cells in response to tumor necrosis factor-alpha: a study of the transcription profile with complementary DNA microarray. *J Biomed Sci.* 2005;12(3):481–502.

Choy YS, Dabora SL, Hall F, et al. Superiority of denaturing high performance liquid chromatography over single stranded conformation and conformation-sensitive gel electrophoresis for mutation detection in TSC2. *Ann Hum Genet.* 1999;63(Pt.5):383–391.

Copeland J.(ed.) *Colossus: The Secrets of Bletchley Park's Code-breaking Computers.* Oxford, University Press; 2006. ISBN-10: 0-19-284055-X, ISBN-13: 978-0-19-284055-4.

Cowan KH, Goldsmith ME, Levine RM, Aitken SC, Douglass E, Clendeninn N, et al. Dihydrofolate reductase gene amplification and possible rearrangement in estrogen-responsive methotrexate-resistant human breast cancer cells. *J Biol Chem.* 1982;257:15079–15086.

Craig JA, Bickmore WA. Chromosome bands–flavours to savour. *Bioessays.* 1993;15(5):349–354.

Curran ME, Splawski I, Timothy KW, Vincent GM, Green ED, Keating MT. A molecular basis for cardiac arrhythmia: HERG mutations cause long QT syndrome. *Cell.* 1995;80(5):795–803.

D'Adamo P, Fassone L, Gedeon A, et al. The X-linked gene G4.5 is responsible for different infantile dilated cardiomyopathies. *Am J Hum Genet.* 1997;61(4):862–867.

Daehmlow S, Erdmann J, Knueppel T, et al. Novel mutations in sarcomeric protein genes in dilated cardiomyopathy. *Biochem Biophys Res Commun.* 2002;298(1):116–120.

Dai G, Kaazempur-Mofrad MR, Natarajan S, et al. Distinct endothelial phenotypes evoked by arterial waveforms derived from atherosclerosis-susceptible and -resistant regions of human vasculature. *Proc Natl Acad Sci USA.* 2004;101(41):14871–14876.

Davis JS, Hassanzadeh S, Winitsky S, et al. The overall pattern of cardiac contraction depends on a spatial gradient of myosin regulatory light chain phosphorylation. *Cell.* 2001;107(5):631–641.

Durand JB, Bachinski LL, Bieling LC, et al. Localization of a gene responsible for familial dilated cardiomyopathy to chromosome 1q32. *Circulation.* 1995;92(12):3387–3389.

Eisenstein M. Putting long-range mapping in reach. *Nat Methods.* 2006;3:239.

Erdmann J, Daehmlow S, Wischke S, et al. Mutation spectrum in a large cohort of unrelated consecutive patients with hypertrophic cardiomyopathy. *Clin Gen.* 2003;64(4):339–349.

Faber BC, Cleutjens KB, Niessen RL, et al. Identification of genes potentially involved in rupture of human atherosclerotic plaques. *Circ Res.* 2001;89(6):547–554.

Fatkin D, MacRae C, Sasaki T, et al. Missense mutations in the rod domain of the lamin A/C gene as causes of dilated cardiomyopathy and conduction-system disease. *N Engl J Med.* 1999;341(23):1715–1724.

Filla A, De Michele G, Cavalcanti F, et al. The relationship between trinucleotide (GAA) repeat length and clinical features in Friedreich ataxia. *Am J Hum Genet.* 1996;59(3):554–560.

Florijn RJ, Bonden LA, Vrolijk H, et al. High-resolution DNA Fiber-FISH for genomic DNA mapping and colour bar-coding of large genes. *Hum Mol Genet.* 1995;4(5):831–836.

Freiburg A, Gautel M. A molecular map of the interactions between titin and myosin-binding protein C. Implications for sarcomeric assembly in familial hypertrophic cardiomyopathy. *Eur J Biochem.* 1996;235(1–2):317–323.

Frueh FW, Noyer-Weidner M. The use of denaturing high-performance liquid chromatography (DHPLC) for the analysis of genetic variations: impact for diagnostics and pharmacogenetics. *Clin Chem Lab Med.* 2003;41(4):452–461.

Galluzzi G, Deidda G, Cacurri S, et al. Molecular analysis of 4q35 rearrangements in fascioscapulohumeral muscular dystrophy (FSHD): application to family studies for a correct genetic advice and a reliable prenatal diagnosis of the disease. *Neuromuscul Disord.* 1999;9:190–198.

García-Castro M, Reguero JR, Batalla A, et al. Hypertrophic cardiomyopathy: low frequency of mutations in the beta-myosin heavy chain (MYH7) and cardiac troponin T (TNNT2) genes among Spanish patients. *Clin Chem.* 2003;49(8):1279–1285.

Garman SC, Garboczi DN. The molecular defect leading to Fabry disease: structure of human alpha-galactosidase. *J Mol Biol.* 2004;337(2):319–335.

Geisterfer-Lowrance AA, Kass S, Tanigawa G, et al. A molecular basis for familial hypertrophic cardiomyopathy: a beta cardiac myosin heavy chain gene missense mutation. *Cell.* 1990;62(5):999–1006.

Genschel J, Schmidt HH. Mutations in the LMNA gene encoding lamin A/C. *Hum Mutat.* 2000;16(6):451–459.

Gerull B, Atherton J, Geupel A, et al. Identification of a novel frameshift mutation in the giant muscle filament titin in a large Australian family with dilated cardiomyopathy. *J Mol Med.* 2006;84(6):478–483.

Gerull B, Gramlich M, Atherton J, et al. Mutations of TTN, encoding the giant muscle filament titin, cause familial dilated cardiomyopathy. *Nat Genet.* 2002;30(2):201–204.

Gollob MH, Green MS, Tang AS, et al. Identification of a gene responsible for familial Wolff-Parkinson-White syndrome. *N Engl J Med.* 2001;344(24):1823–1831.

Gregori D, Rocco C, Miocic S, Mestroni L. Estimating the frequency of familial dilated cardiomyopathy in the presence of misclassification errors. *J Appl Stat.* 2001;28:53–62.

Gribble SM, Fiegler H, Burford DC, Prigmore E, Yang F, Carr P, et al. Applications of combined DNA microarray and chromosome sorting technologies. *Chromosome Res.* 2004;12(1):35–43.

Gronostajski RM, Adhya S, Nagata K, Guggenheimer RA, Hurwitz J. Site-specific DNA binding of nuclear factor I: analyses of cellular binding sites. *Mol Cell Biol.* 1985;5:964–671.

Gross E, Arnold N, Goette J, Schwarz-Boeger U, Kiechle M. A comparison of BRCA1 mutation analysis by direct sequencing, SSCP and DHPLC. *Hum Gen.* 1999;105(1–2):72–78.

Grünig E, Tasman JA, Kücherer H, Franz W, Kübler W, Katus HA. Frequency and phenotypes of familial dilated cardiomyopathy. *J Am Coll Cardiol.* 1998;31(1):186–194.

Haghighi K, Kolokathis F, Pater L, et al. Human phospholamban null results in lethal dilated cardiomyopathy revealing a critical difference between mouse and human. *J Clin Invest.* 2003;111(6):869–876.

Hanson EL, Jakobs PM, Keegan H, et al. Cardiac troponin T lysine 210 deletion in a family with dilated cardiomyopathy. *J Card Fail.* 2002;8(1):28–32.

Hayashi T, Arimura T, Itoh-Satoh M, et al. Tcap gene mutations in hypertrophic cardiomyopathy and dilated cardiomyopathy. *J Am Coll Cardiol.* 2004;44(11):2192–2201.

Healy AM, Pickard MD, Pradhan AD, et al. Platelet expression profiling and clinical validation of myeloid-related protein-14 as a novel determinant of cardiovascular events. *Circulation.* 2006;113(19):2278–2284.

Heeschen C, van Den Brand MJ, Hamm CW, Simoons ML. Angiographic findings in patients with refractory unstable angina according to troponin T status. *Circulation.* 1999;100(14):1509–1514.

Helgadottir A, Thorleifsson G, Manolescu A, et al. A common variant on chromosome 9p21 affects the risk of myocardial infarction. *Science.* 2007;316(5830):1491–1493.

Hershberger RE, Hanson EL, Jakobs PM, et al. A novel lamin A/C mutation in a family with dilated cardiomyopathy, prominent conduction system disease, and need for permanent pacemaker implantation. *Am Heart J.* 2002;144(6):1081–1086.

Hoffmann B, Schmidt-Traub H, Perrot A, Osterziel KJ, Gessner R. First mutation in cardiac troponin C, L29Q, in a patient with hypertrophic cardiomyopathy. *Hum Mutat.* 2001;17(6):524.

Hogervorst FB, Nederlof PM, Gille JJ, et al. Large genomic deletions and duplications in the BRCA1 gene identified by a novel quantitative method. *Cancer Res.* 2003;63:1449–1453.

ISCN 2005: an international system for human cytogenetic nomenclature (2005): recommendations of the International Standing Committee on Human Cytogenetic Nomenclature. International Standing Committee on Human Cytogenetic Nomenclature. Editors: Lisa G. Shaffer, Niels Tommerup. Karger Publishers, 2005. ISBN 3805580193, 9783805580199.

Isnard R, Kalotka H, Dürr A, et al. Correlation between left ventricular hypertrophy and GAA trinucleotide repeat length in Friedreich's ataxia. *Circulation.* 1997;95(9):2247–2249.

Itoh-Satoh M, Hayashi T, Nishi H, et al. Titin mutations as the molecular basis for dilated cardiomyopathy. *Biochem Biophys Res Commun.* 2002;291(2):385–393.

Jääskeläinen P, Kuusisto J, Miettinen R, et al. Mutations in the cardiac myosin-binding protein C gene are the predominant cause of familial hypertrophic cardiomyopathy in eastern Finland. *J Mol Med.* 2002;80(7):412–422.

Jarcho JA, McKenna W, Pare JA, et al. Mapping a gene for familial hypertrophic cardiomyopathy to chromosome 14q1. *N Engl J Med.* 1989;321(20):1372–1378.

Jeffreys AJ. DNA sequence variants in the G gamma-, A gamma-, delta- and beta-globin genes of man. *Cell.* 1979;18:1–10.

Jones KW. Chromosomal and nuclear location of mouse satellite DNA in individual cells. *Nature.* 1970;225(5236):912–915.

Kamisago M, Sharma SD, DePalma SR, et al. Mutations in sarcomere protein genes as a cause of dilated cardiomyopathy. *N Engl J Med.* 2000;343(23):1688–1696.

Karkkainen S, Helio T, Jääskeläinen P, et al. Two novel mutations in the beta-myosin heavy chain gene associated with dilated cardiomyopathy. *Eur J Heart Fail.* 2004a;6(7):861–868.

Kärkkäinen S, Heliö T, Miettinen R, et al. A novel mutation, Ser143Pro, in the lamin A/C gene is common in Finnish patients with familial dilated cardiomyopathy. *Eur Heart J.* 2004b;25(10):885–893.

Karkkainen S, Peuhkurinen K. Genetics of dilated cardiomyopathy. *Ann Med.* 2007;39(2):91–107.

Karkkainen S, Reissell E, Heliö T, et al. Novel mutations in the lamin A/C gene in heart transplant recipients with end stage dilated cardiomyopathy. *Heart.* 2006;92(4):524–526.

Keeling PJ, Gang Y, Smith G, et al. Familial dilated cardiomyopathy in the United Kingdom. *Br Heart J.* 1995;73(5):417–421.

Kim JB, Porreca GJ, Song L, et al. Polony multiplex analysis of gene expression (PMAGE) in mouse hypertrophic cardiomyopathy. *Science.* 2007;316(5830):1481–1484.

Kimura A, Harada H, Park JE, et al. Mutations in the cardiac troponin I gene associated with hypertrophic cardiomyopathy. *Nat Genet.* 1997;16(4):379–382.

Klockars T, Savukoski M, Isosomppi J, et al. Efficient construction of a physical map by fiber-FISH of the CLN5 region: refined assignment and long-range contig covering the critical region on 13q22. *Genomics.* 1996;35:71–78.

Knoll R, Hoshijima M, Hoffman HM, et al. The cardiac mechanical stretch sensor machinery involves a Z disc complex that is defective in a subset of human dilated cardiomyopathy. *Cell.* 2002;111(7):943–955.

Komajda M, Charron P, Tesson F. Genetic aspects of heart failure. *Eur J Heart Fail.* 1999;1(2):121–126.

Koo SH, Ho WF, Lee EJ. Genetic polymorphisms in KCNQ1, HERG, KCNE1 and KCNE2 genes in the Chinese, Malay and Indian populations of Singapore. *Br J Pharmacol.* 2006;61(3):301–308.

Koopmann TT, Alders M, Jongbloed RJ, et al. Long QT syndrome caused by a large duplication in the KCNH2 (HERG) gene undetectable by current polymerase chain reaction-based exon-scanning methodologies. *Heart Rhythm.* 2006;3(1):52–55.

Lander ES, Linton LM, Birren B, et al. Initial sequencing and analysis of the human genome. *Nature.* 2001;409(6822):860–921.

Le Caignec C, Boceno M, Saugier-Veber P, et al. Detection of genomic imbalances by array based comparative genomic hybridisation in fetuses with multiple malformations. *J Med Genet.* 2005;42(2):121–128.

Le Caignec C, Spits C, Sermon K, De Rycke M, Thienpont B, Debrock S, et al. Single-cell chromosomal imbalances detection by array CGH. *Nucleic Acids Res.* 2006;34(9):e68.

Li D, Czernuszewicz GZ, Gonzalez O, et al. Novel cardiac troponin T mutation as a cause of familial dilated cardiomyopathy. *Circulation.* 2001;104(18):2188–2193.

Li D, Tapscoft T, Gonzalez O, et al. Desmin mutation responsible for idiopathic dilated cardiomyopathy. *Circulation.* 1999;100(5):461–464.

Li YY, Maisch B, Rose ML, Hengstenberg C. Point mutations in mitochondrial DNA of patients with dilated cardiomyopathy. *J Mol Cell Cardiol.* 1997;29(10):2699–2709.

Licka M, Zimmermann R, Zehelein J, Dengler TJ, Katus HA, Kübler W. Troponin T concentrations 72 hours after myocardial infarction as a serological estimate of infarct size. *Heart.* 2002;87(6):520–524.

Lindblad-Toh K, Tanenbaum DM, Daly MJ, Winchester E, Lui WO, Villapakkam A, et al. Loss-of-heterozygosity analysis of small-cell lung carcinomas using single-nucleotide polymorphism arrays. *Nat Biotechnol.* 2000;18(9):1001–1005.

Locke DP, Segraves R, Carbone L, et al. Large-scale variation among human and great ape genomes determined by array comparative genomic hybridization. *Genome Res.* 2003;13(3):347–357.

Locke DP, Segraves R, Nicholls RD, et al. BAC microarray analysis of 15q11-q13 rearrangements and the impact of segmental duplications. *J Med Genet.* 2004;41(3):175–182.

MacLeod HM, Culley MR, Huber JM, McNally EM. Lamin A/C truncation in dilated cardiomyopathy with conduction disease. *BMC Med Genet.* 2003;4:4.

Mantripragada KK, Buckley PG, Benetkiewicz M, et al. High-resolution profiling of an 11 Mb segment of human chromosome 22 in sporadic schwannoma using array-CGH. *Int J Oncol.* 2003;22(3):615–622.

Mantripragada KK, Buckley PG, de Ståhl TD, Dumanski JP. Genomic microarrays in the spotlight. *Trends Genet.* 2004a;20(2):87–94.

Mantripragada KK, Tapia-Páez I, Blennow E, Nilsson P, Wedell A, Dumanski JP. DNA copy-number analysis of the 22q11 deletion-syndrome region using array-CGH with genomic and PCR-based targets. *Int J Mol Med.* 2004b;13(2):273–279.

Mantripragada KK, Thuresson AC, Piotrowski A, et al. Identification of novel deletion breakpoints bordered by segmental duplications in the NF1 locus using high resolution array-CGH. *J Med Genet.* 2006;43(1):28–38.

Marcaud L, Reynaud CA, Therwath A, Scherrer K. Modification of the methylation pattern in the vicinity of the chicken globin genes in avian erythroblastosis virus transformed cells. *Nucleic Acids Res.* 1981;9:1841–1851.

Marian AJ. On genetic and phenotypic variability of hypertrophic cardiomyopathy: nature versus nurture. *J Am Coll Cardiol.* 2001;38(2):331–334.

Marin-Garcia J, Goldenthal MJ, Ananthakrishnan R, et al. Specific mitochondrial DNA deletions in idiopathic dilated cardiomyopathy. *Cardiovasc Res.* 1996;31(2):306–313.

Maron BJ. Hypertrophic cardiomyopathy: a systematic review. *JAMA.* 2002;287(10):1308–1320.

Matsuzawa F, Aikawa S, Doi H, Okumiya T, Sakuraba H. Fabry disease: correlation between structural changes in alpha-galactosidase, and clinical and biochemical phenotypes. *Hum Genet.* 2005;117(4):317–328.

McConnell BK, Jones KA, Fatkin D, et al. Dilated cardiomyopathy in homozygous myosin-binding protein-C mutant mice. *J Clin Invest.* 1999;104(12):1771.

McNair WP, Ku L, Taylor MR, et al. SCN5A mutation associated with dilated cardiomyopathy, conduction disorder, and arrhythmia. *Circulation.* 2004;110(15):2163–2167.

McPherson R, Pertsemlidis A, Kavaslar N, et al. A common allele on chromosome 9 associated with coronary heart disease. *Science.* 2007;316(5830):1488–1491.

Medeiros-Domingo A, Kaku T, Tester DJ, et al. SCN4B-encoded sodium channel beta4 subunit in congenital long-QT syndrome. *Circulation.* 2007;116(2):134–142.

Mestroni L, Rocco C, Gregori D, et al. Familial dilated cardiomyopathy: evidence for genetic and phenotypic heterogeneity. Heart Muscle Disease Study Group. *J Am Coll Cardiol.* 1999;34(1):181–190.

Michalatos-Beloin S, Tishkoff SA, Bentley KL, Kidd KK, Ruano G. Molecular haplotyping of genetic markers 10 kb apart by allele-specific long-range PCR. *Nucleic Acids Res.* 1996;24:4841–4843.

Michele DE, Albayya FP, Metzger JM. Direct, convergent hypersensitivity of calcium-activated force generation produced by hypertrophic cardiomyopathy mutant alpha-tropomyosins in adult cardiac myocytes. *Nat Med.* 1999;5(12):1413–1417.

Miller DT, Ridker PM, Libby P, Kwiatkowski DJ. The path from genomics to therapeutics. *J Am Coll Cardiol.* 2007a;49(15):1589–1599.

Miller TE, You L, Myerburg RJ, Benke PJ, Bishopric NH. Whole blood RNA offers a rapid, comprehensive approach to genetic diagnosis of cardiovascular diseases. *Genet Med.* 2007b;9(1):23–33.

Min GL, Martiat P, Pu GA, Goldman J. Use of pulsed field gel electrophoresis to characterize BCR gene involvement in CML patients lacking M-BCR rearrangement. *Leukemia.* 1990;4:650–656.

Mogensen J, Klausen IC, Pedersen AK, et al. Alpha-cardiac actin is a novel disease gene in familial hypertrophic cardiomyopathy. *J Clin Invest.* 1999;103(10): R39–R43.

Mogensen J, Kubo T, Duque M, et al. Idiopathic restrictive cardiomyopathy is part of the clinical expression of cardiac troponin I mutations. *J Clin Invest.* 2003;111(2):209–216.

Mogensen J, Murphy RT, Shaw T, et al. Severe disease expression of cardiac troponin C and T mutations in patients with idiopathic dilated cardiomyopathy. *J Am Coll Cardiol.* 2004;44(10):2033–2040.

Mohapatra B, Jimenez S, Lin JH, et al. Mutations in the muscle LIM protein and alpha-actinin-2 genes in dilated cardiomyopathy and endocardial fibroelastosis. *Mol Genet Metab.* 2003;80(1–2):207–215.

Mohler PJ, Schott JJ, Gramolini AO, et al. Ankyrin-B mutation causes type 4 long-QT cardiac arrhythmia and sudden cardiac death. *Nature.* 2003;421(6923):634–639.

Mohler PJ, Splawski I, Napolitano C, et al. A cardiac arrhythmia syndrome caused by loss of ankyrin-B function. *Proc Natl Acad Sci USA.* 2004;101(24):9137–9142.

Moolman-Smook JC, Mayosi B, Brink P, Corfield VA. Identification of a new missense mutation in MyBP-C associated with hypertrophic cardiomyopathy. *J Med Genet.* 1998;35(3):253–254.

Mörner S, Richard P, Kazzam E, et al. Identification of the genotypes causing hypertrophic cardiomyopathy in northern Sweden. *J Mol Cell Cardiol.* 2003;35(7):841–849.

Moss AJ, Zareba W, Benhorin J, et al. ECG T-wave patterns in genetically distinct forms of the hereditary long QT syndrome. *Circulation.* 1995;92(10):2929–2934.

Mundle SD, Koska RJ. *Fluorescence In Situ Hybridization.* Chapter 15 In: Coleman WD, Tsongalis TJ, ed. *Molecular Diagnostics for the Clinical Laboratorian.* 2nd ed. NJ: Humana Press. 2005:189–202.

Muntoni F, Cau M, Ganau A, et al. Brief report: deletion of the dystrophin muscle-promoter region associated with X-linked dilated cardiomyopathy. *N Engl J Med.* 1993;329(13):921–925.

Murphy RT, Mogensen J, Shaw A, Kubo T, Hughes S, McKenna WJ. Novel mutation in cardiac troponin I in recessive idiopathic dilated cardiomyopathy. *Lancet.* 2004;363(9406):371–372.

Murthy SK, Demetrick DJ. New approaches to fluorescence in situ hybridization. *Methods Mol Biol.* 2006;319:237–259.

Napolitano C, Priori SG, Schwartz PJ, et al. Genetic testing in the long QT syndrome: development and validation of an efficient approach to genotyping in clinical practice. *J Am Med Assoc.* 2005;294(23):2975–2980.

Newby LK, Goldmann BU, Ohman EM. Troponin: an important prognostic marker and risk-stratification tool in non-ST-segment elevation acute coronary syndromes. *J Am Coll Cardiol.* 2003;41(4 suppl S): 31S–36S.

Newton-Cheh C, Larson MG, Corey DC, et al. QT interval is a heritable quantitative trait with evidence of linkage to chromosome 3 in a genome-wide linkage analysis: the Framingham Heart Study. *Heart Rhythm.* 2005;2(3):277–284.

Niimura H, Bachinski LL, Sangwatanaroj S, et al. Mutations in the gene for cardiac myosin-binding protein C and late-onset familial hypertrophic cardiomyopathy. *N Engl J Med.* 1998;338(18):1248–1257.

Niimura H, Patton KK, McKenna WJ, et al. Sarcomere protein gene mutations in hypertrophic cardiomyopathy of the elderly. *Circulation.* 2002;105(4):446–451.

O'Cochlain DF, Perez-Terzic C, Reyes S, et al. Transgenic overexpression of human DMPK accumulates into hypertrophic cardiomyopathy, myotonic myopathy and hypotension traits of myotonic dystrophy. *Hum Mol Genet.* 2004;13(20):2505–2518.

Okagaki T, Weber FE, Fischman DA, Vaughan KT, Mikawa T, Reinach FC. The major myosin-binding domain of skeletal muscle MyBP-C (C protein) resides in the COOH-terminal, immunoglobulin C2 motif. *J Cell Biol.* 1993;123(3):619–626.

Olson TM, Doan TP, Kishimoto NY, Whitby FG, Ackerman MJ, Fananapazir L. Inherited and de novo mutations in the cardiac actin gene cause hypertrophic cardiomyopathy. *J Mol Cell Cardiol.* 2000;32(9): 1687–1694.

Olson TM, Illenberger S, Kishimoto NY, et al. Metavinculin mutations alter actin interaction in dilated cardiomyopathy. *Circulation.* 2002;105(4):431–437.

Olson TM, Keating MT. Mapping a cardiomyopathy locus to chromosome 3p22-p25. *J Clin Invest.* 1996;97(2):528–532.

Olson TM, Kishimoto NY, Whitby FG, Michels VV. Mutations that alter the surface charge of alpha-tropomyosin are associated with dilated cardiomyopathy. *J Mol Cell Cardiol.* 2001;33(4):723–732.

Olson TM, Michels VV, Thibodeau SN, Tai YS, Keating MT. Actin mutations in dilated cardiomyopathy, a heritable form of heart failure. *Science.* 1998;280(5364):750–752.

Oostra BA, Willemsen R. Diagnostic tests for fragile X syndrome. *Expert Rev Mol Diagn.* 2001;1:226–232.

Ophoff RA, Terwindt GM, Vergouwe MN, et al. Familial hemiplegic migraine and episodic ataxia type-2 are caused by mutations in the Ca2+ channel gene CACNL1A4. *Cell.* 1996;87(3):543–552.

Orita M, Iwahana H, Kanazawa H, Hayashi K, Sekiya T. Detection of polymorphisms of human DNA by gel electrophoresis as single-strand conformation polymorphisms. *Proc Natl Acad Sci USA.* 1989;86(8):2766–2770.

Panteghini M, Cuccia C, Bonetti G, Giubbini R, Pagani F, Bonini E. Single-point cardiac troponin T at coronary care unit discharge after myocardial infarction correlates with infarct size and ejection fraction. *Clin Chem.* 2002;48(9):1432–1436.

Patsalis PC, Kousoulidou L, Sismani C, Mannik K, Kurg A. MAPH: from gels to microarrays. *Eur J Med Genet.* 2005;48:241–249.

Pe'er I, de Bakker PI, Maller J, Yelensky R, Altshuler D, Daly MJ. Evaluating and improving power in whole-genome association studies using fixed marker sets. *Nat Gen.* 2006;38(6):663–667.

Peters DG, Zhang XC, Benos PV, Heidrich-O'Hare E, Ferrell RE. Genomic analysis of immediate/early response to shear stress in human coronary artery endothelial cells. *Physiol Gen.* 2002;12(1):25–33.

Pfeufer A, Jalilzadeh S, Perz S, et al. Common variants in myocardial ion channel genes modify the QT interval in the general population: results from the KORA study. *Circ Res.* 2005;96(6):693–701.

Pinkel D, Segraves R, Sudar D, et al. High resolution analysis of DNA copy number variation using comparative genomic hybridization to microarrays. *Nat Genet.* 1998;20(2):207–211.

Pinkel D, Straume T, Gray JW. Cytogenetic analysis using quantitative, high-sensitivity, fluorescence hybridization. *Proc Natl Acad Sci USA.* 1986;83(9):2934–2938.

Plaster NM, Tawil R, Tristani-Firouzi M, et al. Mutations in Kir2.1 cause the developmental and episodic electrical phenotypes of Andersen's syndrome. *Cell.* 2001;105(4):511–519.

Poetter K, Jiang H, Hassanzadeh S, et al. Mutations in either the essential or regulatory light chains of myosin are associated with a rare myopathy in human heart and skeletal muscle. *Nat Genet.* 1996;13(1):63–69.

Pollack JR, Perou CM, Alizadeh AA, et al. Genome-wide analysis of DNA copy-number changes using cDNA microarrays. *Nat Genet.* 1999;23(1):41–46.

Prabhakar R, Boivin GP, Grupp IL, et al. A familial hypertrophic cardiomyopathy alpha-tropomyosin mutation causes severe cardiac hypertrophy and death in mice. *J Mol Cell Cardiol.* 2001;33(10):1815–1828.

Priori SG, Napolitano C, Schwartz PJ, et al. Association of long QT syndrome loci and cardiac events among patients treated with beta-blockers. *J Am Med Assoc.* 2004;292(11):1341–1344.

Priori SG, Schwartz PJ, Napolitano C, et al. Risk stratification in the long-QT syndrome. *N Eng J Med.* 2003;348(19):1866–1874.

Pritchard JK. Are rare variants responsible for susceptibility to complex diseases? *Am J Hum Genet.* 2001;69(1):124–137.

Randi AM, Biguzzi E, Falciani F, et al. Identification of differentially expressed genes in coronary atherosclerotic plaques from patients with stable or unstable angina by cDNA array analysis. *J Thromb Haemost.* 2003;1(4):829–835.

Remes AM, Hassinen IE, Ikäheimo MJ, et al. Mitochondrial DNA deletions in dilated cardiomyopathy: a clinical study employing endomyocardial sampling. *J Am Coll Cardiol.* 1994;23(4):935–942.

Ren H, Francis W, Boys A, et al. BAC-based PCR fragment microarray: high-resolution detection of chromosomal deletion and duplication breakpoints. *Hum Mutat.* 2005;25(5):476–482.

Richard P, Charron P, Carrier L, et al. Hypertrophic cardiomyopathy: distribution of disease genes, spectrum of mutations, and implications for a molecular diagnosis strategy. *Circulation.* 2003;107(17):2227–2232.

Richardson P, McKenna W, Bristow M, et al. Report of the 1995 World Health Organization/International Society and Federation of Cardiology Task Force on the Definition and Classification of Cardiomyopathies. *Circulation.* 1996;93(5):841–842.

Rickman L, Fiegler H, Carter NP, Bobrow M. Prenatal diagnosis by array-CGH. *Eur J Med Genet.* 2005;48(3):232–240.

Rickman L, Fiegler H, Shaw-Smith C, et al. Prenatal detection of unbalanced chromosomal rearrangements by array CGH. *J Med Genet.* 2006;43(4):353–361.

Risch N. Linkage strategies for genetically complex traits. I. Multilocus models. *Am J Hum Genet.* 1990;46(2):222–228.

Risch N, Merikangas K. The future of genetic studies of complex human diseases. *Science.* 1996;273(5281):1516–1517.

Roberts R. Genomics and Cardiac Arrhythmias. *J Am Coll Cardiol.* 2006;47(1):9–21.

Robin NH, Tabereaux PB, Benza R, Korf BR. Genetic testing in cardiovascular disease. *J Am Coll Cardiol.* 2007;50(8):727–737.

Sabbir MG, Dasgupta S, Roy A, et al. Genetic alterations (amplification and rearrangement) of D-type cyclins loci in head and neck squamous cell carcinoma of Indian patients: prognostic significance and clinical implications. *Diagn Mol Pathol.* 2006:15:7–16.

Satoh M, Takahashi M, Sakamoto T, Hiroe M, Marumo F, Kimura A. Structural analysis of the titin gene in hypertrophic cardiomyopathy: identification of a novel disease gene. *Biochem Biophys Res Commun.* 1999;262(2):411–417.

Schmitt JP, Kamisago M, Asahi M, et al. Dilated cardiomyopathy and heart failure caused by a mutation in phospholamban. *Science.* 2003;299(5611):1410–1413.

Schouten JP, McElgunn CJ, Waaijer R, Zwijnenburg D, Diepvens F, Pals G. Relative quantification of 40 nucleic acid sequences by multiplex ligation-dependent probe amplification. *Nucleic Acids Res.* 2002;30:e57.

Schröck E, du Manoir S, Veldman T, et al. Multicolor spectral karyotyping of human chromosomes. *Science.* 1996;273(5274):494–497.

Schröck E, Veldman T, Padilla-Nash H, et al. Spectral karyotyping refines cytogenetic diagnostics of constitutional chromosomal abnormalities. *Hum Genet.* 1997;101(3):255–262.

Schulze-Bahr E, Wang Q, Wedekind H, et al. KCNE1 mutations cause Jervell and Lange-Nielsen syndrome. *Nat Gen.* 1997;17(3):267–268.

Schwartz DC, Cantor CR. Separation of yeast chromosome-sized DNAs by pulsed field gradient gel electrophoresis. *Cell.* 1984;37:67–75.

Schwartz PJ. The congenital long QT syndromes from genotype to phenotype: clinical implications. *J Int Med.* 2006;259:39–47.

Schwartz PJ, Priori SG, Cerrone M, et al. Left cardiac sympathetic denervation in the management of high-risk patients affected by the long-QT syndrome. *Circulation.* 2004;109(15):1826–1833.

Schwartz PJ, Priori SG, Locati EH, et al. Long QT syndrome patients with mutations of the SCN5A and HERG genes have differential responses to Na+ channel blockade and to increases in heart rate. Implications for gene-specific therapy. *Circulation.* 1995;92(12):3381–3386.

Schwartz PJ, Priori SG, Spazzolini C, et al. Genotype–phenotype correlation in the long-QT syndrome: gene-specific triggers for life-threatening arrhythmias. *Circulation.* 2001;103(1):89–95.

Seabright, M. The use of proteolytic enzymes for the mapping of structural rearrangements in the chromosomes of man. *Chromosoma.* 1972;36:204–210.

Sebillon P, Bouchier C, Bidot LD, et al. Expanding the phenotype of LMNA mutations in dilated cardiomyopathy and functional consequences of these mutations. *J Med Genet.* 2003;40(8):560–567.

Seliem MA, Mansara KB, Palileo M, Ye X, Zhang Z, Benson DW. Evidence for autosomal recessive inheritance of infantile dilated cardiomyopathy: studies from the Eastern Province of Saudi Arabia. *Pediatr Res.* 2000;48(6):770–775.

Selzer RR, Richmond TA, Pofahl NJ, et al. Analysis of chromosome breakpoints in neuroblastoma at sub-kilobase resolution using fine-tiling oligonucleotide array CGH. *Genes Chromosomes Cancer.* 2005;44(3):305–319.

Sharp AJ, Locke DP, McGrath SD, et al. Segmental duplications and copy-number variation in the human genome. *Am J Hum Genet.* 2005;77(1):78–88.

Shaw-Smith C, Redon R, Rickman L, et al. Microarray based comparative genomic hybridisation (array-CGH) detects submicroscopic chromosomal deletions and duplications in patients with learning disability/mental retardation and dysmorphic features. *J Med Genet.* 2004;41(4):241–248.

Silvestri G, Santorelli FM, Shanske S, et al. A new mtDNA mutation in the tRNA(Leu(UUR)) gene associated with maternally inherited cardiomyopathy. *Hum Mutat.* 1994;3(1):37–43.

Siu BL, Niimura H, Osborne JA, et al. Familial dilated cardiomyopathy locus maps to chromosome 2q31. *Circulation.* 1999;99(8):1022–1026.

Solomon E, Bobrow M, Goodfellow PN, et al. Human gene mapping using an X/autosome translocation. *Somatic Cell Genet.* 1976;2:125–140.

Solomon E, Voss R, Hall V, et al. Chromosome 5 allele loss in human colorectal carcinomas. *Nature.* 1987;328:616–619.

Solomon SD, Geisterfer-Lowrance AA, Vosberg HP, et al. A locus for familial hypertrophic cardiomyopathy is closely linked to the cardiac myosin heavy chain genes, CRI-L436, and CRI-L329 on chromosome 14 at q11-q12. *Am J Hum Genet.* 1990;47(3):389–394.

Southern E. Tools for genomics. *Nat Med.* 2005;11:1029–1034.

Southern EM. Detection of specific sequences among DNA fragments separated by gel electrophoresis. *J Mol Biol.* 1975;98:503–517.

Southern EM, Anand R, Brown WR, Fletcher DS. A model for the separation of large DNA molecules by crossed field gel electrophoresis. *Nucleic Acids Res.* 1987;15:5925–5943.

Southern EM. Blotting at 25. *Trends Biochem. Sci.* 2000;25:585–588.

Splawski I, Shen J, Timothy KW, et al. Spectrum of mutations in long-QT syndrome genes. KVLQT1, HERG, SCN5A, KCNE1, and KCNE2. *Circulation.* 2000;102(10):1178–1185.

Splawski I, Timothy KW, Decher N, et al. Severe arrhythmia disorder caused by cardiac L-type calcium channel mutations. *Proc Nat Acad Sci USA.* 2005;102(23):8089–8096.

Splawski I, Timothy KW, Sharpe LM, et al. Ca(V)1.2 calcium channel dysfunction causes a multisystem disorder including arrhythmia and autism. *Cell.* 2004;119(1):19–31.

Splawski I, Tristani-Firouzi M, Lehmann MH, Sanguinetti MC, Keating MT. Mutations in the hKCNE1 gene cause long QT syndrome and suppress IKs function. *Nat Gen.* 1997;17:338–340.

Stark GR, Wahl GM. Gene amplification. *Annu Rev Biochem.* 1984;53:447–491.

Stefanelli CB, Rosenthal A, Borisov AB, Ensing GJ, Russell MW. Novel troponin T mutation in familial dilated cardiomyopathy with gender-dependant severity. *Mol Genet Metab.* 2004;83(1–2):188–196.

Strachan T, Read AP. *Human Molecular Genetics 2.* New York: John Wiley & Sons, Inc.; 1999.

Suomalainen A, Paetau A, Leinonen H, et al. Inherited idiopathic dilated cardiomyopathy with multiple deletions of mitochondrial DNA. *Lancet.* 1992;340(8831):1319–1320.

Taylor MR, Fain PR, Sinagra G, et al. Natural history of dilated cardiomyopathy due to lamin A/C gene mutations. *J Am Coll Cardiol.* 2003;41(5):771–780.

Taylor MR, Slavov D, Gajewski A, et al. Thymopoietin (lamina-associated polypeptide 2) gene mutation associated with dilated cardiomyopathy. *Hum Mutat.* 2005;26(6):566–574.

Taylor RW, Giordano C, Davidson MM, et al. A homoplasmic mitochondrial transfer ribonucleic acid mutation as a cause of maternally inherited hypertrophic cardiomyopathy. *J Am Coll Cardiol.* 2003;41(10):1786–1796.

Tester DJ, Will ML, Ackerman MJ. Mutation detection in congenital long QT syndrome: cardiac channel gene screen using PCR, dHPLC, and direct DNA sequencing. In: Wang QK, ed. *Cardiovascular Disease—Methods and Protocols.* Totowa, NJ: Humana Press. 2006;128:181–207.

The Wellcome Trust Case Control Consortium. Genome-wide association study of 14,000 cases of seven common diseases and 3,000 shared controls. *Nature.* 2007;447:661–678.

Towbin JA, Hejtmancik JF, Brink P, et al. X-linked dilated cardiomyopathy. Molecular genetic evidence of linkage to the Duchenne muscular dystrophy (dystrophin) gene at the Xp21 locus. *Circulation.* 1993;87(6):1854–1865.

Trask B, van den Engh G, Pinkel D, et al. Fluorescence in situ hybridization to interphase cell nuclei in suspension allows flow cytometric analysis of chromosome content and microscopic analysis of nuclear organization. *Hum Genet.* 1988;78(3):251–259.

Trask BJ. DNA sequence localization in metaphase and interphase cells by fluorescence in situ hybridization. *Methods Cell Biol.* 1991;35:3–35.

Tsongalis GJ, Silverman LM. Molecular pathology of the fragile X syndrome. *Arch Pathol Lab Med.* 1993;117:1121–1125.

Tsubata S, Bowles KR, Vatta M, et al. Mutations in the human delta-sarcoglycan gene in familial and sporadic dilated cardiomyopathy. *J Clin Invest.* 2000;106(5):655–662.

Underhill PA, Jin L, Lin AA, et al. Detection of numerous Y chromosome biallelic polymorphisms by denaturing high-performance liquid chromatography. *Gen Res.* 1997;7(10):996–1005.

Underhill PA, Jin L, Zemans R, Oefner PJ, Cavalli-Sforza LL. A pre-Columbian Y chromosome-specific transition and its implications for human evolutionary history. *Proc Nat Acad USA.* 1996;93(1):196–200.

Ungaro P, Christian SL, Fantes JA, et al. Molecular characterisation of four cases of intrachromosomal triplication of chromosome 15q11-q14. *J Med Genet.* 2001;38(1):26–34.

Urban AE, Korbel JO, Selzer R, et al. High-resolution mapping of DNA copy alterations in human chromosome 22 using high-density tiling oligonucleotide arrays. *Proc Natl Acad Sci USA.* 2006;103(12):4534–4539.

van Berlo JH, de Voogt WG, van der Kooi AJ, et al. Meta-analysis of clinical characteristics of 299 carriers of LMNA gene mutations: do lamin A/C mutations portend a high risk of sudden death? *J Mol Med.* 2005;83(1):79–83.

Van Driest SL, Ackerman MJ, Ommen SR, et al. Prevalence and severity of benign mutations in the beta-myosin heavy chain, cardiac troponin T, and alpha-tropomyosin genes in hypertrophic cardiomyopathy. *Circulation.* 2002a;106(24):3085–3090.

Van Driest SL, Ommen SR, Tajik AJ, Gersh BJ, Ackerman MJ. Sarcomeric genotyping in hypertrophic cardiomyopathy. *Mayo Clin Proc.* 2005a;80(4):463–469.

Van Driest SL, Ommen SR, Tajik AJ, Gersh BJ, Ackerman MJ. Yield of genetic testing in hypertrophic cardiomyopathy. *Mayo Clin Proc.* 2005b;80(6):739–744.

Van Driest SL, Will ML, Atkins DL, Ackerman MJ. A novel TPM1 mutation in a family with hypertrophic cardiomyopathy and sudden cardiac death in childhood. *J Am Coll Cardiol.* 2002b;90(10):1123–1127.

van Ommen GJ, Breuning MH, Raap AK. FISH in genome research and molecular diagnostics. *Curr Opin Genet Dev.* 1995;5(3):304–308.

Vatta M, Ackerman MJ, Ye B, et al. Mutant caveolin-3 induces persistent late sodium current and is associated with long-QT syndrome. *Circulation.* 2006;114(20):2104–2112.

Vatta M, Mohapatra B, Jimenez S, et al. Mutations in Cypher/ZASP in patients with dilated cardiomyopathy and left ventricular non-compaction. *J Am Coll Cardiol.* 2003;42(11):2014–2027.

Veltman JA, Schoenmakers EF, Eussen BH, et al. High-throughput analysis of subtelomeric chromosome rearrangements by use of array-based comparative genomic hybridization. *Am J Hum Genet.* 2002;70(5):1269–1276.

Verga L, Concardi M, Pilotto A, et al. Loss of lamin A/C expression revealed by immuno-electron microscopy in dilated cardiomyopathy with atrioventricular block caused by LMNA gene defects. *Virchows Arch.* 2003;443(5):664–671.

Villard E, Duboscq-Bidot L, Charron P, et al. Mutation screening in dilated cardiomyopathy: prominent role of the beta myosin heavy chain gene. *Eur Heart J.* 2005;26(8):794–803.

Waggott W, Lo YM, Bastard C, et al. Detection of NPM-ALK DNA rearrangement in CD30 positive anaplastic large cell lymphoma. *Br J Haematol.* 1995;89:905–907.

Wang Q, Curran ME, Splawski I, et al. Positional cloning of a novel potassium channel gene: KVLQT1 mutations cause cardiac arrhythmias. *Nat Gen.* 1996;12(1):17–23.

Wang Q, Shen J, Splawski I, et al. SCN5A mutations associated with an inherited cardiac arrhythmia, long QT syndrome. *Cell.* 1995;80(5): 805–811.

Wang Y, Makedon F, Pearlman J. Tumor classification based on DNA copy number aberrations determined using SNP arrays. *Oncol Rep.* 2006;15,1057–1059.

Ward JR, Cottrell S, Jones TA, et al. A long-range restriction map of human chromosome 5q21-q23. *Genomics.* 1993;17:15–24.

Wasserman SM, Mehraban F, Komuves LG, et al. Gene expression profile of human endothelial cells exposed to sustained fluid shear stress. *Physiol Gen.* 2002;12(1):13–23.

Watkins H, Conner D, Thierfelder L, et al. Mutations in the cardiac myosin binding protein-C gene on chromosome 11 cause familial hypertrophic cardiomyopathy. *Nat Genet.* 1995a;11(4):434–437.

Watkins H, McKenna WJ, Thierfelder L, et al. Mutations in the genes for cardiac troponin T and alpha-tropomyosin in hypertrophic cardiomyopathy. *N Engl J Med.* 1995b;332(16):1058–1064.

Watkins H, Rosenzweig A, Hwang DS, et al. Characteristics and prognostic implications of myosin missense mutations in familial hypertrophic cardiomyopathy. *N Engl J Med.* 1992;326(17):1108–1114.

Watkins H, Thierfelder L, Anan R, et al. Independent origin of identical beta cardiac myosin heavy-chain mutations in hypertrophic cardiomyopathy. *Am J Hum Genet.* 1993;53(6):1180–1185.

Wigle ED. Cardiomyopathy: the diagnosis of hypertrophic cardiomyopathy. *Heart.* 2001;86(6):709–714.

Wijmenga C, Wright TJ, Baan MJ, et al. Physical mapping and YAC-cloning connects four genetically distinct 4qter loci (*D4S163, D4S139, D4F35S1* and *D4F104S1*) in the FSHD gene-region. *Hum Mol Genet.* 1993;2:1667–1672.

Wilde AA, Jongbloed RJ, Doevendans PA, et al. Auditory stimuli as a trigger for arrhythmic events differentiate HERG-related (LQTS2) patients from KVLQT1-related patients (LQTS1). *J Am Coll Cardiol.* 1999;33(2):327–332.

Wolf SF, Migeon BR. Studies of X chromosome DNA methylation in normal human cells. *Nature.* 1982;295:667–671.

Wu WM, Tsai HJ, Pang JH, et al. Linear allele-specific long-range amplification: a novel method of long-range molecular haplotyping. *Hum Mutat.* 2005;26:393–394.

Yamauchi-Takihara K, Nakajima-Taniguchi C, et al. Clinical implications of hypertrophic cardiomyopathy associated with mutations in the alpha-tropomyosin gene. *Heart.* 1996;76(1):63–65.

Yu B, Sawyer NA, Caramins M, et al. Denaturing high performance liquid chromatography: high throughput mutation screening in familial hypertrophic cardiomyopathy and SNP genotyping in motor neurone disease. *J Clin Pathol.* 2005;58(5):479–485.

Zareba W, Moss AJ, Schwartz PJ, et al. Influence of genotype on the clinical course of the long-QT syndrome. International Long-QT Syndrome Registry Research Group. *N Eng J Med.* 1998;339(14):960–965.

Zareba W, Moss AJ, Sheu G, et al. Location of mutation in the KCNQ1 and phenotypic presentation of long QT syndrome. *J Cardiovasc Electrophysiol.* 2003;14(11):1149–1153.

Zeller R, Ivandic BT, Ehlermann P, et al. Large-scale mutation screening in patients with dilated or hypertrophic cardiomyopathy: a pilot study using DGGE. *J Mol Med.* 2006;84(8):682–691.

Zhang L, Timothy KW, Vincent GM, et al. Spectrum of ST-T-wave patterns and repolarization parameters in congenital long-QT syndrome: ECG findings identify genotypes. *Circulation.* 2000;102(23):2849–2855.

Zhou X, Rao NP, Cole SW, Mok SC, Chen Z, Wong DT. Progress in concurrent analysis of loss of heterozygosity and comparative genomic hybridization utilizing high density single nucleotide polymorphism arrays. *Cancer Genet Cytogenet.* 2005;159(1):53–57.

7

Cardiac Magnetic Resonance Imaging in Cardiovascular Genetics

James Moon

Introduction

Over the past decade, rapid advances in cardiovascular magnetic resonance, (CMR, also known as cardiac MRI) have resulted in its emergence as a key technology for phenotyping inherited cardiac diseases, and one that is likely to play an increasing role in refining the diagnosis and management. CMR provides multiple techniques in combination to build up a sophisticated picture of cardiac function, morphology, blood flow, and the state of tissue, particularly vessel wall and myocardium (Pennell et al. 2004). This means the technique has utility across the clinical disease spectrum, including cardiovascular diseases with polygenic etiology (e.g., coronary artery disease), monogenic (e.g., Marfan's), or multisystem effects (thalassemia and cardiac iron overload). However, for this chapter, the focus will be on monogenic disease of heart muscle: hypertrophic cardiomyopathy (HCM), arrhythmogenic right ventricular cardiomyopathy (ARVC), and dilated cardiomyopathy (DCM). Unclassified conditions such as left ventricular noncompaction (LVNC) will also be discussed.

An Overview of CMR

CMR is a medical imaging technology for the noninvasive assessment of the function and structure of the cardiovascular system. It is based on the same basic principles as magnetic resonance imaging (MRI), but with optimization for use in the cardiovascular system. These optimizations are principally the use of ECG gating and rapid imaging techniques or sequences. By combining a variety of such techniques into protocols, key functional and morphological features of the cardiovascular system can be assessed. CMR is highly reproducible and accurate with lower interobserver variation than other techniques. There is the ability to assess a variety of different clinically relevant parameters within the same scan—for example, function, flow, and myocardial health (ischemia, fatty infiltration, or scar). The major disadvantages of CMR are that some individuals cannot be scanned—either because they have implanted devices [e.g., pacemakers and implantable cardioverter defibrillators (ICD)] (Levine et al. 2007; Anonymous 2008) or because of claustrophobia. At or below a 3T (3 Tesla magnet strength), all currently used heart valves are now considered safe for MRI—the force exerted on them by the magnet is less than the beat-to beat forces of the beating heart. Similarly, no current endovascular stents or sternal wires are known to present a problems. Effective clinical processes can minimize claustrophobia and, for some individuals, a sedation protocol may reduce problems further (Francis et al. 2000).

Sequences—Cine Imaging

The main functional CMR imaging technique is a breath-hold ECG-gated cine sequence that shows the heart beating. This sequence is now nearly always based on a *steady-state free precession* (SSFP) sequence (Oppelt et al. 1986), implemented by different manufacturers under different names (e.g., FISP, bFFE, Fiesta). It has the advantages of high blood to myocardial contrast, making the blood appear bright. Endomyocardial structures (e.g., trabeculae) are well delineated and the image contrast is relatively flow independent so that, although swirling flow may be seen (as in poor ventricles) or flow acceleration (e.g., in outflow tract obstruction), the detection of the blood/myocardial interface is independent of flow rate. This sequence is run in a "segmented" way—so, like 3D echocardiography, the cardiac cycle is built up over a number of heartbeats in a breath-hold. Occasional patients have arrhythmia with very early QRS complexes for which arrhythmia rejection systems fail. For these, a nongated real-time imaging, familiar from echocardiography, may be needed, but this imaging modality sacrifices frame rate and resolution. Rapid advances in hardware suggest that this technique will become more widely used over time.

Sequences—Flow

Phase velocity mapping is a technique that permits the measurement of velocity (either in-plane or through-plane) of blood (Kilner et al. 2007). This can be performed and precisely orientated across, say, the aorta or left ventricular (LV) outflow tract to derive peak velocities and, if pixel values are integrated, flow and stroke volume. This may be used in ways familiar from echocardiography—for example, to determine the degree of mitral regurgitation (stroke volume from ventricular analysis minus aortic flow) and shunts. A significant disadvantage of CMR velocity mapping compared to echocardiography is that accurate peak velocity measurement may require a cohesive laminar jet core, which is often absent in dynamic obstruction. Furthermore, high temporal resolution features such as characterization of the Doppler envelope and beat-to-beat variation (post-ectopic, during Valsalva) in peak velocities may not be achievable with CMR.

Tissue Characterization—Intrinsic (No Contrast)

Specific CMR sequences can detect abnormalities in heart muscle. If these are detected without the use of any contrast agent, the sequence is detecting "intrinsic" differences in tissue. The sequences used may detect fat that appears bright. To confirm the presence of fat, the sequence is repeated with a modification that nulls the chemical signature of fat and fat becomes dark. This technique can present difficulties at times, for example, in ARVC patients with a high ectopic burden or when differentiating free wall right ventricular fat from overlying epicardial fat.

Under certain circumstances, other pathological processes can be detected, for example, edema (acute infarction/myocarditis) or cardiac iron (iatrogenic overload, e.g., in β-thalassemia major).

Tissue Characterization—Extrinsic (Contrast)

Contrast agents are used in CMR. Typically these are gadolinium based, with gadolinium (Gd^{3+}) bound to a chelator such as DTPA. Gd-DTPA is an inert, extravascular, and extracellular contrast agent that rapidly diffuses out of blood vessels, but it is limited in its distribution to the spaces between cells. It cannot cross intact cell membranes and thus its distribution in the body is defined by kinetics and the volume of distribution. This defines several different types of tissue that can be detected. The sequences chosen for this imaging, particularly for delayed enhancement, the *Inversion Recovery* technique, is very sensitive to subtle regional differences in Gd-DTPA concentration and detects focal interstitial expansion such as occurs in scar or focal interstitial expansion of endocardial amyloid deposition. But it does not detect a global interstitial expansion such as that found in severe hypertension, for example. Furthermore, the sequence requires operator training and the recognition/exclusion of artifact for optimal sensitivity (Table 7–1). Gd-DTPA is not currently recommended in individuals with severe renal failure and a glomerular filtration rate (GFR) of less than 30mls/min because of a condition called nephrogenic systemic fibrosis (Mitka et al. 2007). This was first identified in patients with severe or end-stage renal failure with very high doses (0.3 mmol/kg) of a specific gadolinium chelate. The belief is that a process called "transmetallation" was occurring with toxic Gd^{3+} becoming unbound to the chelator. Accordingly, there is a move toward cyclic chelators and a GFR limit.

CMR in Hypertrophic Cardiomyopathy

HCM—Early Disease

The first signs of phenotypic expression in HCM may be difficult to detect. When an individual has a parent or sibling with established HCM, they have a pretest probability of 50% of carrying the disease causing mutation. This has led to proposed familial criteria where even minor abnormalities of ECG or echo suggest the presence of early HCM. CMR may help the detection of hypertrophy missed by echo. This is established in apical HCM (Moon et al. 2004; Figure 7–1), but other, particularly, concentric or localized hypertrophy may be overlooked by echo (Figure 7–2; Moon et al. 2005; Rickers et al. 2005). Crypts or recesses, particularly in the LV inferior wall near the RV insertion point may be noted in HCM, but at this time, the significance is controversial (Kuribayashi et al. 1992; Germans et al. 2006; Johansson et al. 2007).

HCM—Established Disease

CMR can clarify wall thickness where there is doubt either because echocardiographic windows are poor or when paraseptal structures make measurement of the left ventricular wall problematic (Figure 7–3). Although CMR is not as good as echo for peak or beat-to-beat variation for gradients in dynamic obstruction, CMR may help with defining complex obstruction, for example, multilevel obstruction or right ventricular outflow tract obstruction that may be difficult to define by echo or postintervention recurrent obstruction, (Figure 7–4) (Lee et al. 2005; Valeti et al. 2007). In apical HCM, near-field effects and rib artifacts may limit non-contrast echocardiography. This could be resolved by CMR or the LV opacification with transpulmonary echo contrast agents. CMR will also detect apical hypertrophy, and apical aneurysms, sometimes containing thrombus, and apical trabeculations.

HCM—Late Gadolinium Enhancement in HCM

Late gadolinium enhancement (LGE) is able to detect fibrosis in vivo bringing this phenomenon into the clinical arena. Fibrosis imaging using CMR is familiar from imaging myocardial infarction (Kim et al. 2000; Wu et al. 2001), but the pathological processes

Table 7–1 Different Types of Myocardium Identifiable Using Gd-DTPA CMR

Tissue Type	Examples	Process	Result
Avascular	Thrombus Microvascular obstruction Areas in acute infarction	No Gd-DTPA reaches the area	**Avascularity imaging** Tissue appears dark as if Gd-DTPA had not been given
Reduced blood flow	Infarction/fibrosis (reduced capillary bed) Ischemic myocardium (after vasodilator stress)	Gd-DTPA arrives slowly in the tissue	**Perfusion imaging** Tissue takes up Gd-DTPA but with transient delay
Interstitial expansion	Replacement scar Interstitial expansion Amyloidosis	Gd-DTPA lingers passively in the tissue due to a larger volume of distribution	**Delayed enhancement** Late relative increases in tissue Gd-DTPA seen as "late gadolinium enhancement" (LGE)

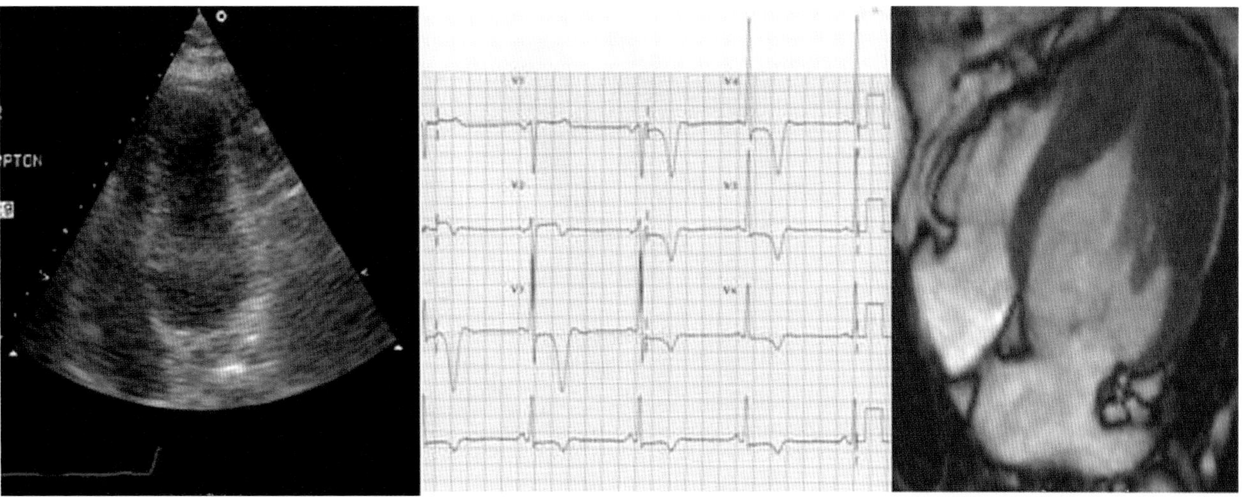

Figure 7–1 Noncontrast echo may miss apical pathology. Here, near-field effects rendered the apical tube like cavity invisible by echo, and the echo demonstrated apical akinesia and diastolic dysfunction. Transpulmonary contrast or CMR are capable of detecting the cavity all the way to the apex.

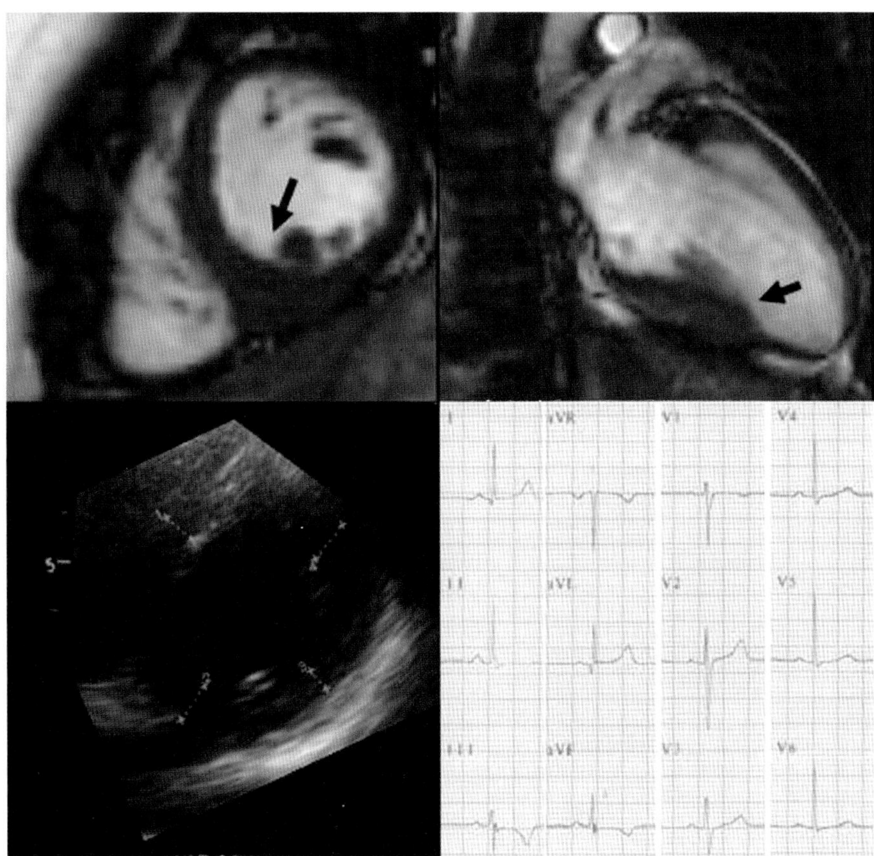

Figure 7–2 CMR detects missed hypertrophy in HCM. Here, an individual fulfilling familial criteria for HCM based on the ECG, is shown by CMR to have localized hypertrophy at the junction of the inferior wall and inferoseptum, which was missed by echo.

occurring in HCM are very different and result in different patterns of fibrosis and detected LGE (Figure 7–5). In myocardial infarction, myocardial necrosis and subsequent fibrosis occur in a wavefront from endo- to epicardium. In HCM, events leading from sarcomeric protein mutation to fibrosis are more complex. There may be a generalized increase in interstitial fibrosis with pericellular, intercellular, and fascicular connective tissue, or fibrosis surrounding vessels (Shirani et al. 2000). Fibrosis associated with disarray, particularly at the RV insertion points may occur (St John Sutton et al. 1980). Replacement scar may also occur leading, if extensive, to heart failure. The hope is that LGE represents *substrate imaging*—that is, by visualizing the abnormalities of myocardium directly, the necessary myocardial abnormalities for the development of malignant arrhythmias and

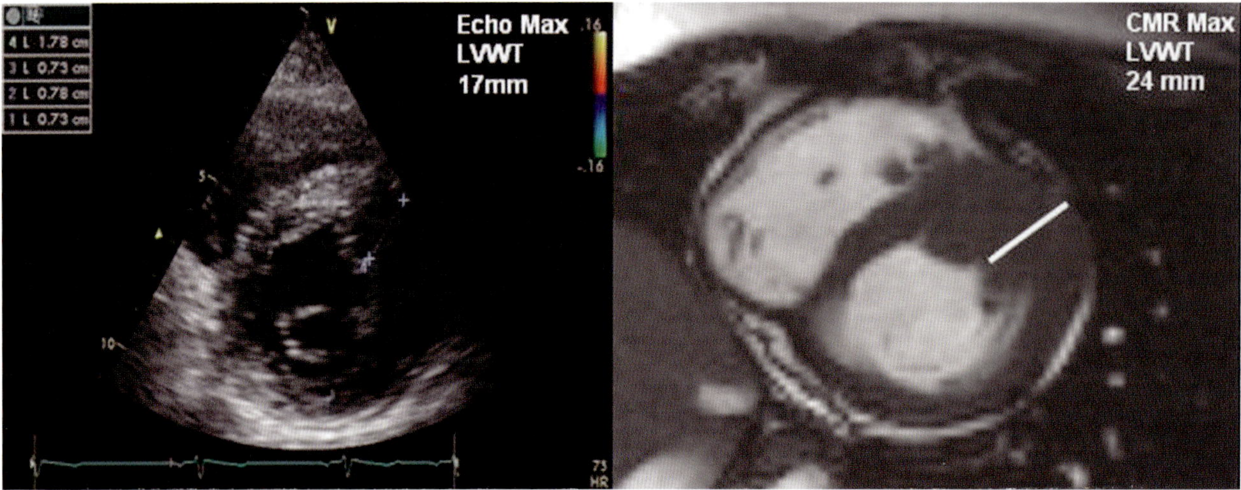

Figure 7–3 Underestimated LVH on echocardiogram compared to CMR. Here, the echocardiographer has drawn an apparently reasonable wall thickness—except the LVH had bulged out unexpectedly into the pericardium, revealed by the CMR.

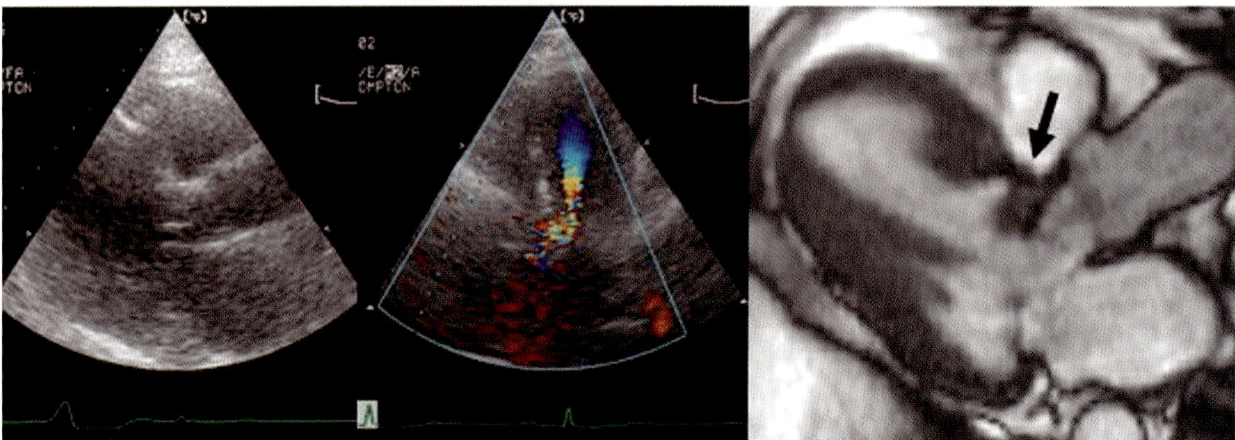

Figure 7–4 Complex anatomy revealed by CMR. A patient presenting with recurrent breathlessness several years after a successful alcohol ablation. Two-dimensional echo and color flow echo revealed obstruction, but not the location, which is apparent on the cine—in this case, due to a residual basal septal bulge (arrow) proximal to the ablation site.

heart failure are detected in advance of these adverse outcomes. However, there are a number of caveats to this and it is fair to say our understanding remains incomplete without outcome data (Moon 2007).

LGE in HCM—Limitations

First, LGE represents regions of focal interstitial expansion. Almost always, this is related to fibrosis, but one example is known where this is not the case, cardiac amyloidosis. In this case, global subendocardial LGE may occur (Figure 7–6a; Maceira et al. 2005). Second, diffuse interstitial expansion will not be visualized. By choosing the scan parameter (TI), the operator scanning for LGE creates a high sensitivity to small regional differences in Gd-DTPA concentrations but sacrifices information on the background Gd-DTPA concentrations. Third, regions of LGE are not necessarily complete replacement fibrosis, but rather a focal increase in the interstitium—for example, more than 15% fibrosis (not 100%) in one published case (Moon et al. 2004).

LGE and Risk of Sudden Death

Up to 80% of patients in some series demonstrate some enhancement, so the presence per se of LGE representing fibrosis is not sufficient to infer risk alone (Choudhury et al. 2002). When found, extensive LGE in young individuals appears to be most significant (Moon et al. 2003a). The potential for an age-dependent significance of LGE could be similar to that of other risk factors, for example, nonsustained VT. There may be specific patterns of LGE with differential significance. For example, RV insertion point fibrosis (see Figure 7–5) may be more benign. Many studies have now linked LGE with the presence of adverse features (Dumont et al. 2007; Pujadas et al. 2007; Dimitrow et al. 2008), but there are no prospective data. One scenario where LGE may be more likely to help, is that occurring in upto 30% of patients where a single sudden death risk factor is present (Elliott et al. 2000). Here, decisions require individualization and the presence of extensive LGE, particularly in a young patient, may be sufficient to influence the decision as to ICD implantation.

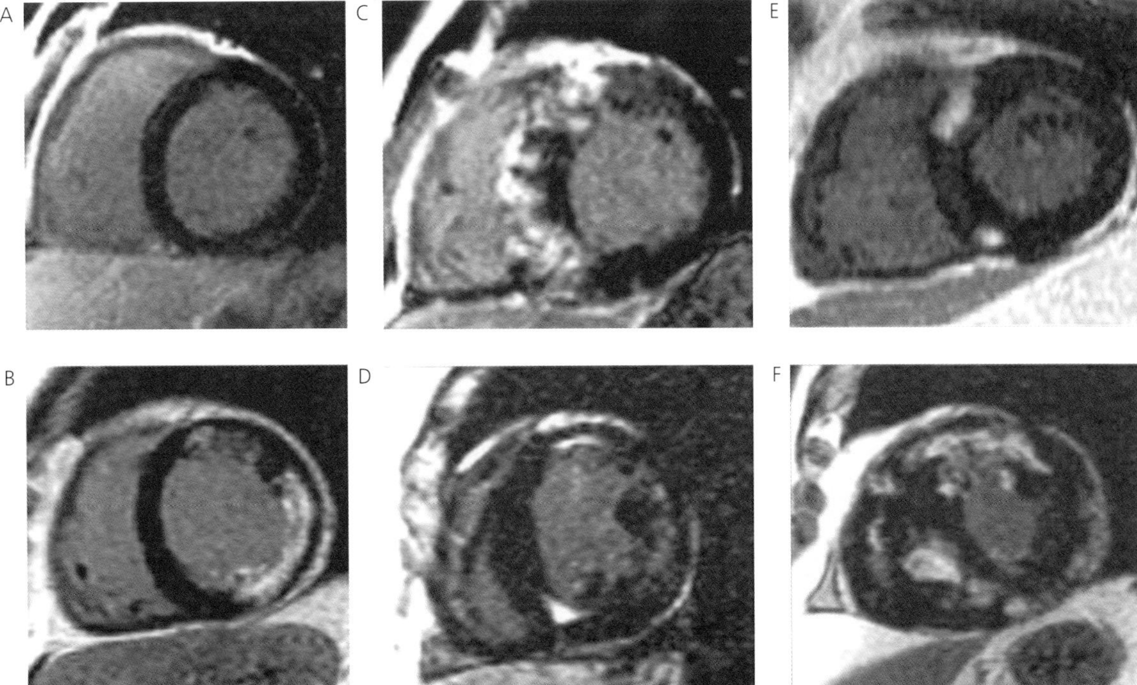

Figure 7–5 Different patterns of LGE in HCM. (a) Normal, (b) an infarct, and (c) to (f) represent different patterns of HCM. (c) extensive LGE, in this case in a high-risk patient, (d) apparent micro infarcts in HCM, (e) RV insertion point pattern (common), and (f) extensive areas, associated with progressive disease.

LGE and Heart Failure

Systolic heart failure is mainly caused by myocyte loss and replacement fibrosis and has a prevalence of around 3%. To date, virtually all reported patients with systolic dysfunction have demonstrated extensive (>25% of total myocardium) LGE. The predictive power of LGE is only now being explored (Maron et al. 2007), but experience of detecting fixed perfusion defects in HCM (Yamada et al. 1998) is positive. This may permit the exploration of disease modifying therapies in HCM before end stage is reached.

HCM—NonSarcomeric Protein Disease

A variety of phenocopies of HCM exist. For some, it is relatively easy to distinguish clinically (e.g., the elite athlete), but others pose significant clinical challenges (say the former elite Afro-Caribbean athlete with hypertension and 16 mm wall thickness). Under these circumstances, CMR provides high-quality imaging and tissue characterization but interpretation may still be complex with a significant "gray zone" of diagnostic uncertainty. Although there may be characteristic features (amyloid, Anderson-Fabry, Figure 7–6), in other circumstances (disease in a progressive disease phase), these may be lost and the diseases may all look similar with fibrosis as a final common pathway.

Athletes

The characteristic CMR features of athletes' heart compared to HCM are familiar from the echo literature. In athletes' heart, wall thicknesses do not exceed 15 mm when appropriately measured, although there are significant unknowns for black athletes or athletes using performance-enhancing drugs. Hypertrophy appears concentric, wall thickening appears supranormal, the hypertrophy is not at the expense of cavity size—cavities are large, and there is no LGE (Petersen et al. 2005a).

Amyloid

Cardiac amyloidosis typically demonstrates concentric hypertrophy, often with RV involvement (Maceira et al. 2005). There may be pleural and/or pericardial effusions, and biventricular long axis function may be visibly and strikingly impaired. After contrast, the Gd kinetics may be very abnormal with a similar peak Gd blood pool signal, but a rapid fall-off and LGE that is difficult to perform, with blood and myocardium nulling simultaneously. There may be extensive subendocardial LGE, although this may be patchy in other patients (Figure 7–6a; Perugini et al. 2006).

Storage Diseases

In the main, storage diseases have not been well documented by CMR. Anderson-Fabry's disease may be a cause for up to 3% of HCM patients, and depending on patient population, features (Sachdev et al. 2002) in the early phase have a typical LGE appearance of basal inferolateral enhancement, caused by fibrosis (Moon et al. 2003, 2006; Figure 7–7). In late disease, storage diseases (glycogen storage disease type IIIa, Anderson-Fabry disease, AMP kinase) all begin to look similar like burnt out sarcomeric HCM.

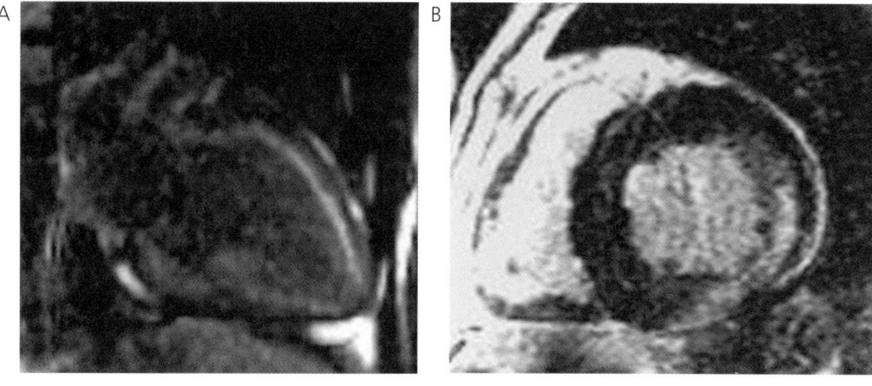

Figures 7–6 Different patterns of LGE in different phenocopies. (a) typical amyloid and (b) Anderson-Fabry disease.

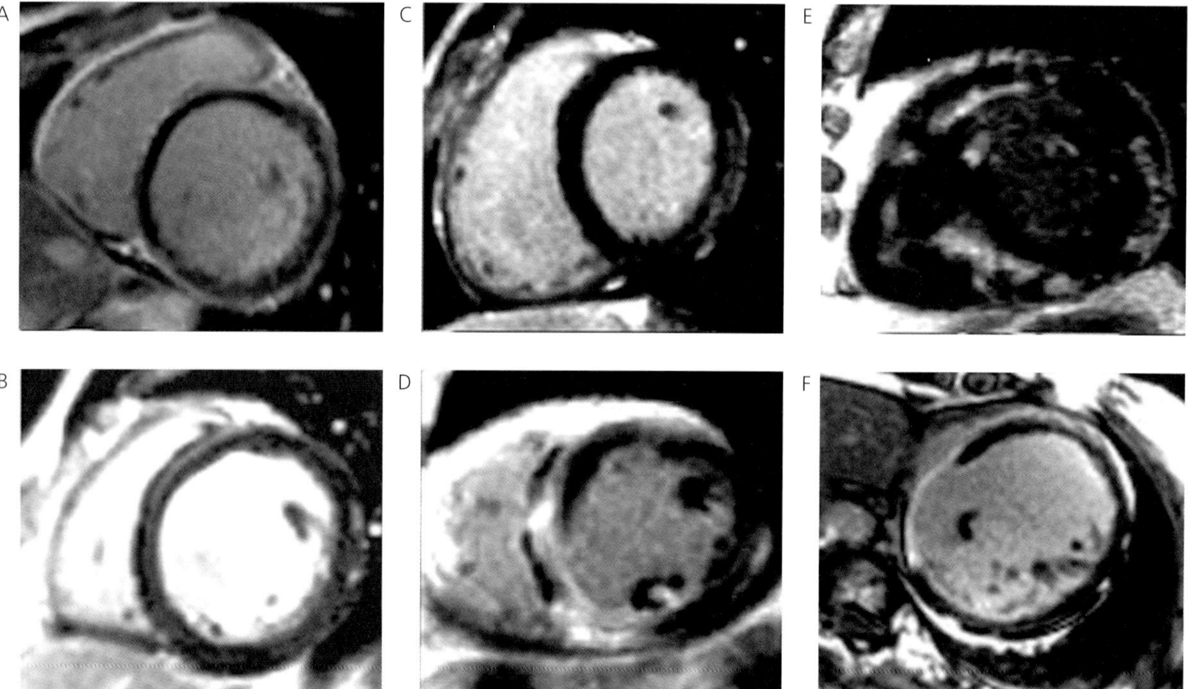

Figure 7–7 Different types of LGE in DCM: (a) none (DCM), (b) mid-myocardial, (c) epicardial (myocarditis, ARVC with LV involvement), (d) sarcoid., (e) burnt out HCM, and (f) DCM with bystander CAD—this ventricle has an LV end diastolic dimension of 8 cm, EF 14%, and single vessel disease.

Dilated Cardiomyopathy (DCM)

DCM is well studied by CMR. Early LV dilatation is quantified volumetrically and can be compared with age-specific reference ranges (Bellenger et al. 2000a; Hudsmith et al. 2005; Maceira et al. 2006). The LV mass increase that is characteristic of DCM at autopsy can be quantified in vivo with the volumetric approach available with CMR, with LV mass increases typical even when there is wall thinning. The size of the heart in relation to the chest is also immediately apparent. An important role of CMR is to distinguish ischemic from nonischemic cardiomyopathy. When ischemic cardiomyopathy is advanced, thinning from infarction, remote remodeling, and subendocardial infarction can make the heart appear very similar to DCM. Other diagnostic tests (clinical examination, ECG, echocardiography, exercise testing, myocardial perfusion) are useful but not definitive—for example, Q waves are nonspecific in heart failure; regional wall motion abnormalities by echocardiography occur in both nonischemic cardiomyopathy and ischemic heart disease, whilst myocardial perfusion imaging in heart failure has poor specificity (50%) for diagnosing the cause of heart failure (Wu et al. 2003; Peter et al. 2004). Overall, autopsy studies have shown that, using conventional clinical techniques for diagnosing the etiology of heart failure in individual patients, ischemic heart disease is underdiagnosed *ante mortem*–for example, 27% of DCM patients were found to have ischemic heart disease, and 17% died of it in one series.

CMR is useful in measuring serial changes in chamber sizes, function, and mass in DCM, and it is able to detect smaller changes over time, for example, by following the anthracycline treatment in both the clinical and research settings (Bellenger et al. 2000b). Additional features may be present and well detected, such as apical or mural thrombus, mitral regurgitation, and RV involvement and a visual or quantitative assessment may be made of dyssynchrony—although here CMR has limits.

DCM—the Use of Gd-DTPA to Detect LGE

CMR in DCM can detect myocardial scarring using Gd-DTPA and the late gadolinium technique. More than half of all DCM patients have no detectable LGE (McCrohon et al. 2003). The commonest types of LGE seen in DCM are described below (Figure 7–7). LGE in DCM may help refine the etiology and may also be a prognostic marker (Assomull et al. 2006).

1. Myocardial Infarction

Always involving the subendocardial, sometimes through to transmural, LGE occurs in locations corresponding to the territory of the epicardial coronary arteries and represent myocardial infarction, making a non-DCM diagnosis likely. They do not, however, mean there will be epicardial coronary artery disease detected at X-ray angiography: coronary artery causes include plaque rupture with downstream embolism without residual narrowing, flush occlusion of branches, healed dissection, embolism, vasospasm, and pharmacologically induced vasospasm (e.g., after cocaine use). Noncoronary artery causes of infarction include coronary artery embolism, Chagas' cardiomyopathy (Rochitte et al. 2005) (although epicardial at autopsy, it often looks like infarction during CMR), and cardiac sarcoidosis (Smedema et al. 2005). Scarring may have impact on treatment options with, for example, some suggestion that posterior scar may be an important factor in determining the response to biventricular pacing for resynchronization (Chalil et al. 2007; Parsai et al. 2007).

2. Mid-Myocardial LGE

Frequently, there is LGE in the mid-myocardium, particularly of the septum. Caution must be taken to ensure this is not artifact induced by technical issues (e.g., having set the TI too short). This may be found in the early phase of inherited cardiomyopathies (Varghese et al. 2004; Raman et al. 2007).

3. LGE Consistent with Burnt-out HCM

In these patients, occasionally mistaken for DCM, there is typically unusual myocardial architecture with residual LVH and very extensive LGE (minimum 25% of the myocardium) in patterns more reminiscent of HCM.

4. LGE Consistent with Previous Myocarditis

Myocarditis is being increasingly recognized both clinically and by CMR. In the late phase, myocarditis is an important differential of DCM and causes a variety of patterns of LGE (Mahrholdt et al. 2004) both in the acute and chronic phase (De Cobelli et al. 2006). Acutely, myocarditis can be associated with very extensive LGE, some of which may resolve as the focal interstitial expansion/edema heals leaving, in some areas, a below-threshold interstitial increase. Myocarditis may demonstrate specific patterns—for example, there is an epicardial predilection, and some evidence for tropism to different areas of the heart with different viruses. Myocardial sarcoid may also affect the heart. Although it is not clear that granuloma are visible by CMR, areas of scarring from sarcoid are sometimes detected, and in some cases, there may be extensive scarring leading to a DCM-like picture (Smedema et al. 2005).

Iron Overload

CMR can be used to detect cardiac iron overload, mainly from transfusion-related iron overload in thalassemia major. Once present, death may occur quickly. In this condition, despite conventional chelation therapy, the majority of patients die in their mid-thirties of an iron-induced cardiomyopathy. CMR can identify patients at higher risk, so chelation therapy can be increased using a T2* measurement to quantify cardiac iron. The results show that the cardiac iron burden is not well related to hepatic overload or ferritin. A reliance on these parameters is therefore unreliable. T2* measurements below 10 ms indicate a high cardiac iron burden and incipient cardiac failure (Anderson et al. 2001).

Arrhythmogenic Right Ventricular Cardiomyopathy (ARVC)

ARVC is an inherited monogenic cardiac condition mainly caused by mutations in genes encoding proteins of the desmosome. Clinically, ventricular tachycardia arising from the right ventricle may cause sudden death. ARVC can be difficult to diagnose before an index event, and currently, the diagnosis relies on a tally of various major and minor criteria based on family history, the ECG, imaging, Holter ectopy, arrhythmia, and the presence of fibrofatty RV myocardial infiltration.

Current imaging criteria, be it CMR or echo/contrast echo, cannot alone diagnose ARVC. They can at most diagnose 1 (of 3) major criterion or 1 (of 3) minor criterion for ARVC (McKenna et al. 1994; Sen-Chowdhry et al. 2004). Fibro-fatty infiltration is an endomyocardial biopsy or autopsy diagnosis and is not at this time an imaging criterion. Using the standardized CMR protocol, severe abnormalities are easily apparent both by echo and CMR. However, the minor criteria can be problematic. Double reading of all cases is recommended (Tandri et al. 2004). In established disease, the abnormalities can be marked (Figure 7–8).

Imaging Challenges of the Right Ventricle

The normal right ventricle is complex and the full range and variation in size structure and function is only beginning to be appreciated. Particular areas such as the free wall insertion point(s) of the moderator band may naturally display apparent contraction abnormalities (Bluemke et al. 2003). A large part of this spectrum is increasingly being recognized as normal variants, and calling these minor wall motion abnormalities is prone to low reproducibility and large interobserver error. Minor musculoskeletal abnormalities (e.g., *pectus excavatum*) make the right ventricle apparently mould or conform itself into the space available, a natural process that may mimic RV pathological abnormalities. The RV free wall is thin and variably trabeculated with overlying pericardial fat and it may be difficult to unequivocally locate the fat signal as either epicardial or myocardial. Even when present, RV fat per se is not pathognomic for ARVC and fatty metaplasia/healing is well recognized in many cardiac pathologies.

All these difficulties make ARVC challenging. Nevertheless, in dedicated centers, particularly when allied to a genotyping program and family screening, even small morphological differences can be linked to gene carriage as early phenotypic expression of ARVC, facilitating clinical management (Sen-Chowdhry et al. 2006).

ARVC—Phenocopies

ARVC has a specific set of possible appearances by CMR, many of which are displayed in Figure 7–9. Nevertheless, a variety of phenocopies can mimic ARVC and these must be distinguished. Examples include RV infarction, RV involvement from sarcoidosis, and cardiac displacement causing abnormal RV morphology and ECG abnormalities. The epicardial, LV-based late enhancement

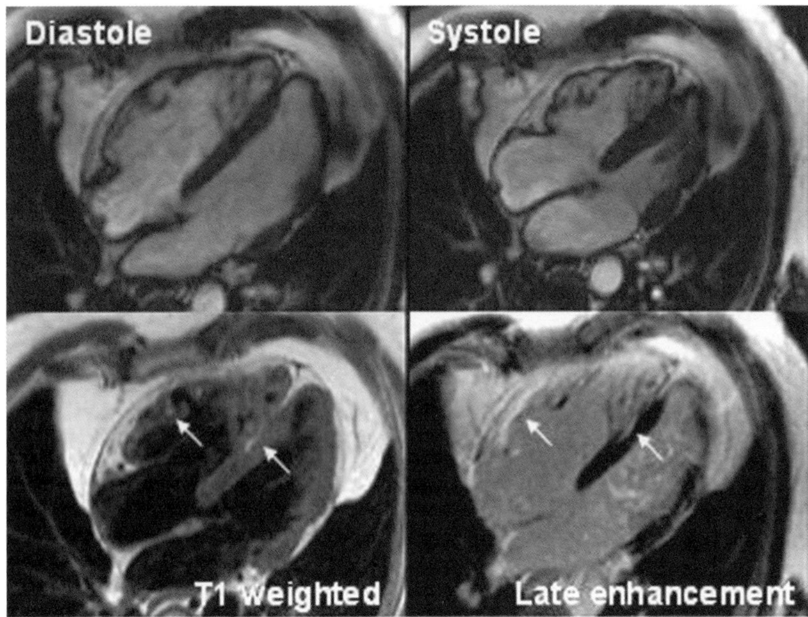

Figure 7–8 Diagnosis of ARVC by CMR. This individual has a plakophilin mutation. There is RV impairment with multiple wall motion abnormalities (micro-aneurysms), discreet areas of LV thinning, extensive fatty infiltration, and RV plus LV LGE.

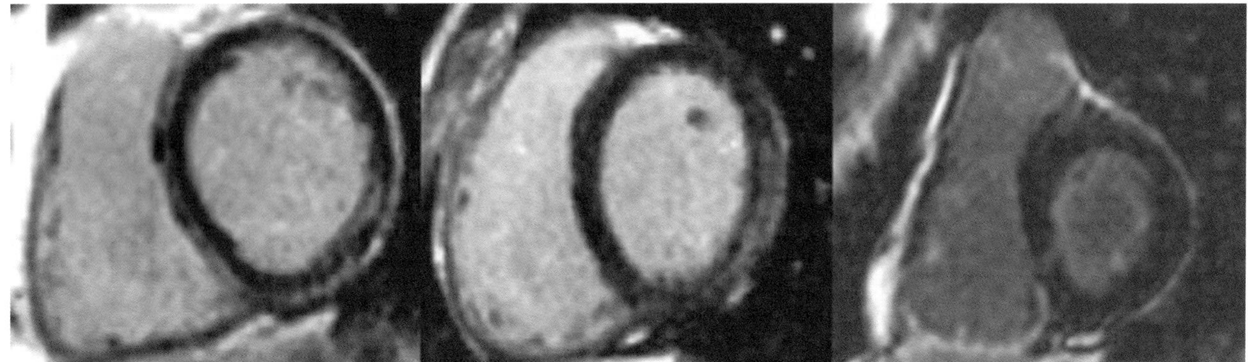

Figure 7–9 ARVC LGE phenocopies. ARVC (left) with RV and LV LGE is difficult to distinguish from myocarditis (middle) and sarcoid with just RV involvement (right).

of old myocarditis may appear indistinguishable from that LV involvement in ARVC—LV involvement in ARVC is being increasingly recognized (Sen-Chowdhry et al. 2007). At times, it can be complex determining whether, as the criteria say, the predominant ventricle involved is the right ventricle or whether there is an overlap syndrome with biventricular involvement.

Left Ventricular Noncompaction

LVNC is a congenital abnormality of LV formation where the spongy myocardium apparently fails to convert to compacted myocardium. As a disease entity, it is currently early in the process of becoming characterized and identified, and a note of caution should be sounded before its diagnosis. The number of papers and citations on the topic are increasing exponentially, and whilst there was clearly underreporting, the impression is that ascertainment bias may also be occurring. With newer, more sophisticated imaging normal variant trabecular architecture is being seen for the first time, and, in some cases, being reported as abnormal. Even tiny alterations in the position of the imaging plane or echo probe may drastically alter the trabecular appearance. The three-dimensional approach to LVNC taken by CMR is important, and the short axis views should be emphasized. With this in mind, LVNC is increasingly being interrogated by CMR, which has particular advantages toward the apex, and key features can be viewed (Figure 7–10). Location-specific analysis of compacted to noncompacted myocardium can be performed, leading to proposed and revised criteria (Petersen et al. 2005). With time, these diagnostic criteria and fundamental answers as to its place in cardiology should be forthcoming.

Summary

CMR as outlined above combines a variety of different techniques for imaging in genetic cardiomyopathy and has established roles in clinical management that range from a useful alternative imaging test to providing new information not previously available. There remain, however, challenges in interpreting some findings and in service delivery and in integrating CMR into clinical practice and guidelines to optimize utility.

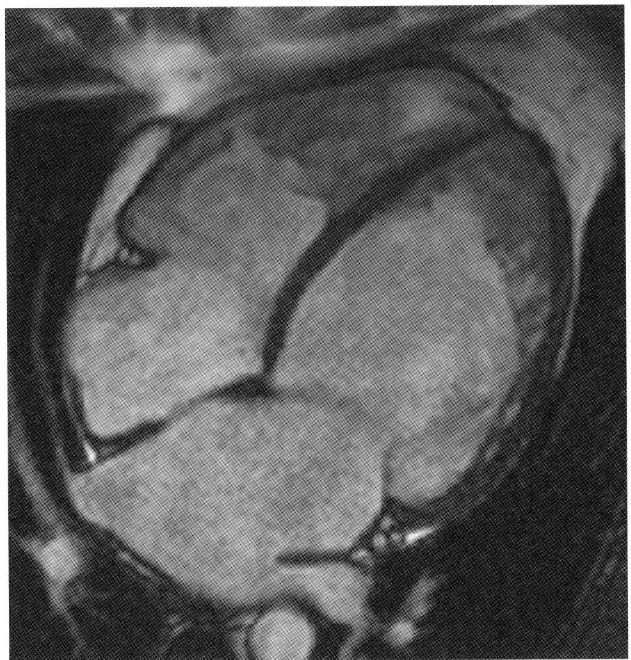

Figure 7–10 Severe abnormalities consistent with LVNC by any current criteria with LV impairment, poorly formed papillary muscles, MR, and biventricular abnormalities (Acknowledgment Dr J Greenwood, Leeds).

References

Anderson LJ, Holden S, Davis B, et al. Cardiovascular T2-star (T2*) magnetic resonance for the early diagnosis of myocardial iron overload. *Eur Heart J.* 2001;22:2171–2179.

Anonymous. "The List"—the list of MRI safe devices, from www.mrisafety.com; 2008.

Assomull RG, Prasad SK, Lyne J, et al. Cardiovascular magnetic resonance, fibrosis, and prognosis in dilated cardiomyopathy. *J Am Coll Cardiol.* 2006;48:1977–1985.

Bellenger NG, Burgess MI, Ray SG, et al. Comparison of left ventricular ejection fraction and volumes in heart failure by echocardiography, radionuclide ventriculography and cardiovascular magnetic resonance; are they interchangeable? *Eur Heart J.* 2000a;21:1387–1396.

Bellenger NG, Davies LC, Francis JM, Coats AJ, Pennell DJ. Reduction in sample size for studies of remodeling in heart failure by the use of cardiovascular magnetic resonance. *J Cardiovasc Magn Reson.* 2000b;2:271–278.

Bluemke DA, Krupinski EA, Ovitt T, et al. MR imaging of arrhythmogenic right ventricular cardiomyopathy: morphologic findings and interobserver reliability. *Cardiology.* 2003;99:153–162.

Chalil S, Foley PW, Muyhaldeen SA, et al. Late gadolinium enhancement-cardiovascular magnetic resonance as a predictor of response to cardiac resynchronization therapy in patients with ischaemic cardiomyopathy. *Europace.* 2007;9:1031–1037.

Choudhury L, Mahrholdt H, Wagner A, et al. Myocardial scarring in asymptomatic or mildly symptomatic patients with hypertrophic cardiomyopathy. *J Am Coll Cardiol.* 2002;40:2156–2164.

De Cobelli F, Pieroni M, Esposito A, et al. Delayed gadolinium-enhanced cardiac magnetic resonance in patients with chronic myocarditis presenting with heart failure or recurrent arrhythmias. *J Am Coll Cardiol.* 2006;47:1649–1654.

Dimitrow PP, Klimeczek P, Vliegenthart R, et al. Late hyperenhancement in gadolinium-enhanced magnetic resonance imaging: comparison of hypertrophic cardiomyopathy patients with and without nonsustained ventricular tachycardia. *Int J Cardiovasc Imaging.* 2008;24:77–83.

Dumont CA, Monserrat L, Soler R, et al. Clinical significance of late gadolinium enhancement on cardiovascular magnetic resonance in patients with hypertrophic cardiomyopathy. *Rev Esp Cardiol.* 2007;60:15–23.

Elliott PM, Poloniecki J, Dickie S, et al. Sudden death in hypertrophic cardiomyopathy: identification of high risk patients. *J Am Coll Cardiol.* 2000;36:2212–2218.

Francis JM, Pennell DJ. Treatment of claustrophobia for cardiovascular magnetic resonance: use and effectiveness of mild sedation. *J Cardiovasc Magn Reson.* 2000;2:139–141.

Germans T, Wilde AA, Dijkmans PA, et al. Structural abnormalities of the inferoseptal LV wall detected by CMR in carriers of HCM mutations. *JACC.* 2006;48:2518–2523.

Hudsmith LE, Petersen SE, Francis JM, Robson MD, Neubauer S. Normal human left and right ventricular and left atrial dimensions using steady state free precession magnetic resonance imaging. *J Cardiovasc Magn Reson.* 2005;7:775–782.

Johansson B, Maceira AM, Babu-Narayan SV, Moon JC, Pennell DJ, Kilner PJ. Clefts can be seen in the basal inferior wall of the LV and the interventricular septum in healthy volunteers as well as patients by CMR. *JACC.* 2007;50:1294–1295.

Kilner PJ, Gatehouse PD, Firmin DN. Flow measurement by magnetic resonance: a unique asset worth optimising. *J Cardiovasc Magn Reson.* 2007;9:723–728.

Kim RJ, Wu E, Rafael A, et al. The use of contrast-enhanced magnetic resonance imaging to identify reversible myocardial dysfunction. *N Engl J Med.* 2000;343:1445–1453.

Kuribayashi T, Roberts WC. Myocardial disarray at junction of ventricular septum and left and right ventricular free walls in hypertrophic cardiomyopathy. *Am J Cardiol.* 1992;70:1333–1340.

Lee J, Moon JC, Clague JR, Sigwart U, Pennell DJ. Late recurrence of outflow tract obstruction seven years after septal ablation in HCM. *Int J Cardiol.* 2005;100:341–342.

Levine GN, Gomes AS, Arai AE, et al. Safety of magnetic resonance imaging in patients with cardiovascular devices. *Circulation.* 2007;116:2878–2891.

Maceira A, Joshi J, Prasad SK, et al. CMR in Cardiac Amyloidosis. *Circulation.* 2005;111:186–193.

Maceira AM, Prasad SK, Khan M, Pennell DJ. Normalized left ventricular systolic and diastolic function by steady state free precession cardiovascular magnetic resonance. *J Cardiovasc Magn Reson.* 2006;8:417–426.

Mahrholdt H, Goedecke C, Wagner A, et al. Cardiovascular magnetic resonance assessment of human myocarditis: a comparison to histology and molecular pathology. *Circulation.* 2004;109:1250–1258.

Maron MS, Appelbaum E, Harrigan C, et al. Significance of delayed enhancement with contrast enhanced CMR in HCM (abstract). *Circulation.* 2007;116:II_694.

McCrohon JA, Moon JC, McKenna WJ, Lorenz CH, Coats ASJ, Pennell DJ. Differentiation of dilated cardiomyopathy from ischemia in heart failure with gadolinium enhanced CMR. *Circulation.* 2003;108:54–59.

McKenna WJ, Thiene G, Nava A, et al. Diagnosis of arrhythmogenic right ventricular dysplasia/cardiomyopathy. *Br Heart J.* 1994;71:215–218.

Mitka M. MRI contrast agents may pose risk for patients with kidney disease. *JAMA.* 2007;297:252–253.

Moon JC. What is late gadolinium enhancement in hypertrophic cardiomyopathy? *Rev Esp Cardiol.* 2007;60:1–4.

Moon JC, Fisher NG, McKenna WJ, Pennell DJ. Detection of apical hypertrophic cardiomyopathy by cardiovascular magnetic resonance in patients with non-diagnostic echocardiography. *Heart.* 2004;90:645–649.

Moon JC, McKenna WJ, McCrohon JA, et al. Toward clinical risk assessment in HCM with gadolinium CMR. *J Am Coll Cardiol.* 2003a;41:1561–1567.

Moon JC, Mogensen J, Elliott PM, et al. Myocardial late gadolinium enhancement cardiovascular magnetic resonance in hypertrophic cardiomyopathy caused by mutations in troponin I. *Heart.* 2005;91:1036–1040.

Moon JC, Reed E, Sheppard M, et al. The histological basis of myocardial hyperenhancement by gadolinium CMR in HCM. *J Am Coll Cardiol.* 2004;43:2260–2264.

Moon JC, Sachdev B, Elkington AG, et al. Gadolinium enhanced CMR in Anderson-Fabry disease: evidence for a disease specific abnormality of the myocardial interstitium. *Eur Heart J.* 2003b;24:2151–2155.

Moon JC, Sheppard M, Reed E, Lee P, Ellitt PM, Pennell DJ. The histological basis of late gadolinium enhancement by cardiovascular magnetic resonance in Anderson-Fabry disease. *JCMR.* 2006;8:479–482.

Oppelt A, Graumann R, Barfuss H. Fisp—a new fast MRI sequence. *Electromedica.* 1986;54:15–18.

Parsai C, Bunce N, Sutherland GR, et al. Does the extent of non viable myocardium, as identified by delayed enhancement cardiac magnetic resonance, preclude response after cardiac resynchronization therapy? (abstract). *Circulation.* 2007;116:II_694.

Pennell DJ, Sechtem UP, Higgins CB, et al. Clinical indications for cardiovascular magnetic resonance (CMR): consensus panel report. *Eur Heart J.* 2004;25:1940–1965.

Perugini E, Rapezzi C, Piva T, et al. Non-invasive evaluation of the myocardial substrate of cardiac amyloidosis by gadolinium cardiac magnetic resonance. *Heart.* 2006;92:343–349.

Peter G, Danias PG, Papaioannou GI, et al. Usefulness of electrocardiographic-gated stress technetium-99m Sestamibi single-photon emission computed tomography to differentiate ischemic from nonischemic cardiomyopathy. *Am J Cardiol.* 2004;94:14–19.

Petersen SE, Selvanayagam JB, Francis JM, et al. Differentiation of athlete's heart from pathological forms of cardiac hypertrophy by means of geometric indices derived from cardiovascular magnetic resonance. *J Cardiovasc Magn Reson.* 2005a;7:551–558.

Petersen SE, Selvanayagam JB, Wiesmann F, et al. Left ventricular noncompaction: insights from cardiovascular magnetic resonance imaging. *J Am Coll Cardiol.* 2005b;46:101–105.

Pujadas S, Carreras F, Arrastio X, et al. Detection and quantification of myocardial fibrosis in hypertrophic cardiomyopathy by contrast-enhanced cardiovascular magnetic resonance. *Rev Esp Cardiol.* 2007;60:10–14.

Raman SV, Sparks EA, Baker PM, McCarthy B, Wooley CF. Mid-myocardial fibrosis by cardiac magnetic resonance in patients with lamin A/C cardiomyopathy: possible substrate for diastolic dysfunction. *J Cardiovasc Magn Reson.* 2007;9:907–913.

Rickers C, Wilke NM, Jerosch-Herold M, et al. Utility of cardiac magnetic resonance imaging in the diagnosis of hypertrophic cardiomyopathy. *Circulation.* 2005;112:855–861.

Rochitte CE, Oliveira PF, Andrade JM, et al. Myocardial delayed enhancement by magnetic resonance imaging in patients with Chagas' disease: a marker of disease severity. *J Am Coll Cardiol.* 2005;46:1553–1558.

Sachdev B, Takenaka T, Teraguchi H, et al. Prevalence of Anderson-Fabry disease in male patients with late onset hypertrophic cardiomyopathy. *Circulation.* 2002;105:1407–1411.

Sen-Chowdhry S, Lowe MD, Sporton SC, McKenna WJ. Arrhythmogenic right ventricular cardiomyopathy: clinical presentation, diagnosis and treatment. *The Am J Med.* 2004;117:685–695.

Sen-Chowdhry S, Prasad SK, Syrris P, et al. Cardiovascular magnetic resonance in arrhythmogenic right ventricular cardiomyopathy revisited: comparison with task force criteria and genotype. *J Am Coll Cardiol.* 2006;48:2132–2140.

Sen-Chowdhry S, Syrris P, Ward D, Asimaki A, Sevdalis E, McKenna WJ. Clinical and genetic characterization of families with arrhythmogenic right ventricular dysplasia/cardiomyopathy provides novel insights into patterns of disease expression. *Circulation.* 2007;115:1710–1720.

Shirani L, Pick R, Roberts WC, Maron BJ. Morphology and significance of the left ventricular collagen network in young patients with hypertrophic cardiomyopathy and sudden cardiac death. *J Am Coll Cardiol.* 2000;35:36–44.

Smedema JP, Snoep G, van Kroonenburgh MP, et al. Evaluation of the accuracy of gadolinium-enhanced cardiovascular magnetic resonance in the diagnosis of cardiac sarcoidosis. *J Am Coll Cardiol.* 2005;45:1683–1690.

St John Sutton MG, Lie JT, Anderson KR, O'Brien PC, Frye RL. Histopathological specificity of hypertrophic obstructive cardiomyopathy. Myocardial fibre disarray and myocardial fibrosis. *Br Heart J.* 1980;44:433–443.

Tandri H, Friedrich MG, Calkins H, Bluemke DA. MRI of arrhythmogenic right ventricular cardiomyopathy/dysplasia. *J Cardiovasc Magn Reson.* 2004;6:557–563.

Valeti US, Nishimura RA, Holmes DR, et al. Comparison of surgical septal myectomy and alcohol septal ablation with cardiac magnetic resonance imaging in patients with hypertrophic obstructive cardiomyopathy. *J Am Coll Cardiol.* 2007;49:350–357.

Varghese A, Pennell DJ. Late gadolinium enhanced cardiovascular magnetic resonance in Becker muscular dystrophy. *Heart.* 2004;90:e59.

Wu E, Judd RM, Vargas JD, Klocke FJ, Bonow RO, Kim RJ. Visualisation of presence, location, and transmural extent of healed Q-wave and non-Q-wave myocardial infarction. *Lancet.* 2001;357:21–28.

Wu YW, Yen RF, Chieng PU, Huang PJ. Tl-201 myocardial SPECT in differentiation of ischemic from nonischemic dilated cardiomyopathy in patients with left ventricular dysfunction. *J Nucl Cardiol.* 2003;10:369–374.

Yamada M, Elliott PM, Kaski JC, et al. Dipyridamole stress thallium-201 perfusion abnormalities in patients with hypertrophic cardiomyopathy. Relationship to clinical presentation and outcome. *Eur Heart J.* 1998;19:500–507.

8

Ultrasound Imaging in Cardiovascular Genetics

Denis Pellerin and Diala Khraiche

Introduction

The major contribution of ultrasound imaging in inherited cardiovascular disease is in the diagnosis and assessment of heart muscle disorders or cardiomyopathies. Cardiac imaging plays a major role in defining the phenotype, determining the correlation between phenotype and genotype, and by identifying patients with higher risk of cardiac death. The distinguishing features of the common forms of cardiomyopathies are easily identified by echocardiography. The role of echo in determining etiology is work in progress, but as with all diagnostic methods requires integration with genetic and clinical information. In patients with left ventricular (LV) hypertrophy, distinction between HCM and phenocopies may be achieved in some cases. For example, amyloidosis is suspected when myocardial texture is heterogeneous and sparkling in combination with pericardial effusion. In patients with DCM, large areas of akinetic and thin myocardial segments corresponding to a coronary artery territory are in favor of an ischemic origin.

The majority of ultrasound data has been obtained using conventional transthoracic echocardiography, which remains the most practical imaging modality in everyday clinical practice. Image quality has been improved by using harmonic imaging and contrast opacification to improve assessment of the endocardial border, wall thickness, and wall thickening in patients with suboptimal image quality on conventional echo. Contrast can also be used for myocardial perfusion assessment. Three-dimensional (3D) echo provides accurate and reproducible calculation of ventricular volumes and ejection fraction and enables views that are unobtainable with two-dimensional (2D) echo. Doppler tissue echocardiography facilitates measurement of myocardial wall motion in real time. Myocardial deformation imaging including Doppler strain and strain rate is measured using data derived from color Doppler myocardial imaging. Non-Doppler strain or speckle tracking is a new method obtained from conventional 2D images used to follow myocardial movement and assess myocardial deformation. Non-Doppler strain can be used to assess long axis function, circumferential and radial deformation and torsion (Helle-Valle et al. 2005; Notomi et al. 2005). Three-dimensional strain is under development. Doppler and non-Doppler deformation parameters imaging have provided new indices of global LV systolic performance that are independent of endocardial definition and less dependent on loading conditions. These modalities are more sensitive than conventional echo in detecting early abnormalities in systolic and diastolic function (Pellerin et al. 2003).

Dilated Cardiomyopathy

Heart failure is rapidly evolving to be a worldwide epidemic. Dilated cardiomyopathy (DCM) is one of the many causes of progressive heart failure and represents the majority of heart transplantation indications (see also Chapter 13). DCM is defined by increased internal diameter of the left or both ventricular chambers, accompanied by systolic contractile dysfunction. Clinical phenotypes include ventricular dysfunction, heart failure, arrhythmia, conduction disease, stroke, sudden death, and skeletal myopathy. DCM can be caused by familial or genetic cardiomyopathies, viral myocarditis, autoimmune myocarditis, peripartum cardiomyopathy, and alcoholic cardiomyopathy or chemotoxicity-induced cardiomyopathy. DCM typically excludes ventricular dilatation caused by myocardial ischemia, valvular dysfunction, pericardial disease, and sustained hypertension. Other exclusion criteria include persistent supraventricular tachyarrhythmia, congenital heart diseases, and cor pulmonale.

Genetic contribution to DCM is likely to be underestimated at the present time. Prevalence ranges from 7% to 25% (Mestroni et al. 1990, 1994). Penetrance is age related and has been evaluated as 10% before 20 years, 34% between 20 and 30 years, 60% between 30 and 40 years, and 90% after 40 years (Michels et al. 1992). Positive family history confers 1.7 times the risk of developing heart failure in offspring (Lee et al. 2006). Familial cases have a younger age of onset but are otherwise clinically indistinguishable from spontaneously occurring nonfamilial cases.

Diagnosis of Familial DCM

The definition of familial DCM is clinically based on the presence of at least two members of the same family proven as affected. Except for the familial history, no clinical, histopathological, or echocardiographic characteristic allows a distinction between familial and nonfamilial cases. Furthermore, some cases considered to be sporadic may be due to de novo mutations and potentially transmissible to descendants.

DCM is characterized by the presence of a dilated LV with impaired ventricular systolic function. In context of familial disease, diagnosis is based on major and minor criteria. Major criteria are (1) LV ejection fraction <45% and/or fractional shortening <25%, as ascertained by echocardiography, radionuclide scan, or angiography; (2) LV end-diastolic diameter >117% of the predicted value corrected for age and body surface area (Henry et al. 1980) corresponds to two standard deviations of the predicted normal limit +5% and can be used in adult and pediatric population, which is useful in family studies. Minor criteria include (1) unexplained supraventricular (atrial fibrillation or sustained arrhythmias) or ventricular arrhythmias, frequent (>1,000/24 h) or repetitive (three or more beats with >120 beats/min) before the age of 50; (2) LV dilatation >112% of the predicted value; (3) LV dysfunction: ejection fraction <50% or fractional shortening <28%; (4) unexplained conduction disease: second- or third-degree atrioventricular conduction defects, complete left bundle branch block, sinus nodal dysfunction; (5) unexplained sudden death or stroke before 50 years of age; and (6) segmental wall motion abnormalities (<1 segment, or 1 if not previously present) in the absence of intraventricular conduction defect or ischemic heart disease.

The diagnosis of familial DCM is made in the presence of two or more affected individuals in a single family or in the presence of a first-degree relative of a DCM patient, with well-documented unexplained sudden death before 35 years of age. Based on the idea that the presence of mild cardiac abnormalities would have a high probability of being the expression of a gene disease in the context of a family, the diagnosis of familial DCM would be fulfilled in a first-degree relative in the presence of the major criteria (LV dilatation and systolic dysfunction) or LV dilatation (>117%) plus one minor criterion or three minor criteria (Mestroni et al. 1999).

Nearly one-third of asymptomatic relatives (29%) have echocardiographic abnormalities, and 27% progress to development of overt DCM. Early identification of preclinical disease is important to permit appropriate intervention that might influence the serious complications and mortality of this disease.

Different forms of familial DCM can be distinguished according to the pattern of transmission and special clinical features. Familial DCM forms related to the pattern of transmission are autosomal dominant (56%) including mutations in the lamin A/C gene and sarcomere gene mutations, autosomal recessive (16%) characterized by worse prognosis, X-linked (10%) due to different mutations of the dystrophin gene including Duchenne muscular dystrophy and Becker muscular dystrophy, and matrilineal transmission. Familial DCM forms related to special clinical features are isolated myocardial forms, dominant conduction defects, neuromuscular involvement, high creatine kinase, and multiorgan involvement (Mestroni et al. 1999).

Echocardiography Examination of Patients with DCM

This includes assessment of global LV volumes and performance, regional LV function, LV diastolic dysfunction, detection, mechanism, and quantification of mitral regurgitation, estimation of right atrial pressure, pulmonary artery pressure and cardiac output, assessment of RV size and function, detection of specific echocardiographic features such as LV noncompaction, and assessment of LV dyssynchrony with selection of potential responders to cardiac resynchronization therapy. These data are mandatory in the report of patients with dilated LV and reduced LV ejection fraction. Echocardiography is useful for the diagnosis, quantification of disease severity, participates in diagnosis of disease etiology, participates in prognostic evaluation, guides therapy, and assesses disease progression during follow-up. Three-dimensional echo, contrast cavity opacification, velocity, and deformation imaging are useful in these matters.

Assessment of LV Volumes and Systolic Performance

Ventricular systolic performance is the ability of the ventricle to pump blood. Ventricular performance varies with heart rate, preload, afterload, and ventricular geometry even in the absence of changes in myocardial contractility. Ventricular contractility is the intrinsic capacity of the myocardium to contract independent of loading conditions. There are no independent clinical measures of contractility. Evaluation of ventricular performance in humans and its changes have been assessed by measurements of pressures, volumes, and pressure–volume loops relating each pressure to the corresponding volume. When echocardiography is used to assess global ventricular performance, most of the indices are load dependent. Using conventional echocardiography, LV systolic performance is often measured by determining end-diastolic and end-systolic diameters from M-mode echo. Normal values of fractional shortening are 36 ± 6 % (>28%). Ventricular volumes (and ejection fraction) can be calculated using the Teicholz formula (volume = $7\ D^3\ /\ 2.4 + D$ where D is end-diastolic diameter).

When there are regional wall motion abnormalities (left bundle branch block, postcardiac surgery, abnormal septal motion, and myocardial infarction) M-mode echo can no longer be used to calculate volumes and derived fractional shortening and ejection fraction. In such cases LV volumes are calculated using bidimensional echo and biplane Simpson's rule. For ventricular volumes intraobserver variability is 4%–6%, interobserver variability is 8.5% for end-diastolic volume, and 16.5% for end-systolic volume. Suboptimal reproducibility is mainly due to lateral wall border visualization. Correct image plane orientation and true long axis of the ventricle are required when using biplane Simpson's rule. Therefore, a variation of 15% for end-diastolic volume, 25% for end-systolic volume, and 10% for LV ejection fraction is required before concluding on a significant change.

Other methods of assessing LV cavity size and systolic function have been described. Visual estimation and regional wall motion score index have showed good correlations with MUGA. Regional wall motion score index is calculated by semiquantification of endocardial motion and wall thickening in each myocardial segment—Normal = 1, Hypokinesia = 2, Akinesia = 3, Dyskinesia = 4. Result is obtained by dividing the sum of all scores by the number of segments analyzed.

Most approaches to measuring ventricular volumes make assumptions about the geometry of the ventricle. Three-dimensional echocardiography has been shown to quantify LV volumes and function more accurately (Siu et al. 1995) and with lower variability than 2D techniques as patients with cardiomyopathy often have alterations in LV shape. Three-dimensional echo has become the gold standard to calculate LV volumes and ejection fraction showing excellent correlations with cardiac MRI. When endocardial border delineation is suboptimal using bi- or tridimensional echo, LV cavity contrast opacification should be used to improve visualization of endocardial border in all segments. Multicenter studies comparing interobserver reliability of several imaging modalities to assess LV ejection fraction reported 0.91 for contrast echo using apical biplane Simpson's rule (95% CI 0.88–0.94), 0.86 for cardiac MRI (95% CI 0.80–0.92), 0.80 for cineventriculography (95% CI 0.74–0.85), and 0.79 for unenhanced echo (95% CI 0.74–0.85) (Hoffmann et al. 2005). When image quality is suboptimal and contrast agents are not available, Dumesnil's formula may be used (Dumesnil et al. 1995). LV ejection fraction is calculated as stroke volume using aortic velocity-time integral divided by end-diastolic volume calculated by Teicholz formula.

LV ejection fraction is underestimated when mitral regurgitation severity is ≥ grade 3. The change in pressure over change in time or dP/dt can be measured by quantifying the slope of the Doppler profile of the mitral regurgitant jet. This is accomplished by measuring the time required for the mitral regurgitant profile to increase from 1 m/s to 3 m/s. Normal value is > 1,000 mmHg/s (Bargiggia et al. 1989).

Assessment of global systolic LV function using conventional echo also includes LV mass and geometry. LV geometry is a surrogate for myocardial fiber orientation. Indices of ventricular geometry include short axis to long axis diameter ratio, mass to volume ratio, relative wall thickness (two posterior wall thickness/cavity dimension), and apical cone. There is interaction between geometry, loading conditions, and function.

Mitral Annular Motion

Mitral annular plane systolic excursion <12 mm determined by M-mode has 90% sensitivity, 88% specificity, and 89% accuracy for the detection of LV ejection fraction <50%. Mitral annular velocity assessment is not dependent on endocardial definition and can be obtained in 77% of patients using conventional echo and in all patients using pulsed wave tissue Doppler measurements (Emilsson et al. 2000). Systolic mitral annular velocity determined by pulsed wave tissue Doppler and averaged over three sites including lateral, septal, and posterior mitral annulus ≤8 cm/s has 94% sensitivity, 93% specificity, and 94% accuracy for the detection of LV ejection fraction <50%. Early diastolic mitral annular velocity (average of three sites) >5.4 cm/s is 88% sensitive and 97% specific for the detection of LV ejection fraction >50% (Gulati et al. 1996). Limitations include prosthetic mitral valve or annulus, mitral annular calcification, primary mitral regurgitation, and ischemia in lateral, septal, and posterior walls. When tissue Doppler velocities are obtained from reconstructed velocity profiles derived from high frame rate color cineloops, 25% should be added to the velocity value to obtain the online spectral Doppler value.

1. Strain, Strain Rate, and Isovolumic Myocardial Acceleration

Doppler-derived myocardial strain and strain rate are measured on high frame rate 2D color Doppler myocardial imaging cineloops and provide noninvasive quantification of myocardial deformation (Heimdal et al. 1998). Myocardial strain is the percentage of shortening or lengthening of a myocardial segment. Strain rate is the rate at which the myocardium shortens or lengthens. These two modalities are relatively independent of cardiac translational motion and tethering from adjacent segments. Systolic strain rate correlates more closely with invasive parameters including peak elastance (Emax = slope of end-systolic pressure–volume relationships during caval occlusion) than systolic tissue velocity (Greenberg et al. 2002). Normal values of peak systolic strain rate in basal posterior wall measured in apical three-chamber range from 2.4 to 3.6/s. However, Doppler strain rate curves are noisy and require very high frame rate and narrow image sector, therefore, separately imaging each wall. Using non-Doppler strain obtained by speckle tracking normal values for longitudinal midseptal strain was 19±4%, normal values for radial basal posterior strain was 37±17%, and normal values for circumferential basal posterior strain was 21±7% (Helle-Valle et al. 2005; Notomi et al. 2005; Hurlburt et al. 2007).

Myocardial acceleration during isovolumic contraction ("isovolumic myocardial acceleration") has been validated as a sensitive noninvasive method of assessing LV and RV performance. Although traditional indices may be less valid for the abnormal RV, the relative insensitivity of isovolumic myocardial acceleration to an abnormal load makes it a potentially powerful clinical tool for the assessment of RV disease (Vogel et al. 2002).

Assessment of Regional LV Function

Regional function is often performed by subjective visual semi-quantitative analysis using assessment of endocardial motion and wall thickening. Better reproducibility of data is obtained with contrast cavity opacification. Quantitative analysis is performed offline using regional myocardial velocity and deformation imaging and regional 3D volumes. Assessment of regional LV function can be performed at rest and during stress. Regional wall motion abnormalities may be observed in patients with DCM. However, a large area of akinetic and thin wall in a coronary artery territory is in favor of an ischemic origin.

Assessment of LV Diastolic Function

A number of factors compromise diastolic filling in DCM including fibrosis and cellular disorganization (increased passive chamber stiffness), asynchrony, abnormal loading, myocardial ischemia, and abnormal cellular flux of calcium (slow relaxation). The result of abnormal diastolic function is increased LV filling pressure. Echo-Doppler can only provide a crude estimation of pressure but this is usually sufficient for patient management. Transmitral inflow is widely used to assess LV diastolic dysfunction. Delayed ventricular relaxation is characterized by decreased transmitral Doppler E/A ratio and prolonged E wave deceleration time (>240 ms). Progressive increase in LV end-diastolic pressure can change this pattern to a pseudonormal pattern. Further increase in left atrial pressure induces a restrictive pattern with E wave deceleration time <150 ms and E/A ratio >2. Delayed ventricular relaxation reflects normal LV filling pressure in most cases. In contrast, LV filling pressure is elevated in the presence of a restrictive pattern in patients with LV ejection fraction <50%. The main problem is to distinguish between normal and pseudonormal patterns. In patients with marked LV cavity dilatation and severely depressed ejection fraction a normal pattern of transmitral inflow is rare. Estimation of LV filling pressure requires the additional recordings of mitral annular tissue Doppler velocity (Sohn et al. 1997), LV flow propagation velocity using color M-mode imaging (Brun et al. 1992; Garcia et al. 1998), and pulmonary venous flow (Rossvoll and Hatle 1993). LV flow propagation velocity (Vp) is inversely correlated to tau (time constant of isovolumic relaxation). Transmitral inflow recording with sample volume at the level of the mitral annulus rather than at the tip of the leaflets, and comparison between tricuspid and mitral inflow velocity curves may also be useful. The ratio of transmitral early diastolic velocity (E) obtained by flow Doppler to mitral annular early diastolic velocity (Ea) obtained by tissue Doppler (E/Ea) has been shown to be correlated to invasive left atrial pressure in patients in sinus rhythm with or without sinus tachycardia (Nagueh et al. 1998b). Correlations between echo and invasive measurements of LV filling pressure are stronger in patients with reduced LV ejection fraction than in patients with normal ejection fraction.

As a general guide, when E/Ea ratio is <8 and LV ejection fraction is >50%, pulmonary capillary wedge pressure is <12 mmHg. When E/Ea ratio is >15, pulmonary capillary wedge pressure is >18 mmHg. When E/Ea ratio is between 8 and 15, other parameters are required (Ommen et al. 2000). The criteria for LV filling pressure >15 mmHg are restrictive filling pattern and LV systolic dysfunction, E/Ea ratio >15, and E/Vp ratio >2.5. Pulmonary venous flow reversal exceeding the duration of the mitral A wave by 30 ms predicts LV end-diastolic pressure >15 mmHg with a sensitivity of 0.85 and a specificity of 0.79. Pulmonary venous systolic fraction <0.4 suggests markedly increased filling pressure (>18 mmHg). Pulmonary venous flow reversal velocity >0.4 m/s may also be useful (Rossvoll and Hatle 1993). Left atrial pressure can also be calculated as the difference between systolic blood pressure and peak LV to left atria pressure gradient from mitral regurgitation. LV end-diastolic pressure can be calculated as the difference between diastolic blood pressure and maximal aortic to LV gradient at end diastole obtained from aortic regurgitation recording. All these indices have been validated in patients with sinus rhythm (Pellerin et al. 1998). In patients with atrial fibrillation, assessment of diastolic function is more difficult. However, several parameters have been described including peak acceleration of isovolumetric relaxation time, E/Ea ratio, and deceleration time of early diastolic of pulmonary venous flow (Nagueh et al. 1996a; Sohn et al. 1999; Matsukida et al. 2001).

Mitral Valve Regurgitation: Mechanisms and Quantification

Mitral regurgitation commonly occurs in patients with congestive heart failure. The diagnosis of functional mitral regurgitation of ventricular origin should be limited to cases of incomplete coaptation without structural anomalies of the leaflets and of other components of the mitral apparatus. The mechanism and quantification of mitral regurgitation can be determined by echo and Doppler.

Different mechanisms have been suggested as the cause of functional regurgitation (Yiu et al. 2000) including: dilatation of the mitral annulus due to dilatation and dysfunction of the LV and the left atrium; dysfunction of the papillary muscles by misalignment due to alteration of the LV shape; reduced closing force of the chordae tendineae due to ventricular dysfunction; and cardiac dyssynchrony. Ratio of length of the anterior mitral leaflet to mitral annulus length >0.9 is normal. A lower ratio shows that the mitral annulus is dilated and the mitral leaflets do not seal. Sphericity of LV cavity is characterized by a decrease in the ratio between the longitudinal and transverse axes and is the cause of increased distance between the papillary muscles. The closure of the leaflets tends to be displaced into the ventricle and is responsible for incomplete valve closure. The presence of functional mitral regurgitation is a marker of adverse LV remodeling and increased sphericity of the chamber.

Mitral regurgitation severity can be estimated by semiquantitative methods including peak E velocity on transmitral inflow >1.5 m/s and reverse systolic wave in two pulmonary venous flows (Enriquez-Sarano et al. 1993; Pu et al. 1999). An extension of the color regurgitant jet into the left atrium and regurgitant jet area has been used for the quantification of mitral regurgitation severity. Using transthoracic echocardiogram, total jet area and ratio of total jet area to left atrium area have been correlated to invasive assessment. Using transesophageal echocardiogram, the aliasing portion of the jet area has been correlated to invasive assessments. Extension of color regurgitant jet into left atrium and regurgitant jet area are unreliable when the regurgitant jet is adherent to the left atrial wall or oblique to the scan plane, are prone to overestimation when the jet is central, and are not reliable markers of severe mitral regurgitation.

However, color flow Doppler provides visualization of the origin of the regurgitant jet and its width (vena contracta). The vena contracta is the narrowest portion of a jet that occurs at or just downstream from the orifice. It is characterized by high velocity, laminar flow, and is slightly smaller than the anatomic regurgitant orifice due to boundary effects. Thus, the cross-sectional area of the vena contracta represents a measure of the effective regurgitant orifice area, which is the narrowest area of actual flow. A vena contracta <0.3 cm usually denotes mild mitral regurgitation whereas the cutoff for severe mitral regurgitation ranges between 0.6 cm to 0.8 cm (Tribouilloy et al. 1992; Heinle et al. 1998). Proximal isovelocity surface area (PISA) or flow convergence is the best quantitative method. The PISA method is derived from the hydrodynamic principle stating that, as blood approaches a regurgitant orifice, its velocity increases forming concentric, roughly hemispheric shells of increasing velocity and decreasing surface area (Bargiggia et al. 1991; Enriquez-Sarano et al. 1995). Color flow mapping offers the ability to image one of these hemispheres that correspond to the Nyquist limit. Effective regurgitant orifice area >0.4 cm^2 is consistent with severe mitral regurgitation, effective regurgitant orifice area between 0.20 and 0.39 cm^2 is consistent with moderate mitral regurgitation, and effective regurgitant orifice area <0.20 cm^2 is consistent with mild mitral regurgitation. Regurgitant volume >50 ml/beat and regurgitant fraction >50% are other criteria of severe mitral regurgitation. These cutoff values are lower in patients after myocardial infarction.

Assessment of LV and left atrium sizes are part of mitral regurgitation severity estimation. Presystolic mitral regurgitation is a marker of atrioventricular dyssynchrony and shortens diastolic filling period with loss of ventricular volume in late diastole. Presystolic mitral regurgitation is related to high LV end-diastolic pressure and long PR interval.

Noninvasive Estimation of Cardiac Output

Cardiac output is calculated in multiplying systolic ejection volume by heart rate. Several measurements should be averaged.

Noninvasive Estimation of Right Atrial Pressure and Pulmonary Artery Pressure

Right atrial pressure is assessed using inferior vena cava diameter and its changes during respiration or sniff. Ratio of the difference between inferior vena cava diameter during expiration and during inspiration to inferior vena cava diameter during expiration is an easy way to estimate right atrial pressure. Right atrial pressure is estimated as 5 mmHg when the ratio is >50%. Right atrial pressure is 10 mmHg when the ratio is 35%–50%. Right atrial pressure is 15 mmHg when the ratio is >35%. Right atrial pressure is 20 mmHg when inferior vena cava is dilated >2.5 cm, hepatic veins are dilated, and inferior vena cava diameter does not change during respiration or sniff. Hepatic vein systolic filling fraction has also been suggested to estimate right atrial pressure (Nagueh et al. 1996b). Relation of invasive mean right atrial pressure to tricuspid E/Ea ratio may also be useful (Nageh et al. 1999).

E/Ea >6 detects right atrial pressure P >10 mmHg with 79% sensibility and 73% specificity.

Systolic pulmonary artery pressure can be calculated as the sum of peak right atrium to RV pressure gradient from tricuspid regurgitation recording and right atrial pressure. Contrast-enhanced tricuspid regurgitation flow may be helpful. This calculation cannot be used when there is severe tricuspid regurgitation with laminar flow.

RV outflow tract flow acceleration time has been shown to be linearly correlated with mean pulmonary artery pressure. Normal value is >120 ms. RV outflow tract flow acceleration time is dependent on cardiac output and valid between 60/min and 100/min. Diastolic pulmonary artery pressure can be calculated as the sum of peak end-diastolic pressure gradient from pulmonary regurgitation recording and right atrial pressure. Mean pulmonary artery pressure can be calculated as peak early diastolic pressure gradient from pulmonary regurgitation, or calculated as two diastolic pulmonary artery pressure + systolic pulmonary artery pressure divided by three.

Assessment of RV Size and Function

Evaluation of right ventricular (RV) performance in humans is limited by complex RV shape, loading conditions, retrosternal position of the RV that is in the near field of the image sector, and complex delineation of trabeculated apical endocardial border. Three-dimensional echo, RV cavity opacification, velocity, and deformation imaging are useful in the evaluation of RV performance. RV cavity size is assessed by RV diameters at basal and mid-lateral segment in apical four-chamber view, RV outflow tract flow diameter in short axis view, and RV to LV diameter ratio. RV cavity size and systolic performance can be assessed by apical fractional area change (normal >35%), volumes using apical monoplane and biplane Simpson's rule combining apical four-chamber and RV inflow views. RV wall thickness and regional wall motion are more easily evaluated with contrast cavity opacification.

Tricuspid annular plane systolic excursion (TAPSE) determined by M-mode, systolic annular velocity of lateral tricuspid annulus determined by pulse wave tissue Doppler imaging (Meluzin et al. 2001) and isovolumic myocardial acceleration are useful in the evaluation of RV performance. RV isovolumic myocardial acceleration is less affected by preload and afterload changes and is correlated with dP/dt max (Vogel et al. 2002).

Right atrial size is best estimated by right atrial area in apical four-chamber view.

Ventricular Noncompaction (also see Chapter 15)

Isolated ventricular noncompaction remains an unclassified form of cardiomyopathy, which is now being recognized with increasing frequency. This cardiomyopathy results from an interruption of the normal process of embryologic myocardial compaction, and is associated with a high risk of systemic embolization, and ventricular arrhythmias and poor prognosis in DCM patients. Accurate recognition requires knowledge of the echocardiographic features showing multiple prominent trabeculations at LV apex with deep intertrabecular recesses communicating with the ventricular cavity. A two-layer structure is seen with a compacted thin epicardial layer and a much thicker noncompacted endocardium of trabecular meshwork with deep endomyocardial spaces (Figure 8–1). There was continuity between LV cavity and intratrabecular recesses using color flow Doppler without evidence of communication to the epicardial coronary artery system. Usual criterion to define noncompaction cardiomyopathy is end-systolic thickness ratio of noncompacted to compacted layer ≥2. The extent of noncompaction is mainly apical segments of posterior and lateral walls. There are no coexisting congenital lesions (Jenni et al. 2001; Sengupta et al. 2004).

Assessment of LV Dyssynchrony and Selection of Potential Responders to Cardiac Resynchronization Therapy

Randomized clinical trials have produced unequivocal support for the use of cardiac resynchronization therapy in patients with refractory heart failure and evidence of LV dyssynchrony. These trials infer LV dyssynchrony from a 12 lead ECG and current guidelines do not include echo criteria. The CARE-HF trial (Cleland et al. 2005) and the COMPANION trial (Bristow et al. 2004) have shown fewer deaths and hospitalizations for heart failure and better improvement of ejection fraction and quality of life scores in the cardiac resynchronization therapy group than in the medical therapy alone group. However, 30% of patients treated by cardiac resynchronization therapy devices do not exhibit LV functional recovery and reverse remodeling. Mechanisms of cardiac resynchronization therapy benefits are incompletely understood and LV lead positioning is limited by venous anatomy. Independent predictors of lack of response to cardiac resynchronization therapy include ischemic heart disease, severe mitral regurgitation, and LV end-diastolic diameter >75 mm. Patients with these three predictors had a probability response of 27% (Diaz-Infante et al. 2005). It is postulated that mechanical dyssynchrony may be better than electrical dyssynchrony for the selection of potential responders and several echo parameters have been suggested. Intraventricular dyssynchrony combining longitudinal and radial parameters (Gorcsan et al. 2007) and atrioventricular dyssynchrony parameters are the main focus. Sensitivity, specificity, and accuracy of these parameters have been high in single center studies, but have poor interinstitutional reproducibility. As a general rule, several parameters must be used and the greater the magnitude of dyssynchrony, the greater the likelihood of positive response to cardiac resynchronization therapy. Echo data are useful in patients with comorbidities or narrow QRS complexes.

Prognostic Markers in DCM

Prognosis of heart failure patients in the general population is usually poor, with 1-year mortality in the range of 25%–30%. However, patients with DCM may have a slightly better outcome but still face 50% mortality over 5 years. DCM accounts for approximately one in three to four of all heart failure cases.

Many echocardiographic predictors of outcome have been reported. LV ejection fraction is a well-established marker of risk in heart failure even in the elderly. However, other parameters such as maximal oxygen uptake during exercise and LV diastolic indices must be used to further stratify patients with low LV ejection fraction. LV contractile reserve has been shown to be an important prognostic indicator of survival in DCM (Dubois-Rande et al. 1992) and predicts systolic recovery and clinical outcome of patients with heart failure (Kitaoka et al. 1999; Naqvi et al. 1999; Pellerin et al. 1999; Pellerin and Brecker 2002b). LV volumes are also markers of risk in heart failure patients.

LV diastolic function plays a role in prognosis evaluation. In symptomatic congestive heart failure patients, the restrictive filling pattern of transmitral Doppler has been shown to be the

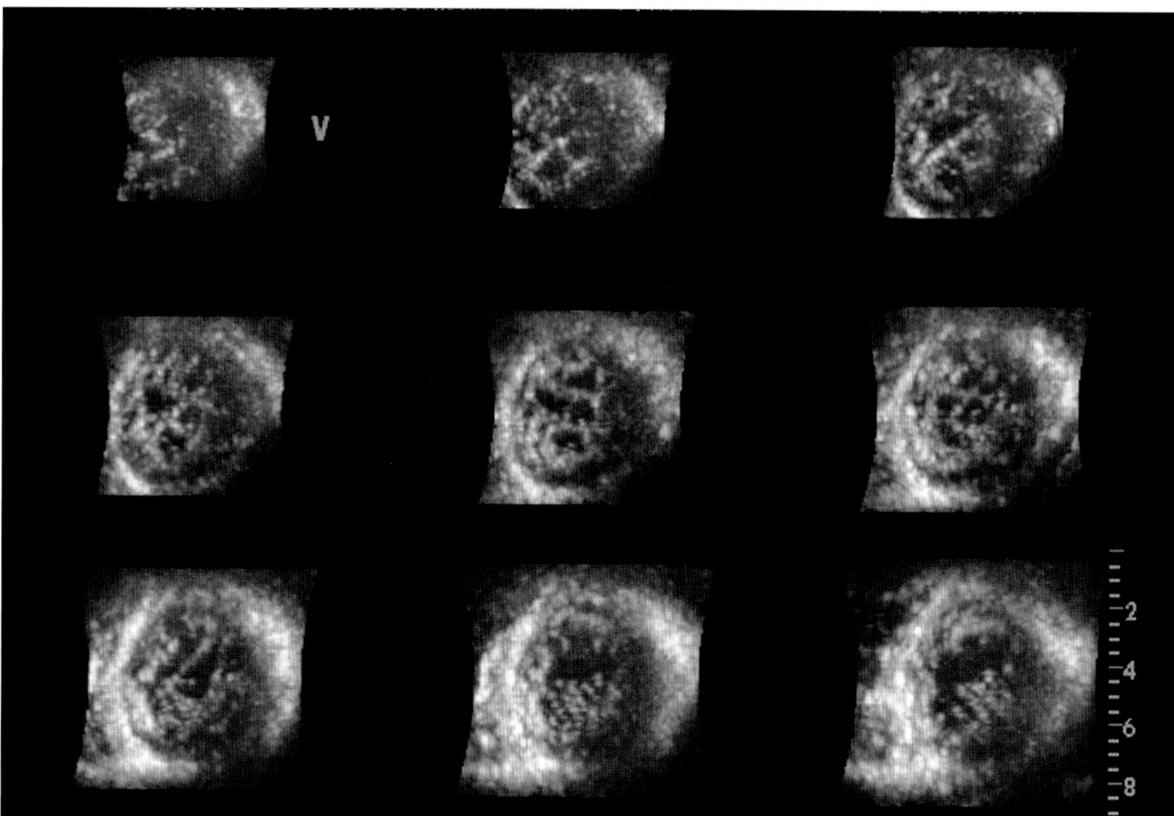

Figure 8–1 Three-dimensional echocardiography showing nine short axis images obtained over a 2 cm distance starting from the LV apex. There are heavy trabeculations in all apical segments extending to posterolateral midsegments.

single best predictor of cardiac death in patients with ischemic and nonischemic DCM and results in a tripling of the mortality rate compared with patients who do not have the restrictive filling pattern. Deceleration time of early diastolic velocity of transmitral flow has been shown to be predictor of functional capacity and correlates with maximum oxygen consumption. Patients with abnormal relaxation patterns appear to have the lowest all cause death and rehospitalization for congestive heart failure compared to those with pseudonormal filling or restrictive filling. Pseudonormal transmitral Doppler filling pattern has been shown to identify patients with intermediate prognosis. Prognostic value of diastolic dysfunction has been assessed by E/Ea ratio, E/Vp ratio, and S/D ratio (Troughton et al. 2005). Prognostic information can also be obtained by changes in transmitral inflow pattern induced by loading manipulations (Pozzoli et al. 1997). There was significant worsening of outcome between patients with stable nonrestrictive pattern, patients with reversible restrictive pattern, and patients with irreversible restrictive pattern.

RV function is also predictive of survival in patients with DCM. Not only do individuals with biventricular dysfunction have a lower New York Heart Association (NYHA) functional class, they also have more severe LV dysfunction and poorer long-term prognosis (La Vecchia et al. 1999). Outcome can be estimated by combining degrees of RV systolic dysfunction and elevated systolic pulmonary artery pressure (Ghio et al. 2001). Other echo markers include severity of mitral regurgitation (Koelling et al. 2002), severe tricuspid regurgitation (Hung et al. 1998; Koelling et al. 2002), left atrial size, reduced coronary flow reserve during vasodilator stress (Rigo et al. 2006), and LV dyssynchrony.

Echocardiography in Specific Causes of DCM

1. Duchenne Muscular Dystrophy

Duchenne muscular dystrophy is the most common X-linked recessive DCM due to mutations of the dystrophin gene transmitted maternally to one half of her male progeny as overt disease and to one half of her female progeny as carrier state. Incidence in the general population is approximately 1/3,500 male births. Echocardiographic findings are DCM (70% of patients develop progressive DCM) and mitral valve prolapse (25% of the patients) (Sanyal et al. 1980). Myocardial fibrosis begins from the epicardial half of the LV posterior wall. Despite normal standard echocardiographic findings in early stage of the disease before onset of the overt cardiomyopathy, myocardial strain imaging can detect early changes such as decreased peak systolic strain of the posterior wall or negative strain value in systole. Mitral regurgitation, which is commonly present in Duchenne muscular dystrophy, is related to dystrophic involvement of posterior papillary muscle and contiguous posterobasal LV wall (Sanyal et al. 1980).

2. Becker Muscular Dystrophy

Becker muscular dystrophy is a X-linked recessive DCM due to mutations of the dystrophin gene that is a milder allelic variant of Duchenne muscular dystrophy. It is generally later in age of onset and slower in progress than Duchenne dystrophy. Most patients remain ambulant into adulthood. Although dystrophin is present in skeletal muscle it has abnormal molecular weight. Cardiac involvement may occur at early age and is unrelated to extent of musculoskeletal disorder. Biventricular dilatation and dysfunction are common. LV hyper trabeculation has more frequently been described in Becker's muscular dystrophy than in other dystrophinopathies (Finsterer and Stollberger 2001a; Finsterer et al. 2001b).

3. Myotonic Muscular Dystrophy (Steinert Disease)

Myotonic muscular dystrophy is a multisystem disorder inherited as an autosomal dominant form associated with myopathy. Estimated incidence is 1/8,000 individuals. Early manifestations include weakness of muscles in face, neck with atrophy of sternocleidomastoid muscles and distal extremities. Myotonic dystrophy is a systemic disease featuring cataracts, testicular atrophy, premature forehead baldness, mental deterioration, and involvement of smooth muscle in esophagus, colon, and uterus. ECG abnormalities include prolongation of PR interval, left anterior fascicular block, and increased QRS duration. Progression to symptomatic atrioventricular block may necessitate pacemaker implantation. Q waves not associated with known myocardial infarction are common, indicating presence of regional myocardial dystrophy.

Although symptoms of cardiac failure or LV systolic dysfunction are relatively rare, LV systolic impairment and hypertrophy are reported on echocardiography. Diastolic dysfunction is consistent with a pattern of impaired LV relaxation (Fragola et al. 1997). Studies using Doppler tissue imaging report subclinical cardiac impairment (lower myocardial diastolic and systolic velocities) in patients compared with normal control subjects (Vinereanu et al. 2004; Parisi et al. 2007). Mitral valve prolapse is reported in up to 30% of patients and is due to geometrical changes of the heart caused by thorax deformities, rather than to structural changes (Streib et al. 1985).

Hypertrophic Cardiomyopathy

HCM is the commonest genetically determined cardiac disorder (Seidman and Seidman 2001) characterized by a wide spectrum of clinical, ECG, echocardiographic, and hemodynamic findings (see also Chapter 13). Genetic, phenotype, and outcome are markedly heterogeneous. Age of expression, penetrance, and risk are unpredictable. Approximately 60%–70% of HCM is caused by mutations in sarcomeric contractile protein genes (Seidman and Seidman 2001; Richard et al. 2003) with autosomal dominant inheritance. No clinical phenotype is mutation specific and similar phenotypes may be caused by different genes. In addition, there is phenotypic heterogeneity within families (Mogensen et al. 2004). HCM is seen in all age and racial groups. Prevalence is approximately 0.2% in the general adult population. Histopathological features include myocyte hypertrophy, myocardial fiber disarray, and interstitial fibrosis.

Role of Echocardiography in Diagnosis

Echocardiography remains the most useful diagnostic method. Diagnosis relies on the echocardiographic demonstration of unexplained LV hypertrophy (Richardson et al. 1996; Maron et al. 2003a). Myocardial wall thickness of more than two standard deviations from the mean, corrected for age, height, and gender is generally accepted as diagnostic. Typically cutoffs in Caucasian adult males and females are 1.5 cm and 1.3 cm respectively, while corrections are applied in children and in very large or small adults. Data from patient history, physical examination, 12-lead ECG, and family history are useful in borderline cases.

Myocardial wall thickness is usually greatest in the anterior septum, but any pattern of diffuse or localized LV hypertrophy distribution, severity, and extent may be seen with or without outflow tract obstruction (Maron et al. 1981; Shapiro and McKenna 1983; Wigle et al. 1985). Sarcomeric contractile protein disease typically exhibits asymmetric septal or other patterns of localized hypertrophy, while true concentric hypertrophy of both ventricles is suggestive of storage or mitochondrial disease.

The pattern of LV hypertrophy impacts on patients' management according to maximal wall thickness, which is a risk factor for sudden cardiac death, and LV obstruction. Conventional echocardiographic measures of ejection fraction and fractional shortening are made from the radial axis at the base of the heart and may be misleading since indices of systolic performance made from the long axis often reveal impairment with reduction of the rotational component. In HCM patients with asymmetric septal hypertrophy, midseptal longitudinal systolic strain has been shown to be markedly decreased, even reversed with paradoxical longitudinal systolic expansion. Midseptal longitudinal systolic strain has been correlated to the degree of septal hypertrophy (Yang et al. 2003). Severe impairment of systolic function is seen in approximately 5% of patients (see paragraph on end-stage HCM).

Pitfalls in the diagnosis of HCM include overmeasurement of wall thickness by inclusion of the moderator band or LV tendons running parallel to the septum and oblique cuts of the LV. HCM can be overlooked when there is poor endocardial definition of the LV apex, unusual pattern of LV hypertrophy, for example, anterolateral wall hypertrophy only and hypertrophy of papillary muscle. LV cavity opacification with contrast provides accurate measurements of LV wall thickness in all segments in patients with suboptimal images. LV cavity contrast opacification enables differential diagnosis between apical HCM and LV noncompaction.

Role of Echocardiography in the Assessment of Symptoms

Shortness of breath, palpitations, syncope, dizziness, and chest pain may be present in HCM patients. The origin of these symptoms is often multifactorial. Echocardiography detects and assesses the severity of LV obstruction, mitral regurgitation, diastolic dysfunction, atrial dilatation, and myocardial ischemia, which participate in the origin of symptoms.

LV Outflow Tract Obstruction

Combination of careful clinical and echo assessments is required as coexistence of symptoms with LV outflow tract obstruction does not imply necessarily causality and significant LV outflow tract gradient is not always associated with symptoms.

HCM patients have LV outflow tract obstruction at rest caused by systolic anterior motion of the mitral valve leaflet (Maron et al. 1983b; Klues et al. 1993). Several factors contribute including narrowing of the LV outflow tract by septal hypertrophy, elongated mitral leaflets coapting in the leaflet body rather than at the tips, anterior displacement of the mitral apparatus, papillary muscles displaced anteriorly and toward one another, and mitral leaflet systolic anterior motion with leaflet-septal contact in early to mid-systole (Spirito and Maron 1983; Klues et al. 1993; Levine et al. 1995). Systolic anterior motion of mitral leaflet may be complete, incomplete, or chordae related. It may be classified as mild when the distance between systolic anterior motion of mitral leaflet and septum is >10 mm, moderate when the distance is ≤10 mm, or when septal contact is brief and as severe when septal contact last ≥30% of systole. Many patients have an echo bright patch of

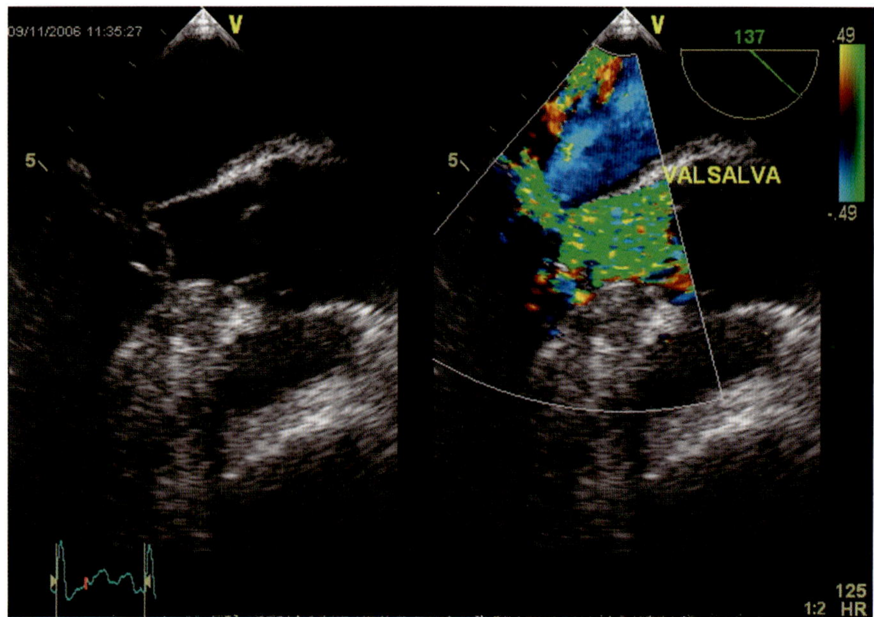

Figure 8–2 TOE study of HCM patient during Valsalva maneuver. The left image shows severe septal hypertrophy, complete systolic anterior motion of the anterior mitral leaflet that is elongated. The right image shows color flow mapping and shows aliasing in LVOT between aortic annulus and mitral leaflet-septal contact related to severe LVOT obstruction (gradient 95mmHg). There is also mitral regurgitation with posteriorly directed jet.

endocardial thickening on the septum in the subaortic region, which reflects repeated contact of the septum with the anterior mitral valve leaflet. Mitral leaflet-septal contact occurs simultaneously with the onset of the pressure gradient (Pollick et al. 1982; Panza et al. 1992).

The severity of obstruction is assessed by continuous wave Doppler signal from the outflow tract, which must be distinguished from that of the mitral regurgitation (Rakowski et al. 1988). Serial studies have shown significant variability in the severity of obstruction. Evaluation of the level of obstruction including detection of midcavity obstruction, subaortic membrane, and accessory mitral valve tissue are crucial for patient management and is performed by pulsed wave Doppler and color flow mapping in transthoracic echocardiogram and transesophageal echocardiogram. LV outflow tract obstruction without systolic anterior motion of mitral leaflet must prompt detection of subaortic membrane and accessory mitral valve tissue (Sharma et al. 2006).

Severe provocable obstruction during exercise may be suspected when a patient with or without resting obstruction describes exercise-related symptoms including shortness of breath, dizziness, and syncope. Valsalva maneuver (Figure 8–2), post-extrasystole recording of the gradient, and use of sublingual nitrates may help in the detection of provoked obstruction. However, exercise echo should be used as gold standard to detect maximal dynamic obstruction (Maron et al. 2006). During the test, symptoms, systolic anterior motion of the mitral valve, LV outflow tract gradient, mitral regurgitation severity and jet direction, and blood pressure response (Maron et al. 2006) are monitored.

HCM is now recognized predominantly as a disease of LV outflow tract obstruction as 70% of HCM patients are predisposed to LV outflow tract obstruction because of systolic anterior motion of mitral leaflet-septal contact, either at rest or with physiological exercise testing. This observation holds major clinical implications for the management of HCM patients, given that subaortic obstruction participates in clinical outcome (Maron et al. 2003b). Patients with severe symptoms refractory to medical therapy may be candidates for major interventions such as surgical septal myectomy or alcohol septal ablation. Response to medical treatment for HCM including a decrease in outflow tract gradient or improvement in diastolic function can be evaluated by serial echocardiographic studies. The decision to proceed with nonmedical therapeutic options is also guided by echocardiography. Patients with mild hypertrophy associated with an angulated septum may have severe exercise-related symptoms. When symptoms are refractory to medical treatment, these patients cannot undergo septal reduction therapy and may benefit from dual-chamber pacing.

Mitral Regurgitation

Mitral regurgitation is related to systolic anterior motion of the mitral valve with leaflet-septal contact and failure of leaflet coaptation in mid-systole, elongated mitral leaflets coapting in the leaflet body rather than at the tip, anterior displacement of the mitral apparatus, and anteriorly displaced papillary muscles. Mitral regurgitation related to LV outflow tract obstruction is posteriorly directed, occurs in mid- to late systole and mitral valve morphology only shows mildly elongated leaflets. The degree of mitral regurgitation correlates with LV outflow tract gradient (Yu et al. 2000). Eliminating LV outflow tract gradient by septal reduction therapy markedly reduces mitral regurgitation (Yu et al. 2000).

Intrinsic and independent mitral valve disease is suspected when mitral regurgitant jet is not posteriorly directed, the jet is pansystolic, and mitral valve morphology shows mitral valve prolapse (Pellerin et al. 2002a), excessive leaflet tissue (Barlow disease), ruptured chordae, annular calcification, or direct papillary muscle insertion into the anterior mitral leaflet (Figure 8–3). These mitral valve abnormalities may occur in up to 10% of patients with obstructive HCM and are important determinants in the selection of septal reduction therapy (Petrone et al. 1992) as these patients require myectomy and mitral valve repair.

Diastolic Dysfunction

Diastolic dysfunction with impaired relaxation and filling is common and secondary to hypertrophy, myocyte disarray, fibrosis, and myocardial ischemia. Delayed relaxation and pseudonormal patterns on transmitral inflow may alternate in the same patient.

A

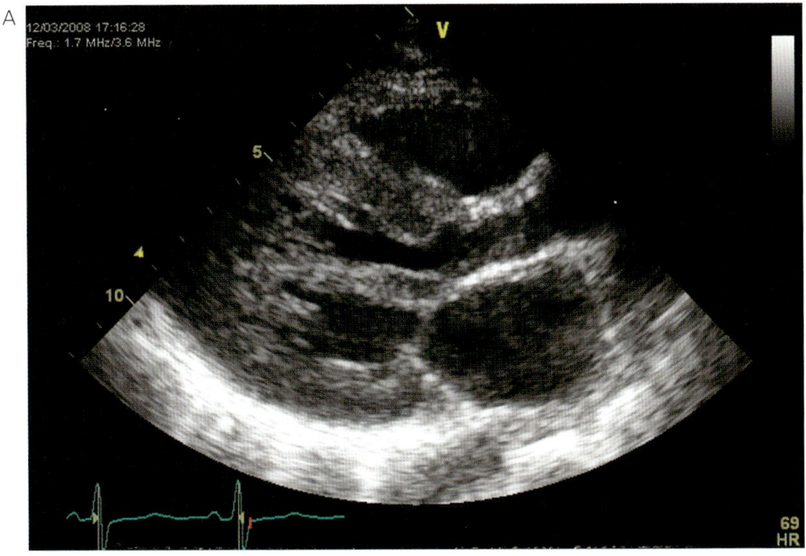

B

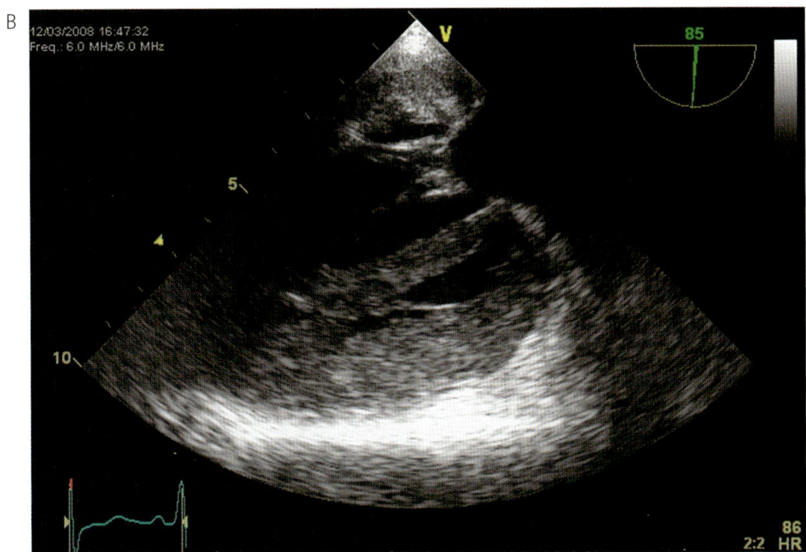

Figure 8–3 a & b (a) PLAX view recorded on TTE in a patient with HCM showing direct insertion of anterior papillary muscle into anterior mitral leaflet. (b) TOE view obtained in the same patient.

In most patients there is elevation of left end-diastolic pressure in association with a flat pressure volume relationship (Nishimura et al. 1996). Diastolic dysfunction is associated with reduced LV stroke volume, increased LV filling pressure, compressive effects on the coronary microcirculation, and progressive atrial enlargement (Spirito and Maron 1990). These factors are involved in the clinical presentation of many patients, including symptoms of fatigue, dyspnea, and angina pectoris.

Conventional Doppler parameters are unreliable for estimating LV filling pressures in HCM (Nishimura et al. 1996; Nagueh et al. 1999b). As transmitral inflow velocities vary with loading conditions, age, and heart rate, Doppler estimation of LV filling pressure in HCM patients requires additional recordings including mitral annular tissue Doppler velocity, LV flow propagation velocity (Vp), and pulmonary venous flow. LV filling pressures can be estimated with reasonable accuracy in HCM patients by measuring E/Ea ratio and E/Vp ratio. These ratios also track changes in filling pressures over time (Nagueh et al. 1999a). Normal, delayed relaxation, and pseudonormal transmitral inflow patterns may be observed in patients with HCM and may alternate in the same patient over time. An important minority up to 5% of patients have restrictive physiology, atrial dilatation, and evidence of right-sided congestion. These patients often mimic those with restrictive cardiomyopathy in that these changes may occur in the absence of significant myocardial hypertrophy.

Atrial Enlargement

The left atrium size is measured at the end of ventricular systole when the left atrium chamber is at its greatest dimension. Left atrium size can be estimated by diameters measured in parasternal long axis view and apical four-chamber view. Left atrium volume can be calculated using a number of formulae. The biplane area-length formula is $8\,(A1)\,(A2)/3\pi\,L$, where A1 and A2 represent left atrium areas acquired from the apical four- and two-chamber views respectively, and L is the shortest left atrium long-axis length measured in both the four- and two-chamber views. Left atrium volume may also be measured using biplane Simpson's rule with biplane left atrium planimetry. Left atrium enlargement is associated with greater LV hypertrophy, more diastolic dysfunction, and higher filling pressures (Yang et al. 2005a). Right atrial size is estimated by right atrium area in apical four-chamber view.

Reduced Coronary Flow Reserve

Echocardiographic assessment of coronary flow reserve using adenosine showed reduced coronary flow reserve in HCM patients. Reduced coronary flow reserve as well as metabolic evidence for myocardial ischemia have been shown during pharmacological provocation, pacing, and exercise (Cannon et al. 1985; Cecchi et al. 2003).

Morphological Variants

Apical Hypertrophic Cardiomyopathy

Apical HCM is a variant of HCM in which hypertrophy is confined to LV apex. This disease entity is also characterized by electrocardiographic pattern of giant negative T wave ≥10 mm most prominent in leads V3 to V6 (Sakamoto 2001). Apical HCM is relatively common in Japan (prevalence of 13%–25% of the total HCM population) as well as in some other Asian countries (Yang et al. 2005b) but seems rare in Western countries (prevalence of 1%–7%). Clinical features of apical HCM were similar between Japan and Western countries except for the prevalence of giant negative T waves (Japan, 64%; United States, 30%). Giant negative T wave is not a specific feature of apical HCM and can also be found in patients with asymmetric septal hypertrophy (Alfonso et al. 1990).

Apical hypertrophy may not be detected on conventional imaging due to poor endocardial definition of the LV apex or may simulate marked hypokinesia or akinesia of the apical region. Low velocity scale color Doppler flow imaging may be helpful although its interpretation is often challenging. LV cavity contrast opacification (Zhu et al. 2002) should be used when apical hypertrophy is suspected (Figure 8–4). When hypertrophy is confined to the apical region of the LV below papillary muscle level, patients show mild clinical symptoms and usually have good prognosis. When there is severe apical hypertrophy extending to midcavity and papillary muscles, apical aneurysms may occur and these too are easily detected by LV cavity contrast opacification. Apical aneurysm or infarction may be associated with ventricular arrhythmia and apical thrombus.

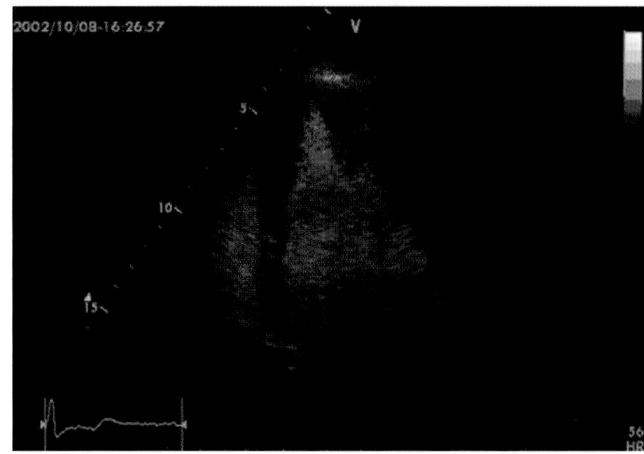

Figure 8–4 Apical 4-chamber view with contrast cavity opacification showing apical HCM. LV apex is in the near field of the image and apical endocardial border is often difficult to visualize using conventional echocardiography. In this patient there was complete apical obliteration in systole.

Hypertrophic Cardiomyopathy with Midventricular Obstruction

Midventricular obstruction is a rare manifestation of HCM. Patients with HCM and midventricular obstruction present with symptoms similar to those with LV outflow tract obstruction such as exertional dyspnea, angina, and palpitation.

Two-dimensional echocardiography and Doppler echocardiography are useful in the diagnosis of midventricular obstruction. Differentiation of midventricular obstruction from outflow tract obstruction requires careful and precise assessment of the site of obstruction and LV hypertrophy. Systolic anterior motion of the mitral valve is not found in patients with midventricular obstruction unless subaortic obstruction coexists. Hypertrophy is prominent at midventricular level, and sometimes accompanied by papillary muscle hypertrophy. Anomalous insertion of the papillary muscles can also produce midventricular obstruction. LV contrast cavity opacification with multiple views is helpful as detection of midventricular hypertrophy is usually difficult using conventional echocardiography. LV systolic function is usually hyperdynamic and LV cavity is obliterated at end systole. Turbulent flow detected by color flow mapping is helpful in the identification of the site of obstruction. Pulsed and continuous wave Doppler recordings are used for the estimation of intraventricular pressure gradients. Special attention should be paid to visualization of LV apex. Apical aneurysm or apical infarction can be observed in the absence of fixed coronary artery disease in patients with midventricular obstruction and is related to high incidence of nonsustained ventricular tachycardia, apical thrombus, and adverse cardiovascular events (Ando et al. 1990; Tse and Ho 2003). Syncope or near-syncope may be related to ventricular tachyarrhythmias originating from LV apical aneurismal segments. Paradoxical early diastolic jet flow is an intraventricular flow from apex to base during isovolumic relaxation and early diastole. Entrapped blood in the apical cavity during ejection flows into the hyperkinetic main chamber in diastole. It suggests high-pressure apical chamber with asynergy (Nakamura et al. 1992). Midventricular obstruction may be responsible for recurrent obstruction after myectomy in obstructive HCM.

Right Ventricular Hypertrophy in HCM

In 30% of HCM patients there is RV hypertrophy. RV wall thickness is measured in subcostal view at the peak of the R wave in basal or midsegments, which provides less measurement variability and closely correlates with RV peak systolic pressure (Matsukubo et al. 1977). Care must be taken to avoid overmeasurement because of the presence of epicardial fat deposition and coarse trabeculations within the RV. RV cavity opacification is useful to confirm suspicion of RV hypertrophy.

Using fundamental imaging, RV hypertrophy is mild when RV wall thickness ≤8 mm, moderate 9–12 mm, and severe >12 mm (McKenna et al. 1988). Using harmonic imaging, these values should be reduced by 1–2 mm. RV hypertrophy may be associated with clinical and echo features of severe disease (short of breath, severe LV hypertrophy, and sustained ventricular tachycardia). However, RV hypertrophy is neither associated with secondary pulmonary hypertension nor with a particular pattern of LV hypertrophy. RV outflow tract obstruction is rare. Presence of severe RV hypertrophy should induce the detection of other causes than sarcomeric HCM including Anderson Fabry disease, amyloidosis, storage disease when RV hypertrophy is severe, and Noonan syndrome.

The spatial orientation of the RV is modified when there is severe LV hypertrophy. This may induce overdetection of RV hypertrophy and myocardial perforation during ventricular lead insertion during PM/ICD implantation. Although the tip of the RV lead may appear close to the spine in anteroposterior fluoroscopy, it may in fact be near the RV apex and pushing the lead may result in ventricular perforation.

Role of Echocardiography in Family Screening

Diagnostic criteria in first-degree relatives of patients with HCM are different from those in probands. Diagnosis depends on a combination of nonspecific or mild abnormalities in several different investigations taken in the context of a positive family history. ECG abnormalities mainly deep Q waves >3 mm (Konno et al. 2004) are sensitive indicator in family members.

Detection of gene carriers without LV hypertrophy has been attempted using mitral annular velocity. Lateral systolic mitral annular velocity <13 cm/s showed 100% sensitivity and 93% specificity, and lateral early diastolic mitral annular velocity <14 cm/s showed 100% sensitivity and 90% specificity in the detection of gene carriers without LV hypertrophy in an initial study (Nagueh et al. 2001). Low early diastolic mitral annular velocity showed a good positive predictive value but a low negative predictive value (Nagueh et al. 2001). In this study ECG abnormalities were not reported. Another study showed that averaged early diastolic mitral annular velocities recorded from various mitral annular sites <13.5 cm/s showed 75% sensitivity and 86% specificity in the detection of gene carriers without LV hypertrophy. Combination of early diastolic mitral annular velocity <15 cm/s and LV ejection fraction ≥68% showed 44% sensitivity and 100% specificity (Ho et al. 2002). Differences in sensitivity and specificity of mitral annular velocity between different reports may relate to the genotype.

Current guidelines recommend that parents, siblings. and offspring of affected individuals undergo history, physical examination, 12 lead ECG, and 2D echo during childhood, annually from age 11 to 18 years, and every 2 to 3 years until the age of 25 years. Thereafter five yearly evaluations are recommended based on the relatively infrequent occurrence of late onset disease (Maron et al. 2004). Other morphological variants in HCM include end-stage HCM (see paragraph on end-stage HCM).

Identification of Patients at Risk of Sudden Death

Sudden death is the leading cause of premature death in patients with HCM (Harris et al. 2006). Individuals who have experienced cardiac arrest and symptomatic sustained ventricular arrhythmia should undergo implantation of a cardioverter defibrillator (Maron et al. 2003a). Patients with prior sustained ventricular arrhythmia have fatal event rates of up to 10% per year. The majority of sudden deaths, however, occur in patients who have not previously experienced arrhythmic symptoms. A number of clinical features are associated with an increased risk of sudden death, including a family history of premature sudden death from HCM, unexplained syncope, the presence of nonsustained ventricular tachycardia during ambulatory ECG monitoring, the finding of an abnormal blood pressure response during upright exercise, and severe LV hypertrophy greater or equal to 3.0 cm (Elliott et al. 2000, 2001; Spirito et al. 2000). LV outflow tract obstruction is also associated with an increase in the risk of sudden death (Maron et al. 2003b). Echocardiography identifies severe LV hypertrophy and obstruction (Spirito et al. 2000; Elliott et al. 2001).

Role of Echocardiography in the Detection of Phenocopies

A wide range of genetic and acquired disorders can cause similar cardiac phenotype to that seen in sarcomeric HCM (Palau 2001; Arad et al. 2005; Limongelli et al. 2007; Figure 8–5). Accurate diagnosis influences genetic counseling, prognosis, and treatment (Richard et al. 2003). Significant RV hypertrophy should induce detection of nonsarcomeric HCM. Renal impairment, skeletal muscle symptoms, and vision or hearing loss provide diagnostic clues for nonsarcomeric HCM.

Anderson Fabry Disease

Anderson Fabry disease is an X-linked recessive disorder of glycosphingolipid metabolism due to deficiency of the lysosomal enzyme α-galactosidase A. It is characterized by intracellular accumulation of glycosphingolipid with prominent involvement of skin and kidneys as well as myocardium. The disease has an estimated incidence up to 1/40,000 live male births. Symptomatic cardiovascular involvement occurs most significantly in affected male carriers, whereas females are usually asymptomatic or minimally symptomatic. Electrocardiogram may show atrioventricular block, short PR interval, LV hypertrophy, QRS prolongation, and ST-segment, and T wave changes. Echo shows LV hypertrophy simulating HCM (Nakao et al. 1995; Teragaki et al. 2004), valvular thickening, and mitral regurgitation caused by deposition of glycolipid in the mitral valve. Mitral valve prolapse and LV dysfunction are seen. Patients with causal mutations for Fabry disease and LV hypertrophy showed significantly lower contraction and relaxation tissue Doppler velocities, lower Ea/Aa ratio, and higher E/Ea ratio than mutation-positive patients without LV hypertrophy (Pieroni et al. 2003).

Enzyme replacement therapy has been shown to enhance micro vascular endothelial globotriaosylceramide clearance in the hearts of patients with Fabry disease. Echocardiography has proven useful in the cardiac assessment after enzyme replacement therapy. Although treatment endpoints mainly rely on symptoms, serial echocardiographic studies have shown reduction of LV mass, LV mass index, and relative wall thickness after 12 months of agalsidase-β. Another group used ultrasonic strain rate imaging to assess radial and longitudinal myocardial deformation. At baseline, both peak systolic strain rate and systolic strain were significantly reduced in the radial and longitudinal direction in patients compared with controls. After 1 year of treatment with 1.0 mg/kg body weight of recombinant α-Gal A (Weidemann et al. 2003) radial peak systolic strain rate increased significantly, and end-diastolic thickness of the posterior wall and myocardial mass decreased. These results suggest that enzyme replacement therapy can decrease LV hypertrophy and improve regional myocardial function. There were however, no significant effects on fractional shortening after 1 and 2 years (Schiffmann et al. 2001).

Cardiac Amyloidosis

Cardiac amyloidosis is caused by deposition of amyloid protein in interstitium of the myocardium resulting in increased ventricular wall thickness and stiffness. Myocardial infiltration by amyloid fibrils can occur in primary, familial, secondary, and senile amyloidosis. Cardiac amyloidosis occurs more commonly in men than

A

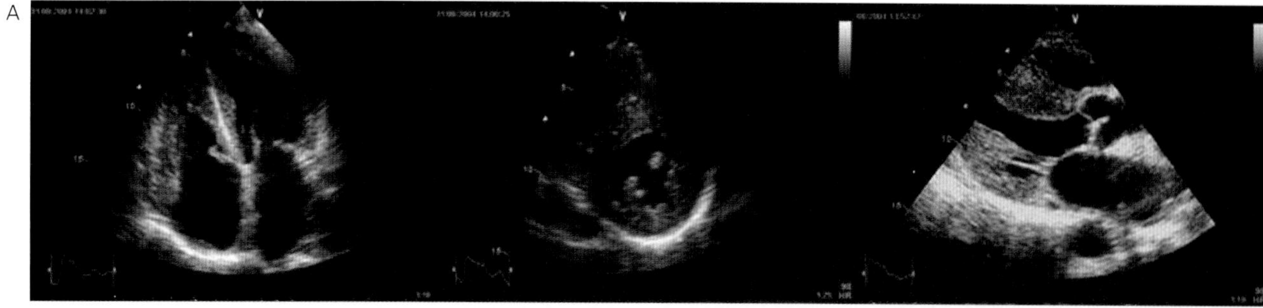

B

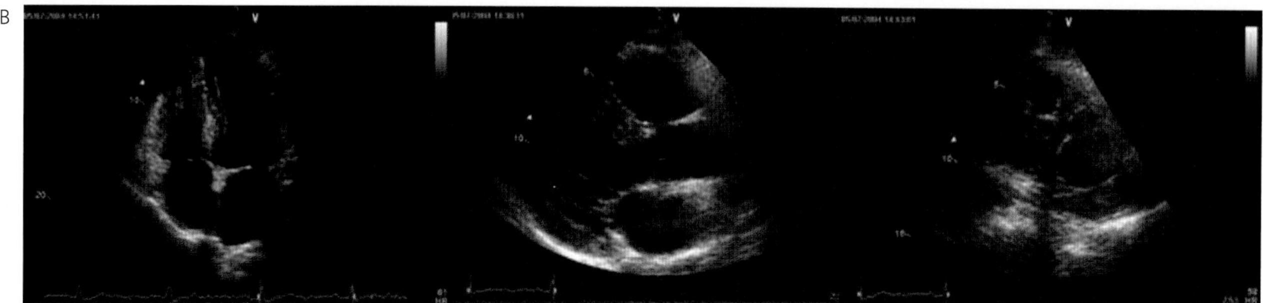

Figure 8–5 Other causes of LV hypertrophy mimicking sarcomeric mutations. Panel A. Concentric LV hypertrophy with normal LV EF and no pericardial effusion in a patient with amyloidosis. Panel B. Asymmetric septal hypertrophy in a male patient with cardiac variant of Fabry disease.

in women, and is rare in individuals before 30 years. ECG features are diminished voltage in the limb leads. Myocardial infarction is often simulated because of small or diminished R waves in the right precordial leads and abnormal Q waves in leads II, III, and aV_F (Gertz et al. 1992).

Two-dimensional echocardiography remains an adequate method for identifying and following individuals with cardiac amyloidosis. Echocardiogram shows concentric LV hypertrophy, small ventricular chambers, dilated atria, thickening of interatrial septum, and thickening and regurgitation of mitral, aortic, and tricuspid valves. Some patients exhibit LV hypertrophy without pericardial effusion and can mimic HCM. The presence of decreased radial LV function would argue against HCM. LV hypertrophy may be associated with granular speckled texture, which is not specific for amyloidosis. Diastolic dysfunction is common. Pericardial effusion is common but rarely results in tamponade probably because of slowly progressive fluid retention. LV hypertrophy with low voltage on ECG appears to distinguish cardiac amyloidosis from HCM. Echocardiography is an effective screening tool for detecting cardiac AL (primary) amyloidosis at early stage using myocardial deformation indices when conventional fractional shortening remains normal (Koyama et al. 2003). The integration of clinical, echocardiographic, electrocardiographic, and tissue biopsy data is essential to make the diagnosis of cardiac amyloidosis. Advanced diastolic dysfunction (grade III to IV restrictive physiology) has been shown to be a stronger predictor of cardiac death than LV wall thickness or systolic function regardless of symptom status (Klein et al. 1991). At a later stage of the disease, restrictive cardiomyopathy or prominent systolic dysfunction occurs with poor response to treatment.

Friedreich's Ataxia

Friedreich ataxia is an autosomal recessive spinocerebellar degenerative disease characterized by ataxia of limb and trunk, dysarthria, loss of deep tendon reflexes, sensory abnormalities, skeletal deformities (kyphoscoliosis), loss of proprioceptive sensations in limbs, diabetes mellitus, and cardiac involvement (Palau 2001). The disease results from a deficiency of functional frataxin, a protein that appears involved in mitochondrial iron homeostasis. The most frequent ECG abnormalities are sinus tachycardia and biphasic or inverted T waves in leads I, II, III, aV_F, and left precordial leads. LV hypertrophy is common. Deep Q waves simulating myocardial infarction often appear in leads II, III, aV_F, and/or precordial leads, probably due to interventricular septal hypertrophy. On echocardiogram concentric LV hypertrophy is more common than asymmetric septal hypertrophy (Gottdiener et al. 1982). Hypertrophy of the papillary muscles and LV outflow gradient may be present although the range of abnormalities appears to be wide. In HCM of Friedreich ataxia systolic function is normal, not supernormal, and diastolic function is not depressed. The cardiomyopathy of Friedreich ataxia in patients who are without cardiac symptoms is associated with reduction in both systolic and early diastolic myocardial velocity gradients across the thickness of the wall. Myocardial velocity gradient is independent of cardiac translation in the chest, and less affected by alterations in preload than Doppler transmitral velocities. Early diastolic myocardial velocity gradient appear to relate closely to the genetic abnormality and the consequential reduction in frataxin protein (Dutka et al. 2000). DCM appears to occur as a progressive transition from HCM.

Noonan Syndrome

Noonan syndrome is an autosomal dominant condition. Patients with Noonan syndrome have short stature, cubitus valgus, webbed neck, congenital lymphedema, and are karyotypically normal. Such patients exhibit an unusual deformity of the sternum, mental retardation, ptosis, low-set ears, ocular hypertelorism (abnormally large space between eyes), and cryptorchidism (Mendez 1985). Patients with this syndrome have tendency to bleeding, and partial deficiency of coagulation factor XI has been reported. A number of cardiac lesions can be observed including valvular pulmonary stenosis and HCM, the latter affecting either ventricle or both (Battiste 1977). Atrial septal defect usually associated with pulmonary stenosis, ventricular septal defect, and patent ductus arteriosus may also occur.

Other Familial Storage Diseases

Mucopolysaccharidoses (e.g., Hunter syndrome, Hurler syndrome, Morquio syndrome) are caused by abnormal lysosomal degradation of proteoglycan and glycosaminoglycan. Short stature, progressive coarsening of facial features, skeletal dysplasia, and corneal clouding are common. Electrocardiogram shows low voltages. Coronary arteries are narrow due to intimal and medial thickening. LV and RV are often hypertrophic and progressive systolic impairment is common. Myocardial infarction is also described. Patients are often too mentally impaired to report typical symptoms. In some forms, the valve leaflets thicken and cause aortic stenosis or mitral regurgitation (Arad et al. 2005). Other familial storage diseases include Gaucher disease (disorder of glucosylceramide metabolism), hemochromatosis, and glycogen storage disease. LEOPARD syndrome is an acronym from its cardinal features such as lentigenes ("L"), ECG conduction defects ("E"), ocular hypertelorism ("O"), pulmonary valvular stenosis ("P"), abnormalities of genitals ("A"), retardation of growth ("R"), and deafness ("D"). Pulmonic stenosis is the most frequent abnormality followed by HCM and endocardial fibroelastosis. LEOPARD syndrome is an autosomal dominant disorder (Arad et al. 2005).

Differentiation Between HCM and Athlete's Heart

HCM is the most common cause of sudden death in athletes in the United States and is often present without symptoms. Sudden death may be the first manifestation of the disease and often occurs during intense exercise. LV wall thickness between 1.3 and 1.6 cm is observed in 2% of male elite athletes (Pelliccia et al. 1991; Pelliccia et al. 1993; Sharma et al. 2002) mainly doing rowing, canoeing, cycling, and cross-country skiing (Spirito et al. 1994). All such athletes have large body size, and have won medals at international or national events. The distinction between HCM and physiologic hypertrophy secondary to athletic training is easily made in most cases. Criteria in favor of HCM are small LV cavity with end-diastolic diameter <45 mm, unusual LV hypertrophy pattern, marked left atrial dilatation, female gender, ECG abnormalities, abnormal LV filling, family history of HCM, and no decrease of wall thickness after deconditioning for 3 months.

However, when distinction is difficult between HCM and Athlete's heart, additional criteria may help. Maximal oxygen uptake <80% of predicted value favors the diagnostic of HCM (Sharma et al. 2000). Early diastolic myocardial velocity gradient across the thickness of the posterior wall ≤7/s measured in subjects between 18 and 45 years old showed 96% sensitivity and 96% specificity in the diagnostic of HCM. There is no similar cutoff value in subjects older than 45 years (Palka et al. 1997). Systolic and early diastolic mitral annular velocities <9 cm/s have 87% sensitivity, 97% specificity, and 92% accuracy in the diagnosis of HCM (Vinereanu et al. 2001). Early diastolic tricuspid annular velocity <16 cm/s has 89% sensitivity and 93% specificity in the diagnostic of HCM (D'Andrea et al. 2003).

Role of Echocardiography in the Management of Outflow Obstruction

Indications for septal reduction therapy in HCM patients include severely symptomatic patients in functional class III and IV with septal thickness >1.8 cm, LV outflow tract gradient >50 mmHg at rest or with provocable gradient >100 mmHg who are unresponsive to medical therapy or experienced side effects. The choice between septal alcohol ablation and surgical myectomy is influenced by age of the patient, severity of hypertrophy, mitral valve abnormalities that are independent of LV outflow tract obstruction, coronary artery anatomy, and other causes of obstruction including midcavity obstruction and subaortic membrane. Comorbidities and patient choice also play a role.

Surgical Myectomy

The most commonly performed surgical procedure is ventricular septal myectomy (Figure 8–6). This either abolishes or significantly reduces the gradient in 95% of cases and is associated with reduced mitral regurgitation and improvement in both exercise capacity and symptoms, which is maintained long term in 70% to 80% of patients (Maron et al. 1983a; Schoendube et al. 1995; McCully et al. 1996). Surgery should be performed in centers where mortality rates are less than 2%.

Before surgery transthoracic and transesophageal echocardiography predicts depth, width, and length of myectomy. The target length of resection is 1 cm below the point of mitral leaflet-septal contact. Quantification and mechanism of obstruction and of mitral regurgitation with detection of independent mitral valve disease and concomitant aortic valve disease are mandatory.

Intraoperative transesophageal echocardiography when off pump detects residual systolic anterior motion of the mitral valve, LV outflow tract gradient, mitral regurgitation as well as complications including ventricular septal defect, and aortic regurgitation. Special caution should be taken in the interpretation of color flow data according to loading and inotropic conditions. Therefore, careful analysis of anatomy of LV outflow tract and mitral leaflets is crucial.

Decision Making during Percutaneous Septal Alcohol Ablation

Percutaneous alcohol ablation is the major nonsurgical approach to gradient reduction. This involves the selective injection of alcohol into a septal perforator branch of the left anterior descending coronary artery to create a localized septal scar. Published data largely arise from a small number of experienced centers, which report similar gradient reduction and improvement in symptoms and exercise capacity to surgery (Sigwart 1995; Lakkis et al. 2000; Park et al. 2002; Chang et al. 2004). Echo participates in the selection of potential candidates. Patients in whom the mechanism of LV outflow tract obstruction does not relate to upper septal hypertrophy will not benefit from alcohol ablation.

In the catheterization laboratory, myocardial contrast echo using intracoronary injection of echo contrast with transthoracic imaging enables identification of myocardial areas supplied by the septal perforator branch and helps selecting the appropriate septal branch (Nagueh et al. 1998a; Faber et al. 2000a, 2000b; Flores-Ramirez et al. 2001). Recording multiple views and identification of the target area are required to avoid damage to papillary muscles and other remote myocardium (Figure 8–7). Myocardial contrast echo identified no target vessel in 8% of patients and a change of target vessel in 11% (Faber et al. 2004).

Patients with LV outflow tract gradients and those with mitral regurgitation are at risk from endocarditis (Faber et al. 2004). Serial echo studies are required during follow-up to assess LV outflow tract gradient, LV remodeling, and mitral regurgitation.

A

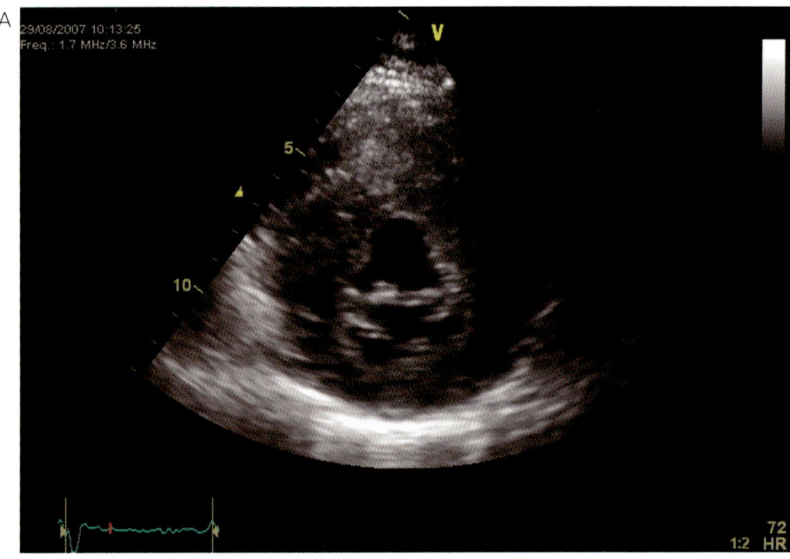

B

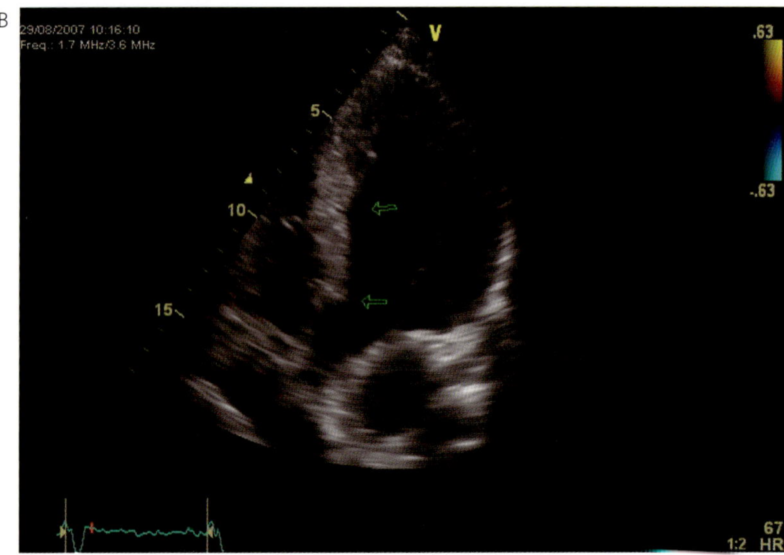

Figure 8–6 a &b (a) SAX view at end systole in HCM patient after septal myectomy showing anteroseptal defect and no systolic anterior motion of mitral leaflet. (b) Apical 4-chamber view in the same patient showing extent of septal myectomy (arrows).

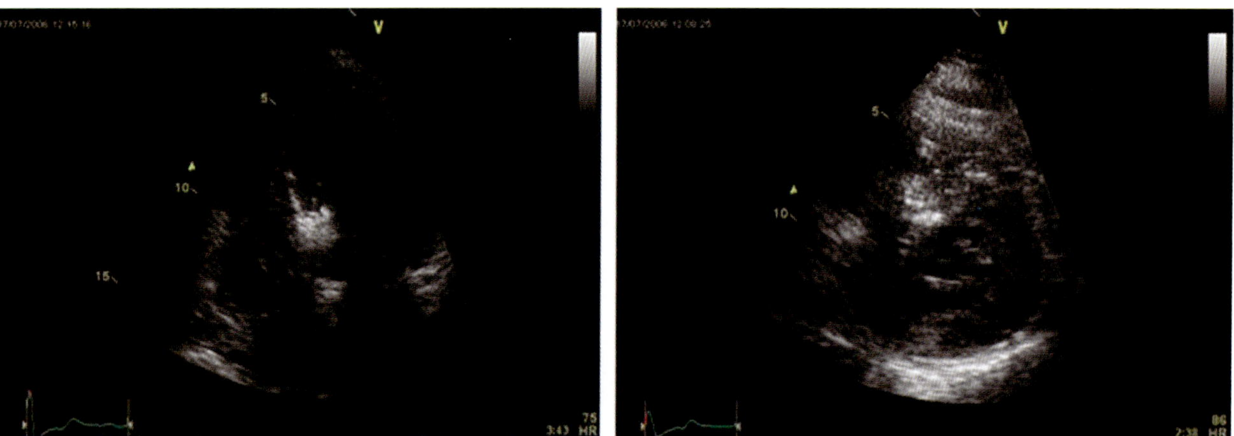

Figure 8–7 Contrast echo during ASA. Contrast echocardiography guiding alcohol septal ablation. The left image is apical 4-chamber view. There is opacification of basal septum in front of the septal contact of the anterior mitral leaflet. No other structure is opacified. The right image is short axis view confirming septal opacification in front of the septal contact of the anterior mitral leaflet.

End-Stage Hypertrophic Cardiomyopathy

Progression to LV dilatation and systolic dysfunction (ejection fraction <50%) with LV remodeling accompanied by wall thinning and cavity dilatation occurs in 5%–10% of patients (Spirito et al. 1987; Maron and Spirito 1998; Maron et al. 2003a). It has been called dilated phase, end stage, and burned-out phase of HCM. Patients with end-stage HCM exhibit congestive heart failure with poor prognosis. Transthoracic echocardiography shows regional wall motion abnormalities, often septal and inferior hypokinesis. These wall motion abnormalities may appear before LV dilatation with apparently normal LV ejection fraction. Since LV cavity size is small and LV systolic function supernormal in most patients with HCM, slightly reduced global LV systolic function and mild LV dilatation may be overlooked. Impaired LV performance precedes cavity dilatation, wall thinning, and heart failure symptoms. End-stage restrictive HCM is characterized by restrictive LV filling pattern with increased chamber stiffness, elevated left atrial and LV end-diastolic pressures. The strongest predictor of end-stage disease is family history of the disease. Serial monitoring and long-term follow-up of HCM patients is required for timely recognition and the necessity for defibrillator implantation and heart transplantation. Alternatively, elderly patients may experience more gradual LV remodeling with regression of wall thickness without systolic dysfunction and clinical deterioration.

Restrictive Cardiomyopathy

Definition and Diagnosis

Although restrictive cardiomyopathies (RCM) are less common than DCM and HCM, they are associated with greater morbidity and mortality. RCM is defined as a disease of the myocardium, which is characterized by restrictive filling, increased LV end-diastolic pressure, marked biatrial dilatation, and reduced diastolic volume of either or both ventricles. Conventional measures of LV systolic function are normal or near normal in the early stage of disease. This condition usually results from increased stiffness of the myocardium that causes pressure within the ventricle (or ventricles) to rise rapidly with only small increase in volume. Since the condition affects either or both ventricles, it may cause symptoms and signs of RV or LV failure.

Severe diastolic dysfunction with restrictive LV filling is a final common pathway for systolic as well as for diastolic failure regardless of origin. All patients with severe cardiomyopathy can have restrictive physiology (Seidman and Seidman 2001). Idiopathic RCM can present at any age with increased incidence in the elderly and women more often than men (Ammash et al. 2000). Affected patients often have signs of pulmonary and systemic congestion (Benotti et al. 1980; Kushwaha et al. 1997; Ammash et al. 2000). Common symptoms are dyspnea, peripheral edema, palpitations, fatigue, weakness, and exercise intolerance due to failure of the cardiac output to increase. Because of impaired ventricular filling, venous return is inhibited with peripheral edema, enlarged liver, ascites, and anasarca in advanced cases.

ECG abnormalities are nonspecific and include atrial fibrillation, ST-T wave abnormalities, premature atrial and ventricular beats, and intraventricular conduction delay. Atrial fibrillation is a common occurrence and causes sudden clinical deterioration. These abnormalities can also be seen in patients with constrictive pericarditis or infiltrative myocardial diseases such as amyloidosis and sarcoidosis. QRS voltage is normal in idiopathic RCM in contrast to low QRS voltages seen in constrictive pericarditis and in amyloidosis (Carroll et al. 1982). A phenotype of RCM and atrioventricular block is common in familial desminopathy. (Arbustini et al. 1998). Chest radiograph usually demonstrates cardiomegaly secondary to significant atrial enlargement with pulmonary venous congestion and pleural effusions.

Echocardiographic examination shows severe diastolic dysfunction with restrictive filling that produces elevated filling pressures and dilated atria. Restrictive filling is defined on transmitral inflow recording as E/A>2, deceleration time of E <150 ms, and isovolumic relaxation time <70 ms (Kushwaha et al. 1997; Ammash et al. 2000). LV systolic function is normal or decreased. Depending on the etiology and phase of the disease, wall thickness is normal or increased. There are no primary valvular diseases.

When there is suspicion of RCM, the first step is the differentiation between RCM and constrictive pericarditis as the treatment is of these two diseases is markedly different. The second step is the detection of specific characteristics related to RCM etiology (Table 8.1).

Table 8–1 Detection of Specific Characteristics Related to RCM Etiology (Kushwaha et al. 1997; Leung and Klein 1998)

Primary RCM
- Idiopathic RCM
- Endomyocardial Fibrosis associated with chronic hypereosinophilia
- Familial RCM

Secondary RCM

Infiltrative Disease
- Amyloidosis
- Sarcoidosis
- Postirradiation therapy
- Gaucher's disease
- Hurler's disease

Storage Disease
- Hemochromatosis
- Glycogen storage disease
- Fabry Disease

Other causes
- Postcardiac surgery
- Carcinoid heart disease
- Metastasis cancers
- Toxic effects of antracycline
- Drugs causing fibrous endocarditis (serotonin, methysergide, ergotamine, mercurial agents, busulfan)

Differentiation between RCM and Constrictive Pericarditis

The problem of distinction only applies to patients with right heart failure who show normal ventricular chamber dimensions and systolic wall motion. Differentiation of RCM and constrictive pericarditis is a difficult clinical problem, but it is important because constrictive pericarditis requires surgical treatment and is usually curable, while the treatment of RCM is medical and is largely aimed at improving symptoms.

Clinical history may be of value in suggesting one of these disorders. History of infiltrative disease that may involve the heart muscle (e.g., amyloidosis or sarcoidosis) favors the diagnosis of restrictive cardiomyopathy. History of tuberculosis, end-stage renal disease, infectious diseases, radiation therapy, or cardiac surgery is useful. RCM is often indistinguishable from constrictive pericarditis using cardiovascular examination. Chest X-ray demonstrates pericardial calcification in about 40% of patients, which is an important diagnostic clue for constrictive pericarditis, and a sign of chronicity and disease severity. It is associated with increased preoperative mortality. However, pericardial calcification is not specific for constrictive pericarditis. There is no single definitive test for diagnosis of RCM/constrictive pericarditis. Three investigations are helpful in distinguishing RCM and constrictive pericarditis including echo-Doppler, BNP, and invasive hemodynamic parameters. Both diagnosis and differentiation of RCM from constrictive pericarditis require the combination of information from these investigations.

Echo-Doppler Parameters in Favor of Pericardial Constriction

In constrictive pericarditis there are exaggerated respiratory variations. Respiratory variations are reciprocal between the two ventricles and reflect ventricular interdependence, as the heart is enclosed within a relatively fixed volume; enlargement of one ventricle tends to be associated with a corresponding decrease in the other ventricular volume. The most useful echo-Doppler parameters are (1) respiratory variation in the velocity of early diastolic velocity of transmitral inflow with respiration (>10%). The tricuspid velocity is increasing in inspiration and the mitral velocity is decreasing; (2) respiratory variation (>18%) in pulmonary vein early diastolic velocity; (3) diastolic flow reversal in hepatic venous flow during expiration; (4) early diastolic mitral annular velocity (Ea) using DTI; (5) color M-mode LV flow propagation velocity >1.00 m/s (Garcia et al. 1996; Rajagopalan et al. 2001). Ventricular interdependence is also seen in the 2D echocardiogram as a movement of the ventricular septum toward the left ventricle with inspiration and toward the right ventricle in expiration in SAX view. Since myocardium is impaired in RCM but not in constrictive cardiomyopathy, the early diastolic mitral annular velocity is notably decreased in RCM, while it is normal in pericardial constriction (Garcia et al. 1996; Rajagopalan et al. 2001). In the same manner, DTI velocity and strain in lateral LV wall and lateral RV wall are normal in constrictive pericarditis but impaired in RCM.

Respiratory variation of the mitral inflow peak early velocity (E) of >10% predicted constrictive pericarditis with 84% sensitivity and 91% specificity and variation in the pulmonary venous early diastolic (D) flow velocity of >18% distinguished constriction with 79% sensitivity and 91% specificity. Using tissue Doppler echocardiography, early velocity of longitudinal expansion (Ea) of >8.0 cm/s differentiated patients with constriction from RCM with 89% sensitivity and 100% specificity. A slope of >100 cm/s for the first aliasing contour in color M-mode LV flow propagation predicted patients with constriction with 74% sensitivity and 91% specificity. Thus, the recent methods of DTI and color M-mode flow propagation are complementary with flow Doppler respiratory variations in distinguishing between constrictive pericarditis and RCM (Garcia et al. 1996; Rajagopalan et al. 2001). Early diastolic myocardial velocity gradient at the posterior wall has been shown to be significantly higher in constrictive pericarditis than in RCM (Palka et al. 2000). However, calculation of myocardial velocity gradient requires specific software that is not commercially available.

BNP levels and invasive hemodynamic measurements participate in the diagnosis of pericardial constriction.

Arrhythmogenic Right Ventricular Cardiomyopathy (see Chapter 14)

ARVC is a myocardial disease in which heart muscle is replaced by scar tissue and fat. Although there is predilection for the RV, LV involvement is well described (Pinamonti et al. 1998; Norman et al. 2005). ARVC is familial in 30%–50%. The most common pattern of inheritance is autosomal dominant, with a penetrance in family members ranging from 20% to 35%. ARVC usually affects males in their late teens to mid-thirties with normal physical examination. Recessive forms have also been described (Naxos disease and Carvajal syndrome). ARVC is now considered as a disease of the desmosomes, which are specialized intercellular junctions of cardiac myocytes.

Right Ventricular Assessment

The normal RV is thin walled with a pyramidal and crescent shape wrapped around the LV. RV systolic pressure and flow are generated by RV free wall thickening and shortening from apex to outflow tract. Low resistance pulmonary circulation, coronary supply, fiber arrangement, small metabolic demand, and asynchronous contraction pattern are specific to the RV. This is in sharp contrast to LV characteristics. LV systolic pressure and flow are generated by a combination of longitudinal, radial, and circumferential motions.

Standardized image acquisition and analysis protocols for the RV have been described (Lindstrom et al. 2001; Lang et al. 2005). The RV is incompletely visualized in any single 2D echocardiographic view. Thus, accurate assessment of RV morphology and function requires multiple echocardiographic views, including parasternal long- and short-axis, RV inflow, apical four-chamber, and subcostal. Assessment of RV includes quantification of RV cavity size, global and regional function, and wall thickness. Conventional echocardiography has several limitations when imaging the RV including a low sensitivity and specificity especially in patients with suboptimal image quality and subtle abnormalities, subjectivity in the interpretation of results, and absence of established quantitative standards for RV dimensions in relation to age, sex, and gender. Evaluation of RV performance in humans is limited by complex RV shape (inflow, body, apex, outflow-infundibulum), loading conditions, the retrosternal position of the RV, which is in the near field of the image sector, and difficult delineation of trabeculated apical endocardial border. Translation and rotation of the heart in the chest apply to all imaging modalities. Indices of global RV systolic performance not dependent on endocardial definition are: TAPSE, velocity of lateral tricuspid annulus, dP/dt on tricuspid regurgitation jet, isovolumic myocardial acceleration, myocardial performance index, and ratio of preejection to ejection duration. RV systolic regional function is more easily evaluated with contrast cavity opacification.

A
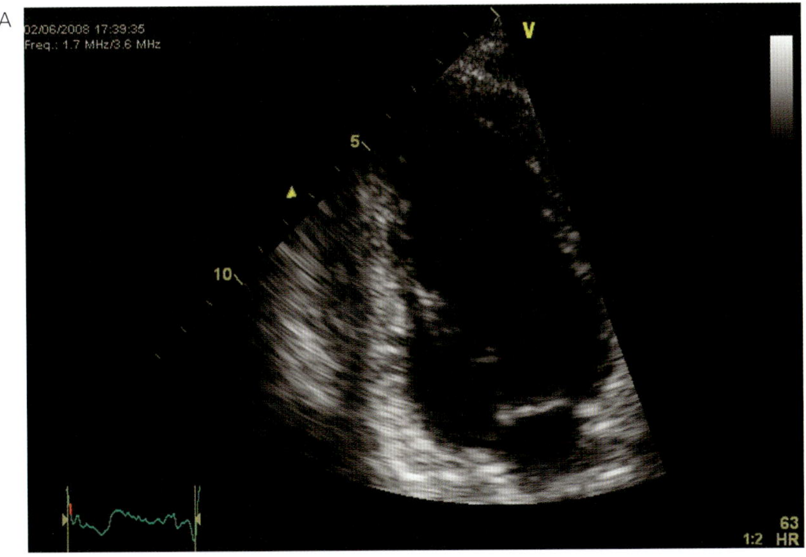

B
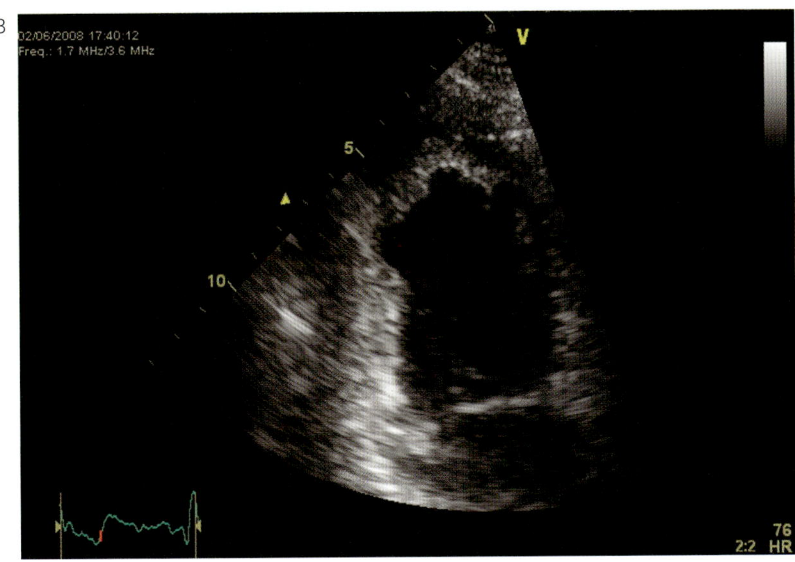

Figure 8–8 a & b (a) Apical two-chamber view in diastole of a patient with LV ARVC. There are no endocardial deformations. (b) Same view of the same patient in systole showing two small areas of dyskinesia, one in apical midinferior LV wall and one at LV apex.

Diagnosis According to Task Force Criteria

Definitive diagnosis relies on histological demonstration of transmural fibro-fatty replacement of the RV myocardium. In view of the variable phenotypic expression of this disease an ESC/ISCF task force has proposed diagnostic criteria for ARVC to enable diagnosis of probands and their asymptomatic relatives (McKenna et al. 1994). No single test is definitive. Multiple investigations (ECG, single-averaged ECG, echo, exercise test, and Holter-ECG) must be combined to facilitate the diagnosis. Task Force criteria for the diagnosis of ARVC in probands include family history, ECG depolarization/conduction abnormalities, ECG repolarization abnormalities, arrhythmias, global or regional dysfunction and structural alterations, and tissue characteristics obtained from endomyocardial biopsy. Global or regional dysfunction and structural alterations have been divided into major criteria including severe dilatation and reduction of RV ejection fraction with no or mild LV involvement; localized RV aneurysms (akinetic or dyskinetic areas with diastolic bulgings), and severe segmental dilatation of the RV. Minor criteria include mild global RV dilatation or ejection fraction reduction with normal LV, mild segmental dilatation, and regional RV hypokinesia. Diagnosis of ARVC would be fulfilled (Marcus et al. 2003) by the presence of two major criteria, one major plus two minor, or four minor criteria(McKenna et al. 1994; Corrado et al. 2000). However, Task Force criteria have limitations in early disease (Nava et al. 2000) and LV involvement.

Diagnosis According to Natural History of ARVC

1. Phase I: Preclinical or Concealed Phase

During this early phase, features are nonspecific and difficult to interpret. Many patients are screened as part of family screening from family with unexplained premature death. Diagnostic criteria in asymptomatic family members include subtle ECG abnormalities. Imaging in ARVC is challenging during the concealed phase and is often negative because the disease often involves only patchy and small areas of abnormal myocardium (Hamid et al. 2002) in the "triangle of dysplasia" (diaphragmatic, infundibular, and apical RV regions) as well as in the LV (Figure 8–8). Combination of multiple views and combination of

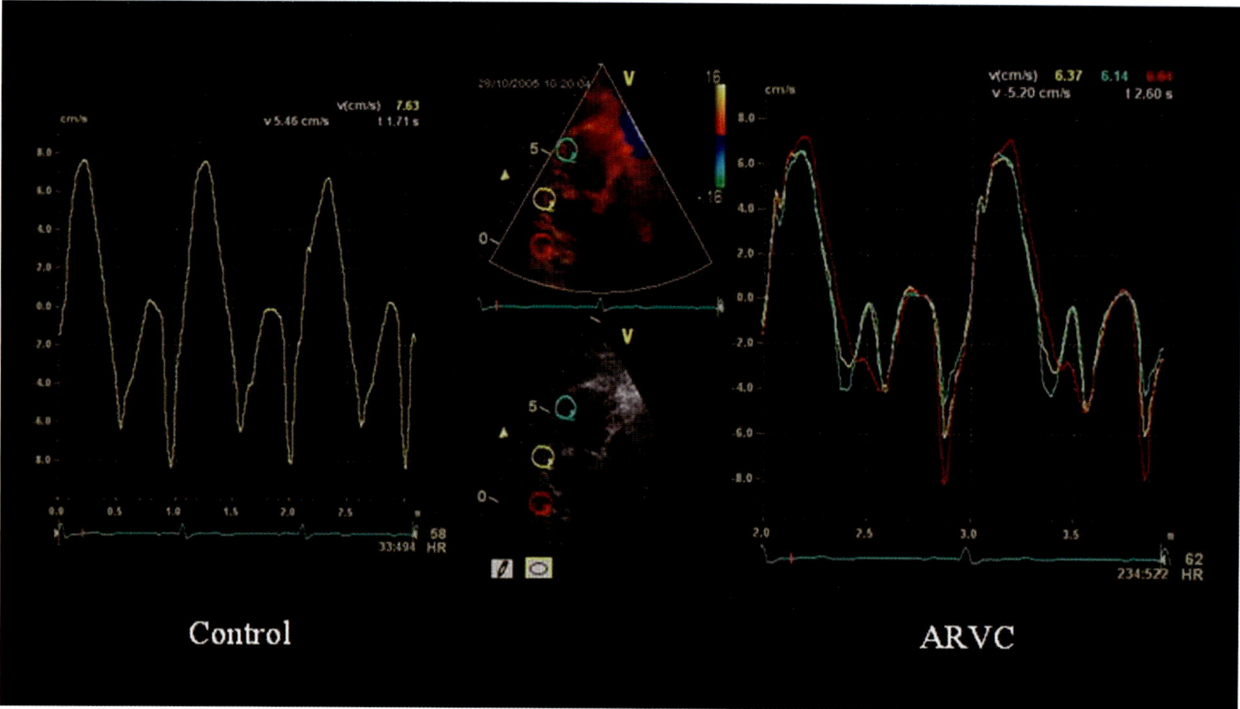

Figure 8–9 Tissue Doppler profiles of the lateral wall of the RV in a normal subject on the right and in ARVC patient on the left. In a normal subject, there is no isovolumic relaxation in the RV in contrast to clear isovolumic relaxation in normal LV segments. There is continuity between end of ejection and early diastolic wave in the RV. In the ARVC patient, there is isovolumic relaxation wave in the RV.

imaging modalities are required. Detection of subtle abnormalities includes RV isovolumic relaxation phase by DTI (Figure 8–9), comparison of systolic mitral and tricuspid annular velocities, and reverse basoapical velocity gradient in RV free wall with highest values in apical segments. According to Laplace Law (LV wall stress = P.R/2WT) wall stress is higher in basal segments, which may be more sensitive to early disease. Double reading of all studies is highly recommended. The main limitation of echocardiography for the diagnosis of ARVC at this early phase is interpretation of small RV wall motion abnormalities, which may be responsible for false-positive interpretation (Figure 8–10). RV regional function is more easily evaluated with contrast cavity opacification (Lopez-Fernandez et al. 2004). However, caution should be taken in the interpretation of RV apical motion due to trabeculations, and interpretation of midapical lateral wall motion due to insertion of the moderator band. In addition, structure of the normal RV is poorly defined. Obese patients have subclinical RV dysfunction (Wong et al. 2006) with fat around the heart. Increasing BMI is associated with increasing severity of RV dysfunction in overweight and obese subjects without overt heart disease, independent of sleep apnea.

Genetic testing will play an increasing role. No risk factors can be identified at this stage except malignant family history and education of patients on hot phase is mandatory.

2. Phase II: Overt Phase

Symptomatic ventricular arrhythmias are common. ARVC is associated with reentrant ventricular tachyarrhythmias of RV origin (left bundle branch morphology) often precipitated by exercise-induced discharge of catecholamine. Differential diagnoses focuses on idiopathic ventricular tachycardia that are benign, nonfamilial, with normal ECG at rest, and normal heart on echocardiography (Calkins 2006).

Patients fulfil Task Force diagnostic criteria at this stage. Echocardiography shows diffuse RV/LV structural abnormalities. Probands with ARVC have right atrial and RV enlargement and decreased RV function. The main problem is to assess the RV with several views during routine examination. When RV cavity dilatation and/or systolic dysfunction are detected, focus is on differential diagnoses including intracardiac shunt and pulmonary embolism.

In patients with ARVC, RV dimensions were significantly increased, and RV fractional area change was significantly decreased versus control patients. The RV outflow tract was the most commonly enlarged dimension in ARVC probands versus controls. RV outflow tract long-axis diastolic dimension >30 mm occurred in 89% of probands and in 14% of controls. The RV morphologic abnormalities were present in many probands (trabecular derangement in 54%, hyper-reflective moderator band in 34%, and sacculations in 17%) but not in controls (Yoerger et al. 2005). Recent studies evaluated the potential utility of 3D echo (Prakasa et al. 2006; Kjaergaard et al. 2007), tissue Doppler, and strain echocardiography (Prakasa et al. 2007) to quantitatively assess RV function and their potential role in diagnosing ARVC. Tissue Doppler peak systolic velocity best correlates with cardiac magnetic resonance—derived RV ejection fraction with high reproducibility and may facilitate simple and quantitative assessment of RV function (Wang et al. 2007). Detection of risk factors for sudden death and evaluation of disease severity are crucial for patient management. Echocardiography assesses disease severity by detecting extensive RV dysfunction with right heart failure and LV involvement (Pinamonti et al. 1998; Wichter et al. 2004).

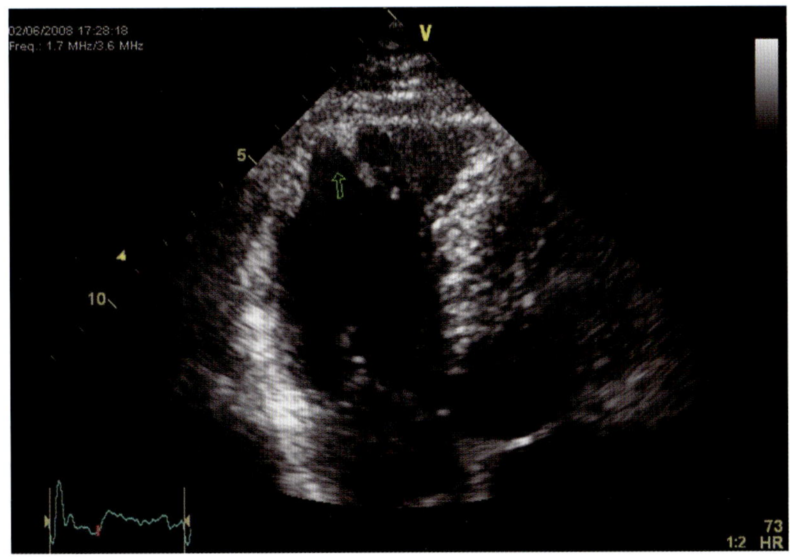

Figure 8-10 Apical four-chamber view at end-systole focusing on the RV. RV apex is heavily trabeculated and there is thick moderator band. Regional wall motion abnormalities close to the junction between lateral RV wall and moderator band should be interpreted with great caution due to tethering effect.

3. Phase III/IV: Advanced Disease

Patients suffer from palpitations, shortness of breath, chest pain, and symptomatic ventricular arrhythmias. Echocardiography shows global RV and LV dilatation and dysfunction with diffuse structural abnormalities that are difficult to distinguish from DCM. Echocardiography also assesses disease severity (Wichter et al. 2004).

Conclusions

Transthoracic echocardiography remains the most practical imaging modality in cardiomyopathies (Wood and Picard 2004). Cardiac imaging plays a major role in inherited cardiovascular disease and participates in diagnosis accuracy, etiology, correlation between phenotype and genotype, and in the identification of patients with higher risk of sudden and total cardiac death. Echocardiography is noninvasive, relatively low cost, does not expose patients to ionizing radiations, and serial studies can be done at the bedside. Massive technical progresses have been made in image quality and recent imaging modalities including cavity contrast opacification, 3D echo, tissue Doppler echocardiography, Doppler and non-Doppler strain. These techniques are complementary, have provided additional information and can be used during any echocardiography examination. Echocardiography data should be interpreted with clinical history, physical examination, family history, and ECG data to optimize patient management. Thus, echocardiography continues to have advantages over competing technologies.

References

Alfonso F, Nihoyannopoulos P, Stewart J, Dickie S, Lemery R, McKenna WJ. Clinical significance of giant negative T waves in hypertrophic cardiomyopathy. *J Am Coll Cardiol.* 1990;15(5):965–971.

Ammash NM, Seward JB, Bailey KR, Edwards WD, Tajik AJ. Clinical profile and outcome of idiopathic restrictive cardiomyopathy. *Circulation.* 2000;101(21):2490–2496.

Ando H, Imaizumi T, Urabe Y, Takeshita A, Nakamura M. Apical segmental dysfunction in hypertrophic cardiomyopathy: subgroup with unique clinical features. *J Am Coll Cardiol.* 1990;16(7):1579–1588.

Arad M, Maron BJ, Gorham JM, et al. Glycogen storage diseases presenting as hypertrophic cardiomyopathy. *N Engl J Med.* 2005;352(4):362–372.

Arbustini E, Morbini P, Grasso M, et al. Restrictive cardiomyopathy, atrioventricular block and mild to subclinical myopathy in patients with desmin-immunoreactive material deposits. *J Am Coll Cardiol.* 1998;31(3):645–653.

Bargiggia GS, Bertucci C, Recusani F, et al. A new method for estimating left ventricular dP/dt by continuous wave Doppler-echocardiography. Validation studies at cardiac catheterization. *Circulation.* 1989;80(5):1287–1292.

Bargiggia GS, Tronconi L, Sahn DJ, et al. A new method for quantitation of mitral regurgitation based on color flow Doppler imaging of flow convergence proximal to regurgitant orifice. *Circulation.* 1991;84(4):1481–1489.

Battiste CE. Congestive cardiomyopathy in Noonan's syndrome. *Mayo Clin Proc.* 1977;52(10):661–664.

Benotti JR, Grossman W, Cohn PF. Clinical profile of restrictive cardiomyopathy. *Circulation.* 1980;61(6):1206–1212.

Bristow MR, Saxon LA, Boehmer J, et al. Cardiac-resynchronization therapy with or without an implantable defibrillator in advanced chronic heart failure. *N Engl J Med.* 2004;350(21):2140–2150.

Brun P, Tribouilloy C, Duvan AM, et al. Left ventricular flow propagation during early filling is related to wall relaxation: a color M-mode Doppler analysis. *J Am Coll Cardiol.* 1992;20(2):420–432.

Calkins H. Arrhythmogenic right-ventricular dysplasia/cardiomyopathy. *Curr Opin Cardiol.* 2006;21(1):55–63.

Cannon RO 3rd, Rosing DR, Maron BJ, et al. Myocardial ischemia in patients with hypertrophic cardiomyopathy: contribution of inadequate vasodilator reserve and elevated left ventricular filling pressures. *Circulation.* 1985;71(2):234–243.

Carroll JD, Gaasch WH, McAdam KP. Amyloid cardiomyopathy: characterization by a distinctive voltage/mass relation. *Am J Cardiol.* 1982;49(1):9–13.

Cecchi F, Olivotto I, Gistri R, Lorenzoni R, Chiriatti G, Camici PG. Coronary microvascular dysfunction and prognosis in hypertrophic cardiomyopathy. *N Engl J Med.* 2003;349(11):1027–1035.

Chang SM, Lakkis NM, Franklin J, Spencer WH 3rd, Nagueh SF. Predictors of outcome after alcohol septal ablation therapy in patients with hypertrophic obstructive cardiomyopathy. *Circulation.* 2004;109(7): 824–827.

Cleland JG, Daubert JC, Erdmann E, et al. The effect of cardiac resynchronization on morbidity and mortality in heart failure. *N Engl J Med.* 2005;352(15):1539–1549.

Corrado D, Fontaine G, Marcus FI, et al. Arrhythmogenic right ventricular dysplasia/cardiomyopathy: need for an international registry. Study Group on Arrhythmogenic Right Ventricular Dysplasia/Cardiomyopathy of the Working Groups on Myocardial and Pericardial Disease and Arrhythmias of the European Society of Cardiology and of the Scientific Council on Cardiomyopathies of the World Heart Federation. *Circulation.* 2000;101(11):E101–E106.

D'Andrea A, Caso P, Severino S, et al. Different involvement of right ventricular myocardial function in either physiologic or pathologic left ventricular hypertrophy: a Doppler tissue study. *J Am Soc Echocardiogr.* 2003;16(2):154–161.

Diaz-Infante E, Mont L, Leal J, et al. Predictors of lack of response to resynchronization therapy. *Am J Cardiol.* 2005;95(12):1436–1440.

Dubois-Rande JL, Merlet P, Roudot F, et al. Beta-adrenergic contractile reserve as a predictor of clinical outcome in patients with idiopathic dilated cardiomyopathy. *Am Heart J.* 1992;124(3):679–685.

Dumesnil JG, Dion D, Yvorchuk K, Davies RA, Chan K. A new, simple and accurate method for determining ejection fraction by Doppler echocardiography. *Can J Cardiol.* 1995;11(11):1007–1014.

Dutka DP, Donnelly JE, Palka P, Lange A, Nunez DJ, Nihoyannopoulos P. Echocardiographic characterization of cardiomyopathy in Friedreich's ataxia with tissue Doppler echocardiographically derived myocardial velocity gradients. *Circulation.* 2000;102(11):1276–1282.

Elliott PM, Gimeno Blanes JR, Mahon NG, Poloniecki JD, McKenna WJ. Relation between severity of left-ventricular hypertrophy and prognosis in patients with hypertrophic cardiomyopathy. *Lancet.* 2001;357(9254):420–424.

Elliott PM, Poloniecki J, Dickie S, et al. Sudden death in hypertrophic cardiomyopathy: identification of high risk patients. *J Am Coll Cardiol.* 2000;36(7):2212–2218.

Emilsson K, Alam M, Wandt B. The relation between mitral annulus motion and ejection fraction: a nonlinear function. *J Am Soc Echocardiogr.* 2000;13(10):896–901.

Enriquez-Sarano M, Bailey KR, Seward JB, Tajik AJ, Krohn MJ, Mays JM. Quantitative Doppler assessment of valvular regurgitation. *Circulation.* 1993;87(3):841–848.

Enriquez-Sarano M, Miller FA Jr, Hayes SN, Bailey KR, Tajik AJ, Seward JB. Effective mitral regurgitant orifice area: clinical use and pitfalls of the proximal isovelocity surface area method. *J Am Coll Cardiol.* 1995;25(3):703–709.

Faber L, Meissner A, Ziemssen P, Seggewiss H. Percutaneous transluminal septal myocardial ablation for hypertrophic obstructive cardiomyopathy: long term follow-up of the first series of 25 patients. *Heart.* 2000a;83(3):326–331.

Faber L, Seggewiss H, Welge D, et al. Echo-guided percutaneous septal ablation for symptomatic hypertrophic obstructive cardiomyopathy: 7 years of experience. *Eur J Echocardiogr.* 2004;5(5):347–355.

Faber L, Ziemssen P, Seggewiss H, et al. Targeting percutaneous transluminal septal ablation for hypertrophic obstructive cardiomyopathy by intraprocedural echocardiographic monitoring. *J Am Soc Echocardiogr.* 2000b;13(12):1074–1079.

Finsterer J, Stollberger C. Spontaneous left ventricular hypertrabeculation in dystrophin duplication based Becker's muscular dystrophy. *Herz.* 2001a;26(7):477–481.

Finsterer J, Stollberger C, Wegmann R, Jarius C, Janssen B. Left ventricular hypertrabeculation in myotonic dystrophy type 1. *Herz.* 2001b;26(4):287–290.

Flores-Ramirez R, Lakkis NM, Middleton KJ, et al. Echocardiographic insights into the mechanisms of relief of left ventricular outflow tract obstruction after nonsurgical septal reduction therapy in patients with hypertrophic obstructive cardiomyopathy. *J Am Coll Cardiol.* 2001;37(1):208–214.

Fragola PV, Calo L, Luzi M, Mammarella A, Antonini G. Doppler echocardiographic assessment of left ventricular diastolic function in myotonic dystrophy. *Cardiology.* 1997;88(6):498–502.

Garcia MJ, Rodriguez L, Ares M, Griffin BP, Thomas JD, Klein AL. Differentiation of constrictive pericarditis from restrictive cardiomyopathy: assessment of left ventricular diastolic velocities in longitudinal axis by Doppler tissue imaging. *J Am Coll Cardiol.* 1996;27(1):108–114.

Garcia MJ, Thomas JD, Klein AL. New Doppler echocardiographic applications for the study of diastolic function. *J Am Coll Cardiol.* 1998; 32(4):865–875.

Gertz MA, Kyle RA, Thibodeau SN. Familial amyloidosis: a study of 52 North American-born patients examined during a 30-year period. *Mayo Clin Proc.* 1992;67(5):428–440.

Ghio S, Gavazzi A, Campana C, et al. Independent and additive prognostic value of right ventricular systolic function and pulmonary artery pressure in patients with chronic heart failure. *J Am Coll Cardiol.* 2001;37(1):183–188.

Gorcsan J 3rd, Tanabe M, Bleeker GB, et al. Combined longitudinal and radial dyssynchrony predicts ventricular response after resynchronization therapy. *J Am Coll Cardiol.* 2007;50(15):1476–1483.

Gottdiener JS, Hawley RJ, Maron BJ, Bertorini TF, Engle WK. Characteristics of the cardiac hypertrophy in Friedreich's ataxia. *Am Heart J.* 1982;103 (4 Pt 1):525–531.

Greenberg NL, Firstenberg MS, Castro PL, et al. Doppler-derived myocardial systolic strain rate is a strong index of left ventricular contractility. *Circulation.* 2002;105(1):99–105.

Gulati VK, Katz WE, Follansbee WP, Gorcsan J 3rd. Mitral annular descent velocity by tissue Doppler echocardiography as an index of global left ventricular function. *Am J Cardiol.* 1996;77(11):979–984.

Hamid MS, Norman M, Quraishi A, et al. Prospective evaluation of relatives for familial arrhythmogenic right ventricular cardiomyopathy/dysplasia reveals a need to broaden diagnostic criteria. *J Am Coll Cardiol.* 2002;40(8):1445–1450.

Harris KM, Spirito P, Maron MS, et al. Prevalence, clinical profile, and significance of left ventricular remodeling in the end-stage phase of hypertrophic cardiomyopathy. *Circulation.* 2006;114(3):216–225.

Heimdal A, Stoylen A, Torp H, Skjaerpe T. Real-time strain rate imaging of the left ventricle by ultrasound. *J Am Soc Echocardiogr.* 1998; 11(11):1013–1019.

Heinle SK, Hall SA, Brickner ME, Willett DL, Grayburn PA. Comparison of vena contracta width by multiplane transesophageal echocardiography with quantitative Doppler assessment of mitral regurgitation. *Am J Cardiol.* 1998;81(2):175–179.

Helle-Valle T, Crosby J, Edvardsen T, et al. New noninvasive method for assessment of left ventricular rotation: speckle tracking echocardiography. *Circulation.* 2005;112(20):3149–3156.

Henry WL, Gardin JM, Ware JH. Echocardiographic measurements in normal subjects from infancy to old age. *Circulation.* 1980;62(5): 1054–1061.

Ho CY, Sweitzer NK, McDonough B, et al. Assessment of diastolic function with Doppler tissue imaging to predict genotype in preclinical hypertrophic cardiomyopathy. *Circulation.* 2002;105(25):2992–2997.

Hoffmann R, von Bardeleben S, ten Cate F, et al. Assessment of systolic left ventricular function: a multi-centre comparison of cineventriculography, cardiac magnetic resonance imaging, unenhanced and contrast-enhanced echocardiography. *Eur Heart J.* 2005;26(6):607–616.

Hung J, Koelling T, Semigran MJ, Dec GW, Levine RA, Di Salvo TG. Usefulness of echocardiographic determined tricuspid regurgitation in predicting event-free survival in severe heart failure secondary to idiopathic-dilated cardiomyopathy or to ischemic cardiomyopathy. *Am J Cardiol.* 1998;82(10):1301–1303, A10.

Hurlburt HM, Aurigemma GP, Hill JC, et al. Direct ultrasound measurement of longitudinal, circumferential, and radial strain using 2-dimensional strain imaging in normal adults. *Echocardiography.* 2007;24(7):723–731.

Jenni R, Oechslin E, Schneider J, Attenhofer Jost C, Kaufmann PA. Echocardiographic and pathoanatomical characteristics of isolated left ventricular non-compaction: a step towards classification as a distinct cardiomyopathy. *Heart.* 2001;86(6):666–671.

Kitaoka H, Takata J, Yabe T, Hitomi N, Furuno T, Doi YL. Low dose dobutamine stress echocardiography predicts the improvement of left ventricular systolic function in dilated cardiomyopathy. *Heart.* 1999;81(5):523–527.

Kjaergaard J, Hastrup Svendsen J, Sogaard P, et al. Advanced quantitative echocardiography in arrhythmogenic right ventricular cardiomyopathy. *J Am Soc Echocardiogr.* 2007;20(1):27–35.

Klein AL, Hatle LK, Taliercio CP, et al. Prognostic significance of Doppler measures of diastolic function in cardiac amyloidosis. A Doppler echocardiography study. *Circulation.* 1991;83(3):808–816.

Klues HG, Roberts WC, Maron BJ. Morphological determinants of echocardiographic patterns of mitral valve systolic anterior motion in obstructive hypertrophic cardiomyopathy. *Circulation.* 1993;87(5):1570–1579.

Koelling TM, Aaronson KD, Cody RJ, Bach DS, Armstrong WF. Prognostic significance of mitral regurgitation and tricuspid regurgitation in patients with left ventricular systolic dysfunction. *Am Heart J.* 2002;144(3):524–529.

Konno T, Shimizu M, Ino H et al. Diagnostic value of abnormal Q waves for identification of preclinical carriers of hypertrophic cardiomyopathy based on a molecular genetic diagnosis. *Eur Heart J.* 2004;25(3):246–251.

Koyama J, Ray-Sequin PA, Faik RH. Longitudinal myocardial function assessed by tissue velocity, strain, and strain rate tissue Doppler echocardiography in patients with AL (primary) cardiac amyloidosis. *Circulation.* 2003;107(19):2446–2452.

Kushwaha SS, Fallon JT, Fuster V. Restrictive cardiomyopathy. *N Engl J Med.* 1997;336(4):267–276.

Lakkis NM, Nagueh SF, Dunn JK, Killip D, Spencer WH 3rd. Nonsurgical septal reduction therapy for hypertrophic obstructive cardiomyopathy: one-year follow-up. *J Am Coll Cardiol.* 2000;36(3):852–855.

Lang RM, Bierig M, Devereux RB, et al. Recommendations for chamber quantification: a report from the American Society of Echocardiography's Guidelines and Standards Committee and the Chamber Quantification Writing Group, developed in conjunction with the European Association of Echocardiography, a branch of the European Society of Cardiology. *J Am Soc Echocardiogr.* 2005;18(12):1440–1463.

La Vecchia L, Paccanaro M, Bonanno C, Varotto L, Ometto R, Vincenzi M. Left ventricular versus biventricular dysfunction in idiopathic dilated cardiomyopathy. *Am J Cardiol.* 1999;83(1):120–122, A9.

Lee DS, Pencina MJ, Benjamin EJ, et al. Association of parental heart failure with risk of heart failure in offspring. *N Engl J Med.* 2006;355(2):138–147.

Leung DY, Klein AL. *Textbook of Cardiovascular Medicine.* JM. Isner, Lippincott-Raven: 1998;604.

Levine RA, Vlahakes GJ, Lefebvre X, et al. Papillary muscle displacement causes systolic anterior motion of the mitral valve. Experimental validation and insights into the mechanism of subaortic obstruction. *Circulation.* 1995;91(4):1189–1195.

Limongelli G, Pacileo G, Marino B, et al. Prevalence and clinical significance of cardiovascular abnormalities in patients with the LEOPARD syndrome. *Am J Cardiol.* 2007;100(4):736–741.

Lindstrom L, Wilkenshoff UM, Larsson H, Wranne B. Echocardiographic assessment of arrhythmogenic right ventricular cardiomyopathy. *Heart.* 2001;86(1):31–38.

Lopez-Fernandez T, Garcia-Fernandez MA, Pérez David E, Moreno Yangüela M. Usefulness of contrast echocardiography in arrhythmogenic right ventricular dysplasia. *J Am Soc Echocardiogr.* 2004;17(4):391–393.

Marcus F, Towbin JA, Zareba W, et al. Arrhythmogenic right ventricular dysplasia/cardiomyopathy (ARVD/C): a multidisciplinary study: design and protocol. *Circulation.* 2003;107(23):2975–2978.

Maron BJ, Epstein SE, Morrow AG. Symptomatic status and prognosis of patients after operation for hypertrophic obstructive cardiomyopathy: efficacy of ventricular septal myotomy and myectomy. *Eur Heart J.* 1983a;4(suppl F):175–185.

Maron BJ, Gottdiener JS, Epstein SE, et al. Patterns and significance of distribution of left ventricular hypertrophy in hypertrophic cardiomyopathy. A wide angle, two dimensional echocardiographic study of 125 patients. *Am J Cardiol.* 1981;48(3):418–428.

Maron BJ, Harding AM, Spirito P, Roberts WC, Waller BF. Systolic anterior motion of the posterior mitral leaflet: a previously unrecognized cause of dynamic subaortic obstruction in patients with hypertrophic cardiomyopathy. *Circulation.* 1983b;68(2):282–293.

Maron BJ, McKenna WJ, Danielson GK, et al. American College of Cardiology/European Society of Cardiology clinical expert consensus document on hypertrophic cardiomyopathy. A report of the American College of Cardiology Foundation Task Force on Clinical Expert Consensus Documents and the European Society of Cardiology Committee for Practice Guidelines. *J Am Coll Cardiol.* 2003;42(9):1687–1713.

Maron BJ, Seidman JG, Seidman CE. Proposal for contemporary screening strategies in families with hypertrophic cardiomyopathy. *J Am Coll Cardiol.* 2004;44(11):2125–2132.

Maron BJ, Spirito P. Implications of left ventricular remodeling in hypertrophic cardiomyopathy. *Am J Cardiol.* 1998;81(11):1339–1344.

Maron MS, Olivotto I, Betocchi S, et al. Effect of left ventricular outflow tract obstruction on clinical outcome in hypertrophic cardiomyopathy. *N Engl J Med.* 2003;348(4):295–303.

Maron MS, Olivotto I, Zenovich AG, et al. Hypertrophic cardiomyopathy is predominantly a disease of left ventricular outflow tract obstruction. *Circulation.* 2006;114(21):2232–2239.

Matsukida K, Kisanuki A, Toyonaga K, et al. Comparison of transthoracic Doppler echocardiography and natriuretic peptides in predicting mean pulmonary capillary wedge pressure in patients with chronic atrial fibrillation. *J Am Soc Echocardiogr.* 2001;14(11):1080–1087.

Matsukubo H, Matsuura T, Endo N, Asayama J, Watanabe T. Echocardiographic measurement of right ventricular wall thickness. A new application of subxiphoid echocardiography. *Circulation.* 1977;56(2):278–284.

McCully RB, Nishimura RA, Bailey KR, Schaff HV, Danielson GK, Tajik AJ. Hypertrophic obstructive cardiomyopathy: preoperative echocardiographic predictors of outcome after septal myectomy. *J Am Coll Cardiol.* 1996;27(6):1491–1496.

McKenna WJ, Kleinebenne A, Nihoyannopoulos P, Foale R. Echocardiographic measurement of right ventricular wall thickness in hypertrophic cardiomyopathy: relation to clinical and prognostic features. *J Am Coll Cardiol.* 1988;11(2):351–358.

McKenna WJ, Thiene G, Nava A, et al. Diagnosis of arrhythmogenic right ventricular dysplasia/cardiomyopathy. Task Force of the Working Group Myocardial and Pericardial Disease of the European Society of Cardiology and of the Scientific Council on Cardiomyopathies of the International Society and Federation of Cardiology. *Br Heart J.* 1994;71(3):215–218.

Meluzin J, Spinarova L, Bakala J, et al. Pulsed Doppler tissue imaging of the velocity of tricuspid annular systolic motion; a new, rapid, and non-invasive method of evaluating right ventricular systolic function. *Eur Heart J.* 2001;22(4):340–348.

Mendez HM. The neurofibromatosis-Noonan syndrome. *Am J Med Genet.* 1985;21(3):471–476.

Mestroni L, Krajinovic M, Severini GM, et al. Familial dilated cardiomyopathy. *Br Heart J.* 1994;72(6 suppl):S35–S41.

Mestroni L, Maisch B, McKenna WJ, et al. Guidelines for the study of familial dilated cardiomyopathies. Collaborative Research Group of the European Human and Capital Mobility Project on Familial Dilated Cardiomyopathy. *Eur Heart J.* 1999;20(2):93–102.

Mestroni L, Miani D, Di Lenarda A, et al. Clinical and pathologic study of familial dilated cardiomyopathy. *Am J Cardiol.* 1990;65(22):1449–1453.

Michels VV, Moll PP, Miller FA, et al. The frequency of familial dilated cardiomyopathy in a series of patients with idiopathic dilated cardiomyopathy. *N Engl J Med.* 1992;326(2):77–82.

Mogensen J, Murphy RT, Kubo T, et al. Frequency and clinical expression of cardiac troponin I mutations in 748 consecutive families with hypertrophic cardiomyopathy. *J Am Coll Cardiol.* 2004;44(12):2315–2325.

Nageh MF, Kopelen HA, Zoghbi WA, Quiñones MA, Nagueh SF. Estimation of mean right atrial pressure using tissue Doppler imaging. *Am J Cardiol.* 1999a;84(12):1448–1451, A8.

Nagueh SF, Bachinski LL, Meyer D, et al. Tissue Doppler imaging consistently detects myocardial abnormalities in patients with hypertrophic cardiomyopathy and provides a novel means for an early diagnosis before and independently of hypertrophy. *Circulation.* 2001;104(2):128–130.

Nagueh SF, Kopelen HA, Quiñones MA. Assessment of left ventricular filling pressures by Doppler in the presence of atrial fibrillation. *Circulation.* 1996a;94(9):2138–2145.

Nagueh SF, Kopelen HA, Zoghbi WA. Relation of mean right atrial pressure to echocardiographic and Doppler parameters of right atrial and right ventricular function. *Circulation.* 1996b;93(6):1160–1169.

Nagueh SF, Lakkis NM, He ZX, et al. Role of myocardial contrast echocardiography during nonsurgical septal reduction therapy for hypertrophic obstructive cardiomyopathy. *J Am Coll Cardiol.* 1998a;32(1):225–229.

Nagueh SF, Lakkis NM, Middleton KJ, Spencer WH 3rd, Zoghbi WA, Quiñones MA. Doppler estimation of left ventricular filling pressures in patients with hypertrophic cardiomyopathy. *Circulation.* 1999b;99(2):254–261.

Nagueh SF, Mikati I, Kopelen HA, Middleton KJ, Quiñones MA, Zoghbi WA. Doppler estimation of left ventricular filling pressure in sinus tachycardia. A new application of tissue doppler imaging. *Circulation.* 1998b;98(16):1644–1650.

Nakamura T, Matsubara K, Furukawa K, et al. Diastolic paradoxic jet flow in patients with hypertrophic cardiomyopathy: evidence of concealed apical asynergy with cavity obliteration. *J Am Coll Cardiol.* 1992;19(3):516–524.

Nakao S, Takenaka T, Maeda M, et al. An atypical variant of Fabry's disease in men with left ventricular hypertrophy. *N Engl J Med.* 1995;333(5):288–293.

Naqvi TZ, Goel RK, Forrester JS, Siegel RJ. Myocardial contractile reserve on dobutamine echocardiography predicts late spontaneous improvement in cardiac function in patients with recent onset idiopathic dilated cardiomyopathy. *J Am Coll Cardiol.* 1999;34(5):1537–1544.

Nava A, Bauce B, Basso C, et al. Clinical profile and long-term follow-up of 37 families with arrhythmogenic right ventricular cardiomyopathy. *J Am Coll Cardiol.* 2000;36(7):2226–2233.

Nishimura RA, Appleton CP, Redfield MM, Ilstrup DM, Holmes DR Jr, Tajik AJ. Noninvasive doppler echocardiographic evaluation of left ventricular filling pressures in patients with cardiomyopathies: a simultaneous Doppler echocardiographic and cardiac catheterization study. *J Am Coll Cardiol.* 1996;28(5):1226–1233.

Norman M, Simpson M, Mogensen J, et al. Novel mutation in desmoplakin causes arrhythmogenic left ventricular cardiomyopathy. *Circulation.* 2005;112(5):636–642.

Notomi Y, Lysyansky P, Setser RM, et al. Measurement of ventricular torsion by two-dimensional ultrasound speckle tracking imaging. *J Am Coll Cardiol.* 2005;45(12):2034–2041.

Ommen SR, Nishimura RA, Appleton CP, et al. Clinical utility of Doppler echocardiography and tissue Doppler imaging in the estimation of left ventricular filling pressures: a comparative simultaneous Doppler-catheterization study. *Circulation.* 2000;102(15):1788–1794.

Palau F. Friedreich's ataxia and frataxin: molecular genetics, evolution and pathogenesis (Review). *Int J Mol Med.* 2001;7(6):581–589.

Palka P, Lange A, Donnelly JE, Nihoyannopoulos P. Differentiation between restrictive cardiomyopathy and constrictive pericarditis by early diastolic doppler myocardial velocity gradient at the posterior wall. *Circulation.* 2000;102(6):655–662.

Palka P, Lange A, Fleming AD, et al. Differences in myocardial velocity gradient measured throughout the cardiac cycle in patients with hypertrophic cardiomyopathy, athletes and patients with left ventricular hypertrophy due to hypertension. *J Am Coll Cardiol.* 1997;30(3):760–768.

Panza JA, Petrone RK, Fananapazir L, Maron BJ. Utility of continuous wave Doppler echocardiography in the noninvasive assessment of left ventricular outflow tract pressure gradient in patients with hypertrophic cardiomyopathy. *J Am Coll Cardiol.* 1992;19(1):91–99.

Parisi M, Galderisi M, Sidiropulos M, et al. Early detection of biventricular involvement in myotonic dystrophy by tissue Doppler. *Int J Cardiol.* 2007;118(2):227–232.

Park TH, Lakkis NM, Middleton KJ, et al. Acute effect of nonsurgical septal reduction therapy on regional left ventricular asynchrony in patients with hypertrophic obstructive cardiomyopathy. *Circulation.* 2002;106(4):412–415.

Pellerin D, Berdeaux A, Cohen L, Giudicelli JF, Witchitz S, Veyrat C. Comparison of 2 myocardial velocity gradient assessment methods during dobutamine infusion with Doppler myocardial imaging. *J Am Soc Echocardiogr.* 1999;12(1):22–31.

Pellerin D, Brecker S, Veyrat C. Degenerative mitral valve disease with emphasis on mitral valve prolapse. *Heart.* 2002a;88(suppl 4):iv20–8.

Pellerin D, Brecker SJ. A step further in inter-institutional agreement in interpretation of dobutamine stress echocardiograms. *Eur Heart J.* 2002b;23(10):768–771.

Pellerin D, Dubourg O, Coisne D, Extramiana F, Witchitz S, Veyrat C. Contribution of doppler imaging of the myocardium to the study of cardiomyopathies. *Arch Mal Coeur Vaiss.* 1998;91(12 suppl):51–58.

Pellerin D, Sharma R, Elliott P, Veyrat C. Tissue Doppler, strain, and strain rate echocardiography for the assessment of left and right systolic ventricular function. *Heart.* 2003;89(suppl 3):iii9–17.

Pelliccia A, Maron BJ, Spataro A, Proschan MA, Spirito P. The upper limit of physiologic cardiac hypertrophy in highly trained elite athletes. *N Engl J Med.* 1991;324(5):295–301.

Pelliccia A, Spataro A, Caselli G, Maron BJ. Absence of left ventricular wall thickening in athletes engaged in intense power training. *Am J Cardiol.* 1993;72(14):1048–1054.

Petrone RK, Klues HG, Panza JA, Peterson EE, Maron BJ. Coexistence of mitral valve prolapse in a consecutive group of 528 patients with hypertrophic cardiomyopathy assessed with echocardiography. *J Am Coll Cardiol.* 1992;20(1):55–61.

Pieroni M, Chimenti C, Ricci R, Sale P, Russo MA, Frustaci A. Early detection of Fabry cardiomyopathy by tissue Doppler imaging. *Circulation.* 2003;107(15):1978–1984.

Pinamonti B, Pagnan L, Bussani R, Ricci C, Silvestri F, Camerini F. Right ventricular dysplasia with biventricular involvement. *Circulation.* 1998;98(18):1943–1945.

Pollick C, Morgan CD, Gilbert BW, Rakowski H, Wigle ED. Muscular subaortic stenosis: the temporal relationship between systolic anterior motion of the anterior mitral leaflet and the pressure gradient. *Circulation.* 1982;66(5):1087–1094.

Pozzoli M, Traversi E, Cioffi G, Stenner R, Sanarico M, Tavazzi L. Loading manipulations improve the prognostic value of Doppler evaluation of mitral flow in patients with chronic heart failure. *Circulation.* 1997;95(5):1222–1230.

Prakasa KR, Dalal D, Wang J, et al. Feasibility and variability of three dimensional echocardiography in arrhythmogenic right ventricular dysplasia/cardiomyopathy. *Am J Cardiol.* 2006;97(5):703–709.

Prakasa KR, Wang J, Tandri H, et al. Utility of tissue Doppler and strain echocardiography in arrhythmogenic right ventricular dysplasia/cardiomyopathy. *Am J Cardiol.* 2007;100(3):507–512.

Pu M, Griffin BP, Vandervoort PM, Stewart WJ, Fan X, Cosgrove DM. The value of assessing pulmonary venous flow velocity for predicting severity of mitral regurgitation: a quantitative assessment integrating left ventricular function. *J Am Soc Echocardiogr.* 1999;12(9):736–743.

Rajagopalan N, Garcia MJ, Rodriguez L, et al. Comparison of new Doppler echocardiographic methods to differentiate constrictive pericardial heart disease and restrictive cardiomyopathy. *Am J Cardiol.* 2001;87(1):86–94.

Rakowski H, Sasson Z, Wigle ED. Echocardiographic and Doppler assessment of hypertrophic cardiomyopathy. *J Am Soc Echocardiogr.* 1988;1(1):31–47.

Richard P, Charron P, Carrier L, et al. Hypertrophic cardiomyopathy: distribution of disease genes, spectrum of mutations, and implications for a molecular diagnosis strategy. *Circulation.* 2003;107(17):2227–2232.

Richardson P, McKenna W, Bristow M, et al. Report of the 1995 World Health Organization/International Society and Federation of Cardiology Task Force on the Definition and Classification of cardiomyopathies. *Circulation.* 1996;93(5):841–842.

Rigo F, Gherardi S, Galderisi M, et al. The prognostic impact of coronary flow-reserve assessed by Doppler echocardiography in non-ischaemic dilated cardiomyopathy. *Eur Heart J.* 2006;27(11):1319–1323.

Rossvoll O, Hatle LK. Pulmonary venous flow velocities recorded by transthoracic Doppler ultrasound: relation to left ventricular diastolic pressures. *J Am Coll Cardiol.* 1993;21(7):1687–1696.

Sakamoto T. Apical hypertrophic cardiomyopathy (apical hypertrophy): an overview. *J Cardiol.* 2001;37(suppl 1):161–178.

Sanyal SK, Johnson WW, Dische MR, Pitner SE, Beard C. Dystrophic degeneration of papillary muscle and ventricular myocardium. A basis for mitral valve prolapse in Duchenne's muscular dystrophy. *Circulation.* 1980;62(2):430–438.

Schiffmann R, Kopp JB, Austin HA 3rd, et al. Enzyme replacement therapy in Fabry disease: a randomized controlled trial. *JAMA.* 2001;285(21):2743–2749.

Schoendube FA, Klues HG, Reith S, Flachskampf FA, Hanrath P, Messmer BJ. Long-term clinical and echocardiographic follow-up after surgical correction of hypertrophic obstructive cardiomyopathy with extended myectomy and reconstruction of the subvalvular mitral apparatus. *Circulation.* 1995;92(9 suppl):II122–27.

Seidman JG, Seidman C. The genetic basis for cardiomyopathy: from mutation identification to mechanistic paradigms. *Cell.* 2001;104(4):557–567.

Sengupta PP, Mohan JC, Mehta V, et al. Comparison of echocardiographic features of noncompaction of the left ventricle in adults versus idiopathic dilated cardiomyopathy in adults. *Am J Cardiol.* 2004;94(3):389–391.

Shapiro LM, McKenna WJ. Distribution of left ventricular hypertrophy in hypertrophic cardiomyopathy: a two-dimensional echocardiographic study. *J Am Coll Cardiol.* 1983;2(3):437–444.

Sharma R, Smith J, Elliott PM, McKenna WJ, Pellerin D. Left ventricular outflow tract obstruction caused by accessory mitral valve tissue. *J Am Soc Echocardiogr.* 2006;19(3):354. e5–354, e8.

Sharma S, Elliott PM, Whyte G, et al. Utility of metabolic exercise testing in distinguishing hypertrophic cardiomyopathy from physiologic left ventricular hypertrophy in athletes. *J Am Coll Cardiol.* 2000;36(3): 864–870.

Sharma S, Maron BJ, Whyte G, Firoozi S, Elliott PM, McKenna WJ. Physiologic limits of left ventricular hypertrophy in elite junior athletes: relevance to differential diagnosis of athlete's heart and hypertrophic cardiomyopathy. *J Am Coll Cardiol.* 2002;40(8):1431–1436.

Sigwart U. Non-surgical myocardial reduction for hypertrophic obstructive cardiomyopathy. *Lancet.* 1995;346(8969):211–214.

Siu SC, Levine RA, Rivera JM, et al. Three-dimensional echocardiography improves noninvasive assessment of left ventricular volume and performance. *Am Heart J.* 1995;130(4):812–822.

Sohn DW, Chai IH, Lee DJ, et al. Assessment of mitral annulus velocity by Doppler tissue imaging in the evaluation of left ventricular diastolic function. *J Am Coll Cardiol.* 1997;30(2):474–480.

Sohn DW, Song JM, Zo JH et al. Mitral annulus velocity in the evaluation of left ventricular diastolic function in atrial fibrillation. *J Am Soc Echocardiogr.* 1999;12(11):927–931.

Spirito P, Bellone P, Harris KM, Bernabo P, Bruzzi P, Maron BJ. Magnitude of left ventricular hypertrophy and risk of sudden death in hypertrophic cardiomyopathy. *N Engl J Med.* 2000;342(24):1778–1785.

Spirito P, Maron BJ. Significance of left ventricular outflow tract cross-sectional area in hypertrophic cardiomyopathy: a two-dimensional echocardiographic assessment. *Circulation.* 1983;67(5):1100–1108.

Spirito P, Maron BJ. Relation between extent of left ventricular hypertrophy and occurrence of sudden cardiac death in hypertrophic cardiomyopathy. *J Am Coll Cardiol.* 1990;15(7):1521–1526.

Spirito P, Maron BJ, Bonow RO, Epstein SE. Occurrence and significance of progressive left ventricular wall thinning and relative cavity dilatation in hypertrophic cardiomyopathy. *Am J Cardiol.* 1987;60(1):123–129.

Spirito P, Pelliccia A, Proschan MA, et al. Morphology of the athlete's heart assessed by echocardiography in 947 elite athletes representing 27 sports. *Am J Cardiol.* 1994;74(8):802–806.

Streib EW, Meyers DG, Sun SF. Mitral valve prolapse in myotonic dystrophy. *Muscle Nerve.* 1985;8(8):650–653.

Teragaki M, Tanaka A, Akioka K, et al. Fabry disease female proband with clinical manifestations similar to hypertrophic cardiomyopathy. *Jpn Heart J.* 2004;45(4):685–689.

Tribouilloy C, Shen WF, Quéré JP, et al. Assessment of severity of mitral regurgitation by measuring regurgitant jet width at its origin with transesophageal Doppler color flow imaging. *Circulation.* 1992;85(4):1248–1253.

Troughton RW, Prior DL, Frampton CM, et al. Usefulness of tissue doppler and color M-mode indexes of left ventricular diastolic function in predicting outcomes in systolic left ventricular heart failure (from the ADEPT study). *Am J Cardiol.* 2005;96(2):257–262.

Tse HF, Ho HH. Sudden cardiac death caused by hypertrophic cardiomyopathy associated with midventricular obstruction and apical aneurysm. *Heart.* 2003;89(2):178.

Vinereanu D, Bajaj BP, Fenton-May J, Rogers MT, Mädler CF, Fraser AG. Subclinical cardiac involvement in myotonic dystrophy manifesting as decreased myocardial Doppler velocities. *Neuromuscul Disord.* 2004;14(3):188–194.

Vinereanu D, Florescu N, Sculthorpe N, Tweddel AC, Stephens MR, Fraser AG. Differentiation between pathologic and physiologic left ventricular hypertrophy by tissue Doppler assessment of long-axis function in patients with hypertrophic cardiomyopathy or systemic hypertension and in athletes. *Am J Cardiol.* 2001;88(1):53–58.

Vogel M, Schmidt MR, Kristiansen SB, et al. Validation of myocardial acceleration during isovolumic contraction as a novel noninvasive index of right ventricular contractility: comparison with ventricular pressure-volume relations in an animal model. *Circulation.* 2002;105(14):1693–1699.

Wang J, Prakasa K, Bomma C, et al. Comparison of novel echocardiographic parameters of right ventricular function with ejection fraction by cardiac magnetic resonance. *J Am Soc Echocardiogr.* 2007;20(9):1058–1064.

Weidemann F, Breunig F, Beer M, et al. Improvement of cardiac function during enzyme replacement therapy in patients with Fabry disease: a prospective strain rate imaging study. *Circulation.* 2003;108(11): 1299–1301.

Wichter T, Paul M, et al. Right ventricular arrhythmias. *Internist (Berl).* 2004;45(10):1125–1135.

Wigle ED, Sasson Z, Henderson MA, et al. Hypertrophic cardiomyopathy. The importance of the site and the extent of hypertrophy. A review. *Prog Cardiovasc Dis.* 1985;28(1):1–83.

Wong CY, O'Moore-Sullivan T, Leano R, Hukins C, Jenkins C, Marwick TH. Association of subclinical right ventricular dysfunction with obesity. *J Am Coll Cardiol.* 2006;47(3):611–616.

Wood MJ, Picard MH. Utility of echocardiography in the evaluation of individuals with cardiomyopathy. *Heart.* 2004;90(6):707–712.

Yang H, Sun JP, Lever HM, et al. Use of strain imaging in detecting segmental dysfunction in patients with hypertrophic cardiomyopathy. *J Am Soc Echocardiogr.* 2003;16(3):233–239.

Yang H, Woo A, Monakier D, et al. Enlarged left atrial volume in hypertrophic cardiomyopathy: a marker for disease severity. *J Am Soc Echocardiogr.* 2005a;18(10):1074–1082.

Yang HS, Song JK, Song JM, et al. Comparison of the clinical features of apical hypertrophic cardiomyopathy versus asymmetric septal hypertrophy in Korea. *Korean J Intern Med.* 2005b;20(2):111–115.

Yiu SF, Enriquez-Sarano M, Tribouilloy C, Seward JB, Tajik AJ. Determinants of the degree of functional mitral regurgitation in patients with systolic left ventricular dysfunction: a quantitative clinical study. *Circulation.* 2000;102(12):1400–1406.

Yoerger DM, Marcus F, Sherrill D, et al. Echocardiographic findings in patients meeting task force criteria for arrhythmogenic right ventricular dysplasia: new insights from the multidisciplinary study of right ventricular dysplasia. *J Am Coll Cardiol.* 2005;45(6):860–865.

Yu EH, Omran AS, Wigle ED, Williams WG, Siu SC, Rakowski H. Mitral regurgitation in hypertrophic obstructive cardiomyopathy: relationship to obstruction and relief with myectomy. *J Am Coll Cardiol.* 2000;36(7):2219–2225.

Zhu H, Muro T, Hozumi T, et al. Usefulness of left ventricular opacification with intravenous contrast echocardiography in patients with asymptomatic negative T waves on electrocardiography. *J Cardiol.* 2002;40(6):259–265.

Part II

Specific Cardiovascular Genetic Disorders

9

Congenital Cardiovascular Malformations

Judith Goodship and Christopher Wren

Cardiovascular malformations (CVMs) affect 7–8 per 1,000 live births and account for 10% of all infant deaths in Western countries and nearly half of all infant deaths from malformation. Around 15% of affected infants die in the first year, 4% of those surviving infancy dying by 16 years (Knowles et al. 2005). Additional noncardiac malformations are present in about a quarter of children with CVMs (Ferencz et al. 1993). The presence of an associated noncardiac malformation suggests the possibility of an underlying chromosomal abnormality or genetic syndrome. Chromosome abnormalities detectable by standard karyotyping are present in 13% of children with CVM (Ferencz et al. 1997). The introduction of routine testing to detect submicroscopic chromosome 22q11 deletions has shown that this chromosomal abnormality accounts for an additional 2% of CVM (Botto et al. 2003). Molecular cytogenetic techniques that detect submicroscopic deletions and duplications across the genome can identify the basis for the CVM in further cases, though the proportion of CVM due to these small deletions and duplications is not yet clear. A syndrome diagnosis can be made in approximately a further 5% of children with CVM. However, the majority of CVMs are isolated abnormalities of unknown cause.

The Genetic Consultation

Whilst the major concern for parents of children with a CVM is the well-being of their child the questions that dominate the genetic consultation are "Why did it happen?" and "Will it happen again?" This is addressed clinically by taking the family history, documenting maternal health and exposures in pregnancy, and assessing whether the child has an isolated CVM or CVM in association with additional abnormalities.

Family History

For some CVMs, families with multiple affected individuals have been reported so a three-generation family history should always be recorded before giving recurrence risks. In addition to providing more accurate information this may identify a family that is large enough to map and identify a new CVM gene. The incidence of CVM is higher in monozygotic twins (Burn and Corney 1984). As it is not uncommon for one of a twin pregnancy to be lost before term one should ask specifically if a first trimester obstetric ultrasound was performed and how many embryos were seen as the family is unlikely to volunteer this information as they will not be aware of its importance.

Maternal History

The maternal illnesses carrying the highest risk of CVM in offspring are rubella (Gregg et al. 1945), phenylketonuria (Lenke and Levy 1980; Levy et al. 2001), and diabetes (Wren et al. 2003). Whilst maternal rubella is rare in countries with vaccination programmes it should still be considered. Untreated maternal phenylketonuria is associated with a greater than sixfold increase in CVM risk, including tetralogy of Fallot (TOF), ventricular septal defect (VSD), patent ductus arteriosus (PDA), and single ventricle. Strict dietary control before conception and in the first seven weeks of gestation reduces this risk. The spectrum of defects for which risk is increased in offspring of diabetics is broad including laterality disturbance, transposition of the great arteries (TGA), atrioventricular septal defect (AVSD), VSD, hypoplastic left heart (HLH), outflow tract defects, and PDA. Good glycemic control before conception and during pregnancy decreases the risk but may be difficult to achieve. Offspring of women with epilepsy are at increased risk of congenital malformations including CVM (Pradat 1992; Hernandez-Diaz et al. 2000); this may be due to a direct teratogenic effect of anticonvulsant therapy or an indirect effect of perturbed folate metabolism. Support for the latter hypothesis comes from the observation that CVM incidence is increased in offspring of mothers who were prescribed trimethoprim in the first trimester but to a lesser extent when mothers also took folic acid supplementation (Czeizel et al. 2001). CVM is also a feature of fetal alcohol syndrome (Clarren and Smith 1978), thalidomide embryopathy (Smithells and Newman 1992), and isoretinoin embryopathy (Geiger et al. 1994).

Examining the Child

CVM may occur in combination with other malformations or dysmorphic features that provide clues to a broader chromosomal or syndromic diagnosis. Making such a diagnosis has implications for the management of the child and possibly of the wider

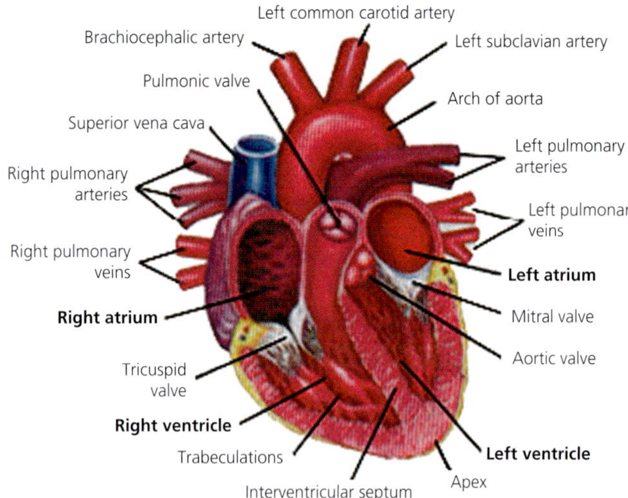

Figure 9–1 Diagram of normal heart.

family. For example, recognition that a baby is likely to have learning, hearing, or visual impairment will lead to screening and early input from relevant agencies. A chromosomal/syndrome diagnosis enables accurate recurrence risks to be given to the couple, for example, reassurance of a low recurrence with a de novo genetic event or the 25% recurrence risk associated with a recessive disorder. As limb abnormalities are present in a number of CVM syndromes, record whether the limbs are normal or the presence of any abnormalities such as polydactyly (and whether pre- or postaxial) and abnormalities of the thumb/radial ray. Record the height, weight, and head circumference and developmental milestones. Note the quality of speech as well as speech development as velopharyngeal insufficiency is common in children who have a chromosome 22q11 deletion. If there are multiple congenital malformations, dysmorphic features, pre- and postnatal retardation of growth, unexplained developmental delay, or any combination of these features in association with CVM, chromosome analysis should be requested unless the pattern is that of a recognizable Mendelian syndrome. The approach to making a syndrome diagnosis and examples of syndromes in which CVMs are common are covered in Chapter 10 and chromosomal abnormalities in which CVMs are common are covered in Chapter 5.

Cardiovascular Malformations

The processes by which the early heart tube is formed, the addition of cells to the ventral end of this linear tube forming the right ventricle and outflow tract, septation of the chambers, and development of the valves to form the normal heart (Figure 9–1) are described in Chapter 1. Perturbations at many points in this finely controlled complex developmental process will lead to a CVM. In this section we describe the commoner CVMs noting some of the syndromes with which they are associated. A recent American Heart Association scientific statement gives more comprehensive listings of associated syndromes and chromosomal abnormalities (Pierpont et al. 2007).

There are a number of approaches to ordering the malformations, for example, by incidence, severity, presentation, or according to the developmental abnormality. Each method has limitations; we have chosen to list the malformations from inflow to outflow tract recognizing that this also has limitations as some malformations affect both the right and left sides of the heart. As CVMs may be isolated or may occur in combination, we have noted common associations between the CVMs in the following subsections.

Total Anomalous Pulmonary Venous Connection

In total anomalous pulmonary venous connection (TAPVC) all four pulmonary veins fail to connect with the left atrium and instead join the systemic venous system. The connection is variable in position and in degree of obstruction. It may be supracardiac to the innominate vein or superior vena cava, infradiaphragmatic to the hepatic or portal vein or intracardiac to the coronary sinus or right atrium. There is an atrial septal defect (ASD) with flow from the right to the left atrium. The timing and mode of presentation depend on whether the anomalous connection is obstructed, infradiaphragmatic connections being most commonly obstructed. Infants present with a combination of cyanosis and heart failure and may be very ill by the time the diagnosis is made. Surgical repair entails reconnection of the pulmonary veins to the left atrium. The long-term outlook for survivors of surgery is very good although in some infants there is recurrent and progressive pulmonary vein stenosis. Medium-term mortality ranges from 8% to 35%, being significantly better if TAPVC is an isolated malformation (Hancock Friesen et al. 2005).

Most cases of TAPVC are sporadic but there have been a few families with multiple affected individuals in more than one generation reported (Bleyl et al. 1995). TAPVC is associated with Cat Eye syndrome, which is caused by an additional marker chromosome derived from chromosome 22. Formation of the marker chromosome is mediated by interchromosomal recombination between inverted low copy repeats on chromosome 22. Thus the marker comprises two centromeres with satellites (ribosomal RNA genes) with two copies of the proximal region of the long arm of chromosome 22 between them. Usually this is a mosaic chromosome abnormality, that is, the marker is present in only a proportion of cells, such that affected individuals have four copies (tetrasomy) of the genes on proximal chromosome 22q11 in a proportion of their cells.

Atrial Septal Defect

ASD is one of the commonest CVMs with a reported prevalence of around 50–100 per 100,000 live births (Hoffman 1987). Children with ASD are usually asymptomatic and present with a murmur. The natural history is development of heart failure in adult life and adult presentation is still fairly common. Treatment involves surgical or transcatheter closure of the defect. The closure of the ASD in childhood leads to a normal life expectancy and quality of life.

ASD is most often an isolated malformation but also frequently occurs in association with other CVMs. It is common in trisomy 21 and trisomy 18, and with a number of chromosome deletions including Wolf Hirschhorn syndrome (4p deletion), Cri du Chat syndrome (5p deletion), and 8p23.1 deletion. It occurs in a number of syndromes including Holt-Oram syndrome, Rubenstein-Taybi syndrome, and Kabuki syndrome. It also occurs in fetal alcohol syndrome. Whilst usually sporadic, dominant families have been described and mutations identified in NKX2.5 (Schott et al. 1998) and GATA4 (Garg et al. 2003).

Complete Atrioventricular Septal Defect

Complete atrioventricular septal defect (CAVSD) is a major malformation of the lower part of the atrial septum, the inlet part of the ventricular septum, and the atrioventricular valve(s). There is a common atrioventricular valve in place of the mitral and tricuspid valves. The common valve usually has five leaflets and is often regurgitant. CAVSD is present in around 30 per 100,000 live births (Hoffman 1987). The majority of infants present with heart failure in infancy if detection of a murmur has not led to investigation earlier. Some infants with a relatively high pulmonary resistance remain well with no murmur and no heart failure in which case the defect may be inoperable when the diagnosis is made. Without treatment, the natural history is premature death from heart failure in infancy, heart failure with an associated infection (such as bronchiolitis) in infancy, or from irreversible pulmonary vascular disease (Eisenmenger's syndrome) in later childhood or early adult life. Surgical repair involves patch closure of the VSD, division of the common atrioventricular valve into left and right atrioventricular valves, and patch closure of the ASD. In most cases postoperative atrioventricular valve function is good although long-term surveillance is required and reoperation for atrioventricular valve regurgitation is sometimes necessary. In the past this was a dangerous operation with high mortality but in recent years the mortality has been close to zero.

Sixty percent of cases of CAVSD occur in the context of Down syndrome and CAVSD accounts for almost half of the CVMs seen in Down syndrome. CAVSD is also associated with trisomies 13 and 18, and chromosomal deletions, for example, chromosome 3p25 deletion. CAVSD occurs in Smith-Lemli-Opitz syndrome and Ellis-van Creveld syndrome. Whilst isolated CAVSD is usually sporadic a few families have been reported that appear to be dominant with partial penetrance (Wilson et al. 1993; Sheffield et al. 1997).

Ventricular Septal Defect

VSD is the commonest CVM with a median reported prevalence of 300 per 100,000 live births (Hoffman 1987). Prevalence figures depend on the technology used to detect them—Doppler ultrasound can detect VSDs too small to produce a murmur, many of which are of no functional or clinical importance and will close spontaneously. Studies in which echocardiograms were performed on every newborn infant identified tiny muscular VSDs in 2%–5%. Recent years have seen a steady increase in the reported prevalence of VSD but the number of significant VSDs that require closure has not changed, being around 60 per 100,000 live births.

Large VSDs cause heart failure in infancy and, untreated, lead to early death or pulmonary vascular disease. Treatment by surgical repair gives a normal life expectancy. Small VSDs are usually asymptomatic and don't require treatment. Many close spontaneously in the first few years of life.

VSDs are most often isolated malformations but they are very common in association with other CVMs and are components of more complex malformation such as TOF and truncus arteriosus. VSDs are associated with many chromosomal abnormalities, for example, trisomies 13, 18, and 21, and syndromes, for example, Cornelia-de Lange syndrome, Rubenstein-Taybi syndrome, Holt-Oram syndrome, and CHARGE association amongst others.

Tetralogy of Fallot

This is the commonest type of cyanotic heart disease in infancy, occurring in around 30 per 100,000 live births. (Hoffman) It is a combination of a large subaortic VSD with anterior displacement of the aorta, which produces complex right ventricular outflow obstruction (Figure 9–2). Most diagnoses are made in infancy after recognition of cyanosis or a heart murmur. Management depends on the severity of the outflow obstruction. Excessive or increasing cyanosis, or hypercyanotic spells, are managed by an early palliative aortopulmonary shunt, which increases the pulmonary artery flow. The eventual aim is definitive repair, with closure of the VSD and relief of the pulmonary outflow obstruction. Surgical repair of TOF was one of the first cardiopulmonary bypass operations and the age at operation has come down dramatically over the years. A generation ago surgery was usually performed at school age; the median age at repair now in many units is around 1 year. Current surgical mortality is low, of the order of 1%. The results of surgery are generally good with relatively few further problems during childhood. The surgery often produces pulmonary regurgitation, which may cause further problems and require further surgery in some patients in adult life.

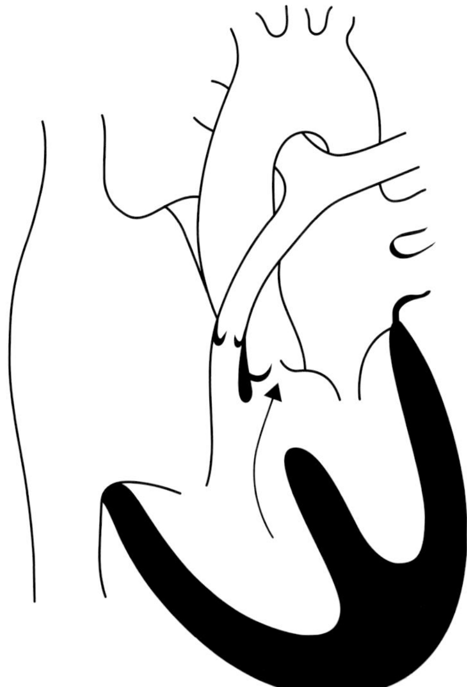

Figure 9–2 Tetralogy of Fallot.

Tetralogy of Fallot is usually an isolated malformation but sometimes occurs in association with other CVMs such as anomalous pulmonary venous connection, AVSD, and so on. It occurs in around 15% of children with 22q11 deletion and this deletion is present in around 5%–10% of infants with TOF (Goldmuntz et al. 1998). TOF also occurs in around 5% of children with trisomy 21 and trisomy 21 accounts for around 5% of infants with TOF. It is also associated with trisomies 13 and 18, and has been documented in a number of syndromes.

Pulmonary Stenosis

This is most often an isolated abnormality, with incomplete opening of the pulmonary valve caused by fusion of the valve cusps. The valve may be bicuspid or dysplastic. The right ventricular pressure is higher to overcome the obstruction and the pressure difference between right ventricle and pulmonary artery is the most accurate measure of the severity of stenosis. Management depends on the severity of the stenosis. Mild stenosis is left untreated because there are no symptoms and the long-term outlook is good. Moderate or severe stenosis is treated with a valvotomy, usually accomplished by a transvenous balloon dilation rather than surgery. The results of valvotomy are good; pulmonary regurgitation may be detectable on echocardiography but is rarely clinically significant.

Pulmonary valve stenosis is most often sporadic but it is associated with Noonan syndrome (25% of Noonan syndrome patients have pulmonary stenosis), Costello syndrome, LEOPARD syndrome, Alagille syndrome, and various chromosome deletions and duplications.

Pulmonary Atresia

The term pulmonary atresia (PA) describes a group of malformations that have in common the absence of a direct connection between the heart and the lungs. The two main types are PA with intact ventricular septum (PA/IVS) (Figure 9–3) and PA with VSD (PA/VSD). In PA/IVS the right ventricle and tricuspid valve are usually severely hypoplastic, and the pulmonary arteries are well developed and supplied by a patent ductus. In PA/VSD, also known as TOF with PA, there are two ventricles with a single subaortic VSD and a very variable pulmonary artery blood supply—sometimes a single ductus, but more often a group of collateral vessels arising from the descending aorta. PA may also be a component of more complex malformations such as double inlet left ventricle, congenitally corrected TGA, or hearts with atrial isomerism. The combined birth prevalence of all types of PA is around 20 per 100,000 live births (Leonard et al. 2000). Almost all affected infants present early in life. In those with PA/IVS, a critically "duct-dependent" malformation, this is usually in the first few hours of life with cyanosis. In those with PA/VSD, which is less often duct dependent, presentation is with cyanosis, perhaps slightly later in infancy. Infants with PA/IVS have a functional single ventricle and the eventual aim is usually some kind of "Fontan" operation, that is, a procedure in which all venous return from the inferior and superior vena cava is directed to the pulmonary arteries. Early palliation involves creating a shunt to replace the ductus. Management of PA/VSD depends on the pulmonary blood supply. About half of those affected will eventually be suitable for definitive surgical repair with closure of the VSD and placement of a conduit to connect the right ventricle to the pulmonary arteries. Leonard and colleagues reported a total mortality of 56% with one-fifth of deaths occurring in the first week and two-thirds within the first year (for infants liveborn in 1980–1995), although the outcome has improved since then.

PA/VSD is seen in 10% of infants with chromosome 22q11 deletion and 20%–30% of cases of PA/VSD occur in the context of chromosome 22q11 deletion (Anaclerio et al. 2001).

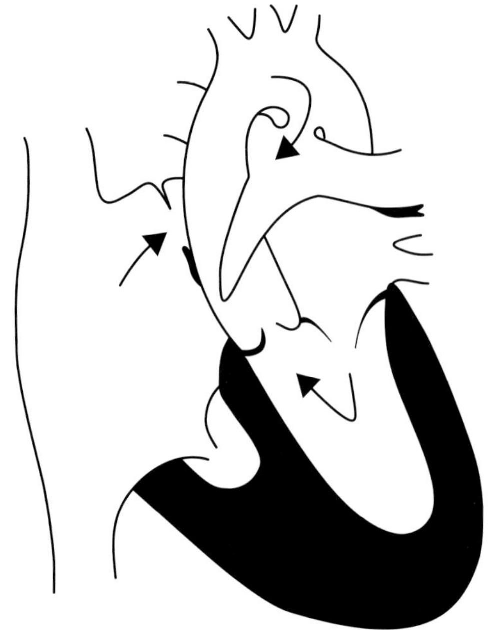

Figure 9–3 Pulmonary atresia with intact interventricular septum.

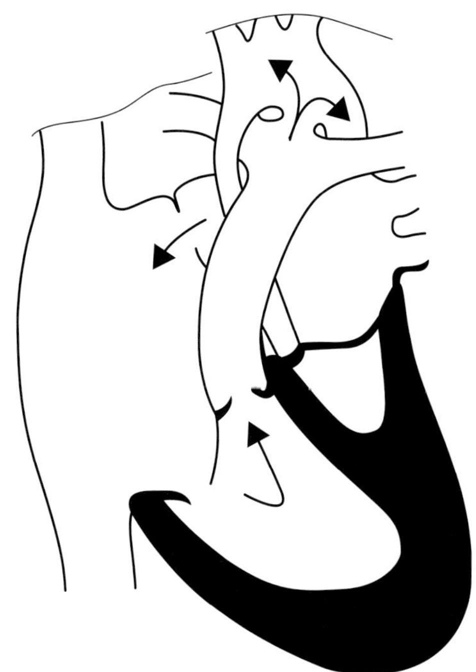

Figure 9–4 Hypoplastic left heart.

Pulmonary Artery Branch Stenosis

Pulmonary artery branch stenosis is a common cause of transient benign murmurs in neonates and is a common finding in TOF and in PA with VSD but as an isolated clinically significant problem it is rare. It may be sporadic but it is commonly associated with Williams-Beuren syndrome and Alagille syndrome.

Hypoplastic Left Heart Syndrome

In hypoplastic left heart syndrome (HLHS) the aortic valve is imperforate, the left ventricle is underdeveloped, and the mitral valve is hypoplastic or atretic (Figure 9–4). Pulmonary venous return enters the right atrium from the left atrium and the only outlet from the heart is through the pulmonary artery. The systemic circulation is duct dependent. The aortic arch is hypoplastic and the ascending aorta is very small, acting simply as a conduit for flow into the coronary arteries. The prevalence at live birth is naturally around 20 per 100,000 but is reduced by antenatal diagnosis and termination of pregnancy. The median age at diagnosis is about 2 days in those diagnosed postnatally (Wren et al. 2008). A prostaglandin infusion is given on presentation and continued after diagnosis pending a management plan. In previous years infants were often allowed to die because of the poor results of intervention. More recently, radical palliative surgery (the Norwood operation and variants that connect the right ventricle to a reconstructed aorta) has become more widespread and results have improved. In the U.K. Birmingham series, infants undergoing a Norwood operation had an actuarial 4-year survival of 44% (Ishino et al. 1999). In another report from the same center there was a 25% 6-month survival among liveborn affected infants (Brackley et al. 2000). In a recent report from Guy's Hospital, London only one-third of antenatally diagnosed infants were liveborn and 50% of the latter survived the first stage of palliation (Andrews et al. 2001).

HLHS is usually a sporadic malformation but there is a familial association with other left-sided malformations (e.g., bicuspid aortic valve and coarctation of the aorta). HLHS is associated with Turner syndrome (45,X) and Jacobsen syndrome (11q23-qter deletion) and also with nonchromosomal syndromes such as Rubenstein-Taybi syndrome.

Transposition of the Great Arteries

This is the commonest type of cyanotic congenital heart disease presenting in newborn infants, occurring in around 30 per 100,000 live births (Hoffman 1987). In "simple" transposition the main abnormality is ventriculoarterial discordance (the aorta arises from the right ventricle and the pulmonary artery from the left ventricle) (Figure 9–5). Separate pulmonary and systemic circulations are incompatible with life and early after birth some cross-flow between the circulations is maintained by patency of the duct and the foramen ovale. Most infants present in the first few days of life with cyanosis, but a few die very early before the diagnosis has been made. On recognition of cyanosis, infants are started on prostaglandin infusion to maintain ductal patency and the situation is stabilized by a balloon atrial septostomy. The normal surgical strategy is early repair with an arterial switch operation, with a surgical mortality of less than 5%. TGA is rarely found in association with genetic syndromes but is one of malformations with highest relative risk in offspring of diabetic mothers (Wren et al. 2003).

Truncus Arteriosus

Truncus arteriosus, or common arterial trunk, is a major malformation of the outflow of the heart occurring in around 10 per 100,000 live births (Hoffman 1987). It results from failure of septation of the ventricular outlets and the proximal arterial segment of the arterial tube (Figure 9–6a & b) to produce a single outlet valve overriding a subarterial VSD. Both left and right ventricular outflow occurs through the valve into a common trunk, which then separates into aorta and pulmonary arteries. The mode of connection of the pulmonary arteries to the trunk is variable. The truncal valve is usually tricuspid or quadricuspid and may be stenosed and/or regurgitant. There is often a right aortic arch and sometimes interruption of the aortic arch. Early primary repair is preferred and involves patching the VSD to the right of the truncal valve and removing the pulmonary arteries from the common trunk to leave the left ventricle connected to the aorta via the truncal valve (neoaortic valve). A conduit is then placed from the right ventricle to the pulmonary arteries to complete a biventricular repair. Results are good but later conduit replacement is inevitable.

About 10% of infants with chromosome 22q11 deletion have truncus (Ryan et al. 1997) and 30%–40% of cases of truncus arteriosus occur in the context of 22q11 deletion (Goldmuntz et al. 1998). Truncus is also associated with maternal diabetes (Loffredo et al. 2001). A recessive pedigree has been reported that was found to have an NKX2.6 mutation (Heathcote et al. 2005).

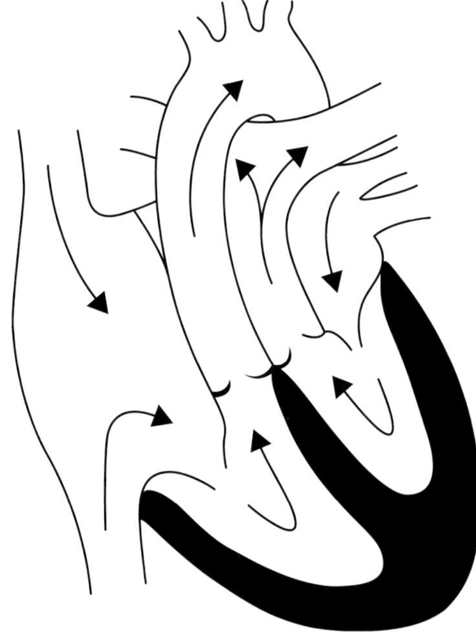

Figure 9–5 Transposition of the great arteries.

Aortic Valve Stenosis (Aortic Stenosis)

Most aortic valve stenosis is relatively mild and presents with a murmur in an asymptomatic infant or child. In neonates with severe stenosis the aortic valve is usually small and dysplastic and the left ventricle may be dilated with poor contraction or hypertrophied with preserved systolic function. Severe stenosis requires valvotomy, which can be achieved surgically or with a balloon catheter.

Isolated bicuspid aortic valve without stenosis or regurgitation is very common, occurring in 10–20 per 1,000 of general population, prevalence higher than all other congenital CVMs put together. The overall natural history of bicuspid valves is difficult to define as most go undetected in early life but around half of adults undergoing aortic valve replacement for calcific aortic stenosis have bicuspid aortic valves.

Aortic valve stenosis is most often an isolated abnormality but it is common in association with other left-sided malformations such as coarctation of the aorta and mitral valve stenosis or regurgitation. It occurs in trisomies 13 and 18, Turner syndrome, and with a variety of chromosomal deletions and duplications.

Supravalvar Aortic Stenosis

Supravalvar aortic stenosis (SVAS) is a rare malformation characterized by stenosis of the ascending aorta just above the aortic valve at the sinutubular junction (Figure 9–7) (Stamm et al. 2001). There may be a more widespread arteriopathy with stenosis of other systemic arteries and of the pulmonary arteries. SVAS is often associated with abnormalities of the immediately adjacent aortic valve producing stenosis and/or regurgitation. Various surgical techniques have been described for relief of SVAS but these have to be tailored to the complexity of the outflow obstruction in the individual patient. Other malformations—mitral valve abnormalities, coarctation of the aorta, VSD, and so on—are also reported in patients with SVAS.

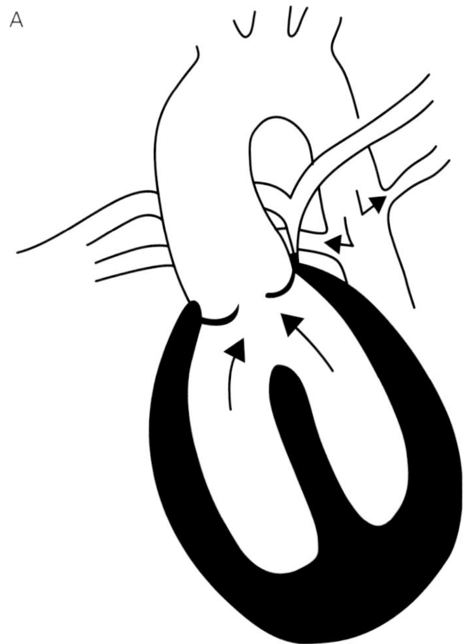

Figure 9–6a Truncus arteriosus—separate origin of pulmonary arteries.

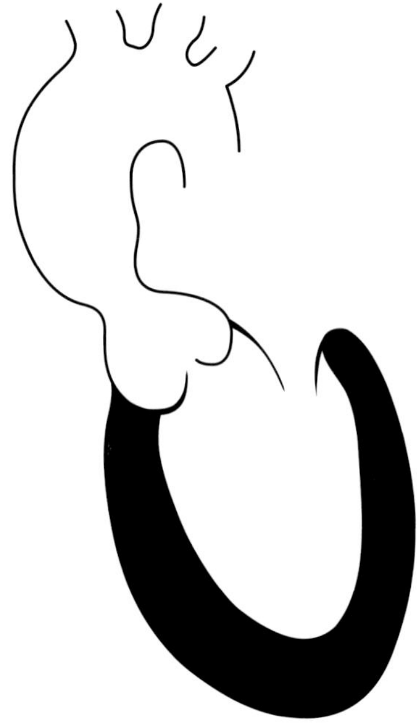

Figure 9–7 Supravalvar aortic stenosis (showing the left heart only).

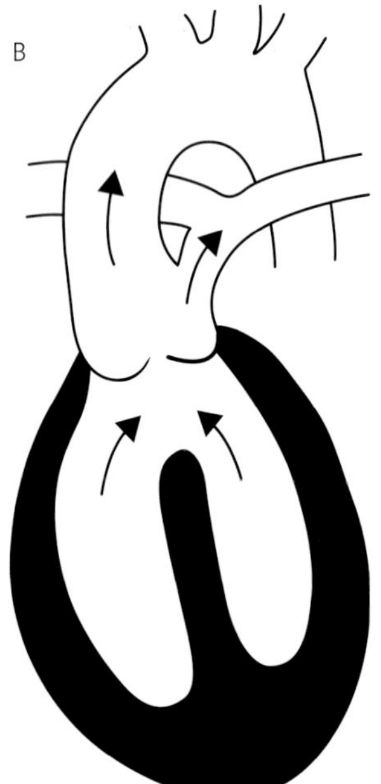

Figure 9–6b Truncus arteriosus—pulmonary artery originating direct from aorta.

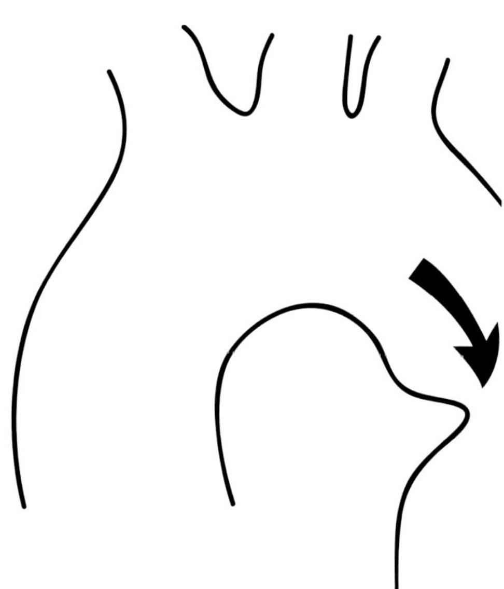

Figure 9–8 Coarctation of the aorta.

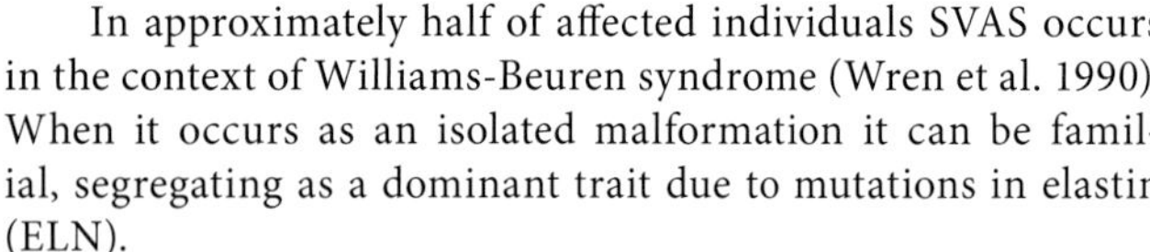

In approximately half of affected individuals SVAS occurs in the context of Williams-Beuren syndrome (Wren et al. 1990). When it occurs as an isolated malformation it can be familial, segregating as a dominant trait due to mutations in elastin (ELN).

Coarctation of the Aorta

Coarctation of the aorta (CoA) can present at any age from prenatal to adult life but most cases are diagnosed in infancy. It is the commonest cause of heart failure or cardiovascular collapse in the newborn infant. There is narrowing of the distal aortic arch adjacent to the ductus (Figure 9–8). It is often accompanied by hypoplasia of the proximal aorta and sometimes of the aortic arch. About 40% of affected infants have an associated cardiac malformation; the commonest association is a VSD or bicuspid aortic valve, but aortic valve stenosis, mitral valve problems, and more complex cardiac malformations are also common. CoA may present with heart failure or collapse in the newborn period, with heart failure or failure to thrive in infancy, and with a murmur or hypertension beyond infancy. The surgical mortality of CoA repair is low and the overall outcome depends on the associated malformations.

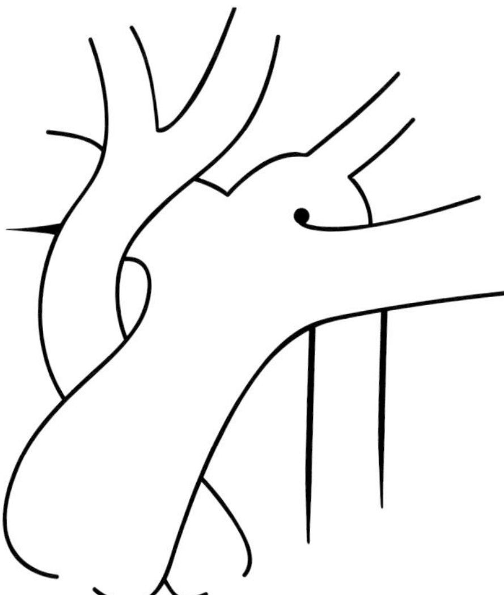

Figure 9–9 Interruption of the aortic arch.

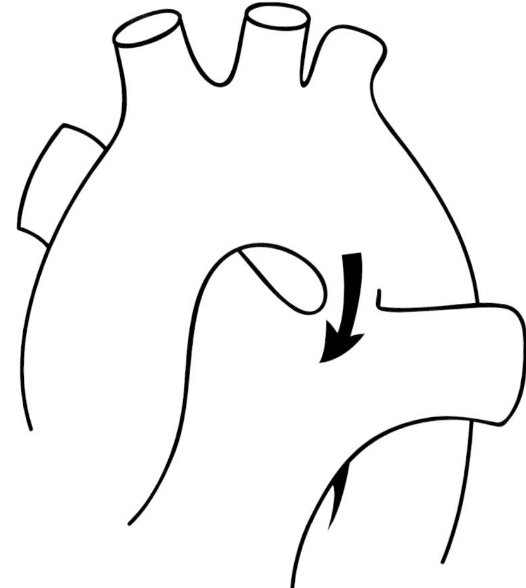

Figure 9–10 Patent ductus arteriosus.

As well as being associated with other CVMs as mentioned above, CoA is associated with Turner syndrome (45,X).

Interruption of the Aortic Arch

In interruption of the aortic arch (IAA) a portion of the aorta fails to develop and the descending aorta is entirely supplied via the ductus. The interruption may be distal to the left subclavian artery (type A) or between the left carotid and the left subclavian arteries (type B) (Figure 9–9). IAA is always associated with a major cardiac abnormality such as VSD, aortopulmonary window, truncus arteriosus, or other complex malformations. Presentation occurs early because the lower half of the body has an entirely duct-dependent circulation and patients with IAA deteriorate very quickly once their duct begins to close, with initial breathlessness, worsening into collapse and death within hours. About half go home without recognition of the problem, but all present with heart failure or death before 6 weeks of age (Wren et al. 1999). The surgical aim is primary repair of the aortic arch and what else is done depends on associated diagnoses. In the presence of an aortopulmonary window, VSD, or truncus, the usual choice would be primary repair of both the arch and the heart problem. In the presence of a double inlet ventricle or complex transposition, it would be more common to perform pulmonary artery banding for palliation. The risks associated with residual or recurrent arch obstruction and with revision procedures will impair life expectancy for this group relative to normal children. Fifty percent of cases of IAA type B occur in the context of chromosome 22q11 deletion and 15% of infants with 22q11 deletion have IAA.

Persistent (Patent) Ductus Arteriosus

The ductus is a normal component of the fetal circulation and usually closes soon after birth. If the ductus remains patent beyond 6–12 weeks postterm, it is described as "persistent" and will not close spontaneously thereafter (Figure 9–10). Patency of the ductus is common in premature infants but is then regarded as a complication of prematurity rather than a malformation. Infants with a large duct present during infancy with heart failure or signs of a significant shunt. If the duct is small the only potential problem is the small risk of infective endarteritis. Surgical or transcatheter closure of the duct is effectively curative, leading to a normal quality of life and life expectancy.

PDA is most often an isolated abnormality but it can occur in association with other CVMs. PDA is seen in trisomies 13 and 21 and is the characteristic CVM of CHAR syndrome.

Recurrence Risks for Isolated Cardiovascular Malformations

CVMs are usually isolated abnormalities and there is no previous family history. When this is the case the recurrence risk in subsequent siblings seems to be of the same order (2%–3%) regardless of the CVM (Campbell and Polani 1961; Campbell 1962, 1965; Zoethout et al. 1964; Nora et al. 1967; Emanuel et al. 1968; Fuhrmann 1968; Wilkins 1969; Williamson 1969; Boon et al. 1972; Zetterqvist 1972; Boon and Roberts 1976; Ando et al. 1977; Child and Dennis 1977; Sanchez-Cascos 1978; Czeizel and Meszaros 1981; Dennis and Warren 1981; Nora and Nora 1983). This empiric recurrence risk can be modified when a maternal factor that can be avoided in a subsequent pregnancy has contributed to the CVM and when the CVM has occurred in a monozygous twin. When a subsequent sibling does have a CVM it is not always the same as that seen in the index case.

Most studies find that the risk of CVM in offspring of affected males and females is likewise in the order of 3% though for AVSD it seems to be higher (10%) (Williamson 1969; Zetterqvist 1972; Taussig et al. 1975; Dennis and Warren 1981; Czeizel et al. 1982; Emanuel et al. 1983; Rose et al. 1985; Nora and Nora 1987; Romano-Zelekha et al. 2001). However, in the British Offspring Study the risk of an affected child was significantly higher if the affected parent was the mother rather than the father ($p = 0.01$)—the figure for offspring of affected males being 2% and of affected females being 6.5% (Burn et al. 1998). Whilst recurrence and offspring risks are low, they are considerably higher than the population risk indicating a genetic component. Although the molecular basis for most CVMs is unknown, studies of unusual pedigrees with multiple affected individuals have led to identification of some causative genes and these are described in the following section.

Molecular Basis of Isolated Cardiovascular Malformations

NKX2.5

Schott and colleagues 1998 (Schott et al. 1998) described mutations in the cardiac transcription factor NKX2.5 in four pedigrees in which secundum ASD segregated as a highly penetrant dominant trait. The first of these families had nine individuals with secundum ASD, one of whom also had SVAS and another a VSD. Two deceased family members, for whom the presence of the mutation could not be tested, had Fallot's tetralogy. All family members for whom records were available had atrioventricular conduction defects. The additional families in this study had isolated ASD with conduction defects. Serial studies in some affected individuals demonstrated progressive conduction defects, 14 affected individuals had pacemakers inserted and 6 individuals who did not have pacemakers died suddenly many years after surgical repair. In these 4 pedigrees all mutation carriers manifest a cardiac abnormality. The group went on to describe another 4 families with NKX2.5 mutations and various combinations of conduction defects, ASD, and VSD, but of interest 4 of the 23 affected individuals in these families had abnormalities of the tricuspid valve, 1 had a small tricuspid valve, and 3 had Ebstein's anomaly (Benson et al. 1999). NKX2.5 mutation screening has been undertaken in sporadic ASD and broader CVM collections but the numbers studied have not been large enough to definitively address its role in sporadic CVM.

GATA4

Garg and colleagues studied another family sufficiently large for mapping studies in which ASD was the predominant CVM (Garg et al. 2003). All 15 affected individuals in this family had an ASD, 8 as an isolated malformation, 2 in conjunction with pulmonary stenosis, 2 associated with pulmonary stenosis and VSD, 1 with VSD and PDA, 1 with atrial and mitral regurgitation, and 1 with AVSD and pulmonary stenosis. None of the family members had a conduction defect. The disorder in the family segregated with a missense change in the cardiac transcription factor *GATA4* that was shown in vitro to have diminished transcriptional activity. GATA4 forms a complex with NKX2.5 and another transcription factor *TBX5*. The GATA4 mutation identified in this family abrogates its physical interaction with *TBX5*, the gene implicated in Holt-Oram syndrome. All mutation carriers in this family had a CVM. Mutation analysis in a second family in which ASD segregated with polymorphisms in the region identified a GATA4 frameshift mutation. All seven living affected individuals in this family have an ASD and again all tested mutation carriers were affected. The role of GATA4 in sporadic CVM is not yet known.

NKX2.6

In one consanguineous pedigree with six individuals with truncus arteriosus in four different branches a homozygous missense change of a highly conserved amino acid was identified in the transcription factor NKX2.6 (Heathcote et al. 2005).

NOTCH1

The aortic valve usually has three cusps but 1% to 2% of individuals have a bicuspid aortic valve, these valves are prone to calcification and aortic stenosis and incompetence may result. Garg and colleagues studied a large family with 11 individuals with CVM, 9 of these had aortic valve disease, 6 bicuspid aortic valve (Garg et al. 2005). Seven individuals in this family developed calcific aortic stenosis, three of whom had a tricuspid aortic valve. One family member had a stenotic mitral valve and VSD; two had a bicuspid pulmonary valve, one with associated VSD, and the other TOF. This family was sufficiently large to undertake genetic mapping and thence to the identification of a nonsense mutation in *NOTCH1*. The presence of aortic calcification in family members with a tricuspid aortic valve suggested that calcification is not simply secondary to hemodynamic changes associated with an abnormal valve but could also be a consequence of NOTCH1 haploinsufficiency. There is evidence to support this hypothesis as NOTCH1 represses RUNX2, a key transcription factor in osteoblast differentiation. Thus NOTCH1 haploinsufficiency causes defects in valve development and there is evidence that it is also associated with osteoblast-specific gene expression leading to the calcium deposition that causes progressive aortic valve disease. Direct sequencing of *NOTCH1* in a second smaller family identified a heterozygous frameshift mutation also predicted to cause haploinsufficiency through nonsense-mediated decay. This second family had three affected family members, the proband had a bicuspid aortic valve, mitral valve atresia, hypoplastic left ventricle, and double outlet right ventricle, and his sibling and mother had aortic valve calcification and stenosis. It is noteworthy that one of the affected individuals in this family had a HLH, as severe aortic valve obstruction is associated with failure of left ventricle growth. There is an increased, 10%, incidence of bicuspid aortic valve in relatives of patients with HLH syndrome suggesting a common genetic etiology with phenotypic variability.

Sarcomere Proteins

In addition to their association with cardiomyopathies, mutations in sarcomere proteins may also be associated with septal defects. A genetic mapping and candidate gene approach in a large pedigree led to identification of a missense substitution in an α-myosin heavy chain (MYH6) that affected the binding of the heavy chain to its regulatory light chain (Ching et al. 2005). There were two obligate carriers in this pedigree who did not have a CVM. In the course of screening for the p.Glu 101 Lys ACTC1 mutation in cardiomyopathy patients in the Galicia region of Spain, Monserrat and colleagues noted mutation carriers with septal defects (Monserrat et al. 2007). They identified 46 mutation carriers, all had increased left ventricular wall thickness, usually with prominent trabeculations and deep invaginations in the thickened segments, half meeting the criteria for left ventricular noncompaction. 9 of the 46 mutation carriers had an ASD or VSD whilst none of the 48 relatives without the mutation had a septal defect ($p = 0.003$). Another ACTC1 missense substitution, affecting binding to myosin, has been identified in two large Swedish ASD families, indicating a founder effect. The phenotype was fully penetrant in these two families (Matsson et al. 2008).

Elastin (ELN)

The genetic basis of SVAS was elucidated through investigation of a family in which SVAS segregated with a balanced chromosome translocation. One of the breakpoints of this reciprocal translocation disrupted the elastin gene (*ELN*) at chromosome 7q11.23 (Curran et al. 1993), a locus that the group had already shown to be linked to SVAS in two unrelated families with autosomal dominant SVAS (Ewart et al. 1993b). There have been a number of subsequent reports of *ELN* mutations in SVAS families. SVAS is present in about 70% of individuals with William's syndrome (Eronen et al. 2002), a disorder that was shown by the same group to be due to chromosome 7q11.23 microdeletion encompassing *ELN* (Ewart et al. 1993a).

Laterality Disturbance and Cardiovascular Malformation

The direction of cardiac looping in early cardiac development is dependent on the left-right axis, which is established at the embryonic node very early in development at the time of gastrulation, just 14 days postfertilization. If the left-right axis is reversed the body plan will be reversed (situs inversus) with dextrocardia, spleen and stomach on the right and liver and gall bladder on the left. The association between primary ciliary dyskinesia and situs inversus has long been recognized. The explanation for the association is that rotating cilia at the embryonic node play a key role in establishing the gene expression differences between the left and right side that are crucial to establishing left and right identity (Nonaka et al. 1998). Primary ciliary dyskinesia (PCD), also known as Kartagener's syndrome, is an autosomal recessive disorder the main features of which are situs inversus, nasal polyps, and bronchiectasis. As establishment of the left-right axis is random in the absence on nodal cilia or when they are immotile, half of affected individuals have situs inversus. However, 6% of affected individuals have a CVM. Two genes encoding ciliary outer dynein arm proteins, *DNAI1* and *DNAH5*, account for 35% of patients with PCD, given the complexity of cilia motility further locus heterogeneity is not surprising.

Heterotaxy and situs ambiguous are interchangeable terms used when there are discrepancies in the situs of the asymmetric organs. Abnormal folding of the intestines with laterality disturbance predisposes to intestinal obstruction. Heterotaxy is often accompanied by a complex CVM. Whilst the ventricles and outflow tracts develop from a single fused tube, the left and right atria are derived from left- and right-sided tubes. As the left and right atria have distinctive morphology the description of CVMs associated with a laterality disorder includes the morphological appearance of the atria. If markers of right-sidedness are expressed bilaterally when the body plan is established we use the term right isomerism. If markers of left-sidedness are expressed bilaterally when the body plan is established we use the term "left isomerism." As lung lobation is asymmetrical in right isomerism sequence there will be bilateral short eparterial bronchi and trilobed lungs, whilst in left isomerism there will be bilateral long hyparterial bronchi and bilobed lungs. In right isomerism the spleen, which arises from the left side of the dorsal mesogastrium, is usually absent predisposing to infection and antibiotic prophylaxis should be given. In left isomerism multiple spleens often develop. Complex CVMs occur in all forms of laterality disturbance with disturbance of atrioventricular connection, septation, and conotruncal anomalies. In right isomerism, in the absence of an atrium with left-sided identity, there is anomalous pulmonary venous return. In right isomerism there are two morphologically right atria, typically with a single ventricle, AVSD, TGA, and anomalous pulmonary venous drainage. In left isomerism sequence there are two morphologically left atria, often an AVSD, development of the sinoatrial node may be affected leading to heart block but usually the CVM is not as severe as in right isomerism sequence.

As the pathway by which left-right is established has been elucidated in animal models, mutation screening of some of the genes has been undertaken in patient cohorts and changes have been identified in a small proportion of affected individuals. When parental samples have been tested these changes have usually been found to be inherited from parents who do not have a heart defect. Individuals with changes in more than one left-right pathway gene have also been reported. It seems likely that the changes identified are contributing to the phenotype but in the absence of certainty of pathogenicity and penetrance these findings do not provide information helpful to parents. Only one of the genes identified thus far in the left-right pathway was discovered through investigation of a family with laterality disturbance, the X chromosome gene *ZIC3* (Gebbia et al. 1997). Midline defects such as sacral agenesis and neural tube defects are frequently seen in association with CVM in individuals with *ZIC3* mutations. Whilst *ZIC3* mutations are a rare cause of laterality disturbance, diagnosis is important as this is an X-linked disorder and carrier females are at risk of an affected son. Unfortunately, even when a *ZIC3* mutation is identified, counseling is not straightforward as both manifesting females (Gebbia et al. 1997) and phenotypically normal males (Megarbane et al. 2000) with a mutation have been reported.

It should also be remembered when taking the history that the incidence of laterality disturbance is increased in the offspring of diabetic women (Splitt et al. 1999). In the absence of family history, consanguinity, and maternal diabetes the empiric recurrence risk is 5% (Rose et al. 1975; Burn et al. 1986).

Conclusion

Known chromosomal, syndromic, and environmental causes account for 20% of CVMs, thus currently the etiology for the majority of CVMs is unknown. Specific recurrence risks can be given if a syndrome diagnosis is made, if a chromosomal abnormality is found, in the presence of a family history or when an environmental factor is identified. A number of studies three decades ago documented the recurrence risk in siblings of patients with isolated CVM and these empiric figures remain the bedrock of counseling today, the recurrence risk being 2%–3% in the absence of previous family history. From a counseling perspective this is a relatively low recurrence risk but it greatly exceeds population risk indicating a genetic component to etiology of nonsyndromic CVM. We hope that ongoing large studies of common and rare variants will lead to improved understanding such that both parents who have a child with a CVM and affected individuals considering having children can be given personalized information based on the cause of the defect rather than continued reliance on population-based figures.

References

Anaclerio S, Marino B, Carotti A, et al. Pulmonary atresia with ventricular septal defect: prevalence of deletion 22q11 in the different anatomic patterns. *Ital Heart J*. 2001;2:384–387.

Ando M, Takao A, Mori K. Genetic and environmental factors in congenital heart disease. In: Inouye E, Nishimura H, eds. *Gene Environmental Interaction in Common Diseases*. University Park Press, Baltimore, USA; 1977:71–88.

Andrews R, Tulloh R, Sharland G, et al. Outcome of staged reconstructive surgery for hypoplastic left heart syndrome following antenatal diagnosis. *Arch Dis Child*. 2001;85:474–477.

Benson DW, Silberbach GM, Kavanaugh-McHugh A, et al. Mutations in the cardiac transcription factor NKX2.5 affect diverse cardiac developmental pathways. *J Clin Invest*. 1999;104:1567–1573.

Bleyl S, Nelson L, Odelberg SJ, et al. A gene for familial total anomalous pulmonary venous return maps to chromosome 4p13-q12. *Am J Hum Genet*. 1995;56:408–415.

Boon AR, Farmer MB, Roberts DF. A family study of Fallot's tetralogy. *J Med Genet*. 1972;9:179–192.

Boon AR, Roberts DF. A family study of coarctation of the aorta. *J Med Genet.* 1976;13:420–433.

Botto LD, May K, Fernhoff PM, et al. A population-based study of the 22q11.2 deletion: phenotype, incidence, and contribution to major birth defects in the population. *Pediatrics.* 2003;112:101–107.

Brackley KJ, Kilby MD, Wright JG, et al. Outcome after prenatal diagnosis of hypoplastic left-heart syndrome: a case series. *Lancet.* 2000;356:1143–1147.

Burn J, Brennan P, Little J, et al. Recurrence risks in offspring of adults with major heart defects: results from first cohort of British collaborative study. *Lancet.* 1998;351:311–316.

Burn J, Coffrey R, Allan LD, Robinson P, Pembrey ME, Macartney FJ. Isomerism: a genetic analysis. *Paediat Cardiol.* 1986;1126–1128.

Burn J, Corney G. Congenital heart defects and twinning. *Acta Genet Med Gemellol (Roma).* 1984;33:61–69.

Campbell M. Factors in the aetiology of pulmonary stenosis. *Br Heart J.* 1962;24:625–632.

Campbell M. Causes of malformations of the heart. *Br Med J.* 1965;5467:895–904.

Campbell M, Polani PE. The aetiology of coarctation of the aorta. *Lancet.* 1961;1:463–468.

Child AH, Dennis NR. The genetics of congenital heart disease. *Birth Defects Orig Artic Ser.* 1977;13:85–91.

Ching YH, Ghosh TK, Cross SJ, et al. Mutation in myosin heavy chain 6 causes atrial septal defect. *Nat Genet.* 2005;37:423–428.

Clarren SK, Smith DW. The fetal alcohol syndrome. *N Engl J Med.* 1978;298:1063–1067.

Curran ME, Atkinson DL, Ewart AK, Morris CA, Leppert MF, Keating MT. The elastin gene is disrupted by a translocation associated with supravalvular aortic stenosis. *Cell.* 1993;73:159–168.

Czeizel A, Meszaros M. Two family studies of children with ventricular septal defect. *Eur J Pediatr.* 1981;136:81–85.

Czeizel A, Pornoi A, Peterffy E, Tarcal E. Study of children of parents operated on for congenital cardiovascular malformations. *Br Heart J.* 1982;47:290–293.

Czeizel AE, Rockenbauer M, Sorensen HT, Olsen J. The teratogenic risk of trimethoprim-sulfonamides: a population based case-control study. *Reprod Toxicol.* 2001;15:637–646.

Dennis NR, Warren J. Risks to the offspring of patients with some common congenital heart defects. *J Med Genet.* 1981;18:8–16.

Emanuel R, Nichols J, Anders JM, Moores EC, Somerville J. Atrioventricular defects a study of 92 families. *Br Heart J.* 1968;30:645–653.

Emanuel R, Somerville J, Inns A, Withers R. Evidence of congenital heart disease in the offspring of parents with atrioventricular defects. *Br Heart J.* 1983;49:144–147.

Eronen M, Peippo M, Hiippala A, et al. Cardiovascular manifestations in 75 patients with Williams syndrome. *J Med Genet.* 2002;39:554–558.

Ewart AK, Morris CA, Atkinson D, et al. Hemizygosity at the elastin locus in a developmental disorder, Williams syndrome. *Nat Gen.* 1993a;5:11–16.

Ewart AK, Morris CA, Ensing GJ, et al. A human vascular disorder, supravalvular aortic stenosis, maps to chromosome 7. *Proc Natl Acad Sci U S A.* 1993b;90:3226–3230.

Ferencz C, Loffredo CA, Correa-Villasenor A, Wilson PD (ed). Genetic and environmental risk factors of major cardiovascular malformations. In: *The Baltimore-Washington Infant Heart Study 1981–1989.* Futura Publishing Co. Inc., New York, USA; 1997.

Ferencz C, Rubin JD, Loffredo CA, Magee CA. Epidemiology of congenital heart disease. In: *The Baltimore-Washington Infant Heart Study 1981–1989.* Futura Publishing Co. Inc., New York, USA; 1993.

Fuhrmann W. A family study in transposition of the great vessels and in tricuspid atresia. *Humangenetik.* 1968;6:148–157.

Garg V, Kathiriya IS, Barnes R, et al. GATA4 mutations cause human congenital heart defects and reveal an interaction with TBX5. *Nature.* 2003;424:443–447.

Garg V, Muth AN, Ransom JF, et al. Mutations in NOTCH1 cause aortic valve disease. *Nature.* 2005;437:270–274.

Gebbia M, Ferrero GB, Pilia G, et al. X-linked situs abnormalities result from mutations in ZIC3. *Nat Gen.* 1997;17:305–308.

Geiger JM, Baudin M, Saurat JH. Teratogenic risk with etretinate and acitretin treatment. *Dermatology.* 1994;189:109–116.

Goldmuntz E, Clark BJ, Mitchell LE, et al. Frequency of 22q11 deletions in patients with conotruncal defects. *J Am Coll Cardiol.* 1998;32:492–498.

Gregg NM, Ramsay, Brevis W, Heseltine M. The occurrence of congenital defects in children following maternal rubella during pregnancy. *Med J Aust.* 1945;2:122–126.

Hancock Friesen CL, Zurakowski D, Thiagarajan RR, et al. Total anomalous pulmonary venous connection: an analysis of current management strategies in a single institution. *Ann Thorac Surg.* 2005;79:596–606; discussion 596–606.

Heathcote K, Braybrook C, Abushaban L, et al. Common arterial trunk associated with a homeodomain mutation of NKX2.6. *Hum Mol Genet.* 2005;14:585–593.

Hernandez-Diaz S, Werler MM, Walker AM, Mitchell AA. Folic acid antagonists during pregnancy and the risk of birth defects. *N Engl J Med.* 2000;343:1608–1614.

Hoffman JI. Incidence, mortality and natural history. In: Anderson RH, Macartney FJ, Shinebourne EA, Tynan M, eds. *Paediatric Cardiology.* Churchill Livingstone, London; 1987.

Ishino K, Stumper O, De Giovanni JJ, et al. The modified Norwood procedure for hypoplastic left heart syndrome: early to intermediate results of 120 patients with particular reference to aortic arch repair. *J Thorac Cardiovasc Surg.* 1999;117:920–930.

Knowles R, Griebsch I, Dezateux C, Brown J, Bull C, Wren C. Newborn screening for congenital heart defects: a systematic review and cost-effectiveness analysis. *Health Technol Assess.* 2005;9:1–152.

Lenke RR, Levy HL. Maternal phenylketonuria and hyperphenylalaninemia. An international survey of the outcome of untreated and treated pregnancies. *N Engl J Med.* 1980;303:1202–1208.

Leonard H, Derrick G, O'Sullivan J, Wren C. Natural and unnatural history of pulmonary atresia. *Heart.* 2000;84:499–503.

Levy HL, Guldberg P, Guttler F, et al. Congenital heart disease in maternal phenylketonuria: report from the Maternal PKU Collaborative Study. *Pediatr Res.* 2001;49:636–642.

Loffredo CA, Wilson PD, Ferencz C. Maternal diabetes: an independent risk factor for major cardiovascular malformations with increased mortality of affected infants. *Teratology.* 2001;64:98–106.

Matsson H, Eason J, Bookwalter CS, et al. Alpha-cardiac actin mutations produce atrial septal defects. *Hum Mol Genet.* 2008;17:256–265.

Megarbane A, Salem N, Stephan E, et al. X-linked transposition of the great arteries and incomplete penetrance among males with a nonsense mutation in ZIC3. *Eur J Hum Genet.* 2000;8:704–708.

Monserrat L, Hermida-Prieto M, Fernandez X, et al. Mutation in the alpha-cardiac actin gene associated with apical hypertrophic cardiomyopathy, left ventricular non-compaction, and septal defects. *Eur Heart J.* 2007;28:1953–1961.

Nonaka S, Tanaka Y, Okada Y, et al. Randomization of left-right asymmetry due to loss of nodal cilia generating leftward flow of extraembryonic fluid in mice lacking KIF3B motor protein. *Cell.* 1998;95:829–837.

Nora JJ, McNamara DG, Fraser FC. Hereditary factors in atrial septal defect. *Circulation.* 1967;35:448–456.

Nora JJ, Nora AH. Genetic epidemiology of congenital heart diseases. *Prog Med Genet.* 1983;5:91–137.

Nora JJ, Nora AH. Maternal transmission of congenital heart diseases: new recurrence risk figures and the questions of cytoplasmic inheritance and vulnerability to teratogens. *Am J Cardiol.* 1987;59:459–463.

Pierpont ME, Basson CT, Benson DW Jr, et al. Genetic basis for congenital heart defects: current knowledge: a scientific statement from the American Heart Association Congenital Cardiac Defects Committee, Council on Cardiovascular Disease in the Young: endorsed by the American Academy of Pediatrics. *Circulation.* 2007;115:3015–3038.

Pradat P. A case-control study of major congenital heart defects in Sweden—1981–1986. *Eur J Epidemiol.* 1992;8:789–796.

Romano-Zelekha O, Hirsh R, Blieden L, Green M, Shohat T. The risk for congenital heart defects in offspring of individuals with congenital heart defects. *Clin Gen.* 2001;59:325–329.

Rose V, Gold RJ, Lindsay G, Allen M. A possible increase in the incidence of congenital heart defects among the offspring of affected parents. *J Am Coll Cardiol.* 1985;6:376–382.

Rose V, Izukawa T, Moes CA. Syndromes of asplenia and polysplenia. A review of cardiac and non-cardiac malformations in 60 cases with special reference to diagnosis and prognosis. *Br Heart J.* 1975;37:840–852.

Ryan AK, Goodship JA, Wilson DI, et al. Spectrum of clinical features associated with interstitial chromosome 22q11 deletions: a European collaborative study. *J Med Genet.* 1997;34:798–804.

Sanchez-Cascos A. The recurrence risk in congenital heart disease. *Eur J Cardiol.* 1978;7:197–210.

Schott JJ, Benson DW, Basson CT, et al. Congenital heart disease caused by mutations in the transcription factor NKX2-5. *Science.* 1998;281:108–111.

Sheffield VC, Pierpont ME, Nishimura D, et al. Identification of a complex congenital heart defect susceptibility locus by using DNA pooling and shared segment analysis. *Hum Mol Genet.* 1997;6:117–121.

Smithells RW, Newman CG. Recognition of thalidomide defects. *J Med Genet.* 1992;29:716–723.

Splitt M, Wright C, Sen D, Goodship J. Left-isomerism sequence and maternal type-1 diabetes. *Lancet.* 1999;354:305–306.

Stamm C, Friehs I, Ho SY, Moran AM, Jonas RA, del Nido PJ. Congenital supravalvar aortic stenosis: a simple lesion? *Eur J Cardiothorac Surg.* 2001;19:195–202.

Taussig HB, Kallman CH, Nagel D, Baumgardner R, Momberger N, Kirk H. Long-time observations on the Blalock-Taussig operation VIII. 20 to 28 year follow-up on patients with a tetralogy of Fallot. *Johns Hopkins Med J.* 1975;137:13–19.

Wilkins JL. Risks of offspring of patients with patent ductus arteriosus. *J Med Genet.* 1969;6:1–4.

Williamson EM. A family study of atrial septal defect. *J Med Genet.* 1969;6:255–265.

Wilson L, Curtis A, Korenberg JR, et al. A large, dominant pedigree of atrioventricular septal defect (AVSD): exclusion from the Down syndrome critical region on chromosome 21. *Am J Hum Genet.* 1993;53:1262–1268.

Wren C, Birrell G, Hawthorne G. Cardiovascular malformations in infants of diabetic mothers. *Heart.* 2003;89:1217–1220.

Wren C, Oslizlok P, Bull C. Natural history of supravalvular aortic stenosis and pulmonary artery stenosis. *J Am Coll Cardiol.* 1990;15:1625–1630.

Wren C, Reinhardt Z, Khawaja K. Twenty-year trends in diagnosis of life-threatening neonatal cardiovascular malformations. *Arch Dis Child Fetal Neonatal Ed.* 2008;93:F33–F35.

Wren C, Richmond S, Donaldson L. Presentation of congenital heart disease in infancy: implications for routine examination. *Arch Dis Child Fetal Neonatal Ed.* 1999;80:F49–F53.

Zetterqvist P. *A Clinical and Genetic Study of Congenital Heart Defects.* Sweden: University of Uppsala; 1972.

Zoethout HE, Carter RE, Carter CO. A Family Study of Aortic Stenosis. *J Med Genet.* 1964;55:2–9.

10

Malformation Syndromes with Heart Disease

Michael A Patton

Most cardiologists concentrate on diagnosing and treating problems in the cardiovascular system, but it is sometimes important to consider the possibility of a multisystem disorder in diagnosis and management. One important example of this principle is where there is a multisystem congenital malformation syndrome. The prognosis of these conditions will often be determined by features outside the cardiovascular system and the diagnosis may rest on the use of a genetic test rather than a cardiac investigation. For example, with supravalvular stenosis in William's syndrome, the key feature in the prognosis may be the associated intellectual disability and the diagnosis is made by considering the other clinical features and confirming the diagnosis by a specialized chromosome test demonstrating a microdeletion of the elastin gene on the long arm of chromosome 7 (Pober et al. 2008).

The word syndrome literally means "to run together" and a malformation syndrome can be defined as a recognizable pattern of malformations. Although many are associated with intellectual disability and have a genetic basis neither of these features are prerequisites to diagnosing a syndrome.

Malformation syndromes are frequently due to single gene mutations and hence may have a high chance of recurrence in future pregnancies. It is important to work with a clinical geneticist in diagnosing the syndromes and advising parents about the possibility or recurrence and prenatal testing.

Although more common in neonates and infants, syndromes can present at any age. In utero the presence of structural heart defect on the fetal scan raises not only the possibility of congenital heart disease but also an associated syndrome that may be associated with intellectual disability. Since few syndromes with intellectual disability have structural brain defects it is important to systematically look for other associated anomalies and to determine if there is a recognizable pattern. It will also be important to undertake prenatal chromosome testing and consider looking for specific chromosomal deletions associated with congenital heart defects such as 22q deletion (DiGeorge syndrome) and trisomy 21 (Down syndrome). The presence of fetal hydrops or increased nuchal edema will increase the likelihood of an underlying chromosome defect. At birth the presence of a heart murmur or heart failure will lead to a full anatomical cardiac diagnosis. At this stage the additional appearance of unusual facial features will assist in the diagnosis of a syndrome. The facial features may change with age and some syndromes are more easily recognized at different ages, for example, Noonan syndrome is an easier facial diagnosis in young children than in adults. Most cardiac syndromes will be diagnosed in childhood but some present later. In Marfan's syndrome it is often the rapid growth in the late teens that alerts the physician to the diagnosis. As most syndromes have been described in children there may be relatively little information on the natural history and long term prognosis. This is now a topic for research (Marsalese et al. 1989; Shaw et al. 2007).

It can sometimes be difficult to determine the relative importance of different clinical features when making a syndrome diagnosis and it can be useful to distinguish between "soft" and "hard" features. A soft dysmorphic feature is one that is relatively common in the general population and is relatively subjective (e.g., prominent nose) whereas a hard sign is a feature that is rare in the general population and clearly defined (e.g., polydactyly). The combination of a structural heart defect and one or more hard signs should suggest a syndrome diagnosis. Table 10-1 gives a list of some of the commoner associations that may assist in making a syndrome diagnosis.

It is important to recognize that each child with a particular syndrome will not have all the associated clinical features, for example, in Down syndrome only 50% of the children will have a structural heart defect (Laursen 1976). There are several scoring systems that define the minimum required features for a diagnosis, for example, Noonan's syndrome (Duncan et al. 1981) and Marfan syndrome (Dean 2007; see also Chapter 11), but increasingly there will be a specific laboratory test to confirm the diagnosis.

Recognition of common disorders such as Down syndrome rarely presents a problem, but with up to 2,000 other malformation syndromes the task of recognizing rarer disorders can be very daunting. One of the most useful aids to syndrome diagnosis is the use of syndrome databases. The London Dysmorphology Database (LDDB) is one example of this. It currently lists 1,017 syndromes that are associated with congenital cardiac malformations. The database may be searched on a combination of features, for example, heart defect and polydactyly will give 77 syndromes whereas the combination of heart defect, polydactyly, and hypospadias will narrow the list down to a manageable list of 17 syndromes including the Smith-Lemli-Opitz (SLO) syndrome for which there is a specific metabolic test (Tint et al. 1994). One of

Table 10–1 Examples of Heart Malformation Syndromes with Associated Noncardiac Malformations

Additional Feature	Associated Heart Malformation Syndromes
Cleft lip/palate	DiGeorge syndrome Goldenhar syndrome CHARGE Kabuki makeup syndrome Fetal alcohol syndrome Smith-Lemli-Opitz syndrome
Polydactyly	Holt Oram syndrome Ellis-van Creveld syndrome Maternal diabetes Fetal valproate syndrome Smith-Lemli-Opitz syndrome
Scoliosis	Williams syndrome VACTERL TAR syndrome Rubenstein-Taybi syndrome Marden Walker syndrome Emery Dreifuss muscular dystrophy
Microphthalmia	CHARGE syndrome Goldenhar syndrome Fetal alcohol syndrome
Ptosis	Noonan syndrome Williams syndrome Fetal alcohol syndrome Smith-Lemli-Opitz syndrome Ohdo syndrome

the strengths of this type of database is that it includes isolated case reports from the literature which would not be easily remembered or searched for in the literature. Importantly this kind of database is not an expert system that defines the differential diagnosis in terms of probability but is rather an information system for experts who will undertake a review of the relevant literature when considering the diagnostic possibilities.

The diagnosis of a syndrome by facial features may appear more of an art than a science and does very much depend on clinical experience. This may change with the development of more sophisticated computing technology. Recently Hammond et al. (2005) have used topographic mapping with computer analysis to study the 3D facial features of Williams syndrome and Noonan syndrome. The trained human eye is still better at the initial diagnosis, but the computer system can highlight features that do not fit neatly into the perceptual model. Computer modeling can also be used to "morph" through the facial features from birth to adulthood giving an insight into the changes in dysmorphic features that occur with time. For clinicians who do not have access to such electronic aids there are a number of atlases (Gorlin 2001; Jones 2008) covering most of the common dysmorphic syndromes.

Etiology

Most dysmorphic syndromes are either due to single gene mutations or to chromosome abnormalities. Hence the recurrence risk is higher than that for isolated heart defects that are usually multifactorial with recurrence risks in the order of 5%.

The family pedigree may give a guide to the likely pattern of inheritance. Autosomal dominant conditions are associated with transmission from generation to generation but reduced expressivity with variability between different individuals in the family may give the appearance of "skipped" generations due to loss of penetrance. Autosomal recessive disorders are found more commonly where there is associated consanguinity and sex-linked inheritance may be considered if the affected individuals are predominantly male.

Chromosome abnormalities may present with early fetal loss or miscarriage. It is useful to ask specifically about recurrent miscarriages when taking the pedigree. For many years the diagnosis of chromosome abnormalities rested on the microscopic analysis of the cultured cell preparation. The standard chromosome karyotype will pick up not only abnormalities of the chromosome number (aneuploidy) but also pick up chromosome rearrangement such as deletions and translocation. However, this technique is complemented by new molecular methods such as CGH microarrays that can carry out gene testing for around 500–1,000 molecular markers across whole genome and as a result can pick up deletions or duplications that would not be visible under the microscope. This will greatly increase the ability to diagnose genetic syndromes associated with congenital heart disease especially where there is associated disability.

Syndromic causes of congenital heart disease can also result from exposure to chemicals or drugs during pregnancy. For women with a chronic disorder that requires medication, such as epilepsy, it is beneficial to review treatment prior to planning a pregnancy as this may reduce the risk of malformation in offspring. Women with epilepsy have around twice the background rate of congenital malformations, but some anticonvulsants such as carbamazepine and lamotrigine are currently thought to be associated with less risk of malformation than phenytoin or sodium valproate. In some cases the use of folic acid in addition to the anticonvulsant therapy may reduce the risk of malformation (Tomson et al. 2004).

Biochemical disorders causing the storage of abnormal metabolites can be associated with cardiomyopathy, skeletal abnormalities, and coarse facial features. As a general rule, these disorders are not a cause of a congenital malformation syndrome as the abnormalities develop after birth with the build up of abnormal metabolites that cannot be cleared by the maternal circulation. The exception to this general rule is when the metabolic defect affects intracellular metabolism , for example, in Zellweger syndrome the defect is within the intracellular peroxisome and features such as dysmorphic facies, enlarged liver, brain abnormalities, epiphyseal stippling, and congenital heart disease may be seen at birth (Brosius et al. 2002).

Specific Syndromes

There are over 1,000 malformation syndromes associated with congenital heart disease and it is clearly not possible to discuss the full range of these syndromes. Some associated with chromosomal or metabolic abnormalities are described elsewhere in the book and the full range of syndromes can be accessed through atlases or databases of malformation syndromes.

Syndromes Associated with Intellectual Disability

1. Williams syndrome

The typical cardiac malformations in Williams Syndrome are supravalvular aortic stenosis and peripheral artery stenosis.

Arterial stenosis can affect other organs (e.g., kidneys). In one study of children with Williams Syndrome, 73% had supravalvular aortic stenosis (SVAS) and 41% had pulmonary arterial stenosis (Brewer et al. 1996; Eronen et al. 2002). Surgery may be required and arterial hypertension may develop in young adults.

There is a characteristic face in Williams syndrome, which is described as "elfin-like." There tends to be periorbital fullness with prominent lips and round cheeks in early childhood but the features become coarser with age. The eye colour is often a striking blue and there may be a stellate pattern in the iris. Short stature, hypercalcemia in infancy and hyperaccusis are also characteristic features. The early development is delayed and intellectual disability is present. These children interact well with adults and may exhibit a "cocktail party" pattern of speech that may mask the degree of intellectual deficit. (Pober et al. 2008).

The cause of Williams syndrome is a submicroscopic deletion on the long arm of chromosome 7 and can be diagnosed with a FISH probe at chromosome analysis. The deleted area includes the gene for elastin and it is this defect in elastin that probably underlies the characteristic cardiac features (Hennekam 2006).

2. Rubenstein-Taybi syndrome

There are a number of distinctive dysmorphic features in Rubenstein-Taybi syndrome(Kline 2007). The facial features include downslanting palpebral fissures, hypertelorism, mild ptosis, and a convex nose with the nasal septum protruding below the alae nasi on lateral view. The facial features become more marked with age. The thumbs and halluces are broad, or occasionally bifid, with medial deviation. Microcephaly and developmental delay are constant features. A number of ocular features have been reported, including congenital glaucoma, cataracts, corneal abnormalities, colobomas, lacrimal duct obstruction, and retinal abnormalities. Around 30% of cases have a cardiac anomaly, the most common being VSD, ASD, and PDA.

In virtually all cases there is no family history as the disorder arises from a de novo mutation in the family. Petrij et al. (1995) demonstrated heterozygous point mutations in the CBP gene, which encodes a protein that binds to the phosphorylated form of the CREB transcription factor . This mutation is found in approximately one-third of affected individuals. Mutations have also been identified in the EP300 gene, which shares homology with CBP. However, as these two genes account for only half of affected cases it seems likely that there are further Rubenstein-Taybi genes to be found.

3. Cornelia De Lange syndrome

This syndrome presents with severe failure to thrive in utero, diaphragmatic hernia, limb defects, and a characteristic facial appearance (Schoumans et al. 2007). The facial appearance shows arched eyebrows that join in the midline (synophrys), a small triangular nose, a broad smooth philtrum, and microcephaly. There may be long eyelashes and a general hirsutism. It is not associated with a specific congenital heart defect but associated heart defects are common. For affected children who survive the neonatal period the effect on psychomotor development is significant and severe intellectual disability is the rule.

It is usually found as a de novo mutation without a family history and recently mutation in the developmental NIPBL gene have been found in 30%–40% of patients (Porter 2008).

4. Smith-Lemli-Opitz syndrome

Smith-Lemli-Opitz syndrome presents as a dysmorphic syndrome with intellectual disability. It is also characterized by microcephaly, failure to thrive, ptosis, anteverted nares, cleft palate, syndactyly of the second and third toes, and postaxial polydactyly. The partial syndactyly of the second and third toes may be a good diagnostic sign but it is also, like a single palmar crease, present as a normal variant in the general population. About a third of patients have congenital heart disease in which AVSD and coarctation of the aorta are most frequent.

The disorder is inherited as an autosomal recessive disorder and is caused by a defect in 7-dehydrocholesterol reductase (Irons et al. 1997). It can be diagnosed by an increase in the precursor metabolite 7-dehydrocholesterol. Smith-Lemli-Opitz syndrome is associated with moderate to severe intellectual disability. Treatment with increased dietary cholesterol may improve behavior but unfortunately does not improve the intellectual disability presumably as the metabolic disruption causes damage to the developing brain in utero (Porter et al. 2008).

5. DiGeorge syndrome

Although this syndrome is now known to be due to a chromosome microdeletion it is usually necessary to make a clinical diagnosis first in order to be in a position to request the specific chromosome test. DiGeorge syndrome may present in many different ways but from the cardiological point of view it characteristically causes complex conotruncal cardiac malformations (Burd et al. 2007). It is due to a submicroscopic deletion of chromosome 22q11 and can be diagnosed by using a specific fluorescent gene probe (TUPLE) to the chromosome karyotype. The degree of intellectual disability is usually mild to moderate and for that reason the deletion may be inherited as an autosomal dominant trait in around 20% of families. In some cases the chromosome defect may be associated with a psychotic illness in addition to the intellectual disability.

This syndrome goes under a number of different names reflecting the diversity of manifestations. It is also known as Sprintzen syndrome, velocardiofacial syndrome, and CATCH 22 syndrome. Submucous cleft palate is one of the frequent findings, which gives a distinctive pattern of speech. There may also be hyporparathyroidism, immune deficiency, and skeletal defects. Ryan et al. presented a useful overview of the clinical features from a European consortium (Ryan et al. 1997).

6. Fetal alcohol syndrome

The consumption of alcohol is widespread and it is controversial whether alcohol in small amounts during pregnancy will cause any fetal harm. However, there is agreement that alcoholism and its associated nutritional deficiencies can cause a characteristic pattern of abnormalities known as the fetal alcohol syndrome. The most significant feature is the presence of microcephaly and intellectual disability in varying degrees. There are also facial features that may assist in the diagnosis. There is usually a smooth underdeveloped philtrum and thin upper lip. The palpebral fissures are short. Congenital heart defects are present in around 30% of cases with VSD, tetralogy of Fallot, and ASD being the most frequent abnormalities (Burd et al. 2007) A wide range of other malformations have been reported on an occasional basis in this syndrome.

Syndromes Associated with Limb Defects

1. Holt Oram syndrome

Holt Oram syndrome characteristically presents to the cardiologist with an atrial septal defect and a limb abnormality (Huang 2002). Around 85% of patients have a heart defect and there are often ECG abnormalities such as long PR interval, bradycardia, and axis deviation. The limb defect is usually an absent or abnormal thumb although more major limb defects are also reported. Radiological examination of the limbs may show other bony defects at the wrist or in the radius. The posture of the shoulders is very characteristic with narrow sloping shoulders and there is often a pectus chest deformity. There is no intellectual disability.

Holt Oram syndrome is an autosomal dominant disorder caused by mutations of the transcription factor *TBX5* on chromosome 12.

2. VATER or VACTERL association

VACTERL is an acronym used to describe children with the following spectrum of abnormalities: Vertebral defects, Anal atresia, Cardiac defects, Tracheo-Esophageal fistula, Renal malformations, and Limb defects (classically radial dysplasia). Dysmorphic features and learning difficulties are not usually present. Ventricular septal defects are the commonest cardiac abnormality. The diagnosis of VACTERL is made from the association of the key features and the diagnosis can be made even without a "full house" of the features.

The cause of this association is not yet known. It may represent a disruption to early fetal development and the combination of features may indicate the structures that are developing at the same stage in fetal development. The recurrence risk for parents of a child with sporadic VACTERL association is 1%.

3. Thrombocytopenia absent radius syndrome

There are a number of syndromes with absent radius or radial hypoplasia. In many of the syndromes with radial hypoplasia there are associated hematological problems. In this syndrome there is an association with thrombocytopenia, which may develop in the neonatal period. In 15% there may be a cardiac defect such as VSD or Tetralogy of Fallot.

Although this was originally described as an autosomal recessive disorder it has now been found to have a rather more complex etiology. It appears there may be an underlying chromosome microdeletion at 1q21 but the syndrome may be an additional inherited modifier gene to be expressed (Klopocki et al. 2007).

4. Fetal valproate syndrome

In around 2%–3% of mothers who take the anticonvulsant sodium valproate in pregnancy there is a characteristic pattern of malformations in the baby. The characteristic facial features are prominent epicanthic folds with a marked infraorbital fold. The eyes are shallow and there may be a high forehead. Limb defects such as polydactyly are common and occasionally there may be more severe malformations such as radial hypoplasia. Various cardiac malformations including an anomalous right pulmonary artery have been reported. There is also a greater risk of having a child with a neural tube defect after taking valproate during pregnancy.

There is an ongoing debate as to whether a higher proportion of infants of mothers on sodium valproate may have minor problems in psychomotor development in the absence of the full recognizable syndrome.

Syndromes with Short Stature

1. Turner syndrome

This abnormality of the sex chromosomes will lead to short stature in girls. It is described with other characteristic clinical features such as webbed neck, broad chest with increased distance between the nipples, cubitus valgus, and renal abnormalities,but it may be diagnosed with short stature alone. The characteristic congenital heart defect is coarctation of the aorta, but bicuspid aortic valves and septal defects may also occur. Long-term cardiac follow-up is required as hypertension and aortic dissection may develop in adult life (Bondy 2008).

2. Noonan syndrome

This autosomal dominant syndrome was inappropriately referred to as the "male Turner syndrome." initially but while both Turner and Noonan syndrome have short stature and webbed neck most of the other features are different and Noonan syndrome affects both males and females. In Noonan syndrome the characteristic heart defect is dysplastic pulmonary stenosis, which occurs in the majority of patients. In about 10% there is a hypertrophic cardiomyopathy that shows myofibrillar disarray and may cause heart failure in infancy (Burch et al. 1993) . The other characteristic features include short stature, ptosis, hypertelorism, low-set anteriorly rotated ears, short neck, pectus excavatum, and cryptorchidism in males (Sharland et al. 1992). The syndrome may have associated haematological complications. It has been associated with defects in the intrinsic coagulation pathway and with a rare form of leukaemia juvenile myelomonocytic leukemia, JMML).

The first gene found for Noonan syndrome was *PTPN11*, which is a cell-signaling gene on chromosome 12 (Tartaglia et al. 2001). It is found in around 50% of patients with the disorder. Subsequently, three other causative genes have been found (SOS1, KRAS and RAF1). The explanation for this is that all the causative genes are in the same cell-signaling pathway (RAS MAPK). Current studies are looking at the genotype–phenotype correlations with the different causative genes and it appears that *PTPN11* correlates with the presence of pulmonary stenosis while RAF1 is more frequently associated with hypertrophic cardiomyopathy (Razzaque et al. 2007).

Another syndrome called LEOPARD syndrome overlaps with some of the features of Noonan syndrome and was until recently thought to be a separate autosomal dominant disorder. The term LEOPARD is an acronym for Lentigines, Electrocardiographic abnormalities, Ocular hypertelorism, Pulmonary stenosis, Abnormalities of genitalia, Retardation of growth, and Deafness (Sarkozy et al. 2004). It has now been found that it is also due to mutations in the same *PTPN11* gene as in Noonan syndrome but the two disorders have a different pattern of mutations.

3. Ellis van Creveld syndome

In about 60% of cases of Ellis van Creveld syndrome there is a congenital cardiac malformation. In most cases it will be an ostium primum ASD or an AVSD malformation.

Ellis van Creveld syndrome is a rare autosomal recessive disorder with extreme short stature due to a skeletal dysplasia with disproportionate short limbs and a small chest with short ribs. Postaxial polydactyly is frequent. In addition, there are oral frenulae, nail dysplasia, and characteristic radiological changes. Affected individuals have normal intelligence.

The disorder is due to homozygous mutations in either of two related genes on chromosome 4 (*EVC* and *EVC2*) (Baujat and Le Merrer 2007). The gene is a developmental gene involved in a pathway referred to as hedgehog signaling. It is a disorder that has been reported in higher frequency in some isolated and consanguineous populations, for example, Amish in North America.

References

Baraitser M, Winter RW. *London Dysmorphology Database [LDDB]* London Medical Databases Ltd London NW1 8YD; 2009.

Baujat G, Le Merrer M. Ellis-van Creveld syndrome. *Orphanet J Rare Dis.* 2007;2:27.

Bondy CA. Congenital cardiovascular disease in Turner Syndrome. *Congenit Heart Dis.* 2008;3(1):2–15.

Brewer CM, Morrison N, Tolmie JL. Clinical and molecular cytogenetic (FISH) diagnosis of Williams syndrome. *Arch Dis Child.* 1996;74(1):59–61.

Brosius U, Gärtner J. Cellular and molecular aspects of Zellweger syndrome and other peroxisome biogenesis disorders. *Cell Mol Life Sci.* 2002;59(6):1058–1069.

Burch M, Sharland M, Shinebourne E, Smith G, Patton M, McKenna W. Cardiologic abnormalities in Noonan syndrome: phenotypic diagnosis and echocardiographic assessment of 118 patients. *J Am Coll Cardiol.* 1993;22(4):1189–1192.

Burd L, Deal E, Rios R, Adickes E, Wynne J, Klug MG. Congenital heart defects and fetal alcohol spectrum disorders. *Congenit Heart Dis.* 2007;2(4):250–255.

Dean JC. Marfan syndrome: clinical diagnosis and management. *Eur J Hum Genet.* 2007;15(7):724–733.

Duncan WJ, Fowler RS, Farkas LG, et al. A comprehensive scoring system for evaluating Noonan syndrome. *Am J Med Genet.* 1981;10(1):37–50.

Eronen M, Peippo M, Hiiplala A, et al. Cardiovascular manifestations in 75 patients with Williams syndrome. *J Med Genet.* 2002;39(8):554–558.

Gorlin RJ, Cohen MM, Hennekam R. *Syndromes of the Head and Neck*, 4th ed. Oxford University Press, NY: New York; 2001.

Hammond P, Hutton TJ, Allanson JE, et al. Discriminating power of localized three-dimensional facial morphology. *Am J Hum Genet.* 2005;77(6):999–1010.

Hennekam RC. Rubinstein-Taybi syndrome. *Eur J Hum Genet.* 2006;14(9):981–985.

Huang T. Current advances in Holt-Oram syndrome. *Curr Opin Pediatr.* 2002;14(6):691–695.

Irons M, Elias ER, Abuelo D, et al. Treatment of Smith-Lemli-Opitz syndrome: results of a multicenter trial. *Am J Med Genet.* 1997;68(3):311–314.

Jones K. *Smith's Patterns of Human Malformation*, 6th ed. Elsevier Philadelphia; 2005.

Kline AD, Krantz ID, Sommer A, et al. Cornelia de Lange syndrome: clinical review, diagnostic and scoring systems, and anticipatory guidance. *Am J Med Genet A.* 2007;143A(12):1287–1296.

Klopocki E, Schulze H, Strauss G, et al. Complex inheritance pattern resembling autosomal recessive inheritance involving a microdeletion in thrombocytopenia-absent radius syndrome. *Am J Hum Genet.* 2007;80(2):232–240.

Laursen HB. Congenital heart disease in Down's syndrome. *Br Heart J.* 1976;38(1):32–38.

Marsalese DL, Moodie DS, Vacante M, et al. Marfan's syndrome: natural history and long-term follow-up of cardiovascular involvement. *J Am Coll Cardiol.* 1989;14(2):422–428.

Petrij F, Giles RH, Dauwerse HG, et al. Rubinstein-Taybi syndrome caused by mutations in the transcriptional co-activator CBP. *Nature.* 1995;376(6538):348–351.

Pober BR, Johnson M, Urban Z. Mechanisms and treatment of cardiovascular disease in Williams-Beuren syndrome. *J Clin Invest.* 2008;118(5):1606–1615.

Porter FD. Smith-Lemli-Opitz syndrome: pathogenesis, diagnosis and management. *Eur J Hum Genet.* 2008;16(5):535–541.

Razzaque MA, Nishizawa T, Komoike Y, et al. Germline gain-of-function mutations in RAF1 cause Noonan syndrome. *Nat Genet.* 2007;39(8):1013–1017.

Ryan AK, Goodship JA, Wilson DI, et al. Spectrum of clinical features associated with interstitial chromosome 22q11 deletions: a European collaborative study. *J Med Genet.* 1997;34(10):798–804.

Sarkozy A, Conti E, Digilio MC, et al. Clinical and molecular analysis of 30 patients with multiple lentigines LEOPARD syndrome. *J Med Genet.* 2004;41(5):e68.

Schoumans J, Wincent J, Barbaro M, et al. Comprehensive mutational analysis of a cohort of Swedish Cornelia de Lange syndrome patients. *Eur J Hum Genet.* 2007;15(2):143–149.

Sharland M, Burch M, McKenna WM, Patton MA. A clinical study of Noonan syndrome. *Arch Dis Child.* 1992;67(2):178–183.

Shaw AC, Kalidas K, Crosby AH, Jeffery S, Patton MA. The natural history of Noonan syndrome: a long-term follow-up study. *Arch Dis Child.* 2007;92(2):128–132.

Tartaglia M, Mehler EL, Goldberg R, et al. Mutations in PTPN11, encoding the protein tyrosine phosphatase SHP-2, cause Noonan syndrome. *Nat Genet.* 2001;29(4):465–468.

Tint GS, Irons M, Elias ER, et al. Defective cholesterol biosynthesis associated with the Smith-Lemli-Opitz syndrome. *N Engl J Med.* 1994;330(2):107–113.

Tomson T, Perucca E, Battino D. Navigating toward fetal and maternal health: the challenge of treating epilepsy in pregnancy. *Epilepsia.* 2004;45(10):1171–1175.

11

Marfan Syndrome and Related Disorders

John CS Dean, Sally J Davies, and Bart Loeys

Introduction

Marfan syndrome is a variable, autosomal dominant connective tissue disorder whose cardinal features affect the cardiovascular system (aortic root dilatation, aortic rupture, aortic and mitral valve disease), the eyes (lens subluxation, myopia), and the skeleton (tall stature, arachnodactyly, joint hypermobility, pectus deformities). There are also important effects on the lungs, the skin, and the dura. The various features are described in the Ghent nosology, which is commonly used to diagnose the condition. The overwhelming majority of cases are associated with mutation in the fibrillin-1 gene on chromosome 15, but recent molecular advances have demonstrated pathogenetic links between the fibrillin-1 protein and other proteins such as the transforming growth factor β receptors (*TGFβR*) 1 and 2. Some Marfan-like cases without lens involvement have been reported to have mutations in one of these genes rather than fibrillin-1. To complicate the picture further, some rare fibrillin-1 mutations appear to have a mild effect and are found in patients who have some features of Marfan syndrome but do not fulfil the accepted diagnostic criteria. Such patients have been described as having a fibrillinopathy, because they do not fulfil the Marfan syndrome diagnostic criteria. Finally, mutations in *TGFβR1* and *TGFβR2* are predominantly found in the related disorders, Loeys-Dietz syndrome types 1 and 2 and occasionally in some cases of isolated familial thoracic aortic aneurysm. In this chapter, we will discuss the diagnosis and management of Marfan syndrome, the overlap with other fibrillinopathies, and with the Loeys-Dietz syndromes.

Historical Background

Marfan syndrome is named after Antoine Bernard-Jean Marfan, a French pediatrician, who described a 5-year-old girl (Gabrielle P) with long thin limbs, particularly noticeable in the fingers and toes, in an article published in Paris in 1896 (Marfan 1896). He named this combination of skeletal findings dolichostenomelia. Gabrielle also had joint contractures and scoliosis. In 1902, Achard described an older patient with some similar features that were familial, and in 1912 and 1914 respectively, cardiac and ocular findings were added to the syndrome (Parish 1960). It is no longer certain whether Marfan's original patient had the condition that bears his name—it is now believed that she suffered from a Marfan-related condition, called Beals syndrome or congenital contractural arachnodactly. In 1955, McKusick described Marfan syndrome as a heritable disorder of connective tissue, and noted its variability (McKusick 1955), laying the foundations for later clinical and molecular descriptions of the condition. Histochemical studies and a positional cloning approach led to the identification of mutation in the fibrillin-1 gene as the usual cause of Marfan syndrome in 1991 (Dietz et al. 1991). In 1993, a large French family with a Marfan-like disorder was described where the condition showed linkage to chromosome 3 rather than fibrillin-1 (Boileau et al. 1993; Collod et al. 1994), but the issue of whether Marfan syndrome displays locus heterogeneity remained controversial. In 2005, coinciding with the discovery of *TGFβR2* mutations in the related Loeys-Dietz syndrome, mutation in *TGFβR2* on chromosome 3 was also found to underlie the so-called nonocular form of Marfan syndrome, sometimes designated Marfan syndrome type 2 (Mizuguchi et al. 2004).

Defining Marfan Syndrome

Marfan syndrome (MIM 154700) as currently defined is a variable, autosomal dominant disorder of connective tissue whose cardinal features affect the cardiovascular system, eyes, and skeleton. The minimal birth incidence is around 1 in 9,800 (Gray et al. 1994), and the prevalence may be around 1 in 5,000 (Dietz and Pyeritz 1995). Progressive aortic dilatation, typically maximal at the sinus of Valsalva, associated with aortic valve incompetence leads to aortic dissection or rupture and is the principal cause of mortality in many cases, but mitral valve prolapse with incompetence may be significant, and lens dislocation, myopia, and arthralgia associated with chronic joint laxity can cause substantial morbidity. The most common clinical presentations are personal or family history of lens subluxation, personal or family history of aortic dissection or rupture, or in a young person with a tall, thin body habitus, long limbs, arachnodactyly, pectus deformities, and sometimes scoliosis (Figures 11–1 and 11–2). In each case, other findings in the clinical picture such as a high arched palate with dental crowding, skin striae distensae, recurrent hernia, or

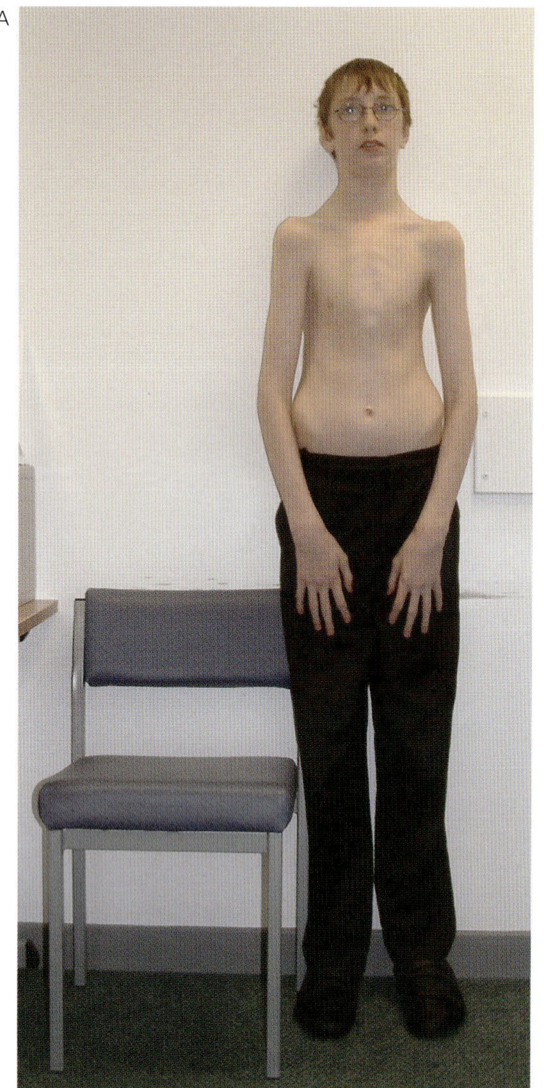

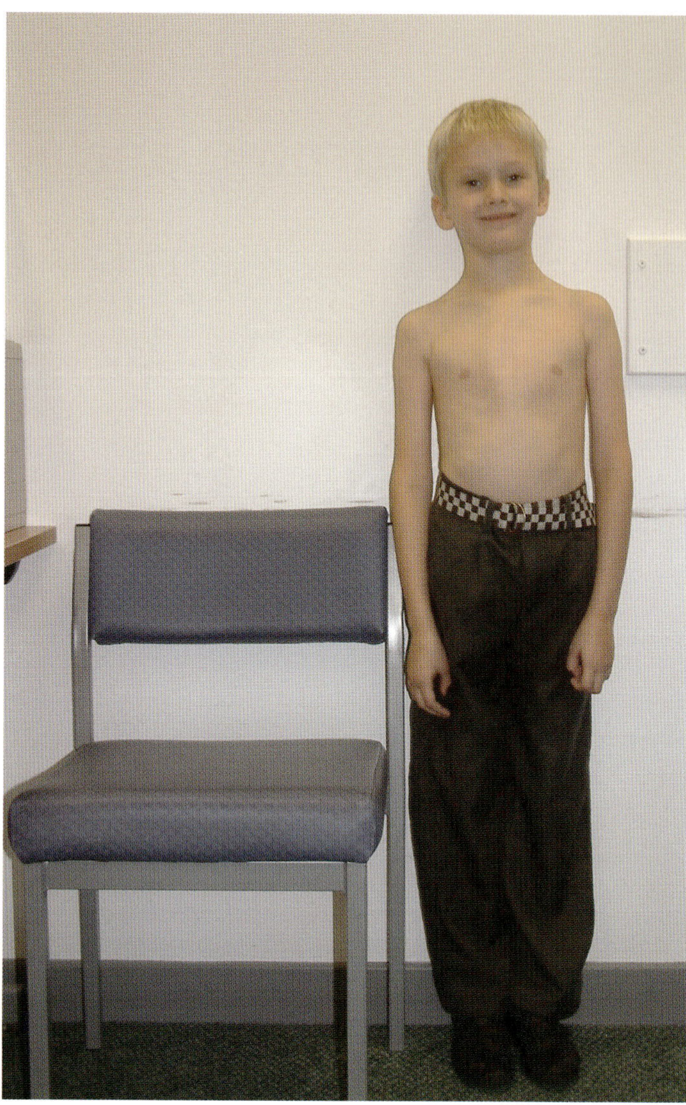

Figure 11–1 Two young people with Marfan syndrome. (a) Thirteen-year-old boy with lens subluxation, skeletal system involvement, and mild aortic root dilatation. He therefore fulfils the Ghent criteria on clinical findings alone. (b) Six-year-old boy with skeletal system involvement and mild aortic root dilatation. His father died from an aortic dissection, but had never been evaluated using the Ghent nosology. A nonsense mutation in exon 54 of fibrillin-1 was detected in the boy allowing a diagnosis of Marfan syndrome to be confirmed, and appropriate follow-up and management to be arranged.

recurrent pneumothorax may increase suspicion. Family history may be helpful, but around 27% of cases arise from new mutation (Gray et al. 1998). Between 66% and 91% of bona fide Marfan syndrome patients have an identifiable fibrillin-1 mutation (Loeys et al. 2001; Loeys et al. 2004), but fibrillin-1 mutations also cause some Marfan-like disorders or fibrillinopathies with a better prognosis, such as MASS phenotype, (MIM 604308, Mitral valve prolapse, mild nonprogressive Aortic dilatation, skin and skeletal features, or isolated ectopia lentis, MIM 129600) (Dietz and Pyeritz 1995). In addition, mutations in the *TGFβR2* gene on chromosome 3 and in the *TGFβR1* gene on chromosome 9 were recently found in some families with apparent Marfan syndrome (Mizuguchi et al. 2004; Sakai et al. 2006; Singh et al. 2006). "Marfan syndrome type 2" (MIM 154705) (Mizuguchi and Matsumoto 2007) families are less likely to have ectopia lentis. *TGFβR2* mutations at the R460 codon have also been described in families with the chromosome 3-linked form of familial thoracic ascending aortic aneurysm (Pannu et al. 2005; Law et al. 2006) (FTAA3, MIM 608967), and *TGFβR1* and *2* mutations are found in Loeys-Dietz syndromes type 1 and 2 (Loeys et al. 2005, 2006). Careful clinical assessment of patients with suspected Marfan syndrome is therefore essential to achieve an accurate diagnosis, provide prognostic information, and decide management options, and to this end, the various features were codified in 1988 into the so-called Berlin criteria, and revised as the Ghent nosology in 1996 (de Paepe et al. 1996). Patients who can be diagnosed as affected using this nosology are likely to be at greater risk of cardiovascular complications, and need regular follow-up with prophylactic medical and surgical treatment, and lifestyle advice. To facilitate use of the nosology in the clinic, an integrated care pathway for clinical diagnosis and

A 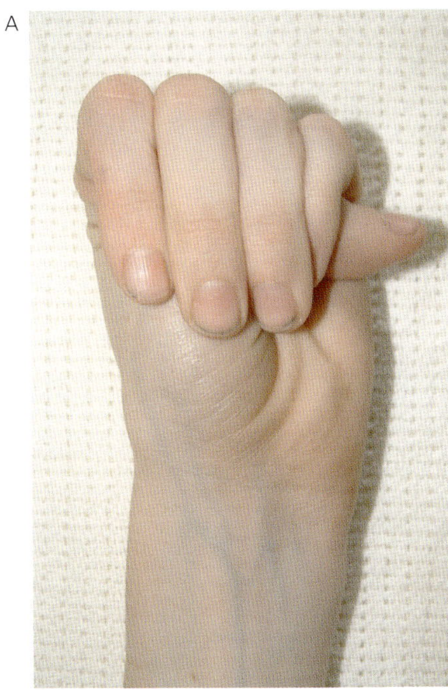

B 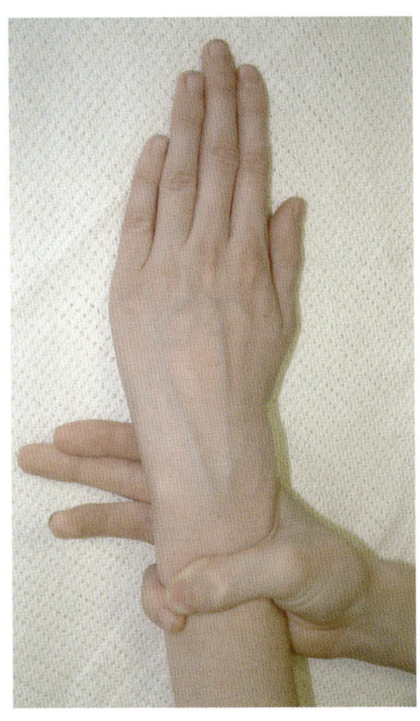

Figure 11–2 Arachnodactyly. (a) Positive Steinberg thumb sign: entire thumbnail protrudes beyond ulnar border of hand. (b) Positive Walker-Murdoch wrist sign: thumb and fifth finger overlap when encircling the wrist. Both signs must be present to diagnose arachnodactyly.

a Scottish clinical guideline for management of Marfan patients was devised by a consensus group in 1999 (Campbell et al. 2000) using SIGN methodology (Scottish Intercollegiate Guidelines Network 2004).

Diagnosis of Marfan Syndrome Using the Ghent Nosology

In the Ghent nosology, clinical features are assessed within seven body "systems," to determine whether that system provides a major criterion, or only system involvement (Table 11–1). In a proband, the diagnosis of Marfan syndrome requires a major criterion in two systems and involvement of a third. The cardiovascular, ocular, and skeletal systems can provide major criteria, or system involvement, the pulmonary system and skin/integument can provide only system involvement, the dura and family/genetic history provide only major criteria. The cardiovascular assessment requires measurement of the aortic diameter at the sinuses of Valsalva, usually by transthoracic echocardiography (Figure 11–3), and comparison with normal values based on age and body surface area, calculated from height and weight (Figure 11–4; Roman et al. 1993; de Paepe et al. 1996). Other imaging techniques such as transoesophageal echocardiography, or MRI scanning (Figure 11–5) may be helpful in some cases (Meijboom et al. 2000), including those with severe pectus deformity. Assessment of the skeletal system should include pelvic X-ray to detect protrusio acetabulae (Yule et al. 1999), only if a positive finding would provide system involvement, or change skeletal system involvement to a major criterion, such that a positive Marfan diagnosis could then be made in conjunction with other system findings. Similarly, lumbar MRI scan for dural ectasia, and genetic testing by linkage or mutation screening should be undertaken where a positive finding would make the diagnosis of Marfan syndrome. Ocular evaluation for myopia (due to increased globe length, measured by ultrasound), corneal flattening (measured by keratometry), hypoplastic iris or iris muscle, and lens subluxation requires ophthalmology assessment. Where there is a family history, the independent fulfilment of the diagnostic criteria in a relative can provide a major criterion. As mutation detection has become more widespread, it seems reasonable to use the detection of a mutation known to cause Marfan syndrome to count as a major criterion also in an index case, so that the same criteria may be applied to both index cases and relatives, as is implicit in the original nosology.

Because many Marfan features (echocardiographic findings [Shores et al. 1994], ectopia lentis, scoliosis, upper–lower segment ratio, protrusio acetabulae) are age dependent in their occurrence (Joseph et al. 1992; Lipscomb et al. 1997), younger patients with a family history of Marfan syndrome who do not fulfil the diagnostic criteria, and younger Marfan-like patients with no family history who fail to meet the diagnostic criteria by one system, should be offered repeat evaluations periodically (e.g., at least at ages 5, 10, and 15 years) until age 18 years.

The differential diagnosis of a tall young person with Marfan-like skeletal features includes homocystinuria (MIM 236300), Beals syndrome or congenital contractural arachnodactyly (MIM 121050), Marshall-Stickler syndrome (MIM 108300, 604841, 184840), Ehlers-Danlos syndrome (EDS) (MIM 130050), and MASS phenotype (MIM 604308). Where there is a family history of aortic aneurysm, familial thoracic aortic aneurysm (FTAA) should be considered (MIM 607086, other features of Marfan syndrome—mainly skeletal—may or may not be present). Additional clinical findings may suggest other disorders—bicuspid aortic valve and FTAA type 1 (MIM 607086), craniosynostosis, intellectual impairment, and Shprintzen-Goldberg syndrome (MIM 182212), arterial tortuosity or widespread aneurysms, hypertelorism, bifid uvula/cleft palate, craniosynostosis and Loeys-Dietz syndrome type 1 (Loeys et al. 2005) (MIM 609192), arterial tortuosity or widespread aneurysms, visceral rupture, joint hypermobility,

Table 11–1 Ghent Diagnostic Nosology

System	Major Criterion	Involvement
Skeletal	At least 4 of the following features: pectus carinatum pectus excavatum requiring surgery ULSR <0.86 or span:height >1.05 wrist and thumb signs scoliosis >20° or spondylolisthesis reduced elbow extension (<170°) pes plenus protrusio acetabulae	2 of the major features, or 1 major feature and 2 of the following: pectus excavatum joint hypermobility high palate with dental crowding characteristic face
Ocular	Lens dislocation (ectopia lentis)	Flat cornea Increased axial length of globe (causing myopia) Hypoplastic iris or ciliary muscle (causing decreased miosis)
Cardiovascular	Dilatation of the aortic root Dissection of the ascending aorta	Mitral valve prolapse Dilatation of the pulmonary artery, below age 40 Calcified mitral annulus, below age 40 Other dilatation or dissection of the aorta
Pulmonary	None	Spontaneous pneumothorax Apical blebs
Skin/Integument	None	Striae atrophicae Recurrent or incisional hernia
Dura	Lumbosacral dural ectasia	None
Genetic findings	Parent, child, or sibling meets these criteria independently Fibrillin-1 mutation known to cause Marfan syndrome Inheritance of DNA marker haplotype linked to Marfan syndrome in the family	None

Notes: ULSR Upper:lower segment ratio. Having one of the features listed constitutes a major criterion or system involvement for all systems except the skeletal system, where more than one feature is needed.

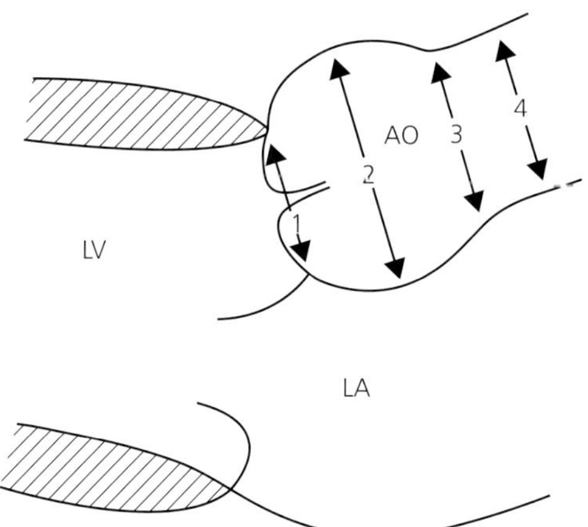

Figure 11–3 Diagram of the aortic root as seen at echocardiography. The aortic diameter should be measured at the aortic annulus (1), the sinuses of Valsalva (2), the supraaortic ridge (3), and the proximal ascending aorta (4). In Marfan syndrome, dilatation usually starts at the sinuses of Valsalva, so this measurement is critical in monitoring the early evolution of the condition. Diameters must be related to normal values for age and body surface area. After Roman et al. (1989) with permission.

thin skin with atrophic scarring, and Loeys-Dietz syndrome type 2 (Loeys et al. 2006) or intellectual impairment, velopharyngeal insufficiency, and Lujan-Fryns syndrome (MIM 309520). The initial evaluation of patients with possible Marfan syndrome requires a multidisciplinary approach including clinical genetics, cardiology, ophthalmology, and radiology.

Using the Ghent Criteria in the Clinic: The Scottish Experience

Assessment of a patient using the Ghent nosology requires evaluation of 30 clinical features. Interpreting the outcome can be complex, yet this nosology is the "gold standard" for clinical diagnosis. A recent study of patients reported to the Fibrillin-1 Universal Marfan Database (Faivre et al. 2008) probably confirms earlier concerns that the Ghent nosology as originally envisaged may be too strict—fibrillin-1 mutations are found in patients who do not apparently fulfil the nosology. However, the clinical information available for the cases reported is incomplete—some may have fulfilled the nosology with more extensive clinical investigation, and the risk of aortic dilatation in these "Ghent negative" cases is uncertain. The Scottish care pathway and clinical guideline were devised to make use of the nosology more practical in the clinic—any degree of scoliosis is accepted in the skeletal system, the presence of myopia is sufficient as a minor ocular criterion (keratometry and eye ultrasound are not required), and X-ray for protrusio acetabulae, MRI for dural ectasia, and fibrillin-1 gene testing are each required only if a positive result would ensure a diagnosis of Marfan syndrome by fulfilling the Ghent nosology (Dean 2007). Of course, fibrillin-1 gene testing also may be offered to enable testing of relatives rather than as a diagnostic test in the proband. Table 11–2 shows the outcome of using this modification of the Ghent criteria in a Marfan clinic in Aberdeen between 1999 and 2008.

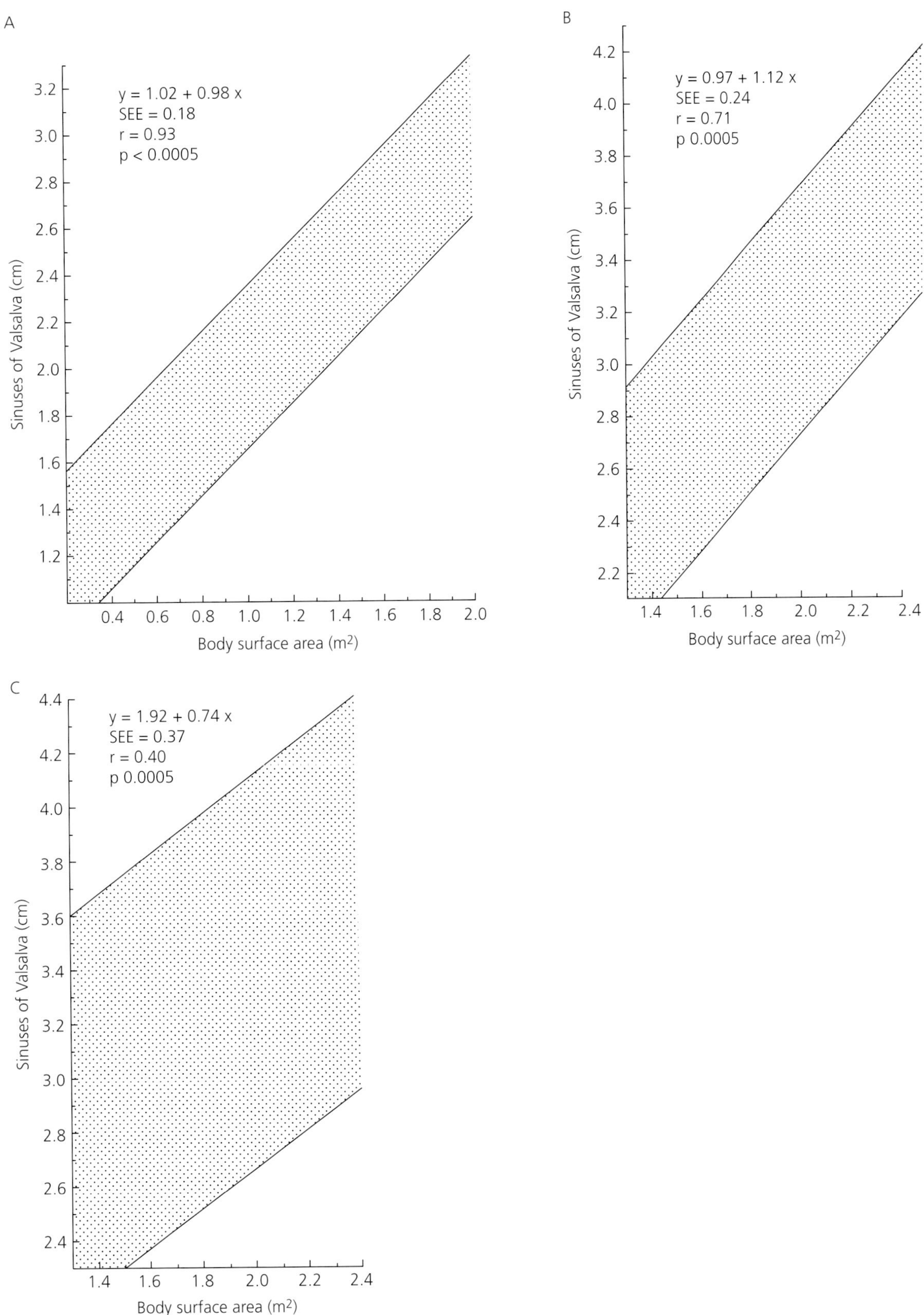

Figure 11–4 Normal ranges for aortic root dimension; 95% confidence interval for sinus of Valsalva diameter versus body surface area for (a) children up to 15 years old, (b) adults <40 years old, and (c) adults 40 years and over. Body surface area is calculated using the Mosteller formula: BSA (m^2) = ([Height (cm) x Weight (kg)]/3600)$^{1/2}$ (Mosteller 1987). Reprinted from Roman et al. (1989). Two-dimensional echocardiographic aortic root dimensions in normal children and adults. *Am J Cardiol*. 64;507–512, with permission.

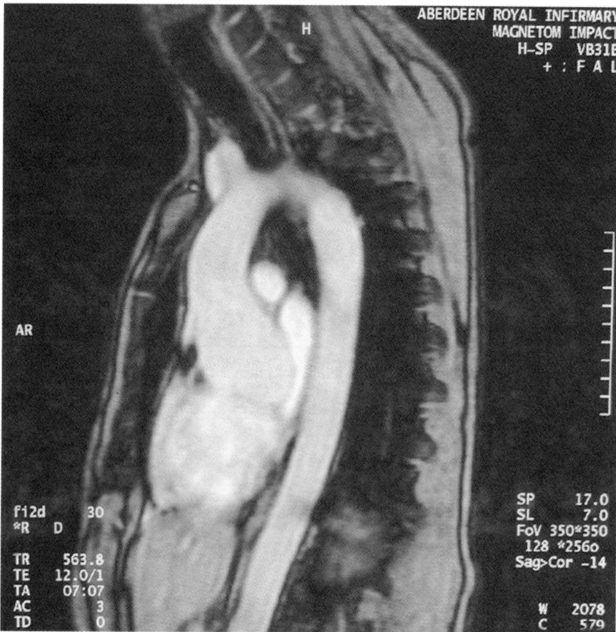

Figure 11–5 MRA. Parasagittal cine magnetic resonance angiogram (MRA) showing dilated aortic root but with normal upper ascending arch and descending aorta in a young adult.

One hundred and forty probands were referred during this period, the three most common presentations being skeletal findings compatible with Marfan syndrome with or without other features, personal and/or family history of aortic aneurysm, and lens subluxation. In 26.5%, Marfan syndrome could be unequivocally diagnosed using the modified Ghent criteria, and in these cases, 69% of those tested (18/26) had fibrillin-1 mutations, and 1 had a *TGFβR1* mutation. In 65%, Marfan could be unequivocally excluded; 18 of these 91 cases had some minor Marfan features (e.g., skeletal system involvement), but no mutations in fibrillin-1, *TGFβR1*, or *TGFβR2* were detected. Five cases (5%) had FTAA, on the basis of a personal or family history or aortic root dilatation or dissection in the absence of other Marfan syndrome features—three of these had *TGFβR1* mutations. Six cases (5%) had isolated ectopia lentis, only one of five tested had a fibrillin-1 mutation. One case of neonatal Marfan syndrome had recurrent pneumothorax, aortic root dilatation, and joint laxity—but no DNA was available for genetic investigation. From this, it can be seen that the Ghent criteria can be used effectively to diagnose or exclude Marfan syndrome in the majority of adult cases, but for those who do not fulfil the criteria, yet have significant clinical features (such as personal or family history of aortic aneurysm or lens subluxation), or are not yet adult, further repeated individual and family investigation should be undertaken (including genotyping) and alternative diagnoses should be considered. It is vital to confirm a reported family history of Marfan syndrome, as the criteria will be misleading in families where other conditions have predisposed to arterial rupture (e.g., Loeys-Dietz syndrome, FTAA). For the Loeys-Dietz syndrome it is important to screen for features that are not included in the Ghent nosology but clinically allow easy distinction from Marfan syndrome. These include bifid uvula/bifid uvula, craniosynostosis, blue sclerae, arterial tortuosity, aneurysms beyond the sinus of Valsalva, and thin skin with atrophic scarring. Molecular testing of an affected family member including fibrillin-1, *TGFβR1*, and *TGFβR2* may help confirm either diagnosis and allows predictive testing for younger family members. The age-dependent penetrance of many Marfan features means that children at risk for whom genetic testing is not possible or is unhelpful must be kept under review, as the criteria will not reliably exclude Marfan syndrome in those under 18 years. This applies both to those at risk by way of a positive family history, and to index cases whose clinical findings do not meet the Ghent criteria by one system (Table 11–3). Although the criteria are very useful for adults in classical Marfan syndrome, the rapidly emerging information about disease phenotypes associated with fibrillin-1, *TGFβR2*, and *TGFβR1* mutations may require some revision to include disorders such as Loeys-Dietz syndrome and FTAA. This would allow their more general use to guide molecular investigation of families and identify individuals at risk of aneurysmal disease. An international expert panel is currently redefining the Ghent nosology to accommodate these concerns.

Molecular Pathology of Marfan Syndrome and Related Disorders

Classical Marfan syndrome is associated with mutation in fibrillin-1, an important component of the elastic microfibril. Fibrillin-1 is a 350-kD glycoprotein, synthesized as a 375-kD precursor, which is processed and secreted into the extracellular matrix (ECM). It polymerizes to form microfibrils and helps to stabilize latent transforming growth factor β binding proteins (LTBPs) in the ECM (Robinson et al. 2006). LTBPs hold TGF-β in an inactive state (Mizuguchi and Matsumoto 2007). A failure of the interaction between fibrillin-1 and LTBPs may result in excess TGF-β signaling (Gelb 2006). Most fibrillin-1 mutations are

Table 11–2 Ghent Nosology and Genetic Testing of Probands in the Aberdeen Marfan Clinic

Ghent Assessment	Final Diagnosis	Cases	% of All Cases	Fibrillin-1 Mutations	*TGFβR1* Mutations	Total Cases Screened
Positive	Marfan	37	26.5%	18 (69%)	1	26
Negative	Not affected	91	65%	0	0	18
	FTAA	5	3.5%	0	3	5
	EL	6	4%	1	0	5
	Neonatal Marfan	1	1%	0	0	0
Total		140	100%	18	4	57

Notes: FTAA, familial thoracic aortic aneurysm; EL, isolated ectopia lentis.

Table 11–3 Key Issues in the Assessment of Marfan Syndrome

- Diagnosis or exclusion of Marfan syndrome in an individual should be based on the Ghent diagnostic nosology.
- The initial assessment should include a personal history, detailed family history, and clinical examination including ophthalmology examination and transthoracic echocardiogram.
- The aortic diameter at the sinus of Valsalva should be related to normal values based on age and body surface area.
- The development of scoliosis and protrusio acetabulae is age dependent, commonly occurring following periods of rapid growth. X-ray for these features, depending on age, if a positive finding would make the diagnosis of Marfan syndrome.
- A pelvic MRI scan to detect dural ectasia is indicated if a positive finding would make the diagnosis of Marfan syndrome.
- The Ghent nosology cannot exclude Marfan syndrome in children, because of the age-dependent penetrance of many features.
- Younger patients with a positive family history but unsuccessful DNA testing and insufficient clinical features to fulfil the diagnostic criteria, and younger patients with no family history who miss fulfilling the diagnostic criteria by one system only, should be offered further clinical evaluations at least until age 18, or until a diagnosis can be made.
- Family history of aortic aneurysm may represent a disorder such as FTAA, where the use of the Ghent nosology to assess risk in relatives is inappropriate.

missense, suggesting a dominant negative effect on microfibrillar assembly. Ectopia lentis tends to be associated with missense mutations causing cysteine substitutions within the epidermal growth factor (EGF)-like domains of the protein, but nonsense and frameshift mutations are seen in other cases, suggesting that while cysteine residues are important to the function of the suspensory ligament of the eye, either abnormal fibrillin or reduced amounts of fibrillin (haploinsufficiency) may cause other aspects of the Marfan phenotype (Judge et al. 2004). In keeping with this hypothesis, protein-truncating mutations tend to be associated with more severe skeletal and skin involvement, but are less common in cases with ectopia lentis (Faivre et al. 2007). Marked variability in severity has been documented—different mutations in the same codon can cause either severe neonatal Marfan syndrome or classical adult Marfan syndrome. Similarly, mutations in the central region of the gene (exons 24–32), sometimes called the "neonatal region," may be associated with phenotypes ranging from severe neonatal Marfan syndrome to isolated ectopia lentis (Dietz and Pyeritz 1995; Loeys et al. 2001; Mizuguchi and Matsumoto 2007), although in general mutations in this region are associated with more severe disease (Faivre et al. 2007). Although it was thought that abnormalities of microfibril structure might play an architectural role in causing the Marfan phenotype, it is now clear that the role of fibrillin-1 in regulation of TGF-β signaling may be more pertinent. The discovery of *TGFβR1* and *TGFβR2* mutations in Loeys-Dietz syndrome, a Marfan-related condition supports this, as does evidence from mouse models (Dietz et al. 2005; Mizuguchi and Matsumoto 2007). *TGFβR1* or *TGFβR2* mutations in humans are also associated with loss of elastin fibers, and fiber disarray. Although the *TGFβR1* and *TGFβR2* mutations described so far are loss-of-function mutations, increased TGF-β signaling was found in patient tissues and Marfan mouse models, and TGF-β blockade by neutralizing antibodies or angiotensin II type 1 (AT1) receptor blockers rescues the model phenotypes (Loeys et al. 2005; Habashi et al. 2006; Mizuguchi and Matsumoto 2007). The pathogenic process must involve a complex disruption of TGF-β signaling yet to be fully elucidated.

Aspects of Clinical Management in Marfan Syndrome

Although clinical management of many genetic disorders is not backed by extensive trials and case series (Campbell et al. 2000), there are a large number of published studies of Marfan syndrome, which were reviewed in the development of the Scottish Marfan guideline. Some of the key studies will now be discussed, to provide a flavor of the evidence and dilemmas that influence Marfan management today.

1. Cardiovascular System in Marfan Syndrome

Cardiovascular complications of Marfan syndrome include mitral valve prolapse and regurgitation, left ventricular dilatation and cardiac failure, and pulmonary artery dilatation, but aortic root dilatation is the most common cause of morbidity and mortality. Aortic valve incompetence usually arises in the context of a dilated aortic root, and the risk of aortic dissection (Figure 11–6) increases when the diameter at the sinus of Valsalva exceeds 5 cm (Roman et al. 1993; Groenink et al. 1999), when the aortic dilatation is more extensive, when the rate of dilatation exceeds 1.5 mm per year, and where there is a family history of aortic dissection (Shores et al. 1994; Legget et al. 1996; Groenink et al. 1999; Meijboom et al. 2005). Myocardial infarction may occur if an aortic root dissection occludes the coronary ostia. Marfan syndrome mortality from aortic complications has decreased (70% in 1972, 48% in 1995) and life expectancy has increased (mean age at death 32±16 years in 1972 versus 45±17 years in 1998) (Gray et al. 1998) associated with increased medical and surgical intervention (Table 11.4).

The Marfan aorta is characterized by elastic fiber fragmentation and disarray, paucity of smooth muscle cells, and deposition of collagen and mucopolysaccharide between the cells of the media. These appearances are sometimes described as "cystic medial degeneration" although there are no true cysts present. This finding is not specific for Marfan syndrome and can also be found in other conditions such as LDS, FTAA, and BAV with FTAA. Mucopolysaccharide deposition in the valves may cause

Table 11–4 Key Issues in Cardiovascular Management

- β-blocker therapy should be considered at any age if the aorta is dilated, but prophylactic treatment may be more effective in those with an aortic diameter of less than 4 cm.
- Risk factors for aortic dissection include aortic diameter greater than 5 cm, aortic dilatation extending beyond the sinus of Valsalva, rapid rate of dilatation (>5% per year, or 1.5 mm/year in adults), and family history of aortic dissection.
- At least annual evaluation should be offered, comprising clinical history, examination, and echocardiography. In children, serial echocardiography at 6–12-month intervals is recommended, the frequency depending on the aortic diameter (in relation to body surface area) and the rate of increase.
- Prophylactic aortic root surgery should be considered when the aortic diameter at the sinus of Valsalva exceeds 5 cm.
- In pregnancy, there is an increased risk of aortic dissection if the aortic diameter exceeds 4 cm. Frequent cardiovascular monitoring throughout pregnancy and into the puerperium is advised.

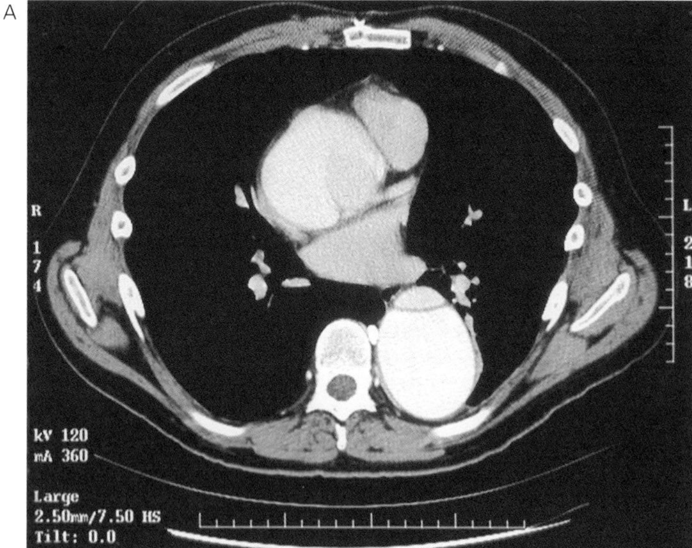

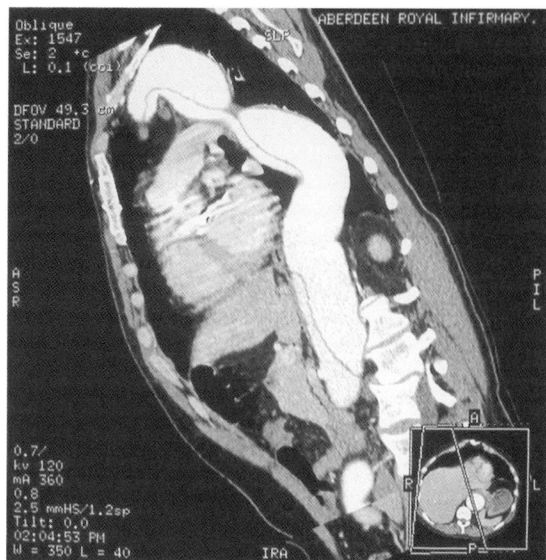

Figure 11–6 MR and CT images. (a) Axial CT scan at T7 of a Marfan patient showing dilated ascending and descending aorta with dissection flap anteriorly in the descending aorta and previous surgery to the ascending aorta. (b) Parasagittal reformatted CT of chest and abdomen in the same patient with contrast showing dilatation of the whole of the aorta with a spiral dissection from the arch through to the lower abdominal aorta. MR and CT images courtesy of Professor J Weir, Department of Radiology, Aberdeen Royal Infirmary.

valve leaflet thickening. Elastic fiber degeneration in the aorta is associated with reduced distensibility in response to the pulse pressure wave. This abnormal aortic compliance can be detected at any age by echocardiography (Rios et al. 1999) or gated MRI scanning (Adams et al. 1995), although it is less marked in children. Reduction of the systolic ejection impulse by β-blockers might be expected to reduce the risk of aortic dissection in Marfan syndrome (Shores et al. 1994). Studies in turkeys prone to aortic dissection showed improved survival with propranolol and two trials in Marfan patients (a randomized trial of propranolol therapy and a retrospective historically controlled trial of propranolol or atenolol therapy) demonstrated a reduced rate of aortic dilatation and fewer aortic complications in the treatment group (Salim et al. 1994; Shores et al. 1994). Some patients respond better than others, responders tending to be younger and showing improved aortic distensibility, reduced pulse wave velocity, and smaller pretreatment aortic diameters (less than 4 cm in one study) (Salim et al. 1994; Shores et al. 1994; Legget et al. 1996; Haouzi et al. 1997; Groenink et al. 1998; Rios et al. 1999). Poor response may be associated with more extensive elastic fiber degeneration, either due to a more severe mutation or more advanced disease. β-blockade should therefore be considered in all Marfan patients, including children. Some patients may not tolerate β-blockers, and alternative drugs that reduce the ejection impulse such as calcium antagonists (Rossi-Foulkes et al. 1999) and angiotensin-converting enzyme (ACE) inhibitors have been considered. ACE inhibitors also reduce vascular smooth muscle cell apoptosis in vitro through an angiotensin II type 2 (AT2) receptor dependent mechanism - [apoptosis is implicated in the cystic medial degeneration seen in the Marfan aorta (Nagashima et al. 2001)]. This theoretical benefit may be in addition to any hemodynamic effects. Enalapril improved aortic distensibility and reduced the rate of aortic dilatation compared with β-blockers in one small clinical trial in children and adolescents (Yetman et al. 2005). In a mouse model, the angiotensin II type 1 (AT1) receptor antagonist losartan reduced aortic growth rate, and prevented elastic fiber degeneration, presumably through effects on TGF-β signaling as well as hemodynamic effects, although angiotensin II also stimulates Smad-2 dependent signaling in vascular smooth muscle cells and vessel wall fibrosis by an AT1 receptor dependent but TGF-β independent mechanism (Habashi et al. 2006). In one small observational study in 18 children with Marfan syndrome, the rate of increase of aortic diameter was significantly reduced after treatment with an AT1 receptor blocker (Brooke et al. 2008)—the outcome of a larger randomized trial is awaited (Lacro et al. 2007). As ACE inhibitors reduce angiotensin II production, they will act on both AT1 and AT2 dependent pathways—the benefit or otherwise of inhibiting both pathways is unknown. Matrix metalloproteinases (MMPs) are large endopeptidases, which degrade matrix proteins including elastin. They may therefore contribute to the elastic fiber degeneration of Marfan syndrome. Their expression is closely regulated at several levels, but increased expression of MMP 2 and MMP 9 has been found in the Marfan aorta. In a mouse model, doxycyline, a nonspecific inhibitor of MMP 2 and 9 prevented thoracic aortic aneurysm, and suppressed upregulation of TGF-β expression (Chung et al. 2008)—no human data has yet been reported. Enalapril is known to decrease MMP 9 activity in non-Marfan patients (Williams et al. 2008). In another study, abnormal flow mediated vasodilation of the brachial artery was demonstrated in Marfan patients, although agonist mediated vasodilation was normal (Wilson et al. 1999). This was attributed to abnormal endothelial cell mechanotransduction associated with abnormal fibrillin. Although losartan is possibly the most promising alternative to β-blockers at present, there may therefore be other molecular targets for future pharmacological intervention.

If medical treatment fails, and the aortic root dilates to 5 cm or more, then prophylactic surgery should be considered (de Paepe et al. 1996; Groenink et al. 1999; Meijboom et al. 2004). One study suggests that the threshold diameter should be 0.5 cm lower in affected women (Meijboom et al. 2005). Other factors such as the rate of aortic growth, and family history of dissection should be taken into account. Numerous studies have shown better survival rates for prophylactic compared with emergency aortic surgery (Groenink et al. 1999; Gott et al. 2002), and improved longevity for Marfan patients who undergo prophylactic surgery compared with their untreated relatives (Finkbohner et al. 1995). Alternative procedures include the Bentall composite graft repair, in which both the aortic root and the aortic valve are replaced, or a valve conserving technique such as reimplantation of the native aortic valve in a Dacron tube (described by David) or remodeling of the aortic root (described by Yacoub) (de Oliveira et al. 2003; Nataf and Lansac 2006). The Bentall procedure has a low mortality in experienced hands with long-term survival of around 80% at 5 years and 60% at 10 years (Treasure 1993), but requires lifelong anticoagulation postoperatively, whereas valve conserving techniques may avoid the need for anticoagulation. Use of a valve-sparing procedure has been controversial as it is suggested that further deterioration of the aortic valve leaflets will require later valve replacement surgery. Recent case series have suggested that in expert hands, and in selected cases such as those where the aortic valve appears structurally normal (incompetence being due to annular dilatation) the medium term outcome is as good as the Bentall procedure, without the hazards of anticoagulation (Bassano et al. 2001; Kallenbach et al. 2005). In longer-term follow-up (8 years), one series suggested a better outcome for valve conserving surgery, although this was attributed to preferential use of the Bentall procedure in higher risk patients. Thromboembolism was more common after the Bentall procedure (9% compared to 1% at 8 years) but reoperation was more common in patients who had undergone valve conserving surgery (6% compared to 2% at 8 years) (Patel et al. 2008). There is certainly a case for considering a valve sparing procedure for children, women of childbearing age, and those in whom anticoagulation may be hazardous. As Marfan patients survive longer, reoperation for new aneurysms developing elsewhere in the arterial tree are becoming common—in one series, 70% developed second aneurysms requiring surgery (Finkbohner et al. 1995). Continuation of long-term medical prophylaxis after surgery is therefore strongly recommended (Treasure 1993) along with follow-up imaging of the descending and abdominal aorta (Nataf and Lansac 2006). Other cardiac valves may also be involved—mitral valve surgery is required in up to 10% of those requiring aortic root surgery (Finkbohner et al. 1995).

2. Ocular System

Ocular features of Marfan syndrome include bilateral ectopia lentis (40%–56%), myopia (28%), and retinal detachment (0.78%) (van den Berg et al. 1996; Loeys et al. 2004). Lens dislocation into the anterior chamber may occur. Subluxation usually develops in early childhood, but may first present in the second decade (Maumenee 1981). Myopia is associated with an increased length of the globe and an increased risk of retinal detachment (Pyeritz and McKusick 1979). Early detection and correction of refractive errors prevents amblyopia—correction after the age of 12 years is less likely to restore visual acuity. Anisotropia (unequal refraction between the two eyes) and the possible anterior chamber abnormalities are further important considerations for management (Pyeritz and McKusick 1979). Ophthalmology assessment is important, and regular orthoptic review is recommended, particularly in childhood. Vitreolensectomy with laser prophylaxis to prevent retinal detachment can be effective in improving visual acuity in some patients (Hubbard et al. 1998).

3. Musculoskeletal System

Skeletal abnormalities develop and may progress during childhood. Scoliosis affects around 60% of Marfan patients and may progress rapidly during growth spurts, leading to marked deformity, pain, and restricted ventilatory deficit. In adults, back pain (associated with scoliosis) is three times more frequent than in the general population (Pyeritz and Francke 1993). Occasionally scoliosis may progress in adult life especially if the angle of curvature is >40°. Back pain is said to be more common in patients with dural ectasia but the evidence for this is problematic. Dural ectasia is present in 69% of Marfan patients by CT scan and 95% by MRI imaging (Fattori et al. 1999; Oosterhof et al. 2001). In a study of 32 patients, dural ectasia was present in 76% of those with back pain and 41% of those without (Ahn et al. 2000). Treatment of dural ectasia to manage back pain remains speculative (Fattori et al. 1999). Similarly, bone mineral density appears to be reduced at the spine and hip in Marfan syndrome (Le Parc et al. 2001; Giampietro et al. 2003), but no associated increase in fracture rate has been observed.

Joint hypermobility is common, affecting 85% of children under 18 years, and 56% of adults with many patients suffering arthralgia, myalgia, or ligamentous injury (Grahame and Pyeritz 1995). A Marfan-related myopathy with abnormal muscle fibrillin was described in one family (Behan et al. 2003) causing skeletal and respiratory muscle weakness. The significance of this for musculoskeletal symptoms in the wider Marfan patient group awaits further study.

4. Respiratory System

Pectus excavatum occurs in approximately two-thirds of patients with Marfan syndrome, and when severe, can be associated with a restrictive ventilatory defect (Streeten et al. 1987; Scherer et al. 1988). It can cause difficulty with cardiac surgical procedures but correction is most often requested for cosmetic reasons. Patients with Marfan syndrome are more likely to have delayed wound healing following repair of pectus excavatum (Golladay et al. 1985; Arn et al. 1989). Surgical correction in children should be avoided, as recurrence is common in this age group (Arn et al. 1989).

Spontaneous pneumothorax occurs in 4%–11% of patients and may be associated with apical bullae (Hall et al. 1984; Wood et al. 1984). Recurrence is common, and there should be a low threshold for surgical intervention. Mechanical ventilation can exacerbate respiratory difficulties in Marfan neonates because of susceptibility to pneumothorax, bullae, and emphysema.

Adult patients with Marfan syndrome have an increased tendency to upper airway collapse during sleep, causing obstructive sleep apnea. This is associated with abnormalities of craniofacial structure. It may contribute to daytime somnolence, sometimes attributed to β-blocker therapy (Cistulli et al. 2001).

5. Central Nervous System

Dural ectasia may reduce the effectiveness of epidural anesthesia (Lacassie et al. 2005), and has been associated with intracranial hypotension-associated headache in some case reports (Rosser et al. 2005). Anterior sacral meningocele has been described rarely as a complication of Marfan syndrome, and may lead to diagnostic confusion when presenting as a pelvic or abdominal mass (Voyvodic et al. 1999). Cerebral hemorrhage and other neurovascular disorders are uncommon in Marfan patients (Wityk et al. 2002), but intracranial aneurysms may be more common in the Loeys-Dietz syndrome (Loeys et al. 2006).

6. Pregnancy in Marfan Syndrome

The risk of aortic dissection during pregnancy is increased, although women with Marfan syndrome who have had children have a similar lifetime risk of aortic dissection to those who have remained childless (Pacini et al. 2008), despite the fact that the rate of aortic dilatation after childbirth may be higher in women who started pregnancy with an aortic root exceeding 4.5 cm in diameter (Meijboom et al. 2006). It has been suggested that pregnancy acts as a "revealer" of those women likely to have dissections. Inhibition of collagen and elastin deposition in the aorta by estrogen, the hyperdynamic hypervolemic circulatory state of pregnancy (Immer et al. 2003) and conditions such as gestational hypertension and preeclampsia may be additional factors (Chow 1993), although these last two conditions are less common in women on β-blockers (Meijboom et al. 2006). Aortic dissection occurs in around 4.5% of pregnancies in women with Marfan syndrome (Chow 1993) and the risk is greater if the aortic root exceeds 4 cm at the start of pregnancy, or if it dilates rapidly (Lind and Wallenburg 2001). More frequent monitoring of aortic diameter in pregnancy is advisable. If the aortic root dilates to 5 cm during the pregnancy, consideration should be given to immediate aortic replacement, early delivery, or termination of pregnancy. There may be an increased risk of spontaneous preterm labour (Meijboom et al. 2006), but the frequencies of spontaneous miscarriage or postpartum hemorrhage are similar to those seen in the general population.

As Marfan syndrome is autosomal dominant, there is a one in two (50%) chance that the child of an affected person will inherit the disorder. Marfan patients seldom ask for prenatal diagnosis, although preimplantation genetic diagnosis has been undertaken for families with prior molecular work up in the genetic clinic (Loeys et al. 2002). Ultrasound diagnosis is unreliable. Marfan patients should be offered genetic counseling before planning a family.

It is often difficult to diagnose Marfan syndrome in a newborn baby, but offspring of Marfan patients should be assessed early in life, with gene testing where possible, so that appropriate follow-up can be organized.

Marfan Syndrome and Sports

Although there have been no trials to investigate the effectiveness of sports limitation to avoid joint damage, common sense suggests that activities likely to stress the joints should be avoided. Heart rate, systolic blood pressure, and cardiac output increase during both dynamic exercise (e.g., running) and static exercise (e.g., weightlifting). Peripheral vascular resistance and diastolic blood pressure tend to fall during dynamic exercise, but increase during static exercise (Salim and Alpert 2001). Marfan patients should therefore avoid high intensity static exercise, but can be encouraged to participate in lower intensity dynamic exercise (Maron et al. 2004). Contact sports are not advised, to protect the aorta and the lens of the eye, and scuba diving should be avoided because of the increased risk of pneumothorax.

Loeys-Dietz Syndrome

Recently, a novel autosomal dominant aortic aneurysm syndrome was identified and this entity is characterized by the triad of hypertelorism, bifid uvula/cleft palate, and arterial tortuosity with ascending aortic aneurysm/dissection. This disorder was first delineated in 10 families and designated Loeys-Dietz syndrome (LDS—MIM 60919) (Loeys et al. 2005) showing multiple additional findings including craniosynostosis, Arnold Chiari type 1 malformation, dural ectasia, pectus deformity, scoliosis, arachnodactyly, club feet, patent ductus arteriosus, atrial septal defect, and bicuspid semilunar valves, but most importantly aneurysms/dissections throughout the arterial tree. Evaluation of a larger series of patients proved that the previously reported triad remains the most specific finding for this diagnosis (Loeys et al. 2006), but also indicated the increased incidence of additional findings including developmental delay, hydrocephalus, congenital hip dislocation, dural ectasia, spondylolisthesis, cervical spine dislocation or instability, submandibular branchial cysts, osteoporosis with multiple fractures at a young age, and defective tooth enamel. When present, developmental delay did not always associate with either craniosynostosis or hydrocephalus, suggesting that learning disability is a rare primary manifestation. LDS patients may share several manifestations of the Marfan syndrome but do not display ectopia lentis or significant dolichostenomelia, findings that are typical in Marfan syndrome.

Based on the central role of TGF-β signaling in cardiovascular, skeletal, and craniofacial development, the genes encoding the *TGF-β* receptors (*TGFβR1* and *TGFβR2*) were considered as candidate genes. Also, a prior report had suggested that heterozygous loss-of-function mutations could cause a *TGFβR2* phenocopy of Marfan syndrome (Mizuguchi et al. 2004), a phenotype significantly overlapping with LDS. In the initial analysis of 10 patients with the classic, severe presentation of LDS (including typical craniofacial features; LDS-I) 6 mutations in *TGFβR2* and 4 in *TGFβR1* were identified (Loeys et al. 2005). While this observation intuitively corroborated the essential role of the TGF-β pathway in the pathogenesis of aortic aneurysm, it was not clear how a loss of function of the receptor for TFG-β could lead to upregulation of TGF-β activity, as had been previously observed in mouse models for Marfan syndrome. The study of fibroblasts derived from heterozygous patients with LDS failed to reveal any defect in the acute phase response to administered ligand and showed an apparent increase in TGF-β signaling after 24 hours of ligand deprivation and a slower decline in the TGF-β signal after restoration of ligand. An even more informative result was the observation of increased expression of TGF-β-dependent gene products such as collagen and CTGF (connective tissue growth factor) and increased nuclear accumulation of pSmad2 in the aortic wall of patients with LDS, as well as in patients with Marfan syndrome.

Following the initial identification of *TGFβR* mutations in the first 10 patients with LDS, a more in-depth clinical and molecular study of 52 affected families, of which 40 had probands with typical clinical manifestations of LDS was published (Loeys et al. 2006). Mutations in *TGFβR1* or *TGFβR2* were found in all probands with typical LDS (referred to as LDS type I). As there is a clear phenotypic overlap between LDS and the vascular EDS type IV, a cohort of 40 patients who presented with a vascular EDS-like syndrome, but did not bear the characteristic type III collagen abnormalities was investigated (Loeys et al. 2006). *TGFβR1* or *TGFβR2* mutations were identified in 12 probands presenting with this condition, which was referred to as LDS type II. The phenotype of these patients was characterized by velvety, translucent skin, easy bruising, atrophic scars, uterine rupture, and arterial aneurysms/dissections within the cerebral, thoracic, and abdominal circulations.

The natural history of both types of LDS was characterized by aggressive arterial aneurysms (mean age at death, 26 years) and a high incidence of pregnancy-related complications. Obviously, the natural history of disease in LDS patients is far more aggressive than that of Marfan syndrome or vascular EDS, including aortic dissection in young childhood and/or at much lower aortic dimensions than in other connective tissue disorders. Patients with LDS type I, as compared with those with LDS type II, had a poorer prognosis toward cardiovascular surgery and life expectancy. Importantly however, aneurysms in LDS appeared to be well amenable to early and aggressive surgical intervention, in contrast to what is observed in vascular EDS, in which intraoperative mortality is very high due to the extreme fragility of the vessel walls.

There are no differences in phenotype between individuals with mutations in *TGFβR1* and *TGFβR2* and no apparent phenotype–genotype correlations that explain the distinction between LDS type I and LDS type II. Furthermore, there are no apparent differences between the mutations that we and others have found in patients with LDS versus those described as causing Marfan syndrome type 2 (Mizuguchi et al. 2004) or familial thoracic aortic aneurysm and dissection (FTAA) (Pannu et al. 2006). Indeed, identical mutations described as causing Marfan syndrome type 2 or FTAA have been identified in patients with typical LDS type I or LDS type II.

All this suggests that comprehensive clinical evaluation is critical for making the diagnostic distinction between the Marfan syndrome, LDS, and the vascular EDS, and that in addition to molecular studies of *FBN1* (fibrillin-1) or *COL3A1* (collagen type III), genotyping of *TGFβR1/2* genes can also be useful in the diagnostic workup and further management of patients presenting with aortic aneurysms.

The management principles are largely based on previous experience with Marfan and vascular EDS but are also guided by the differences between these diseases and Loeys-Dietz syndrome. Two important management differences distinguish patients with *FBN1/COL3A1* mutations from *TGFβR1/2* positive patients. In the latter, more extensive imaging of the arterial tree (from head to pelvis) is indicated and earlier surgery at smaller aortic root dimensions is justifiable. β-adrenergic blockers or other medications are used to reduce hemodynamic stress. Angiotensin receptor blockers have been used in LDS but no randomized trials exist to prove their benefit. Aneurysms in LDS are amenable to early and aggressive surgical intervention (in contrast to vascular EDS, in which surgery is used as a last resort because of the extremely high rate of intraoperative complications and death). Many individuals can receive a valve-sparing procedure that precludes the need for chronic anticoagulation. Given the safety and the increasing availability of the valve-sparing procedure, this method is preferred. For young children with severe systemic findings of LDS, surgical repair of the ascending aorta should be considered once the maximal dimension exceeds the 99th percentile and the aortic annulus exceeds 1.8 cm, allowing the placement of a graft of sufficient size to accommodate growth.

For adolescents and adults, surgical repair of the ascending aorta should be considered once the maximal dimension approaches 4 cm. This recommendation is based on both numerous examples of documented aortic dissection in adults with aortic root dimensions at or below 4 cm and the excellent response to prophylactic surgery. An extensive family history of larger aortic dimension without dissection could alter this practice for individual patients. This practice may not eliminate risk of dissection and death, and earlier intervention based on family history or the patient's personal assessment of risk versus benefit may be indicated.

Conclusion

The Ghent nosology remains the most effective way of diagnosing or excluding Marfan syndrome, providing its limitations with respect to children are not forgotten. It can help to identify families with aortic dissection who do not have Marfan syndrome, but it should not be used to assess risk in such families. Despite the morbidity and mortality associated with Marfan syndrome and related disorders, appropriate medical and surgical management can improve and extend the lives of many patients, and advancing research holds the promise of further improvements in the future.

Acknowledgments

The Scottish Marfan Guideline was developed in conjunction with colleagues from many disciplines as part of a project funded by the Clinical Resources and Audit Group of the Scottish Executive Department of Health. Bart Loeys is a senior clinical investigator of the Fund for Scientific Research—Flanders.

References

Adams JN, Brooks M, Redpath TW, et al. Aortic distensibility and stiffness index measured by magnetic resonance imaging in patients with Marfan's syndrome. *Br Heart J.* 1995;73:265–269.

Ahn NU, Sponseller PD, Ahn UM, et al. Dural ectasia is associated with back pain in Marfan syndrome. *Spine.* 2000;25:1562–1568.

Arn PH, Scherer LR, Haller JA Jr, et al. Outcome of pectus excavatum in patients with Marfan syndrome and in the general population. *J Pediatr.* 1989;115:954–958.

Bassano C, De Matteis GM, Nardi P, et al. Mid-term follow-up of aortic root remodelling compared to Bentall operation. *Eur J Cardiothorac Surg.* 2001;19:601–605.

Behan WM, Longman C, Petty RK, et al. Muscle fibrillin deficiency in Marfan's syndrome myopathy. *J Neurol Neurosurg Psychiatry.* 2003;74: 633–638.

Boileau C, Jondeau G, Babron MC, et al. Autosomal dominant Marfan-like connective-tissue disorder with aortic dilation and skeletal anomalies not linked to the fibrillin genes. *Am J Hum Genet.* 1993;53:46–54.

Brooke BS, Habashi JP, Judge DP, et al. Angiotensin II blockade and aortic-root dilation in Marfan's syndrome. *N Engl J Med.* 2008;358:2787–2795.

Campbell H, Bradshaw N, Davidson R, et al. Evidence based medicine in practice: lessons from a Scottish clinical genetics project. *J Med Genet.* 2000;37:684–691.

Chow SL. Acute aortic dissection in a patient with Marfan's syndrome complicated by gestational hypertension. *Med J Aust.* 1993;159:760–762.

Chung AW, Yang HH, Radomski MW, et al. Long-term doxycycline is more effective than atenolol to prevent thoracic aortic aneurysm in Marfan syndrome through the inhibition of matrix metalloproteinase-2 and -9. *Circ Res.* 2008;102:e73–e85.

Cistulli PA, Gotsopoulos H, Sullivan CE. Relationship between craniofacial abnormalities and sleep-disordered breathing in Marfan's syndrome. *Chest.* 2001;120:1455–1460.

Collod G, Babron MC, Jondeau G, et al. A second locus for Marfan syndrome maps to chromosome 3p24.2-p25. *Nat Genet.* 1994;8:264–268.

Dean JC. Marfan syndrome: clinical diagnosis and management. *Eur J Hum Genet.* 2007;15:724–733.

de Oliveira NC, David TE, Ivanov J, et al. Results of surgery for aortic root aneurysm in patients with Marfan syndrome. *J Thorac Cardiovasc Surg.* 2003;125:789–796.

de Paepe AM, Devereux RB, Dietz HC, et al. Revised diagnostic criteria for the Marfan syndrome. *Am J Med Genet.* 1996;62:417–426.

Dietz HC, Cutting GR, Pyeritz RE, et al. Marfan syndrome caused by a recurrent de novo missense mutation in the fibrillin gene. *Nature.* 1991;352:337–339.

Dietz HC, Loeys B, Carta L, et al. Recent progress towards a molecular understanding of Marfan syndrome. *Am J Med Genet C Semin Med Genet.* 2005;139C:4–9.

Dietz HC, Pyeritz RE. Mutations in the human gene for fibrillin-1 (FBN1) in the Marfan syndrome and related disorders. *Hum Mol Genet.* 1995;4 Spec No:1799–1809.

Faivre L, Collod-Beroud G, Child A, et al. Contribution of molecular analyses in diagnosing Marfan syndrome and type I fibrillinopathies: an international study of 1009 probands. *J Med Genet.* 2008;45:384–390.

Faivre L, Collod-Beroud G, Loeys BL, et al. Effect of mutation type and location on clinical outcome in 1,013 probands with Marfan syndrome or related phenotypes and FBN1 mutations: an international study. *Am J Hum Genet.* 2007;81:454–466.

Fattori R, Nienaber CA, Descovich B, et al. Importance of dural ectasia in phenotypic assessment of Marfan's syndrome. *Lancet.* 1999;354:910–913.

Finkbohner R, Johnston D, Crawford ES, et al. Marfan syndrome. Long-term survival and complications after aortic aneurysm repair. *Circulation.* 1995;91:728–733.

Gelb BD. Marfan's syndrome and related disorders—more tightly connected than we thought. *N Engl J Med.* 2006;355:841–844.

Giampietro PF, Peterson M, Schneider R, et al. Assessment of bone mineral density in adults and children with Marfan syndrome. *Osteoporos Int.* 2003;14:559–563.

Golladay ES, Char F, Mollitt DL. Children with Marfan's syndrome and pectus excavatum. *South Med J.* 1985:78:1319–1323.

Gott VL, Cameron DE, Alejo DE, et al. Aortic root replacement in 271 Marfan patients: a 24-year experience. *Ann Thorac Surg.* 2002;73:438–443.

Grahame R, Pyeritz RE. The Marfan syndrome: joint and skin manifestations are prevalent and correlated. *Br J Rheumatol.* 1995;34:126–131.

Gray JR, Bridges AB, Faed MJ, et al. Ascertainment and severity of Marfan syndrome in a Scottish population. *J Med Genet.* 1994;31:51–54.

Gray JR, Bridges AB, West RR, et al. Life expectancy in British Marfan syndrome populations. *Clin Genet.* 1998;54:124–128.

Groenink M, de RA, Mulder BJ, et al. Changes in aortic distensibility and pulse wave velocity assessed with magnetic resonance imaging following beta-blocker therapy in the Marfan syndrome. *Am J Cardiol.* 1998;82:203–208.

Groenink M, Lohuis TA, Tijssen JG, et al. Survival and complication free survival in Marfan's syndrome: implications of current guidelines. *Heart.* 1999;82:499–504.

Habashi JP, Judge DP, Holm TM, et al. Losartan, an AT1 antagonist, prevents aortic aneurysm in a mouse model of Marfan syndrome. *Science.* 2006;312:117–121.

Hall JR, Pyeritz RE, Dudgeon DL, et al. Pneumothorax in the Marfan syndrome: prevalence and therapy. *Ann Thorac Surg.* 1984;37:500–504.

Haouzi A, Berglund H, Pelikan PC, et al. Heterogeneous aortic response to acute beta-adrenergic blockade in Marfan syndrome. *Am Heart J.* 1997;133:60–63.

Hubbard AD, Charteris DG, Cooling RJ. Vitreolensectomy in Marfan's syndrome. *Eye.* 1998;12(Pt 3a):412–416.

Immer FF, Bansi AG, Immer-Bansi AS, et al. Aortic dissection in pregnancy: analysis of risk factors and outcome. *Ann Thorac Surg.* 2003;76:309–314.

Joseph KN, Kane HA, Milner RS, et al. Orthopedic aspects of the Marfan phenotype. *Clin Orthop Relat Res.* 1992;251–261.

Judge DP, Biery NJ, Keene DR, et al. Evidence for a critical contribution of haploinsufficiency in the complex pathogenesis of Marfan syndrome. *J Clin Invest.* 2004;114:172–181.

Kallenbach K, Karck M, Pak D, et al. Decade of aortic valve sparing reimplantation: are we pushing the limits too far? *Circulation.* 2005;112:I253–I259.

Lacassie HJ, Millar S, Leithe LG, et al. Dural ectasia: a likely cause of inadequate spinal anaesthesia in two parturients with Marfan's syndrome. *Br J Anaesth.* 2005;94:500–504.

Lacro RV, Dietz HC, Wruck LM, et al. Rationale and design of a randomized clinical trial of beta-blocker therapy (atenolol) versus angiotensin II receptor blocker therapy (losartan) in individuals with Marfan syndrome. *Am Heart J.* 2007;154:624–631.

Law C, Bunyan D, Castle B, et al. Clinical features in a family with an R460H mutation in transforming growth factor beta receptor 2 gene. *J Med Genet.* 2006;43:908–916.

Legget ME, Unger TA, O'Sullivan CK, et al. Aortic root complications in Marfan's syndrome: identification of a lower risk group. *Heart.* 1996;75:389–395.

Le Parc JM, Molcard S, Tubach F. Bone mineral density in Marfan syndrome. *Rheumatology (Oxford).* 2001;40:358–359.

Lind J, Wallenburg HC. The Marfan syndrome and pregnancy: a retrospective study in a Dutch population. *Eur J Obstet Gynecol Reprod Biol.* 2001;98:28–35.

Lipscomb KJ, Clayton-Smith J, Harris R. Evolving phenotype of Marfan's syndrome. *Arch Dis Child.* 1997;76:41–46.

Loeys B, De BJ, Van AP, et al. Comprehensive molecular screening of the FBN1 gene favors locus homogeneity of classical Marfan syndrome. *Hum Mutat.* 2004;24:140–146.

Loeys B, Nuytinck L, Delvaux I, et al. Genotype and phenotype analysis of 171 patients referred for molecular study of the fibrillin-1 gene FBN1 because of suspected Marfan syndrome. *Arch Intern Med.* 2001;161:2447–2454.

Loeys B, Nuytinck L, Van AP, et al. Strategies for prenatal and preimplantation genetic diagnosis in Marfan syndrome (MFS). *Prenat Diagn.* 2002;22:22–28.

Loeys BL, Chen J, Neptune ER, et al. A syndrome of altered cardiovascular, craniofacial, neurocognitive and skeletal development caused by mutations in TGFBR1 or TGFBR2. *Nat Genet.* 2005;37:275–281.

Loeys BL, Schwarze U, Holm T, et al. Aneurysm syndromes caused by mutations in the TGF-beta receptor. *N Engl J Med.* 2006;355:788–798.

Marfan AB-J. Un cas de déformation congénitgale des quatres membres, plus prononcée aux extremités, caractérisée par l'allongement des os avec un certain degré d'amincissiment. *Bulletins et memoires de la Société medicale des hôpitaux de Paris.* 1896;13:220–228.

Maron BJ, Chaitman BR, Ackerman MJ, et al. Recommendations for physical activity and recreational sports participation for young patients with genetic cardiovascular diseases. *Circulation.* 2004;109:2807–2816.

Maumenee IH. The eye in the Marfan syndrome. *Vasc Dis Prev.* 1981;79:684–733.

McKusick VA. Heritable disorders of connective tissue III. The Marfan syndrome. *J Chronic Dis.* 1955;2:609–644.

Meijboom LJ, Drenthen W, Pieper PG, et al. Obstetric complications in Marfan syndrome. *Int J Cardiol.* 2006;110:53–59.

Meijboom LJ, Groenink M, Van Der Wall EE, et al. Aortic root asymmetry in Marfan patients: evaluation by magnetic resonance imaging and comparison with standard echocardiography. *Int J Card Imaging.* 2000;16:161–168.

Meijboom LJ, Nollen GJ, Mulder BJM. Prevention of cardiovascular complications in Marfan syndrome. *Vasc Dis Prev.* 2004;1:79–86.

Meijboom LJ, Timmermans J, Zwinderman AH, et al. Aortic root growth in men and women with the Marfan's syndrome. *Am J Cardiol.* 2005;96:1441–1444.

Mizuguchi T, Collod-Beroud G, Akiyama T, et al. Heterozygous TGFBR2 mutations in Marfan syndrome. *Nat Genet.* 2004;36:855–860.

Mizuguchi T, Matsumoto N. Recent progress in genetics of Marfan syndrome and Marfan-associated disorders. *J Hum Genet.* 2007;52:1–12.

Mosteller RD. Simplified calculation of body-surface area. *N Engl J Med.* 1987;317:1098.

Nagashima H, Sakomura Y, Aoka Y, et al. Angiotensin II type 2 receptor mediates vascular smooth muscle cell apoptosis in cystic medial degeneration associated with Marfan's syndrome. *Circulation.* 2001;104:I282–I287.

Nataf P, Lansac E. Dilation of the thoracic aorta: medical and surgical management. *Heart.* 2006;92:1345–1352.

Oosterhof T, Groenink M, Hulsmans FJ, et al. Quantitative assessment of dural ectasia as a marker for Marfan syndrome. *Radiology.* 2001;220:514–518.

Pacini L, Digne F, Boumendil A, et al. Maternal complication of pregnancy in Marfan syndrome. *Int J Cardiol.* 2008;136(2):156–161.

Pannu H, Avidan N, Tran-Fadulu V, et al. Genetic basis of thoracic aortic aneurysms and dissections: potential relevance to abdominal aortic aneurysms. *Ann N Y Acad Sci*. 2006;1085:242–255.

Pannu H, Fadulu VT, Chang J, et al. Mutations in transforming growth factor-beta receptor type II cause familial thoracic aortic aneurysms and dissections. *Circulation*. 2005;112:513–520.

Parish JG. Skeletal syndromes associated with arachnodactyly. *Proc R Soc Med*. 1960;53:515–518.

Patel ND, Weiss ES, Alejo DE, et al. Aortic root operations for Marfan syndrome: a comparison of the Bentall and valve-sparing procedures. *Ann Thorac Surg*. 2008;85:2003–2010.

Pyeritz RE, Francke U. The Second International Symposium on the Marfan Syndrome. *Am J Med Genet*. 1993;47:127–135.

Pyeritz RE, McKusick VA. The Marfan syndrome: diagnosis and management. *N Engl J Med*. 1979;300:772–777.

Rios AS, Silber EN, Bavishi N, et al. Effect of long-term beta-blockade on aortic root compliance in patients with Marfan syndrome. *Am Heart J*. 1999;137:1057–1061.

Robinson PN, Arteaga-Solis E, Baldock C, et al. The molecular genetics of Marfan syndrome and related disorders. *J Med Genet*. 2006;43:769–787.

Roman MJ, Devereux RB, Kramer-Fox R, et al. Two-dimensional echocardiographic aortic root dimensions in normal children and adults. *Am J Cardiol*. 1989;64:507–512.

Roman MJ, Rosen SE, Kramer-Fox R, et al. Prognostic significance of the pattern of aortic root dilation in the Marfan syndrome. *J Am Coll Cardiol*. 1993;22:1470–1476.

Rosser T, Finkel J, Vezina G, et al. Postural headache in a child with Marfan syndrome: case report and review of the literature. *J Child Neurol*. 2005;20:153–155.

Rossi-Foulkes R, Roman MJ, Rosen SE, et al. Phenotypic features and impact of beta blocker or calcium antagonist therapy on aortic lumen size in the Marfan syndrome. *Am J Cardiol*. 1999;83:1364–1368.

Sakai H, Visser R, Ikegawa S, et al. Comprehensive genetic analysis of relevant four genes in 49 patients with Marfan syndrome or Marfan-related phenotypes. *Am J Med Genet A*. 2006;140:1719–1725.

Salim MA, Alpert BS. Sports and Marfan syndrome—awareness and early diagnosis can prevent sudden death. *Phys Sportsmed*. 2001;29:80–93.

Salim MA, Alpert BS, Ward JC, et al. Effect of beta-adrenergic blockade on aortic root rate of dilation in the Marfan syndrome. *Am J Cardiol*. 1994;74:629–633.

Scherer LR, Arn PH, Dressel DA, et al. Surgical management of children and young adults with Marfan syndrome and pectus excavatum. *J Pediatr Surg*. 1988;23:1169–1172.

Scottish Intercollegiate Guidelines Network SIGN—Guideline Development Handbook (SIGN 50). Scottish Intercollegiate Guidelines Network: 2004.

Shores J, Berger KR, Murphy EA, et al. Progression of aortic dilatation and the benefit of long-term beta-adrenergic blockade in Marfan's syndrome. *N Engl J Med*. 1994;330:1335–1341.

Singh KK, Rommel K, Mishra A, et al. TGFBR1 and TGFBR2 mutations in patients with features of Marfan syndrome and Loeys-Dietz syndrome. *Hum Mutat*. 2006;27:770–777.

Streeten EA, Murphy EA, Pyeritz RE. Pulmonary function in the Marfan syndrome. *Chest*. 1987;91:408–412.

Treasure T. Elective replacement of the aortic root in Marfan's syndrome. *Br Heart J*. 1993;69:101–103.

van den Berg JS, Limburg M, Hennekam RC. Is Marfan syndrome associated with symptomatic intracranial aneurysms? *Stroke*. 1996;27:10–12.

Voyvodic F, Scroop R, Sanders RR. Anterior sacral meningocele as a pelvic complication of Marfan syndrome. *Aust NZJ Obstet Gynaecol*. 1999;39:262–265.

Williams A, Davies S, Stuart AG, et al. Medical treatment of Marfan syndrome: a time for change. *Heart*. 2008;94:414–421.

Wilson DG, Bellamy MF, Ramsey MW, et al. Endothelial function in Marfan syndrome: selective impairment of flow-mediated vasodilation. *Circulation*. 1999;99:909–915.

Wityk RJ, Zanferrari C, Oppenheimer S. Neurovascular complications of Marfan syndrome: a retrospective, hospital-based study. *Stroke*. 2002;33:680–684.

Wood JR, Bellamy D, Child AH, et al. Pulmonary disease in patients with Marfan syndrome. *Thorax*. 1984;39:780–784.

Yetman AT, Bornemeier RA, McCrindle BW. Usefulness of enalapril versus propranolol or atenolol for prevention of aortic dilation in patients with the Marfan syndrome. *Am J Cardiol*. 2005;95:1125–1127.

Yule SR, Hobson EE, Dean JC, et al. Protrusio acetabuli in Marfan's syndrome. *Clin Radiol*. 1999;54:95–97.

12

Thoracic and Abdominal Aortic Aneurysms

Susan L Drinkwater, Dhavendra Kumar, and Peter Taylor

Introduction

Aortic aneurysms involving the thoracic and abdominal aorta are increasing in incidence. The majority of these occur sporadically, but a small proportion has a family history of a close relative either dying unexpectedly due to ruptured aortic aneurysm or having had emergency life-saving surgery. The family history is important for all patients presenting with an aortic aneurysm. Aortic dissection may present acutely with rupture or end-organ ischemia. In the long term about 30%–40% of these patients develop aneurysms. Apart from several environmental factors, hereditary factors are also associated with aneurysmal dilatation and/or rupture of both thoracic and abdominal aorta and as well as peripheral arteries (Ward et al. 1992).

Although aortic aneurysms have a complex multifactorial/polygenic etiology, mutations in a few major genes are known to result in familial thoracic aortic aneurysms following the autosomal dominant inheritance pattern. Some of the Mendelian forms of thoracic aneurysms may be part of a recognizable multisystem disorder, such as Marfan syndrome, Ehlers-Danlos syndrome type IV (EDSIV), and Loeys-Dietz syndrome. These are discussed in detail elsewhere in this book (see Table of Contents). This chapter describes the genetic and clinical features of both thoracic and abdominal aortic aneurysms and aortic dissection.

Anatomy of the Aorta

The aorta runs from the aortic valve to its bifurcation into the common iliac arteries. It is divided into several parts, the ascending aorta, the arch, the descending thoracic aorta, and the abdominal aorta, which starts where it crosses the diaphragm (Figure 12–1). It is a large, elastic artery that is composed of three layers: an intima, media, and adventitia. The intima is the innermost layer, which has a luminal surface of endothelium and a subendothelial extracellular matrix, which lies on the internal elastic lamina. The media is bounded by the internal and external elastic laminae, and it contains lamellar units composed of layers of smooth muscle cells (SMCs) with their surrounding matrix, including a meshwork of collagen (types I and III), and a layer of elastin. There

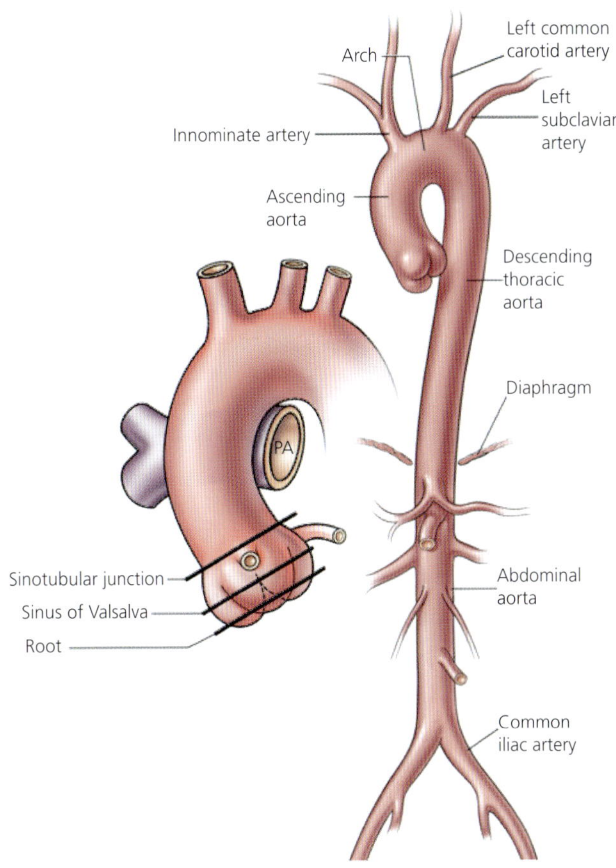

Figure 12–1 The anatomy of the aortic root, ascending aorta, descending aorta, abdominal aorta and major branches. (Adapted from Textbook of Cardiovascular Medicine, Third Ed., Eric J Topol (Ed.) with permission.)

are more than 28 lamellar units in the aortic wall. The number of lamellar units in the aortic wall correlates with radius, and there are more in the thoracic aorta than the abdominal aorta, with an abrupt decrease below the renal arteries. The adventitia lies outside the external elastic lamina and consists of loose connective tissue, fibroblasts, capillaries, and nerve fibers. A microvasculature (the vasa vasorum) penetrates the media from the adventitial side in order to provide a nutrient supply to the deep layers of the media. The inner layers are perfused by blood directly from the lumen.

Aortic Aneurysms

An aneurysm is a permanent localized dilatation of an artery with an increase in diameter of greater than 50% (1.5 times) its normal diameter, involving all layers of the arterial wall (intima, media, and adventitia) (Johnston et al. 1991). The normal diameter of the aorta is variable, depending on age, height, gender, and blood pressure, and is larger in the thorax than the abdomen.

Aneurysms may form anywhere in the aorta (Figure 12–1), but the most common location is below the renal arteries and above the bifurcation of the iliac arteries. This occurs three to seven times more commonly than in the thoracic portion. Aortic aneurysms often coexist with aneurysms of other arteries including the common and internal iliac arteries (20%–30%) and the femoral and popliteal arteries (15%). Interestingly, aneurysms of the external iliac are exceptionally rare, and some authorities attribute this to the embryology of the fetal circulation. Overall, multiple aneurysms occur in 3.4%–13% of patients with thoracic aneurysms and in about 12% of those with abdominal aortic aneurysms (Crawford and Cohen 1982). Up to 25% of patients with a large thoracic aortic aneurysm (TAA) will also have an AAA (Bickerstaff et al. 1982; Crawford and Cohen 1982; Pressler and McNamara 1985). The incidence of aneurysms increases with age and is more common in men.

1. Thoracic Aortic Aneurysms

The annual incidence of thoracic aortic aneurysm is estimated to be around 6 cases per 100,000 (Bickerstaff et al. 1982). Thoracic aneurysms occur most commonly in the sixth and seventh decade of life. In contrast to the infrarenal abdominal aorta, aneurysms of the thoracic aorta have an almost equal gender distribution. Hypertension is an important risk factor, being present in over 60% of patients.

Aneurysms of the thoracic aorta can be classified into four general anatomic categories:

1. Ascending aortic aneurysms arise anywhere from the aortic valve to the innominate artery.
2. Aortic arch aneurysms include any thoracic aneurysm that involves the brachiocephalic vessels.
3. Descending thoracic aneurysms arise anywhere distal to the left subclavian artery and are confined to the thoracic aorta.
4. Thoracoabdominal aneurysms arise anywhere distal to the left subclavian artery, but also extend to the abdominal aorta. These aneurysms are subdivided by the Crawford classification (Figure 12–2) (Svensson et al. 1993):
   a. Involves all or most of the descending thoracic aorta and the upper abdominal aorta above the renal arteries
   b. Involves all or most of the descending thoracic aorta and all or most of the abdominal aorta below the renal arteries
   c. Involves the distal half or less of the descending thoracic aorta (usually below T6) with varying segments of the abdominal aorta
   d. Involves all or most of the abdominal aorta, including the segment from which the visceral vessels arise

Beyond distinguishing thoracic aneurysms by anatomic position, the four broad categories further provide guidance as to the likely etiology, indications for intervention, operative approach to repair the aneurysm, and outcome.

2. Abdominal Aortic Aneurysms

An autopsy series from Sweden found abdominal aortic aneurysms in 4.3% of men and 2.1% of women, and screening of the population over the age of 55 years in Rotterdam found a prevalence of 4.1% in men and 0.7% in women (2.1% overall) (Pleumeekers et al. 1995). Prevalence is higher in high-risk populations and increases with age (Lucarotti et al. 1993; Ashton et al. 2002), affecting 7%–8% of men over the age of 65 years (Lucarotti et al. 1993; Norman et al. 2004b). Abdominal aortic aneurysms are six times more common in men (Vardulaki et al. 2000) and in women tend to present a

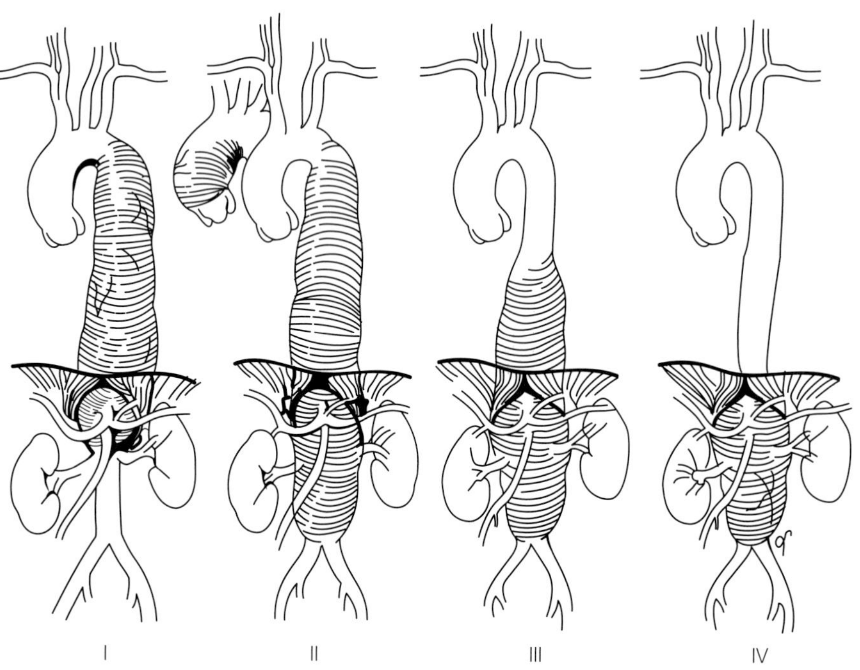

Figure 12–2 Crawford classification of thoracoabdominal aortic aneurysms type I to IV.

decade later. The incidence has increased over the past 30 years (Melton et al. 1984; Fowkes et al. 1989). There is an 8:1 preponderance of aneurysms in cigarette smokers compared with nonsmokers (Singh et al. 2001). Up to 40% of patients with abdominal aortic aneurysms are hypertensive (Vardulaki et al. 2000). There is also a hereditary component in 15%–25%.

Abdominal aortic aneurysms are often classified according to their relationship to the renal arteries. They may be infrarenal, juxtarenal, pararenal, or suprarenal.

3. Aortic Dissection

An aortic dissection occurs when blood separates the inner and outer layers of the vessel, producing a false lumen or double-barreled aorta, which can reduce blood flow to the major arteries arising from the aorta (Figure 12–3). Dissections can weaken the outer wall, resulting in rupture or formation of an aneurysm. Aortic dissection affects around 10 per 100, 000 of the population per year (Svensson and Crawford 1992), and it has high mortality. If left untreated, 62%–91% of patients will be dead in 1 week.

Pathogenesis of Aortic Aneurysms and Dissections

1. Aortic Dissection

This was originally thought to be the result of a tear in the inner layer (intimal layer) of the aortic wall allowing blood to enter the middle layer (media). However, evidence from cross-sectional imaging has shown that dissection can result from intramural hematoma and is now thought to result from a bleed into the media from the vasa vasorum. Penetrating ulcers may also evolve into aortic dissections.

2. Aortic Aneurysms

The pathogenesis of abdominal aortic aneurysms has been studied in great detail; however, thoracic aneurysms have not been subjected to the same intense scrutiny and the exact process remains one of conjecture rather than knowledge.

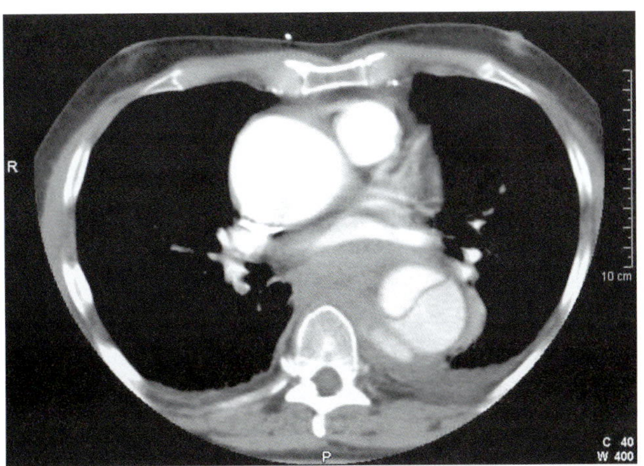

Figure 12–3 CT scan showing an acute type B aortic dissection with rupture.

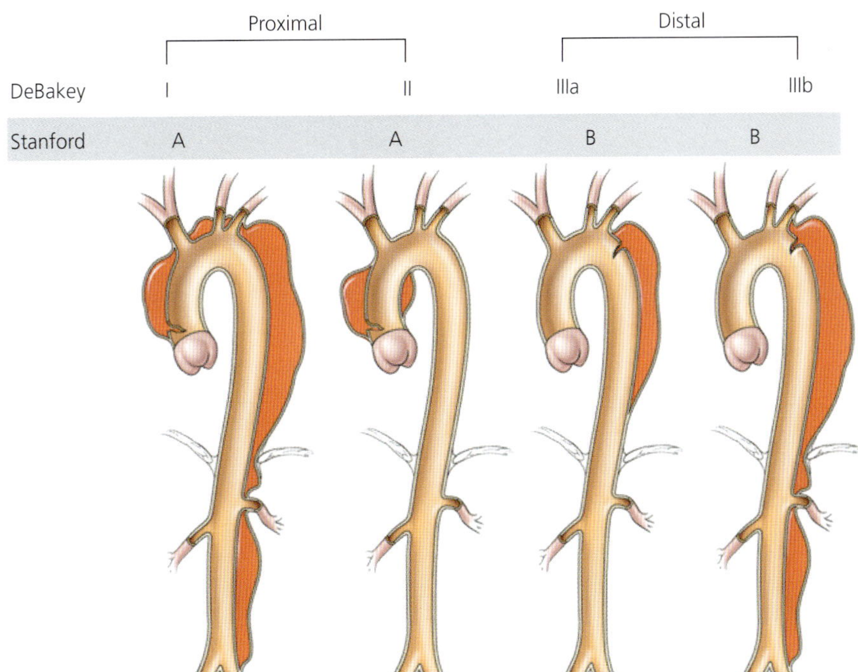

Figure 12–4 DeBakey and Stanford types of aortic dissections. Figure 12–4 illustrates the DeBakey (DeBakey et al. 1965) and Stanford (Daily et al. 1970) types of aortic dissections. They are classified according to the part of the aorta that has been affected by the dissection. A proximal dissection (DeBakey types I and II, Stanford type A) involves the ascending aorta, whilst a distal dissection (DeBakey type III, Stanford type B) only affects the aorta distal to the left subclavian artery. Dissections are classified as acute if they present within 14 days and chronic if the presentation is longer than this. Early death is more common with proximal dissections affecting the ascending aorta and arch compared with distal dissections involving the descending thoracic aorta. Reprinted from Doroghazi RM, Slater EE, DeSanctis RW, Buckley MJ, Austen WG, Rosenthal S. Long-term survival of patients with treated aortic dissection. *J Am Coll Cardiol.* 1984;3(4):1026–1034.

Histological features of aneurysms are of a thin dilated wall, replacement and fragmentation of elastin in the media with a much thinner layer of collagen, loss of SMCs, and remodeling of the extracellular matrix. This thinned wall usually contains calcium as well as atherosclerotic lesions, rendering the wall brittle. Laminated thrombus lines the lumen concentrically, resulting in a nearly normal flow channel, but possibly making the inner layers of the aortic wall relatively hypoxic.

Aneurysms elongate as they enlarge, causing them to become bowed and tortuous (Dobrin 1989). It is believed that both expansion and tortuosity is related to weakening and fragmentation of the elastic lamellae, which are known to break down with age. Elastin depletion occurs early in aneurysm development and is one of the most consistent biochemical and histochemical findings in human aortic aneurysms (Dobrin et al. 1984) related to increased elastase activity (Cohen et al. 1988). Collagen depletion occurs to a lesser extent. Collagen makes up about 25% of the wall of an atherosclerotic aorta, but only 6%–18% of an aneurysmal aortic wall.

The predilection of aneurysms to form in the infrarenal aorta may be explained by the fewer elastic lamellae present there compared to the thoracic aorta.

Aortic aneurysms are associated with a combination of factors, including age, atherosclerosis, hypertension, chronic inflammation due to infection, and autoimmune processes. The majority of thoracoabdominal and abdominal aortic aneurysms are termed "atherosclerotic" or "degenerative" (82%) (Panneton and Hollier 1995). Although aneurysms and occlusive atherosclerosis share most of the same risk factors (e.g., aging, smoking, hypertension, and male gender) and atherosclerosis is present in the wall of aneurysms, only 25% of patients with aortic aneurysms have significant occlusive disease. This has led to speculation that atherosclerosis is a coincidental or facilitating process rather than a primary cause, which is why the term "degenerative" is often used instead.

Occasionally, an inflammatory or infectious process may cause an aortic aneurysm. This includes giant cell arteritis, syphilitic aortitis, mycotic aneurysm often due to bacterial endocarditis, Takayasu's disease, rheumatoid arthritis, psoriatic arthritis, ankylosing spondylitis, reactive arthritis, Wegener's granulomatosis, and Reiter's syndrome. The pathophysiological process leading to aortic dilatation and aneurysm formation is thought to be due to intramural inflammation and degeneration either in response to spirochete infection as in syphilitic aortitis or as a manifestation of a systemic autoimmune process. Thoracic aneurysm formation is a particular problem in patients with giant cell arteritis, who are 17 times as likely as other subjects to develop this complication (Evans et al. 1995) and they may also develop dissection or AAA (Evans et al. 1995). It can be caused by chronic or late recrudescent aortitis resulting in elastin and collagen disruption, or dilatation may develop due to mechanical stress on an aortic wall that was weakened in the early active phase of the disease.

Aneurysms can also develop as a late consequence of aortic dissection, in 30%–40% of cases. This accounts for 17% of all thoracoabdominal aortic aneurysms (TAAAs).

Presentation of Aortic Aneurysm

1. Asymptomatic

Patients with aortic aneurysms are often asymptomatic at the time of presentation (Pressler and McNamara 1985), with approximately 75% of infrarenal aneurysms being symptom free when diagnosed. Most are found during the investigation of unrelated symptoms, such as back pain or urinary symptoms. Some are discovered by routine abdominal examination, but infrarenal aneurysms need to be at least 4 cm to be palpable in a thin patient. Obesity, ascites, or other abdominal pathology may prevent an aneurysm being detected until too late. They may be picked up during surgery for other pathology. A thoracic aneurysm may be found on a routine chest X-ray or CT scan for unrelated pathology.

2. Rupture

The most serious complication of aortic aneurysm is rupture, which is fatal without intervention. This is a sudden catastrophic event that presents with severe chest/abdominal/flank pain (depending on the location of the rupture) and circulatory collapse. If the rupture is contained in the retroperitoneal space, the patient may make it to hospital and be treated. Free rupture is immediately fatal with approximately 50%–75% of patients with ruptured aneurysms dying before they reach hospital. Approximately 5% of infrarenal aneurysms rupture into the inferior vena cava. The classic triad of lower limb edema, pulsatile expansile abdominal mass, and a continuous abdominal bruit present throughout both systole and diastole, and it usually depends on the maintenance of an adequate blood pressure. Rarely rupture may occur into the gastrointestinal tract, in the esophagus or duodenum. Such primary aortoenteric fistulae usually result in death from massive hemorrhage but some are preceded by an initial small "herald" bleed.

3. Pain/Tenderness

Sudden expansion of an aneurysm may produce pain in the chest, back, flank, or abdomen. Chronic abdominal pain with tenderness over the aneurysm could represent an inflammatory aneurysm. Acute abdominal pain and tenderness in the absence of rupture could signify that rupture is imminent. Such patients should be treated within 24 hours of presentation.

4. Cardiac Symptoms

Ascending aneurysms can present with congestive heart failure due to aortic regurgitation from aortic root dilatation and annular distortion. They can also lead to local compression of a coronary artery, resulting in myocardial ischemia or infarction, while a sinus of Valsalva aneurysm can rupture into the right side of the heart, producing a continuous murmur and, in some cases, congestive heart failure.

5. Compression or Erosion of Other Structures

Ascending and arch aneurysms can erode into the mediastinum. Such patients can present with one or more of the following: hoarseness due to compression of left vagus or left recurrent laryngeal nerve; hemidiaphragmatic paralysis due to compression of the phrenic nerve; wheezing, cough, hemoptysis, dyspnea, or pneumonitis if there is compression of the tracheobronchial tree; dysphagia due to esophageal compression; or superior vena cava syndrome. Aneurysmal compression of other intrathoracic structures or erosion into adjacent bone may cause chest or back pain.

Abdominal aortic aneurysms may cause back pain or nerve root compression. Stretching of the duodenum may lead to weight loss, abdominal pain, and early satiety.

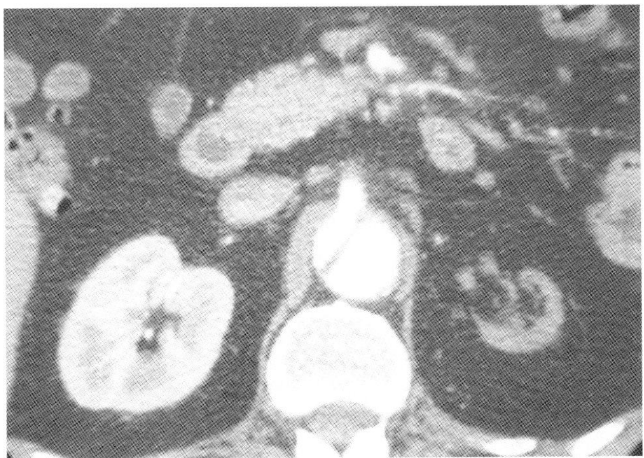

Figure 12–5 CT Scan showing aortic dissection associated with atrophy of the left kidney.

6. Thrombosis/Embolism

This is a rare mode of presentation of an aortic aneurysm. Aneurysmal compression of branch vessels or the occurrence of embolism to various peripheral arteries due to thrombus within the aneurysm can cause coronary, cerebral, renal, mesenteric, lower extremity, and rarely, spinal cord ischemia and resultant symptoms. Patients presenting with emboli to the toes of both feet who usually have palpable pedal pulses should have a CT scan performed of the whole of the abdominal and thoracic aorta to exclude an aneurysm.

Presentation of Aortic Dissection

Aortic dissection typically presents with severe, ripping chest pain radiating to the intrascapular region. Rupture may occur into the mediastinum, pleura, or abdomen. A Stanford type A dissection (involving the ascending aorta) may cause stroke, myocardial infarction, aortic valve regurgitation, and cardiac tamponade and is a life-threatening emergency requiring immediate intervention. Distal extension may present with paraplegia, visceral and renal ischemia, and acute limb ischemia.

Branch vessel ischemia complicates 30%–50% of all dissections, resulting in myocardial ischemia (3%), stroke (3%–7%), paraplegia (3%), peripheral limb ischemia (24%), visceral ischemia (5%), and renal ischemia (8%) (Figure 12–5) (Fann et al. 1990).

Diagnosis of Aortic Aneurysm and Dissection

Physical examination of AAA is not reliable and for thoracic aortic aneurysms is impossible. Imaging modalities therefore need to be employed for diagnosis, surveillance, and procedure planning.

Imaging of Aortic Aneurysms

Plain Radiography

A common way in which asymptomatic aneurysms are detected is on routine radiography. A thoracic aneurysm produces a widening of the mediastinal silhouette, enlargement of the aortic knob, or displacement of the trachea from midline on a chest X-ray. However, smaller aneurysms may not be apparent. An AAA may be detectable on a plain abdominal X-ray if there is calcification in the wall in 67%–75% of cases.

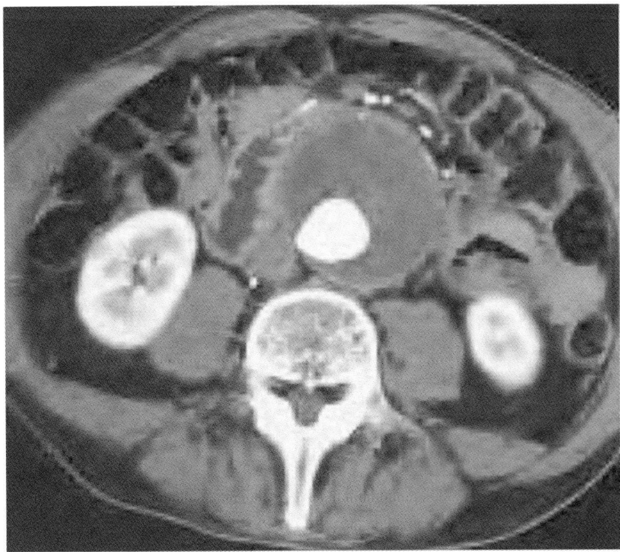

Figure 12–6 CT scan demonstrating infrarenal abdominal aortic aneurysm.

Ultrasound Scanning

Real-time B-mode ultrasonography is the most common way to assess the size of an AAA as it is noninvasive, is widely available, employs no ionizing radiation, and can easily measure aneurysm size. It is not reliable in assessing the relationship of the aneurysm to the renal arteries, or for determining whether the aneurysm has ruptured. It is the modality of choice for establishing diagnosis and for surveillance of abdominal aortic aneurysms. It is not useful for imaging the thoracic or suprarenal aorta, however, because of the overlying air-containing lungs and viscera.

CT Scanning

Computed tomography (CT) with intravenous contrast is an accurate diagnostic tool for evaluating both thoracic and abdominal aortic aneurysms (Figure 12–6) (Rubin 1997). It can accurately assess the extent of the aneurysm and the amount of thrombus in the wall and is necessary for planning if stent grafting is to be considered. It is the modality of choice for assessing the thoracic aorta and is the best method for evaluating branch vessel pathology. It can also identify rupture. It does involve a substantial dose of ionizing radiation and uses contrast that may provoke anaphylaxis or renal failure in susceptible patients. The advent of multidetector (or multislice) CT scans allows a faster acquisition time with a lower dose of radiation. Software programmes are now widely available to reconstruct the aorta in three dimension, and centerline reconstruction allows planning for complex endovascular reconstruction.

Magnetic Resonance Angiography

Magnetic resonance angiography offers noninvasive angiography with multiplanar image reconstruction and visualization of extraluminal structures (Figure 12–7) (Alley et al. 1998). This imaging technique has the disadvantage of limited availability, increased cost, and slower acquisition time compared to multidetector CT scan. The latest software allows very high resolution images to be reconstructed in three dimensions. It cannot detect calcification but it can detect direction of flow, which may be an

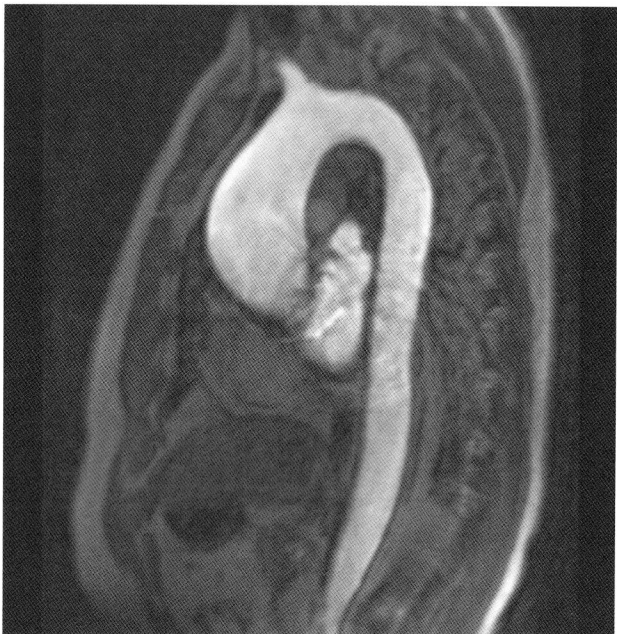

Figure 12–7 Gadolinium-enhanced magnetic resonance angiogram showing an ascending thoracic aortic aneurysm in the saggital plane. The aneurysm occupies the tubular part of the ascending aorta sparing the sinuses of Valsalva and aortic arch. This is a common location for ascending thoracic aortic aneurysm without Marfan syndrome and may be associated with bicuspid aortic valve. Reprinted from *Textbook of Cardiovascular Medicine*, Third Ed., Eric J Topol (Ed.) with permission.

advantage over CT scan in patients with acute aortic dissection, when accurate detection of the primary tear may allow endovascular treatment to seal this, so treating the complications resulting from pressurization of the false lumen. It is contraindicated if the patient has metal clips or a stent made of ferrous material. The patient may not be able to tolerate the test if claustrophobic. Gadolinium contrast is also nephrotoxic and can also cause deterioration in renal function secondary to nephrogenic systemic fibrosis in patients with preexisting renal failure.

Echocardiography

Transthoracic echocardiography can demonstrate dilation of the ascending aorta and abnormalities such as a bicuspid aortic valve (Pachulski et al. 1991). It is of limited value in assessing the descending thoracic aorta, because of nonconductance of the signal by lung air. However, imaging within the mediastinum using transesophageal echocardiography can be extremely useful, particularly when dissection is suspected.

Aortography

Historically, conventional aortography has been the gold standard for the evaluation of the aorta and its branches. However, it is invasive, uses nephrotoxic contrast, and only delineates the lumen. It may still be useful when accurate information is required about aortic branch vessels particularly for planning a procedure involving the aortic arch and proximal descending aorta. However, this imaging modality has largely been replaced by the use of multislice CT scanning.

Familial Thoracic Aortic Aneurysms and Dissections

Approximately 20% of thoracic aortic aneurysms and dissections result from a genetic predisposition (Biddinger et al. 1997; Coady et al. 1999). There is no known increased predisposition in any ethnic or racial group. Associated multisystem physical abnormalities often occur in patients with aneurysms involving the ascending thoracic aorta. Examples include microfibrillinopathies, such as Marfan syndrome and contractural arachnodactyly syndrome (see Chapter 11). Conversely, aneurysms involving the descending thoracic aorta are commonly sporadic, although familial forms are described (Table 12–1). This section only deals with the nonsyndromal forms of familial thoracic aortic aneurysms (TAA). Appropriate references to syndromal forms of thoracic aneurysms are made, for example, Marfan's syndrome and related syndromes that are covered elsewhere in the book.

Several forms of familial TAAs are listed in the late Victor McKusick's online catalog of Mendelian inheritance in man (OMIM) (Table 12–1). Inheritance in most familial forms follows an autosomal dominant pattern of incomplete penetrance with considerable variable expression. Acute aortic dissection may also occur in patients with these familial disorders, and they are often designated as thoracic aortic aneurysm with dissection (TAAD). Clearly this is a single clinically useful label for a heterogeneous group of disorders. This section deals with the clinical and genetic aspects of familial thoracic aortic aneurysms and dissections.

Clinical Features

The primary manifestations of familial aortic aneurysms and dissections are either (1) dilatation of the ascending aorta at the level of the ascending aorta or at the level of the sinuses of

Table 12–1 Familial Thoracic Aortic Aneurysms

Designation Synonyms/Symbol OMIM# Inheritance Locus Gene Allelic Variants

Familial thoracic aortic annuloaortic ectasia 607086 AD 11q23.3-q24?

Aneurysm type 1; familial aortic dissection

Erdhein cystic medial necrosis AAT1; FAA1

Familial thoracic aortic AAT2; FAA2 607087 AD 5q13-q14 ?

Aneurysm type 2 TAAD1

Familial thoracic aortic AAT4; FAA4; TAAD2 132900 AD 16p13.13-p13.12 MYH11 IVS32 + 1G;

Aneurysm type 4; aortic aneurysm/dissection 160745 ARG1758GLN; with patent ductus arteriosus del72exon28

Familial thoracic aortic AAT6; familial thoracic 611788 AD 10q22-q24 ACTA2 ARG149CYS;

Aneurysm type 6; aortic aneurysm with livido ARG258HIS; reticularis and iris flocculi; ARG258CYS thoracic aortic aneurysm with aortic dissections (TAAD3)

Familial arterial tortuosity LDS1A 609192 AD 9q33-q34 TGFBR1 MET318ARG; ascending aortic dissections ASP400GLY

Loeys-Dietz syndrome THR200ILE; ARG487PRO; SER241LEU LDS2A 608967 AD 9q33-q34 TGFBR1 ARG487GLN; ARG487TRP; GLY174VAL LDS1B 610168 AD 3p22 TGFBR2 YR336ASN; ALA355PRO; GLY357TRP; ARG528HIS; ARG528CYS; IVS1, A-G, -2 LDS2B 610380 AD 3p22 TGFBR2 GLN508GLN; LEU308PRO; SER449PHE; ARG537CYS; ARG460CYS; ARG460HIS

Valsalva or (2) dissection of the ascending aorta (type A dissection), or (3) both. Although dissections or aneurysms may occur in isolation, enlargement of the ascending aorta typically precedes dissection in the majority of individuals (Milewicz et al. 1998). As an aneurysm enlarges, the aortic annulus can become stretched, leading to secondary aortic regurgitation. Death usually results from aortic rupture. The onset and rate of progression of aortic dilatation is highly variable even within families. The variable expression of the disorder means that one individual in the family may present with an aneurysm at a young age, whereas another individual may present at an elderly age. The mean age of presentation of individuals with familial thoracic aneurysms with dissection is younger than that of individuals with sporadic aneurysms or dissections, but older than the mean age of presentation of individuals with Marfan syndrome (Coady et al. 1999).

Aortic dissection is exceedingly rare in early childhood but aortic dilatation may be present in childhood. In most adults, the risk of aortic rupture becomes significant when the maximal aortic dimension reaches about 5.5 cm, although individuals with *TGFBR2* mutations may rupture prior to enlargement to 5 cm (Loeys et al. 2005; Milewicz, unpublished data). A minority of affected family members present with dissections of the descending aorta not associated with prior aortic dilation.

With proper management, including medical therapy and prophylactic repair of aneurysmal dilatation, the life expectancy of an individual with a thoracic aortic aneurysm should approach that of the general population. It is assumed that those family members who are screened because of family history will have a better prognosis than relatives who present with symptoms.

There may be rapid progression of aortic root enlargement and aortic dissection or rupture during pregnancy, delivery, or the postpartum period. Data obtained from women with Marfan syndrome indicate a low complication risk if the aortic root diameter does not exceed 4 cm.

Although aneurysms and dissections of the ascending thoracic aorta may occur as an isolated abnormality without other phenotypic effects, other manifestations are occasionally observed:

Inguinal hernia. An observation of six families with aortic aneurysms and dissections found inguinal hernias in 10 of 16 affected men over age 30 years; none of the affected women had inguinal hernias.

Scoliosis. Four of eight affected women had scoliosis; none of the affected men had scoliosis.

Other cardiovascular abnormalities. Aneurysms in other portions of the aorta may occur in as many as 20% of individuals. In some families with familial thoracic aortic aneurysms with dissection, associated anatomic abnormalities are encountered including bicuspid aortic valve (Roberts and Roberts 1991; Loscalzo et al. 2007), dilatation of the ascending aorta, abnormal ascending aortic wall, coarctation of aorta, and patent ductus arteriosus (McKusick 1972; Gale et al. 1977; Lindsay 1988). Mutations in *MYH11* have been identified in two families with thoracic aortic aneurysms with dissection, and in one family this was associated with patent ductus arteriosus. Peripheral arterial dilatation is also known to be associated.

Surveillance of Patients with Familial TAAD

Echocardiography should be performed at frequent intervals to monitor the status of the ascending aorta. The entire aorta should be imaged every few years, as the incidence of aneurysms in other portions of the aorta may be as high as 20%. After repair of the ascending aorta, the remaining portion of the aorta needs to be routinely imaged for enlargement of the distal aorta, whether the individual had a type A dissection initially or underwent prophylactic repair of the ascending aorta. Periodic imaging of the cerebral circulation in individuals with a *TGFBR2* mutation to evaluate for cerebral aneurysms is recommended as these aneurysms may occur later in life.

Molecular Genetics

Although Erdheim's medial cystic necrosis is more commonly seen in thoracic aortic aneurysms, this is known to occur in certain familial connective tissue syndromes (OMIM 154700) and Ehlers-Danlos syndrome type IV. Molecular genetic studies using genetic linkage and whole-genome scanning have helped in mapping several genes associated with aneurysms and dissections of the thoracic aorta (Table 12–1). Candidate genes are only known for three types of thoracic aortic aneurysm including TAAD2.

Mutations in *TGFBR1* (MIM 190181), *TGFBR2* (MIM 190182), and *MYH11* (MIM 160745) cause the phenotype of TAAD2. Mutations in *TGFBR1* may also be associated with thoracic aortic aneurysms, but the phenotype in such cases is usually complex including other physical abnormalities as in Loeys-Dietz syndrome. Recently mutations in the actin gene (*ACTA2*) have been described in AAT6 (MIM 61178), provisionally designated TAAD3. The other two major loci include FAA1 (11q23.3-q24) and TAAD1 (5q13-q14); no candidate genes have yet been identified.

TGFBR1

One of the two receptors for the most potent serine/threonine kinases transmembrane growth factors, transforming growth factor β (TGFB1), is *TGFBR1*. This receptor together with *TGFBR2* regulated most activities of TGFB. While *TGFBR2* inhibits the proliferative activity of TGF-β, *TGFBR1* mediates the induction of several genes involved in cell–matrix interactions. The *TGFBR1* protein contains single peptide that is made up of 503 amino acids weighing 53 kD with a single N-glycosylation site, a transmembrane region, and a putative cytoplasmic protein kinase domain. The *TGFBR1* gene was localized to 9q22 using polymerase chain reaction with a hybrid cell DNA panel and FISH (Kuan and Kono 1998; Pasche et al. 1998) mapped the *TGFBR1* gene to mouse chromosome 4. The *TGFBR1* gene is approximately 31 kb long and contains 9 exons. The organization of the segment of the gene that encodes the C-terminal portion of the serine/threonine kinase domain appears to be highly conserved among members of the gene family. The membrane-bound protein encoded by *TGFBR1* binds TGF-β and forms a heterodimeric complex with the TGF-β II receptor (Franzen et al. 1993; Johnson et al. 1995). Ligand binding by TGF-β I receptors is dependent on coexpression with type II receptors. Type II receptors alone can bind ligand, but require association with type I receptors for activation of their kinase (signaling) function.

In patients with phenotypes classified as type II Marfan syndrome, Loeys-Dietz syndrome (Loeys et al. 2006), or TAAD (see LDS2A), Matyas et al. (2006) detected three novel mutations in the *TGFBR1* gene. Singh et al. (2006) searched for *TGFBR1* and *TGFBR2* mutations in 41 unrelated patients fulfilling the diagnostic criteria of the Ghent nosology (De Paepe et al. 1996) or with a tentative diagnosis of Marfan syndrome, in whom mutations in the FBN1 coding region were not identified. In *TGFBR1*, two mutations and two polymorphisms were detected. In *TGFBR2*, five mutations and six polymorphisms were identified. Reexamination of patients with a *TGFBR1* or *TGFBR2* mutation revealed extensive clinical overlap between these patients.

TGFBR2

The coding region of *TGFBR2* consists of eight exons. Two isoforms are transcribed from the gene as a result of alternative splicing of a coding exon located between the exons designated exon 1 and exon 2. Two recurrent missense mutations affecting the kinase domain that lead to familial TAAD have been described (Pannu et al. 2005). Several missense mutations that cause syndromic TAAD in association with Marfan syndrome, Loeys-Dietz aortic aneurysm syndrome, or related syndromes have been described (Mizuguchi et al. 2004; Ki et al. 2005; Loeys et al. 2005; Ades et al. 2006; Disabella et al. 2006). *TGFBR2* is a ubiquitously expressed type II transmembrane receptor protein with serine-threonine kinase activity. *TGFBR2* binds TGF-β and transduces the TGF-β signal intracellularly by recruitment and phosphorylation of the type I transmembrane receptor, *TGFBR1*. TGF-β signaling plays an important role in cellular proliferation, differentiation, and extracellular matrix production.

TGFBR2 mutations leading to aneurysms and dissections occur predominantly in the functionally important kinase domain and are predicted to cause loss of function. This has been demonstrated by structural analysis of some mutations and functional analysis of mutant *TGFBR2* in cell lines (Mizuguchi et al. 2004; Pannu et al. 2005). However, evidence also suggests that the TGF-β pathway might be upregulated in aortic tissue from individuals with *TGFBR2* mutations (Loeys et al. 2005). The precise function of the abnormal gene product is currently under investigation.

MYH11

The coding region of *MYH11* consists of 41 exons. Two alternatively spliced transcripts, SM1 and SM2, are generated by alternate usage of a 3' coding exon 41. Two splicing and one missense mutation in the C-terminal coiled-coil region of *MYH11* have been described in two families with TAAD and patent ductus arteriosus (PDA) (Zhu et al. 2006). *MYH11*, or smooth muscle myosin heavy chain, is a smooth muscle cell-specific protein. Smooth muscle myosin, the major contractile protein in these cells, is composed of a *MYH11* dimer along with two pairs of nonidentical light chains. Deletion and missense mutations located in the C-terminal domain of *MYH11* are predicted to affect the structure and assembly of myosin thick filaments.

Evidence suggests that mutant *MYH11* acts in a dominant negative manner by altering the stability of the coiled-coil structure in the rod region of the protein through its interaction with wild type *MYH11* (Zhu et al. 2006).

ACTA2

Actin is one of the major constituent proteins of all forms of muscle tissue. Six different actin isoforms are known distributed in skeletal muscle, cardiac muscle, SMCs, and in the cytoplasm (Vandekerckhove and Weber 1979). The SMC actin is important for the vascular structure. Ueyama et al. (1984) isolated and characterized the human aortic smooth muscle actin. The aortic smooth muscle actin (ACTSA) contains two more introns (between codons 84/85 and 121/122) than the skeletal and cardiac muscle actin genes. The gene was mapped by Southern blot analysis to 10q22-q24 (Ueyama et al. 1990) and further specifically to 10q23.3 (Ueyama et al. 1995). The α-2 actin is the main component of the aortic smooth muscle (*ACTA2*).

The major function of vascular SMCs is contraction to regulate blood pressure and flow. SMC contractile force requires cyclic interactions between *ACTA2* and the β-myosin heavy chain, encoded by the *MYH11* gene (MIM 160745). Recently missense *ACTA2* mutations are shown to be responsible for about 14% cases of inherited TAAD (Guo et al. 2007). This is assigned a separate MIM number (AAT6; 611788). In the family described by Guo et al. (2007) with thoracic aortic aneurysms and dissections and livedo reticularis linked to 10q23-q24, identified an arg149-to-cys substitution in the *ACTA2* gene (R149C). The mutation segregated with livedo reticularis in the family with a lod score of 5.85. These results suggested that the R149C *ACTA2* mutation was responsible for both thoracic aortic aneurysm and livedo reticularis in the initially studied family. Sequencing of the *ACTA2* gene in 97 unrelated families with a similar phenotype identified 14 additional families with *ACTA2* mutations. A total of five families carried the R149C mutation, which was shown by haplotype analysis to have arisen de novo in each. The authors commented that another form of TAAD (AAT4; 132900), caused by mutations in another component of the SMC contractile unit, *MYH11* (MIM 160745), is also associated with PDA in some affected individuals. Structural analyses and immunofluorescence of actin filaments in SMCs derived from individuals heterozygous for *ACTA2* mutations illustrated that these mutations interfere with actin filament assembly and are predicted to decrease SMC contraction. Aortic tissues from affected individuals showed aortic medial degeneration, focal areas of medial SMC hyperplasia and disarray, and stenotic arteries in the vasa vasorum due to medial SMC proliferation. These data, along with the previously reported *MYH11* mutations causing familial thoracic aortic aneurysm, indicate the importance of SMC contraction in maintaining the structural integrity of the ascending aorta.

Genetic Counseling

Genetic counseling for familial TAAD is recommended in all cases. This should follow the standard format as for any other incompletely penetrant and clinically variable autosomal dominant inherited disorder (see Chapter 36). The following guidelines may assist the genetic counselor or clinician dealing with the affected person or a close relative.

The majority of individuals diagnosed with familial TAAD have an affected parent. It is appropriate to evaluate both parents for manifestations of thoracic aortic aneurysms by performing a comprehensive clinical examination and an echocardiogram to image the ascending aorta, the sinuses of Valsalva, and cardiac valves. The risk to the siblings of the proband depends upon the status of the parents. If a parent is affected, the risk to the sibling of inheriting the disease-causing mutation is 50% (1 in 2); however, because of reduced penetrance, the likelihood that the sibling will develop TAAD is slightly reduced, with increasing risk as the individual increases in age. If there are other affected individuals in the extended family, reduced penetrance and variable expression of the disease raise the possibility that siblings could be at risk even if the parents are unaffected.

The children of an affected parent are at 50% risk of inheriting the mutant allele and the disorder. Since the penetrance of TAAD is reduced, the offspring who inherit a mutant allele from a parent may or may not develop thoracic aortic aneurysms. The risk to other family members depends upon the status of the proband's parents, siblings, and offspring. If a parent is found to be affected, his or her family members are at risk.

DNA banking from the affected person is an important issue that should be addressed in genetic counseling. It is important that this is discussed in accordance with the local guidelines for DNA banking, such as Human Tissue Act 2006 in the United Kingdom. DNA banking is the storage of DNA (typically extracted from white blood cells) for possible future use. In the event of coroner's autopsy due to sudden unexplained death, it is important that a suitable tissue (e.g., a small piece of spleen in normal saline) or any other pathological material should be salvaged at the time of autopsy. This would require careful discussion with the Coroner's pathologist and the relevant family member, possibly next of kin (see Chapter 38). Since it is likely that testing methodology and our understanding of genes, mutations, and diseases will improve in the future, consideration should be given to banking DNA of affected individuals. DNA banking is particularly relevant in situations in which the sensitivity of currently available testing is less than 100% or molecular genetic testing is available on a research basis only.

Predictive Genetic Testing

First-degree relatives of an affected person and members of the extended family may wish to undergo predictive genetic testing. This would only be possible if a disease-causing mutation in either *TGFBR2* or *MYH11* was confirmed. Mutations in other genes, such as *ACTA2,* should be verified for pathogenicity prior to being accepted for predictive genetic testing. Genetic counseling to any such "at-risk" family member should focus on prior recurrence risk (50% in a first-degree relative), reliability of the known mutation, sensitivity of the mutation, clinical predictability based on evidence for genotype–phenotype correlation, availability of long-term multidisciplinary cardiology surveillance including option for prophylactic aortic reconstructive surgery (see section on *Surveillance*), appreciating and understanding the psychosocial implications, and implications for employment, mortgage, life insurance, and any other ethical or legal related issues.

Prenatal and Preimplantation Genetic Testing

Prenatal diagnosis for pregnancies at increased risk for TAA/TAAD may be the preferred option should one of the parents be affected. This should be possible if a disease-causing mutation in either *TGFBR2* or *MYH11* was confirmed. The disease-causing allele of an affected family member must be identified before prenatal testing can be performed by the mutation analysis of DNA extracted from fetal cells obtained by amniocentesis usually performed at about 15–18 weeks' gestation or preferably chorionic villus sampling (CVS) at about 10–12 weeks' gestation. No genetic laboratory is offering molecular genetic testing for prenatal diagnosis for TAAD caused by mutations in other genes listed in Table 10–1. However, prenatal testing may be available for families in which the disease-causing mutation has been identified in an affected family member in a research or clinical laboratory. In such a situation a thorough search for suitable laboratories can be made through accessing online resources (e.g., UKGTN, EDNAL, GeneTests, etc.). Ultrasound examination in the first two trimesters is insensitive for detecting manifestations of thoracic aortic aneurysm.

Preimplantation genetic diagnosis (PGD) may be available for families in which the disease-causing mutation has been identified in an affected family member in a research or clinical laboratory. Where this option is considered then enquiries may be made to relevant IVF/fertility clinics. For example, in the United Kingdom, an application would be required for permission from the statutory Human Fertilization and Embryology authority (HFEA).

Surveillance of the "At-Risk"

Family members at risk for inheriting the genetic predisposition for TAA/TAAD should be examined serially throughout their lifetime by transthoracic echocardiogram to evaluate the size of the ascending aorta and sinuses of Valsalva. Other imaging modalities, such as MRA and/or CT, to view the entire aorta should be used every 4 to 5 years. The frequency of imaging may vary from 2 to 3 years, but preferably should be carried out annually. The following general recommendations may be useful and should be incorporated in most cases:

- The variable age of onset of the aortic disease in familial TAAD makes it necessary to begin imaging the aorta of individuals at risk at a relatively young age.
- The ultrasound imaging should begin 10 years before the earliest age of onset in the family. In a child this should commence when the child can undergo an echocardiogram without sedation, usually around age 6–7 years.
- Because penetrance may be reduced in TAAD, it is appropriate to image any first-degree relative of an affected individual with a familial form of TAAD, whether they are the parents, siblings, or offspring of the proband.
- Imaging of sons of women who are at risk but who have a normal echocardiogram should be considered because of the decreased penetrance of TAAD in women.
- Isometric exercise and competitive sports that lead to significant blows to the chest should be avoided because they may accelerate aortic root dilatation.
- Women with TAAD are advised to obtain prepregnancy counseling from a medical geneticist, a genetic counselor, a cardiologist familiar with this condition, and a high-risk obstetrician.
- It is recommended that women who have TAAD be followed up during pregnancy by a cardiologist and a high-risk obstetrician. Serial monitoring of the aorta may be warranted, depending on the prepregnancy assessment of the aorta.

Disorders Complicating TAAD

Several clinically distinct malformation syndromes may present with thoracic aortic aneurysms and aortic dissections. These are discussed in other sections in this book (Chapters 11 & 28). The reader may find the following commentaries helpful:

Marfan Syndrome

Marfan syndrome is a systemic disorder of connective tissue involving the ocular, skeletal, and cardiovascular systems (see Chapter 11). Myopia is the most common ocular feature; displacement of the lens from the center of the pupil is seen in about 60% of affected individuals. The skeletal system involvement includes joint laxity, disproportionately long extremities for the size of the trunk, pectus excavatum or pectus carinatum, and scoliosis.

Cardiovascular manifestations include dilatation of the aorta at the level of the sinuses of Valsalva, a predisposition for aortic tear and rupture, mitral valve prolapse with or without regurgitation, triscuspid valve prolapse, and enlargement of the proximal pulmonary artery. Mutations of the *FBN1* gene are causative. Inheritance is autosomal dominant.

FBN1 Mutations without Marfan Syndrome

Rarely, familial TAAD results from *FBN1*mutations. In these families, affected individuals do not have the ocular complications of Marfan syndrome and do not have sufficient skeletal features to fulfil the diagnostic criteria for Marfan syndrome (Francke et al. 1995; Milewicz et al. 1996).

Congenital Contractural Arachnodactyly (CCA)

This disorder is characterized by a Marfan-like appearance with a tall, slender habitus in which arm span exceeds height and long, slender fingers and toes (arachnodactyly). At birth, most affected individuals have contractures of the major joints (knees and ankles) and the proximal interphalangeal joints of the fingers and toes (i.e., camptodactyly). Hip contractures, adducted thumbs, and clubfoot may occur. Contractures usually improve with time. Kyphosis/scoliosis, present in about half of all affected individuals, begins as early as infancy, is progressive, and causes the greatest morbidity in CCA. Dilatation of the aorta is present in some individuals and can progressively enlarge over time (Gupta et al. 2004). Dilatation progressing to aortic dissection has not been reported. Mutations of the *FBN2* gene are causative. Inheritance is autosomal dominant.

Ehlers-Danlos Syndrome, Vascular Type (EDS type IV)

Cardinal features are thin, translucent skin; easy bruising; characteristic facial appearance; and arterial, intestinal, and/or uterine fragility. Affected individuals are at risk for arterial rupture, aneurysm, and/or dissection; gastrointestinal perforation or rupture; and uterine rupture during pregnancy. The diagnosis of EDS, vascular type is based on compatible clinical findings and confirmed by biochemical testing demonstrating the production of structurally abnormal collagen III by dermal fibroblasts or by molecular genetic testing demonstrating a mutation in the *COL3A1* gene. Inheritance is autosomal dominant.

Loeys-Dietz Syndrome (LDS)

Features of this syndrome include cardiovascular abnormalities (aortic aneurysms, dissection, and tortuousity; PDA), craniofacial abnormalities (including cleft palate, ocular hypertelorism, craniosynostosis, broad or bifid uvula, proptosis), and skeletal abnormalities (arachnodactyly, dolichostenomelia, pectus deformity, camptodactyly, scoliosis, and joint laxity). The diagnosis of LDAS can be confirmed through molecular testing for *TGFBR2* and *TGFBR1* mutations. Inheritance is autosomal dominant.

Abdominal Aortic Aneurysm

Abdominal aortic aneurysm (AAA) is a multifactorial disorder resulting from complex interaction of hereditary and environmental factors (Table 12–2). The disorder is commonly sporadic but the heritable form may be familial (Loosemore et al. 1988; OMIM 10070). Two distinct heritable forms are recognized, AAA1 mapped to 19q13 (OMIM 609781) and AAA2 mapped to 4q31 (OMIM 609782).

Inheritance

In the majority of cases, AAA occurs sporadically. Some multiplex families exhibit clustering of affected individuals indicating the autosomal dominant inheritance pattern of incomplete penetrance and variable clinical expression (Tilson and Seashore 1984). In one study, the segregation analysis with the mixed model gave single-gene effect with dominant inheritance as the most likely explanation for the familial occurrence (Verloes et al. 1995). The frequency of mutated allele was estimated to be 1 in 250 with an age-related penetrance of around 0.4.

Several studies report complex pedigrees indicating multifactorial inheritance pattern attributed to mutations in several genes with a combined pathogenic effect (Johansen and Koepsell 1986; Baird et al. 1995). Higher prevalence of AAA and subsequent risk of rupture is reported in several studies among first-degree relatives (Lawrence et al. 1995; Kuivaniemi et al. 2003). These studies favour the multifactorial/polygenic model. One study involving first-degree relatives of 91 probands rejected the nongenetic model and suggested that the susceptibility for AAA was related to a recessive gene at an autosomal diallelic major locus (Majumder et al. 1991).

One large study identified 233 families with at least 2 individuals diagnosed with AAA (Kuivaniemi et al. 2003). Although families originated from different geographic regions but these were all white and included 633 affected individuals with an average of 2.8 cases per family. Most families had on average 2 affected cases, six families had 6, three with 7, and one with 8 affected cases. Most of the probands and their affected relatives were male, commonly a brother. About two-third families appeared to show an autosomal recessive inheritance pattern, whereas autosomal dominant pattern appeared likely in about one-fourth families. Eight families showed autosomal dominant inheritance pattern with incomplete inheritance pattern. In 66 families indicating an autosomal dominant inheritance pattern, 141 transmissions of the diseases from an affected parent were recorded following male-to-male (46%), male-to-female (11%), female-to-male (32%), and female-to-female (11%) transmissions. However, this study (Kuivaniemi et al. 2003) concluded that AAAs are a multifactorial disorder with multiple genetic and environmental factors.

Genetic counseling should be offered to close relatives of an affected person with AAA. The lifetime risks for a first-degree male relative is about 15%, probably slightly less for a female relative. Serial screening for AAA should be offered from 10 years before the age of onset in the affected relative.

Pathogenesis and Molecular Genetics

The pathogenesis of AAA is complex (Table 12–2). As previously mentioned, AAAs are characterized by histological signs of chronic inflammation, destructive remodeling of the extracellular matrix (ECM), and depletion of vascular smooth cells (Steinmetz et al. 2003). Matrix metalloproteinases (MMPs) are connective tissue degrading enzymes with a key role in structural changes to the arterial wall leading to aneurysm formation. MMPs are involved in late stages of aneurysm development (Newman et al. 1994). Several different forms of MMPs are known, for example, MMP3, MMP8, MMP9, and MMP13 (Tromp et al. 2004). Activity of MMPs is closely related to its bioactivators, such as plasmin and its inhibitors like plasminogen activator inhibitor (PAI1). Increased levels of MMP3, MMP9, and PAI1 are shown in AAA (Yoon et al. 1999). Promoters of these genes contain polymorphisms with alleles that exhibit different in vitro transcriptional activities. A higher level of phosphorylated MMP8 (also called JNK) is observed in the

Table 12–2 Abdominal Aortic Aneurysm—Key Points

Abdominal aortic aneurysms (AAAs) usually occur sporadically
It is much more common in men and presents later in women
Familial cases of AAAs are also encountered; associated peripheral arterial aneurysms are likely in some familial cases
Some families may follow autosomal dominant inheritance pattern
Diallelic autosomal recessive inheritance pattern is likely
Most familial clustering indicate multifactorial/polygenic etiology
Histological changes indicate chronic inflammation, destructive remodeling of extracellular matrix, and depletion of vascular smooth muscle cells
Activation of matrix metalloproteinases (MMPs) is the end stage of in the pathogenesis of AAA
Important candidate genes involved in AAA include plasminogen activator inhibitor (PAI1), tissue inhibitor of metalloproteinase (TIMP1; TIMP3), elastin (ELN), and type III procollagen (COL3A1)
4G allele polymorphism in PAI1 gene is considered to offer a protective advantage while 5G allele may increase genetic susceptibility
Genetic risks may be guided by the family history alone as no reliable molecular tests exist
Clinical assessment and long-term surveillance may be applicable and should be carried out by the specialist vascular team

arterial wall of AAA. It is postulated that JNK controls the gene expression program that cooperatively enhances ECM degradation (Yoshimura et al. 2005). In mouse models, selective inhibition of JNK in vivo not only prevented the development of AAA but also caused regression of established AAA. It is believed that JNK is a proximal signaling molecule and plays an active role by promoting abnormal ECM metabolism.

Several candidate genes have been hypothesized to be associated with AAA (Ogata et al. 2005). These essentially result in structural alterations in the vascular smooth muscle and ECM leading to formation of aneurysms. Apart from type III procollagen, other protein molecules implicated in AAA include tissue inhibitor of metalloproteinase-1 (TIMP1), TIMP3, matrix metalloproteinase-10 (MMP10), and elastin (ELN). Ogata et al. (2005) have identified DNA sequence changes in the genes encoding these proteins.

Earlier molecular genetic studies in familial aortic aneurysms (FAAs) reported mutation in the COL3A1 gene (Kontusaari et al. 1989, 1990). Detailed DNA sequencing of the triple-helical domain of type III procollagen on cDNA prepared from 54 patients with FAA only revealed single amino acid substitution (gly136-to-arg) of possible functional significance. The study concluded that only 2% of FAA possibly results from mutations in type III procollagen.

The PAI1 is another important candidate gene studied at length. Mutation in this gene results in an increased activity of tissue plasminogen activator (PLAT) that in turn leads to conversion of inactive plasminogen to active form plasmin and activation of MMPs. This cascade of activities results in structural alterations of ECM, which is a major step in the molecular changes leading to aneurysm formation.

Molecular genetic studies in FAAs and AAAs have shown a 4G/5G nucleotide insertion/deletion polymorphism-675 upstream from the initiation of transcription in the PAI1 gene (Dawson et al. 1993). The 4G allele binds only an activator, whereas the 5G allele binds an activator and a repressor and is associated with a relatively reduced transcription of PAI1. The 5G polymorphism is associated with minimal inhibition of plasminogen activators and, consequently, increased conversion of plasminogen to plasmin and increased activation of MMPs. These patients are likely to be more susceptible for developing AAA. In a large study on 190 patients (163 age- and sex-matched controls) with AAA, including 39 with a strong family history, the frequency of 4G:5G in the AAA population compared to the control population was 06:04 (Rossaak et al. 2000). However, 26% of patients with familial AAA were homozygous 5G compared to 13% of the control sample. In the same study, the 4G allele frequency was 0.47 in the familial AAA compared to 0.62 in the nonfamilial patients ($p = 0.02$) and 0.61 in the control population ($p = 0.03$). Importance of 5G allele is argued along with other confounding factors including atherosclerosis and diabetes mellitus. It is postulated that 4G allele probably offers protective advantage for AAA.

Genetic association studies involving 47 AAA patients, 57 intracranial aneurysm (IA) patients, and 174 controls employed polymorphisms in the MMP3, MMP9, and PAI1 genes (Yoon et al. 1999). The study did not find any appreciable higher frequency of 5A MMP3 allele in IA patients, but significantly higher frequency was observed among AAA patients suggesting its importance as a potential genetic risk factor among Finns. This study supported the previous observation of higher MMP3 expression in AAA than in control tissues (Yoon et al. 1999; Trump et al. 2004).

The evidence for genetic heterogeneity in familial AAA (OMIM 100070) is provided from whole-genome scans in 36 families with AAA (Shibumura et al. 2004). Using affected relative-pair (ARP) linkage analysis, strong evidence for linkage (lod = 4.64) has emerged for a region near marker D19S433 at 51.88 cM on19q13. This region is further clarified in a large genetic linkage analysis in 83 families (lod = 4.75) mapped to D19S416 at 58.69 cM. The study was designed allowing for age, sex, number of affected first-degree relatives, and their interaction as covariates. Another potential region for AAA has emerged on chromosome 4q31 (AAA2; OMIM 609782) with a lod score of 3.73 ($p = 0.0012$) near marker D4S1644 using the same covariate model as for chromosome (Shibumura et al. 2004).

Prognosis and Indications for Treatment

Thoracic Aortic Aneurysms

The likelihood of a thoracic aortic aneurysm to rupture is dependent in part on the etiology (Table 12–3). There was a 24%–28.7% 2-year survival in patients with untreated thoracic and TAAAs who had serious comorbidity rendering them unfit for surgery (Bickerstaff et al. 1982; Crawford and DeNatale 1986). Half of the deaths resulted from rupture (Crawford and DeNatale 1986).

The prognosis for dissecting aneurysms is much worse than for degenerative aneurysms (7% versus 19.2% 5-year survival) with rupture being the major cause of death for both (Bickerstaff et al. 1982). In a series of patients with degenerative, nondissecting aneurysms, the overall risk of rupture with nonoperative treatment was 12% at 2 years and 32% at 4 years. Aneurysms larger than 5 cm had an 18% rupture rate at 2 years (Cambria et al. 1995). The overall median expansion of degenerative aneurysms is 1.4 mm/year, but increases with increasing aortic diameter in an exponential manner (Bonser et al. 2000). Intraluminal thrombus, previous stroke, smoking, and peripheral vascular disease are important factors associated with aneurysm growth.

Table 12–3 Thoracic Aortic Aneurysms–Key Points

Familial thoracic aortic aneurysms (TAA) are a genetically heterogeneous group of inherited cardiovascular disorders
Several clinically recognizable syndromes exist manifesting with TAA; notable examples include Marfan syndrome and type IV Ehlers-Danlos syndrome
Inheritance pattern is commonly autosomal dominant with incomplete pentrance and variable clinical manifestations
Medical cystic necrosis is the common pathological sequelae common to most forms of TAA
Aortic dissection, commonly involving the ascending aorta is a recognized life-threatening complication
Associated structural abnormalities may include bicuspid aortic valve, abnormal aortic annulus, and dilatation of the ascending aorta
Dilatation and aneurysms involving the medium/small-sized peripheral arteries may be accompanied with AAT manifesting with myocardial infarction, stroke, rupture, and paralysis
Several gene loci are mapped on different chromosomal locations
Mutations in *TGFBR1, TGFBR2, MYH11,* and *ACTA2* account for a large proportion of familial AAT, including those manifesting with aortic dissections (TAAD); *TGFBR1* is less likely to be causative for nonsyndromal TAA/TAAD
Some mutations may predispose to aortic dissections but there are no acceptable genotype-phenotype correlations
Genetic counseling is necessary and should include discussion on inheritance pattern, genetic risks, need for long-term surveillance of "at-risk" close relatives, option for predictive genetic testing, and reproductive choices
Clinical management and surveillance should be coordinated and supervised by a dedicated multidisciplinary team consisting of cardiologist, specialist cardiac nurse, clinical geneticist, cardiac genetic counselor, cardiothoracic surgeon, imaging experts, and counseling support to deal with psychosocial implications

References: Ades et al. (2006).

The mortality from aneurysms associated with acute dissections is higher than for chronic dissections (Fann and Miller 1995), with 83% deaths from aortic rupture in acute type B dissecting aneurysms compared to 52% in chronic dissecting aneurysms (Pressler and McNamara 1980).

The indications for treatment of a thoracic aortic aneurysm therefore depend on the pathology (Table 12–3). A type A dissection requires immediate surgical treatment. A type B dissection requires treatment if it is associated with acute aneurysmal expansion or complications, but can usually be managed with antihypertensive medical therapy. A chronic type B dissecting aneurysm or a degenerative thoracic aneurysm requires treatment if causing symptoms, presenting with rupture, or if greater than 5.5 cm in diameter, but comorbidity must be taken into account. The aim of elective surgery is to prevent fatal aneurysm rupture and is therefore only of benefit if the gain in life expectancy exceeds the risk of the operation and must be assessed on an individual basis.

Aneurysms of the ascending aorta are repaired when the rate of dilation approaches 1 cm per year, or when aortic regurgitation progresses, or when the aortic diameter reaches 5.5 cm. In patients with familial TAAD caused by *TGFBR2* mutations or associated with a bicuspid aortic valve, intervention is recommended when the ascending aorta reaches 5 cm in diameter although some authorities now recommend intervention at 4.5 cm.

Abdominal Aortic Aneurysms

The size of an AAA is the most important factor that determines the risk of rupture. The annual risk of rupture for an AAA between 4 cm and 5.4 cm in size is 0.5%–1% (Collin et al. 1998; NEJM 2002; Lederle et al. 2002; Prinssen et al. 2004). This increases to 6.6% for aneurysms between 6 cm and 7 cm in size, and 19% for those larger than 7 cm. There is a 5-year rupture rate of 25% for aneurysms with a diameter of 5–5.9 cm, 35% for diameters of 6–6.9 cm, and 75% for diameters over 7 cm (Szilagyi et al. 1972). Following the publication of the UK small aneurysm trial and the ADAM trial, current consensus is that aneurysms under 5.5 cm should be kept under surveillance in combination with best medical therapy, whilst those over 5.5 cm should be considered for intervention (1998). Infrarenal aneurysms expand by an average of 34 mm per year. An aneurysm less than 3 cm in diameter in a man above 65 years is unlikely to ever rupture and does not require monitoring (Couto et al. 2002). However some may expand rapidly, and as a result, annual surveillance is recommended until the aneurysm reaches 4.5 cm in diameter, when it should be performed every six months. This is best done by ultrasound, with a CT scan when the aneurysm reaches 5 cm in diameter, with a view to planning intervention. Infrarenal abdominal aortic aneurysms rupture at smaller diameters in women, and treatment may therefore be considered when the diameter reaches 5 cm.

Aortic Dissections

Proximal dissections require urgent intervention, but distal dissections are usually managed with medical therapy (aggressive blood pressure control) unless they have ongoing symptoms, branch vessel ischemia or aneurysmal formation. Chronic type B dissection may cause aneurysms associated with progressive dilatation of the false lumen, which occurs in 30%–40% of patients, requiring later intervention. 17% of TAAAs result from aortic dissection (Panneton and Hollier 1995).

Medical Therapy

The diagnosis of an aortic aneurysm carries with it an increased risk of cardiovascular death, which increases with aneurysm diameter (Crawford and DeNatale 1986; Brady et al. 2001; Norman et al. 2004a). The presence of an aortic aneurysm, even if small and unlikely to rupture, should therefore be an indication for medical therapy including statins and antiplatelet drugs, in order to reduce the risk of death from atherosclerotic complications.

Smoking cessation and blood pressure control can reduce the rate of expansion of a small aneurysm. β-blockers, particularly propanolol have been used with varying results (Gadowski et al. 1994; Bonser et al. 2000; NEJM 2002). β-blockers are routinely prescribed for individuals with the Marfan syndrome, and similar treatment is recommended for individuals with familial TAAD (Shores et al. 1994). Hypertension should be aggressively treated and controlled in individuals with TAAD. ACE inhibitors may also be of benefit in slowing sac expansion (Moran 2005). Use of statins has also been associated with a 50% reduction in aneurysm growth rate (Schouten 2006).

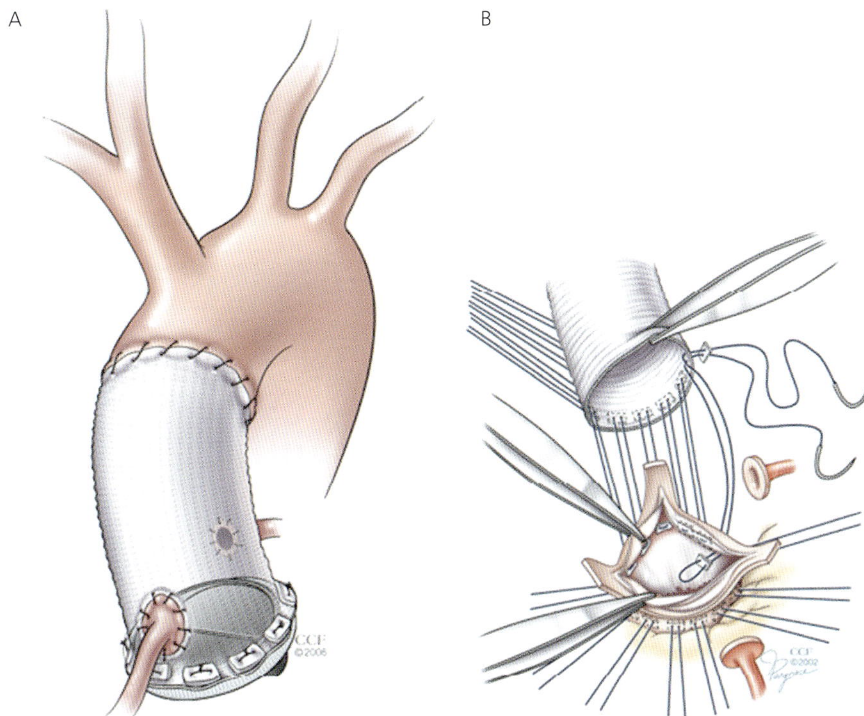

Figure 12–8 Open repair of a thoracoabdominal aortic aneurysm.

Surgical Intervention for Aortic Aneurysms and Dissections

Open Surgical Repair

The majority of patients with aortic aneurysms have coexisting conditions associated with generalized atherosclerosis. Risk factors for death include impaired renal function, coronary artery disease, chronic lung disease, and advanced age. Open repair of a thoracic or TAAA requires a thoracotomy. An AAA requires a large incision for access. There are also the physiological insults of aortic cross-clamping, massive blood loss, hypothermia, and visceral ischemia/reperfusion to contend with. Complications include respiratory failure, renal impairment, paraplegia, myocardial infarction, and multiple organ dysfunction.

Open aortic aneurysm repair usually requires general anesthesia, although abdominal aortic aneurysms can sometimes be performed under epidural anesthesia in patients with severe respiratory disease.

Aortic Root and Ascending Aortic Aneurysms/ Type A Dissections

In the Bentall procedure, the most common operation for repair of an ascending aortic aneurysm (Gott et al. 1999), both the ascending aorta and the aortic valve are replaced with a composite valve and a Dacron graft (Figure 12–8). Following replacement of the aortic valve using this procedure, affected individuals must be placed on lifelong anticoagulation therapy and must have the remainder of their aorta routinely imaged. More recently, a valve-sparing procedure has been developed that precludes the need for chronic anticoagulation (David et al. 1999). More aggressive surgical repair may be indicated for individuals with a family history of aortic dissection without significant aortic root enlargement and in individuals with *TGFBR2* mutations.

Thoracoabdominal Aortic Aneurysms

The patient is positioned into a right lateral decubitus position (Figure 12–9). The thoracoabdominal incision is made in the fifth intercostal space for a type I or a high type II TAAA or in the seventh to ninth intercostal space for a type III or type IV TAAA. The abdominal incision is then carried down the midline or paramedian line. Distal aortic perfusion is maintained by a shunt and CSF drainage and hypothermia are used to protect against paraplegia. The crus of the diaphragm is divided to the left of the aorta and the visceral and renal arteries are identified and selectively reperfused. Clamps are applied to the proximal and distal aorta above and below the aneurysm, the sac is opened, and a graft made from Dacron or polytetrafluoroethylene (PTFE) is inlayed. The mesenteric, renal and large intercostal vessels are reimplanted using Dacron grafts or a Carrel patch. The use of left heart bypass and selective visceral reperfusion is associated with a reduced incidence of renal failure and paraplegia. 30-day mortality rates are 4.3%–15% in specialist units but may be as high as 22% (Cowan et al. 2003).

Abdominal Aortic Aneurysms

The abdominal aorta is approached from a long midline incision, or a transverse incision. Clamps are applied to the proximal and distal aorta, the sac is opened, and an inlay graft placed. Approximately 60% to 70% of infrarenal aneurysms can be repaired using a simple tube graft anastomosed to the infrarenal neck proximally and to the aortic bifurcation distally. In the remaining 30% to 40% of cases, a bifurcated graft is used with anastomoses to the common iliac bifurcation or the common femoral artery in the groin

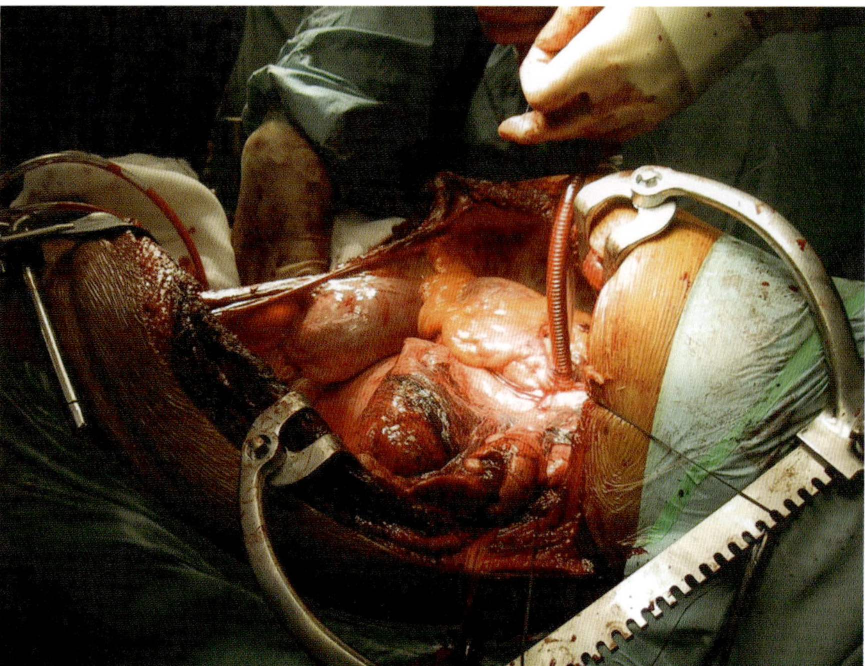

Figure 12–9 Surgical approaches for repair of ascending thoracic aortic aneurysm. (a) The modified Bentall procedure. (b) The aortic valve-sparing David procedure. Reprinted from *Textbook of Cardiovascular Medicine*, Third Ed., Eric J Topol (Ed.) with permission.

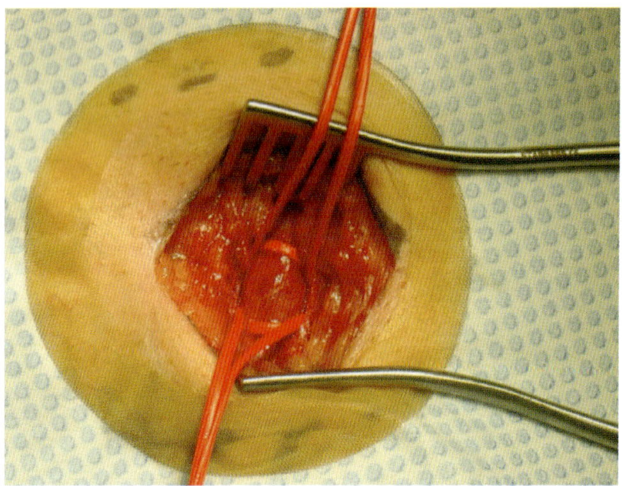

Figure 12–10 Demonstrating the small incision required for access to the femoral artery.

For repair of juxtarenal aneurysms, suprarenal clamping is necessary. There is a risk of renal failure from embolization of thrombus at the neck of the aneurysm or from renal ischemia during clamping. Complications such as paraplegia are very rare from infrarenal aneurysm repair (1/250). Mortality rates vary from 4% to 10%.

Endovascular Surgery

Aortic Aneurysms

The first case of endovascular aneurysm repair (EVAR) was reported in 1991 (Parodi et al. 1991) and this has subsequently revolutionized the treatment of patients with aortic aneurysms. The aneurysm is repaired by a stent graft, made of an expandable metal such as stainless steel or nitinol (a nickel titanium alloy) covered with fabric, (expanded polytetrafluoroethylene or ePTFE), and usually composed of modular units. The stent graft is positioned under radiological control, over a wire inserted into the artery. The femoral artery is usually used for access. The only incisions required are therefore cut downs to the femoral artery (Figure 12–10), although in time these will become percutaneous procedures. A general anesthetic is not usually required; the procedure is usually performed under epidural anesthesia. This avoids the need for a large incision and extensive tissue dissection and blood loss associated with open surgical repair, as well as the physiological insult of aortic cross-clamping.

Stent grafts can be used to treat aortic aneurysms from the distal arch to the iliac arteries, but not all aneurysms are suitable for endoluminal treatment. There needs to be a suitable landing zone for the device in nonaneurysmal aorta proximally and distally. This needs to be at least 2 cm in the thoracic aorta and 1 cm below the renal arteries. The landing zone needs to be relatively straight with parallel sides in order to achieve a seal. The device needs to negotiate the iliac arteries, which may not be possible if they are narrowed by atherosclerosis, too tortuous or calcified. It may be possible to gain access by the anastomosis of a polyester tube conduit to the common iliac artery if the external iliac artery is too narrow.

When treating thoracic aneurysms, the landing zone may include the left subclavian artery. It is possible to cover the left subclavian artery without prior reconstruction but there is an increased risk of left arm ischemia, stroke, or paraplegia (particularly if there is a dominant left vertebral artery). Some authors recommend bypass or transposition from the left subclavian to the left common carotid artery to reduce this risk prior to covering the origin or the left subclavian artery (Figure 12–11). For distal arch aneurysms, it is possible to also cover the orifice of the left common carotid artery if a prior bypass from the left to the right

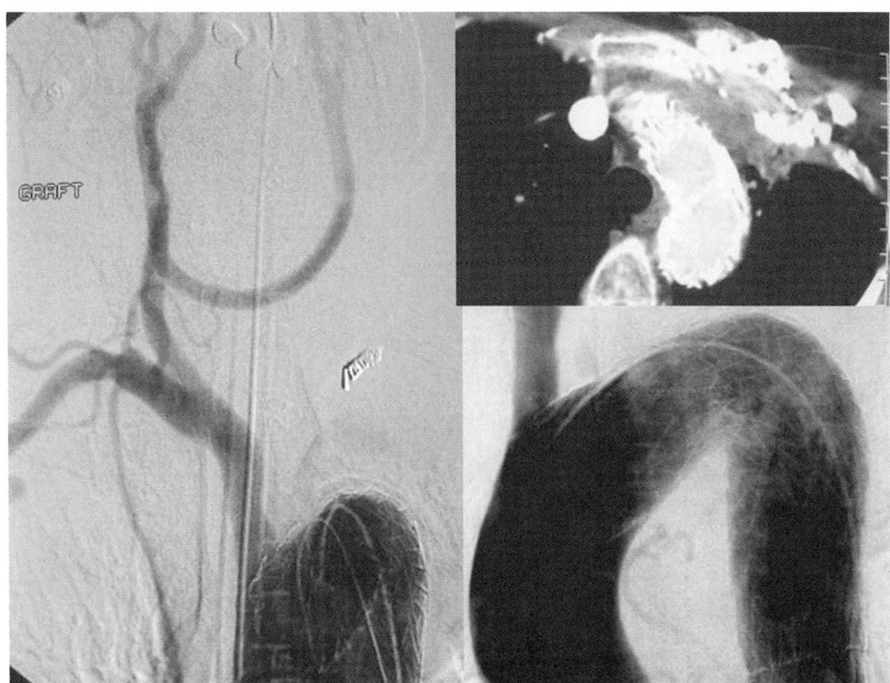

Figure 12–11 Angiographic and CT scan appearances of a thoracic aortic stent graft covering both the left common carotid and left subclavian arteries. Prior to stenting, a carotid-carotid bypass has been performed.

common carotid arteries is made. This may be combined with revascularization of the left subclavian artery.

With thoracoabdominal aortic aneurysms where the arteries to the kidneys and viscera are involved, stent grafting may be performed after a prior revascularization of the visceral and renal arteries with bypass grafts from the iliac arteries (Figure 12–12). This "hybrid" procedure avoids the need for a thoracotomy, but is a lengthy procedure associated with morbidity. Alternatively, one of the newer branched or fenestrated devices may be used. These have to be custom-made and are more difficult to deploy. However, some excellent results have been published with mortality rates of 5%.

During the procedure, the patient has to lie flat for several hours, which may exacerbate a lung complaint even if epidural anesthesia is used. There is a risk of perioperative stroke or myocardial infarction. The iliac vessels may be damaged by passage of the sheath, leading to hemorrhage. There may be technical difficulties resulting in a conversion to an open procedure. Covering of the intercostal vessels and/or left subclavian arteries may lead to paraplegia, particularly if other parts of the aorta have been repaired, or if there is iliac disease. This is treated with urgent CSF drainage and avoidance of hypotension and requires that patients are closely monitored after stenting. Some pain and pyrexia in the first 36 hours after stent graft placement is common and reflects thrombosis occurring in the sac. This may be associated with a rise in inflammatory markers.

The patient usually leaves hospital after a couple of days. However, there is a risk of late complications, and they may need additional procedures. The main complication requiring reintervention is the persistence of blood flow in the aneurysm sac after endovascular repair, termed "endoleak." These may result from an inadequate seal at either the proximal or distal landing zone (type I); retrograde flow into the aneurysm sac from aortic side branches (lumbar, intercostal, or inferior mesenteric arteries) (type II); a leak between the modular components the stent graft or a hole in the fabric (type III); or porosity of the graft wall (type IV). A further situation may arise where high pressure may persist in the aneurysm sac without evidence of an endoleak, leading to sac expansion, termed "endotension." Endoleaks can be associated with aneurysm enlargement and eventual rupture. This is most commonly seen with type I and type III endoleaks, which involve high pressure flow, and these almost always require intervention.

Other complications are migration, which may lead to a type I or III endoleak, stent fractures, and graft thrombosis—presenting with acute limb ischemia. Overall, with the latest devices, approximately 8% of patients require secondary procedures, which are similar to open surgery.

The short and mid term results from EVAR compare favourably with open repair. The EVAR1 trial of infrarenal aneurysms fit for open surgery reported 30 day mortality rates of 1.7% after endovascular stent grafting compared with 4.7% with open repair (Lancet 2005) Long-term results are awaited. There is however a slightly higher reintervention rate with endovascular repair compared with open surgery and the patient needs to be kept under continued surveillance to diagnose late complications. This is usually either annual CT or a combination of abdominal duplex scans to diagnose endoleak and plain abdominal X-rays to diagnose fractures of the stent and migration.

Aortic Dissections

There are several solutions for treating branch vessel ischemia associated with an acute type B dissection. A conventional aortic stent may be placed in the true aortic lumen, in order to maintain patency, or a stent could be placed in the occluded branch vessel to improve flow from either the true or false lumen. If a branch vessel is ischemic as a result of poor flow in the lumen from which it arises, a "fenestration" may be performed, where a balloon is passed over a wire between the lumina, enabling perfusion from both sides. This may be used in association with branch vessel or aortic stents.

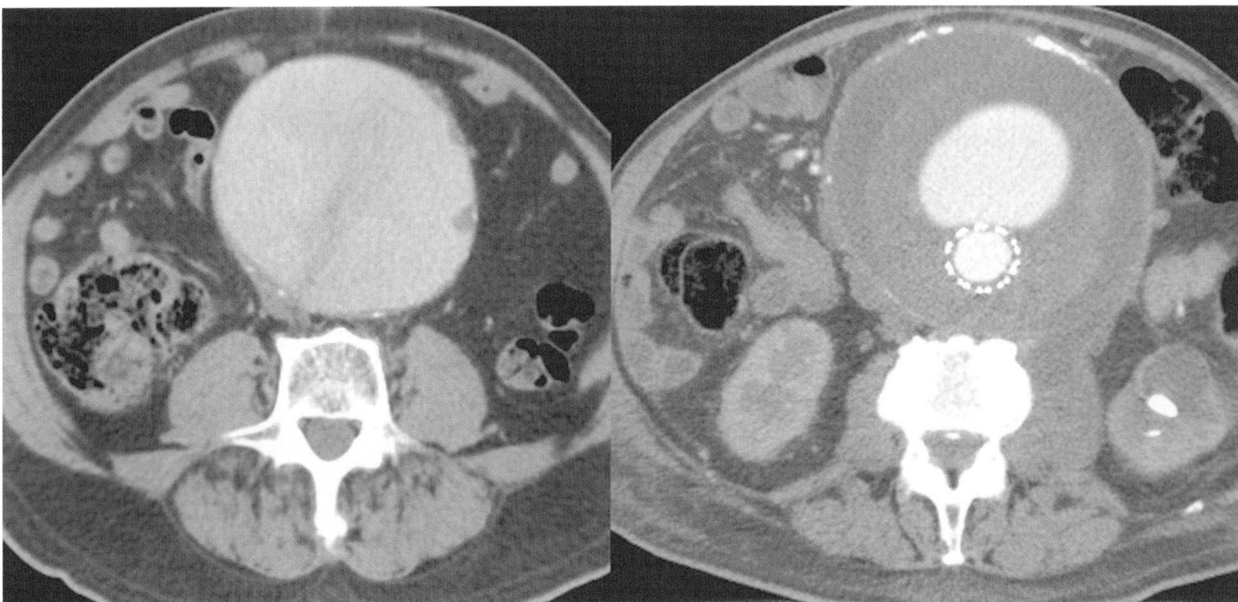

Figure 12–12 CT scan appearances of a large aortic aneurysm prior- and post-stenting. On the right hand picture there is evidence of an endoleak with contrast both within the stent, and outside the stent in the aneurysm sac.

An alternative approach is to use an endovascular approach by deploying an aortic stent graft to cover the primary entry tear. This allows the pressure in the true lumen to increase and that in the false lumen to fall, which encourages the false lumen to thrombose. This combination is often sufficient to overcome ischemia caused by compression of important branches by the pressure in the false lumen. Endovascular repair may also prevent long-term complications such as rupture from continued aortic dilatation. The length of aorta covered in covering the primary tear may influence the outcome; however, the corollary of this is an increase in the risk of paraplegia. The risk of paraplegia with endoluminal treatment of acute complicated type B aortic dissection is however very low and at 1% is much lower than open surgical procedures that carry a risk of between 5% and 20%.

Chronic type B dissections may be treated by aortic stent grafts in the same fashion as aortic aneurysms, when they are greater than 5.5 cm or continue to expand with pain. The use of endoluminal repair for uncomplicated chronic type B dissection was shown to be associated with a higher risk of death at 10% compared with hypotensive medication (3%) by the INSTEAD trial, which is yet to be published.

The advent of newer technologies has allowed certain types of acute type A dissections to be treated with endovascular aortic stent grafts.

Conclusions

Aneurysms of the aorta are increasing in incidence and prevalence. This is due to several factors including an ageing population, aneurysm screening programmes, widespread availability and use of ultrasound and CT scans, and improved education of both patient and doctor. The past decade has seen an endovascular revolution, which has made the treatment of aortic aneurysms much safer. However, there are still concerns about the durability of endovascular devices and long-term follow-up is required. The further understanding of the etiology of degenerative aneurysms will hopefully lead to the development of an effective medical treatment in the future. Patients who are identified genetically to be at high risk of developing aortic dilatation, dissection or an aneurysm are likely to benefit from regular clinical surveillance, medical prophylaxis, (β blockers and ACE-inhibitors or ACE-receptor blockers) and preventive surgical intervention.

References

Ades LC, Sullivan K, Biggin A, et al. FBN1, TGFBR1, and the Marfan-craniosynostosis/mental retardation disorders revisited. *Am J Med Genet*. 2006;140A:1047–1058.

Alley MT, Shifrin RY, Pelc NJ, Herfkens RJ. Ultrafast contrast-enhanced three-dimensional MR angiography: state of the art. *Radiographics*. 1998;18(2):273–285.

Ashton HA, Buxton MJ, Day NE, et al. The Multicentre Aneurysm Screening Study (MASS) into the effect of abdominal aortic aneurysm screening on mortality in men: a randomised controlled trial. *Lancet*. 2002;360(9345):1531–1539.

Baird PA, Sadovnick AD, Yee IML, Cole CW, Cole L. Sibling risks of abdominal aortic aneurysm. *Lancet*. 1995;346:601–604.

Bickerstaff LK, Pairolero PC, Hollier LH, et al. Thoracic aortic aneurysms: a population-based study. *Surgery*. 1982;92(6):1103–1108.

Biddinger A, Rocklin M, Coselli J, Milewicz DM. Familial thoracic aortic dilatations and dissections: a case control study. *J Vasc Surg*. 1997;25:506–511.

Bonser RS, Pagano D, Lewis ME, et al. Clinical and patho-anatomical factors affecting expansion of thoracic aortic aneurysms. *Heart*. 2000; 84(3):277–283.

Brady AR, Fowkes FG, Thompson SG, Powell JT. Aortic aneurysm diameter and risk of cardiovascular mortality. *Arterioscler Thromb Vasc Biol*. 2001;21(7):1203–1207.

Cambria RA, Gloviczki P, Stanson AW, et al. Outcome and expansion rate of 57 thoracoabdominal aortic aneurysms managed nonoperatively. *Am J Surg*. 1995;170(2):213–217.

Coady MA, Davies RR, Roberts M, et al. Familial patterns of thoracic aortic aneurysms. *Arch Surg*. 1999;134:361–367.

Cohen JR, Mandell C, Chang JB, Wise L. Elastin metabolism of the infrarenal aorta. *J Vasc Surg.* 1988;7(2):210–214.

Collin J, Araujo L, Walton J, Lindsell D. Oxford screening programme for abdominal aortic aneurysm in men aged 65 to 74 years. *Lancet.* 1988;II:613–615.

Couto E, Duffy SW, Ashton HA, et al. Probabilities of progression of aortic aneurysms: estimates and implications for screening policy. *J Med Screen.* 2002;9(1):40–42.

Cowan JA Jr, Dimick JB, Henke PK, Huber TS, Stanley JC, Upchurch GR Jr. Surgical treatment of intact thoracoabdominal aortic aneurysms in the United States: hospital and surgeon volume-related outcomes. *J Vasc Surg.* 2003;37(6):1169–1174.

Crawford ES, Cohen ES. Aortic aneurysm: a multifocal disease. Presidential address. *Arch Surg.* 1982;117(11):1393–1400.

Crawford ES, DeNatale RW. Thoracoabdominal aortic aneurysm: observations regarding the natural course of the disease. *J Vasc Surg.* 1986;3(4):578–582.

Daily PO, Trueblood HW, Stinson EB, Wuerflein RD, Shumway NE. Management of acute aortic dissections. *Ann Thorac Surg.* 1970; 10(3):237–247.

David TE, Armstrong S, Ivanov J, Webb GD. Aortic valve sparing operations: an update. *Ann Thorac Surg.* 1999;67:1840–1842.

Dawson SJ, Wiman B, Hamsten A, Green F, Humphries S, Henney AM. The two allele sequences of a common polymorphism in the promoter of the plasminogen activator inhibitor-1 (PAI-1) gene respond differently to interleukin-1 in HepG2 cells. *J Biol Chem.* 1993;268:10739–10745.

DeBakey ME, Henly WS, Cooley DA, Morris GC Jr, Crawford ES, Beall AC Jr. Surgical managment of dissecting aneurysms of the aorta. *J Thorac Cardiovasc Surg.* 1965;49:130–149.

De Paepe A, Devereux RB, Dietz HC, Hennekam RCM, Pyeritz RE. Revised diagnostic criteria for the Marfan syndrome. *Am J Med Genet.* 1996;62:417–426.

Disabella E, Grasso M, Marziliano N, et al. Two novel and one known mutation of the TGFBR2 gene in Marfan syndrome not associated with FBN1 gene defects. *Eur J Hum Genet.* 2006;14:34–38.

Dobrin PB. Pathophysiology and pathogenesis of aortic aneurysms. Current concepts. *Surg Clin North Am.* 1989;69(4):687–703.

Dobrin PB, Baker WH, Gley WC. Elastolytic and collagenolytic studies of arteries. Implications for the mechanical properties of aneurysms. *Arch Surg.* 1984;119(4):405–409.

Doroghazi RM, Slater EE, DeSanctis RW, Buckley MJ, Austen WG, Rosenthal S. Long-term survival of patients with treated aortic dissection. *J Am Coll Cardiol.* 1984;3(4):1026–1034.

Evans JM, O'Fallon WM, Hunder GG. Increased incidence of aortic aneurysm and dissection in giant cell (temporal) arteritis. A population-based study. *Ann Intern Med.* 1995;122(7):502–507.

Fann JI, Miller DC. Aortic dissection. *Ann Vasc Surg.* 1995;9(3):311–323.

Fann JI, Sarris GE, Mitchell RS, et al. Treatment of patients with aortic dissection presenting with peripheral vascular complications. *Ann Surg.* 1990;212(6):705–713.

Fowkes FG, Macintyre CC, Ruckley CV. Increasing incidence of aortic aneurysms in England and Wales. *BMJ.* 1989;298(6665):33–35.

Francke U, Berg MA, Tynan K, et al. A Gly1127Ser mutation in an EGF-like domain of the fibrillin-1 gene is a risk factor for ascending aortic aneurysm and dissection. *Am J Hum Genet.* 1995;56:1287–1296.

Franzen P, ten Dijke P, Ichijo H, et al. Cloning of a TGF-beta type I receptor that forms a heteromeric complex with the TGF-beta type II receptor. *Cell.* 1993;75:681–692.

Gadowski GR, Pilcher DB, Ricci MA. Abdominal aortic aneurysm expansion rate: effect of size and beta-adrenergic blockade. *J Vasc Surg.* 1994;19(4):727–731.

Gale AN, McKusick VA, Hutchins GM, Gott VL. Familial congenital bicuspid aortic valve: secondary calcific aortic stenosis and aortic aneurysm. *Chest.* 1977;72:668–670.

Gott VL, Greene PS, Alejo DE, et al. Replacement of the aortic root in patients with Marfan's syndrome. *N Engl J Med.* 1999; 340:1307–1313.

Guo D-C, Pannu H, Tran-Fadulu V, et al. Mutations in smooth muscle alpha-actin (ACTA2) lead to thoracic aortic aneurysms and dissections. *Nat Gen.* 2007;39:1488–1493.

Gupta PA, Wallis DD, Chin TO, et al. FBN2 mutation associated with manifestations of Marfan syndrome and congenital contractural arachnodactyly. *J Med Genet.* 2004;41:e56.

Johansen K, Koepsell T. Familial tendency for abdominal aortic aneurysms. *JAMA.* 1986;256:1934–1936.

Johnson DW, Qumsiyeh M, Benkhalifa M, Marchuk DA. Assignment of human transforming growth factor-beta type I and type III receptor genes (TGFBR1 and TGFBR3) to 9q33-q34 and 1p32-p33, respectively. *Genomics.* 1995;28:356–357.

Johnston KW, Rutherford RB, Tilson MD, Shah DM, Hollier L, Stanley JC. Suggested standards for reporting on arterial aneurysms. Subcommittee on Reporting Standards for Arterial Aneurysms, Ad Hoc Committee on Reporting Standards, Society for Vascular Surgery and North American Chapter, International Society for Cardiovascular Surgery. *J Vasc Surg.* 1991;13(3):452–458.

Ki CS, Jin DK, Chang SH, et al. Identification of a novel TGFBR2 gene mutation in a Korean patient with Loeys-Dietz aortic aneurysm syndrome; no mutation in TGFBR2 gene in 30 patients with classic Marfan's syndrome. *Clin Genet.* 2005;68:561–563.

Kontusaari S, Kuivaniemi H, Tromp G, Grimwood R, Prockop DJ. A single base mutation in the type III procollagen gene (COL3A1) on chromosome 2q that causes familial aneurysms (Abstract). *Cytogenet Cell Genet.* 1989;51:1024–1025.

Kontusaari S, Tromp G, Kuivaniemi H, Romanic AM, Prockop DJ. A mutation in the gene for type III procollagen (COL3A1) in a family with aortic aneurysms. *J Clin Invest.* 1990;86:1465–1473.

Kuan J, Kono DH. Tgfbr1 maps to chromosome 4. *Mamm Genome.* 1998; 9:95–96.

Kuivaniemi H, Shibamura H, Arthur C, et al. Familial abdominal aortic aneurysms: collection of 233 multiplex families. *J Vasc Surg.* 2003; 37:340–345.

Lancet. Mortality results for randomised controlled trial of early elective surgery or ultrasonographic surveillance for small abdominal aortic aneurysms. The UK Small Aneurysm Trial Participants. *Lancet.* 1998;352(9141):1649–1655.

Lancet. Endovascular aneurysm repair versus open repair in patients with abdominal aortic aneurysm (EVAR trial 1): randomised controlled trial. *Lancet.* 2005;365(9478):2179–2186.

Lawrence PF, Lorenzo-Rivero S, Lyon JL. The incidence of iliac, femoral, and popliteal artery aneurysms in hospitalized patients. *J Vasc Surg.* 1995;22:409–415.

Lederle FA, Wilson SE, Johnson GR. Immediate repair compared with surveillance of small abdominal aortic aneurysms. *N Engl J Med.* 2002;346(19):1437–1444.

Lindsay J Jr. Coarctation of the aorta, bicuspid aortic valve and abnormal ascending aortic wall. *Am J Cardiol.* 1988;61:182–184.

Loeys BL, Chen J, Neptune ER, et al. A syndrome of altered cardiovascular, craniofacial, neurocognitive and skeletal development caused by mutations in TGFBR1 or TGFBR2. *Nat Genet.* 2005;37:275–281.

Loeys BL, Schwarze U, Holm, T, et al. Aneurysm syndromes caused by mutations in the TGF-beta receptor. *N Eng J Med.* 2006;355:788–798.

Loosemore TM, Child AH, Dormandy JA. Familial abdominal aortic aneurysms. *J Roy Soc Med.* 1988;81:472–473.

Loscalzo ML, Goh DLM, Loeys B, Kent KC, Spevak PJ, Dietz HC. Familial thoracic aortic dilation and bicommissural aortic valve: a prospective analysis of natural history and inheritance. *Am J Med Genet.* 2007;143A:1960–1967.

Lucarotti M, Shaw E, Poskitt K, Heather B. The Gloucestershire Aneurysm Screening Programme: the first 2 years' experience. *Eur J Vasc Surg.* 1993; 7(4):397–401.

Majumder PP, St. Jean PL, Ferrell RE, Webster MW, Steed DL. On the inheritance of abdominal aortic aneurysm. *Am J Hum Genet.* 1991;48:164–170.

Matyas G, Arnold E, Carrel T, et al. Identification and in silico analyses of novel TGFBR1 and TGFBR2 mutations in Marfan syndrome-related disorders. *Hum Mutat.* 2006;27:760–769.

McKusick VA. Association of aortic valvular disease and cystic medial necrosis (Letter). *Lancet I.* 1972;1026–1027.

Melton LJ III, Bickerstaff LK, Hollier LH, et al. Changing incidence of abdominal aortic aneurysms: a population-based study. *Am J Epidemiol.* 1984;120(3):379–386.

Milewicz DM, Chen H, Park ES, et al. Reduced penetrance and variable expressivity of familial thoracic aortic aneurysms/dissections. *Am J Cardiol.* 1998;82:474–479.

Milewicz DM, Michael K, Fisher N, Coselli JS, Markello T, Biddinger A. Fibrillin-1 (FBN1) mutations in patients with thoracic aortic aneurysms. *Circulation.* 1996;94:2708–2711.

Mizuguchi T, Collod-Beroud G, Akiyama T, et al. Heterozygous TGFBR2 mutations in Marfan syndrome. *Nat Genet.* 2004;36:855–860.

NEJM. Long-term outcomes of immediate repair compared with surveillance of small abdominal aortic aneurysms. *N Engl J Med.* 2002;346(19):1445–1452.

Newman KM, Malon AM, Shin RD, Scholes JV, Ramey WG, Tilson MD. Matrix metalloproteinases in abdominal aortic aneurysm: characterization, purification, and their possible sources. *Connect Tissue Res.* 1994;30:265–276.

Norman P, Le M, Pearce C, Jamrozik K. Infrarenal aortic diameter predicts all-cause mortality. *Arterioscler Thromb Vasc Biol.* 2004a; 24(7):1278–1282.

Norman PE, Jamrozik K, Lawrence-Brown MM, et al. Population based randomised controlled trial on impact of screening on mortality from abdominal aortic aneurysm. *BMJ.* 2004b;329(7477):1259.

Ogata T, Shibamura H, Tromp G, et al. Genetic analysis of polymorphisms in biologically relevant candidate genes in patients with abdominal aortic aneurysms. *J Vasc Surg.* 2005;41:1036–1042.

Pachulski RT, Weinberg AL, Chan K-L. Aortic aneurysm in patients with functionally normal or minimally stenotic bicuspid aortic valve. *Am J Cardiol.* 1991;67:781–782.

Panneton JM, Hollier LH. Nondissecting thoracoabdominal aortic aneurysms: part I. *Ann Vasc Surg.* 1995;9(5):503–514.

Pannu H, Fadulu VT, Chang J, et al. Mutations in transforming growth factor-beta receptor type II cause familial thoracic aortic aneurysms and dissections. *Circulation.* 2005;112:513–520.

Parodi JC, Palmaz JC, Barone, HD. Transfemoral intraluminal graft implantation for abdominal aortic aneurysms. *Ann Vasc Surg.* 1991; 5(6):491–499.

Pasche B, Luo Y, Rao PH, et al. Type I transforming growth factor beta receptor maps to 9q22 and exhibits a polymorphism and a rare variant within a polyalanine tract. *Cancer Res.* 1998;58:2727–2732.

Pleumeekers HJ, Hoes AW, van der DE, et al. Aneurysms of the abdominal aorta in older adults. The Rotterdam Study. *Am J Epidemiol.* 1995; 142(12):1291–1299.

Pressler V, McNamara JJ. Thoracic aortic aneurysm: natural history and treatment. *J Thorac Cardiovasc Surg.* 1980;79(4):489–498.

Pressler V, McNamara JJ. Aneurysm of the thoracic aorta. Review of 260 cases. *J Thorac Cardiovasc Surg.* 1985;89(1):50–54.

Prinssen M, Verhoeven EL, Buth J, et al. A randomized trial comparing conventional and endovascular repair of abdominal aortic aneurysms. *N Engl J Med.* 2004;351(16):1607–1618.

Roberts CS, Roberts WC. Dissection of the aorta associated with congenital malformation of the aortic valve. *J Am Coll Cardiol.* 1991;17:712–716.

Rossaak JI, van Rij AM, Jones GT, Harris EL. Association of the 4G/5G polymorphism in the promoter region of plasminogen activator inhibitor-1 with abdominal aortic aneurysms. *J Vasc Surg.* 2000;31:1026–1032.

Rubin GD. Helical CT angiography of the thoracic aorta. *J Thorac Imaging,* 1997;12(2):128–149.

Shibamura H, Olson JM, van Vlijmen-van Keulen C, et al. Genome scan for familial abdominal aortic aneurysm using sex and family history as covariates suggests genetic heterogeneity and identifies linkage to chromosome 19q13. *Circulation.* 2004;109:2103–2108.

Shores J, Berger KR, Murphy EA, Pyeritz RE. Progression of aortic dilatation and the benefit of long-term beta-adrenergic blockade in Marfan's syndrome. *N Engl J Med.* 1994;330:1335–1341.

Singh K, Bonaa KH, Jacobsen BK, Bjork L, Solberg S. Prevalence of and risk factors for abdominal aortic aneurysms in a population-based study: the Tromso Study. *Am J Epidemiol.* 2001;154(3):236–244.

Singh KK, Rommel K, Mishra A, et al. TGFBR1 and TGFBR2 mutations in patients with features of Marfan syndrome and Loeys-Dietz syndrome. *Hum Mutat.* 2006;27:770–777.

Steinmetz EF, Buckley C, Thompson RW. Prospects for the medical management of abdominal aortic aneurysms. *Vasc Endovasc Surg.* 2003;37:151–163.

Svensson LG, Crawford ES. Aortic dissection and aortic aneurysm surgery: clinical observations, experimental investigations, and statistical analyses. Part II. *Curr Probl Surg.* 1992;29(12):913–1057.

Svensson LG, Crawford ES, Hess KR, Coselli JS, Safi HJ. Experience with 1509 patients undergoing thoracoabdominal aortic operations. *J Vasc Surg.* 1993;17(2):357–368.

Szilagyi DE, Elliott JP, Smith RF. Clinical fate of the patient with asymptomatic abdominal aortic aneurysm and unfit for surgical treatment. *Arch Surg.* 1972;104(4):600–606.

Tilson MD, Seashore MR. Fifty families with abdominal aortic aneurysms in two or more first-order relatives. *Am J Surg.* 1984;147: 551–553.

Tromp G, Gatalica Z, Skunca M, et al. Elevated expression of matrix metalloproteinase-13 in abdominal aortic aneurysms. *Ann Vasc Surg.* 2004; 18:414–420.

Ueyama H, Bruns G, Kanda N. Assignment of the vascular smooth muscle actin gene ACTSA to human chromosome 10. *Jpn J Hum Genet.* 1990;35:145–150.

Ueyama H, Hamada H, Battula N, Kakunaga T. Structure of a human smooth muscle actin gene (aortic type) with a unique intron site. *Molec Cell Biol.* 1984;4:1073–1078.

Ueyama H, Inazawa J, Ariyama T, et al. Reexamination of chromosomal loci of human muscle actin genes by fluorescence in situ hybridization. *Jpn J Hum Genet.* 1995;40:145–148.

Vandekerckhove J, Weber K. The complete amino acid sequence of actins from bovine aorta, bovine heart, bovine fast skeletal muscle, and rabbit slow skeletal muscle. *Differentiation.* 1979,14:123–133.

Vardulaki KA, Walker NM, Day NE, Duffy SW, Ashton HA, Scott RA. Quantifying the risks of hypertension, age, sex and smoking in patients with abdominal aortic aneurysm. *Br J Surg.* 2000;87(2):195–200.

Verloes A, Sakalihasan N, Koulischer L, Limet R. Aneurysms of the abdominal aorta: familial and genetic aspects in three hundred thirteen pedigrees. *J Vas Surg.* 1995;21:646–655.

Ward AS. Aortic aneurysmal disease: a generalized dilating diathesis? *Arch Surg.* 1992;127:990–991.

Yoon S, Tromp G, Vongpunsawad S, Ronkainen A, Juvonen T, Kuivaniemi H. Genetic analysis of MMP3, and PAI-1 in Finnish patients with abdominal aortic or intracranial aneurysms. *Biochem Biophys Res Commun.* 1999;265:563–568.

Yoshimura K, Aoki H, Ikeda Y, et al. Regression of abdominal aortic aneurysm by inhibition of c-Jun N-terminal kinase. *Nat Med.* 2005;11: 1330–1338.

Zhu L, Vranckx R, Khau Van Kien P, et al. Mutations in myosin heavy chain 11 cause a syndrome associating thoracic aortic aneurysm/aortic dissection and patent ductus arteriosus. *Nat Gen.* 2006;38:343–349.

13

Hypertrophic, Dilated, and Restrictive Cardiomyopathies

Juan Pablo-Kaski and Perry Elliott

Cardiomyopathies are defined as myocardial disorders in which the heart is structurally and functionally abnormal, in the absence of coronary artery disease, valvular heart disease, hypertension, or congenital heart disease sufficient to cause the observed myocardial abnormality (Elliott et al. 2008). Cardiomyopathies are classified into four main subtypes, based on ventricular morphology and physiology: hypertrophic cardiomyopathy (HCM); dilated cardiomyopathy (DCM); restrictive cardiomyopathy (RCM); and arrhythmogenic right ventricular cardiomyopathy (ARVC) (see Chapter 14). Those cases that do not fit readily into these subtypes are termed "unclassified cardiomyopathies," and include left ventricular (LV) noncompaction (see Chapter 15), endocardial fibroelastosis, and Tako-Tsubo cardiomyopathy. Each subtype of cardiomyopathy is subdivided into familial/genetic and nonfamilial/nongenetic forms (Elliott et al. 2008).

Hypertrophic Cardiomyopathy

HCM is defined as LV hypertrophy in the absence of abnormal loading conditions (valve disease, hypertension, congenital heart defects) sufficient to explain the degree of hypertrophy (Elliott et al. 2008). Studies in North America, Europe, Japan, and China consistently report a prevalence of unexplained LV hypertrophy of approximately 1 in 500 adults (Hada et al. 1987; Codd et al. 1989; Maron et al. 1994, 1995; Zou et al. 2004; Morita et al. 2006). The prevalence of HCM in children is unknown, but population-based studies have reported an annual incidence of 0.3 to 0.5 per 100,000 (Lipshultz et al. 2003; Nugent et al. 2003).

Etiology

In most adolescents and adults, HCM is an autosomal dominant trait caused by mutations in cardiac sarcomere protein genes (Marian and Roberts 2001; Seidman and Seidman 2001; Richard et al. 2003). In less than 10% of infants and children, and in an even smaller proportion of adults, HCM can be associated with inborn errors of metabolism, neuromuscular disorders, and malformation syndromes (Schwartz et al. 1996; Elliott and McKenna 2004; Nugent et al. 2005; Elliott et al. 2008). Patients with cardiomyopathy associated with metabolic disorders or malformation syndromes are often diagnosed earlier in life (infancy or early childhood), whereas patients with neuromuscular diseases tend to be diagnosed as teenagers (Nugent et al. 2005).

1. Sarcomere Protein Disease

Genetic studies have shown that 50%–60% of adults with HCM have mutations in 1 of 11 genes that encode the proteins of the cardiac sarcomere: β-myosin heavy chain (*MYH7*, chromosome 14); myosin-binding protein C (*MYBPC3*, chromosome 11); cardiac troponin T (*TNNT2*, chromosome 1); cardiac troponin I (*TNNI3*, chromosome 19); α-tropomyosin (*TPM1*, chromosome 15); α-cardiac actin (*ACTC*, chromosome 15); essential myosin light chain (*MYL3*, chromosome 3); regulatory myosin light chain (*MYL2*, chromosome 12); cardiac troponin C (*TNNC1*, chromosome 3); α-myosin heavy chain (*MYH6*, chromosome 14) (Marian and Roberts 2001; Seidman and Seidman 2001; Richard et al. 2003; Ahmad et al. 2005); and titin (*TTN*, chromosome 2) (Satoh et al. 1999). Recently, mutations in genes encoding z-disc proteins have been shown to cause HCM in a very small proportion of patients. The genes implicated to date are myozenin (*MYOZ2*) and telethonin (*TCAP*) (Bos et al. 2006; Osio et al. 2007).

There is considerable genetic heterogeneity, with over 400 different mutations identified to date, as well as marked variation in disease penetrance and clinical expression (Arad et al. 2002). The mechanisms through which mutations in the sarcomere protein genes result in the characteristic pathophysiological features of HCM are not completely understood. It has been speculated that the disease phenotype results from reduced contractile function, but studies of myocyte function in patients who harbor mutations in the sarcomere protein genes are inconsistent (Redwood et al. 1999). Some biophysical studies of HCM mutant proteins have shown an increase in calcium sensitivity, leading to increases in tension generation and ATPase activity (Michele et al. 1999; Bing et al. 2000; Harada et al. 2000; Redwood et al. 2000; Elliott et al. 2000a; Szczesna et al. 2000, 2001; Deng et al. 2001; Lang et al. 2002; Morimoto et al. 2002; Westfall et al. 2002; Heller et al. 2003; Kohler et al. 2003; Roopnarine 2003; Harada and Potter 2004; Kobayashi et al. 2004; Palmer et al. 2004). Animal studies have confirmed calcium as a key agent in the pathophysiologic processes that lead to the development of LV hypertrophy. Murine models of sarcomeric HCM have increased calcium sensitivity and altered calcium cycling between the sarcomere and the sarcoplasmic reticulum. In vitro studies using purified myosin filaments and skinned papillary muscle from mice with the Arg403Gly mutation in the *MYH6* gene demonstrated increased calcium sensitivity of force development, which would result in impaired ventricular relaxation in vivo (Blanchard et al. 1999; Palmiter et al. 2000). Similarly, several studies in murine models of *TNNT2* and *TPM1* disease have demonstrated an increase in calcium sensitivity of force development (Oberst et al. 1998; Tardiff et al. 1998, 1999; Miller et al. 2001; Prabhakar et al. 2001; Michele et al. 2002; Prabhakar et al. 2003). *TNNT2* mouse models show varying degrees of myocyte disarray and fibrosis with little LV hypertrophy, in common with *TNNT2* disease in humans (Oberst et al. 1998; Tardiff et al. 1998, 1999). Troponin-mutated mice exhibit severely impaired myocardial relaxation, independent of the degree of fibrosis, and consistent with the finding of increased calcium sensitivity at myofilament level (Oberst et al. 1998; Tardiff et al. 1998, 1999). Some HCM mutations may result in inefficient use of ATP at the myofilament level, suggesting that cardiac myocytes in HCM have greater energy requirements than normal cells (Ahmad et al. 2005). This is supported by findings from murine models of HCM, where mutations in *MYH6*, *MYBPC3*, *TNNT2*, and *TNNI3* result in increased contractility but at the expense of increased work (Blanchard et al. 1999; Tyska et al. 2000; Chandra et al. 2001; Miller et al. 2001). Furthermore, mice harboring the Arg403Gly mutation in *MYH6* have reduced basal energy stores and abnormal ATP/ADP ratios (Spindler et al. 1998; Redwood et al. 1999; Tyska et al. 2000; Palmer et al. 2004).

Abnormal calcium kinetics may also contribute to the high incidence of sudden death in patients with mutations in the *TNNT2* gene. In support of this, ventricular myocytes from mice harboring the I79N mutation in *TNNT2* have abnormal calcium transients and slowed decay kinetics, significantly increased diastolic calcium concentrations with isoprotenerol treatment, and stress-induced nonsustained ventricular tachycardia (NSVT) (Knollmann et al. 2003).

The downstream events resulting from altered calcium signaling and increased myocyte energy requirements are incompletely understood. In particular, it is unknown whether transcription factors known to play a role in the development of load-induced cardiac hypertrophy are also important in HCM.

The majority of sarcomeric protein gene mutations have a dominant negative effect on sarcomere function, that is, the mutant protein is incorporated into the sarcomere, but its interaction with the normal wild-type protein disrupts normal sarcomeric assembly and function. Allelic heterogeneity may be explained by the effect of different mutations on the structure and function of the complete peptide. β-myosin heavy chain, for example, consists of a globular head, an α-helical rod, and a hinge region. The globular head contains binding sites for ATPase and actin as well as interaction sites for regulatory and essential light chains in the head-rod region. Most mutations in the β-myosin gene are missense DNA nucleotide substitutions that change a single amino acid in the polypeptide sequence. The majority of disease causing β-myosin heavy chain mutations is found in one of four locations: the actin binding site, the nucleotide binding pocket, a region in the hinge region adjacent to the binding site for two reactive thiols, and the α-helix close to the essential light chain interaction site. Therefore, depending on the position of the mutation, changes might be expected in ATPase activity, actin–myosin interaction, and protein conformation during contraction.

There is substantial variation in the expression of identical mutations indicating that other genetic and possibly environmental factors influence disease expression. The effect of age is perhaps the best characterized factor, most patients developing ECG and echocardiographic manifestations of the disease after puberty and before the age of 30 Years Gender also appears to influence disease expression in sarcomere protein disease. Studies on the Arg403Gly *MYH6* mouse model show the development of LV dilatation and systolic impairment in male but not female mice (Olsson et al. 2001), and there is evidence to suggest that, in humans, males are at greater risk of developing end-stage disease than females (Harris et al. 2006). Other potential modifying factors include renin-angiotensin-aldosterone system gene polymorphism and the occurrence of homozygosity and compound heterozygotes (Marian et al. 1993; Lechin et al. 1995).

The importance of sarcomeric protein gene mutations in childhood HCM is unknown. The observation that the development of LV hypertrophy in individuals with familial disease often occurs during the period of somatic growth in adolescence (Maron et al. 1986a) has led to the suggestion that sarcomeric protein disease in very young children is rare (Maron 2004). However, recent studies of children with HCM have shown that, like in adults, sarcomeric protein gene mutations account for approximately 50% of cases of idiopathic HCM, even in infants and young children (Morita et al. 2008; Kaski et al. 2009).

2. Metabolic Cardiomyopathies

A number of inheritable inborn errors of metabolism are associated with LV hypertrophy (Table 13–1) (see also Chapter 26).

Anderson-Fabry disease is a lysosomal storage disorder caused by mutations in the α-galactosidase A gene. It is inherited as an X-linked dominant trait and the resultant enzyme deficiency causes progressive accumulation of glycosphingolipid in the skin, nervous system, kidneys, and heart (Linhart and Elliott 2007). Cardiac manifestations include progressive LV hypertrophy, valve disease, conduction abnormalities, and supraventricular and ventricular arrhythmias. Disease expression in the heart begins after adolescence in males and females (Linhart et al. 2000; Mehta et al. 2004; Shah et al. 2005; Linhart and Elliott 2007). Treatment with recombinant α-galactosidase A improves renal and neurological manifestations as well as quality of life, but its effect on the cardiac manifestations is still not determined (Linhart and Elliott 2007).

Danon disease is an X-linked lysosomal storage disorder, characterized clinically by cardiomyopathy, skeletal myopathy, and developmental delay. It is caused by mutations in the gene encoding the lysosome-associated membrane protein-2 (LAMP-2) (Nishino et al. 2000) that result in intracytoplasmic accumulation of autophagic material and glycogen within vacuoles in cardiac and skeletal myocytes (Danon et al. 1981). Males develop symptoms during childhood and adolescence, whereas female carriers usually develop HCM and DCM during adulthood (Sugie et al. 2002). The prognosis is generally poor, with most patients dying from cardiac failure, although sudden death is also reported, even in female carriers (Sugie et al. 2002). Other features of Danon disease include Wolff-Parkinson-White syndrome, elevated serum creatine kinase, and retinitis pigmentosa (Prall et al. 2006).

Pompe disease (glycogen storage disease type IIa*)* is an autosomal recessive disorder caused by a deficiency in the enzyme acid maltase. Infantile, juvenile, and adult variants are recognized, differing in their age of onset, rate of disease progression, and organ involvement. The infantile and childhood forms are characterized by myocardial glycogen deposition, massive cardiac hypertrophy, and heart failure. The infantile form presents in the first few months of life with severe skeletal muscle hypotonia, progressive weakness, cardiomegaly, hepatomegaly, and macroglossia and is

Table 13–1 Classification and Etiology of Hypertrophic Cardiomyopathy

Familial	Nonfamilial
Familial, unknown gene	Obesity
Sarcomeric protein disease	Infants of diabetic mothers
β-myosin heavy chain	Athletic training
Cardiac myosin-binding protein C	Amyloid (AL/prealbumin)
Cardiac troponin I	
Troponin-T	
Alpha Tropomyosin	
Essential myosin light chain	
Regulatory myosin light chain	
Cardiac actin	
alpha myosin heavy chain	
Titin	
Troponin C	
Muscle LIM protein	
Glycogen storage disease [e.g., GSD II (Pompe's disease); GSD III (Forbes' disease), AMP kinase (WPW, HCM, conduction disease)]	
Danon disease	
Lysosomal storage diseases (e.g., Anderson-Fabry disease, Hurler's syndrome)	
Disorders of fatty acid metabolism	
Carnitine deficiency	
Phosphorylase B kinase deficiency	
Mitochondrial cytopathies (e.g., MELAS, MERFF, LHON)	
Syndromic HCM	
Noonan's syndrome	
LEOPARD syndrome	
Friedreich's ataxia	
Beckwith-Wiedermann syndrome	
Swyer's syndrome (pure gonadal dysgenesis)	
Costello syndrome	
Other:	
Phospholamban promoter	
Familial amyloid	

Data from Elliott et al. Classification of the cardiomyopathies: a position statement from the European Society of Cardiology working group on myocardial and pericardial diseases. *Eur Heart J*. 2008;29:270–276.

usually fatal before 2 years of age due to cardiorespiratory failure. The ECG typically shows broad high-voltage QRS complexes and ventricular preexcitation. In the juvenile and adult onset variants, disease is usually limited to skeletal muscle, with a slowly progressive proximal myopathy and respiratory muscle weakness. Recombinant enzyme replacement in the infantile and childhood forms appears to cause regression of LV hypertrophy and is associated with improved survival (Klinge et al. 2005).

Mutations in the gene encoding the *γ_2 subunit of the adenosine monophosphate-activated protein kinase* (*PRKAG2*) (Blair et al. 2001) are responsible for a syndrome of HCM, conduction abnormalities, and Wolff-Parkinson-White syndrome. Histologically, there is accumulation of glycogen within cardiac myocytes and conduction tissue. A skeletal myopathy is present in many individuals and skeletal muscle biopsy shows excess mitochondria and ragged red fibers (Murphy et al. 2005). Patients develop progressive conduction disease and LV hypertrophy and atrial arrhythmias are common. Electrocardiographic expression is universal by the age of 18 years (Murphy et al. 2005). Disease-related mortality is related to thromboembolic stroke (resulting from atrial fibrillation) and sudden death (Murphy et al. 2005). Recent studies suggest that *PRKAG2* mutations account for no more than 1% of cases of HCM (Murphy et al. 2005).

3. Mitochondrial Cardiomyopathies

Primary mitochondrial disorders are caused by sporadic or inherited mutations in nuclear or mitochondrial DNA that may be transmitted as autosomal dominant, autosomal recessive, X-linked or maternal traits (see also Chapter 31). The most frequent abnormalities occur in genes that encode the respiratory chain protein complexes, leading to impaired oxygen utilization and reduced energy production. The clinical presentation of mitochondrial disease is variable in age at onset, symptoms, and the range and severity of organ involvement. Data on the prevalence of cardiac disease in primary mitochondrial disorders are mostly derived from pediatric populations. Cardiac involvement is a feature in up to 40% of mitochondrial encephalomyopathies (Scaglia et al. 2004), and usually takes the form of a HCM (Holmgren et al. 2003), although other cardiomyopathies, including dilated and LV noncompaction, are reported (Scaglia et al. 2004). Children with mitochondrial disease and cardiac involvement present earlier than those with noncardiac disease (Holmgren et al. 2003; Scaglia et al. 2004) and have a much worse prognosis (Scaglia et al. 2004). The cardiac phenotype is usually concentric LV hypertrophy without outflow tract obstruction, and rapid progression to LV dilatation, systolic impairment, and heart failure are described (Holmgren et al. 2003; Scaglia et al. 2004). Sudden arrhythmic death has also been reported (Holmgren et al. 2003; Scaglia et al. 2004).

I. Friedreich's Ataxia Friedreich's ataxia is an autosomal recessive condition caused by mutations in the frataxin gene. Cardiac involvement is very common, and is usually (but not exclusively) characterized by concentric LV hypertrophy without LV outflow tract obstruction (Child et al. 1986). Patients are usually asymptomatic from a cardiac viewpoint, but progression to LV dilatation and heart failure is described (Casazza et al. 1990). Treatment with the antioxidant idebenone appears to reduce the degree of LV hypertrophy (Hausse et al. 2002) but further studies are needed to assess the long-term effects.

4. Malformation Syndromes Associated with LV Hypertrophy

A number of malformation syndromes, most of which present in childhood, are associated with HCM (Table 13–1) (see also Chapter 10). Noonan syndrome is characterized by short stature, dysmorphic facies, skeletal malformations, and a webbed neck (Noonan and Ehmke 1963; Noonan 1968; Tartaglia and Gelb 2005). Cardiac involvement is present in up to 90% of patients with Noonan syndrome and most commonly takes the form of pulmonary valve stenosis and HCM (Sharland et al. 1992). Some cases present with congestive cardiac failure in infancy and may be associated with biventricular hypertrophy and bilateral ventricular outflow tract obstruction (Sharland et al. 1992). The cardiac histological findings in Noonan syndrome are indistinguishable from idiopathic HCM (Burch et al. 1992). Noonan syndrome is inherited as an autosomal dominant trait with variable penetrance and expression. Mutations in the *PTPN11* gene, encoding the protein tyrosine phosphatase SHP-2 [a protein with a critical role in RAS-ERK-mediated intracellular signal transduction pathways controlling diverse developmental processes (Chen et al. 2000)], have been shown to cause Noonan syndrome (Tartaglia et al. 2001). To date, at least 39 different mutations have been identified, accounting for approximately 50% of cases of Noonan syndrome (Tartaglia and Gelb 2005). It is noteworthy that only 5%–9% of all individuals with mutations in the *PTPN11* gene have HCM (Tartaglia et al. 2002; Zenker et al. 2004). LEOPARD syndrome (Lentigines, ECG abnormalities, Ocular hypertelorism, Pulmonary stenosis, Abnormalities of the genitalia, Retardation of growth, and Deafness) shares many phenotypic features with Noonan syndrome, and recent studies have shown that most patients with LEOPARD syndrome also have mutations in the *PTPN11* gene (Digilio et al. 2002). Other genes implicated in Noonan syndrome include *SOS1* (Tartaglia et al. 2007) (encoding a RAS-specific guanine nucleotide exchange factor), which accounts for up to 28% of cases (Roberts et al. 2007; Zenker et al. 2007); *KRAS* (which encodes a GTP-binding protein in the RAS-ERK pathway) in less than 5% of cases (Schubbert et al. 2006); and *RAF1* (a downstream effector of RAS) (Pandit et al. 2007; Razzaque et al. 2007).

Pathology

The most common pattern of myocardial hypertrophy in sarcomeric HCM is asymmetric septal hypertrophy (Davies and McKenna 1995; Hughes 2004). However, other patterns also occur, including concentric, midventricular [sometimes associated with a LV apical diverticulum (Maron et al. 1996)] and apical (Maron et al. 1982a; Wigle et al. 1985; Webb et al. 1990). Coexistent right ventricular hypertrophy is common but rarely, if ever, occurs in isolation (Davies and McKenna 1995). The papillary muscles are often displaced anteriorly and may have abnormal insertion into the mitral valve. There is often an area of endocardial fibrosis on the septum beneath the aortic valve caused by repeated contact with the anterior leaflet during systolic anterior motion of the anterior mitral valve leaflet (Davies and McKenna 1995; Hughes 2004). The mitral valve itself is often structurally abnormal with elongation of one or more mitral valve cusps (Klues et al. 1992). Myocardial bridging of the left anterior descending coronary artery has been observed in adults and children with HCM (Kitazume et al. 1983; Yetman et al. 1998).

Histologically, familial HCM is characterized by a triad of myocyte hypertrophy, myocyte disarray (architectural disorganization of the myocardium, with adjacent myocytes aligned obliquely or perpendicular to each other in association with increased interstitial collagen), and interstitial fibrosis (Davies and McKenna 1995; Hughes 2004) (Figure 13–1). Although myocyte disarray occurs in many pathologies, the presence of extensive disarray (more than 10% of the ventricular myocardium) is generally thought to be a highly specific marker for HCM (Davies and McKenna 1995; Hughes 2004). Small intramural coronary arteries are often dysplastic and narrowed due to wall thickening by smooth muscle cell hyperplasia (Maron et al. 1986b).

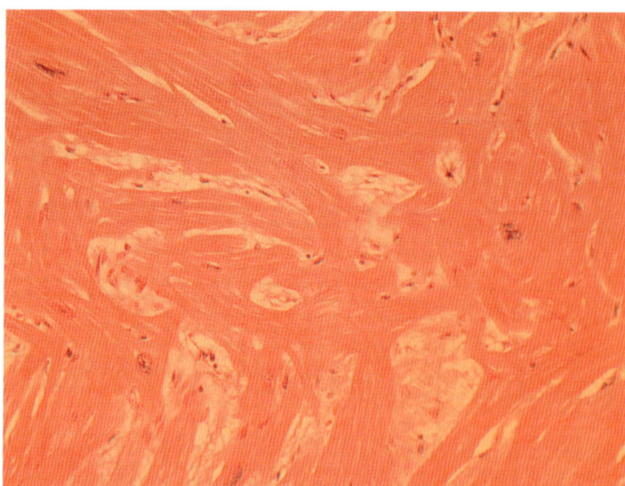

Figure 13–1 High power hematoxylin and eosin sections of ventricular myocardium showing the typical swirling and splayed pattern of myocytes in myocyte disarray. The enlarged and hyperchromatic nuclei indicate myocyte hypertrophy. There is an increase in interstitital fibrous tissue. *Courtesy*: Dr Michael Ashworth, Great Ormond Street Hospital, London, U.K.

Clinical Presentation

1. Symptoms

Most individuals with HCM have few if any symptoms. The initial diagnosis is often made during family screening or following the incidental detection of a heart murmur or an abnormal ECG. The most common symptoms are dyspnea and chest pain, which is commonly exertional, but may also occur at rest or following large meals. Typically, there is day-to-day variation in the amount of activity required to produce symptoms (McKenna et al. 1981a; McKenna and Deanfield 1984). Syncope is a relatively common symptom for which there are multiple mechanisms including LV outflow tract obstruction, abnormal vascular responses, and atrial and ventricular arrhythmias (Counihan et al. 1991; Elliott and McKenna 2004; Tome Esteban and Kaski 2007). Unexplained or exertional syncope is associated with increased risk of sudden death in children and adolescents. Infants can present with symptoms of heart failure, such as breathlessness, poor feeding, excessive sweating, and failure to thrive (Maron et al. 1976, 1982c; Schaffer et al. 1983; Skinner et al. 1997; Bruno et al. 2002). These symptoms usually occur in the presence of apparently normal LV systolic function and are often caused by outflow tract obstruction or diastolic dysfunction.

2. Clinical Examination

General examination may provide important diagnostic clues in patients with syndromic or metabolic HCM. Paradoxically, cardiovascular examination is often normal, but in patients with LV outflow tract obstruction, a number of typical features may be identified. The arterial pulse has a rapid upstroke and downstroke, caused by rapid ejection during the initial phase of systole followed by a sudden decrease in cardiac output during midsystole. Occasionally, this is followed by a palpable reflected wave, resulting in a bisferiens pulse. The jugular venous pulsation may have a prominent "a" wave, caused by reduced right ventricular compliance. Palpation of the precordium may reveal a sustained, or double, apical pulsation, reflecting an atrial impulse followed by LV contraction; rarely, an additional late systolic impulse, resulting in a triple apex beat, may be felt. Auscultatory findings in patients with obstructive HCM include an ejection systolic murmur at the left sternal edge radiating to the right upper sternal edge and apex, but usually not to the carotid arteries or axilla. This murmur may be associated with a palpable precordial thrill. As the obstruction in HCM is a dynamic phenomenon, the intensity of the murmur is increased by maneuvers that reduce the preload or afterload, such as standing from a squatting position and the Valsalva maneuver. Most patients with LV outflow tract obstruction also have mitral regurgitation (caused by abnormal coaptation of the mitral valve leaflets during systole). This may result in a pansystolic, high-frequency murmur at the apex, radiating to the axilla.

Natural History

HCM can present at any age, from infancy to old age (Maron et al. 2003c). Many patients follow a stable and benign course, with a low risk of adverse events, but a large number may experience progressive symptoms, caused by gradual deterioration in LV systolic and diastolic function and atrial arrhythmias. A proportion of individuals die suddenly, whereas others may die from progressive heart failure, thromboembolism, and rarely, infective endocarditis.

Recent studies in adults with HCM report annual sudden death rates of 1% or less in adults (Maron et al. 1999a, 2003c) and 1%–1.5% per year in children and adolescents. In the United States, HCM accounts for 36% of cases of sudden death in competitive athletes younger than 35 years of age (Maron et al. 2003a) but in European populations other causes, including coronary artery disease and ARVC, predominate (Corrado et al. 2001).

Progression to a "burnt out" phase is a well-recognized complication of HCM (Ten Cate and Roelandt 1979; Beder et al. 1982; Fujiwara et al. 1984; Yutani et al. 1985; Fighali et al. 1987; Spirito et al. 1987; Hecht et al. 1993; Bingisser et al. 1994; Seiler et al. 1995; Maron and Spirito 1998; Thaman et al. 2004, 2005; Biagini et al. 2005; Harris et al. 2006), with a reported prevalence ranging from 2% to 15% in adults (Spirito et al. 1987; Thaman et al. 2005; Harris et al. 2006). This end stage is characterized by progressive LV dilatation, wall thinning, and systolic impairment (Cohn et al. 2000) and is associated with a poor prognosis (Thaman et al. 2005), with an overall mortality rate of up to 11% per year (Harris et al. 2006). Presentation in infancy can also be associated with severe and intractable heart failure (Maron et al. 1974, 1982c; Schaffer et al. 1983; Skinner et al. 1997).

Atrial fibrillation (AF) is the commonest sustained arrhythmia in HCM, occurring in up to 25% of patients (Robinson et al. 1990; Spirito et al. 1992; Olivotto et al. 2001). Its development is related to left atrial dilatation, and its incidence increases with age. Although well tolerated in many cases, AF can result in acute and severe hemodynamic deterioration and is associated with a high risk of thromboembolism. Furthermore, the presence of AF is independently associated with heart-failure-related death and long-term disease progression, but not sudden death (Robinson et al. 1990; Spirito et al. 1992; Olivotto et al. 2001).

Investigations

1. Electrocardiography

The resting 12-lead ECG is abnormal in 95% of individuals with HCM. Common features include repolarization abnormalities, pathological Q waves (most frequently in the inferolateral leads), and left atrial enlargement. Voltage criteria for LV hypertrophy alone are not specific for HCM, and are often seen in normal, healthy teenagers and young adults. In infants, right ventricular hypertrophy is commonly found. Giant negative T waves in the mid-precordial leads are characteristic of apical HCM (Yamaguchi et al. 1979). Some patients have a short PR interval (not associated with Wolff-Parkinson-White syndrome). Atrioventricular conduction delay (including first-degree block) is rare except in particular subtypes of HCM (e.g., in association with PRKAG2 mutations and mitochondrial disease) (Krikler et al. 1980; Fananapazir et al. 1989).

2. Echocardiography

The presence on echocardiography of LV wall thickness greater than two standard deviations above the body surface area-corrected mean in any myocardial segment (or greater than 13 mm in adults) is sufficient for the diagnosis of HCM (Maron et al. 2003c) (see also Chapter 8). Although the focus of early M-mode echocardiographic studies was on the detection of asymmetrical septal hypertrophy, two-dimensional echocardiography has shown that any pattern of LV hypertrophy is consistent with the diagnosis of HCM, including concentric (equal hypertrophy across all segments of the left ventricle), eccentric (with the lateral and posterior walls more affected than the septum), distal (distal segments more affected than basal segments), and apical (hypertrophy confined to the LV apex) (Maron et al. 1981a; Shapiro and McKenna 1983; Wigle et al. 1985; Klues et al. 1995) patterns.

Approximately 25% of patients have obstruction to the LV outflow tract at rest, and as many as 70% may have latent, or provokable, LV outflow tract obstruction caused by contact between the anterior mitral valve leaflet and the ventricular septum during systole (Maron et al. 2006; Shah et al. 2007). Dynamic obstruction in the LV outflow tract is associated with midsystolic closure of the aortic valve, often associated with coarse fluttering of the aortic valve on M-mode echocardiography. LV outflow tract obstruction is detected using color flow Doppler and quantified using continuous wave Doppler. Most patients with systolic anterior motion of the mitral valve and LV outflow tract obstruction have a posteriorly directed jet of mitral regurgitation, which can be detected using color Doppler imaging. The presence of complex mitral regurgitant jets (e.g., anteriorly directed or central) should prompt a search for other mitral valve abnormalities. In some patients, systolic obliteration of the ventricular cavity may produce a high velocity gradient in the midventricle. RV outflow tract obstruction may be seen in infants with HCM, and in older children and adults with cardiomyopathy associated with Noonan syndrome and some metabolic disorders.

LV global systolic function, as assessed from change in ventricular volume during the cardiac cycle, is typically increased. However, regional and long-axis function is often reduced, and cardiac output responses during exercise may be impaired (Perrone-Filardi et al. 1993; Okeie et al. 2000; Tabata et al. 2000). A proportion of adults with HCM develop progressive myocardial thinning, global LV systolic impairment, and cavity dilatation.

Diastolic function is often impaired in patients with HCM. Characteristically, patients with HCM and diastolic LV impairment demonstrate reduced early diastolic (Ea) velocities in the mitral annulus and septum, and reversal of the ratio of early to late diastolic velocities (Ea/Aa). In addition, the ratio of mitral inflow E wave to annular early diastolic velocity (E/Ea) can be used as a measure of LV end-diastolic pressure, and predicts exercise capacity in adults (Matsumura et al. 2002) and children (McMahon et al. 2004) with HCM. Tissue Doppler imaging may be useful in detecting mild disease in otherwise phenotypically normal gene carriers (Nagueh et al. 2001; Poutanen et al. 2006).

3. Ambulatory Electrocardiography

The frequency of supraventricular and ventricular arrhythmias in HCM increases with age (Maron et al. 1981b; McKenna et al. 1981b, 1988; Robinson et al. 1990). Ambulatory ECG monitoring reveals supraventricular arrhythmias in 30%–50% and NSVT in

25% of individuals. Most episodes of NSVT are relatively slow, asymptomatic, and occur during periods of increased vagal tone. Sustained ventricular tachycardia is uncommon, but may occur in association with apical aneurysms (Alfonso et al. 1989).

4. Cardiopulmonary Exercise Testing

Individuals with HCM usually have a reduced peak oxygen consumption compared with healthy age-matched controls, even when asymptomatic (Jones et al. 1998; Sharma et al. 2000). In addition, one quarter of adults with HCM have an abnormal blood pressure response to exercise, with the blood pressure falling or failing to rise by more than 25 mmHg from baseline (Sadoul et al. 1997; Olivotto et al. 1999). This results from abnormal vasodilatation of the nonexercising vascular beds, possibly triggered by inappropriate firing of LV baroreceptors (Counihan et al. 1991) and impaired cardiac output responses (Ciampi et al. 2002). An abnormal blood pressure response to exercise is associated with an increased risk of sudden death in young adults (Sadoul et al. 1997; Elliott et al. 2000b).

5. Cardiac Magnetic Resonance Imaging

Cardiac magnetic resonance imaging (MRI) is used to evaluate the distribution and severity of LV hypertrophy and can provide functional measurements of systolic and diastolic function (see Chapter 7). In addition, MRI can be used to assess myocardial tissue characteristics in vivo with gadolinium contrast agents. Many patients with HCM have areas of patchy gadolinium hyperenhancement, and studies suggest that the extent of gadolinium enhancement correlates with risk factors for sudden death and with progressive LV remodeling (Choudhury et al. 2002; Moon et al. 2003).

Management

The management of individuals with HCM focuses on three main areas: the counseling of patients and relatives; symptom management; and the prevention of disease-related complications.

1. Family Evaluation

All patients with HCM should be counseled on the implications of the diagnosis for their families. Careful pedigree analysis can reassure relatives who are not at risk of inheriting the disease (Maron et al. 2003c). For those who may be at risk, clinical screening with ECG and echocardiography may be appropriate after counseling. Current guidelines recommend screening at intervals of 12–18 months, usually starting at the age of 12 years (unless there is a "malignant" family history of premature sudden death, the child is symptomatic or a competitive athlete in intensive training, or there is a clinical suspicion of LV hypertrophy) until full growth and maturation is achieved (usually by the age of 18–21 years). Following this, if there are no signs of phenotypic expression, screening approximately every 5 years is advised, as the onset of LV hypertrophy may be delayed until well into adulthood in some families (McKenna et al. 1997; Charron et al. 1998; Niimura et al. 1998; Maron et al. 2001; Ackerman et al. 2002; Van Driest et al. 2002; Richard et al. 2003).

It is now possible to offer relatively rapid genetic testing to individuals with unequivocal disease. If a disease-causing mutation is identified, relatives can be offered predictive testing. However, it is paramount that this is performed only after appropriate genetic counseling and consideration of issues relating to patient autonomy, confidentiality, and psychosocial harm (including loss of self-esteem, stigmatization or discrimination, and guilt).

2. Treatment of Symptoms Caused by LV Outflow Tract Obstruction

The firstline strategy for symptom control of patients with obstructive HCM is medical therapy with β-adrenergic receptor blockers. At standard doses, β-blockers can reduce symptoms of chest pain, dyspnea, and presyncope on exertion, but it is unlikely that they reduce outflow obstruction at rest. Studies using very large doses of propranolol (up to 23 mg/kg per day) in children and adolescents have reported improved long-term survival (Ostman-Smith et al. 1999), but side effects are common, and even moderate doses can affect growth and school performance in young children or trigger depression in children and adolescents (Maron et al. 2003c). In adults, the addition of the class I antiarrhythmic disopyramide to a β-blocker can reduce obstruction and improve symptoms (Pollick 1988; Pollick et al. 1988; Sherrid et al. 1988), an effect exerted through its negative inotropic action. Disopyramide is usually well tolerated, but initiation at a low dose is recommended, as some patients (particularly the elderly) may experience marked anticholinergic side effects. As disopyramide causes accelerated atrioventricular node conduction and may increase the ventricular rate during atrial fibrillation, it should ideally not be administered without drugs that slow atrioventricular conduction. In addition, disopyramide causes prolongation of the QT interval and so the ECG must be monitored regularly and other drugs that prolong QT interval avoided.

The calcium antagonist verapamil improves symptoms caused by outflow tract obstruction, probably by relieving myocardial ischemia and reducing myocardial contractility (Bonow et al. 1985; Udelson et al. 1989). However, in patients with severe symptoms caused by large (>100 mmHg) gradients and pulmonary hypertension verapamil can cause rapid hemodynamic deterioration (Epstein and Rosing 1981; Wigle et al. 1995) and therefore must be used with caution in this group.

Several options are available to patients with obstructive HCM who do not tolerate drugs or whose symptoms are refractory to medical therapy. The gold standard (Morrow et al. 1975; Williams et al. 1987; Schulte et al. 1993; Theodoro et al. 1996; Ommen et al. 2005) is septal myotomy-myectomy, in which a trough of muscle is removed from the interventricular septum through an aortic incision. In the hands of experienced surgeons, the mortality is less than 1% and the success rate is high, with complete and permanent abolition of the outflow gradient and a marked improvement in symptoms and exercise capacity in over 90% of patients. Complications include complete heart block requiring permanent pacemaker insertion in less than 5% of patients and small ventricular septal defects.

Atrioventricular pacing has been shown to reduce LV outflow gradients in uncontrolled observational studies (Fananapazir et al. 1994; Posma et al. 1996; Rishi et al. 1997) and two randomized controlled clinical trials (Nishimura et al. 1997; Maron et al. 1999b). However, the randomized trials showed no objective improvement in exercise capacity and a symptomatic effect no better than placebo (Nishimura et al. 1997; Maron et al. 1999b) except possibly in a subgroup of elderly patients with relatively mild hypertrophy.

An alternative to surgery for adult patients with obstructive disease is alcohol ablation of the interventricular septum. Ninety-five percent alcohol is injected into a septal perforator coronary artery branch to produce an area of localized myocardial necrosis within the basal septum (Knight et al. 1997; Lakkis et al. 2000). Myocardial damage is kept to a minimum by first visualizing the area supplied by the perforator branch using echocardiographic contrast injection (Faber et al. 1998). Although short-term results are promising, the long-term effects are unknown, and there is potential for the resulting myocardial scar to act as a substrate for ventricular arrhythmia and sudden death.

3. Management of Symptoms in Nonobstructive Disease

In patients without LV outflow tract obstruction, chest pain and dyspnea are usually caused by LV diastolic impairment and myocardial ischemia. Treatment in this group of patients is empiric and often suboptimal. Both β-blockers and calcium antagonists can ameliorate symptoms by improving LV relaxation and filling, reducing LV contractility, and relieving myocardial ischemia. Other drugs such as nitrates and angiotensin-converting enzyme (ACE) inhibitors may be beneficial in some patients, but should be avoided in patients with provokable outflow tract obstruction. Individuals who develop end-stage disease should receive conventional heart failure treatment, including ACE inhibitors, angiotensin II receptor antagonists, spironolactone, β-blockers such as carvedilol or bisoprolol, digoxin, and if necessary, cardiac transplantation. A recent study has shown that biventricular pacing improves heart failure symptoms and results in reverse atrial and ventricular remodeling in up to 40% of patients with end-stage HCM (Rogers et al. 2008).

4. Pregnancy

Serious complications during pregnancy in women with HCM are rare, occurring in less than 2% of pregnancies. Increased risk of maternal mortality appears to be confined to women with high-risk profiles (Autore et al. 2002; Thaman et al. 2003). The vasodilation associated with standard epidural analgesia may worsen LV outflow tract obstruction, and care must be taken when administering cardioactive drugs. In general, most pregnant women with HCM undergo normal vaginal delivery without the need for cesarean section, although women considered to be at high risk should be offered specialized obstetric antenatal and perinatal care.

5. Prevention of Sudden Cardiac Death

Although, the overall risk of sudden death in patients with HCM is only approximately 1% per year, a minority of individuals have a much greater risk of ventricular arrhythmia and sudden death (Maron et al. 2003b). The mechanism of sudden death is thought to be ventricular arrhythmia in the majority of patients, sometimes triggered by atrial arrhythmia, myocardial ischemia, and exercise (Maron et al. 1982b). The most reliable predictor of sudden cardiac death in HCM is a history of previous cardiac arrest (Cecchi et al. 1989; Elliott et al. 1999). In patients without such a history, the most clinically useful markers of risk are a family history of sudden cardiac death (Maron et al. 1978; McKenna et al. 1981a); unexplained syncope (unrelated to neurocardiogenic mechanisms); an abnormal blood pressure response to upright exercise (Frenneaux et al. 1990; Sadoul et al. 1997; Elliott et al. 2000b); NSVT on ambulatory electrocardiographic monitoring or during exercise (Maron et al. 1981b; Elliott et al. 2000b; Monserrat et al. 2003); and severe LV hypertrophy on echocardiography (defined as a maximal LV wall thickness of 30 mm or more) (Spirito et al. 2000; Elliott et al. 2001). Patients with none of these features have a low risk of sudden death (less than 1% per year), whereas those with two or more risk factors are at substantially higher risk of dying suddenly (estimated annual mortality rates of 3% for those with two risk factors rising to 6% in those with three or more risk factors) (Elliott et al. 2000b). Patients with a single risk factor represent a more difficult group as the annual death rate in this group is low (1.2%), but the confidence intervals are wide (0.2%–2.2%), suggesting that some individuals with a single risk factor may be twice more likely to die suddenly than patients without risk factors. Therefore, the risk evaluation of these patients has to take into account the significance of the individual risk factor (e.g., a particularly malignant family history may be sufficient to consider primary preventative measures in the absence of a second risk factor) as well as patient-specific variables such as age (Elliott et al. 2000b; McKenna and Behr 2002). Several studies have shown that LV outflow tract obstruction is associated with increased cardiovascular mortality, including sudden death (Maron et al. 2003d; Elliott et al. 2006). The absolute risk of sudden death associated with outflow tract obstruction in isolation is low, but it may represent an incremental risk factor in combination with other conventional markers (Elliott et al. 2006).

In patients considered to be at high risk of sudden death, insertion of an implantable cardioverter-defibrillator (ICD) should be regarded as the treatment of choice (Maron et al. 2003c). Retrospective registry data demonstrate that ICDs prevent sudden death in patients with HCM, with annual appropriate discharge rates of 11% in the secondary prevention patients (those with a history of cardiac arrest or sustained ventricular arrhythmia) and 3%–5% in the primary prevention group (Maron et al. 2000, 2007). In children with HCM, appropriate discharge rates are higher in the secondary prevention group (Silka et al. 1993; Kaski et al. 2007b).

Prior to the advent of implantable cardioverter-defibrillators, amiodarone was used to prevent sudden death in high-risk HCM patients (McKenna et al. 1985). However, amiodarone does not prevent sudden cardiac death in this high-risk group (Kaski et al. 2007b). Amiodarone does, however, remain a useful drug for the treatment of atrial fibrillation in patients with HCM.

6. Prevention of Infective Endocarditis

Patients with obstructive HCM have an increased risk of developing infective endocarditis, usually on the anterior mitral valve leaflet (Spirito et al. 1999). Therefore, patients with HCM and LV outflow tract obstruction should receive antibiotic prophylaxis at times of potential bacteremia, according to current AHA guidelines (Wilson et al. 2008).

Summary

HCM is the commonest inherited cardiovascular disorder, occurring in approximately 1 in 500 individuals (Box 13–1). Most cases are caused by mutations in genes encoding proteins of the cardiac sarcomere. The pathophysiologic mechanisms underlying the development of the clinical phenotype in patients with sarcomeric

Box 13–1 Key Points

- HCM is a heterogeneous condition that can affect patients at any age.
- Most cases are caused by autosomal dominant mutations in cardiac sarcomere protein genes.
- Other causes include inherited errors of metabolism, mitochondrial disease, malformation syndromes, and neuromuscular disorders.
- The management of HCM includes evaluation of family members, symptom management, and identification and prevention of disease-related complications, including sudden death, heart failure, and thromboembolism.

protein disease are incompletely understood, but are thought to be related to abnormal calcium sensitivity of force development and altered bioenergetics. Other causes of HCM include metabolic, syndromic, and neuromuscular diseases. Common symptoms include chest pain, palpitation, dyspnea, and syncope. Some patients with HCM are at increased risk of sudden cardiac death. The management of HCM requires a multidisciplinary approach, encompassing genetic and psychological counseling, pharmacological and surgical therapies, family screening, and risk stratification and prevention of sudden cardiac death.

Dilated Cardiomyopathy

DCM is defined as a myocardial disorder characterized by the presence of LV dilatation and LV systolic impairment in the absence of abnormal loading conditions (e.g., hypertension, valve disease) or coronary artery disease sufficient to cause global systolic dysfunction (Elliott et al. 2008). Right ventricular dilatation and dysfunction may also be present. The prevalence of DCM is thought to be in the range of 1 in 2,500 adults, with an annual incidence of between 5 and 8 per 100,000 (Codd et al. 1989). In children, the incidence is much lower (0.5–0.8 per 100,000 per year), but DCM is the commonest cardiomyopathy in the pediatric population (Lipshultz et al. 2003; Nugent et al. 2003).

Etiology

DCM is caused by many disorders including neuromuscular disorders, inborn errors of metabolism, and malformation syndromes (Table13–2), but in the majority of patients, no identifiable cause is found (Elliott 2000). Nevertheless, up to 35% of individuals with DCM have familial disease, in which at least one other first-degree relative is affected (Grunig et al. 1998), and a further 20% of family members have isolated LV enlargement with preserved systolic function, 10% of whom subsequently develop overt DCM (Baig et al. 1998; Mahon et al. 2005).

1. Familial/Genetic DCM

Familial disease occurs in over a third of adult patients with DCM (Grunig et al. 1998). The reported prevalence of familial DCM in pediatric population studies is much lower (up to 17%) (Daubeney et al. 2006; Towbin et al. 2006), although this is likely to be an underestimate. A number of genetic mutations can cause DCM (Ahmad et al. 2005). In many cases, these are transmitted as an autosomal dominant trait, but other forms of inheritance, including autosomal recessive, X-linked, and mitochondrial are also recognized.

II. Autosomal Dominant DCM Autosomal dominant inheritance accounts for approximately 23% of all cases of DCM (Bowles et al. 2000). Two major forms of autosomal dominant DCM are recognized: isolated (or pure) DCM and DCM associated with cardiac conduction system disease. In many cases, there may also be a skeletal myopathy. Genes implicated in isolated DCM include cytoskletal [δ-sarcoglycan (Tsubata et al. 2000), β-sarcoglycan (Barresi et al. 2000), and desmin] and sarcomere protein genes [including α-cardiac actin (Olson et al. 1998), troponin T (Kamisago et al. 2000), β-myosin heavy chain (Kamisago et al. 2000), troponin C (Mogensen et al. 2004; Kaski et al. 2007a), and α-tropomyosin (Olson et al. 2001)].

The pathophysiological mechanism through which cytoskeletal mutations cause DCM is impaired transmission of the contractile force generated by the sarcomere. In many cases, sarcomeric protein gene mutations associated with DCM are located in functional domains involved in force propagation, suggesting a common pathophysiological mechanism with cytoskeletal mutations. However, troponin T mutations can cause DCM by altering calcium sensitivity and contractility. As in HCM, altered myocyte bioenergetic processes also play a role in the development of DCM associated with sarcomeric and cytoskeletal mutations.

Several genes associated with isolated DCM and conduction disease have been mapped (Towbin and Bowles 2002; Ahmad et al. 2005), but only one, lamin A/C, which encodes a nuclear envelope intermediate filament protein, has been identified. Mutations in lamin A/C result in atrial arrhythmia and progressive atrioventricular conduction disease that frequently precede the development of LV dilatation and systolic dysfunction by several years (Kass et al. 1994; Fatkin et al. 1999; Brodsky et al. 2000) (see also Chapter 27). Some mutations in lamin A/C result in DCM and conduction disease alone (Fatkin et al. 1999), whereas others lead to juvenile-onset muscular dystrophies (including Emery-Dreiffus muscular dystrophy) (Bonne et al. 1999; Muchir et al. 2000) or familial partial lipodystrophy with insulin-resistant diabetes (Shackleton et al. 2000). The pathophysiological mechanisms underlying disease in lamin A/C remain poorly understood, but several hypotheses have been proposed. These include nuclear fragility with disruption of the nuclear architecture; alterations in cellular signaling or gene expression, resulting in abnormal interaction between lamins and other nuclear proteins such as desmin; and interference with the processing of prelamin A, which results in abnormal lamin function and nuclear abnormalities (Capell and Collins 2006; Worman and Bonne 2007). Cardiac myocytes from mice deficient in lamin A/C have abnormalities of the nucleus and desmin cytoskeletal network and impaired mechanotransduction and activation of transcriptional programmes in response to mechanical stress (Sullivan et al. 1999; Broers et al. 2004; Lammerding et al. 2004).

III. X-linked Dilated Cardiomyopathy X-linked inheritance accounts for between 2% and 5% of familial cases of DCM (Muntoni et al. 1993; Towbin et al. 1993; Cohen and Muntoni 2004; Towbin et al. 2006). Most cases are caused by Duchenne, Becker, and Emery-Dreifuss muscular dystrophies. Isolated X-linked DCM, also caused by mutations in the dystrophin gene, was first described in 1987 in young males with severe disease and rapid progression of congestive cardiac failure to death or transplantation (Berko and Swift 1987). The condition is characterized by raised serum creatine kinase muscle isoforms, but does not result in the clinical features of muscular dystrophy seen in Duchenne or Becker muscular dystrophies. Female carriers of Duchenne and Becker muscular dystrophies, as well as female carriers of X-linked DCM, develop DCM later in life, usually in their 50s, that is, milder in severity than that in their male counterparts. Cardiac muscle biopsies in female carriers show a mosaic pattern of dystrophin expression (Politano et al. 1996).

Barth syndrome (DCM, skeletal myopathy, and neutropenia) is an X-linked disorder caused by mutations in the *G4.5* gene, which encodes the protein tafazzin (Barth et al. 1983; Kelley et al. 1991). The condition typically presents in male neonates or young infants with congestive heart failure, neutropenia, and 3-methylgutaconic aciduria. Although some children die in infancy (due to progressive heart failure, sudden death, or sepsis), most survive into childhood and beyond, but the DCM persists. Mutations in the *G4.5* gene also cause isolated DCM, endocardial fibroelastosis, and LV noncompaction, with or without the other features of Barth syndrome (Bleyl et al. 1997; D'Adamo et al. 1997).

Table 13–2 Classification and Etiology of Dilated Cardiomyopathy

Familial	Nonfamilial
Familial, unknown gene	Myocarditis (infective/toxic/immune)
Sarcomeric protein mutations (see HCM)	Kawasaki disease
Z band:	Eosinophilic (Churg Strauss syndrome)
ZASP	Viral persistence
Muscle LIM protein	Drugs
TCAP	Pregnancy
Cytoskeletal genes:	Endocrine
Dystrophin	Nutritional—thiamine, carnitine, selenium, hypophosphatemia, hypocalcemia.
Desmin	Alcohol
Metavinculin	Tachycardiomyopathy
Sarcoglycan complex	
CRYAB	
Epicardin	
Nuclear membrane	
Lamin A/C	
Emerin	
Intercalated disc protein mutations (see ARVC)	
Mitochondrial cytopathy	

Data from Elliott et al. Classification of the cardiomyopathies: a position statement from the European Society of Cardiology working group on myocardial and pericardial diseases. *Eur Heart J.* 2008;29:270–276.

2. Nonfamilial/Nongenetic DCM

While numerous causes of nonfamilial DCM are recognized (Table 13–2) in most patients, no obvious environmental or endogenous trigger for disease is found. In animal models, acute myocarditis caused by viral infection results in an initial phase of myocyte necrosis and macrophage activation, which in turn results in the release of numerous cytokines including interleukin-1, tumor necrosis factor, and interferon gamma. These stimulate the infiltration of mononuclear cells and production of neutralizing antibodies, resulting in viral clearance. Following this viral clearance phase, hearts may recover completely or may enter a chronic phase of fibrosis, LV dilatation, and heart failure. This chronic phase occurs as a consequence of secondary activation of neurohumoral systems.

Many studies have examined the prevalence of myocardial inflammation and viral particles in DCM. In early studies utilizing the Dallas criteria for myocarditis, the prevalence of positive biopsy results varied widely (between 9% and 70% of patients), reflecting patient selection and the highly subjective nature of the criteria (Feldman and McNamara 2000). More recent studies have used immunocytochemical techniques to detect myocardial inflammation in patients with DCM, showing that up to two-thirds of patients have an inflammatory cardiomyopathy with inflammatory endothelial activation (Noutsias et al. 1999; Maisch et al. 2005). This is associated with increased expression of HLA class II major histocompatibility antigens as well as cell adhesion molecules (Noutsias et al. 1999).

The underlying cause of the inflammation seen in DCM remains incompletely understood. There is circumstantial evidence that some of the inflammation relates to autoimmune processes: there is an association between DCM and HLA-DR4 antigen; many patients have elevated levels of circulating cytokines and cardiac-specific antibodies; there is evidence for familial aggregation of autoimmune diseases in some individuals with DCM; and relatives of patients with DCM also have increased levels of circulating cytokines and antiheart antibodies (Caforio et al. 1994, 2002).

A second hypothesis is that the inflammation is secondary to the persistence of viral particles in the myocardium. Studies in children suggest that 20% of patients with DCM have evidence for viral persistence compared to 1.4% of normal controls (Schowengerdt et al. 1997). In adults, the prevalence varies from 0% to as much as 80% of patients (Baboonian and Treasure 1997; Wessely et al. 1998; Kuhl et al. 2005). There are several reasons for the variability, including differences related to the size and number of the biopsy samples or to laboratory technique and processing. Furthermore, the patients included in many studies had normal ejection fractions and were suspected of having a viral myocarditis on the basis of arrhythmia, the presence of regional wall motion abnormalities, or atypical cardiac symptoms particularly in the context of local epidemics of viral infections (Kuhl et al. 2005).

Until recently, the most commonly implicated virus in myocarditis has been the Coxsackie B enterovirus (Baboonian and McKenna 2003). The Coxsackie viral protease cleaves dystrophin and thus disrupts the cytoskeletal structural integrity of the cardiac myocyte (Badorff et al. 1999). More recently, adenovirus DNA has been identified using polymerase chain reaction in 9%–39% of samples from explanted hearts or endomyocardial biopsies in children with acute myocarditis (Martin et al. 1994; Shimizu et al. 1995; Akhtar et al. 1999; Calabrese and Thiene 2003), and in some studies, adenovirus was identified more frequently than enterovirus in both children and adults with myocarditis (Baboonian and McKenna 2003; Bowles et al. 2003). Parvovirus infection has been reported in up to 11% of adults with histological evidence of myocardial inflammation or LV dysfunction (Klein et al. 2004). Childhood parvovirus myocarditis has also been reported (Munro et al. 2003), including four cases of sudden cardiac death (Murry et al. 2001; Rohayem et al. 2001; Dettmeyer et al. 2003; Zack et al. 2005). Many other viruses have been implicated in myocarditis, including cytomegalovirus, hepatitis C virus, and herpes simplex virus. In addition, the human immunodeficiency virus has been associated with myocarditis and LV dysfunction (Hofman et al. 1993; Herskowitz et al. 1994; Barbaro et al. 1998).

IV. Other Causes of Dilated Cardiomyopathy in Childhood Inborn errors of metabolism account for only 4% of cases of DCM. Of these, mitochondrial disorders are the commonest (46% of cases), followed by Barth syndrome (24%) and primary or systemic carnitine deficiency (11%) (Towbin et al. 2006). Patients with DCM in association with metabolic disease typically present in infancy and there is a male predominance. Malformation syndromes are rarely associated with DCM in 1% of cases (Towbin et al. 2006). Hypocalcemic rickets can present as an isolated DCM in infancy (Labrune et al. 1986; Yaseen et al. 1993; Abdullah et al. 1999; Gulati et al. 2001; Price et al. 2003; Maiya et al. 2008).

Pathology

The characteristic macroscopic features of DCM are the presence of a globular shaped heart with ventricular (and often also atrial) chamber dilatation and diffuse endocardial thickening (Hughes and McKenna 2005). Thrombus may be present in the atrial appendages and within the ventricular cavity. Overall, myocardial mass is increased, but ventricular wall thickness is reduced.

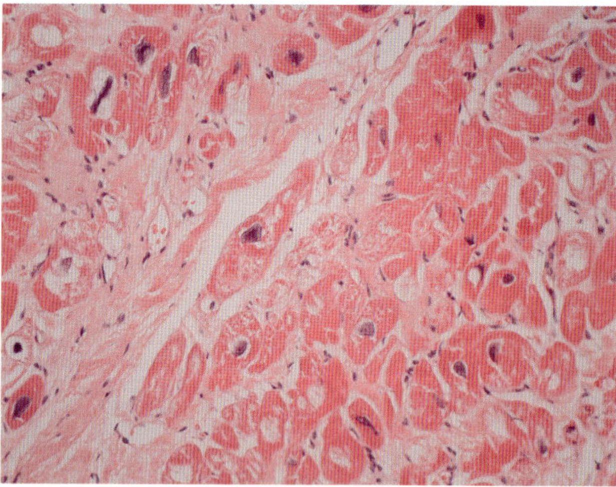

Figure 13–2 Histology of dilated cardiomyopathy. Histology of DCM: This section shows myocyte morphology in DCM, individual myocytes showing hypertrophy with some vacuolation and enlarged, irregular hyperchormatic dark blue nuclei. Some myocytes are trapped in fibrous tissue (light pink). *Courtesy*: Dr Margaret Burke, Harefield Hospital, London, U.K.

The histological features of DCM are nonspecific and include myocyte degeneration, interstitial fibrosis, myocyte nuclear hypertrophy, and pleomorphism (Figure 13–2). There is often extensive myofibrillary loss, resulting in a vacuolated appearance of the myocytes. In addition, there is frequently an increase in interstitial T lymphocytes and focal accumulations of macrophages associated with individual myocyte death (Hughes and McKenna 2005).

Clinical Presentation

The symptoms and signs associated with DCM are highly variable and dependent on the degree of LV dysfunction. Whilst sudden death or a thromboembolic event may be the initial presentation, the majority of patients present with symptoms of high pulmonary venous pressure and/or low cardiac output. This presentation can be acute [often precipitated by intercurrent illness or arrhythmia (Elliott 2000)] or chronic, preceding the diagnosis by many months or years. Increasingly, DCM is diagnosed incidentally in asymptomatic individuals as a result of family screening.

1. Symptoms

Older children and adults often present initially with reduced exercise tolerance and dyspnea on exertion. As LV function deteriorates, dyspnea at rest, orthopnea, paroxysmal nocturnal dyspnea, peripheral edema, and ascites may develop. Infants with DCM typically present with poor feeding, tachypnea, respiratory distress, diaphoresis during feeding, and failure to thrive. In children, symptoms related to mesenteric ischemia may occur, such as abdominal pain after meals, nausea, vomiting, and anorexia. Symptoms related to arrhythmia such as palpitation, presyncope, and syncope occur at any age.

2. Physical Examination

Multisystem examination is important in patients with DCM, as it may guide the physician toward a possible etiology. In particular, examination of the neuromuscular system may reveal features of mild or subclinical skeletal myopathy; ophthalmological examination for retinitis pigmentosa is important if mitochondrial disorders are suspected. Features of low cardiac output include persistent sinus tachycardia, weak peripheral pulses, and, in advanced disease, hypotension. The jugular venous pressure may be elevated. There may also be signs of respiratory distress, particularly in infants and younger children. Palpation of the precordium usually reveals a displaced apical impulse. Hepatomegaly and ascites are common in patients with congestive cardiac failure. Peripheral and sacral edema may also be seen. Auscultation of the heart may reveal the presence of a third (and sometimes fourth) heart sound. There may be a pansystolic murmur at the apex radiating to the axilla caused by functional mitral regurgitation. Auscultation of the chest may reveal basal crackles; infants may present with wheeze that is difficult to distinguish from asthma or bronchiolitis.

Natural History

The prognosis of DCM is variable and depends on the presentation and etiology. Early survival studies suggested a mortality in symptomatic adults with idiopathic DCM approaching 25% at 1 year and 50% at 5 years (Abelmann and Lorell 1989). More recent reports have shown better outcomes, with 5-year survival rates of approximately 20%, perhaps reflecting earlier disease recognition and advances in medical therapy. Most patients die of progressive congestive cardiac failure, but thromboembolism and sudden death are also important. In children, actuarial rates of freedom from death or transplantation range from 70% to 80% at 1 year and 55% to 65% at 5 years (Burch et al. 1994; Daubeney et al. 2006; Towbin et al. 2006), including patients with viral myocarditis. In the pediatric population, predictors of poor outcome include older age at diagnosis, reduced fractional shortening (expressed as a function of body surface area or age), congestive cardiac failure at presentation, and familial, idiopathic, or neuromuscular disease (Daubeney et al. 2006; Towbin et al. 2006).

Investigations

1. Electrocardiography

The 12-lead ECG in DCM may be normal, but more typically shows sinus tachycardia and nonspecific ST segment and 'T' wave changes (usually in the inferior and lateral leads). In patients with extensive LV fibrosis, abnormal Q waves (particularly in the septal leads) may be present. Evidence of atrial enlargement and voltage criteria for ventricular hypertrophy (usually left, but occasionally bilateral ventricular hypertrophy) is common. All degrees of atrioventricular block may be seen, and should raise the possibility of mutations in the lamin A/C gene. Supraventricular (particularly atrial fibrillation) and ventricular arrhythmias are common in DCM. Studies have shown a prevalence of NSVT as high as 43% (Zecchin et al. 2005); in the pediatric population, ventricular tachycardia is less common, occurring in 9.5% of cases (Friedman et al. 1991).

2. Chest Roentgenography

The chest radiograph is often abnormal in patients with DCM. Typically, there is an increased cardiothoracic ratio, reflecting LV and left atrial dilatation. Patients with pulmonary edema have signs of increased pulmonary vascular markings on the chest radiograph, and pleural effusions may be present.

3. Echocardiography

In general, the presence of a LV end-diastolic dimension greater than two standard deviations above body surface area-corrected means (or greater than 112% of predicted dimension) and fractional shortening less than 25% (ejection fraction less than 55%) are sufficient to make the diagnosis (Henry et al. 1980; Richardson et al. 1996; Elliott 2000). Two-dimensional echocardiography can be very useful in determining whether thrombus is present within the ventricular or atrial cavities. The presence and severity of functional mitral (and tricuspid) regurgitation can be assessed using color flow Doppler. In addition, pulsed-wave and continuous wave Doppler can be used to estimate pulmonary artery pressures. Although primarily regarded as a disease of impaired systolic LV function, patients with DCM frequently have abnormalities of diastolic LV function, which can be evaluated and quantified using mitral inflow and pulmonary venous pulsed-wave Doppler velocities and tissue Doppler imaging.

4. Cardiac Biomarkers

Levels of serum creatine kinase should be measured in all patients with DCM, as this may provide important clues to the etiology of the condition (e.g., elevated in patients with dystrophin and lamin A/C mutations). Other cardiac biomarkers, such as troponin I and troponin T, may also be elevated in DCM, and suggest possible inflammatory or ischemic etiology. Plasma B-type natriuretic peptide levels are elevated in children and adults with chronic heart failure and predict survival, hospitalization rates, and listing for cardiac transplantation (Price et al. 2006).

5. Exercise Testing

Symptom-limited exercise testing combined with respiratory gas analysis is a useful technique to assess functional limitation and disease progression in patients with stable DCM. Typically, patients with DCM have lower exercise duration, peak oxygen consumption, and systolic blood pressure at peak exercise than normal controls (Guimaraes et al. 2001). The detection of respiratory markers of severe lactic acidemia during metabolic exercise testing can point toward mitochondrial or metabolic causes for the DCM.

6. Cardiac Catheterization

Cardiac catheterization with endomyocardial biopsy may be a useful adjunct in the investigation of some patients with DCM, but its use is declining with improved noninvasive techniques. In particular, hemodynamic assessment of LV end-diastolic and pulmonary artery pressures has been superseded by echocardiographic techniques. Cardiac catheterization is still used to assess hemodynamics prior to consideration for cardiac transplantation.

Endomyocardial biopsy may be diagnostic for myocarditis and for some metabolic or mitochondrial disorders. Recent guidelines recommend that endomyocardial biopsy should be performed in the setting of new onset heart failure of less than 2 weeks duration with normal or enlarged LV dimensions and hemodynamic compromise, or between 2 weeks and 3 months in the presence of LV dilatation and ventricular arrhythmias or higher degree heart block (Cooper et al. 2007). The Dallas criteria define myocarditis according to the presence of histological evidence of myocyte injury with degeneration or necrosis, and an inflammatory infiltrate not due to ischemia (Aretz et al. 1987). Four forms of myocarditis are recognized: (1) *active myocarditis*, defined by the presence of both myocyte degeneration or necrosis and definite cellular infiltrate, with or without fibrosis; (2) *borderline myocarditis*, observed when there is a definite cellular infiltrate but no evidence of myocardial cellular injury; (3) *persistent myocarditis*, defined as continued active myocarditis on repeat biopsy; and (4) *resolving/resolved myocarditis*, determined by diminished or absent infiltrate with evidence of connective tissue healing on repeat biopsy (Aretz et al. 1987). Despite their widespread use, the Dallas criteria have many limitations, including a low specificity and sensitivity, with a diagnostic yield as low as 10%–20% in some series (Magnani and Dec 2006). In addition, studies have shown a poor association between histological evidence of myocarditis and the presence of autoantibodies in patients with clinically suspected myocarditis (Caforio et al. 1997), and studies in large cohorts of patients with clinically suspected myocarditis have failed to demonstrate associated positive biopsy findings (Fowles and Mason 1984; Parrillo et al. 1984).

7. Cardiac Magnetic Resonance Imaging

Cardiac MRI is a useful alternative imaging technique in patients with poor echocardiographic windows (see Chapter 7). In addition, the detection of fibrosis with gadolinium contrast enhancement may provide an imaging-guided method to improve the diagnostic yield of endomyocardial biopsies (De Cobelli et al. 2006).

Management

Therapy aims to improve symptoms and prevent complications such as progressive cardiac failure, sudden death, and thromboembolism. Loop and thiazide diuretics are used in all heart failure patients with fluid retention to achieve a euvolemic state. However, they should not be used as monotherapy as they exacerbate neurohormonal activation, which may contribute to disease progression. Spironolactone, a specific aldosterone antagonist, reduces relative mortality by 30% in adults with severe heart failure (NYHA class IV and ejection fraction less than 35%) (Pitt et al. 1999b). Side effects include hyperkalemia (although this is infrequent in the presence of normal renal function) and gynecomastia.

1. ACE Enzyme Inhibitors and Angiotensin Receptor Blockers

Activation of the renin-angiotensin-aldosterone system is central to the pathophysiology of heart failure, regardless of the underlying etiology (Elliott 2000; Rosenthal et al. 2004). Numerous randomized trials have shown that ACE inhibitors improve symptoms, reduce hospitalizations, and reduce cardiovascular mortality in adults with heart failure (1987; 1991; 1992 ; Cohn et al. 1991). Furthermore, they also reduce the rate of disease progression in asymptomatic patients. A substantial proportion of patients taking ACE inhibitors in clinical practice are not titrated up to the target doses reported in many trials, but there is evidence to suggest that higher doses are associated with a greater reduction in the combined risk of death or transplantation (Packer et al. 1999). Most patients tolerate ACE inhibitors well. The most common side effects are dry cough and symptomatic hypotension (particularly following the initial dose), which can be prevented with careful uptitration of doses.

Angiotensin receptor blockers block the cell surface receptor for angiotensin II and have similar hemodynamic effects to ACE inhibitors but with a better side-effect profile. Clinical trials in adults with heart failure have shown similar hemodynamic effects, efficacy, and safety between angiotensin receptor blockers and ACE inhibitors (Pitt et al. 1997, 1999a). Angiotensin receptor blockers are currently recommended in adults who do not tolerate ACE inhibitors. Several studies have suggested that combination treatment using both ACE inhibitors and angiotensin receptor blockers may be better at preventing ventricular remodeling and reducing symptoms than either drug alone, although there was no additional survival benefit (Hamroff et al. 1999; McKelvie et al. 1999; Cohn and Tognoni 2001; Pfeffer et al. 2003).

2. β-Blockers

Excess sympathetic activity contributes to heart failure, and multicenter, placebo controlled trials using carvedilol (Packer et al. 1996, 2001; Cleland et al. 2006a), metoprolol (1999a), and bisoprolol (1999b) have shown substantial reductions in mortality (from sudden death and progressive heart failure) in adults with predominantly NYHA class II and III heart failure symptoms. β-blockers are usually well tolerated; side effects include bradycardia, hypotension, and fluid retention. β-blockers should be started at low doses and carefully uptitrated, and they should not be initiated in patients with decompensated heart failure. A recent trial has suggested that they can be started safely before ACE inhibitors in stable heart failure (Willenheimer et al. 2005). In children, the results of the first randomized controlled trial in pediatric cardiomyopathy, from the multicenter Pediatric Carvedilol Study Group, were published recently (Shaddy et al. 2007). This showed a trend toward benefit in the carvedilol group in terms of all-cause mortality, cardiovascular mortality, and heart failure hospitalization; although due to the low number of events in the study and the heterogeneous study population, this was not statistically significant.

3. Digoxin

Digoxin improves symptoms in patients with heart failure (Packer et al. 1993), but no survival benefit has been demonstrated in large study cohorts (Rosenthal et al. 2004). In fact, high serum digoxin levels may be associated with increased mortality in some patients (Rathore et al. 2003). Although digoxin is still widely used to treat heart failure in infants and children, there are very few data in the pediatric population.

4. Anticoagulation

The annual risk of thromboembolism in patients with DCM is low. In adults with DCM, the prevalence of mural thrombi ranges between 3% and 50% (reflecting the insensitivity of echocardiography), with an incidence of systemic thromboembolism between 1.5% and 3.5% per year (Sirajuddin et al. 2002). Anticoagulation with warfarin is advised in patients in whom an intracardiac thrombus is identified echocardiographically and in those with a history of thromboembolism. There are no trial data to guide prophylactic anticoagulation in DCM, but patients with severe ventricular dilatation and moderate to severe systolic impairment may benefit from warfarin therapy.

5. Novel Pharmacological Therapies

Nesiritide, a recombinant B-type natriuretic peptide with diuretic, natriuretic, and vasodilator effects, has been used in adults with decompensated heart failure, and has recently been shown to be safe in children with decompensated cardiac failure, associated with improvements in urine output and functional status (Mahle et al. 2005; Jefferies et al. 2006). Its value compared with more conventional therapies remains to be determined. Metabolic modulators such as perhexiline shift adenosine triphosphate production from free fatty acids to glucose, thus optimizing energy utilization by the myocardium (Abozguia et al. 2006). Agents that target contractility, such as the ATP-dependent sodium-potassium transmembrane pump inhibitor istaroxime, provide inotropic support without proarrhythmic effects (Micheletti et al. 2007). The 3-hydroxyl-3-methyglutaryl coenzyme A (HMG-CoA) reductase inhibitors ("statins"), routinely used in the treatment of ischemic heart disease, have a number of nonlipid-lowering effects, including effects on angiogenesis, LV remodeling, neurohormonal activation, and antiarrhythmic effects, which render them potentially useful for the treatment of heart failure (Ramasubbu et al. 2008). A number of retrospective studies and one meta-analysis have suggested that statins reduce mortality in patients with ischemic and nonischemic cardiomyopathy; the CORONA study, a prospective study of over 5,000 patients with heart failure of ischemic origin, showed a nonsignificant reduction in all-cause mortality (Kjekshus et al. 2007).

6. Treatment of Arrhythmia in DCM

Whilst arrhythmias are common in DCM, the use of many commonly used antiarrhythmic agents is limited by their negative chronotropic and proarrhythmic effects. Data on the effect of amiodarone on survival in DCM are contradictory (Doval et al. 1994; Massie et al. 1996). The largest study to date, the Sudden Cardiac Death in Heart Failure Trial (SCD-HeFT), showed no survival benefit of amiodarone (compared with a 23% reduction in overall mortality with implantable cardioverter-defibrillators) (Bardy et al. 2005). However, amiodarone appears to be safe in patients with DCM, and may be effective at preventing or treating atrial arrhythmias. Implantation of an internal cardioverter-defibrillator is recommended for patients with symptomatic ventricular arrhythmia and in those with heart failure symptoms and an ejection fraction less than 35% (Bardy et al. 2005), to prevent sudden death or as a bridge to transplantation.

7. Nonpharmacological Treatment of Advanced DCM

Cardiac transplantation remains the mainstay of management of children and adults with intractable heart failure symptoms and end-stage disease. However, its use is limited by a shortage of donor organs and the development of graft vasculopathy. Therefore, a number of other approaches aimed at improving symptoms and stabilizing the disease or delaying transplantation have emerged. In some cases, mechanical assist devices, such as LV assist devices, the Berlin heart, or extracorporeal membrane oxygenation may be required (Hetzer et al. 1998; Duncan et al. 1999; Levi et al. 2002). Studies in children have shown good results with aggressive management of end-stage DCM, including bridging to recovery (McMahon et al. 2003).

V. Cardiac Resynchronization Therapy Many patients with DCM have abnormal LV activation that in turn results in prolonged and incoordinate ventricular relaxation. Cardiac resynchronization therapy (biventricular or multisite pacing) attempts to reestablish synchronous atrioventricular, interventricular, and intraventricular contraction to maximize ventricular efficiency. Studies in adults with severe heart failure and left bundle branch block have shown marked symptomatic improvement in some patients (Auricchio et al. 1999) and reduced mortality from heart failure or sudden death (Bristow et al. 2004; Cleland et al. 2005, 2006b).

Summary

DCM is characterized by the presence of LV dilatation and systolic dysfunction (Box 13–2). Most cases are idiopathic, but a family history is present in as many as 35% of individuals with DCM. Inheritance can be autosomal dominant, autosomal recessive, X-linked, or mitochondrial. The genes implicated in familial DCM include genes that encode proteins of the myocardial cytoskeleton,

Box 13–2 Key Points

- Most cases of DCM are idiopathic.
- Familial disease occurs in up to 35% of individuals.
- Inheritance can be autosomal dominant, autosomal recessive, X-linked, or mitochondrial.
- Genes implicated in familial disease include myocardial cytoskeletal, sarcomere protein, and nuclear envelope genes.
- Advances in pharmacologic and nonpharmacologic therapy have improved survival and quality of life, but the prognosis in many cases remains poor.

nuclear envelope, or sarcomere. Advances in medical therapy over the past two decades have improved survival and quality of life, but the prognosis in many cases remains poor. Novel pharmacological and device therapies may provide further improvements in long-term outcome.

Table 13–3 Classification and Etiology of Restrictive Cardiomyopathy

Familial	Nonfamilial
Familial, unknown gene	Idiopathic
Sarcomeric protein mutations:	Amyloid (AL/prealbumin)
Troponin I (RCM+/–HCM)	Sclerodermia
Essential light chain of myosin	Endomyocardial fibrosis
Familial Amyloidosis	Hypereosinophilic syndrome
Transthyretin (RCM+neuropathy)	Drugs: serotonin, methysergide, ergotamine, mercurial agents, busulfan
Apolipoprotein (RCM+nephropathy)	
Desminopathy	Carcinoid heart disease
Pseuxanthoma elasticum	Metastatic cancers
Hemochromatosis	Radiation
Anderson-Fabry disease	Drugs: anthracyclines
Glycogen storage disease	

Data from Elliott et al. Classification of the cardiomyopathies: a position statement from the European Society of Cardiology working group on myocardial and pericardial diseases. *Eur Heart J.* 2008;29:270–276.

Restrictive Cardiomyopathy

RCM is characterized by a pattern of ventricular filling in which increased stiffness of the myocardium causes ventricular pressure to rise precipitously with only small increases in volume in the presence of normal or reduced diastolic volumes of one or both ventricles, normal or reduced systolic volumes, and normal ventricular wall thickness (Elliott et al. 2008). Restrictive ventricular physiology can also occur in a number of different pathologies, including HCM and DCM. RCM is the least common of all the cardiomyopathies.

Etiology

RCM is associated with several conditions (Table 13–3), including infiltrative and storage disorders, and endomyocardial disease (Kushwaha et al. 1997). In adults, RCM is most commonly caused by amyloidosis in the Western world (Saraiva 1995; McCarthy and Kasper 1998), while in the tropics, endomyocardial fibrosis is the commonest cause in adults and probably also in children (Kushwaha et al. 1997). Outside the tropics, most cases of RCM in children are idiopathic (Kushwaha et al. 1997).

1. Idiopathic Restrictive Cardiomyopathy

Many cases of RCM in adults, and the majority in children, remain idiopathic. Familial disease is described in approximately 30% of patients with idiopathic RCM (Mogensen 2009). Mutations in the gene encoding desmin (an intermediate filament protein with key structural and functional roles within skeletal and cardiac myocyte myofibrils) cause RCM associated with skeletal myopathy and cardiac conduction system abnormalities (Dalakas et al. 2000). Desmin mutations are inherited in an autosomal dominant manner, but sporadic mutations are not infrequent (Dalakas et al. 2000).

More recently, mutations in cardiac sarcomere protein genes have been found to cause RCM. The initial report identified mutations in the gene encoding cardiac troponin I in over 50% of adults with idiopathic RCM (Mogensen et al. 2003). Subsequently, mutations in β-myosin heavy chain gene were identified in adults with familial HCM with a restrictive phenotype and little or no hypertrophy. In children with idiopathic RCM, mutations in the genes encoding troponin I, troponin T, α-cardiac actin, and β-myosin heavy chain have been recently reported (Mogensen et al. 2003; Peddy et al. 2006; Karam et al. 2008; Kaski et al. 2008).

2. Endomyocardial Fibrosis and Eosinophilic Cardiomyopathy (Löffler's Endocarditis)

Restrictive ventricular physiology can be caused by endocardial pathology (fibrosis, fibroelastosis, and thrombosis). These disorders are subclassified according to the presence of eosinophilia into endomyocardial diseases with hypereosinophilia [or hypereosinophilic syndromes (HES)] and endomyocardial disease without hypereosinophilia (e.g., endomyocardial fibrosis). Parasitic infection, drugs such as methysergide, inflammatory and nutritional factors are implicated in acquired forms of endomyocardial fibrosis.

Endomyocardial fibrosis is endemic in tropical and subtropical parts of Africa, India, Asia, and South and Central America, and may account for up to 25% of cardiac-related deaths in equatorial Africa (Goodwin 1992). It is rare outside the tropics (Kushwaha et al. 1997). Adolescents and young adults are most frequently affected. Disease onset is usually insidious, with progressive biventricular failure in most cases. The overall prognosis is poor, with a 44% mortality rate at 1 year, increasing to nearly 90% at 3 years (Shaper et al. 1968). Typically, fibrous endocardial lesions in the RV and/or LV inflow tract cause incompetence of the atrioventricular valves leading to pulmonary congestion and right heart failure.

3. Amyloidosis

Cardiac amyloidosis (see Chapter 30) is classified according to the precursor protein. Cardiac involvement is most common in primary amyloidosis, occurring in as many as 60% of cases, and associated with a poor prognosis; at least 50% of patients with primary amyloidosis die from cardiac-related causes (heart failure or arrhythmia) (Kyle and Gertz 1995). Cardiac involvement is typically less severe in secondary and senile systemic amyloidosis. Hereditary amyloidosis is caused by mutations in the transthyretin (TTR) and apolipoprotein I genes; over 80 point mutations in TTR have been identified to date, including several known to be associated with significant cardiac disease (Shah et al. 2006). The primary manifestation of TTR mutations is a peripheral and autonomic neuropathy, known as familial amyloid polyneuropathy. One mutation, transyrethin Ile122, has been reported to cause cardiac disease without any neurological involvement in elderly black people (Jacobson et al. 1997).

4. Other Infiltrative and Storage Disorders Associated with Restrictive Cardiomyopathy

Several infiltrative and storage disorders cause RCM (see Table 13–3). These include lysosomal storage disorders such as mucopolysaccharidosis (Hurler's syndrome) and Anderson-Fabry disease, which is more commonly associated with HCM (Kushwaha et al. 1997).

Cardiac sarcoidosis can present with RCM progressing to systolic impairment, and is also typically associated with conduction disease and a risk of sudden death. The diagnostic tests for sarcoidosis (elevated serum ACE levels and the presence of noncaseating granuloma on endomyocardial biopsy) may be normal, and a high index of suspicion is required to diagnose it. Cardiac MRI and PET are the most sensitive imaging techniques, and changes appear to correlate with disease activity. Treatment includes corticosteroids, implantable cardioverter-defibrillators for patients with a history of NSVT, and cardiac transplantation. However, sarcoid granulomatous lesions may recur in the transplanted cardiac allograft (Doughan and Williams 2006).

Pathology

The macroscopic features of RCM include biatrial dilatation in the presence of normal heart weight, a small ventricular cavity, and no LV hypertrophy. However, the morphologic spectrum of primary RCM includes mild ventricular hypertrophy with increased heart weight and mild ventricular dilatation without hypertrophy (Angelini et al. 1997). In many hearts, there is thrombus in the atrial appendages and patchy endocardial fibrosis (Kushwaha et al. 1997).

The histological features of idiopathic RCM are classically nonspecific with patchy interstitial fibrosis, which may range in extent from very mild to severe (Kushwaha et al. 1997). There may also be fibrosis of the sinoatrial and atrioventricular nodes (Fitzpatrick et al. 1990). Myocyte disarray is not uncommon in patients with pure RCM, even in the absence of macroscopic ventricular hypertrophy (Angelini et al. 1997). In patients with infiltrative and metabolic cardiomyopathies, there will be specific findings appropriate to the disorder (Hughes and McKenna 2005).

Pathophysiology

The finding that mutations in the sarcomere protein genes cause RCM has provided new insights into the pathophysiology of restrictive LV physiology. In vitro studies have suggested that troponin I mutations that cause RCM have a greater increase in calcium ion sensitivity than those that cause HCM, resulting in more severe diastolic dysfunction and potentially accounting for the restrictive phenotype in humans (Gomes et al. 2005; Yumoto et al. 2005). In addition, the hearts of troponin I-mutated transgenic mice show increased contractility and impaired relaxation (James et al. 2000). Similar findings have been observed in mice with disease-causing α-myosin heavy chain mutations (Tyska et al. 2000). These results suggest that altered calcium sensitivity may play a role in the development of RCM. However, the fact that the same mutation within the same family can result in both restrictive and hypertrophic phenotypes suggests that other genetic and environmental factors are likely to also be involved in the pathogenesis of RCM (Kubo et al. 2007).

Clinical Features

1. Symptoms

The presentation of RCM is usually with symptoms and signs of cardiac failure and arrhythmia. In children, disease progression is rapid, with over 50% of children dying within 2 years of diagnosis and most children requiring cardiac transplantation within 4 years (Russo and Webber 2005; Fenton et al. 2006). The presentation and natural history in adults is more variable. Common symptoms include dyspnea on exertion, recurrent respiratory tract infections, and general fatigue and weakness. This may progress rapidly to dyspnea at rest, orthopnea, and paroxysmal nocturnal dyspnea. Symptoms related to increased right-sided pressures may include peripheral edema and abdominal distension due to ascites. Many patients complain of chest pain and symptoms suggestive of arrhythmia such as palpitation. Syncope is a presenting symptom in 10% of children with RCM (Gewillig et al. 1996; Rivenes et al. 2000). Rarely, sudden death may be the initial manifestation of the disease.

2. Physical Examination

Clinical examination typically reveals signs of left- and right-sided cardiac failure. Tachypnea, signs of respiratory distress, and failure to thrive are seen in infants and young children. In older children and adults, the jugular venous pressure is elevated, with a prominent y descent, and fails to fall (or may even rise) during inspiration (Kussmaul's sign). Peripheral edema, ascites, and hepatomegaly are common. The apical impulse is usually normal. Cardiac auscultation reveals a normal first heart sound and normal splitting of the second heart sound. The pulmonary component of the second heart sound may be loud, if pulmonary vascular resistance is high. There is usually a third heart sound (and occasionally a fourth heart sound) giving rise to a gallop rhythm. The murmurs of atrioventricular valve regurgitation may be heard.

Investigations

1. Electrocardiography

The resting 12-lead ECG is abnormal in the majority of patients with RCM. The most frequent abnormalities include p-mitrale and p-pulmonale, nonspecific ST segment and T wave abnormalities, ST segment depression and T wave inversion, usually in the inferolateral leads. Voltage criteria for LV and RV hypertrophy may also be present, although in patients with amyloidosis, low voltage QRS complexes are seen. Conduction abnormalities, including intraventricular conduction delay, and abnormal Q waves may also be seen.

2. Chest Roentgenography

The chest radiograph may show cardiomegaly caused by atrial enlargement, and pulmonary venous congestion. Interstitial edema, manifest by the presence of Kerley B lines, may be seen in severe cases.

3. Echocardiography

Typically, there is marked dilatation of both atria, often dwarfing the size of the ventricles, in the presence of normal or mildly reduced systolic function, and a nonhypertrophied, nondilated left ventricle. In children, severe impairment of LV systolic function (fractional shortening less than 25%) may develop in as many as 30% of cases (Gewillig et al. 1996; Denfield et al. 1997; Chen et al. 2001; Weller et al. 2002). Many patients with a clinical label of

RCM also have mild LV hypertrophy (Lewis 1992; Gewillig et al. 1996; Denfield et al. 1997; Chen et al. 2001; Weller et al. 2002), which may represent part of the spectrum of sarcomere protein disease.

The pattern of mitral inflow pulsed-wave Doppler velocities in RCM is typically one of increased early diastolic filling velocity, decreased atrial filling velocity, an increased ratio of early diastolic filling to atrial filling, a decreased E wave deceleration time, and a decreased isovolumic relaxation time. Pulmonary vein and hepatic vein pulsed-wave Doppler velocities demonstrate higher diastolic than systolic velocities, increased atrial reversal velocities, and an atrial reversal duration greater than mitral atrial filling duration. Tissue Doppler imaging shows reduced diastolic annular velocities, and an increased ratio of early diastolic tissue Doppler annular velocity to mitral early diastolic filling velocity, reflecting elevated LV end-diastolic pressures.

4. Cardiopulmonary Exercise Testing

Symptom-limited exercise testing with respiratory gas analysis provides a useful objective measure of exercise limitation, which can help in symptom management and is an important component of the pretransplantation assessment. Peak oxygen consumption is usually reduced. Exercise testing may also reveal ischemic electrocardiographic changes at higher heart rates, which may correlate with symptoms such as chest pain (Rivenes 2000; Lewis 1992).

5. Cardiac Catheterization

The characteristic hemodynamic feature on cardiac catheterization is a rapid early decline in ventricular pressure at the onset of diastole, with a rapid rise to a plateau in early diastole, the so-called "dip-and-plateau" or "square root sign" (Kushwaha et al. 1997). LV end-diastolic, left atrial, and pulmonary capillary wedge pressures are markedly elevated, and usually 5 mmHg or more, greater than right atrial and right ventricular end-diastolic pressures. Volume loading and exercise accentuate the difference between left- and right-sided pressures.

In children, pulmonary hypertension is frequently present during initial cardiac catheterization. Elevated pulmonary vascular resistance indices are commonly found, and tend to progress during follow-up (Kimberling et al. 2002; Weller et al. 2002; Fenton et al. 2006). Elevated pulmonary vascular resistance may initially be reversible with nitric oxide or prostacyclin (Kimberling et al. 2002; Fenton et al. 2006), but it is usually not possible to predict the development of fixed pulmonary vascular resistance (Weller et al. 2002). Endomyocardial biopsy is usually nondiagnostic, but it may be useful in some of the storage and infiltrative causes of RCM.

Management

1. Symptomatic Therapy

Diuretics are useful in patients with symptoms and signs of pulmonary or systemic venous congestion. Overdiuresis, however, should be avoided as it may result in excessive preload reduction and hemodynamic collapse. Careful fluid management is an important aspect of the treatment of patients with RCM. In view of atrial enlargement and propensity to atrial arrhythmia, prophylactic anticoagulation with warfarin or antiplatelet agents is recommended. As the atrial contribution to ventricular filling in patients with RCM is important, efforts to maintain sinus rhythm with β-blockers and amiodarone may be appropriate. Treatment with afterload-reducing agents, such as ACE inhibitors, calcium channel blockers, and nitrates rarely improves symptoms and can cause deterioration (Bengur et al. 1991).

Box 13–3 Key Points

- RCM is the rarest of the cardiomyopathies.
- Most cases are idiopathic.
- Familial disease is recognized in up to 50% of individuals with idiopathic RCM.
- Genes implicated in idiopathic RCM include sarcomere protein genes and desmin.
- Other causes include infiltrative and storage disorders.
- Prognosis is poor, especially in infants and children, in whom transplantation is usually the only therapeutic option.

2. Specific Therapies

For patients with amyloidosis, treatment options include chemotherapy and autologous stem cell transplantation, although patients with cardiac involvement are not usually optimum candidates for this. Steroid and cytotoxic therapy are used in the early stages of Löffler's endocarditis. Patients with sarcoidosis commonly present with ventricular arrhythmias or conduction disease, which may require treatment with implantable defibrillator or pacemaker therapy.

3. Optimization of Hemodynamics Prior to Transplantation

Transplantation is the only definitive treatment for children with RCM, and for adults with advanced disease that is unresponsive to medical therapy. In children, whilst fixed, irreversible elevations in pulmonary vascular resistance preclude orthotopic cardiac transplantation (Weller et al. 2002), short-term pretransplantation treatment with prostacyclin (for a mean duration of 57 days) has been shown to reduce transpulmonary gradients sufficiently to allow orthotopic heart transplantation (Fenton et al. 2006). While on the waiting list for transplantation, patients should undergo serial Holter monitoring; implantable cardioverter-defibrillators may be offered to patients with evidence of ventricular arrhythmia as a bridge to transplantation.

Summary

RCM is uncommon and most cases are idiopathic (Box 13–3). A large proportion of cases may be familial due to diverse genetic etiology. Mutations in sarcomere and desmin genes are implicated in idiopathic RCM. Some infiltrative and storage disorders may complicate with RCM. Prognosis is variable but in particular poor in infants and children where cardiac transplantation may be helpful.

References

(1987). Effects of enalapril on mortality in severe congestive heart failure. Results of the Cooperative North Scandinavian Enalapril Survival Study (CONSENSUS). The CONSENSUS Trial Study Group. *N Eng J Med*. 316:1429–1435.

(1991). Effect of enalapril on survival in patients with reduced left ventricular ejection fractions and congestive heart failure. The SOLVD Investigators. *N Eng J Med*. 325:293–302.

(1992). Effect of enalapril on mortality and the development of heart failure in asymptomatic patients with reduced left ventricular ejection fractions. The SOLVD Investigattors. *N Eng J Med*. 327:685–691.

(1999a). Effect of metoprolol CR/XL in chronic heart failure: Metoprolol CR/XL randomised intervention trial in congestive heart failure (MERIT-HF). *Lancet.* 353:2001–2007.

(1999b). The Cardiac Insufficiency Bisoprolol Study II (CIBIS-II): a randomised trial. *Lancet.* 353:9–13.

Abdullah M, Bigras JL, McCrindle BW. Dilated cardiomyopathy as a first sign of nutritional vitamin D deficiency rickets in infancy. *Can J Cardiol.* 1999;15:699–701.

Abelmann WH, Lorell BH. The challenge of cardiomyopathy. *J Am Coll Cardiol.* 1989;13:1219–1239.

Abozguia K, Clarke K, Lee L, Frenneaux M. Modification of myocardial substrate use as a therapy for heart failure. *Nat Clin Pract.* 2006;3:490–498.

Ackerman MJ, VanDriest SL, Ommen SR, et al. Prevalence and age-dependence of malignant mutations in the beta-myosin heavy chain and troponin T genes in hypertrophic cardiomyopathy: a comprehensive outpatient perspective. *J Am Coll Cardiol.* 2002;39:2042–2048.

Ahmad F, Seidman JG, Seidman CE. The genetic basis for cardiac remodeling. *Annu Rev Genomics Hum Genet.* 2005;6:185–216.

Akhtar N, Ni J, Stromberg D, Rosenthal GL, Bowles NE, Towbin JA. Tracheal aspirate as a substrate for polymerase chain reaction detection of viral genome in childhood pneumonia and myocarditis. *Circulation.* 1999;99:2011–2018.

Alfonso F, Frenneaux MP, McKenna WJ. Clinical sustained uniform ventricular tachycardia in hypertrophic cardiomyopathy: association with left ventricular apical aneurysm. *Br Heart J.* 1989;61:178–181.

Angelini A, Calzolari V, Thiene G, et al. Morphologic spectrum of primary restrictive cardiomyopathy. *Am J Cardiol.* 1997;80:1046–1050.

Arad M, Seidman JG, Seidman CE. Phenotypic diversity in hypertrophic cardiomyopathy. *Hum Mol Genet.* 2002;11:2499–2506.

Aretz HT, Billingham ME, Edwards WD, et al. Myocarditis. A histopathologic definition and classification. *Am J Cardiovasc Pathol.* 1987;1:3–14.

Auricchio A, Stellbrink C, Block M, et al. Effect of pacing chamber and atrioventricular delay on acute systolic function of paced patients with congestive heart failure. The Pacing Therapies for Congestive Heart Failure Study Group. The Guidant Congestive Heart Failure Research Group. *Circulation.* 1999;99:2993–3001.

Autore C, Conte MR, Piccininno M, et al. Risk associated with pregnancy in hypertrophic cardiomyopathy. *J Am Coll Cardiol.* 2002;40:1864–1869.

Baboonian C, McKenna W. Eradication of viral myocarditis: is there hope? *J Am Coll Cardiol.* 2003;42:473–476.

Baboonian C, Treasure T. Meta-analysis of the association of enteroviruses with human heart disease. *Heart (BCS).* 2003;78:539–543.

Badorff C, Lee GH, Lamphear BJ, et al. Enteroviral protease 2A cleaves dystrophin: evidence of cytoskeletal disruption in an acquired cardiomyopathy. *Nat Med.* 1999;5:320–326.

Baig MK, Goldman JH, Caforio AL, Coonar AS, Keeling PJ, McKenna WJ. Familial dilated cardiomyopathy: cardiac abnormalities are common in asymptomatic relatives and may represent early disease. *J Am Coll Cardiol.* 1998;31:195–201.

Barbaro G, Di LG, Grisorio B, Barbarini G. Incidence of dilated cardiomyopathy and detection of HIV in myocardial cells of HIV-positive patients. Gruppo Italiano per lo Studio Cardiologico dei Pazienti Affetti da AIDS. *N Engl J Med.* 1998;339:1093–1099.

Bardy GH, Lee KL, Mark DB, et al. Amiodarone or an implantable cardioverter-defibrillator for congestive heart failure. *N Eng J Med.* 2005;352:225–237.

Barresi R, Di Blasi C, Negri T, et al. Disruption of heart sarcoglycan complex and severe cardiomyopathy caused by beta sarcoglycan mutations. *J Med Genet.* 2000;37:102–107.

Barth PG, Scholte HR, Berden JA, et al. An X-linked mitochondrial disease affecting cardiac muscle, skeletal muscle and neutrophil leucocytes. *J Neurol Sci.* 1983;62:327–355.

Beder SD, Gutgesell HP, Mullins CE, McNamara DG. Progression from hypertrophic obstructive cardiomyopathy to congestive cardiomyopathy in a child. *Am Heart J.* 1982;104:155–156.

Bengur AR, Beekman RH, Rocchini AP, Crowley DC, Schork MA, Rosenthal A. Acute hemodynamic effects of captopril in children with a congestive or restrictive cardiomyopathy. *Circulation.* 1991;83:523–527.

Berko BA, Swift M. X-linked dilated cardiomyopathy. *N Eng J Med.* 1987;316:1186–1191.

Biagini E, Coccolo F, Ferlito M, et al. Dilated-hypokinetic evolution of hypertrophic cardiomyopathy: prevalence, incidence, risk factors, and prognostic implications in pediatric and adult patients. *J Am Coll Cardiol.* 2005;46:1543–1550.

Bing W, Knott A, Redwood C, et al. Effect of hypertrophic cardiomyopathy mutations in human cardiac muscle alpha -tropomyosin (Asp175Asn and Glu180Gly) on the regulatory properties of human cardiac troponin determined by in vitro motility assay. *J Mol Cell Cardiol.* 2000;32:1489–1498.

Bingisser R, Candinas R, Schneider J, Hess OM. Risk factors for systolic dysfunction and ventricular dilatation in hypertrophic cardiomyopathy. *Int J Cardiol.* 1994;44:225–233.

Blair E, Redwood C, Ashrafian H, et al. Mutations in the gamma(2) subunit of AMP-activated protein kinase cause familial hypertrophic cardiomyopathy: evidence for the central role of energy compromise in disease pathogenesis. *Hum Mol Genet.* 2001;10:1215–1220.

Blanchard E, Seidman C, Seidman JG, LeWinter M, Maughan D. Altered crossbridge kinetics in the alphaMHC403/+ mouse model of familial hypertrophic cardiomyopathy. *Circ Res.* 1999;84:475–483.

Bleyl SB, Mumford BR, Thompson V, et al. Neonatal, lethal noncompaction of the left ventricular myocardium is allelic with Barth syndrome. *Am J Hum Gen.* 1997;61:868–872.

Bonne G, Di Barletta MR, Varnous S, et al. Mutations in the gene encoding lamin A/C cause autosomal dominant Emery-Dreifuss muscular dystrophy. *Nat Gen.* 1999;21:285–288.

Bonow RO, Dilsizian V, Rosing DR, Maron BJ, Bacharach SL, Green MV. Verapamil-induced improvement in left ventricular diastolic filling and increased exercise tolerance in patients with hypertrophic cardiomyopathy: short- and long-term effects. *Circulation.* 1985;72:853–864.

Bos JM, Poley RN, Ny M, et al. Genotype-phenotype relationships involving hypertrophic cardiomyopathy-associated mutations in titin, muscle LIM protein, and telethonin. *Mol Genet Metab.* 2006;88:78–85.

Bowles NE, Bowles KR, Towbin JA. The "final common pathway" hypothesis and inherited cardiovascular disease. The role of cytoskeletal proteins in dilated cardiomyopathy. *Herz.* 2000;25:168–175.

Bowles NE, Ni J, Kearney DL, et al. Detection of viruses in myocardial tissues by polymerase chain reaction. evidence of adenovirus as a common cause of myocarditis in children and adults. *J Am Coll Cardiol.* 2003;42:466–472.

Bristow MR, Saxon LA, Boehmer J, et al. Cardiac-resynchronization therapy with or without an implantable defibrillator in advanced chronic heart failure. *N Eng J Med.* 2004;350:2140–2150.

Brodsky GL, Muntoni F, Miocic S, Sinagra G, Sewry C, Mestroni L. Lamin A/C gene mutation associated with dilated cardiomyopathy with variable skeletal muscle involvement. *Circulation.* 2000;101:473–476.

Broers JL, Peeters EA, Kuijpers HJ, et al. Decreased mechanical stiffness in LMNA/cells is caused by defective nucleo-cytoskeletal integrity: implications for the development of laminopathies. *Hum Mol Genet.* 2004;13:2567–2580.

Bruno E, Maisuls H, Juaneda E, Moreyra E, Alday LE. Clinical features of hypertrophic cardiomyopathy in the young. *Cardiol Young.* 2002;12:147–152.

Burch M, Mann JM, Sharland M, Shinebourne EA, Patton MA, McKenna WJ. Myocardial disarray in Noonan syndrome. *Br Heart J.* 1992;68:586–588.

Burch M, Siddiqi SA, Celermajer DS, Scott C, Bull C, Deanfield JE. Dilated cardiomyopathy in children: determinants of outcome. *Br Heart J.* 1994;72:246–250.

Caforio AL, Goldman JH, Baig MK, et al. Cardiac autoantibodies in dilated cardiomyopathy become undetectable with disease progression. *Heart (BCS).* 1997;77:62–67.

Caforio AL, Keeling PJ, Zachara E, et al. Evidence from family studies for autoimmunity in dilated cardiomyopathy. *Lancet.* 1994;344:773–777.

Caforio AL, Mahon NJ, Tona F, McKenna WJ. Circulating cardiac autoantibodies in dilated cardiomyopathy and myocarditis: pathogenetic and clinical significance. *Eur J Heart Fail.* 2002;4:411–417.

Calabrese F, Thiene G. Myocarditis and inflammatory cardiomyopathy: microbiological and molecular biological aspects. *Cardiovasc Res.* 2003;60:11–25.

Capell BC, Collins FS. Human laminopathies: nuclei gone genetically awry. *Nat Rev.* 2006;7:940–952.

Casazza F, Ferrari F, Piccone U, Maggiolini S, Capozi A, Morpurgo M. Progression of cardiopathology in Friedreich ataxia: clinico-instrumental study. *Cardiologia (Rome, Italy).* 1990;35:423–431.

Cecchi F, Maron BJ, Epstein SE. Long-term outcome of patients with hypertrophic cardiomyopathy successfully resuscitated after cardiac arrest. *J Am Coll Cardiol.* 1989;13:1283–1288.

Chandra M, Rundell VL, Tardiff JC, Leinwand LA, De Tombe PP, Solaro RJ. Ca(2+) activation of myofilaments from transgenic mouse hearts expressing R92Q mutant cardiac troponin T. *Am J Physiol.* 2001;280, H705–H713.

Charron P, Dubourg O, Desnos M, et al. Clinical features and prognostic implications of familial hypertrophic cardiomyopathy related to the cardiac myosin-binding protein C gene. *Circulation.* 1998;97:2230–2236.

Chen B, Bronson RT, Klaman LD, et al. Mice mutant for Egfr and Shp2 have defective cardiac semilunar valvulogenesis. *Nat Gen.* 2000;24:296–299.

Chen SC, Balfour IC, Jureidini S. Clinical spectrum of restrictive cardiomyopathy in children. *J Heart Lung Transplant.* 2001;20:90–92.

Child JS, Perloff JK, Bach PM, Wolfe AD, Perlman S, Kark RA. Cardiac involvement in Friedreich's ataxia: a clinical study of 75 patients. *J Am Coll Cardiol.* 1986;7:1370–1378.

Choudhury L, Mahrholdt H, Wagner A, et al. Myocardial scarring in asymptomatic or mildly symptomatic patients with hypertrophic cardiomyopathy. *J Am Coll Cardiol.* 2002;40:2156–2164.

Ciampi Q, Betocchi S, Lombardi R, et al. Hemodynamic determinants of exercise-induced abnormal blood pressure response in hypertrophic cardiomyopathy. *J Am Coll Cardiol.* 2002;40:278–284.

Cleland JG, Charlesworth A, Lubsen J, et al. A comparison of the effects of carvedilol and metoprolol on well-being, morbidity, and mortality (the "patient journey") in patients with heart failure: a report from the Carvedilol Or Metoprolol European Trial (COMET). *J Am Coll Cardiol.* 2006a;47:1603–1611.

Cleland JG, Daubert JC, Erdmann E, et al. The effect of cardiac resynchronization on morbidity and mortality in heart failure. *N Eng J Med.* 2005;352:1539–1549.

Cleland JG, Daubert JC, Erdmann E, et al. Longer-term effects of cardiac resynchronization therapy on mortality in heart failure the CArdiac REsynchronization-Heart Failure (CARE-HF) trial extension phase. *Eur Heart J.* 2006b;27:1928–1932.

Codd MB, Sugrue DD, Gersh BJ, Melton LJ 3rd. Epidemiology of idiopathic dilated and hypertrophic cardiomyopathy. A population-based study in Olmsted County, Minnesota, 1975–1984. *Circulation.* 1989;80:564–572.

Cohen N, Muntoni F. Multiple pathogenetic mechanisms in X linked dilated cardiomyopathy. *Heart (BCS).* 2004;90:835–841.

Cohn JN, Ferrari R, Sharpe N. Cardiac remodeling—concepts and clinical implications: a consensus paper from an international forum on cardiac remodeling. Behalf of an International Forum on Cardiac Remodeling. *J Am Coll Cardiol.* 2000;35:569–582.

Cohn JN, Johnson G, Ziesche S, et al. A comparison of enalapril with hydralazine-isosorbide dinitrate in the treatment of chronic congestive heart failure. *N Eng J Med.* 1991;325:303–310.

Cohn JN, Tognoni G. A randomized trial of the angiotensin-receptor blocker valsartan in chronic heart failure. *N Eng J Med.* 2001;345: 1667–1675.

Cooper LT, Baughman KL, Feldman AM, et al. The role of endomyocardial biopsy in the management of cardiovascular disease: a scientific statement from the American Heart Association, the American College of Cardiology, and the European Society of Cardiology Endorsed by the Heart Failure Society of America and the Heart Failure Association of the European Society of Cardiology. *Eur Heart J.* 2007;28: 3076–3093.

Corrado D, Basso C, Thiene G. Sudden cardiac death in young people with apparently normal heart. *Cardiovas Res.* 2001;50:399–408.

Counihan PJ, Frenneaux MP, Webb DJ, McKenna WJ. Abnormal vascular responses to supine exercise in hypertrophic cardiomyopathy. *Circulation.* 1991;84:686–696.

D'Adamo P, Fassone L, Gedeon A, et al. The X-linked gene G4.5 is responsible for different infantile dilated cardiomyopathies. *Am J Hum Gen.* 1997;61:862–867.

Dalakas MC, Park KY, Semino-Mora C, Lee HS, Sivakumar K, Goldfarb LG. Desmin myopathy, a skeletal myopathy with cardiomyopathy caused by mutations in the desmin gene. *N Engl J Med.* 2000;342:770–780.

Danon MJ, Oh SJ, DiMauro S, et al. Lysosomal glycogen storage disease with normal acid maltase. *Neurology.* 1981;31:51–57.

Daubeney PE, Nugent AW, Chondros P, et al. Clinical features and outcomes of childhood dilated cardiomyopathy: results from a national population-based study. *Circulation.* 2006;114:2671–2678.

Davies MJ, McKenna WJ. Hypertrophic cardiomyopathy—pathology and pathogenesis. *Histopathology.* 1995;26:493–500.

De Cobelli F, Pieroni M, Esposito A, et al. Delayed gadolinium-enhanced cardiac magnetic resonance in patients with chronic myocarditis presenting with heart failure or recurrent arrhythmias. *J Am Coll Cardiol.* 2006;47:1649–1654.

Denfield SW, Rosenthal G, Gajarski RJ, et al. Restrictive cardiomyopathies in childhood. Etiologies and natural history. *Tex Heart Inst J.* 1997;24:38–44.

Deng Y, Schmidtmann A, Redlich A, Westerdorf B, Jaquet K, Thieleczek R. Effects of phosphorylation and mutation R145G on human cardiac troponin I function. *Biochemistry.* 2001;40:14593–14602.

Dettmeyer R, Kandolf R, Baasner A, Banaschak S, Eis-Hubinger AM, Madea B. Fatal parvovirus B19 myocarditis in an 8-year-old boy. *J Forensic Sci.* 2003;48:183–186.

Digilio MC, Conti E, Sarkozy A, et al. Grouping of multiple-lentigines/LEOPARD and Noonan syndromes on the PTPN11 gene. *Am J Hum Gen.* 2002;71:389–394.

Doughan AR, Williams BR. Cardiac sarcoidosis. *Heart (BCS).* 2006;92:282–288.

Doval HC, Nul DR, Grancelli HO, Perrone SV, Bortman GR, Curiel R. Randomised trial of low-dose amiodarone in severe congestive heart failure. Grupo de Estudio de la Sobrevida en la Insuficiencia Cardiaca en Argentina (GESICA). *Lancet.* 1994;344:493–498.

Duncan BW, Hraska V, Jonas RA, et al. Mechanical circulatory support in children with cardiac disease. *J Thorac Cardiovasc Surg.* 1999;117:529–542.

Elliott K, Watkins H, Redwood CS. Altered regulatory properties of human cardiac troponin I mutants that cause hypertrophic cardiomyopathy. *J Biol Chem.* 2000a;275:22069–22074.

Elliott P. Cardiomyopathy. Diagnosis and management of dilated cardiomyopathy. *Heart (BCS).* 2000;84:106–112.

Elliott P, Andersson B, Arbustini E, et al. Classification of the cardiomyopathies: a position statement from the European Society Of Cardiology Working Group on Myocardial and Pericardial Diseases. *Eur Heart J.* 2008;29:270–276.

Elliott P, McKenna WJ. Hypertrophic cardiomyopathy. *Lancet.* 2004;363:1881–1891.

Elliott PM, Gimeno Blanes JR, Mahon NG, Poloniecki JD, McKenna WJ. Relation between severity of left-ventricular hypertrophy and prognosis in patients with hypertrophic cardiomyopathy. *Lancet.* 2001;357:420–424.

Elliott PM, Gimeno JR, Tome MT, et al. Left ventricular outflow tract obstruction and sudden death risk in patients with hypertrophic cardiomyopathy. *Eur Heart J.* 2006;27:1933–1941.

Elliott PM, Poloniecki J, Dickie S, et al. Sudden death in hypertrophic cardiomyopathy: identification of high risk patients. *J Am Coll Cardiol.* 2000b;36:2212–2218.

Elliott PM, Sharma S, Varnava, A, Poloniecki, J, Rowland, E, McKenna WJ. Survival after cardiac arrest or sustained ventricular tachycardia in patients with hypertrophic cardiomyopathy. *J Am Coll Cardiol.* 1999;33:1596–1601.

Epstein SE, Rosing DR. Verapamil: its potential for causing serious complications in patients with hypertrophic cardiomyopathy. *Circulation.* 1981;64:437–441.

Faber L, Seggewiss H, Gleichmann U. Percutaneous transluminal septal myocardial ablation in hypertrophic obstructive cardiomyopathy: results with respect to intraprocedural myocardial contrast echocardiography. *Circulation.* 1998;98:2415–2421.

Fananapazir L, Epstein ND, Curiel RV, Panza JA, Tripodi D, McAreavey D. Long-term results of dual-chamber (DDD) pacing in obstructive hypertrophic cardiomyopathy. Evidence for progressive symptomatic and hemodynamic improvement and reduction of left ventricular hypertrophy. *Circulation.* 1994;90:2731–2742.

Fananapazir L, Tracy CM, Leon MB, et al. Electrophysiologic abnormalities in patients with hypertrophic cardiomyopathy. A consecutive analysis in 155 patients. *Circulation.* 1989;80:1259–1268.

Fatkin D, MacRae C, Sasaki T, et al. Missense mutations in the rod domain of the lamin A/C gene as causes of dilated cardiomyopathy and conduction-system disease. *N Eng J Med.* 1999;341:1715–1724.

Feldman AM, McNamara D. Myocarditis. *N Engl J Med.* 2000;343:1388–1398.

Fenton MJ, Chubb H, McMahon AM, Rees P, Elliott MJ, Burch M. Heart and heart-lung transplantation for idiopathic restrictive cardiomyopathy in children. *Heart (BCS).* 2006;92:85–89.

Fighali S, Krajcer Z, Edelman S, Leachman RD. Progression of hypertrophic cardiomyopathy into a hypokinetic left ventricle: higher incidence in patients with midventricular obstruction. *J Am Coll Cardiol.* 1987;9:288–294.

Fitzpatrick AP, Shapiro LM, Rickards AF, Poole-Wilson PA. Familial restrictive cardiomyopathy with atrioventricular block and skeletal myopathy. *Br Heart J.* 1990;63:114–118.

Fowles RE, Mason JW. Role of cardiac biopsy in the diagnosis and management of cardiac disease. *Prog Cardiovasc Dis.* 1984;27:153–172.

Frenneaux MP, Counihan PJ, Caforio AL, Chikamori T, McKenna WJ. Abnormal blood pressure response during exercise in hypertrophic cardiomyopathy. *Circulation.* 1990;82:1995–2002.

Friedman RA, Moak JP, Garson A Jr. Clinical course of idiopathic dilated cardiomyopathy in children. *J Am Coll Cardiol.* 1991;18:152–156.

Fujiwara H, Onodera T, Tanaka M, et al. Progression from hypertrophic obstructive cardiomyopathy to typical dilated cardiomyopathy-like features in the end stage. *Jpn Circ J.* 1984;48:1210–1214.

Gewillig M, Mertens L, Moerman P, Dumoulin M. Idiopathic restrictive cardiomyopathy in childhood. A diastolic disorder characterized by delayed relaxation. *Eur Heart J.* 1996;17:1413–1420.

Gomes AV, Liang J, Potter JD. Mutations in human cardiac troponin I that are associated with restrictive cardiomyopathy affect basal ATPase activity and the calcium sensitivity of force development. *J biol Chem.* 2005;280:30909–30915.

Goodwin JF. Cardiomyopathies and specific heart muscle diseases. Definitions, terminology, classifications and new and old approaches. *Postgrad Med J.* 1992;68(Suppl 1):S3–S6.

Grunig E, Tasman JA, Kucherer H, Franz W, Kubler W, Katus HA. Frequency and phenotypes of familial dilated cardiomyopathy. *J Am Coll Cardiol.* 1998;31:186–194.

Guimaraes GV, Bellotti G, Mocelin AO, Camargo PR, Bocchi EA. Cardiopulmonary exercise testing in children with heart failure secondary to idiopathic dilated cardiomyopathy. *Chest.* 2001;120: 816–824.

Gulati S, Bajpai A, Juneja R, Kabra M, Bagga A, Kalra V. Hypocalcemic heart failure masquerading as dilated cardiomyopathy. *Indian J Pediatr.* 2001;68:287–290.

Hada Y, Sakamoto T, Amano K, et al. Prevalence of hypertrophic cardiomyopathy in a population of adult Japanese workers as detected by echocardiographic screening. *Am J Cardiol.* 1987;59:183–184.

Hamroff G, Katz SD, Mancini D, et al. Addition of angiotensin II receptor blockade to maximal angiotensin-converting enzyme inhibition improves exercise capacity in patients with severe congestive heart failure. *Circulation.* 1999;99:990–992.

Harada K, Potter JD. Familial hypertrophic cardiomyopathy mutations from different functional regions of troponin T result in different effects on the pH and Ca2+ sensitivity of cardiac muscle contraction. *J Biol Chem.* 2004;279:14488–14495.

Harada K, Takahashi-Yanaga F, Minakami R, Morimoto S, Ohtsuki I. Functional consequences of the deletion mutation deltaGlu160 in human cardiac troponin T. *J Biochem.* 2000;127:263–268.

Harris KM, Spirito P, Maron MS, et al. Prevalence, clinical profile, and significance of left ventricular remodeling in the end-stage phase of hypertrophic cardiomyopathy. *Circulation.* 2006;114:216–225.

Hausse AO, Aggoun Y, Bonnet D, et al. Idebenone and reduced cardiac hypertrophy in Friedreich's ataxia. *Heart (BCS).* 2002;87:346–349.

Hecht GM, Klues HG, Roberts WC, Maron BJ. Coexistence of sudden cardiac death and end-stage heart failure in familial hypertrophic cardiomyopathy. *J Am Coll Cardiol.* 1993;22:489–497.

Heller MJ, Nili M, Homsher E, Tobacman LS. Cardiomyopathic tropomyosin mutations that increase thin filament Ca2+ sensitivity and tropomyosin N-domain flexibility. *J Biol Chem.* 2003;278: 41742–41748.

Henry WL, Gardin JM, Ware JH. Echocardiographic measurements in normal subjects from infancy to old age. *Circulation.* 1980;62:1054–1061.

Herskowitz A, Wu TC, Willoughby SB, et al. Myocarditis and cardiotropic viral infection associated with severe left ventricular dysfunction in late-stage infection with human immunodeficiency virus. *J Am Coll Cardiol.* 1994;24:1025–1032.

Hetzer R, Loebe M, Potapov EV, et al. Circulatory support with pneumatic paracorporeal ventricular assist device in infants and children. *Ann Thorac Surg.* 1998;66:1498–1506.

Hofman P, Drici MD, Gibelin P, Michiels JF, Thyss A. Prevalence of toxoplasma myocarditis in patients with the acquired immunodeficiency syndrome. *Br Heart J.* 1993;70:376–381.

Holmgren D, Wahlander H, Eriksson BO, Oldfors A, Holme E, Tulinius M. Cardiomyopathy in children with mitochondrial disease; clinical course and cardiological findings. *Eur Heart J.* 2003;24:280–288.

Hughes SE. The pathology of hypertrophic cardiomyopathy. *Histopathology.* 2004;44:412–427.

Hughes SE, McKenna WJ. New insights into the pathology of inherited cardiomyopathy. *Heart (BCS).* 2005;91:257–264.

Jacobson DR, Pastore RD, Yaghoubian R, et al. Variant-sequence transthyretin (isoleucine 122) in late-onset cardiac amyloidosis in black Americans. *N Eng J Med.* 1997;336:466–473.

James J, Zhang Y, Osinska H, et al. Transgenic modeling of a cardiac troponin I mutation linked to familial hypertrophic cardiomyopathy. *Circ Res.* 2000;87.805–811.

Jefferies JL, Denfield SW, Price JF, et al. A prospective evaluation of nesiritide in the treatment of pediatric heart failure. *Pediatr Cardiol.* 2006;27:402–407.

Jones S, Elliott PM, Sharma S, McKenna WJ, Whipp BJ. Cardiopulmonary responses to exercise in patients with hypertrophic cardiomyopathy. *Heart (BCS).* 1998;80:60–67.

Kamisago M, Sharma SD, DePalma SR, et al. Mutations in sarcomere protein genes as a cause of dilated cardiomyopathy. *N Eng J Med.* 2000;343:1688–1696.

Karam S, Raboisson MJ, Ducreux C, et al. A de novo mutation of the beta cardiac myosin heavy chain gene in an infantile restrictive cardiomyopathy. *Congenit Heart Dis.* 2008;3:138–143.

Kaski JP, Burch M, Elliott PM. Mutations in the cardiac Troponin C gene are a cause of idiopathic dilated cardiomyopathy in childhood. *Cardiol Young.* 2007a;17:675–677.

Kaski JP, Syrris P, Tome Esteban MT, et al. Idiopathic restrictive cardiomyopathy in children is caused by mutations in cardiac sarcomere protein genes. *Heart (BCS).* 2008;94(11):1478–1484.

Kaski JP, Syrris P, Tome Esteban MT, et al. Prevalence of sarcomere protein gene mutations in pre-adolescent children with hypertrophic cardiomyopathy. *Circulation: Cardiovascular Genetics.* 2009;2: 436–441.

Kaski JP, Tome Esteban MT, Lowe M, et al. Outcomes after implantable cardioverter-defibrillator treatment in children with hypertrophic cardiomyopathy. *Heart (BCS).* 2007b;93:372–374.

Kass S, MacRae C, Graber HL, et al. A gene defect that causes conduction system disease and dilated cardiomyopathy maps to chromosome 1p1–1q1. *Nat Gen.* 1994;7:546–551.

Kelley RI, Cheatham JP, Clark BJ, et al. X-linked dilated cardiomyopathy with neutropenia, growth retardation, and 3-methylglutaconic aciduria. *J Pediatr.* 1991;119:738–747.

Kimberling MT, Balzer DT, Hirsch R, Mendeloff E, Huddleston CB, Canter CE. Cardiac transplantation for pediatric restrictive cardiomyopathy: presentation, evaluation, and short-term outcome. *J Heart Lung Transplant.* 2002;21:455–459.

Kitazume H, Kramer JR, Krauthamer D, El Tobgi S, Proudfit WL, Sones FM. Myocardial bridges in obstructive hypertrophic cardiomyopathy. *Am Heart J.* 1983;106:131–135.

Kjekshus J, Apetrei E, Barrios V, et al. Rosuvastatin in older patients with systolic heart failure. *N Eng J Med.* 2007;357:2248–2261.

Klein RM, Jiang H, Niederacher D, et al. Frequency and quantity of the parvovirus B19 genome in endomyocardial biopsies from patients with suspected myocarditis or idiopathic left ventricular dysfunction. *Z Kardiol.* 2004;93:300–309.

Klinge L, Straub V, Neudorf U, et al. Safety and efficacy of recombinant acid alpha-glucosidase (rhGAA) in patients with classical infantile Pompe disease: results of a phase II clinical trial. *Neuromuscul Disord.* 2005;15:24–31.

Klues HG, Maron BJ, Dollar AL, Roberts WC. Diversity of structural mitral valve alterations in hypertrophic cardiomyopathy. *Circulation.* 1992;85:1651–1660.

Klues HG, Schiffers A, Maron BJ. Phenotypic spectrum and patterns of left ventricular hypertrophy in hypertrophic cardiomyopathy: morphologic observations and significance as assessed by two-dimensional echocardiography in 600 patients. *J Am Coll Cardiol.* 1995;26:1699–1708.

Knight C, Kurbaan AS, Seggewiss H, et al. Nonsurgical septal reduction for hypertrophic obstructive cardiomyopathy: outcome in the first series of patients. *Circulation.* 1997;95:2075–2081.

Knollmann BC, Kirchhof P, Sirenko SG, et al. Familial hypertrophic cardiomyopathy-linked mutant troponin T causes stress-induced ventricular tachycardia and Ca2+-dependent action potential remodeling. *Circ Res.* 2003;92:428–436.

Kobayashi T, Dong WJ, Burkart EM, Cheung HC, Solaro RJ. Effects of protein kinase C dependent phosphorylation and a familial hypertrophic cardiomyopathy-related mutation of cardiac troponin I on structural transition of troponin C and myofilament activation. *Biochemistry.* 2004;43:5996–6004.

Kohler J, Chen Y, Brenner B, et al. Familial hypertrophic cardiomyopathy mutations in troponin I (K183D, G203S, K206Q) enhance filament sliding. *Physiol Genomics.* 2003;14:117–128.

Krikler DM, Davies MJ, Rowland E, Goodwin JF, Evans RC, Shaw DB. Sudden death in hypertrophic cardiomyopathy: associated accessory atrioventricular pathways. *Br Heart J.* 1980;43:245–251.

Kubo T, Gimeno JR, Bahl A, et al. Prevalence, clinical significance, and genetic basis of hypertrophic cardiomyopathy with restrictive phenotype. *J Am Coll Cardiol.* 2007;49:2419–2426.

Kuhl U, Pauschinger M, Noutsias M, et al. High prevalence of viral genomes and multiple viral infections in the myocardium of adults with "idiopathic" left ventricular dysfunction. *Circulation.* 2005;111:887–893.

Kushwaha SS, Fallon JT, Fuster V. Restrictive Cardiomyopathy. *N Eng J Med.* 1997;336:267–276.

Kyle RA, Gertz MA. Primary systemic amyloidosis: clinical and laboratory features in 474 cases. *Semin Hematol.* 1995;32:45–59.

Labrune P, Bader B, Devictor D, Madelin JC, Huault G. Hypocalcemia, cardiac failure and ventricular tachycardia in an infant with rickets. *Arch Fr Pediatr.* 1986;43:413–415.

Lakkis NM, Nagueh SF, Dunn JK, Killip D, Spencer WH 3rd. Nonsurgical septal reduction therapy for hypertrophic obstructive cardiomyopathy: one-year follow-up. *J Am Coll Cardiol.* 2000;36:852–855.

Lammerding J, Schulze PC, Takahashi T, et al. Lamin A/C deficiency causes defective nuclear mechanics and mechanotransduction. *J Clin Invest.* 2004;113:370–378.

Lang R, Gomes AV, Zhao J, Housmans PR, Miller T, Potter JD. Functional analysis of a troponin I (R145G) mutation associated with familial hypertrophic cardiomyopathy. *J Biol Chem.* 2002;277:11670–11678.

Lechin M, Quinones MA, Omran A, et al. Angiotensin-I converting enzyme genotypes and left ventricular hypertrophy in patients with hypertrophic cardiomyopathy. *Circulation.* 1995;92:1808–1812.

Levi D, Marelli D, Plunkett M, et al. Use of assist devices and ECMO to bridge pediatric patients with cardiomyopathy to transplantation. *J Heart Lung Transplant.* 2002;21:760–770.

Lewis AB. Clinical profile and outcome of restrictive cardiomyopathy in children. *Am Heart J.* 1992;123:1589–1593.

Linhart A, Elliott PM. The heart in Anderson-Fabry disease and other lysosomal storage disorders. *Heart (BCS).* 2007;93:528–535.

Linhart A, Palecek T, Bultas J, et al. New insights in cardiac structural changes in patients with Fabry's disease. *Am Heart J.* 2000;139:1101–1108.

Lipshultz SE, Sleeper LA, Towbin JA, et al. The incidence of pediatric cardiomyopathy in two regions of the United States. *N Engl J Med.* 2003;348:1647–1655.

Magnani JW, Dec GW. Myocarditis: current trends in diagnosis and treatment. *Circulation.* 2006;113:876–890.

Mahle WT, Cuadrado AR, Kirshbom PM, Kanter KR, Simsic JM. Nesiritide in infants and children with congestive heart failure. *Pediatr Crit Care Med.* 2005;6:543–546.

Mahon NG, Murphy RT, MacRae CA, Caforio AL, Elliott PM, McKenna WJ. Echocardiographic evaluation in asymptomatic relatives of patients with dilated cardiomyopathy reveals preclinical disease. *Ann Intern Med.* 2005;143:108–115.

Maisch B, Richter A, Sandmoller A, Portig I, Pankuweit S. Inflammatory dilated cardiomyopathy (DCMI). *Herz.* 2005;30:535–544.

Maiya S, Sullivan I, Allgrove J, et al. Hypocalcaemia and vitamin D deficiency: an important, but preventable, cause of life-threatening infant heart failure. *Heart (BCS).* 2008;94:581–584.

Marian AJ, Roberts R. The molecular genetic basis for hypertrophic cardiomyopathy. *J Mol Cell Cardiol.* 2001;33:655–670.

Marian AJ, Yu QT, Workman R, Greve G, Roberts R. Angiotensin-converting enzyme polymorphism in hypertrophic cardiomyopathy and sudden cardiac death. *Lancet.* 1993;342:1085–1086.

Maron BJ. Hypertrophic cardiomyopathy in childhood. *Pediatr Clin North Am.* 2004;51:1305–1346.

Maron BJ, Bonow RO, Seshagiri TN, Roberts WC, Epstein SE. Hypertrophic cardiomyopathy with ventricular septal hypertrophy localized to the apical region of the left ventricle (apical hypertrophic cardiomyopathy). *Am J Cardiol.* 1982a;49:1838–1848.

Maron BJ, Carney KP, Lever HM, et al. Relationship of race to sudden cardiac death in competitive athletes with hypertrophic cardiomyopathy. *J Am Coll Cardiol.* 2003a;41:974–980.

Maron BJ, Casey SA, Poliac LC, Gohman TE, Almquist AK, Aeppli DM. Clinical course of hypertrophic cardiomyopathy in a regional United States cohort. *JAMA.* 1999a;281:650–655.

Maron BJ, Edwards JE, Henry WL, Clark CE, Bingle GJ, Epstein SE. Asymmetric septal hypertrophy (ASH) in infancy. *Circulation.* 1974;50:809–820.

Maron BJ, Estes NA 3rd, Maron MS, Almquist AK, Link MS, Udelson JE. Primary prevention of sudden death as a novel treatment strategy in hypertrophic cardiomyopathy. *Circulation.* 2003b;107:2872–2875.

Maron BJ, Gardin JM, Flack JM, Gidding SS, Kurosaki TT, Bild DE. Prevalence of hypertrophic cardiomyopathy in a general population of young adults. Echocardiographic analysis of 4111 subjects in the CARDIA Study. Coronary Artery Risk Development in (Young) Adults. *Circulation.* 1995;92:785–789.

Maron BJ, Gottdiener JS, Epstein SE. Patterns and significance of distribution of left ventricular hypertrophy in hypertrophic cardiomyopathy. A wide angle, two dimensional echocardiographic study of 125 patients. *Am J Cardiol.* 1981a;48:418–428.

Maron BJ, Hauser RG, Roberts WC. Hypertrophic cardiomyopathy with left ventricular apical diverticulum. *Am J Cardiol.* 1996;77:1263–1265.

Maron BJ, Henry WL, Clark CE, Redwood DR, Roberts WC, Epstein SE. Asymetric septal hypertrophy in childhood. *Circulation.* 1976;53:9–19.

Maron BJ, Lipson LC, Roberts WC, Savage DD, Epstein SE. "Malignant" hypertrophic cardiomyopathy: identification of a subgroup of families with unusually frequent premature death. *Am J Cardiol.* 1978;41:1133–1140.

Maron BJ, McKenna WJ, Danielson GK, et al. American College of Cardiology/European Society of Cardiology Clinical Expert Consensus Document on Hypertrophic Cardiomyopathy. A report of the American College of Cardiology Foundation Task Force on Clinical Expert Consensus Documents and the European Society of Cardiology Committee for Practice Guidelines. *Eur Heart J.* 2003c;24:1965–1991.

Maron BJ, Niimura H, Casey SA, et al. Development of left ventricular hypertrophy in adults in hypertrophic cardiomyopathy caused by cardiac myosin-binding protein C gene mutations. *J Am Coll Cardiol.* 2001;38:315–321.

Maron BJ, Nishimura RA, McKenna WJ, Rakowski H, Josephson ME, Kieval RS. Assessment of permanent dual-chamber pacing as a treatment for drug-refractory symptomatic patients with obstructive hypertrophic cardiomyopathy. A randomized, double-blind, crossover study (M-PATHY). *Circulation.* 1999b;99:2927–2933.

Maron BJ, Peterson EE, Maron MS, Peterson JE. Prevalence of hypertrophic cardiomyopathy in an outpatient population referred for echocardiographic study. *Am J Cardiol.* 1994;73:577–580.

Maron BJ, Roberts WC, Epstein SE. Sudden death in hypertrophic cardiomyopathy: a profile of 78 patients. *Circulation.* 1982b;65:1388–1394.

Maron BJ, Savage DD, Wolfson JK, Epstein SE. Prognostic significance of 24 hour ambulatory electrocardiographic monitoring in patients with hypertrophic cardiomyopathy: a prospective study. *Am J Cardiol.* 1981b;48:252–257.

Maron BJ, Shen WK, Link MS, et al. Efficacy of implantable cardioverter-defibrillators for the prevention of sudden death in patients with hypertrophic cardiomyopathy. *N Eng J Med.* 2000;342:365–373.

Maron BJ, Spirito P. Implications of left ventricular remodeling in hypertrophic cardiomyopathy. *Am J Cardiol.* 1998;81:1339–1344.

Maron BJ, Spirito P, Shen WK, et al. Implantable cardioverter-defibrillators and prevention of sudden cardiac death in hypertrophic cardiomyopathy. *JAMA.* 2007;298:405–412.

Maron BJ, Spirito P, Wesley Y, Arce J. Development and progression of left ventricular hypertrophy in children with hypertrophic cardiomyopathy. *N Eng J Med.* 1986a;315:610–614.

Maron BJ, Tajik AJ, Ruttenberg HD, et al. Hypertrophic cardiomyopathy in infants: clinical features and natural history. *Circulation.* 1982c;65:7–17

Maron BJ, Wolfson JK, Epstein SE, Roberts WC. Intramural ("small vessel") coronary artery disease in hypertrophic cardiomyopathy. *J Am Coll Cardiol.* 1986b;8:545–557.

Maron MS, Olivotto I, Betocchi S, et al. Effect of left ventricular outflow tract obstruction on clinical outcome in hypertrophic cardiomyopathy. *N Eng J Med.* 2003d;348:295–303.

Maron MS, Olivotto I, Zenovich AG, et al. Hypertrophic cardiomyopathy is predominantly a disease of left ventricular outflow tract obstruction. *Circulation.* 2006;114:2232–2239.

Martin AB, Webber S, Fricker FJ, et al. Acute myocarditis. Rapid diagnosis by PCR in children. *Circulation.* 1994;90:330–339.

Massie BM, Fisher SG, Radford M, et al. Effect of amiodarone on clinical status and left ventricular function in patients with congestive heart failure. CHF-STAT Investigators. *Circulation.* 1996;93:2128–2134.

Matsumura Y, Elliott PM, Virdee MS, Sorajja P, Doi Y, McKenna WJ. Left ventricular diastolic function assessed using Doppler tissue imaging in patients with hypertrophic cardiomyopathy: relation to symptoms and exercise capacity. *Heart (BCS).* 2002;87:247–251.

McCarthy RE 3rd, Kasper EK. A review of the amyloidoses that infiltrate the heart. *Clin Cardiol.* 1998;21:547–552.

McKelvie RS, Yusuf S, Pericak D, et al. Comparison of candesartan, enalapril, and their combination in congestive heart failure: randomized evaluation of strategies for left ventricular dysfunction (RESOLVD) pilot study. The RESOLVD Pilot Study Investigators. *Circulation.* 1999;100:1056–1064.

McKenna W, Deanfield J, Faruqui A, England D, Oakley C, Goodwin J. Prognosis in hypertrophic cardiomyopathy: role of age and clinical, electrocardiographic and hemodynamic features. *Am J Cardiol.* 1981a;47:532–538.

McKenna WJ, Behr ER. Hypertrophic cardiomyopathy: management, risk stratification, and prevention of sudden death. *Heart (BCS).* 2002;87:169–176.

McKenna WJ, Deanfield JE. Hypertrophic cardiomyopathy: an important cause of sudden death. *Arch Dis Child.* 1984;59:971–975.

McKenna WJ, England D, Doi YL, Deanfield JE, Oakley C, Goodwin JF. Arrhythmia in hypertrophic cardiomyopathy. I: influence on prognosis. *Br Heart J.* 1981b;46:168–172.

McKenna WJ, Franklin RC, Nihoyannopoulos P, Robinson KC, Deanfield JE. Arrhythmia and prognosis in infants, children and adolescents with hypertrophic cardiomyopathy. *J Am Coll Cardiol.* 1988;11:147–153.

McKenna WJ, Oakley CM, Krikler DM, Goodwin JF. Improved survival with amiodarone in patients with hypertrophic cardiomyopathy and ventricular tachycardia. *Br Heart J.* 1985;53:412–416.

McKenna WJ, Spirito P, Desnos M, Dubourg O, Komajda M. Experience from clinical genetics in hypertrophic cardiomyopathy: proposal for new diagnostic criteria in adult members of affected families. *Heart (BCS).* 1997;77:130–132.

McMahon AM, van DC, Burch M, et al. Improved early outcome for end-stage dilated cardiomyopathy in children. *J Thorac Cardiovasc Surg.* 2003;126:1781–1787.

McMahon CJ, Nagueh SF, Pignatelli RH, et al. Characterization of left ventricular diastolic function by tissue Doppler imaging and clinical status in children with hypertrophic cardiomyopathy. *Circulation.* 2004;109:1756–1762.

Mehta A, Ricci R, Widmer U, et al. Fabry disease defined: baseline clinical manifestations of 366 patients in the Fabry Outcome Survey. *Eur J Clin Inves.* 2004;34:236–242.

Michele DE, Albayya FP, Metzger JM. Direct, convergent hypersensitivity of calcium-activated force generation produced by hypertrophic cardiomyopathy mutant alpha-tropomyosins in adult cardiac myocytes. *Nat Med.* 1999;5:1413–1417.

Michele DE, Gomez CA, Hong KE, Westfall MV, Metzger JM. Cardiac dysfunction in hypertrophic cardiomyopathy mutant tropomyosin mice is transgene-dependent, hypertrophy-independent, and improved by beta-blockade. *Circ Res.* 2002;91:255–262.

Micheletti R, Palazzo F, Barassi P, et al. Istaroxime, a stimulator of sarcoplasmic reticulum calcium adenosine triphosphatase isoform 2a activity, as a novel therapeutic approach to heart failure. *Am J Cardiol.* 2007;99:24A–32A.

Miller T, Szczesna D, Housmans PR, et al. Abnormal contractile function in transgenic mice expressing a familial hypertrophic cardiomyopathy-linked troponin T (I79N) mutation. *J Biol Chem.* 2001;276:3743–3755.

Mogensen J, Kubo T, Duque M, et al. Idiopathic restrictive cardiomyopathy is part of the clinical expression of cardiac troponin I mutations. *J Clin Invest.* 2003;111:209–216.

Mogensen J, Murphy RT, Shaw T, et al. Severe disease expression of cardiac troponin C and T mutations in patients with idiopathic dilated cardiomyopathy. *J Am Coll Cardiol.* 2004;44:2033–2040.

Mogensen J, Arbustini E. Restrictive cardiomyopathy. *Curr Opin Cardiol.* 2009;24(3):214–220.

Monserrat L, Elliott PM, Gimeno JR, Sharma S, Penas-Lado M, McKenna WJ. Non-sustained ventricular tachycardia in hypertrophic cardiomyopathy: an independent marker of sudden death risk in young patients. *J Am Coll Cardiol.* 2003;42:873–879.

Moon JC, McKenna WJ, McCrohon JA, Elliott PM, Smith GC, Pennell DJ. Toward clinical risk assessment in hypertrophic cardiomyopathy with gadolinium cardiovascular magnetic resonance. *J Am Coll Cardiol.* 2003;41:1561–1567.

Morimoto S, Lu QW, Harada K, et al. Ca(2+)-desensitizing effect of a deletion mutation Delta K210 in cardiac troponin T that causes familial dilated cardiomyopathy. *Proc Natl Acad Sci USA.* 2002;99:913–918.

Morita H, Larson MG, Barr SC, et al. Single-gene mutations and increased left ventricular wall thickness in the community: the Framingham Heart Study. *Circulation.* 2006;113:2697–2705.

Morita H, Rehm HL, Menesses A, et al. Shared genetic causes of cardiac hypertrophy in children and adults. *N Eng J Med.* 2008;358:1899–1908.

Morrow AG, Reitz BA, Epstein SE, et al. Operative treatment in hypertrophic subaortic stenosis. Techniques, and the results of pre and postoperative assessments in 83 patients. *Circulation.* 1975;52:88–102.

Muchir A, Bonne G, van der Kooi AJ, et al. Identification of mutations in the gene encoding lamins A/C in autosomal dominant limb girdle muscular dystrophy with atrioventricular conduction disturbances (LGMD1B). *Hum Mol Genet.* 2000;9:1453–1459.

Munro K, Croxson MC, Thomas S, Wilson NJ. Three cases of myocarditis in childhood associated with human parvovirus (B19 virus). *Pediatr Cardiol.* 2003;24:473–475.

Muntoni F, Cau M, Ganau A, et al. Brief report: deletion of the dystrophin muscle-promoter region associated with X-linked dilated cardiomyopathy. *N Eng J Med.* 1993;329:921–925.

Murphy RT, Mogensen J, McGarry K, et al. Adenosine monophosphate-activated protein kinase disease mimicks hypertrophic cardiomyopathy and Wolff-Parkinson-White syndrome: natural history. *J Am Coll Cardiol.* 2005;45:922–930.

Murry CE, Jerome KR, Reichenbach DD. Fatal parvovirus myocarditis in a 5-year-old girl. *Hum Pathol.* 2001;32:342–345.

Nagueh SF, Bachinski LL, Meyer D, et al. Tissue Doppler imaging consistently detects myocardial abnormalities in patients with hypertrophic cardiomyopathy and provides a novel means for an early diagnosis before and independently of hypertrophy. *Circulation.* 2001;104:128–130.

Niimura H, Bachinski LL, Sangwatanaroj S, et al. Mutations in the gene for cardiac myosin-binding protein C and late-onset familial hypertrophic cardiomyopathy. *N Eng J Med.* 1998;338:1248–1257.

Nishimura RA, Trusty JM, Hayes DL, et al. Dual-chamber pacing for hypertrophic cardiomyopathy: a randomized, double-blind, crossover trial. *J Am Coll Cardiol.* 1997;29:435–441.

Nishino I, Fu J, Tanji K, et al. Primary LAMP-2 deficiency causes X-linked vacuolar cardiomyopathy and myopathy (Danon disease). *Nature.* 2000;406:906–910.

Noonan JA. Hypertelorism with Turner phenotype. A new syndrome with associated congenital heart disease. *Am J Dis Child (1960).* 1968;116:373–380.

Noonan JA, Ehmke DA. Associated Noncardiac Malformations in Children with Congenital Heart Disease. *J Pediatr.* 1963;63:468.

Noutsias M, Seeberg B, Schultheiss HP, Kuhl U. Expression of cell adhesion molecules in dilated cardiomyopathy: evidence for endothelial activation in inflammatory cardiomyopathy. *Circulation.* 1999;99:2124–2131.

Nugent AW, Daubeney PE, Chondros P, et al. The epidemiology of childhood cardiomyopathy in Australia. *N Engl J Med.* 2003;348:1639–1646.

Nugent AW, Daubeney PE, Chondros P, et al. Clinical features and outcomes of childhood hypertrophic cardiomyopathy: results from a national population-based study. *Circulation.* 2005;112:1332–1338.

Oberst L, Zhao G, Park JT, et al. Dominant-negative effect of a mutant cardiac troponin T on cardiac structure and function in transgenic mice. *J Clin Invest.* 1998;102:1498–1505.

Okeie K, Shimizu M, Yoshio H, et al. Left ventricular systolic dysfunction during exercise and dobutamine stress in patients with hypertrophic cardiomyopathy. *J Am Coll Cardiol.* 2000;36:856–863.

Olivotto I, Cecchi F, Casey SA, Dolara A, Traverse JH, Maron BJ. Impact of atrial fibrillation on the clinical course of hypertrophic cardiomyopathy. *Circulation.* 2001;104:2517–2524.

Olivotto I, Maron BJ, Montereggi A, Mazzuoli F, Dolara A, Cecchi F. Prognostic value of systemic blood pressure response during exercise in a community-based patient population with hypertrophic cardiomyopathy. *J Am Coll Cardiol.* 1999;33:2044–2051.

Olson TM, Kishimoto NY, Whitby FG, Michels VV. Mutations that alter the surface charge of alpha-tropomyosin are associated with dilated cardiomyopathy. *J Mol Cell Cardiol.* 2001;33:723–732.

Olson TM, Michels VV, Thibodeau SN, Tai YS, Keating MT. Actin mutations in dilated cardiomyopathy, a heritable form of heart failure. *Science (New York).* 1998;280:750–752.

Olsson MC, Palmer BM, Leinwand LA, Moore RL. Gender and aging in a transgenic mouse model of hypertrophic cardiomyopathy. *Am J Physiol.* 2001;280:H1136–H1144.

Ommen SR, Maron BJ, Olivotto I, et al. Long-term effects of surgical septal myectomy on survival in patients with obstructive hypertrophic cardiomyopathy. *J Am Coll Cardiol.* 2005;46:470–476.

Osio A, Tan L, Chen SN, et al. Myozenin 2 is a novel gene for human hypertrophic cardiomyopathy. *Circ Res.* 2007;100:766–768.

Ostman-Smith I, Wettrell G, Riesenfeld T. A cohort study of childhood hypertrophic cardiomyopathy: improved survival following high-dose beta-adrenoceptor antagonist treatment. *J Am Coll Cardiol.* 1999;34:1813–1822.

Packer M, Bristow MR, Cohn JN, et al. The effect of carvedilol on morbidity and mortality in patients with chronic heart failure. U.S. Carvedilol Heart Failure Study Group. *N Eng J Med.* 1996;334:1349–1355.

Packer M, Coats AJ, Fowler MB, et al. Effect of carvedilol on survival in severe chronic heart failure. *N Eng J Med.* 2001;344:1651–1658.

Packer M, Gheorghiade M, Young JB, et al. Withdrawal of digoxin from patients with chronic heart failure treated with angiotensin-converting-enzyme inhibitors. RADIANCE Study. *N Eng J Med.* 1993;329:1–7.

Packer M, Poole-Wilson PA, Armstrong PW, et al. Comparative effects of low and high doses of the angiotensin-converting enzyme inhibitor, lisinopril, on morbidity and mortality in chronic heart failure. ATLAS Study Group. *Circulation.* 1999;100:2312–2318.

Palmer BM, Fishbaugher DE, Schmitt JP, et al. Differential cross-bridge kinetics of FHC myosin mutations R403Q and R453C in heterozygous mouse myocardium. *Am J Physiol.* 2004;287:H91–H99.

Palmiter KA, Tyska MJ, Haeberle JR, Alpert NR, Fananapazir L, Warshaw DM. R403Q and L908V mutant beta-cardiac myosin from patients with familial hypertrophic cardiomyopathy exhibit enhanced mechanical performance at the single molecule level. *J Muscle Res Cell Motil.* 2000;21:609–620.

Pandit B, Sarkozy A, Pennacchio LA, et al. Gain-of-function RAF1 mutations cause Noonan and LEOPARD syndromes with hypertrophic cardiomyopathy. *Nat Gen.* 2007;39:1007–1012.

Parrillo JE, Aretz HT, Palacios I, Fallon JT, Block PC. The results of transvenous endomyocardial biopsy can frequently be used to diagnose myocardial diseases in patients with idiopathic heart failure. Endomyocardial biopsies in 100 consecutive patients revealed a substantial incidence of myocarditis. *Circulation.* 1984;69:93–101.

Peddy SB, Vricella LA, Crosson JE, et al. Infantile restrictive cardiomyopathy resulting from a mutation in the cardiac troponin T gene. *Pediatrics.* 2006;117:1830–1833.

Perrone-Filardi P, Bacharach SL, Dilsizian V, Panza JA, Maurea S, Bonow RO. Regional systolic function, myocardial blood flow and glucose uptake at rest in hypertrophic cardiomyopathy. *Am J Cardiol.* 1993;72:199–204.

Pfeffer MA, Swedberg K, Granger CB, et al. Effects of candesartan on mortality and morbidity in patients with chronic heart failure: the CHARM-Overall programme. *Lancet.* 2003;362:759–766.

Pitt B, Poole-Wilson P, Segal R, et al. Effects of losartan versus captopril on mortality in patients with symptomatic heart failure: rationale, design, and baseline characteristics of patients in the Losartan Heart Failure Survival Study—ELITE II. *J Card Fail.* 1999a;5:146–154.

Pitt B, Segal R, Martinez FA, et al. Randomised trial of losartan versus captopril in patients over 65 with heart failure (Evaluation of Losartan in the Elderly Study, ELITE). *Lancet.* 1997;349:747–752.

Pitt B, Zannad F, Remme WJ, et al. The effect of spironolactone on morbidity and mortality in patients with severe heart failure. Randomized Aldactone Evaluation Study Investigators. *N Eng J Med.* 1999b;341:709–717.

Politano L, Nigro V, Nigro G, et al. Development of cardiomyopathy in female carriers of Duchenne and Becker muscular dystrophies. *JAMA.* 1996;275:1335–1338.

Pollick C. Disopyramide in hypertrophic cardiomyopathy. II. Noninvasive assessment after oral administration. *Am J Cardiol.* 1988;62:1252–1255.

Pollick C, Kimball B, Henderson M, Wigle ED. Disopyramide in hypertrophic cardiomyopathy. I. Hemodynamic assessment after intravenous administration. *Am J Cardiol.* 1988;62:1248–1251.

Posma JL, Blanksma PK, Van Der Wall EE, Vaalburg W, Crijns HJ, Lie KI. Effects of permanent dual chamber pacing on myocardial perfusion in symptomatic hypertrophic cardiomyopathy. *Heart (BCS)*. 1996;76:358–362.

Poutanen T, Tikanoja T, Jaaskelainen P, et al. Diastolic dysfunction without left ventricular hypertrophy is an early finding in children with hypertrophic cardiomyopathy-causing mutations in the beta-myosin heavy chain, alpha-tropomyosin, and myosin-binding protein C genes. *Am Heart J*. 2006;151:725 e721–725, e729.

Prabhakar R, Boivin GP, Grupp IL, et al. A familial hypertrophic cardiomyopathy alpha-tropomyosin mutation causes severe cardiac hypertrophy and death in mice. *J Mol Cell Cardiol*. 2001;33:1815–1828.

Prabhakar R, Petrashevskaya N, Schwartz A, et al. A mouse model of familial hypertrophic cardiomyopathy caused by a alpha-tropomyosin mutation. *Mol Cell Biochem*. 2003;251:33–42.

Prall FR, Drack A, Taylor M, et al. Ophthalmic manifestations of Danon disease. *Ophthalmology*. 2006;113:1010–1013.

Price DI, Stanford LC Jr, Braden DS, Ebeid MR, Smith JC. Hypocalcemic rickets: an unusual cause of dilated cardiomyopathy. *Pediatr Cardiol*. 2003;24:510–512.

Price JF, Thomas AK, Grenier M, et al. B-type natriuretic peptide predicts adverse cardiovascular events in pediatric outpatients with chronic left ventricular systolic dysfunction. *Circulation*. 2006;114:1063–1069.

Ramasubbu K, Estep J, White DL, Deswal A, Mann DL. Experimental and clinical basis for the use of statins in patients with ischemic and nonischemic cardiomyopathy. *J Am Coll Cardiol*. 2008;51:415–426.

Rathore SS, Curtis JP, Wang Y, Bristow MR, Krumholz HM. Association of serum digoxin concentration and outcomes in patients with heart failure. *JAMA*. 2003;289:871–878.

Razzaque MA, Nishizawa T, Komoike Y, et al. Germline gain-of-function mutations in RAF1 cause Noonan syndrome. *Nat Gen*. 2007; 39:1013–1017.

Redwood C, Lohmann K, Bing W, et al. Investigation of a truncated cardiac troponin T that causes familial hypertrophic cardiomyopathy: Ca(2+) regulatory properties of reconstituted thin filaments depend on the ratio of mutant to wild-type protein. *Circ Res*. 2000;86:1146–1152.

Redwood CS, Moolman-Smook JC, Watkins H. Properties of mutant contractile proteins that cause hypertrophic cardiomyopathy. *Cardiovasc Res*. 1999;44:20–36.

Richard P, Charron P, Carrier L, et al. Hypertrophic cardiomyopathy: distribution of disease genes, spectrum of mutations, and implications for a molecular diagnosis strategy. *Circulation*. 2003;107:2227–2232.

Richardson P, McKenna W, Bristow M, et al. Report of the 1995 World Health Organization/International Society and Federation of Cardiology Task Force on the Definition and Classification of cardiomyopathies. *Circulation*. 1996;93:841–842.

Rishi F, Hulse JE, Auld DO, et al. Effects of dual-chamber pacing for pediatric patients with hypertrophic obstructive cardiomyopathy. *J Am Coll Cardiol*. 1997;29:734–740.

Rivenes SM, Kearney DL, Smith EOB, Towbin JA, Denfield SW. Sudden Death and Cardiovascular Collapse in Children With Restrictive Cardiomyopathy. *Circulation*. 2000;102:876–882.

Roberts AE, Araki T, Swanson KD, et al. Germline gain-of-function mutations in SOS1 cause Noonan syndrome. *Nat Gen*. 2007;39:70–74.

Robinson K, Frenneaux MP, Stockins B, Karatasakis G, Poloniecki JD, McKenna WJ. Atrial fibrillation in hypertrophic cardiomyopathy: a longitudinal study. *J Am Coll Cardiol*. 1990;15:1279–1285.

Rogers DP, Marazia S, Chow AW, et al. Effect of biventricular pacing on symptoms and cardiac remodelling in patients with end-stage hypertrophic cardiomyopathy. *Eur J Heart Fail*. 2008;10(5):507–513.

Rohayem J, Dinger J, Fischer R, Klingel K, Kandolf R, Rethwilm A. Fatal myocarditis associated with acute parvovirus B19 and human herpesvirus 6 coinfection. *J Clin Microbiol*. 2001;39:4585–4587.

Roopnarine O. Mechanical defects of muscle fibers with myosin light chain mutants that cause cardiomyopathy. *Biophys J*. 2003;84:2440–2449.

Rosenthal D, Chrisant MR, Edens E, et al. International Society for Heart and Lung Transplantation: practice guidelines for management of heart failure in children. *J Heart Lung Transplant*. 2004;23:1313–1333.

Russo LM, Webber SA. Idiopathic restrictive cardiomyopathy in children. *Heart (BCS)*. 2005;91:1199–1202.

Sadoul N, Prasad K, Elliott PM, Bannerjee S, Frenneaux MP, McKenna WJ. Prospective prognostic assessment of blood pressure response during exercise in patients with hypertrophic cardiomyopathy. *Circulation*. 1997;96:2987–2991.

Saraiva MJ. Transthyretin mutations in health and disease. *Hum Mut*. 1995;5:191–196.

Satoh M, Takahashi M, Sakamoto T, Hiroe M, Marumo F, Kimura A. Structural analysis of the titin gene in hypertrophic cardiomyopathy: identification of a novel disease gene. *Biochem Biophys Res Commun*. 1999;262:411–417.

Scaglia F, Towbin JA, Craigen WJ, et al. Clinical spectrum, morbidity, and mortality in 113 pediatric patients with mitochondrial disease. *Pediatrics*. 2004;114:925–931.

Schaffer MS, Freedom RM, Rowe RD. Hypertrophic cardiomyopathy presenting before 2 years of age in 13 patients. *Pediatr Cardiol*. 1983;4:113–119.

Schowengerdt KO, Ni J, Denfield SW, et al. Association of parvovirus B19 genome in children with myocarditis and cardiac allograft rejection: diagnosis using the polymerase chain reaction. *Circulation*. 1997;96:3549–3554.

Schubbert S, Zenker M, Rowe SL, et al. Germline KRAS mutations cause Noonan syndrome. *Nat Gen*. 2006;38:331–336.

Schulte HD, Bircks WH, Loesse B, Godehardt EA, Schwartzkopff B. Prognosis of patients with hypertrophic obstructive cardiomyopathy after transaortic myectomy. Late results up to twenty-five years. *J Thorac Cardiovasc Surg*. 1993;106:709–717.

Schwartz ML, Cox GF, Lin AE, et al. Clinical approach to genetic cardiomyopathy in children. *Circulation*. 1996;94:2021–2038.

Seidman JG, Seidman C. The genetic basis for cardiomyopathy: from mutation identification to mechanistic paradigms. *Cell*. 2001;104:557–567.

Seiler C, Jenni R, Vassalli G, Turina M, Hess OM. Left ventricular chamber dilatation in hypertrophic cardiomyopathy: related variables and prognosis in patients with medical and surgical therapy. *Br Heart J*. 1995;74:508–516.

Shackleton S, Lloyd DJ, Jackson SN, et al. LMNA, encoding lamin A/C, is mutated in partial lipodystrophy. *Nat Gen*. 2000;24:153–156.

Shaddy RE, Boucek MM, Hsu DT, et al. Carvedilol for children and adolescents with heart failure: a randomized controlled trial. *JAMA*. 2007;298:1171–1179.

Shah JS, Esteban MT, Thaman R, et al. Prevalence of Exercise Induced Left Ventricular Outflow Tract Obstruction in Symptomatic Patients with Non-obstructive Hypertrophic Cardiomyopathy. *Heart (BCS)*. 2008;94(10):1288–1294.

Shah JS, Hughes DA, Sachdev B, et al. Prevalence and clinical significance of cardiac arrhythmia in Anderson-Fabry disease. *Am J Cardiol*. 2005;96:842–846.

Shah KB, Inoue Y, Mehra MR. Amyloidosis and the heart: a comprehensive review. *Arch Intern Med*. 2006;166:1805–1813.

Shaper AG, Hutt MS, Coles RM. Necropsy study of endomyocardial fibrosis and rheumatic heart disease in Uganda 1950–1965. *Br Heart J*. 1968;30:391–401.

Shapiro LM, McKenna WJ. Distribution of left ventricular hypertrophy in hypertrophic cardiomyopathy: a two-dimensional echocardiographic study. *J Am Coll Cardiol*. 1983;2:437–444.

Sharland M, Burch M, McKenna WM, Paton MA. A clinical study of Noonan syndrome. *Arch Dis Child*. 1992;67:178–183.

Sharma S, Elliott P, Whyte G, et al. Utility of cardiopulmonary exercise in the assessment of clinical determinants of functional capacity in hypertrophic cardiomyopathy. *Am J Cardiol*. 2000;86:162–168.

Sherrid M, Delia E, Dwyer E. Oral disopyramide therapy for obstructive hypertrophic cardiomyopathy. *Am J Cardiol*. 1988;62:1085–1088.

Shimizu C, Rambaud C, Cheron G, et al. Molecular identification of viruses in sudden infant death associated with myocarditis and pericarditis. *Pediatr Infect Dis J*. 1995;14:584–588.

Silka MJ, Kron J, Dunnigan A, Dick M 2nd. Sudden cardiac death and the use of implantable cardioverter-defibrillators in pediatric patients. The Pediatric Electrophysiology Society. *Circulation*. 1993;87:800–807.

Sirajuddin RA, Miller AB, Geraci SA. Anticoagulation in patients with dilated cardiomyopathy and sinus rhythm: a critical literature review. *J Card Fail*. 2002;8:48–53.

Skinner JR, Manzoor A, Hayes AM, Joffe HS, Martin RP. A regional study of presentation and outcome of hypertrophic cardiomyopathy in infants. *Heart (BCS).* 1997;77:229–233.

Spindler M, Saupe KW, Christe ME, et al. Diastolic dysfunction and altered energetics in the alphaMHC403/+ mouse model of familial hypertrophic cardiomyopathy. *J Clin Invest.* 1998;101:1775–1783.

Spirito P, Bellone P, Harris KM, Bernabo P, Bruzzi P, Maron BJ. Magnitude of left ventricular hypertrophy and risk of sudden death in hypertrophic cardiomyopathy. *N Eng J Med.* 2000;342:1778–1785.

Spirito P, Lakatos E, Maron BJ. Degree of left ventricular hypertrophy in patients with hypertrophic cardiomyopathy and chronic atrial fibrillation. *Am J Cardiol.* 1992;69:1217–1222.

Spirito P, Maron BJ, Bonow RO, Epstein SE. Occurrence and significance of progressive left ventricular wall thinning and relative cavity dilatation in hypertrophic cardiomyopathy. *Am J Cardiol.* 1987;60:123–129.

Spirito P, Rapezzi C, Bellone P, et al. Infective endocarditis in hypertrophic cardiomyopathy: prevalence, incidence, and indications for antibiotic prophylaxis. *Circulation.* 1999;99:2132–2137.

Sugie K, Yamamoto A, Murayama K, et al. Clinicopathological features of genetically confirmed Danon disease. *Neurology.* 2002;58:1773–1778.

Sullivan T, Escalante-Alcalde D, Bhatt H, et al. Loss of A-type lamin expression compromises nuclear envelope integrity leading to muscular dystrophy. *J Cell Biol.* 1999;147:913–920.

Szczesna D, Ghosh D, Li Q, et al. Familial hypertrophic cardiomyopathy mutations in the regulatory light chains of myosin affect their structure, Ca2+ binding, and phosphorylation. *J Biol Chem.* 2001;276:7086–7092.

Szczesna D, Zhang R, Zhao J, Jones M, Guzman G, Potter JD. Altered regulation of cardiac muscle contraction by troponin T mutations that cause familial hypertrophic cardiomyopathy. *J Biol Chem.* 2000;275:624–630.

Tabata T, Oki T, Yamada H, Abe M, Onose Y, Thomas JD. Subendocardial motion in hypertrophic cardiomyopathy: assessment from long- and short-axis views by pulsed tissue Doppler imaging. *J Am Soc Echocardiogr.* 2000;13:108–115.

Tardiff JC, Factor SM, Tompkins BD, et al. A truncated cardiac troponin T molecule in transgenic mice suggests multiple cellular mechanisms for familial hypertrophic cardiomyopathy. *J Clin Invest.* 1998;101:2800–2811.

Tardiff JC, Hewett TE, Palmer BM, et al. Cardiac troponin T mutations result in allele-specific phenotypes in a mouse model for hypertrophic cardiomyopathy. *J Clin Invest.* 1999;104:469–481.

Tartaglia M, Gelb BD. Noonan syndrome and related disorders: genetics and pathogenesis. *Annu Rev Genomics Hum Genet.* 2005;6:45–68.

Tartaglia M, Kalidas K, Shaw A, et al. PTPN11 mutations in Noonan syndrome: molecular spectrum, genotype-phenotype correlation, and phenotypic heterogeneity. *Am J Hum Gen.* 2002;70:1555–1563.

Tartaglia M, Mehler EL, Goldberg R, et al. Mutations in PTPN11, encoding the protein tyrosine phosphatase SHP-2, cause Noonan syndrome. *Nat Gen.* 2001;29:465–468.

Tartaglia M, Pennacchio LA, Zhao C, et al. Gain-of-function SOS1 mutations cause a distinctive form of Noonan syndrome. *Nat Gen.* 2007;39:75–79.

ten Cate FJ, Roelandt J. Progression to left ventricular dilatation in patients with hypertrophic obstructive cardiomyopathy. *Am Heart J.* 1979;97:762–765.

Thaman R, Gimeno JR, Murphy RT, et al. Prevalence and clinical significance of systolic impairment in hypertrophic cardiomyopathy. *Heart (BCS).* 2005;91:920–925.

Thaman R, Gimeno JR, Reith S, et al. Progressive left ventricular remodeling in patients with hypertrophic cardiomyopathy and severe left ventricular hypertrophy. *J Am Coll Cardiol.* 2004;44:398–405.

Thaman R, Varnava A, Hamid MS, et al. Pregnancy related complications in women with hypertrophic cardiomyopathy. *Heart (BCS).* 2003;89:752–756.

Theodoro DA, Danielson GK, Feldt RH, Anderson BJ. Hypertrophic obstructive cardiomyopathy in pediatric patients: results of surgical treatment. *J Thorac Cardiovasc Surg.* 1996;112:1589–1597; discussion 1597–1589.

Tome Esteban MT, Kaski JP. Hypertrophic cardiomyopathy in children. *Paediatr Child Health.* 2007;17:19–24.

Towbin JA, Bowles NE. The failing heart. *Nature.* 2002;415:227–233.

Towbin JA, Hejtmancik JF, Brink P, et al. X-linked dilated cardiomyopathy. Molecular genetic evidence of linkage to the Duchenne muscular dystrophy (dystrophin) gene at the Xp21 locus. *Circulation.* 1993;87:1854–1865.

Towbin JA, Lowe AM, Colan SD, et al. Incidence, causes, and outcomes of dilated cardiomyopathy in children. *JAMA.* 2006;296:1867–1876.

Tsubata S, Bowles KR, Vatta M, et al. Mutations in the human delta-sarcoglycan gene in familial and sporadic dilated cardiomyopathy. *J Clin Invest.* 2000;106:655–662.

Tyska MJ, Hayes E, Giewat M, Seidman CE, Seidman JG, Warshaw DM. Single-molecule mechanics of R403Q cardiac myosin isolated from the mouse model of familial hypertrophic cardiomyopathy. *Circ Res.* 2000;86:737–744.

Udelson JE, Bonow RO, O'Gara PT, et al. Verapamil prevents silent myocardial perfusion abnormalities during exercise in asymptomatic patients with hypertrophic cardiomyopathy. *Circulation.* 1989;79:1052–1060.

Van Driest SL, Ackerman MJ, Ommen SR, et al. Prevalence and severity of "benign" mutations in the beta-myosin heavy chain, cardiac troponin T, and alpha-tropomyosin genes in hypertrophic cardiomyopathy. *Circulation.* 2002;106:3085–3090.

Webb JG, Sasson Z, Rakowski H, Liu P, Wigle ED. Apical hypertrophic cardiomyopathy: clinical follow-up and diagnostic correlates. *J Am Coll Cardiol.* 1990;15:83–90.

Weller RJ, Weintraub R, Addonizio LJ, Chrisant MR, Gersony WM, Hsu DT. Outcome of idiopathic restrictive cardiomyopathy in children. *Am J Cardiol.* 2002;90:501–506.

Wessely R, Klingel K, Santana LF, et al. Transgenic expression of replication-restricted enteroviral genomes in heart muscle induces defective excitation-contraction coupling and dilated cardiomyopathy. *J Clin Invest.* 1998;102:1444–1453.

Westfall MV, Borton AR, Albayya FP, Metzger JM. Myofilament calcium sensitivity and cardiac disease: insights from troponin I isoforms and mutants. *Circ Res.* 2002;91:525–531.

Wigle ED, Rakowski H, Kimball BP, Williams WG. Hypertrophic cardiomyopathy. Clinical spectrum and treatment. *Circulation.* 1995;92:1680–1692.

Wigle ED, Sasson Z, Henderson MA, et al. Hypertrophic cardiomyopathy. The importance of the site and the extent of hypertrophy. A review. *Prog Cardiovasc Dis.* 1985;28:1–83.

Willenheimer R, van Veldhuisen DJ, Silke B, et al. Effect on survival and hospitalization of initiating treatment for chronic heart failure with bisoprolol followed by enalapril, as compared with the opposite sequence: results of the randomized Cardiac Insufficiency Bisoprolol Study (CIBIS) III. *Circulation.* 2005;112:2426–2435.

Williams WG, Wigle ED, Rakowski H, Smallhorn J, LeBlanc J, Trusler GA. Results of surgery for hypertrophic obstructive cardiomyopathy. *Circulation.* 1987;76:V104–V108.

Wilson W, Taubert KA, Gewitz M, et al. Prevention of infective endocarditis: guidelines from the American Heart Association: a guideline from the American Heart Association Rheumatic Fever, Endocarditis and Kawasaki Disease Committee, Council on Cardiovascular Disease in the Young, and the Council on Clinical Cardiology, Council on Cardiovascular Surgery and Anesthesia, and the Quality of Care and Outcomes Research Interdisciplinary Working Group. *J Am Dent Assoc (1939).* 2008;139(Suppl):3S–24S.

Worman HJ, Bonne G. "Laminopathies": a wide spectrum of human diseases. *Exp Cell Res.* 2007;313:2121–2133.

Yamaguchi H, Ishimura T, Nishiyama S, et al. Hypertrophic nonobstructive cardiomyopathy with giant negative T waves (apical hypertrophy): ventriculographic and echocardiographic features in 30 patients. *Am J Cardiol.* 1979;44:401–412.

Yaseen H, Maragnes P, Gandon-Laloum S, et al. A severe form of vitamin D deficiency with hypocalcemic cardiomyopathy. *Pediatrie.* 1993;48:547–549.

Yetman AT, McCrindle BW, MacDonald C, Freedom RM, Gow R. Myocardial bridging in children with hypertrophic cardiomyopathy—a risk factor for sudden death. *N Eng J Med.* 1998;339:1201–1209.

Yumoto F, Lu QW, Morimoto S, et al. Drastic Ca2+ sensitization of myofilament associated with a small structural change in troponin I in inherited restrictive cardiomyopathy. *Biochem Biophys Res Commun.* 2005;338:1519–1526.

Yutani C, Imakita M, Ishibashi-Ueda H, et al. Three autopsy cases of progression to left ventricular dilatation in patients with hypertrophic cardiomyopathy. *Am Heart J.* 1985;109:545–553.

Zack F, Klingel K, Kandolf R, Wegener R. Sudden cardiac death in a 5-year-old girl associated with parvovirus B19 infection. *Forensic Sci Int.* 2005;155:13–17.

Zecchin M, Di Lenarda A, Gregori D, et al. Prognostic role of non-sustained ventricular tachycardia in a large cohort of patients with idiopathic dilated cardiomyopathy. *Ital Heart J.* 2005;6:721–727.

Zenker M, Buheitel G, Rauch R, et al. Genotype-phenotype correlations in Noonan syndrome. *J Pediatr.* 2004;144:368–374.

Zenker M, Horn D, Wieczorek D, et al. SOS1 is the second most common Noonan gene but plays no major role in cardio-facio-cutaneous syndrome. *J Med Genet.* 2007;44:651–656.

Zou Y, Song L, Wang Z, et al. Prevalence of idiopathic hypertrophic cardiomyopathy in China: a population-based echocardiographic analysis of 8080 adults. *Am J Med.* 2004;116:14–18.

14

Arrhythmogenic Right Ventricular Cardiomyopathy

Petros Syrris and William J McKenna

Introduction

Arrhythmogenic right ventricular cardiomyopathy (ARVC) is an inherited cardiac disorder characterized histologically by progressive myocyte loss and replacement of the right ventricular myocardium by fibrous and/or fibrofatty tissue (Figure 14–1). Clinically the disorder presents with ventricular arrhythmias originating from the right ventricle (RV) that may result in sudden death, especially in young individuals or athletes (Thiene et al. 1988; Corrado et al. 2003). Patients often experience dizzy spells, palpitation, and syncope or may be completely asymptomatic. Fontaine et al. (1977) first reported 6 cases with sustained ventricular tachycardia (VT) of RV origin and enlarged RV who had normal pulmonary vasculature and subsequently Marcus et al. (1982) used the term "arrhythmogenic right ventricular dysplasia" (ARVD) to describe the condition in a report of 24 cases. ARVC is now the preferred term as it is an abnormality of heart muscle rather than a developmental defect of the RV. Subsequent pathological and clinical studies identified ARVC as a progressive heart muscle disease, which was recognized in the reclassification of cardiomyopathies by the World Health Organisation/International Society and Federation of Cardiology Task force on the Definition and Classification of Cardiomyopathies (Richardson et al. 1996).

Natural History

ARVC is a progressive heart muscle disease that initially affects the RV and subsequently advances to the left ventricle (LV) causing biventricular failure. Based on observations from clinical studies the natural history of ARVC has been divided into four distinct phases (Corrado et al. 2000a). In the early phase ("concealed phase") patients are often free of symptoms but may nevertheless be at risk of sudden death, especially during physical exertion. This phase is characterized by subtle RV structural and electrical changes and clinical investigations often reveal no significant abnormalities. During the "overt" arrhythmic phase, which is characterized by RV arrhythmias the patients experience palpitation and syncope. Structural abnormalities are present and are detectable by cardiac imaging. In the later phases ("right ventricular failure phase") the progression of disease through the RV leads to impaired contractility and global RV dysfunction with relatively preserved LV function while in the final stage LV involvement is accompanied by biventricular failure, which may be clinically indistinguishable from dilated cardiomyopathy (DCM) (Corrado et al. 1997; Nemec et al. 1999; Corrado et al. 2000b).

It is believed that ARVC moves from quiescent to active phases of disease, which may be recognized by the onset of symptoms of chest pain, palpitation, and impaired consciousness (Sen-Chowdhry et al. 2004). Such active phases, termed "hot phases," may indicate the advancement of disease to previously unaffected regions of the myocardium, which may coincide with a transient arrhythmic activity. Even though, in many cases, "hot phases" are clinically silent or mildly symptomatic, patients appear to be at higher risk of sudden cardiac death (Sen-Chowdhry et al. 2004).

Epidemiology

The prevalence of ARVC in the general population is frequently quoted as 1 in 5,000 (Norman and McKenna 1999) but this is likely to be an underestimate due to difficulties in making a diagnosis. There is some evidence that the prevalence of the disease could be significantly higher in some subpopulations: Rampazzo et al. (1994) reported 4.4/1,000 cases in a region of Italy. Other studies reported a prevalence of 1 in 1,000 individuals (Peters et al. 2004). Undiagnosed ARVC was the cause of sudden death in 12.5%–25% of young people and athletes under the age of 35 years in Italy (Thiene et al. 1988; Corrado et al. 1990, 1998) whilst this figure rose to 17% of sudden death cases aged 20–40 years in the United States (Shen et al. 1994).

ARVC is typically transmitted in an autosomal dominant manner with approximately a 3:1 male/female gender ratio. A familial background of disease was initially estimated at approximately 30% (Laurent et al. 1987; Nava et al. 1988a) of autosomal dominant ARVC cases but it is likely to be >50% (Corrado and Thiene 2006).

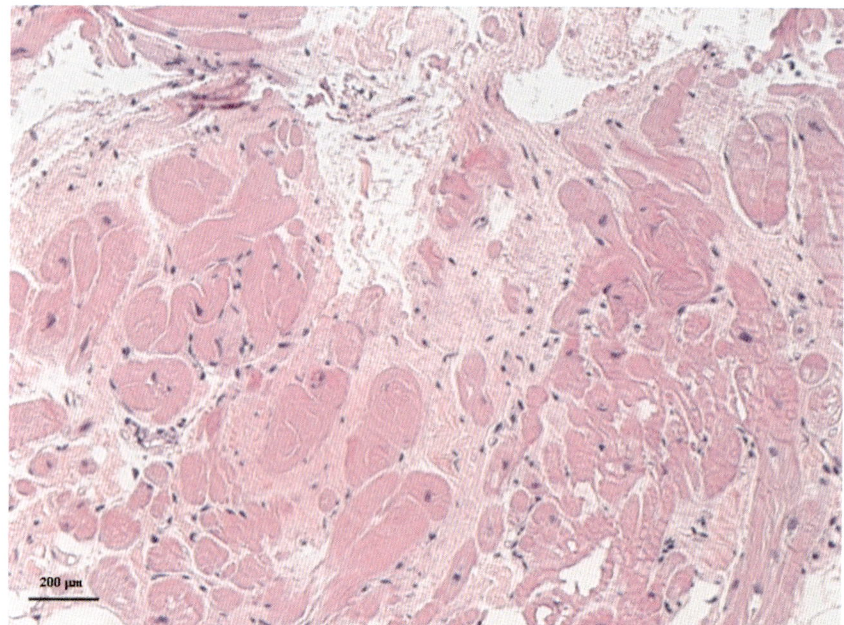

Figure 14–1 Histology of an endomyocardial biopsy of the RV from an ARVC patient showing characteristic loss of myocardium and fibroadipose substitution (hematoxylin and eosin staining). Reprinted from Syrris P, Ward D, Asimaki A, et al. Desmoglein-2 mutations in arrhythmogenic right ventricular cardiomyopathy: a genotype–phenotype characterization of familial disease. *Eur Heart J.* 2007;28:581–588, with permission.

Histology

Histologically the disorder is characterized by fibrofatty replacement of myocardium mainly in the apex, the RV inflow tract and the RV outflow tract (named the triangle of dysplasia) (Marcus et al. 1982). Initially there were considered to be two different morphological patterns of ARVC: the fatty form and the fibrofatty form (Corrado et al. 2000a). The fatty form was confined to the RV, mainly in the apical and infundibular areas. It involved replacement of the myocytes with adipose tissue without fibrosis or wall thinning. Conversely, the fibrofatty form involves large areas of fibrosis with or without adipose infiltration (Figure 14–1). It is mainly found in the inferoposterior wall and is also associated with thinning of the RV wall, aneurysmal dilatation, and inflammatory infiltrates (Corrado et al. 2000a). Differentiation of "normal" fatty involvement of the RV is problematic and the diagnosis is only made when there is myocyte loss with fibrous replacement with or without fatty infiltration.

Diagnosis

Clinical manifestations of ARVC typically include ECG depolarization/repolarization abnormalities, ventricular arrhythmias with left bundle branch block (LBBB) morphology, structural alterations, and dysfunction of the RV. However, diagnosis of ARVC is hindered by the phenotypic variability and incomplete penetrance of the disease. Patients can present with a range of severe to mild symptoms and clinical manifestations or can be completely asymptomatic. This poses a problem in diagnosing ARVC at both extremes of the disease spectrum: asymptomatic patients may remain undiagnosed (but still be at risk of sudden death, i.e., "concealed phase") and patients with end-stage ARVC (e.g., congestive heart failure) are often misdiagnosed as suffering from DCM (Corrado et al. 1997).

Clinical diagnosis of ARVC has been standardized by the introduction of a diagnostic algorithm based on a constellation of major and minor criteria, derived from 12-lead ECG, imaging (echocardiography, angiography, or magnetic resonance), ECG monitoring and exercise testing (arrhythmia), histology (biopsy, explant, or postmortem), and the presence of familial disease (Table 14–1) (McKenna et al. 1994). Application of this set of criteria, proposed by the Task Force of the Working Group on Myocardial and Pericardial Disease of the European Society of Cardiology and of the Scientific Council on Cardiomyopathies of the International Society and Federation of Cardiology, can provide a definite diagnosis of ARVC if a patient fulfils two major criteria or one major and two minor or four minor criteria from different categories (see Table 14–1) (McKenna et al. 1994).

Electrocardiographic Abnormalities

Depolarization/conduction and repolarization abnormalities include a wide spectrum of ECG changes and can be detected in up to 90% of ARVC cases (Nava et al. 1997). The most common of them is T-wave inversion in the right precordial leads (V1–V3) (Figure 14–2), which, in one report, was present in 54% of confirmed cases (Peters and Trummel 2003). However, due to their nonspecific nature, such changes were initially considered to be only minor diagnostic criteria (McKenna et al. 1994). For example, T-wave inversion with ST segment elevation can be naturally occurring in children and young adolescents (Sharma et al. 1999) and newly recognized ECG abnormalities such as poor R-wave progression from leads V1 to V4 (Wichter et al. 2004) may be positional or due to a condition mimicking ARVC (phenocopies).

Delayed depolarization changes with prolongation of the right precordial QRS duration (>110 ms) and postexcitation epsilon waves are believed to reflect a delayed RV activation and are considered major diagnostic criteria (Table 14–1). In the abovementioned study, when QRS prolongation was redefined as QRS duration in (V1 + V2 + V3)/(V4 + V5 + V6) ≥1.2, this finding had a sensitivity of 98% in ARVC patients without the need to exclude ECGs with complete or incomplete RBBB (Peters and Trummel 2003). Epsilon waves, on the other hand, in the right precordial leads are highly suggestive of ARVC and can be detected in >30%

Table 14–1 Task Force Criteria for Diagnosis of ARVC

Disease Features	Criteria	
	Major	Minor
Global or regional dysfunction and structural abnormalities	Severe dilatation and reduction of RV ejection fraction with no (or only mild) LV impairment Localized RV aneurysms (akinetic or dyskinetic areas with diastolic bulging) Severe segmental dilatation of the RV	Mild global RV dilatation and/or ejection fraction reduction with normal LV Mild segmental dilatation of the RV Regional RV hypokinesia
Tissue characterization	Fibrofatty replacement of myocardium on endocardial biopsy	
Repolarization abnormalities		Inverted T-waves in right precordial leads (V2 and V3) in persons >12 yrs and in absence of right bundle branch block (RBBB)
Depolarization conduction abnormalities	Epsilon waves or localized prolongation (>110ms) of the QRS complex in the right precordial leads (V1–V3)	Late potentials on signal-averaged ECG
Arrhythmias		Sustained or nonsustained left bundle branch block type VT (ECG, Holter, exercise testing) Frequent ventricular extrasystoles (>1,000/24 h on Holter)
Family history	Familial disease confirmed at necropsy or surgery	Familial history of premature sudden death (<35 yrs) due to suspected right ventricular dysplasia Familial history (clinical diagnosis based on present criteria)

Notes: Diagnostic criteria were proposed by the Working Group on Myocardial and Pericardial Disease of the European Society of Cardiology and of the Scientific Council on Cardiomyopathies of the International Society and Federation of Cardiology (McKenna et al. 1994). Diagnosis of ARVC is fulfilled by the presence of two major criteria or one major plus two minor or four minor criteria from different categories.

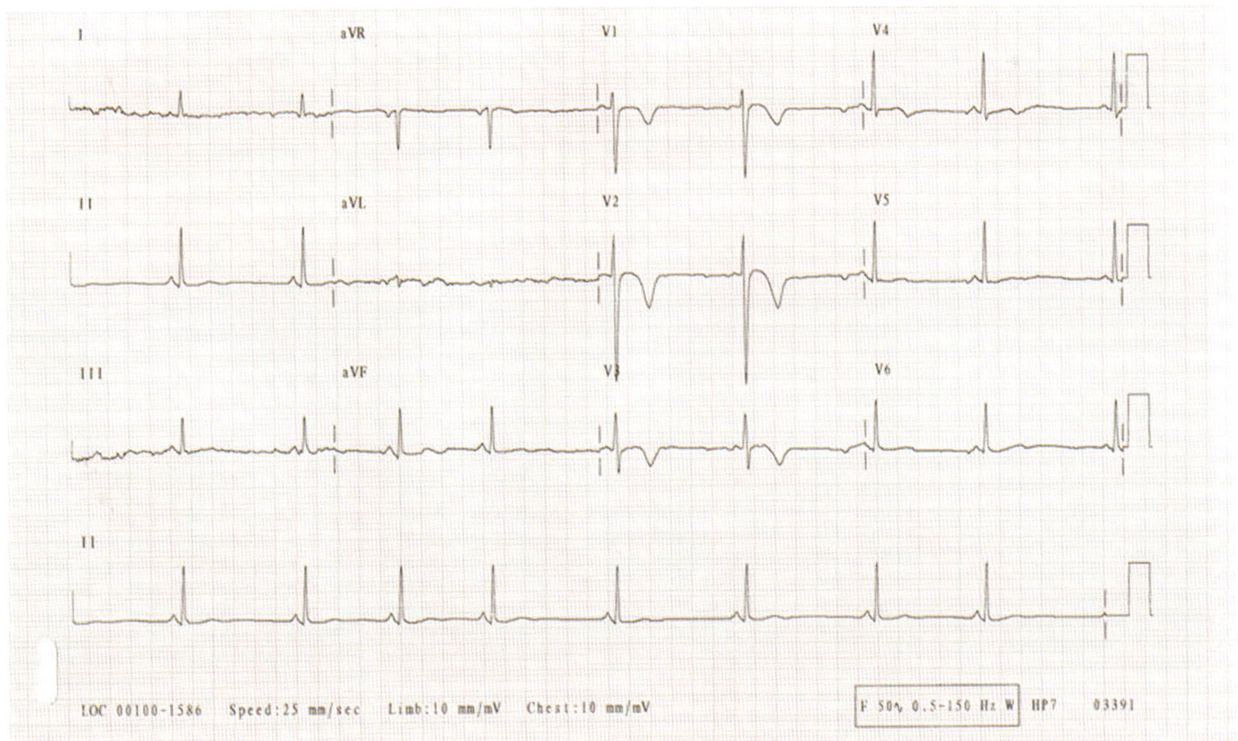

Figure 14–2 Electrocardiogram from an ARVC patient showing sinus rhythm with prominent T-wave inversion in right precordial leads. Reprinted with permission.

of patients as late potentials on high-resolution or signal-averaged ECG (Corrado et al. 2000a).

A recent clinical study found that prolongation of the right precordial S-wave ≥55 ms was present in 95% of ARVC patients without RBBB and correlated with disease severity and induction of VT on electrophysiological testing. Based on these findings the authors proposed a "prolonged S-wave upstroke in V1 through V3" as a new diagnostic criterion (Nasir et al. 2004).

Arrhythmia

Symptomatic ventricular arrhythmias of RV origin are the most common clinical manifestation of ARVC, typically presenting during physical exertion. They range from isolated premature ventricular beats to sustained VT of LBBB morphology or ventricular fibrillation (VF). In a study of 67 index cases and 298 family members sustained VT was seen in 64% and nonsustained VT in 29% of index patients whilst frequent ventricular extrasystoles (>1,000/24 h) on Holter monitoring were detected in 42% (Hamid et al. 2002).

Imaging

Detection of RV morphological and structural abnormalities by imaging techniques such as echocardiography, angiography, and cardiac magnetic resonance (CMR) is considered a major criterion for the diagnosis of ARVC (McKenna et al. 1994). These abnormalities include localized wall thinning and segmental dilatation (often with aneurysms), global dilatation of the RV with or without ejection fraction reduction and LV involvement, and regional wall motion abnormalities (dyskinesia, hypokinesia). Echocardiography is considered as "the first-line imaging approach" in evaluating suspected ARVC cases or their relatives (Corrado et al. 2000a). Using this technique Hamid et al. found severe RV dilatation and reduced ejection fraction in 45% of index cases whilst mild RV dilatation was present in 26% (Hamid et al. 2002). RV angiography has a high specificity in detecting regional bulgings or aneurysms in the "triangle of dysplasia" (Daliento et al. 1990) and is regarded as the best method to evaluate RV function by some experts (Marcus and Fontaine 1995).

However, all imaging techniques have serious limitations in accurately identifying pathological changes in the RV. For example, visualization of the RV by echocardiography is often unsatisfactory and measurement of right ventricular volumes, dimensions, and function has been problematic.

Use of CMR for the diagnosis of ARVC has caused considerable controversy. CMR can detect fatty tissue infiltration and allow assessment of volumes, function, and regional wall motion abnormalities. Nevertheless, studies have demonstrated a high degree of interobserver variability and subjectivity with respect to interpreting wall thinning, localized contraction abnormalities and fatty deposition (Bluemke et al. 2003; Tandri et al. 2003; White et al. 2004). In addition it is often difficult to distinguish pathological fatty infiltration of the RV from normal epicardial and pericardial fat. A recent study, which aimed at assessing the utility of CMR in ARVC in relation to diagnostic criteria and genotype, concluded that this method can be a valuable tool in evaluating ARVC patients provided that it is performed using a dedicated protocol by experienced specialists in analysis of volumes, RV wall motion, and delayed-enhancement imaging (Sen-Chowdhry et al. 2006).

Histological Findings

Demonstration of the hallmark histological characteristic of ARVC, that is, myocyte loss and replacement by fibrous or fibrofatty tissue at postmortem can provide a definitive diagnosis of the disorder and is considered a major diagnostic criterion (McKenna et al. 1994). However, adequate myocardial tissue is rarely available for histological analysis and the diagnosis is often missed even at postmortem.

An endomyocardial biopsy can also detect such morphological alterations but is less accurate and has a number of diagnostic limitations. RV biopsies are most safely taken from the septum that is rarely involved whereas the triangle of dysplasia and RV free wall that are often affected are more difficult and less safe to biopsy. It may be difficult on biopsy to distinguish ARVC from other conditions presenting with fibrous or fibrofatty infiltration of the RV myocardium including chronic alcoholism and cardiomyopathic disorders (Corrado et al. 2000a). Furthermore, nonpathological subepicardial adipose tissue can also be found in healthy individuals. For these reasons a myocardial biopsy has limitations as a routine diagnostic tool but in some cases may confirm the diagnosis of ARVC. It is recommended that upon morphometric analysis of a specimen of the RV myocardium, observed reduction of myocytes <60% should be considered a major diagnostic criterion whilst numbers of myocytes between 60% and 75% are considered a minor diagnostic criterion (Table 14–2; Marcus et al. 2008).

Proposed Modification of Diagnostic Criteria

Use of the Task Force diagnostic criteria for ARVC over the years has demonstrated that they are specific for diagnosis in those who present with ventricular arrhythmias (T-wave inversion in RV leads, regional wall motion abnormalities in the RV) but are insensitive, particularly in the setting of familial disease. As ARVC shows considerable phenotypic heterogeneity, frequently, relatives of affected ARVC patients have only mild disease features that do not fulfil the original diagnostic criteria. Nevertheless these individuals have a high probability of carrying the causative mutation responsible for ARVC in their affected relative (50% for first-degree relatives). Hamid et al. (2002) investigated family members of ARVC probands to ascertain the prevalence and mode of expression of familial disease. They reported that 10% of relatives had disease features fulfilling ARVC diagnostic criteria and a further 11% had isolated minor criteria insufficient to diagnose ARVC but who could, nevertheless, be affected too. The authors, therefore, proposed a modification of the Task Force criteria for first-degree relatives of confirmed ARVC patients (Table 14–3). According to that the presence of a single disease feature (right precordial T-wave inversion, late potentials on signal-averaged ECG, VT with LBBB morphology, and minor functional and structural abnormalities of the RV on imaging) in a relative should be considered diagnostic of ARVC.

As intended application of the proposed modified criteria can improve diagnostic yield in the setting of familial ARVC but can also lead to a false-positive diagnosis (Syrris et al. 2006a).

Left Ventricular Involvement

ARVC was believed to affect only the RV (Marcus et al. 1982); however, it is now recognized that LV involvement is common. A review of pathological findings of 47 heart specimens examined at

Table 14–2 Updated Criteria for Diagnosis of ARVC

Disease Features	Criteria: Major	Criteria: Minor
Global and/or regional dysfunction and structural alterations	Severe RV global dilatation and impaired contraction in the absence of severe LV dysfunction Localized RV or LV aneurysms (akinetic or dyskinetic areas with diastolic distortion of normal wall motion)	Moderate RV global dilatation and impaired contraction LV late enhancement in epicardium and/or mid-myocardium
Tissue Characterization on endomyocardial biopsy (fibrous replacement of the RV free wall myocardium in at least 1 sample, with or without fatty tissue)	Residual myocytes <60% with morphometric analysis, or <50% if estimated	Residual myocytes 60%–75% with morphometric analysis, or 50%–65% if estimated
ECG—repolarization abnormalities	Inverted T-waves in leads V1, V2, and V3 in people >14 years in the absence of typical complete RBBB	Inverted T-waves in leads V1 and V2 in the absence of typical complete RBBB Inverted T-waves in leads, II, III, aVF, and/or V4, V5, and V6
ECG—Depolarization abnormalities	Delayed conduction with QRS >110 ms in V1, V2, or V3 and/or terminal activation duration ≥55 ms in the absence of typical complete RBBB	Late potentials on signal-averaged ECG
Arrhythmias	Nonsustained or sustained VT of LBBB morphology excluding typical, inferior QRS axis, RVOT tachycardia	Nonsustained or sustained VT of LBBB morphology of unknown axis or inferior QRS axis, RVOT tachycardia Frequent ventricular extrasystoles (VES >500 during 24 h ECG)
Family History—Genetics	Familial disease confirmed at necropsy or surgery Familial disease confirmed in a first-degree relative	Familial history of premature sudden death (<40 yr) due to suspected ARVC

Source: Marcus et al. (2009).
Notes: Diagnosis of ARVC is fulfilled by the presence of two major criteria or one major plus two minor or four minor criteria from different categories. Fulfilment of fewer criteria is considered as follows: Borderline: 1 major and 1 minor or 3 minor; Suspected: 1 major or 2 minor; Unlikely: 1 minor.

Table 14–3 Proposed Modified Criteria for Diagnosis of ARVC

Right Ventricular Dysplasia in a First-Degree Relative Plus One of the Following:	
ECG	Inverted T-waves in right precordial leads (V2 and V3)
Signal-averaged ECG	Late potentials on signal-averaged ECG
Arrhythmias	Left bundle branch block type VT on ECG, signal-averaged ECG, Holter monitoring, or during exercise testing Extrasystoles >200/24 h
Structural or functional abnormality of the RV	Mild global right ventricular dilatation or ejection fraction reduction with normal LV Mild segmental dilatation of the RV Regional RV hypokinesia

Notes: Modification of Task Force diagnostic criteria was proposed by Hamid et al. (2002) for the diagnosis of familial ARVC. These criteria apply to first-degree relatives who do not fulfil the original Task Force recommendations.

autopsy or cardiac transplantation found macroscopic and microscopic evidence of LV involvement in 76% (Corrado et al. 1997). A number of genetic studies have demonstrated LV abnormalities in ARVC cases with or without RV disease (Bauce et al. 2005; Syrris et al. 2006a, 2006b, 2007). Histopathology studies have also reported postmortem findings of subepicardial and mediomural fibroadipose replacement confined to the LV as a cause of sudden unexpected cardiac death in the young (Gallo et al. 1992; Pinamonti et al. 1992; Michalodimitrakis et al. 2002). The family of a proband with isolated LV fibrofatty findings on postmortem was recently investigated (Norman et al. 2005). All affected individuals had prominent LV disease on imaging and left precordial variants of ECG patterns associated with ARVC. This variant of ARVC was designated arrhythmogenic left ventricular cardiomyopathy (ALVC) (Norman et al. 2005; Sen-Chowdhry et al. 2005). A recent study of 200 ARVC patients detected biventricular involvement in 56% and predominant left-sided disease in 5% of cases and, with respect to LV disease, recognized three distinct disease patterns: classic, left-sided (ALVC), and biventricular (Sen-Chowdhry et al. 2007).

In order to increase the specificity of the original Task Force diagnostic criteria it was considered appropriate to define the finding of structural and functional abnormalities of the RV as diagnostic only in the absence of any more than mild LV systolic impairment (McKenna et al. 1994). However, as it was detailed above, LV involvement is part of the phenotypic spectrum of ARVC and can be present even at the early stages of the disease rather than in the final "biventricular pump failure phase" alone. This feature has been recognized in the most recent modification of the diagnostic criteria (see Table 14–2) (Marcus et al. 2009).

Management

The main goal of management of ARVC is control of arrhythmias and the prevention of sudden cardiac death in patients at risk. An unfavorable prognosis has been associated with a number of risk factors such as a previous cardiac arrest, early onset of symptoms, syncope, severe RV dilatation, and LV involvement (Sen-Chowdhry et al. 2004). However, currently there are no prospective studies assessing these clinical markers as prognostic indicators. Due to the peculiar natural history of ARVC (asymptomatic "concealed phase," etc.) sudden death may be the first manifestation of the disease. Therefore it is vital to identify and clinically follow up individuals at risk of sudden cardiac death. It is recommended that clinical evaluation of suspected index cases and relatives (symptomatic or not) should include detailed clinical history, ECG, signal-averaged ECG, 24-h ECG monitoring, and exercise testing in addition to at least one imaging modality (Corrado et al. 2000a).

Treatment of ARVC aims to prevent arrhythmias and sudden death. Extreme physical exertion in the form of competitive sports or endurance training is not recommended as this represents a risk of disease progression as well as sudden death. β-blockers are the mainstay of pharmaceutical treatment. Evidence suggests that sotalol or amiodarone are the most effective antiarrhythmic drugs. For example, in a study of 81 patients with ARVC or RV outflow tachycardia sotalol prevented VT in 68% of patients (Wichter et al. 1992).

Use of the implantable cardioverter-defibrillator (ICD) is recommended for patients at high risk of sudden death. It is usually offered to those who survived a cardiac arrest caused by rapid VT or VF, have a history of syncope, LV involvement, or drug resistant VT. Although ICD implantation certainly has a beneficial impact on survival—a study reported 0% 5-year mortality rate after ICD implantation in males compared to 28% in controls (Hodgkinson et al. 2005)—it is not free of potential implications, particularly in the young (Dubin et al. 1996; Sears and Conti 2004; Wichter et al. 2004). They include risks of damaging the RV myocardium during implantation, requirement of multiple generator replacements, potential improper ICD function and failure (Fontaine 1997). In addition, the significant cost of implantation and the psychological burden associated with the device cannot be underestimated.

In summary, diagnosis of ARVC remains problematic for several reasons, including lack of symptoms or clinical manifestations, problems imaging the RV, and the lack of specific ECG disease manifestations. Therefore, there is a need for an updated set of diagnostic criteria and establishment of natural history, risk evaluation, and management algorithms for affected asymptomatic or mildly symptomatic family members who represent the majority of ARVC patients.

Molecular Genetics of ARVC

Chromosomal Loci

In the past 13 years studies have documented eight types of ARVC based on data obtained by genetic linkage analysis of affected families (Table 14–4). The first report of this kind studied two families with a total of 19 affected individuals and mapped the locus responsible for the disorder on 14q23-q24 (ARVD1) (Rampazzo et al. 1994). A second locus was mapped to chromosome 1q42-q43 in patients with effort-induced polymorphic ventricular tachyarrhytmias and minimal structural abnormalities of the RV (Rampazzo et al. 1995; Bauce et al. 2000). In the next 2 years two more loci (ARVD3 and ARVD4) were discovered on chromosomes 14 and 2, respectively (Severini et al. 1996; Rampazzo et al. 1997). The locus responsible for a familial form of ARVC with heterogeneous clinical presentation was then mapped to chromosome 3p23 (ARVD5) (Ahmad et al. 1998). Some patients in those families presented with RV dilatation and VT with LBBB morphology whilst others had only nonspecific electrocardiographic changes.

Subsequent linkage studies described a further three loci with autosomal dominant mode of inheritance: ARVD6, 10p12-p14 (Li et al. 2000); ARVD7, 10q22 (Melberg et al. 1999); ARVD8, 6p24 (Rampazzo et al. 2002), and one locus with autosomal recessive transmittance, Naxos disease, 17q21 (Coonar et al. 1998). However, at present, only four genes corresponding to these chromosomal locations have been identified, namely ARVD1, ARVD2, ARVD8, and Naxos disease, and are discussed below in more detail. For the rest the genes responsible for these particular types of ARVC remain unknown.

Syndromic ARVC

The first gene responsible for ARVC was identified in families with a recessive syndromic variant of the disease, Naxos disease. Affected individuals presented with ARVC, nonepidermolytic palmoplantar keratoderma and woolly hair (Protonotarios et al. 1986). The disease can be, almost exclusively, found in the genetically isolated Greek island of Naxos and was named after it. Genetic linkage of nine affected families with autosomal recessive inheritance and 100% penetrance mapped Naxos disease to chromosome 17q21 (Coonar et al. 1998) and the gene responsible for it, plakoglobin, was discovered soon after by the candidate-gene approach (McKoy et al. 2000). Plakoglobin (JUP) is a key component of the desmosomes and adherens junctions, structures important for cell adhesion in various tissues including cardiac muscle and skin. Affected individuals were homozygous for a two-base pair deletion (Pk2175del2), which leads to a premature termination of translation and truncation of the plakoglobin protein (McKoy et al. 2000). Clinically homozygous children have diffuse palmoplantar keratoderma and woolly hair from infancy while the typical ARVC cardiac phenotype is usually present by puberty. Heterozygotes appear asymptomatic but around 10% have minor ECG abnormalities (Protonotarios et al. 2001).

A second desmosomal gene, desmoplakin, was found responsible for a recessive syndromic form identified in three Ecuadorian families (Norgett et al. 2000). This form was named Carvajal syndrome after the dermatologist, Luis Carvajal-Huerta, who first described it (Carvajal-Huerta 1998). Affected individuals have left ventricular DCM, keratoderma, and woolly hair at infancy and progress to cardiac enlargement and heart failure in their adolescent years. Genetic analysis studies first mapped the

Table 14–4 Chromosomal Loci, Genes, and Mutations in ARVC

Locus	Chromosomal Location	Mode of Inheritance	Additional Clinical Features	Gene	Number of Mutations
ARVD1	14q23-q24	Autosomal dominant		Transforming growth factor β3 (*TGFB3*)	2
ARVD2	1q42-q43	Autosomal dominant	Catecholaminergic polymorphic VT	Cardiac ryanodine receptor (*RYR2*)	<10
ARVD3	14q12-q22	Autosomal dominant			
ARVD4	2q32.1-q32.3	Autosomal dominant			
ARVD5	3p23	Autosomal dominant			
ARVD6	10p12-p14	Autosomal dominant			
ARVD7	10q22	Autosomal dominant	Myofibrillar myopathy		
ARVD8	6p24	Autosomal dominant Autosomal recessive Autosomal recessive	 DCM, keratoderma and woolly hair (Carvajal syndrome) Pemphigous-like skin disorder, woolly hair	Desmoplakin (*DSP*)	<15 1 1
ARVD9	12p11	Autosomal dominant Autosomal recessive		Plakophilin-2 (*PKP2*)	>50 1
Naxos Disease	17q21	Autosomal recessive	Nonepidermolytic palmoplantar keratoderma and woolly hair	Plakoglobin (*JUP*)	1
	18q12	Autosomal dominant		Desmoglein-2 (*DSG2*)	<25
	18q12	Autosomal dominant		Desmocollin-2 (*DSC2*)	<5
	17q21	Autosomal dominant		Plakoglobin (*JUP*)	1

Notes: Loci ARVD1–ARVD8 and Naxos disease were mapped by genetic linkage analysis in families with ARVC. PKP2, DSG2, and DSC2 were identified by a candidate-gene approach.

disease to chromosome 6p24 and mutational screening of desmoplakin (*DSP*) detected a single nucleotide deletion that segregated with disease. All affected individuals were homozygous for this mutation (7901delG), which resulted in truncation of the desmoplakin protein (Norgett et al. 2000). Histopathologic examination of the heart of a deceased patient showed features more consistent with a diagnosis of biventricular ARVC (Kaplan et al. 2004a).

Using the same experimental approach Alcalai et al. (2003) detected a missense mutation (G2375R) as the cause of a syndromic form in a family of Arab origin. Affected individuals, homozygous for G2375R, presented with classic ARVC (T-wave inversion with localized QRS prolongation in the right precordial leads, V1–V3, etc.), a pemphigus-like skin disorder and woolly hair (Alcalai et al. 2003).

Interestingly, *DSP* has also been implicated in several cutaneous disorders with apparently no cardiac involvement, for example, acantholytic epidermolysis bullosa, skin fragility/woolly hair syndrome, and so on (reviewed by Lai Cheong et al. 2005).

Dominant ARVC

1. Desmoplakin

In 2002 Rampazzo et al. analyzing an Italian family with typical ARVC mapped the disease locus to chromosome 6p24 and subsequently identified desmoplakin as the gene responsible for the condition. Affected family members were heterozygous for a missense mutation (S299S), which was predicted to modify a putative phosphorylation site in the N-terminal domain of DSP where binding of plakoglobin occurs (Rampazzo et al. 2002). Patients showed a phenotype of variable severity (ranging from severe to mild) with classic ECG and echocardiography ARVC abnormalities. Sudden death was also reported in the family. Three other studies have also reported mutations in *DSP* (Bauce et al. 2005; Norman et al. 2005; Yang et al. 2006) but the total number of known mutations in this gene remains small (Table 14–4). Bauce et al. (2005) detected 4 mutations in 25 index cases whilst a larger study reported a much lower percentage (4 in 66 patients) (Yang et al. 2006). Evidence suggests that mutations in *DSP* are associated with a high rate of sudden death and broad range of clinical manifestations. LV involvement is also present with one family presenting with predominant LV disease (ALVC), arrhythmias of LV origin, and lateral T-wave inversion (Norman et al. 2005). In the latter, affected family members carried a truncating insertion (T586fsX594) predicted to disrupt the binding of DSP to desmin.

The implication of plakoglobin and desmoplakin in the pathogenesis of ARVC, either in a syndromic variant or in isolation, was a breakthrough in understanding the pathophysiological mechanisms of the condition. Since JUP and DSP are vital components of the desmosome, evidence suggested that ARVC might be a disease of cell adhesion (Sen-Chowdhry et al. 2005). In turn that pointed toward a possible involvement of other genes encoding desmosomal proteins with plakophilin-2, desmoglein-2, and desmocollin-2 as major candidates. Indeed several genetic studies, almost simultaneously, performed mutational screening of key desmosomal genes in patients with ARVC and their families.

2. Plakophilin-2

Gerull et al. (2004) first showed that mutations in plakophilin-2 (*PKP2*) are a major cause of ARVC. Their study examined 120 probands who fulfilled ARVC diagnostic criteria and detected *PKP2* mutations in 32 (Gerull et al. 2004). Disease was incompletely penetrant in most mutation carriers, a finding that has been confirmed in all subsequent studies. Syrris et al. (2006a) provided, for the first time, a systematic evaluation of *PKP2* mutation carriers and their families. The authors using both Task Force and proposed modified diagnostic criteria found a high degree of penetrance for *PKP2* mutations and highlighted the need for a more accurate set of criteria, especially with respect to LV disease (Syrris et al. 2006a). To date more than 50 mutations in plakophilin-2—mainly nonsense mutations and small deletions and insertions—have been reported (Table 14–4) in several genetic and clinical studies (Antoniades et al. 2006; Dalal et al. 2006; Kannankeril et al. 2006; Nagaoka et al. 2006; van Tintelen et al. 2006; Awad et al. 2006b). Generally, there appear to be no particular disease features associated with a specific mutation with patients exhibiting a high phenotypic variability even when carrying an identical pathogenic sequence change. This is particularly highlighted by findings in studies where *PKP2* mutations have been found in around 5% of cases not fulfilling Task Force diagnostic criteria (van Tintelen et al. 2006; Syrris et al. 2006a). At present *PKP2* is the most frequently mutated gene in ARVC with a mutation yield of up to 43% in patients fulfilling Task Force diagnostic criteria (van Tintelen et al. 2007). This type of ARVC caused by *PKP2* mutations is often referred to as ARVD9 (Table 14–4).

3. Desmoglein-2

Mutations in desmoglein-2 only account for approximately 10% of typical ARVC (Pilichou et al. 2006; Awad et al. 2006a; Syrris et al. 2007). In a series of 80 ARVC index cases 9 heterozygous mutations in *DSG2* were found in 8 patients (Pilichou et al. 2006). Clinical presentation was indistinguishable to that due to mutations in other desmosomal genes with LV disease in half of the index cases. This was confirmed in a separate study that provided a genotype–phenotype characterization of familial disease. The authors found 8 novel mutations in 9 probands in a cohort of 86 Caucasian ARVC patients (Syrris et al. 2007). RV morphological abnormalities were found in 66% of gene carriers and LV involvement in 25% whilst classical right precordial T-wave inversion only in 26%. Interestingly there was a high percentage of gene-positive individuals with a family history of sudden death/aborted sudden death (66%) (Syrris et al. 2007).

4. Desmocollin-2

Desmocollin-2 (*DSC2*) has been the latest desmosomal gene implicated in ARVC and mutations in it appear to be infrequent. Syrris et al. (2006b) reported 4 *DSC2* mutations in 77 probands who were negative for mutations in *JUP*, *DSP*, *PKP2*, and *DSG2*. Disease expression was variable and most mutations carriers had LV involvement (Syrris et al. 2006b). A splice site mutation has also been identified in 1 patient of 88 probands free of *PKP2* and *DSG2* mutations (Heuser et al. 2006).

5. Plakoglobin

Recently, the first dominant mutation in plakoglobin was described in a German family with typical ARVC (Asimaki et al. 2007). Affected individuals carried an insertion of a serine residue in the N-terminus of *JUP* (S39_K40insS), which may increase plakoglobin turnover via proteasomal degradation (Asimaki et al. 2007).

Nondesmosomal ARVC

1. Cardiac Ryanodine Receptor

Two studies mapped a distinct clinical type of familial ARVC to chromosome 1q42-q43 (ARVD2) (Rampazzo et al. 1995; Bauce et al. 2000). In contrast to typical ARVC, patients with ARVD2 type of disease showed effort-induced polymorphic VT without the characteristic ECG features of the disease (Nava et al. 1988b). Furthermore, ARVD2 exhibited a high rate of juvenile sudden cardiac death and a high penetrance with a 1:1 sex ratio. Pathogenic mutations were then detected in the cardiac ryanodine receptor gene (*RYR2*), which codes for an important calcium release channel of the sarcoplasmic reticulum in myocytes (Tiso et al. 2001; Bauce et al. 2002).

Interestingly *RYR2* mutations have also been found in families with isolated catecholaminergic polymorphic VT (CPVT) (Laitinen et al. 2001; Priori et al. 2001). In both conditions mutations in *RYR2* are thought to disrupt the regulation of the calcium channel leading to Ca^{+2} leaking into the cytoplasm, which in turn may provoke ventricular arrhythmias (Tiso et al. 2002). However, this disease mechanism cannot provide an explanation for the structural changes seen in the RV in ARVC. It is likely that ARVD2 is a primary form of inherited arrhythmia rather than an ARVC.

Transforming Growth Factor β3

Mutational screening of the coding regions of several positional candidates for ARVD1 on chromosome 14q23-q24 failed to identify the causative gene for this particular type of the disorder (Rampazzo et al. 2003; Rossi et al. 2004). In 2005, Beffagna et al. found two sequence changes in the promoter and untranslated regions of the transforming growth factor β3 gene (*TGF-β3*) in an ARVD1-linked family and an unrelated index case respectively (Beffagna et al. 2005). TGF-β3 as a member of a large family of regulatory cytokines is important in tissue development and homeostasis. Based on data from functional studies on murine cells expressing the *TGF-β3* mutations, the authors proposed a novel disease mechanism for ARVC involving overexpression of this molecule. It was also postulated that the identified mutations in *TGF-β3* could promote myocardial fibrosis in vivo, a known substrate for reentrant ventricular arrhythmias (Weber et al. 1992). However, no pathogenic changes in *TGF-β3* were found in two other families with ARVD1, which raises questions about the putative involvement of *TGF-β3* in ARVC.

Pathophysiological Mechanisms of ARVC

Early Hypotheses

In early attempts to explain the mechanisms underlying the pathophysiology of ARVC three main theories were proposed (Basso et al. 1996):

a. Apoptosis or programmed myocyte death: Mallat et al. reported evidence of apoptosis in the RV myocardium of six of eight ARVC patients in contrast to normal subjects (Mallat et al. 1996).
b. Inflammatory heart disease (e.g., myocarditis): This theory was based on reports of inflammatory infiltrates detected in heart specimens from ARVC patients (Fontaine et al. 1990) and enteroviral RNA being present in some patients with ARVC, myocarditis, and DCM (Pinamonti et al. 1996). More recent studies have showed that myocarditis can mimic

ARVC and that it may be superimposed on an existing disease progression in the affected heart muscle rather than being involved in the actual etiology of the disorder (Chimenti et al. 2004).

c. Transdifferentation of myocardial cells: This hypothesis assumes that myocardial cells can change from muscle to adipose tissue and is based on observations on one patient (d' Amati et al. 2000).

Desmosomal Disease

Current knowledge indicates that ARVC is a disease of the desmosome. Desmosomes are major intercellular junctions that connect intermediate filaments to the cell surface and mediate cell–cell adhesion (Huber 2003). They provide cells with mechanical strength and also play an important role in tissue morphogenesis and differentiation. Desmosomes are present in tissues that experience routine mechanical stress like the epidermis and the myocardium and consist of proteins belonging to three families: plakins, armadillo proteins, and cadherins (Green and Gaudry 2000). The major desmosomal components of each family present in the cardiac muscle are desmoplakin (plakin); plakoglobin and plakophilin-2 (armadillo proteins); desmoglein-2 and desmocollin-2 (cadherins). Desmosomes are complex three-dimensional structures whose integrity and functionality rely on numerous protein–protein interactions. In cardiac desmosomes the C-terminus of desmoplakin binds to desmin intermediate filaments whilst the N-terminus interacts with plakoglobin and plakophilin. Desmoglein and desmocollin are transmembrane molecules that mediate strong adhesion by binding to each other through their N-terminus whilst the C-terminus has binding sites for plakoglobin and plakophilin (Garrod et al. 2002; Huber 2003). A simplified schematic representation of the molecular organization of the cardiac desmosome is shown in Figure 14–3.

The recent discovery of mutations in desmosomal genes in ARVC patients has provided the basis for the desmosomal disease model. It has been proposed that impairment of desmosomal function due to genetic defects would result in myocyte detachment and death under conditions of mechanical stress, possibly followed by inflammation (Sen-Chowdhry et al. 2005). As regeneration of cardiac myocytes is very limited in the adult heart, cells are replaced by fibrous or fibrofatty tissue, a hallmark histological finding in ARVC hearts. This hypothesis also explains why ARVC shows a predilection for the thin-walled areas of the RV (triangle of dysplasia) and the postlateral wall of the LV, which are structurally more vulnerable to prolonged physical stress.

As desmosomes are abundant in various tissues mutations in desmosomal genes may also result in a more generalized phenotype with or without cardiac abnormalities (Huber 2003; Lai Cheong et al. 2005). The cutaneous disease manifestations of Naxos disease and Carvajal syndrome are good examples of such widespread disease. ARVC patients with mutations in *PKP2*, *DSG2*, and *DSC2* are free of cutaneous disease manifestations, which is most likely due to the fact that these isoforms are solely expressed in the heart. Skin and hair are spared as functional substitution of PKP2, DSG2, and DSC2 by other isoforms may take place.

To date there is a very limited number of studies investigating the effects of specific desmosomal gene mutations on the ultrastructure of the myocardium in ARVC but existing evidence provides support to the aforementioned model. Theoretically such mutations may result in incorporation of defective proteins in the desmosome; affect key domains in protein–protein interactions; disrupt the correct targeting of proteins to desmosomes (mislocalization) or even lead to insufficient incorporation of a protein. Kaplan et al. (2004b) studied the effects of the Naxos disease mutation in *JUP* in cardiac samples from affected individuals. The authors reported that mutant JUP was expressed in heart but failed to localize properly to intercalated disks (Kaplan et al. 2004b). Similarly, another study showed marked reduction in desmoplakin and plakoglobin in heart specimens of a patient with Carvajal syndrome. Electron microscopy of the same samples showed the presence of elongated desmosomes and unusual junctional structures (Kaplan et al. 2004a). Basso et al. (2006)

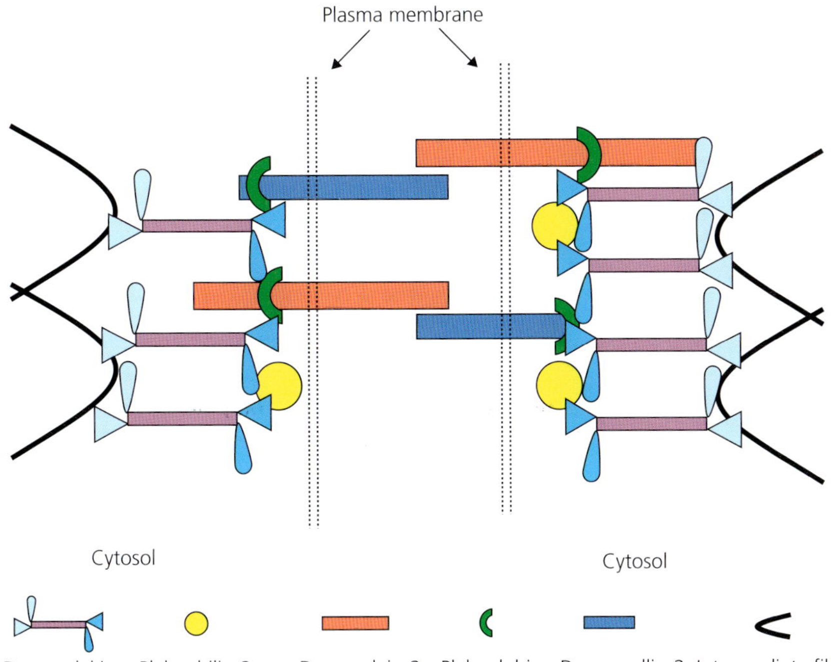

Figure 14–3 The molecular organization of the cardiac desmosome. Adapted from Green KJ, Gaudry CA. Are desmosomes more than tethers for intermediate filaments? *Nat Rev Mol Cell Biol.* 2000;1:208–216.

investigated heart specimens from 21 ARVC patients (10 of whom had desmosomal gene mutations) by electron microscopy and detected increased desmosome lengths and decreased desmosome numbers in mutation carriers.

Remodeling of Intercalated Disks

It has been shown that there is extensive remodeling of intercalated disks in diseased hearts. In particular, Basso et al. (2006) found evidence of mislocalization and decreased number of D type of intercellular junctions (responsible for the mechanical stability between cells) in hearts of ARVC patients. Similarly, heart samples from a Carvajal syndrome patient also had "atypical, highly convoluted intercalated disks" (Kaplan et al. 2004a). Furthermore, it is intriguing that destabilization of desmosomes by defective desmosomal proteins may have a direct effect on the gap junctions too. A gap junction is a type of intercellular junction that mediates ion transfer and is responsible for both electrical and mechanical coupling of the myocardial syncytium (Jamora and Fuchs 2002). Immunofluorescence microscopy and immunohistochemistry experiments with hearts from Naxos disease patients found marked reduction of connexin43 (a major gap junction protein) expression in both ventricles and prominent remodeling of myocyte gap junctions in the RV (Kaplan et al. 2004b). The authors hypothesized that this phenomenon is due to abnormal linkage between mechanical junctions and cytoskeleton and, in combination with mild structural abnormalities, may provide a substrate for arrhythmias. At present it is unclear if this mechanism can generate fatal tachycardias in the absence of myocardial abnormalities.

Suppression of Wnt/β-Catenin Signaling

Recently, a novel molecular disease mechanism based on signaling defects involving plakoglobin has been proposed by Garcia-Gras et al. (2006). The authors showed that suppression of the expression of desmoplakin in atrial myocyte cell lines resulted in nuclear localization of plakoglobin and a twofold reduction in canonical Wnt/β-catenin signaling (Garcia-Gras et al. 2006). The Wnt/β-catenin signaling pathway plays a key role in development and homeostasis (Huelsken et al. 2001). It also regulates the cytoplasmic concentration of β-catenin, an armadillo repeat protein closely related to plakoglobin. There is evidence that competition between these two proteins disrupts Wnt/β-catenin signaling, which is sufficient to cause transdifferentiation of myoblasts into adipocytes in vitro (Ross et al. 2000). Therefore, it is likely that DSP deficiency may inhibit the canonical Wnt/β-catenin signaling and thus trigger a shift from a myocyte fate to an adipocyte fate for cardiac cells (Garcia-Gras et al. 2006).

It should be noted that the mechanisms detailed above do not necessarily preclude each other. It is, therefore, likely that ARVC can be the outcome of several different pathogenic processes that may act synergistically. In the future identification of novel ARVC genes and functional studies of mutations in known genes will undoubtedly shed more light on the pathophysiology of the disorder.

Genetic Testing in ARVC

Genetic testing in ARVC is still at an early stage as until very recently the genetic causes of the disease were unknown. In the last few years the discovery of pathogenic mutations in desmosomal genes has made a possible incorporation of genetic analysis in the clinical management of the disorder an exciting new prospect.

Mutational Yield in Known ARVC Genes

A review of the current literature on ARVC suggests that up to 40% of patients have a mutation in one of the five desmosomal genes (*JUP, DSP, PKP2, DSG2,* and *DSC2*) implicated in the disease. This is an estimate that is difficult to verify as publications vary in their study design and screening cohorts have substantial differences. Ideally, to obtain comparable data, ARVC patients should be genotyped for all known disease genes. However, this has not been the case, either because new genes were discovered after a study was published or the authors concentrated on a specific gene. A recent study of 69 patients screened for the five desmosomal genes identified mutations in 20 (~30%) (Sen-Chowdhry et al. 2007) whilst another study of 80 cases analyzed for mutations in all known ARVC genes except *DSC2* reported an overall mutation rate of 42.5% (in particular 16%, 14%, 10%, and 2.5% for *DSP, PKP2, DSG2,* and *TGF-β3* respectively) (Pilichou et al. 2006).

Undoubtedly, the most important gene in ARVC is *PKP2* with mutations in it accounting for approximately 25%–30% of all ARVC cases. Again, mutation rates in *PKP2* vary substantially between studies ranging from >40% (van Tintelen et al. 2006) to just 11% of genotyped patients (Syrris et al. 2006a). These discrepancies can be attributed to variation in cohort size, geographic factors, and differences in patient selection. For example, the high percentage of *PKP2* mutations in the Dutch population is most likely due to a founder effect (van Tintelen et al. 2006) and unlike in other clinical centers, U.K.-based studies routinely use the proposed modified set of criteria for diagnosing ARVC (Syrris et al. 2006a, 2007).

There could be a number of reasons why the remaining approximately 60% of ARVC patients do not have an identifiable gene mutation. Possible involvement of some minor desmosomal genes or even other unknown nondesmosomal genes in the pathogenesis of ARVC is one of them. Furthermore, patients may have mutations in noncoding parts of genes (e.g., promoter region, etc.) that are not routinely screened for sequence changes. Also, the presence of phenocopies should not be underestimated. A characteristic example is given by Syrris et al. (2006a): two relatives of patients with *PKP2* mutations who were considered as probable mutation carriers on the basis of isolated RV enlargement in one and isolated high volume ventricular ectopy in the other, were found to be negative for that particular mutation. The ARVC phenotype can sometimes be similar to other conditions; for example, ventricular arrhythmias of LBBB morphology can be present in RV outflow tract tachycardia and RV ectopy (>1,000/24 h) in ischemic heart disease or other conditions (Gaita et al. 2001). In addition, in some cases, the presence of LV disease can lead to a misdiagnosis of DCM.

Feasibility, Recommended Strategy, and Benefits of Genetic Testing

As it is the case with other types of inherited cardiac disorders and in particular cardiomyopathies, such as hypertrophic cardiomyopathy (HCM), clinical application of DNA analysis in ARVC is technically feasible, but it is hindered by a variety of reasons related to cost, availability, and allocation of resources and accessibility to patients.

From a technical point of view the most accurate and rapid method of genetic testing is arguably automated direct sequencing. However, screening of large ARVC cohorts with this method can be very expensive as the five known desmosomal genes are large, in particular desmoplakin, with a combined genomic region that requires screening of approximately 40 kb. The cost can be prohibitive if *RYR2* with over 100 exons has to be screened too. As a result, many laboratories usually employ other more cost-effective techniques (e.g., denaturing high performance liquid chromatography, etc.) as a first screening step to identify samples with possible mutations that are then subjected to direct sequencing.

Mutation analysis of ARVC patients should commence from plakophilin-2 that accounts for the highest rate of mutations, followed by desmoplakin, desmoglein-2, desmocollin-2, and plakoglobin in order of importance. *RYR2* should only be targeted if a patient has catecholaminergic polymorphic VT that is associated with mutations in this gene and screening of *TGF-β3* should be reserved for cases showing linkage to ARVD1. With respect to desmosomal genes, despite the occurrence of some recurrent mutations, mainly in *PKP2*, mutations can be found throughout the coding regions with a number of "private" mutations having been detected in families. Therefore, screening cannot be limited to any specific exons.

Completion of screening of the five desmosomal genes is recommended even after the identification of a mutation. There is evidence that a percentage of ARVC patients may be carrying more than one mutation (Sen-Chowdhry et al. 2007), which is consistent with current knowledge of other cardiomyopathies such as HCM (Richard et al. 2003).

To date genetic/clinical experience has shown that there is no clear correlation between genotype and phenotype in ARVC patients carrying different mutations in the same gene or even an identical mutation. The same is true between patients harboring an identified mutation and those without. A typical example is given in a study of familial disease caused by desmoglein-2 mutations (Syrris et al. 2007). A deletion in this gene was detected in a severely affected proband (possibly due to occupational strenuous physical activity) who needed implantation of an ICD. Both her mother (79 years) and daughter (11 years) were mutation carriers but their clinical presentation was markedly different. The former was asymptomatic with normal ECG and echocardiography whilst the latter had T-wave inversion in V1, V2, a biphasic T-wave in V3, and RV wall motion abnormalities even at such a young age (Syrris et al. 2007). These findings, unfortunately, preclude targeting of any specific genes for screening based on clinical findings. Furthermore, comparisons between patients positive and negative for *PKP2* mutations have shown that there was no difference in the percentage of patients who received an ICD or the incidences of appropriate discharge (Dalal et al. 2006; van Tintelen et al. 2006). These observations suggest that genetic testing for *PKP2* mutations is unlikely to contribute substantially to risk assessment of patients.

However, genetic analysis has a number of clear benefits. Undoubtedly, the greatest of them is the identification of individuals at risk of sudden death. It has been well documented that ARVC patients can be completely asymptomatic or mildly symptomatic but still be at risk of life-threatening ventricular arrhythmias. This is highlighted by the findings that sudden cardiac death is the first clinical manifestation in >50% of probands (Nava et al. 2000; Hamid et al. 2002). Therefore, early detection of a pathogenic mutation in a young family member can be potentially life saving.

When a mutation is found in an index case predictive testing should be offered to family members who are potentially at risk (cascade screening) and especially to first-degree relatives who have a 50% probability of carrying the mutation. Such a strategy will not only identify silent mutation carriers who can then be managed clinically but will also distinguish gene-negative individuals with no need for clinical evaluation and repeat follow-ups.

Genetic screening can be important in facilitating a diagnosis of ARVC in "borderline" cases. Because of the nonspecific nature of the manifestations of ARVC, often the presence of arrhythmia of RV origin or RV aneurysms can be highly indicative of ARVC but may also be due to other conditions. A positive genetic test can, therefore, confirm the diagnosis in such cases although a negative result cannot unequivocally exclude ARVC.

Identification of a deleterious mutation can have a profound effect on a patient's life. In many cases a change in lifestyle is required as it is considered prudent for mutation carriers to avoid intensive physical activity and competitive sports (Sen-Chowdhry et al. 2005). Gene-positive individuals should have regular follow-up examinations in an attempt to detect the onset of characteristic disease features that may indicate the entry into a potentially fatal "hot phase." Finally, where appropriate, prophylactic measures can be taken including antiarrhythmic drugs and ICD implantation. Such steps can have a favorable clinical outcome; one study reported a 0.08 annual mortality rate in a cohort of patients under long-term follow-up and treatment (Nava et al. 2000).

A positive genetic finding in a family member can often raise a number of delicate issues including clinical, financial, social, legal, and psychological. Therefore, as standard practice, information obtained by genetic testing should be discussed with the family during genetic counseling.

In conclusion, despite a number of obstacles, genetic testing in ARVC has an important role to play, mainly as a means of identifying gene-positive individuals at risk of sudden death and confirming diagnosis. At this stage, however, it appears to have a limited impact on risk stratification and therapy.

Conclusions

ARVC is an inherited cardiac muscle disease associated with ventricular arrhythmias, heart failure, and sudden cardiac death. It affects primarily the RV but biventricular involvement is common and in some cases there is predominant LV disease. Its histological hallmark is myocyte loss in the myocardium and replacement by fibrous and fibrofatty tissue. In its early phase ("concealed phase") patients may be completely free of symptoms but still be at risk of fatal ventricular arrhythmias.

Diagnosis of ARVC is currently problematic as the disorder exhibits a nonspecific nature of clinical manifestations, phenotypic variability, and incomplete penetrance. Diagnosis is based on the Task Force criteria that have proved to be specific but not sensitive in diagnosing all forms of ARVC, especially when LV disease is present. So there is a need for modification of the original criteria based on our current knowledge of the disorder and its clinical presentation.

ARVC is considered a disease of cell adhesion and approximately 40% of patients have a mutation in one of five desmosomal genes: plakoglobin, desmoplakin, plakophilin-2, desmoglein-2, and desmocollin-2. This suggests that other yet unknown genes, desmosomal or not, may also be involved in the pathogenesis of ARVC. Genetic testing in ARVC is a valuable tool in identifying mutation carriers at risk of sudden death and confirming diagnosis. However, it currently has little prognostic value as there appears to be no clear correlation between genotype (either at the mutation or gene level) with phenotypic expression.

References

Ahmad F, Li D, Karibe A, et al. Localization of a gene responsible for arrhythmogenic right ventricular dysplasia to chromosome 3p23. *Circulation.* 1998;98:2791–2795.

Alcalai R, Metzger S, Rosenheck S, Meiner V, Chajek-Shaul T. A recessive mutation in desmoplakin causes arrythmogenic right ventricular dysplasia, skin disorder, and woolly hair. *J Am Coll Cardiol.* 2003;42:319–327.

Antoniades L, Tsatsopoulou A, Anastasakis A, et al. Arrhythmogenic right ventricular cardiomyopathy caused by deletions in plakophilin-2 and plakoglobin (Naxos disease) in families from Greece and Cyprus: genotype–phenotype relations, diagnostic features and prognosis. *Eur Heart J.* 2006;27:2208–2216.

Asimaki A, Syrris P, Wichter T, Matthias P, Saffitz JE, McKenna WJ. A novel dominant mutation in plakoglobin causes arrhythmogenic right ventricular cardiomyopathy. *Am J Hum Genet.* 2007;81:964–973.

Awad MM, Dalal D, Cho E, et al. DSG2 mutations contribute to arrhythmogenic right ventricular dysplasia/cardiomyopathy. *Am J Hum Genet.* 2006a;79:136–142.

Awad MM, Dalal D, Tichnell C, et al. Recessive arrhythmogenic right ventricular dysplasia due to novel cryptic splice mutation in PKP2. *Hum Mutat.* 2006b;27:1157.

Basso C, Czarnowska E, Della Barbera M, et al. Ultrastructural evidence of intercalated disc remodelling in arrhythmogenic right ventricular cardiomyopathy: an electron microscopy investigation on endomyocardial biopsies. *Eur Heart J.* 2006;27:1847–1854.

Basso C, Thiene G, Corrado D, Angelini A, Nava A, Valente M. Arrhythmogenic right ventricular cardiomyopathy. Dysplasia, dystrophy, or myocarditis? *Circulation.* 1996;94:983–991.

Bauce B, Basso C, Rampazzo A, et al. Clinical profile of four families with arrhythmogenic right ventricular cardiomyopathy caused by dominant desmoplakin mutations. *Eur Heart J.* 2005;26:1666–1675.

Bauce B, Nava A, Rampazzo A, et al. Familial effort polymorphic ventricular arrhythmias in arrhythmogenic right ventricular cardiomyopathy map to 1q42–43. *Am J Cardiol.* 2000;85:573–579.

Bauce B, Rampazzo A, Basso C, et al. Screening for ryanodine receptor type 2 mutations in families with effort-induced polymorphic ventricular arrhythmias and sudden death: early diagnosis of asymptomatic carriers. *J Am Coll Cardiol.* 2002;40:341–349.

Beffagna G, Occhi G, Nava A, et al. Regulatory mutations in transforming growth factor-β3 gene cause arrhythmogenic right ventricular cardiomyopathy type 1. *Cardiovasc Res.* 2005;65:366–373.

Bluemke DA, Krupinski EA, Ovitt T, et al. Imaging of arrhythmogenic right ventricular cardiomyopathy: morphologic findings and interobserver reliability. *Cardiology.* 2003;99:153–162.

Carvajal-Huerta L. Epidermolytic palmoplantar keratoderma with woolly hair and dilated cardiomyopathy. *J Am Acad Dermatol.* 1998;39:418–421.

Chimenti C, Pieroni M, Maseri A, Frustaci A. Histologic findings in patients with clinical and instrumental diagnosis of sporadic arrhythmogenic right ventricular dysplasia. *J Am Coll Cardiol.* 2004;43:2305–2313.

Coonar AS, Protonotarios N, Tsatsopoulou A, et al. Gene for arrhythmogenic right ventricular cardiomyopathy with diffuse nonepidermolytic palmoplantar keratoderma and woolly hair (Naxos disease) maps to 17q21. *Circulation.* 1998;97:2049–2058.

Corrado D, Basso C, Rizzoli G, Schiavon M, Thiene G. Does sports activity enhance the risk of sudden death in adolescents and young adults? *J Am Coll Cardiol.* 2003;42:1959–1963.

Corrado D, Basso C, Schiavon M, Thiene G. Screening for hypertrophic cardiomyopathy in young athletes. *N Engl J Med.* 1998;339:364–369.

Corrado D, Basso C, Thiene G. Arrhythmogenic right ventricular cardiomyopathy: diagnosis, prognosis, and treatment. *Heart.* 2000a;83:588–595.

Corrado D, Basso C, Thiene G, et al. Spectrum of clinicopathologic manifestations of arrhythmogenic right ventricular cardiomyopathy/dysplasia: a multicenter study. *J Am Coll Cardiol.* 1997;30:1512–1520.

Corrado D, Thiene G. Arrhythmogenic right ventricular cardiomyopathy/dysplasia. Clinical impact of molecular genetic studies. *Circulation.* 2006;113:1634–1637.

Corrado D, Fontaine G, Marcus FI, et al. Arrhythmogenic right ventricular dysplasia/cardiomyopathy: need for an international registry. European Society of Cardiology and the Scientific Council on Cardiomyopathies of the World Heart Federation. *J Cardiovasc Electrophysiol.* 2000b;11:827–832.

Corrado D, Thiene G, Nava A, Rossi L, Pennelli N. Sudden death in young competitive athletes: clinicopathologic correlations in 22 cases. *Am J Med.* 1990;89:588–596.

Dalal D, Molin LH, Piccini J, et al. Clinical features of arrhythmogenic right ventricular dysplasia/cardiomyopathy associated with mutations in plakophilin-2. *Circulation.* 2006;113:1641–1649.

Daliento L, Rizzoli G, Thiene G, et al. Diagnostic accuracy of right ventriculography in arrhythmogenic right ventricular cardiomyopathy. *Am J Cardiol.* 1990;66:741–745.

d' Amati G, di Gioia CR, Giordano C, Gallo P. Myocyte transdifferentiation: a possible pathogenetic mechanism for arrhythmogenic right ventricular cardiomyopathy. *Arch Pathol Lab Med.* 2000;124:287–290.

Dubin AM, Batsford WP, Lewis RJ, Rosenfeld LE. Quality-of-life in patients receiving implantable cardioverter defibrillators at or before age 40. *Pacing Clin Electrophysiol.* 1996;19:1555–1559.

Fontaine G. The use of ICDs for the treatment of patients with Arrhythmogenic Right Ventricular Dysplasia (ARVD). *J Interv Card Electrophysiol.* 1997;1:329–330.

Fontaine G, Fontaliran F, Lascault G, et al. Congenital and acquired right ventricular dysplasia. *Arch Mal Coeur Vaiss.* 1990;83:915–920.

Fontaine G, Frank R, Vedel J, Grosgogeat Y, Cabrol C, Facquet J. Stimulation studies and epicardial mapping in ventricular tachycardia: study of mechanisms and selection for surgery. In: Kulbertus HE, ed. *Reentrant Arrhythmias: Mechanisms and Treatment.* Lancaster, PA: MTP Publishing; 1977:334–350.

Gaita F, Giustetto C, Di Donna P, et al. Long-term follow-up of right ventricular monomorphic extrasystoles. *J Am Coll Cardiol.* 2001;38:364–370.

Gallo P, d'Amati G, Pelliccia F. Pathologic evidence of extensive left ventricular involvement in arrhythmogenic right ventricular cardiomyopathy. *Hum Pathol.* 1992;23:948–952.

Garcia-Gras E, Lombardi R, Giocondo MJ, et al. Suppression of canonical Wnt/beta-catenin signaling by nuclear plakoglobin recapitulates phenotype of arrhythmogenic right ventricular cardiomyopathy. *J Clin Invest.* 2006;116:2012–2021.

Garrod DR, Merritt AJ, Nie Z. Desmosomal cadherins. *Curr Opin Cell Biol.* 2002;14:537–545.

Gerull B, Heuser A, Wichter T, et al. Mutations in the desmosomal protein plakophilin-2 are common in jmarrhythmogenic right ventricular cardiomyopathy. *Nat Genet.* 2004;36:1162–1164.

Green KJ, Gaudry CA. Are desmosomes more than tethers for intermediate filaments? *Nat Rev Mol Cell Biol.* 2000;1:208–216.

Hamid MS, Norman M, Quraishi A, et al. Prospective evaluation of relatives for familial arrhythmogenic right ventricular cardiomyopathy/dysplasia reveals a need to broaden diagnostic criteria. *J Am Coll Cardiol.* 2002;40:1445–1450.

Heuser A, Plovie ER, Ellinor PT, et al. Mutant desmocollin-2 causes arrhythmogenic right ventricular cardiomyopathy. *Am J Hum Genet.* 2006;79:1081–1088.

Hodgkinson KA, Parfrey PS, Bassett AS, et al. The impact of implantable cardioverter-defibrillator therapy on survival in autosomal dominant arrhythmogenic right ventricular cardiomyopathy (ARVD5). *J Am Coll Cardiol.* 2005;45:400–408.

Huber O. Structure and function of desmosomal proteins and their role in development and disease. *Cell Mol Life Sci.* 2003;60:1872–1890.

Huelsken J, Birchmeier W. New aspects of Wnt signaling pathways in higher vertebrates. *Curr Opin Genet Dev.* 2001;11:547–553.

Jamora C, Fuchs E. Intercellular adhesion, signalling and the cytoskeleton. *Nat Cell Biol.* 2002;4:E101–E108.

Kannankeril PJ, Bhuiyan ZA, Darbar D, Mannens MM, Wilde AA, Roden DM. Arrhythmogenic right ventricular cardiomyopathy due to a novel plakophilin 2 mutation: wide spectrum of disease in mutation carriers within a family. *Heart Rhythm.* 2006;3:939–944.

Kaplan SR, Gard JJ, Carvajal-Huerta L, Ruiz-Cabezas JC, Thiene G, Saffitz JE. Structural and molecular pathology of the heart in Carvajal syndrome. *Cardiovasc Pathol.* 2004a;13:26–32.

Kaplan SR, Gard JJ, Protnotarios N, et al. Remodeling of myocyte gap junctions in arrhythmogenic right ventricular cardiomyopathy due to a deletion in plakoglobin (Naxos disease). *Heart Rhythm.* 2004b; 1:3–11.

Lai Cheong JE, Wessagowit V, McGrath JA. Molecular abnormalities of the desmosomal protein desmoplakin in human disease. *Clin Exp Dermatol.* 2005;30:261–266.

Laitinen PJ, Brown KM, Piippo K, et al. Mutations of the cardiac ryanodine receptor (RyR2) gene in familial polymorphic ventricular tachycardia. *Circulation.* 2001;103:485–490.

Laurent M, Descaves C, Biron Y, Deplace C, Almange C, Daubert JC. Familial form of arrhythmogenic right ventricular dysplasia. *Am Heart J.* 1987;113:827–829.

Li D, Ahmad F, Gardner MJ, et al. The locus of a novel gene responsible for arrhythmogenic right-ventricular dysplasia characterized by early onset and high penetrance maps to chromosome 10p12-p14. *Am J Hum Genet.* 2000;66:148–156.

Mallat Z, Tedgui A, Fontaliran F, Frank R, Durigon M, Fontaine G. Evidence of apoptosis in arrhythmogenic right ventricular dysplasia. *N Engl J Med.* 1996;335:1190–1196.

Marcus FI, Fontaine G. Arrhythmogenic right ventricular dysplasia/cardiomyopathy: a review. *Pacing Clin Electrophysiol.* 1995;18:1298–1314.

Marcus FI, Fontaine GH, Guiraudon G, et al. Right ventricular dysplasia: a report of 24 adult cases. *Circulation.* 1982;65:384–398.

Marcus FI, McKenna WJ, Sherrill D, et al. Diagnosis of arrhythmogenic right ventricular cardiomyopathy (ARVC). 2009; (In press).

McKenna WJ, Thiene G, Nava A, et al. Diagnosis of arrhythmogenic right ventricular dysplasia/cardiomyopathy. Task Force of the Working Group Myocardial and Pericardial Disease of the European Society of Cardiology and of the Scientific Council on Cardiomyopathies of the International Society and Federation of Cardiology. *Br Heart J.* 1994;71:215–218.

McKoy G, Protonotarios N, Crosby A, et al. Identification of a deletion in plakoglobin in arrhythmogenic right ventricular cardiomyopathy with palmoplantar keratoderma and woolly hair (Naxos disease). *Lancet.* 2000;355:2119–2124.

Melberg A, Oldfors A, Blomstrom-Lundqvist C, et al. Autosomal dominant myofibrillar myopathy with arrhythmogenic right ventricular cardiomyopathy linked to chromosome 10q. *Ann Neurol.* 1999;46:684–692.

Michalodimitrakis M, Papadomanolakis A, Stiakakis J, Kanaki K. Left side right ventricular cardiomyopathy. *Med Sci Law.* 2002;42:313–317.

Nagaoka I, Matsui K, Ueyama T, et al. Novel mutation of plakophilin-2 associated with arrhythmogenic right ventricular cardiomyopathy. *Circ J.* 2006;70:933–935.

Nasir K, Bomma C, Tandri H, et al. Electrocardiographic features of arrhythmogenic right ventricular dysplasia/cardiomyopathy according to disease severity: a need to broaden diagnostic criteria. *Circulation.* 2004;110:1527–1534.

Nava A, Bauce B, Basso C, et al. Clinical profile and long-term follow-up of 37 families with arrhythmogenic right ventricular cardiomyopathy. *J Am Coll Cardiol.* 2000;36:2226–2233.

Nava A, Canciani B, Daliento L, et al. Juvenile sudden death and effort ventricular tachycardias in a family with right ventricular cardiomyopathy. *Int J Cardiol.* 1988b;21:111–126.

Nava A, Rossi L, Thiene G. *Arrhythmogenic Right Ventricular Cardiomyopathy-Dysplasia.* Elsevier, Amsterdam; 1997.

Nava A, Thiene G, Canciani B, et al. Familial occurrence of right ventricular dysplasia: a study involving nine families. *J Am Coll Cardiol.* 1988a;12:1222–1228.

Nemec J, Edwards BS, Osborn MJ, Edwards WD. Arrhythmogenic right ventricular dysplasia masquerading as dilated cardiomyopathy. *Am J Cardiol.* 1999;84:237–239.

Norgett EE, Hatsell SJ, Carvajal-Huerta L, et al. Recessive mutation in desmoplakin disrupts desmoplakin-intermediate filament interactions and causes dilated cardiomyopathy, woolly hair and keratoderma. *Hum Mol Genet.* 2000;9:2761–2766.

Norman M, Simpson M, Mogensen J, et al. Novel mutation in desmoplakin causes arrhythmogenic left ventricular cardiomyopathy. *Circulation.* 2005;112:636–642.

Norman MW, McKenna WJ. Arrhythmogenic right ventricular dysplasia/cardiomyopathy: perspectives on disease. *Z Kardiol.* 1999;88:550–554.

Peters S, Trummel M. Diagnosis of arrhythmogenic right ventricular dysplasia-cardiomyopathy: value of standard ECG revisited. *Ann Noninvasive Electrocardiol.* 2003;8:238–245.

Peters S, Trummel M, Meyners W. Prevalence of right ventricular dysplasia-cardiomyopathy in a non-referral hospital. *Int J Cardiol.* 2004;97:499–501.

Pilichou K, Nava A, Basso C, et al. Mutations in desmoglein-2 gene are associated with arrhythmogenic right ventricular cardiomyopathy. *Circulation.* 2006;113:1171–1179.

Pinamonti B, Miani D, Sinagra G, Bussani R, Silvestri F, Camerini F. Familial right ventricular dysplasia with biventricular involvement and inflammatory infiltration. Heart Muscle Disease Study Group. *Heart.* 1996;76:66–69.

Pinamonti B, Sinagra G, Salvi A, et al. Left ventricular involvement in right ventricular dysplasia. *Am Heart J.* 1992;123:711–724.

Priori SG, Napolitano C, Tiso N, et al. Mutations in the cardiac ryanodine receptor gene (hRyR2) underlie catecholaminergic polymorphic ventricular tachycardia. *Circulation.* 2001;103:196–200.

Protonotarios N, Tsatsopoulou A, Anastasakis A, et al. Genotype-phenotype assessment in autosomal recessive arrhythmogenic right ventricular cardiomyopathy (Naxos disease) caused by a deletion in plakoglobin. *J Am Coll Cardiol.* 2001;38:1477–1484.

Protonotarios N, Tsatsopoulou A, Patsourakos P, et al. Cardiac abnormalities in familial palmoplantar keratosis. *Br Heart J.* 1986;56:321–326.

Rampazzo A, Beffagna G, Nava A, et al. Arrhythmogenic right ventricular cardiomyopathy type 1 (ARVD1): confirmation of locus assignment and mutation screening of four candidate genes. *Eur J Hum Genet.* 2003;11:69–76.

Rampazzo A, Nava A, Danieli GA, et al. The gene for arrhythmogenic right ventricular cardiomyopathy maps to chromosome 14q23-q24. *Hum Mol Genet.* 1994;3:959–962.

Rampazzo A, Nava A, Erne P, et al. A new locus for arrhythmogenic right ventricular cardiomyopathy (ARVD2) maps to chromosome 1q42-q43. *Hum Mol Genet.* 1995;4:2151–2154.

Rampazzo A, Nava A, Malacrida S, et al. Mutation in human desmoplakin domain binding to plakoglobin causes a dominant form of arrhythmogenic right ventricular cardiomyopathy. *Am J Hum Genet.* 2002;71:1200–1206.

Rampazzo A, Nava A, Miorin M, et al. ARVD4, a new locus for arrhythmogenic right ventricular cardiomyopathy, maps to chromosome 2 long arm. *Genomics.* 1997;45:259–263.

Richard P, Charron P, Carrier L, et al. Hypertrophic cardiomyopathy: distribution of disease genes, spectrum of mutations, and implications for a molecular diagnosis strategy. *Circulation.* 2003;107:2227–2232.

Richardson P, McKenna W, Bristow M, et al. Report of the 1995 World Health Organization/International Society and Federation of Cardiology Task Force on the Definition and Classification of Cardiomyopathies. *Circulation.* 1996;93:841–842.

Ross SE, Hemati N, Longo KA, et al. Inhibition of adipogenesis by Wnt signaling. *Science.* 2000;289:950–953.

Rossi V, Beffagna G, Rampazzo A, Bauce B, Danieli GA. TAIL1: an isthmin-like gene, containing type 1 thrombospondin-repeat and AMOP domain, mapped to ARVD1 critical region. *Gene.* 2004;335:101–108.

Sears SF, Conti JB. Implantable cardioverter-defibrillators for children and young adolescents: mortality benefit confirmed—what's next? *Heart.* 2004;90:241–242.

Sen-Chowdhry S, Lowe MD, Sporton SC, McKenna WJ. Arrhythmogenic right ventricular cardiomyopathy: clinical presentation, diagnosis, and management. *Am J Med.* 2004;117:685–695.

Sen-Chowdhry S, Prasad SK, Syrris P, et al. Cardiovascular magnetic resonance in arrhythmogenic right ventricular cardiomyopathy revisited: comparison with task force criteria and genotype. *J Am Coll Cardiol.* 2006;48:2132–2140.

Sen-Chowdhry S, Syrris P, McKenna WJ. Genetics of arrhythmogenic right ventricular cardiomyopathy. *J Cardiovasc Electrophysiol.* 2005;16:927–935.

Sen-Chowdhry S, Syrris P, Ward D, Asimaki A, Sevdalis E, McKenna WJ. Clinical and genetic characterization of families with arrhythmogenic right ventricular dysplasia/cardiomyopathy provides novel insights into patterns of disease expression. *Circulation.* 2007;115:1710–1720.

Severini GM, Krajinovic M, Pinamonti B, et al. A new locus for arrhythmogenic right ventricular dysplasia on the long arm of chromosome 14. *Genomics.* 1996;31:193–200.

Sharma S, Whyte G, Elliott P, et al. Electrocardiographic changes in 1000 highly trained junior elite athletes. *Br J Sports Med.* 1999;33:319–324.

Shen WK, Edwards WD, Hammill SC, Gersh BJ. Right ventricular dysplasia: a need for presice pathological definition for interpretation of sudden death [abstract]. *J Am Coll Cardiol.* 1994;23:24.

Syrris P, Ward D, Asimaki A, et al. Clinical expression of plakophilin-2 mutations in familial arrhythmogenic right ventricular cardiomyopathy. *Circulation.* 2006a;113:356–364.

Syrris P, Ward D, Asimaki A, et al. Desmoglein-2 mutations in arrhythmogenic right ventricular cardiomyopathy: a genotype-phenotype characterization of familial disease. *Eur Heart J.* 2007;28:581–588.

Syrris P, Ward D, Evans A, et al. Arrhythmogenic right ventricular dysplasia/cardiomyopathy associated with mutations in the desmosomal gene desmocollin-2. *Am J Hum Genet.* 2006b;79:978–984.

Tandri H, Calkins H, Marcus FI. Controversial role of magnetic resonance imaging in the diagnosis of arrhythmogenic right ventricular dysplasia. *Am J Cardiol.* 2003;92:649.

Thiene G, Nava A, Corrado D, Rossi L, Pennelli N. Right ventricular cardiomyopathy and sudden death in young people. *N Eng J Med.* 1988;318:119–133.

Tiso N, Salamon M, Bagattin A, Danieli GA, Argenton F, Bortolussi M. The binding of the RyR2 calcium channel to its gating protein FKBP12.6 is oppositely affected by ARVD2 and VTSIP mutations. *Biochem Biophys Res Commun.* 2002;299:594–598.

Tiso N, Stephan DA, Nava A, et al. Identification of mutations in the cardiac ryanodine receptor gene in families affected with arrhythmogenic right ventricular cardiomyopathy type 2 (ARVD2). *Hum Mol Genet.* 2001;10:189–194.

van Tintelen JP, Entius MM, Bhuiyan ZA, et al. Plakophilin-2 mutations are the major determinant of familial arrhythmogenic right ventricular dysplasia/cardiomyopathy. *Circulation.* 2006;113:1650–1658.

van Tintelen JP, Hofstra RM, Wiesfeld AC, van den Berg MP, Hauer RN, Jongbloed RD. Molecular genetics of arrhythmogenic right ventricular cardiomyopathy: emerging horizon? *Curr Opin Cardiol.* 2007;22:185–192.

Weber KT, Brilla CG, Campbell SE, Zhou G, Matsubara L, Guarda E. Pathologic hypertrophy with fibrosis: the structural basis for myocardial failure. *Blood Press.* 1992;1:75–85.

White JB, Razmi R, Nath H, Kay GN, Plumb VJ, Epstein AE. Relative utility of magnetic resonance imaging and right ventricular angiography to diagnose arrhythmogenic right ventricular cardiomyopathy. *J Interv Card Electrophysiol.* 2004;10:19–26.

Wichter T, Borggrefe M, Haverkamp W, Chen X, Breithardt G. Efficacy of antiarrhythmic drugs in patients with arrhythmogenic right ventricular disease. Results in patients with inducible and noninducible ventricular tachycardia. *Circulation.* 1992;86:29–37.

Wichter T, Paul M, Wollmann C, et al. Implantable cardioverter/defibrillator therapy in arrhythmogenic right ventricular cardiomyopathy: single-center experience of long-term follow-up and complications in 60 patients. *Circulation.* 2004;109:1503–1508.

Yang Z, Bowles NE, Scherer SE, et al. Desmosomal dysfunction due to mutations in desmoplakin causes arrhythmogenic right ventricular dysplasia/cardiomyopathy. *Circ Res.* 2006;99:646–655.

15

Ventricular Noncompaction

Girish Dwivedi, Ibrar Ahmed, Zaheer Yousef, and Michael Frenneaux

Introduction

Noncompaction of the ventricular myocardium (NVM) is a rare congenital cardiomyopathy, characterized by prominent ventricular trabeculae and deep intertrabecular recesses (Dusek et al. 1975; Chin et al. 1990; Maron et al. 2006). It is thought to be related to arrest of myocardial development (Dusek et al. 1975; Jenni et al. 1986; Chin et al. 1990) and is classified as a primary cardiomyopathy of genetic origin by the American Heart Association (Maron et al. 2006). Although it is often associated with other congenital cardiac anomalies (Lauer et al. 1964; Dusek et al. 1975; Ozkutlu et al. 2002), it can also be seen in the absence of other cardiac defects (Ritter et al. 1997). The etiology in most cases remains elusive and the major genetic determinants remain to be determined. Clinical manifestations are variable, ranging from no symptoms to disabling congestive heart failure, arrhythmias, and systemic thromboembolism. Echocardiography is the diagnostic procedure of choice, but the diagnosis is often missed or delayed because of lack of knowledge about this condition and its similarity to other diseases of the myocardium. Diagnosis in the modern day is facilitated by the introduction of specific morphologic criteria on echocardiography and magnetic resonance imaging (MRI). Treatment centers on the management of heart failure, arrhythmias, and prevention of thromboembolic events.

Cardiac Embryology and Development

A number of studies have shown that the development of the human heart involves precisely regulated molecular and embryogenetic events (Srivastava and Olson 2000; Harvey 2002) (see also Chapters 1 & 2). Each event is initiated by a specific signaling molecule and mediated by tissue-specific transcription factor(s). It was initially thought that all the cells that comprise the muscle of the mature heart originate from bilaterally distributed mesodermal fields that were established during early gastrulation (Agmon et al. 1999). However, it is now known that the cellular components that ultimately develop in to the myocardium have multiple origins (Agmon et al. 1999). Furthermore, addition of myocardial cells to the developing heart occurs at various stages during embryogenesis (Eisenberg and Markwald 2004). Myocardial development involves the formation of two different myocardial layers within the ventricular wall, the trabecular layer, and the subepicardial compact layer. The endocardium constitutes the cellular base of the trabecular layer while the compact layer is formed underneath the epicardium. The process of ventricular trabeculation is considered a highly synchronized developmental process that changes at every stage of cardiac development. Prior to the development of the coronary circulation, the embryonic myocardium consists of a "spongy" meshwork of interwoven myocardial fibers forming trabeculae with deep intertrabecular recesses, which communicate with the left ventricular (LV) cavity (Agmon et al. 1999; Bernanke and Velkey 2002; Freedom et al. 2005). These intertrabecular spaces are responsible for blood supply to the myocardium at this stage of cardiac development. Cardiac trabeculation is dependent on the secretion of various factors during development such as neuregulin, serotonin 2B receptor, vascular endothelial growth factor, and angiopoietin (Srivastava and Olson 2000; Harvey 2002). During weeks 5 to 8 of human fetal development, the ventricular myocardium undergoes a gradual process of compaction, from the epicardium toward endocardium, from base to apex, with transformation of the relatively large intertrabecular spaces into capillaries with gradual disappearance of the large spaces within the trabecular meshwork and completion of compaction (Agmon et al. 1999; Bernanke and Velkey 2002; Freedom et al. 2005). Occurring parallel to this process of compaction of the ventricular myocardium is the formation of the coronary vessels ending with the establishment of the coronary circulation (Agmon et al. 1999; Bernanke and Velkey 2002; Freedom et al. 2005).

Noncompaction of the Ventricular Myocardium

NVM is believed to be the result of arrested endomyocardial morphogenesis (Chin et al. 1990; Ritter et al. 1997; Zambrano et al. 2002). It was first described in association with other congenital anomalies, such as obstruction of the right or left ventricular outflow tracts, complex cyanotic congenital heart diseases, and coronary artery anomalies (Lauer et al. 1964; Dusek et al. 1975; Ritter et al. 1997; Table 15–1). Although the abnormal compaction process in these cases is still not completely understood, it has been suggested that pressure overload or myocardial ischemia associated with these conditions prevents regression of the embryonic myocardial sinusoids. Arrest of the regression of the embryonic

Table 15–1 Structural Heart Diseases Associated with Noncompaction

Absent aortic valve
Anomalous origin of right subclavian artery
Anomalous pulmonary venous return
Aortic stenosis
Aortico-left ventricular tunnel
Arteriovenous block
Atrial isomerism
Atrial septal aneurysm
Atrial septal defect
Atrioventricular diverticulum
Bicuspid aortic valve
Coarctation of the aorta
Congenital mitral valve stenosis
Coronary osteal stenosis
Dextrocardia
Double orifice mitral valve
Ebstein's anomaly
Heterotaxy
Histiocyte cardiomyopathy
Hypoplastic left heart syndrome
Hypoplastic right ventricle
Malposed great arteries
Mitral valve cleft
Patent ductus arteriosus
Polyvalvular dysplasia
Pulmonary hypertension
Pulmonary stenosis
Right ventricular muscle bands
Tetralogy of Fallot
Transposition of the great arteries
Ventricular inversion
Ventricular septal defect

Source: Adapted from Finsterer et al. 2006.

myocardial sinusoids results in the persistence of deep intertrabecular recesses in communication with both the ventricular cavity and the coronary circulation (Öechslin et al. 2000).

Isolated noncompaction of the ventricular myocardium (INVM), first described by Chin et al. in 1990, is characterized by persistent embryonic myocardial morphology found in the absence of other cardiac anomalies (Chin et al. 1990). The deep recesses in INVM communicate only with the ventricular cavity and not with the coronary circulation, as is the case with NVM (Rigopoulos et al. 2002).

NVM of the right ventricle (RV) may coexist with LV involvement in less than 50% of patients (Lauer et al. 1964; Ritter et al. 1997; Öechslin et al. 2000), but due to the difficulty encountered in distinguishing NVM from normal RV trabeculations, several authors challenge the existence of isolated RV noncompaction (Öechslin et al. 2000; Jenni et al. 2001). Furthermore, some authors have recommended the term "LV hypertrabeculation" instead of "isolated noncompaction," as coexisting cardiac abnormalities have been described in "isolated" cases, and the latter term suggests that the pathogenesis is proven (Finsterer et al. 2002; Stöllberger et al. 2002).

It should be noted that there has been no definitive proof of an arrest in embryonic endomyocardial morphogenesis. In an interesting series, the Bleyl team did not find any characteristic features of noncompaction on fetal echocardiography in three infants who were subsequently diagnosed with INVM (Bleyl et al. 1997a). These findings challenge the theory of arrested embryonic development as the pathogenesis of LV noncompaction (Bleyl et al. 1997b; Stöllberger et al. 2002) and suggest an acquired condition rather than congenital. Alternatively, these findings may reflect limitations of fetal echocardiography (Bleyl et al. 1997). Other investigators (Stöllberger et al. 2002) have postulated that other pathogenetic processes could account for noncompaction such as dissection of myocardium, frustrated attempts of myocardial hypertrophy, myocardial tearing caused by dilatation, a metabolic defect, or compensatory hypervascularization.

Pathology

In addition to the first necropsy findings described by Chin et al. (1990), many other studies published in cases with INVM reveal prominent trabecular meshwork and numerous intertrabecular recesses in the ventricular myocardium (Dusek et al. 1975; Jenni et al. 1986; Ritter et al. 1997). The recesses, lined with endothelium in continuity with the ventricular myocardium, have been described to extend deep into the trabecular meshwork, and to end blindly at the compact outer layer, without communication with the coronary circulation (Allenby et al. 1988; Chin et al. 1990). Thus, the term "INVM" (Chin et al. 1990) seems more apt than "isolated myocardial sinusoids" (Engberding and Bender 1984).

In an autopsy series of 474 normal hearts by Boyd et al. (1987), upto 70% had prominent trabeculations in the LV cavity, but only 4% of these had more than three trabeculations (Figure 15–1). Based on this, Stöllberger et al. defined pathological LV hypertrabeculation (LVHT) when more than three trabeculations were identified on echocardiography (Stöllberger and Finsterer 2004b).

As previously mentioned, histologically, INVM is distinct from noncompaction associated with other congenital heart diseases, in that the deep intertrabecular recesses communicate only with the LV cavity in the former and may communicate with both the coronary circulation and the LV cavity in the latter (Öechslin et al. 2000).

Pathophysiology

There are no abnormal findings on coronary angiography in patients with INVM (Engberding and Bender 1984; Chin et al. 1990; Junga et al. 1999). Positron emission tomography has demonstrated a decrease in coronary flow reserve in noncompacted and compacted segments of the LV. It is likely that microcirculatory dysfunction might contribute to LV contractile dysfunction and be responsible for the subendocardial fibrosis found on histology as most of the compacted segments have evidence of reduced coronary flow reserve as demonstrated by wall motion abnormalities (Junga et al. 1999; Jenni et al. 2001, 2007; Soler et al. 2002). Indeed, a case report showing impaired aerobic fatty acid metabolism in noncompacted ventricular segments support the putative mechanism that in INVM, myocardial failure, and remodeling are the result of ischemia (Toyono et al. 2001). Clinical symptoms

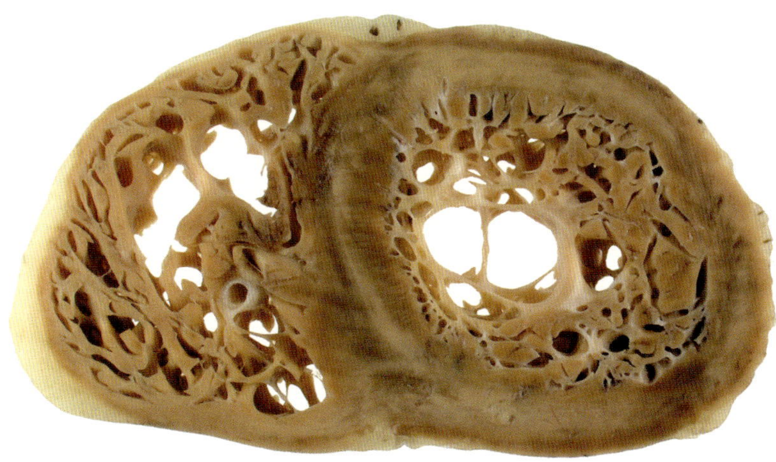

Figure 15.1 Gross appearance of the cut section of heart removed from an 18-year-old woman who had a successful cardiac transplantation. She developed chronic progressive heart failure diagnosed with familial dilated cardiomyopathy (father similarly affected). Note marked biventricular distortion of the cadiac musculature filled with trabeculae and variable size cysts characteristic of the ventricular non-compaction (with permission from the patient and Department of Cardiac Transplantation, Bimingham University Hospital, Birmingham, UK).

of cardiac failure that are seen in the majority of the patients with INVM are probably secondary to both systolic as well as diastolic LV dysfunction.

Genetics

Our understanding of the molecular signaling pathways governing the morphogenesis of the cardiovascular system has increased significantly in recent years. A number of candidate genes have been identified that are thought to be involved in myocardial morphogenesis. Indeed, recent studies have suggested that the genetic etiology underlying previously hitherto considered "distinct" cardiomyopathies may be shared, with commonality in genetic origin being found in ventricular noncompaction, hypertrophic cardiomyopathy (HCM) and dilated cardiomyopathy (DCM) (Hoedemaekers et al. 2007; Klaassen et al. 2008). However, despite the progress made in genomics the precise mechanisms underlying myocardial noncompaction are unclear.

The inheritance of NVM may either be sporadic or familial. An autosomal dominant mode of inheritance is considered to be more common than X-linked inheritance for familial cases (Bleyl et al. 1997; Sasse-Klaassen et al. 2004; Xing et al. 2006) although autosomal recessive inheritance has also been suggested (Digilio et al. 1999). Increased occurrence of NVM in family members of the affected individual is widely observed since the initial description of NVM (Chin et al. 1990; Ritter et al. 1997). In two of the largest series of patients (Aras et al. 2006; Xing et al. 2006), the frequency of familial noncompaction was found to be 25% and 33%. Such a high rate of occurrence in family members warrants a detailed pedigree analysis and careful clinical and cardiac evaluation of all first-degree family members of affected individuals.

Up till now, mutations in seven noncompaction-associated loci have been discovered. TAZ is the only confirmed disease-causing locus identified till now. As mentioned previously, NVM may be seen as a cardiac feature in a variety of metabolic diseases and genetic syndromes (Table 15–2).

Genes Linked to Noncompaction

The NVM associated loci have been classified according to the amount of evidence in the literature demonstrating them to be primary disease-causing genes (Zaragoza et al. 2007).

Confirmed Genes

TAZ which is located on Xq28 and encodes for taffazin (G4.5 protein) involved in the biosynthesis of cardiolipin, an essential component of the mitochondrial inner membrane, was the first locus discovered to be associated with NVM (Bleyl et al. 1997). Barth syndrome, a metabolic condition with DCM, with or without noncompaction, 3-methylglutaconic aciduria, skeletal myopathy, and neutropenia is also described with mutation in TAZ (Bione et al. 1996). In total, six different mutations in TAZ have been described in children with NVM (Bleyl et al. 1997; Ichida et al. 2001; Chen et al. 2002; Xing et al. 2006; Marziliano et al. 2007).

Nonconfirmed Genes

DTNA (ADB) that is located on 18q12.1 and encodes for dystrobrevin-(α), a dystrophin-associated protein involved in maintaining the structural integrity of the muscle membrane, was the second locus described with NVM (Ichida et al. 2001). Although one mutation in DTNA was identified in a single affected family several affected individuals also had congenital heart disease, including ventricular septal defect and hypoplastic left heart (Ichida et al. 2001). Therefore, DTNA as a primary disease-causing locus is still to be confirmed. Interestingly, no other conditions have been associated with mutations in DTNA.

Speculative Genes

Four different mutations in LDB3 (ZASP), which is located on 10q23.2 and encodes for the LIM domain binding 3 protein (ZASP or Cypher), a muscle sarcomeric Z-band protein, have been identified in four affected families and two sporadic cases. Most of these individuals with LDB3 mutations had myocardium with features of noncompaction and/or DCM (Vatta et al. 2003; Xing et al. 2006; Marziliano et al. 2007). *SCN5A*, *MYH7*, and *MYBPC3* are more recently recognized noncompaction-associated genes. *SCN5A* is located on 3p22.2 and encodes for the cardiac sodium channel (α)-subunit that mediates the membrane action potential required for normal heart rhythm. Two mutations in *SCN5A* have been identified in families with NVM (Makita 2008). *MYH7* and *MYBPC3* are located on 14q12 and 11p11.2 respectively and encode for sarcomeric proteins involved in cardiomyocyte contraction. A mutation in LMNA, which is located on 1q22 encoding for lamin A/C, was identified in a single family consisting of an individual with NVM and three mutation carriers had a DCM or mild LV

Table 15–2 Syndromes Associated with Noncompaction of the Left Ventricle

Syndrome	Locus	Clinical Characteristics
Barth syndrome	Xq28	Dilated cardiomyopathy, neutropenia, skeletal myopathy
Beals syndrome	5q23-q31	Congenital contractures, delayed motor development, Marfanoid
Beckers muscular dystrophy	Xp21.2	Muscle wastage, cardiomyopathy, arrhythmias
Charcot-Marie-Tooth Disease type 1A	17p11.2	Peripheral neuropathy, muscle atrophy
Duchenne muscular dystrophy	Xp21.2	Muscle degeneration, cardiomyopathy, arrhythmias
Melnick-needles syndrome	Xq28	Skeletal abnormalities, craniofacial dysmorphogenesis
Myotonic dystrophy	19q13.2-q13.3	Myotonia, distal weakness, cognitive impairment
Myoadenylate-deaminase deficiency	1p21-p13	Exercise intolerance, myalgia
Nail-patella syndrome	9q34.1	Nail dysplasia, patellar hypoplasia
Noonan syndrome	12q24.1	Failure to thrive, cardiomyopathy, septal defects
Roifman syndrome	X	Dysgammablobulinemia, skeletal dysplasia
Trisomy 13		Cognitive impairment, polydactyly, skeletal abnormalities

Source: Adapted from Zaragoza et al. 2007.

enlargement (Hermida-Prieto et al. 2004). Emery–Dreifuss muscular dystrophy, limb girdle muscular dystrophy1B, Hutchinson–Gilford progeria syndrome, and atypical Werner syndrome have also been found to be associated with mutations in LMNA.

Large studies screening for mutations in the known loci (Ritter et al. 1997; Chen et al. 2002; Pignatelli et al. 2003; Kenton et al. 2004; Xing et al. 2006) find that most affected individuals do not have mutations detected in either TAZ or DTNA. The contribution of LMNA, SCNA, MYH7, and MYBP3 to the etiology of NVM is not known. Therefore, it would not be unreasonable to conclude that the genetic etiology of most NVM is still unknown.

Loci and Chromosomal Regions Associated with NVM

A newborn girl with facial dysmorphism, multiple ventricular septal defects, and epilepsy (Thienpont et al. 2007), array-CGH detected up to a 5.9 Mb terminal deletion at 1p36, was shown to have NVM. Although NVM had not been previously reported in other patients described with 1q43 deletion syndrome, in a recent report, a newborn girl with NVM, facial dysmorphism, hypotonia, and cardiac septal defects was found to have an interstitial 5.4 Mb deletion of 1q43 (Kanemoto et al. 2006). The authors contemplated that haploinsufficiency of 1q43 containing the cardiac ryanodine receptor gene is the cause of NVM. It is possible that chromosome 1 may contain two noncompaction associated loci at 1p36 and 1q43. Patients with 1p36 deletion syndrome can also develop DCM.

NKX2–5 is a potential locus associated with NVM on the chromosome 5. The *NKX2–5* gene encodes for a key transcription factor in cardiogenesis. Mutations of this gene are associated with a variety of congenital heart diseases such as atrial septal defect, double-outlet right ventricle, tetralogy of Fallot, arteriovenous block, and Ebstein's anomaly (Schott et al. 1998; Benson et al. 1999). Deletion of 5q35, which includes the *NKX2–5* gene, was detected in a girl with an atrial septal defect, patent ductus arteriosus, minor dysmorphism, developmental delay, heart block, DCM, and NVM (Pauli et al. 1999). Furthermore features of NVM are notable in the *NKX2–5* mutant mouse model (Pashmforoush et al. 2004). These findings add weight, but are not conclusive, of the link between *NKX2–5* mutations and NVM.

Metabolic Diseases and Genetic Syndromes Associated with Noncompaction of the LV

Mutations in the Tafazzin gene, an X-linked condition, lead to Barth Syndrome. Tafazzin is a proposed signaling molecule regulating apoptosis and a known component of the inner mitochondrial membrane (Schlame and Ren 2006). Barth syndrome is associated with DCM. However, in a recent publication, Schlame and colleagues described features of NVM in 15 of the 30 patients with Barth syndrome (Schlame and Ren 2006). Interestingly one child was noted to have NVM at birth but NVM disappeared by the age of 6 years (Schlame and Ren 2006). Indeed, it is possible that such remodeling may cause underestimation of the true incidence of NVM amongst patients with Barth syndrome.

NVM may also be seen as a feature of mitochondrial diseases. In two large studies of pediatric patients with mitochondrial disorder NVM was seen as one of the cardiac features (Scaglia et al. 2004; Yaplito-Lee et al. 2007). Similarly in adults, out of 62 patients with NVM, 13 were found to have metabolic myopathy, a condition described with respiratory chain abnormalities (Stöllberger et al. 2002). Succinate dehydrogenase deficiency, a mitochondrial disorder, has been found to be associated with NVM (Davili et al. 2007). Mitochondrial DNA (mtDNA) mutations found in patients with NVM include G3460A, which is also found in Leber's hereditary optic neuropathy (Finsterer et al. 2001), and A3243G, a skeletal muscle heteroplasmic mutation in a patient with complete heart block, myopathy, and nail-patella syndrome (Finsterer et al. 2007b). Additional reports include a man with ragged red fibers, complex partial seizures, limb wasting, and an A8381G mtDNA change in the MT-ATP8 gene (Finsterer et al. 2004b), and a patient with hearing impairment, ophthalmoplegia, central nervous system abnormalities, polyneuropathy, diabetes mellitus, and multiple mtDNA changes (A15662G, T3398C, T4216C, and G15812A) in the *MT-ND1* (NADH dehydrogenase subunit 1) and *MT-CYB* genes (Finsterer et al. 2000).

The specific role of mitochondrial dysfunction in the etiology of noncompacted myocardium is not known. As the mitochondrion is essential for cardiac development and function, providing most of the energy for contraction and ion transport through mitochondrial oxidative phosphorylation, generating most of the endogenous reactive oxygen species as a toxic byproduct, and regulating programmed cell death (Wallace 1999), it follows that defects in mtDNA mutations, and/or other aspects of mitochondrial metabolism, would be likely to impact cardiac development, leading to noncompaction.

Other metabolic diseases described with NVM include myoadenylate-deaminase deficiency described in a man who was found to have a mutation in the myoadenylate-deaminase deficiency disease-causing locus *AMPD1* (Finsterer et al. 2004a). Also NVM has been described in a 2-year-old girl with vitamin B12 (cobalamin) deficiency and a homozygous mutation in *MMACHC* associated with combined methylmalonic aciduria and homocystinuria (cobalamin C type) (Tanpaiboon et al. 2006).

Neuromuscular disorders are often associated with various types of cardiomyopathy. Duchenne and Becker muscular dystrophy, and limb-girdle muscular dystrophy have been noted to be associated with cardiomyopathy and are classified as dystrophinopathies (Stöllberger et al. 1996; Lofiego et al. 2007; Finsterer et al. 2007a). These dystrophinopathies may also demonstrate features of NVM (Finsterer et al. 2007a). Other neuromuscular disorders described with NVM include Charcot-Marie-Tooth disease and myotonic dystrophy (Finsterer et al. 2005; Corrado et al. 2006).

Many other genetic syndromes describe NVM as one of their features (OMIM 2008). There has been a recent spurt of publications and the ever-expanding list includes Turner syndrome (van Heerde et al. 2003; OMIM 2008), trisomy 13 (McMahon et al. 2005), and 22q11.2 deletion syndrome (Pignatelli et al. 2003), malformations syndromes—microphthalmia with linear skin defects (Kherbaoui-Redouani et al. 2003), Roifman syndrome (Mandel et al. 2001), Melnick-Needles syndrome (Wong and Bofinger 1997), nail-patella syndrome (Finsterer et al. 2007b), Noonan syndrome (Amann and Sherman 1992), and congenital contractural arachnodactyly (Beals syndrome) (Matsumoto et al. 2006).

Epidemiology and Demographics

NVM has been diagnosed in all age groups. In the original case series of isolated noncompaction by Chin et al., the median age at the time of diagnosis was 7 years (range: 11 months–22 years) (Chin et al. 1990). The true echocardiographic prevalence of INVM is difficult to ascertain, mainly due to the referral bias to specialist centers. In the largest echocardiographic series of patients with INVM, the prevalence was 0.014% of patients referred to the echocardiography laboratory (Öechslin et al. 2000). Men appear to be affected more frequently than women, with males accounting for 56%–82% of cases in the four largest reported series (Chin et al. 1990; Ritter et al. 1997; Maltagliati and Pepi 2000; Öechslin et al. 2000).

Clinical Presentation

Noncompaction is identified incidentally or is found to be present in patients presenting with one or a combination of three major clinical manifestations (Chin et al. 1990; Ritter et al. 1997; Agmon et al. 1999).

1. Heart failure
2. Arrhythmias
3. Embolic events.

Clinical characteristics of patients from five study populations with NVM are presented in Table 15–3.

A patient with noncompaction can present with findings that can range from asymptomatic LV dysfunction to severe disabling congestive heart failure. In the cohort with INVM described in the initial report by Chin et al., depressed ventricular systolic function was noted in 63% of patients (Chin et al. 1990). Over 70% of the patients in the largest series with INVM had symptomatic heart failure (Öechslin et al. 2000). In children with INVM, the initial presentation of INVM may be as that of a restrictive cardiomyopathy (Hook et al. 1996; Ichida et al. 1999). In a prospective case series of Japanese children with INVM followed for up to 17 years, irrespective of the presence or absence of symptoms at the time of initial diagnosis, LV dysfunction developed in the majority (Ichida et al. 1999).

The origin of systolic dysfunction in noncompaction remains unclear but of the available evidence, consensus is emerging that suggests that subendocardial hypoperfusion and microcirculatory dysfunction, even in the absence of epicardial coronary artery disease, probably play important roles in ventricular dysfunction and arrhythmogenesis. It has been suggested that in the presence of prominent and numerous trabeculae, subendocardial ischemia may result from isometric contraction of the endocardium and myocardium within the deep intertrabecular recesses.

Diastolic dysfunction has been described in patients with ventricular noncompaction and is thought to be related to both abnormal relaxation and restrictive filling caused by the numerous prominent trabeculae (Agmon et al. 1999).

Sudden cardiac death accounted for half of the deaths in the larger series of patients with INVM (Chin et al. 1990; Ritter et al. 1997; Öechslin et al. 2000; Rigopoulos et al. 2002). Although ventricular arrhythmias occurred in nearly 40% of patients in the initial description of INVM by Chin et al. (1990), Ichida et al. (1999) described no cases of ventricular tachycardia or sudden death in the largest series of pediatric patients with INVM. Rhythm disturbances including paroxysmal supraventricular tachycardia and complete heart block have been reported in patients with INVM (Ichida et al. 1999). Nonspecific findings on the resting electrocardiography (ECG) are found in the majority of patients with NVM. ECG changes include LV hypertrophy, abnormal Q-waves, repolarization changes, T-waves changes, ST-segment abnormalities, axis shifts, intraventricular conduction abnormalities, and AV block (Chin et al. 1990; Reynen et al. 1997; Ritter et al. 1997; Ichida et al. 1999; Öechslin et al. 2000; Table 15–4). ECG findings consistent with Wolff-Parkinson-White syndrome have been described in up to 15% of pediatric patients (Ichida et al. 1999; Yasukawa et al. 2001) but it was not observed in the two largest series of adults with isolated noncompaction (Ritter et al. 1997; Öechslin et al. 2000).

In three series of patients with IVNM, the occurrence of thromboembolic events, including cerebrovascular accidents, transient ischemic attacks, pulmonary embolism, and mesenteric infarction, ranged from 21% to 38% (Chin et al. 1990; Ritter et al. 1997; Öechslin et al. 2000). Embolic complications are possibly related to development of thrombi due to combination of factors that alter flow through the ventricle including an extensively trabeculated ventricle, depressed systolic function, and development of atrial fibrillation (Ritter et al. 1997; Agmon et al. 1999). Of note, however, is that no systemic embolic events were reported in the largest pediatric series with INVM (Ichida et al. 1999).

An association between INVM and facial dysmorphisms, including a prominent forehead, low-set ears, strabismus, high-arching palate, and micrognathia, was described by Chin et al. (1990).

Table 15–3 Clinical Characteristics of Patients from Five Study Populations with Noncompaction of the Ventricular Myocardium

Patient Characteristics	Öechslin et al. 2000	Ritter et al. 1997	Ichida et al. 1999	Stllberger et al. 2002	Chin et al. 1990
Patients	34	17	27	62	8
Females %	26	18	44	30	37
Age (years)	16–71	18–71	0–15	50 mean	0.9–22.5
Noncompacted segments %					
Apex	94	100	100	98	Most common
Inferior wall	84	100	70	8	—
Lateral wall	100		41	19	—
Mural thrombi %	9	6	0	—	25
Impaired LV function %	82	76	60	58	63
Abnormal ECG %	94	88	88	92	88
Ventricular tachycardia %	41	47	0	18	38
Atrial fibrillation %	26	29	—	5	—
Systemic embolism %	21	24	0	—	38
Sudden death %	18	18	7	—	13

Source: Adapted from Weiford et al. 2004.

Table 15–4 Electrocardiographic Abnormalties Associated with Noncompaction

Axis shifts
Abnormal Q-waves
Intraventricular conduction abnormalities
AV block
Repolarization changes
LV hypertrophy
ST-segment abnormalities
T-wave changes
Atrial fibrillation
Paroxysmal supraventricular tachycardia
WPW-syndrome
Bigemini ventricular extrasystoles
Ventricular tachycardia
Ventricular fibrillation

Source: Adapted from Finsterer et al. 2006.

One-third of children with INVM in the series by Ichida et al. had similar dysmorphic facial features (Ichida et al. 1999). No associated dysmorphic facial features were observed in two adult populations with INVM (Ritter et al. 1997; Öechslin et al. 2000). An association between noncompaction and neuromuscular disorders has also been described with as many as 82% of patients having some form of neuromuscular disorder (Stöllberger et al. 1996, 2002).

Diagnostic Criteria of Ventricular Noncompaction

The diagnosis of NVM can be accurately made by two-dimensional echocardiography in combination with color Doppler technique (Figure 15–2). Two-dimensional echocardiography is used to demonstrate multiple prominent ventricular trabeculations with deep intertrabecular recesses. Color Doppler imaging is used to demonstrate the flow of blood through the deep recesses in continuity with the ventricular cavity (Agmon et al. 1999). As previously mentioned, INVM is diagnosed when the above criteria are satisfied and there are no coexisting cardiac lesions.

Echocardiographic studies have shown that noncompaction is found predominantly in the apical and inferior wall region (Ritter et al. 1997). RV apex has been described in over 40% of patients in one case series (Ritter et al. 1997). Noncompaction is often found in association with depressed ventricular systolic function (Öechslin et al. 2000) that may coexist with impaired diastolic function. Furthermore, impaired diastolic function is not confined to segments of affected myocardium but may also affect what appears to be macroscopically normal myocardium (Öechslin et al. 2000).

In order to standardize the diagnosis, various echocardiographic criteria have been proposed. Chin et al. were the first to describe a quantitative approach to diagnose noncompaction using a trabeculation peak to trough ratio (Chin et al. 1990). However, this criteria has not been widely accepted into clinical practice (Agmon et al. 1999; Rigopoulos et al. 2002). Later on, Öechslin et al. described the abnormally thickened myocardium as a two-layered structure, with a normally compacted epicardial layer and a thickened endocardial layer (Öechslin et al. 2000). They proposed a quantitative evaluation for the diagnosis of INVM by determining the ratio of maximal thickness of the noncompacted to compacted layers (measured at end systole in a parasternal short axis view), with a ratio >2 being diagnostic of INVM. One advantage of this criterion is that it allows differentiation of the trabeculations of INVM from that observed with DCM or hypertensive cardiomyopathy (Jenni et al. 2001). Stöllberger et al. have proposed that LVHT is characterized by the presence of three or more coarse, prominent trabeculations apical to the papillary muscles, which have the same echogenicity as the myocardium, move synchronously with it, are not connected to the papillary muscles, and are

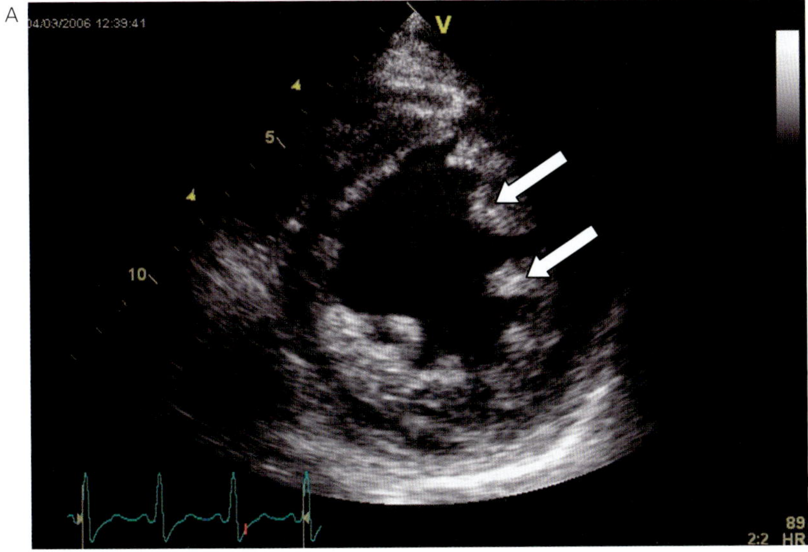

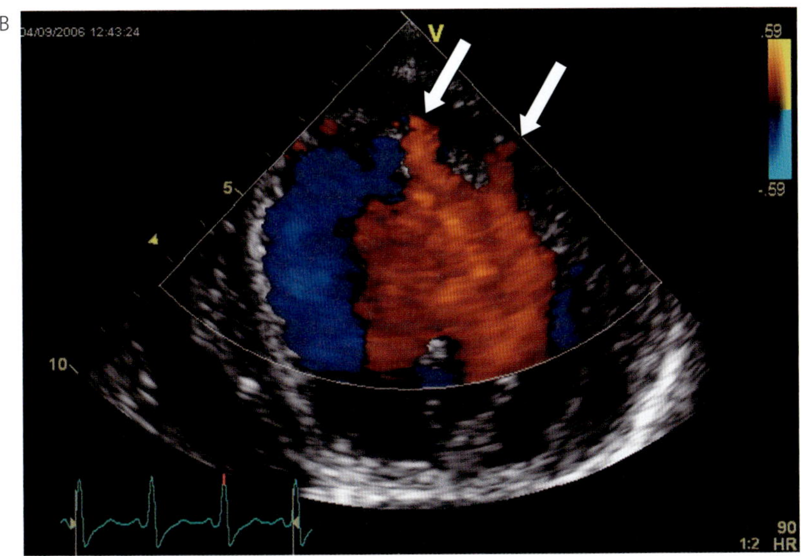

Figure 15–2 Transthoracic echocardiography demonstrating prominent trabeculation (a) with color flow mapping demonstrating blood flow into the deep intertrabecular recesses in the left ventricle (b).

surrounded by intertrabecular spaces that are perfused from the ventricular cavity (Stöllberger et al. 2002). Similarities between the definitions of Öechslin et al. and Stöllberger et al. comprise the description of trabeculation and intertrabecular recesses communicating with and perfused from the ventricular cavity. Differences between these two definitions are the absence of an anatomic landmark to differentiate between trabeculations and papillary muscles in Öechslin's definition and the absence of the number of trabeculations as a criterion of LVHT (Öechslin et al. 2000). Stöllberger's definition, on the contrary, uses the anatomical landmark apically to the papillary muscles and requires the number of trabeculations (Stöllberger et al. 2002). A further difference between the two definitions includes the ratio of noncompacted to compacted layer at end systole, which is a key criterion in Öechslin's definition and not included in Stöllberger's definition. To unify the two definitions, in a recent review, Stöllberger et al. have proposed that for future echocardiographic studies and clinical applications, it would be useful to differentiate between definite, probable, and possible LVHT (Finsterer and Stöllberger 2008). Definite LVHT is said to present if both definitions are completely fulfilled. Probable LVHT is present if only either Öechslin's or only Stöllberger's criteria are fulfilled. Possible LVHT is present if the number of trabeculations is <4 or if the ratio noncompacted to compacted layer is <2. Limitations of these modified criteria are that they are not yet anatomically confirmed. Future studies on LVHT, however, will profit concerning their accuracy if both definitions are applied together and if the findings are assessed as proposed above.

Similarity with other defects, as well as nonspecific clinical manifestations, can make the diagnosis of noncompaction difficult. Ichida et al. reported that the diagnosis of INVM was missed in 89% of children (Ichida et al. 1999). Ritter et al. observed a mean time from onset of symptoms to correct diagnosis of more than 3 years in one adult population with INVM (Ritter et al. 1997). Transesophageal echocardiography and contrast echocardiography may be used when transthoracic studies cannot reliably exclude other processes (Maltagliati and Pepi 2000; Koo et al. 2002). One report described the use of contrast echocardiography with sonicated albumin in a patient with INVM (Koo et al. 2002).

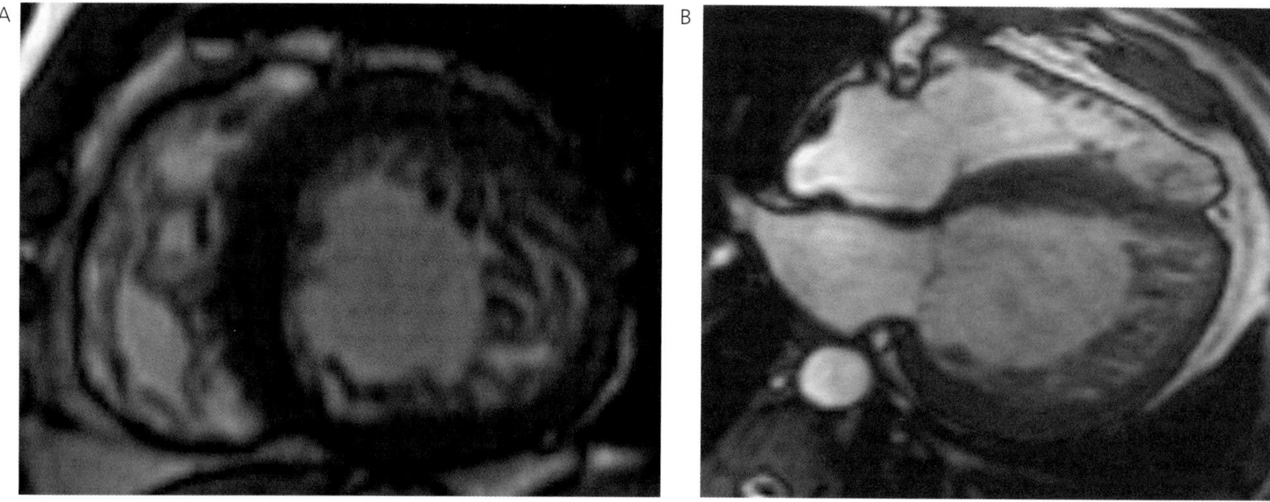

Figure 15–3 MRI images demonstrating noncompacted fibers in short axis (a) and long axis views (b). Note that noncompacting fibers are mainly confined to posterior and lateral walls.

Although echocardiography has been the diagnostic test of choice for noncompaction, other modalities have been used for the diagnosis, including contrast ventriculography (Engberding and Bender 1984; Conces et al. 1991; Koo et al. 2002), computed tomography (Conces et al. 1991; Hamamichi et al. 2001), and MRI (Junga et al. 1999; Daimon et al. 2002; Soler et al. 2002). MRI in particular has shown a good correlation with echocardiography for localization and extent of noncompaction (Junga et al. 1999; Figure 15–3). Furthermore, it is proposed that the differences in MRI signal intensity in noncompacted myocardium can be used to identify substrate for potentially lethal arrhythmias (Daimon et al. 2002). It is now possible with modern MRI techniques such as gradient echo sequences to differentiate NVM accurately from noncompacted areas of the LV as observed in healthy volunteers and in patients with cardiomyopathies and concentric LV hypertrophy. The cut-off value for distinction was given by a diastolic ratio of noncompacted to compacted layer of greater than 2.3 (Petersen et al. 2005).

Tests such as invasive electrophysiological studies have not been widely used in patients with INVM. However, signal-averaged electrocardiography in five children with INVM showed late potentials in three and prolonged QT dispersion in one (Junga et al. 1999). It is proposed that similar tests can be used to identify individuals at increased risk for ventricular arrhythmias and sudden death.

Differential Diagnosis

Any condition that results in prominent trabeculae with or without deep recesses may mimic NVM. Apical HCM, DCM, arrhythmogenic RV dysplasia, endocardial fibroelastosis, cardiac metastases, and LV thrombus are some of the more common causes that should be borne in mind when considering the diagnosis of NVM (Boyd et al. 1987; Agmon et al. 1999; Maltagliati and Pepi 2000; Stöllberger et al. 2002). However, one should be wary of making the diagnosis too readily, especially in the presence of impaired ventricular function (Kohli et al. 2008).

Patients with LV hypertrophy secondary to pressure overload from systemic hypertension or congenital LV outflow tract obstruction are known to demonstrate excessive trabeculae (Jenni et al. 2001; Pignatelli et al. 2003). The existing trabeculae appear abnormally prominent with deep intertrabecular recesses as the myocardial hypertrophy involves the trabeculae as well as the outer compact layer. However, this can be distinguished from NVM by the preservation of the ratio of the noncompacted to compacted layer of myocardium (Chin et al. 1990; Jenni et al. 2001). That is not to say that patients with NVM cannot develop myocardial hypertrophy as a compensatory mechanism (Bleyl et al. 1997; Ritter et al. 1997; Mizuno et al. 2001; Lengyel 2002; Zambrano et al. 2002; Weiford et al. 2004), though the ratio of noncompacted to compacted myocardium is not preserved. In addition, myocardial thickening in cases with primary noncompaction of the myocardium has been described to spare the regions of hypertrabeculation (Finsterer et al. 2002).

As previously mentioned, the absence of sinusoids (direct communications between the ventricular cavity and the coronary circulation) is another criterion that has frequently been cited for diagnosing primary myocardial noncompaction. These sinusoids develop as a means of decompression of the ventricular cavity in cases with semilunar valve atresia with an intact ventricular septum and are never present in otherwise structurally normal hearts (Calder et al. 1987; Emmanouilides et al. 1995a). They are mostly found in patients with pulmonary atresia and only rarely involve the LV (Emmanouilides et al. 1995b). In these instances, excessive myocardial trabeculations, if present, are secondary to myocardial hypertrophy and not a form of primary myocardial disease.

Prognosis

The clinical course and prognosis of patients with noncompaction of the myocardium is highly variable. It can range from a prolonged asymptomatic course to rapidly progressive heart failure with resultant heart transplantation or death (Conces et al. 1991; Bleyl et al. 1997; Ichida et al. 1999; Rigopoulos et al. 2002; Pignatelli et al. 2003; Murphy et al. 2005). Transient recovery of ventricular function followed by later deterioration has been reported in infants (Pignatelli et al. 2003), but the usual clinical course is one of rapid deterioration once symptoms develop (Hook et al. 1996;

Ritter et al. 1997; Mizuno et al. 2001). In a group of children with myocardial noncompaction followed for up to 17 years, LV dysfunction developed in the vast majority, regardless of the presence of symptoms at initial diagnosis (Hook et al. 1996). Ritter et al. followed 17 symptomatic adults for 6 years. Of which 8 patients had died (47.1%) and 2 underwent heart transplantation (Ritter et al. 1997). In another series of 34 adults with myocardial noncompaction, 47% either died or underwent cardiac transplantation during the follow-up period of 44±39 months (Öechslin et al. 2000).

The occurrences of ventricular arrhythmias, systemic emboli, and death were considerably lower in a large pediatric series from Japan (Ichida et al. 1999) compared with those of adults. Increased age, higher LV end-diastolic diameter at presentation, symptoms of New York Heart Association Class III or IV, permanent or persistent atrial fibrillation, bundle branch block, and the association with neuromuscular disease have been found to be predictors for increased mortality (Öechslin et al. 2000; Stöllberger et al. 2007). Patients with these high-risk features are candidates for early and aggressive therapeutic interventions.

Box 15–1 Key Points

- NVM is an uncommon cause of cardiomyopathy.
- It is widely thought to be related to arrested myocardial development.
- The genetic origin as well as the underlying pathogenesis remains unclear.
- It has a classical histopathological pattern and distinctive appearance on echocardiography and MRI, which allows differentiation from other cardiomyopathies.
- NVM is clinically characterized by a high prevalence of heart failure, thromboembolic complications, and arrhythmias.
- Management of NVM centers on these three major clinical manifestations.
- The clinical course and the prognosis of NVM patients are highly variable.
- Increasing age, a dilated LV, symptoms of New York Heart Association Class III or IV severity, atrial fibrillation, bundle branch block, and the association with neuromuscular disease should lower the threshold for more aggressive management.
- The high incidence of familial occurrence warrants echocardiographic familial screening.

Management

Management of NVM centers on the management of the three major clinical manifestations: heart failure, arrhythmias, and systemic embolic events. Systolic and diastolic ventricular dysfunctions are treated with standard medical therapy (Weiford et al. 2004). Although there are no large trials in patients with noncompaction, there is anecdotal evidence of the beneficial effects of the β-blocker carvedilol on LV dysfunction, mass, and neurohormonal dysfunction (Toyono et al. 2001). Biventricular pacemakers may have a role to play in the treatment of patients with severely symptomatic heart failure, poor LV function, and prolonged intraventricular conduction (Weiford et al. 2004). Cardiac transplantation should be given consideration for those with refractory congestive heart failure (Conraads et al. 2001; Stamou et al. 2004).

Due to the high incidence of arrhythmias in patients with NVM, annual ambulatory ECG monitoring is prudent. With the availability of automated implantable defibrillator technology, it is likely that this will play a greater role in the management of myocardial noncompaction, although more work is required on stratifying patients according to risk of sudden cardiac death (Weiford et al. 2004). Although implantation of implantable defibrillator is currently not recommended as primary prophylaxis, its use may be justifiable for secondary prophylaxis after documented hemodynamically compromising sustained ventricular tachycardia or aborted sudden death, with the appreciation that the primary event may be the terminal event.

Use of long-term prophylactic anticoagulant therapy for all patients with ventricular noncompaction remains a controversial topic as the true prevalence of embolic phenomenon has not been established and hence the risk–benefit analysis cannot be done. However, the prevention of embolic complications remains an important issue. Whilst some authors recommend long-term prophylactic anticoagulation for all patients with ventricular noncompaction (Ritter et al. 1997; Öechslin et al. 2000), others advise anticoagulation only for patients with additional risk factors such as atrial fibrillation, evidence of thrombus, or associated ventricular dysfunction (Stöllberger and Finsterer 2004a).

Due to association of neuromuscular disorders and facial dysmorphism with noncompaction, their evaluation and treatment are required to complete the management (Weiford et al. 2004; Finsterer et al. 2006; Box 15–1). In addition, because of the familial association described with noncompaction, screening echocardiography of first-degree relatives is recommended.

References

Agmon Y, Connolly HM, Olson LJ, Khandheria BK, Seward JB. Noncompaction of the ventricular myocardium. *J Am Soc Echocardiogr.* 1999;12(10):859–863.

Allenby PA, Gould NS, Schwartz MF, Chiemmongkoltip P. Dysplastic cardiac development presenting as cardiomyopathy. *Arch Pathol Lab Med.* 1988;112(12):1255–1258.

Amann G, Sherman FS. Myocardial dysgenesis with persistent sinusoids in a neonate with Noonan's phenotype. *Pediatr Pathol.* 1992;12(1):83–92.

Aras D, Tufekcioglu O, Ergun K, et al. Clinical features of isolated ventricular noncompaction in adults long-term clinical course, echocardiographic properties, and predictors of left ventricular failure. *J Card Fail.* 2006;12(9):726–733.

Benson DW, Silberbach GM, Kavanaugh-McHugh A, et al. Mutations in the cardiac transcription factor NKX2.5 affect diverse cardiac developmental pathways. *J Clin Invest.* 1999;104(11):1567–1573.

Bernanke DH, Velkey JM. Development of the coronary blood supply: changing concepts and current ideas. *Anat Rec.* 2002;269(4):198–208.

Bione S, D'Adamo P, Maestrini E, Gedeon AK, Bolhuis PA, Toniolo D. A novel X-linked gene, G4.5, is responsible for Barth syndrome. *Nat Genet.* 1996; 12(4):385–389.

Bleyl SB, Mumford BR, Brown-Harrison MC, et al. Xq28-linked noncompaction of the left ventricular myocardium: prenatal diagnosis and pathologic analysis of affected individuals. *Am J Med Genet.* 1997a;72(3): 257–265.

Bleyl SB, Mumford BR, Thompson V, et al. Neonatal, lethal noncompaction of the left ventricular myocardium is allelic with Barth syndrome. *Am J Hum Genet.* 1997b;61(4):868–872.

Boyd MT, Seward JB, Tajik AJ, Edwards WD. Frequency and location of prominent left ventricular trabeculations at autopsy in 474 normal human hearts: implications for evaluation of mural thrombi by two-dimensional echocardiography. *J Am Coll Cardiol.* 1987;9(2):323–326.

Calder AL, Co EE, Sage MD. Coronary arterial abnormalities in pulmonary atresia with intact ventricular septum. *Am J Cardiol.* 1987;59(5):436–442.

Chen R, Tsuji T, Ichida F, et al. Mutation analysis of the G4.5 gene in patients with isolated left ventricular noncompaction. *Mol Genet Metab.* 2002;77(4):319–325.

Chin TK, Perloff JK, Williams RG, Jue K, Mohrmann R. Isolated noncompaction of left ventricular myocardium. A study of eight cases. *Circulation.* 1990;82(2):507–513.

Conces DJ Jr, Ryan T, Tarver RD. Noncompaction of ventricular myocardium: CT appearance. *AJR Am J Roentgenol.* 1991;156(4):717–718.

Conraads V, Paelinck B, Vorlat A, Goethals M, Jacobs W, Vrints C. Isolated non-compaction of the left ventricle: a rare indication for transplantation. *J Heart Lung Transplant.* 2001;20(8):904–907.

Corrado G, Checcarelli N, Santarone M, Stollberger C, Finsterer J. Left ventricular hypertrabeculation/noncompaction with PMP22 duplication-based Charcot-Marie-Tooth disease type 1A. *Cardiology.* 2006;105(3):142–145.

Daimon Y, Watanabe S, Takeda S, Hijikata Y, Komuro I. Two-layered appearance of noncompaction of the ventricular myocardium on magnetic resonance imaging. *Circ J.* 2002;66(6):619–621.

Davili Z, Johar S, Hughes C, Kveselis D, Hoo J. Succinate dehydrogenase deficiency associated with dilated cardiomyopathy and ventricular noncompaction. *Eur J Pediatr.* 2007;166(8):867–870.

Digilio MC, Marino B, Bevilacqua M, Musolino AM, Giannotti A, Dallapiccola B. Genetic heterogeneity of isolated noncompaction of the left ventricular myocardium. *Am J Med Genet.* 1999;85(1):90–91.

Dusek J, Ostadal B, Duskova M. Postnatal persistence of spongy myocardium with embryonic blood supply. *Arch Pathol.* 1975;99(6):312–317.

Eisenberg LM, Markwald RR. Cellular recruitment and the development of the myocardium. *Dev Biol.* 2004;274(2):225–232.

Emmanouilides GC, Riemenschneider TA, Allen HD, Gutgesell HP. Hypoplastic left heart syndrome. In: *Moss and Adams Heart Disease in Infants, Children and Adolescents.* Williams and Wilkins, Baltimore; 1995a:1133–1153.

Emmanouilides GC, Riemenschneider TA, Allen HD, Gutgesell HP. Pulmonary atresia and intact ventricular septum. In: *Moss and Adams Heart Disease in Infants, Children, and Adolescents.* Williams and Wilkins, Baltimore; 1995b:962–983.

Engberding R, Bender F. Identification of a rare congenital anomaly of the myocardium by two-dimensional echocardiography: persistence of isolated myocardial sinusoids. *Am J Cardiol.* 1984;53(11):1733–1734.

Finsterer J, Bittner R, Bodingbauer M, Eichberger H, Stollberger C, Blazek G. Complex mitochondriopathy associated with 4 mtDNA transitions. *Eur Neurol.* 2000;44(1):37–41.

Finsterer J, Schoser B, Stollberger C. Myoadenylate-deaminase gene mutation associated with left ventricular hypertrabeculation/non-compaction. *Acta Cardiol.* 2004a;59(4):453–456.

Finsterer J, Stolberger C, Kopsa W. Noncompaction in myotonic dystrophy type 1 on cardiac MRI. *Cardiology.* 2005;103(3):167–168.

Finsterer J, Stollberger C. Definite, probable, or possible left ventricular hypertrabeculation/noncompaction. *Int J Cardiol.* 2008;123(2): 175–176.

Finsterer J, Stollberger C, Blazek G. Neuromuscular implications in left ventricular hypertrabeculation/noncompaction. *Int J Cardiol.* 2006;110(3): 288–300.

Finsterer J, Stollberger C, Feichtinge H. Histological appearance of left ventricular hypertrabeculation/noncompaction. *Cardiology.* 2002;98(3): 162–164.

Finsterer J, Stollberger C, Feichtinger H. Non-compaction on autopsy in Duchenne muscular dystrophy. *Cardiology.* 2007a;108(3):161–163.

Finsterer J, Stollberger C, Kopsa W, Jaksch M. Wolff-Parkinson-White syndrome and isolated left ventricular abnormal trabeculation as a manifestation of Leber's hereditary optic neuropathy. *Can J Cardiol.* 2001;17(4):464–466.

Finsterer J, Stollberger C, Schubert B. Acquired left ventricular hypertrabeculation/noncompaction in mitochondriopathy. *Cardiology.* 2004b;102(4):228–230.

Finsterer J, Stollberger C, Steger C, Cozzarini W. Complete heart block associated with noncompaction, nail-patella syndrome, and mitochondrial myopathy. *J Electrocardiol.* 2007b;40(4):352–354.

Freedom RM, Yoo SJ, Perrin D, Taylor G, Petersen S, Anderson RH. The morphological spectrum of ventricular noncompaction. *Cardiol Young.* 2005;15(4):345–364.

Hamamichi Y, Ichida F, Hashimoto I, et al. Isolated noncompaction of the ventricular myocardium: ultrafast computed tomography and magnetic resonance imaging. *Int J Cardiovasc Imaging.* 2001;17(4):305–314.

Harvey RP. Patterning the vertebrate heart. *Nat Rev Genet.* 2002;3(7): 544–556.

Hermida-Prieto M, Monserrat L, Castro-Beiras A, et al. Familial dilated cardiomyopathy and isolated left ventricular noncompaction associated with lamin A/C gene mutations. *Am J Cardiol.* 2004;94(1):50–54.

HoedemaekersYM, Caliskan K, Majoor-Krakauer D, et al. Cardiac beta-myosin heavy chain defects in two families with non-compaction cardiomyopathy: linking non-compaction to hypertrophic, restrictive, and dilated cardiomyopathies. *Eur Heart J.* 2007;28(22):2732–2737.

Hook S, Ratliff NB, Rosenkranz E, Sterba R. Isolated noncompaction of the ventricular myocardium. *Pediatr Cardiol.* 1996;17(1):43–45.

Ichida F, Hamamichi Y, Miyawaki T, et al. Clinical features of isolated noncompaction of the ventricular myocardium: long-term clinical course, hemodynamic properties, and genetic background. *J Am Coll Cardiol.* 1999;34(1):233–240.

Ichida F, Tsubata S, Bowles KR, et al. Novel gene mutations in patients with left ventricular noncompaction or Barth syndrome. *Circulation.* 2001;103(9):1256–1263.

Jenni R, Goebel N, Tartini R, Schneider J, Arbenz U, Oelz O. Persisting myocardial sinusoids of both ventricles as an isolated anomaly: echocardiographic, angiographic, and pathologic anatomical findings. *Cardiovasc Intervent Radiol.* 1986;9(3):127–131.

Jenni R, Oechslin E, Schneider J, Attenhofer Jost C, Kaufmann PA. Echocardiographic and pathoanatomical characteristics of isolated left ventricular non-compaction: a step towards classification as a distinct cardiomyopathy. *Heart.* 2001;86(6):666–671.

Jenni R, Oechslin EN, van der Loo B. Isolated ventricular non-compaction of the myocardium in adults. *Heart.* 2007;93(1):11–15.

Junga G, Kneifel S, Von Smekal A, Steinert H, Bauersfeld U. Myocardial ischaemia in children with isolated ventricular non-compaction. *Eur Heart J.* 1999;20(12):910–916.

Kanemoto N, Horigome H, Nakayama J, et al. Interstitial 1q43-q43 deletion with left ventricular noncompaction myocardium. *Eur J Med Genet.* 2006;49(3):247–253.

Kenton AB, Sanchez X, Coveler KJ, et al. Isolated left ventricular noncompaction is rarely caused by mutations in G4.5, alpha-dystrobrevin and FK Binding Protein-12. *Mol Genet Metab.* 2004;82(2):162–166.

Kherbaoui-Redouani L, Eschard C, Bednarek N, Morville P. Cutaneous aplasia, non compaction of the left ventricle and severe cardiac arrhythmia. a new case of MLS syndrome (microphtalmia with linear skin defects). *Arch Pediatr.* 2003;10(3):224–226.

Klaassen S, Probst S, Oechslin E, et al. Mutations in sarcomere protein genes in left ventricular noncompaction. *Circulation.* 2008;117(22):2893–2901.

Kohli SK, Pantazis AA, Shah JS, et al. Diagnosis of left-ventricular noncompaction in patients with left-ventricular systolic dysfunction: time for a reappraisal of diagnostic criteria? *Eur Heart J.* 2008;29(1):89–95.

Koo BK, Choi D, Ha JW, Kang SM, Chung N, Cho SY. Isolated noncompaction of the ventricular myocardium: contrast echocardiographic findings and review of the literature. *Echocardiography.* 2002;19(2):153–156.

Lauer RM, Fink HP, Petry EL, Dunn MI, Diehl AM. Angiographic demonstration of intramyocardial sinusoids in pulmonary-valve atresia with intact ventricular septum and hypoplastic right ventricle. *N Engl J Med.* 1964;271:68–72.

Lengyel M. Isolated left ventricular noncompaction—first description in a Hungarian patient. *Orv Hetil.* 2002;143(27):1651–1653.

Lofiego C, Biagini E, Pasquale F, et al. Wide spectrum of presentation and variable outcomes of isolated left ventricular non-compaction. *Heart.* 2007;93(1):65–71.

Makita N, Sasaki K, Yokoshiki H, et al. Left ventricular noncompaction associated with mutations in cardiac Na channel gene SCN5A. Programme and abstracts of the American Heart Association Scientific Sessions; 2008. Ref Type: abstract.

Maltagliati A, Pepi M. Isolated noncompaction of the myocardium: multiplane transesophageal echocardiography diagnosis in an adult. *J Am Soc Echocardiogr.* 2000;13(11):1047–1049.

Mandel K, Grunebaum E, Benson L. Noncompaction of the myocardium associated with Roifman syndrome. *Cardiol Young.* 2001;11(2):240–243.

Maron BJ, Towbin JA, Thiene G, et al. Contemporary definitions and classification of the cardiomyopathies: an American Heart Association Scientific Statement from the Council on Clinical Cardiology, Heart Failure and Transplantation Committee; Quality of Care and Outcomes Research and Functional Genomics and Translational Biology Interdisciplinary Working Groups; and Council on Epidemiology and Prevention. *Circulation.* 2006;113(14):1807–1816.

Marziliano N, Mannarino S, Nespoli L, et al. Barth syndrome associated with compound hemizygosity and heterozygosity of the TAZ and LDB3 genes. *Am J Med Genet A.* 2007;143(9):907–915.

Matsumoto T, Watanabe A, Migita M, et al. Transient cardiomyopathy in a patient with congenital contractural arachnodactyly (Beals syndrome). *J Nippon Med Sch.* 2006;73(5):285–288.

McMahon CJ, Chang AC, Pignatelli RH, et al. Left ventricular noncompaction cardiomyopathy in association with trisomy 13. *Pediatr Cardiol.* 2005;26(4):477–479.

Mizuno Y, Thompson TG, Guyon JR, et al. Desmuslin, an intermediate filament protein that interacts with alpha—dystrobrevin and desmin. *Proc Natl Acad Sci USA.* 2001;98(11):6156–6161.

Murphy RT, Thaman R, Gimeno Blanes J. Natural history and familial characteristics of isolated left ventricular non-compaction. *Eur Heart J.* 2005;26(2):187–192.

Oechslin EN, Attenhofer Jost CH, Rojas JR, Kaufmann PA, Jenni R. Long-term follow-up of 34 adults with isolated left ventricular noncompaction: a distinct cardiomyopathy with poor prognosis. *J Am Coll Cardiol.* 2000;36(2):493–500.

OMIM Online Mendelian Inheritance in Man. 2008. Ref Type: Internet Communication.

Ozkutlu S, Ayabakan C, Celiker A, Elshershari H. Noncompaction of ventricular myocardium: a study of twelve patients. *J Am Soc Echocardiogr.* 2002;15(12):1523–1528.

Pashmforoush M, Lu JT, Chen H, et al. Nkx2-5 pathways and congenital heart disease; loss of ventricular myocyte lineage specification leads to progressive cardiomyopathy and complete heart block. *Cell.* 2004;117(3):373–386.

Pauli RM, Scheib-Wixted S, Cripe L, Izumo S, Sekhon GS. Ventricular noncompaction and distal chromosome 5q deletion. *Am J Med Genet.* 1999;85(4):419–423.

Petersen SE, Selvanayagam JB, Wiesmann F, et al. Left ventricular noncompaction: insights from cardiovascular magnetic resonance imaging. *J Am Coll Cardiol.* 2005;46(1):101–105.

Pignatelli RH, McMahon CJ, Dreyer WJ, et al. Clinical characterization of left ventricular noncompaction in children: a relatively common form of cardiomyopathy. *Circulation.* 2003;108(21):2672–2678.

Reynen K, Bachmann K, Singer H. Spongy myocardium. *Cardiology.* 1997;88(6):601–602.

Rigopoulos A, Rizos IK, Aggeli C, et al. Isolated left ventricular noncompaction: an unclassified cardiomyopathy with severe prognosis in adults. *Cardiology.* 2002;98(1-2):25–32.

Ritter M, Oechslin E, Sutsch G, Attenhofer C, Schneider J, Jenni R. Isolated noncompaction of the myocardium in adults. *Mayo Clin Proc.* 1997;72(1):26–31.

Sasse-Klaassen S, Probst S, Gerull B, et al. Novel gene locus for autosomal dominant left ventricular noncompaction maps to chromosome 11p15. *Circulation.* 2004;109(22):2720–2723.

Scaglia F, Towbin JA, Craigen WJ, et al. Clinical spectrum, morbidity, and mortality in 113 pediatric patients with mitochondrial disease. *Pediatrics.* 2004;114(4):925–931.

Schlame M, Ren M. Barth syndrome, a human disorder of cardiolipin metabolism. *FEBS Lett.* 2006;580(23):5450–5455.

Schott JJ, Benson DW, Basson CT, et al. Congenital heart disease caused by mutations in the transcription factor NKX2–5. *Science.* 1998;281(5373):108–111.

Soler R, Rodriguez E, Monserrat L, Alvarez N. MRI of subendocardial perfusion deficits in isolated left ventricular noncompaction. *J Comput Assist Tomogr.* 2002;26(3):373–375.

Srivastava D, Olson EN. A genetic blueprint for cardiac development. *Nature.* 2000;407(6801):221–226.

Stamou SC, Lefrak EA, Athari FC, Burton NA, Massimiano PS. Heart transplantation in a patient with isolated noncompaction of the left ventricular myocardium. *Ann Thorac Surg.* 2004;77(5):1806–1808.

Stollberger C, Finsterer J. Thrombi in left ventricular hypertrabeculation/noncompaction—review of the literature. *Acta Cardiol.* 2004a;59(3):341–344.

Stollberger C, Finsterer J. Trabeculation and left ventricular hypertrabeculation/noncompaction. *J Am Soc Echocardiogr.* 2004b;17(10): 1120–1121.

Stollberger C, Finsterer J, Blazek G. Left ventricular hypertrabeculation/noncompaction and association with additional cardiac abnormalities and neuromuscular disorders. *Am J Cardiol.* 2002;90(8):899–902.

Stollberger C, Finsterer J, Blazek G, Bittner RE. Left ventricular noncompaction in a patient with becker's muscular dystrophy. *Heart.* 1996;76(4):380.

Stollberger C, Winkler-Dworak M, Blazek G, Finsterer J. Prognosis of left ventricular hypertrabeculation/noncompaction is dependent on cardiac and neuromuscular comorbidity. *Int J Cardiol.* 2007;121(2): 189–193.

Tanpaiboon P, Callahan PF, Sloan J, et al. Noncompaction of the ventricular myocardium and hydrops fetalis in cobalamin C deficiency. Programme and abstracts of the American Society of Human Genetics Annual Meeting. 2006. Ref Type: abstract.

Thienpont B, Mertens L, Buyse G, Vermeesch JR, Devriendt K. Left-ventricular non-compaction in a patient with monosomy 1p36. *Eur J Med Genet.* 2007;50(3):233–236.

Toyono M, Kondo C, Nakajima Y, Nakazawa M, Momma K, Kusakabe K. Effects of carvedilol on left ventricular function, mass, and scintigraphic findings in isolated left ventricular non-compaction. *Heart.* 2001;86(1):E4.

van Heerde M, Hruda J, Hazekamp MG. Severe pulmonary hypertension secondary to a parachute-like mitral valve, with the left superior caval vein draining into the coronary sinus, in a girl with Turner's syndrome. *Cardiol Young.* 2003;13(4):364–366.

Vatta M, Mohapatra B, Jimenez S, et al. Mutations in Cypher/ZASP in patients with dilated cardiomyopathy and left ventricular non-compaction. *J Am Coll Cardiol.* 2003;42(11):2014–2027.

Wallace DC. Mitochondrial diseases in man and mouse. *Science.* 1999;283(5407):1482–1488.

Weiford BC, Subbarao VD, Mulhern KM. Noncompaction of the ventricular myocardium. *Circulation.* 2004;109(24):2965–2971.

Wong JA, Bofinger MK. Noncompaction of the ventricular myocardium in Melnick-Needles syndrome. *Am J Med Genet.* 1997;71(1):72–75.

Xing Y, Ichida F, Matsuoka T, et al. Genetic analysis in patients with left ventricular noncompaction and evidence for genetic heterogeneity. *Mol Genet Metab.* 2006;88(1):71–77.

Yaplito-Lee J, Weintraub R, Jamsen K, Chow CW, Thorburn DR, Boneh A. Cardiac manifestations in oxidative phosphorylation disorders of childhood. *J Pediatr.* 2007;150(4):407–411.

Yasukawa K, Terai M, Honda A, Kohno Y. Isolated noncompaction of ventricular myocardium associated with fatal ventricular fibrillation. *Pediatr Cardiol.* 2001;22(6):512–514.

Zambrano E, Marshalko SJ, Jaffe CC, Hui P. Isolated noncompaction of the ventricular myocardium: clinical and molecular aspects of a rare cardiomyopathy. *Lab Invest.* 2002;82(2):117–122.

Zaragoza MV, Arbustini E, Narula J. Noncompaction of the left ventricle: primary cardiomyopathy with an elusive genetic etiology. *Curr Opin Pediatr.* 2007;(4):619–627.

16

Molecular Genetics of Arrhythmias

Seo-Kyung Chung, Jonathan R Skinner, and Mark I Rees

Introduction

Inherited heart disorders are the most common causes of sudden cardiac death (SCD) in young people (Roberts 2006; Behr et al. 2008; Knollmann and Roden 2008). The usual mode of death is ventricular tachycardia or fibrillation. Sudden death in young athletes is most commonly due to inherited heart diseases with a structural component, particularly hypertrophic cardiomyopathy (HCM) or arrhythmogenic right ventricular cardiomyopathy (ARVC). However, population-based autopsy series have revealed that it is more common for sudden death in 0–35-year-olds to occur in individuals with a structurally normal heart (Doolan et al. 2004; Puranik et al. 2005). Molecular autopsies, and/or cardiological investigation of family members, have revealed that the "cardiac channelopathies" long QT syndrome, Brugada syndrome, and catecholaminergic polymorphic ventricular tachycardia (CPVT) lie behind up to 35% of such deaths in 1–40-year-olds (Tan et al. 2005; Tester and Ackerman 2007) and at least 10% in infants (Arnestad et al. 2007). These disorders of the cardiac ion channels result in disturbance of the cardiac action potential, and generally these hearts appear normal under the microscope.

Arrhythmic disorders can also be secondary to congenital, acquired, or sporadic disorders. However, recent research demonstrates that even acquired arrhythmias may be associated with genetic variants in specific cardiac channels (Lehnart et al. 2007; Roden 2008). Even atrial fibrillation, the commonest arrhythmia in the human and commonly associated with other cardiac and noncardiac disease, can have a genetic basis.

More than 30 genes have been identified in association with arrhythmic syndromes. However, the relation between genotype and phenotype is not straightforward in most genetic disorders, due to the incomplete penetrance of the mutation and the variability in clinical manifestations. Even within a family, the same genetic mutation may result in striking phenotype variance, from sudden death of an infant or young child to asymptomatic carriage in the elderly.

In this chapter, the molecular genetics and cell biology underlying primary arrhythmic disorders are introduced in overview (Table 16–1; Figure 16–1) while Chapters 17 to 19 cover individual disorders in more detail. This chapter also refers to inherited cardiomyopathies that are covered in Chapters 13 and 14.

Molecular Genetics of Arrhythmias: Long QT Syndrome (LQTS)

For decades, after its initial description in 1957 (Jervell and Lange-Nielsen 1957), LQTS was regarded as a very rare disease, but it is now apparent that LQTS was frequently unrecognized (Roden 2008).

Current estimates are that the prevalence of LQTS mutation carriers is 1 in 1,000–3,000 (Yang et al. 2002).

The typical symptoms of LQTS are episodic dizziness, syncope (abrupt loss of consciousness), apneic seizures, and SCD (Wehrens et al. 2000). The symptoms typically occur during physical activity or emotional stress, but can occur during sleep and may be confused with epilepsy (Towbin and Vatta 2001).

LQTS can be congenital, acquired, or a sporadic disorder (Towbin and Vatta 2001). Congenital LQTS exits in two forms, Romano-Ward Syndrome (RWS) (Romano et al. 1963) and Jervell and Lange-Nielsen Syndrome (JLNS) (Jervell and Lange-Nielsen 1957). RWS is the most common form of inherited LQTS and is transmitted as an autosomal dominant trait (Dumaine and Antzelevitch 2002). In contrast, JLNS is rare, and inherited in an autosomal recessive manner with a more malignant course with congenital deafness (Dumaine and Antzelevitch 2002).

LQTS has been found in a small number of near-miss sudden infant death syndrome (SIDS) cases (Schwartz et al. 2001; Towbin 2001) and diagnosed posthumously from genetic material in both infants and 1–40-year-olds dying suddenly without any apparent cause (Schwartz et al. 2000a, 2001; Ackerman et al. 2001; Tester and Ackerman 2005).

The risk of cardiac events is higher in males until teenage years, but higher in females during adulthood (Locati et al. 1998; Hobbs et al. 2006; Sauer et al. 2007; Goldenberg et al. 2008). Syncope and sudden death are due to ventricular arrhythmia particularly torsades-de-pointes tachycardia and ventricular fibrillation (Keating and Sanguinetti 2001).

LQTS can be acquired as a result of side effects from medications such as antibiotics and antiarrhythmics, heart disease, or metabolic abnormalities (Roden et al. 1996) (see also Chapter 18). Recent studies have indicated that acquired LQTS, the most common form of LQTS, also has a predisposing genetic basis in genes associated with congenital LQTS. Specific examples have been identified in individuals with drug-induced LQTS

Table 16–1 Inherited Cardiac Arrhythmias

Inherited Heart Disease	Cardiac Arrhythmias	Inheritance	Gene(s)
Long QT syndrome (LQTS)	Ventricular tachycardia (torsade de pointes)	AD/AR	*KCNQ1, KCNH2, SCN5A, ANK2, KCNE1, KCNE2, KCNJ2, CACNA1C, SCN4B*
Brugada syndrome (BrS)	Ventricular fibrillation, Atrial fibrillation	AD	*SCN5A, GPD1L*
Dilated cardiomyopathy (DCM)	Atrial fibrillation, ventricular tachycardia/ventricular fibrillation		*KCNH2, PLN*
Catecholaminergic polymorphic ventricular tachycardia (CPVT)	Bidirectional ventricular tachycardia, polymorphic ventricular tachycardia	AD/AR	*RyR2, CASQ2*
Short QT syndrome (SQTS)	ventricular fibrillation	AD	*KCNH2, KCNQ1, KCNJ2*
Leve-Lenegre disease	Sinus bradycardia/sinus arrest	AD/AR	*SCN5A, HCN4*
SSS			
Atrial fibrillation (AF)	Atrial fibrillation	AD	*KCNQ1, KCNE2, KCNJ2, GJA5, KCNE1, KCNA5, ANK2, KCNH2, ABCC9*
Timothy syndrome (TS)	Ventricular tachycardia (torsade de pointes), 2:1 atrioventricular block		*CACNA1C*
Cardiomyopathies			
ARVC	Ventricular tachycardia/ventricular fibrillation		*PKP2, DSP, JUP, DSG2, DSC2, DES*
HCM	Ventricular tachycardia/ventricular fibrillation/atrial fibrillation		*MYH7, MYBPC3, TNNT2, TNNI3, TPM1, MYL2, MYL3, ACTC1, TTN*
Wolff-Parkinson-White (WPW) syndrome	Supraventricular tachycardia, atrial fibrillation with rapid atrioventricular conduction		*PRKAG2, LAMP2*

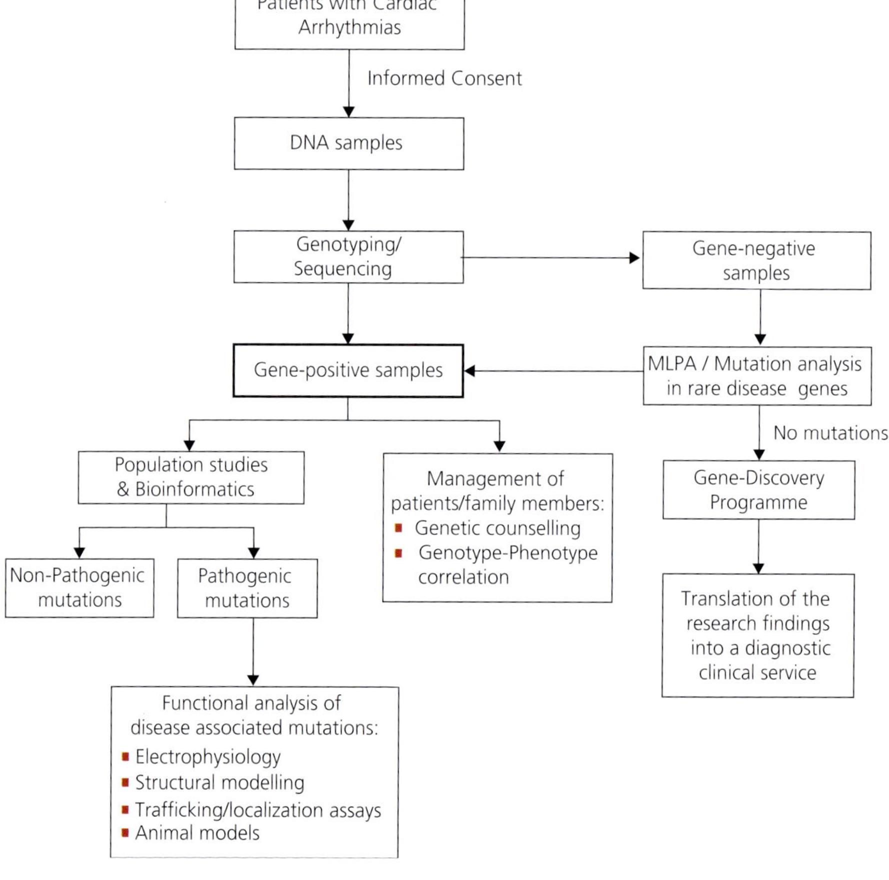

Figure 16–1 Flowchart of the mutation analysis scheme. Using DNA samples from patients with cardiac arrhythmia, mutations underlying the disorders can be identified through various genotyping techniques. On identifying the disease-linked mutations, management of patients and functional confirmation of the mutations are required. For those patients with unclassified variants or those who are gene negative in the major disease-associated genes, follow-up studies are necessary to uncover the specific mechanism underlying the arrhythmia or identify new genes respectively.

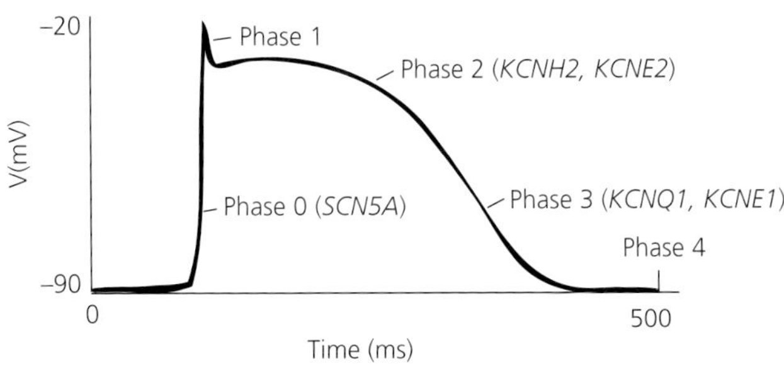

Figure 16–2 Cardiac action potential. The rapid depolarization (phase 0) is mediated by influx of Na^+ current. Phase 1 repolarization is mediated by transient K^+ efflux (Ito). The plateau (phase 2) is due to a balance of the L-type inward Ca^{2+} current and outward K^+ current. Phase 3 repolarization is caused predominantly by outward I_{Ks} current.

(Sesti et al. 2000; Makita et al. 2002; Yang et al. 2002; Harrison-Woolrych et al. 2006). Sporadic LQTS is also recognized when diagnostic features of LQTS occurs in the patient, but with no family history and are devoid of mutations in the typical LQTS candidate genes (Towbin and Vatta 2001).

Congenital LQTS is a disorder of cardiac ion channels joining a long list of channelopathies in medicine (Morita et al. 2008; Roden 2008). To date, more than 700 mutations have been identified in 10 genes encoding subunit components of cardiac ion channels that coordinate the cardiac action potential (Figure 16–2). Dominant mutations in five of these genes are typically associated with RWS, whereas homozygous or heterozygous compound mutations of either *KCNQ1* or *KCNE1* are linked to JLNS (Neyroud et al. 1997; Schulze-Bahr et al. 1997; Splawski et al. 1997; Tyson et al. 1997). There are also examples where two mutations in two different LQTS genes coexist and often leading to severe and complex arrhythmia (Kobori et al. 2004; Lupoglazoff et al. 2004; Yamaguchi et al. 2005). It is apparent that different genotypes tend to cause typical phenotypes; syncope and sudden death are most commonly triggered by exercise in *KCNQ1* mutations, but occur mostly at rest with *SCN5A* mutations. Boys and young men are at high risk of sudden death in *KCNQ1* and *SCN5A* mutations, but young women are at highest risk with HERG mutations (Hobbs et al. 2006; Sauer et al. 2007; Goldenberg et al. 2008). Mutations situated in the transmembrane position tend to be more malignant, and large deletions and insertions in LQTS genes are an emerging diagnostic consideration (Koopmann et al. 2006; Eddy et al. 2008).

Mutations in the genes encoding inward rectifier potassium channel 2 gene (*KCNJ2*) and Caveolin-3 (*CAV3*) are rare cases of congenital LQTS with the latter being implicated in SIDS cases (Vatta et al. 2006; Cronk et al. 2007; Garcia-Touchard et al. 2007).

Brugada Syndrome

Brugada syndrome (BrS) is a hereditary cardiac disorder characterized by elevation of the ST segment on the precordial ECG leads and ventricular fibrillation, most commonly in young males during sleep. BrS may cause up to 20% of sudden deaths in young people with postmortem structurally normal hearts (Brugada and Brugada 1992). Mutations in the sodium channel subunit, *SCN5A* have been identified in 25%–30% of Brugada patients (Lehnart et al. 2007), the majority of which are dominant missense mutations. A second locus of BrS has been mapped to chromosome 3, and other genes are pending identification for Brugada syndrome (Roberts 2006).

Atrial Fibrillation

Atrial fibrillation (AF) is the most common arrhythmia and accounts for 30% of all strokes in adults over the age of 60 years (Roberts 2006) and is most commonly an acquired disorder associated with other cardiac pathology. Several chromosomal loci and four specific genes have been associated with AF; *KCNQ1, KCNE2, KCNJ2,* and *CJA5* (Table 16–2) (Chen et al. 2003; Yang et al. 2004; Xia et al. 2005; Gollob et al. 2006). In contrast to commonly occurring germline variations in cardiac conditions, a rare somatic mutation has been revealed in *GJA5* in atrial cells but absent from the germline (Gollob et al. 2006). The *SCN5A* gene product is expressed in atria and ventricles, and in Brugada syndrome both ventricular and atrial fibrillation may occur (Kusano et al. 2008).

Wolff-Parkinson-White Syndrome

Wolff-Parkinson-White (WPW) syndrome is one of the most common causes of paroxysmal supraventricular tachycardia and is caused by the extra electrical pathway between atria and ventricles (Roberts 2006). WPW syndrome is caused by genetic defects; however, it is mostly sporadic rather than congenital and not all genes have been discovered. Mutations in *PRKAG2*, encoding the gamma 2 subunit of the ATP-sensor enzyme adenosine monophosphate-activated protein kinase (AMPK) have been identified in some WPW syndrome families (Gollob et al. 2001).

Catecholaminergic Polymorphic Ventricular Tachycardia

Catecholaminergic polymorphic ventricular tachycardia (CPVT) is characterized by ventricular tachycardia triggered by emotional or physical stress. Patients with structurally normal hearts and normal QT intervals present with recurrent syncope, seizures, and sudden death (Leenhardt et al. 1995; Tester et al. 2004; Liu et al. 2007; Mohamed et al. 2007). It tends to have a higher malignancy than LQTS, and though much rarer, presents in similar numbers in the molecular autopsy of young sudden death victims, particularly teenagers (Tester and Ackerman 2007). Mutations in two genes have been identified in CPVT cases: *RYR-2* is the major CPVT gene (CPVT1), and encodes for the ryanodine receptor responsible for release of intracellular $Ca2^+$ in sarcomeric reticullum (SR) of cardiomyocytes (Laitinen et al. 2001; Priori et al. 2001). A *RYR-2* mutation has also been associated with a SIDS case (Tester et al. 2007). The *CASQ2* gene is the second CPVT locus (CPVT2) and encodes a $Ca2^+$ buffering protein of the SR, calsequestrin-2A, which represents a rare recessive form of CPVT with several homozygous mutations in the literature (Lahat et al. 2001, 2004; di Barletta et al. 2006).

Short QT Syndrome

Short QT sydrome (SQTS) is characterized by syncope, paroxysmal AF, and cardiac arrhythmias. SQTS is presented either as familial or sporadic cases usually in a young population without structural heart disease (Lehnart et al. 2007). Mutations have been identified in three LQTS associated genes, *KCNH2, SCN5A,* and *KCNJ2* (Bellocq et al. 2004; Brugada et al. 2004; Hong et al. 2005; Priori et al. 2005). Evidence is emerging that SQTS is more common than previously expected, but it still remains rare. SQTS has been implicated in ventricular fibrillation and SCD cases that previously were considered idiopathic (Bjerregaard and Gussak 2005).

Sick Sinus Syndrome

Sick sinus syndrome (SSS) is characterized by abnormal sinus node function resulting in bradyarrhythmias. SSS can be congenital or acquired. Mutations in the cardiac Na^+ channel, *SCN5A*, can result

Table 16–2 Genes Associated with Cardiac Ion Channelopathies

Gene	Locus	Protein	Disease	Incidence of Cases	Mode of Inheritance	Functional Consequences
K^+ Channel						
KCNQ1	11p15.5	Kv7.1α	LQT1, SIDS JLNS1 SQT2 AF1	45%–50% Rare Rare Rare	AD Recessive Unknown AD	Loss of function Loss of function Gain of function Gain of function (AP shortens)
KCNH2	7q35	Kv11.1α	LQT2, SIDS SQT1 AF8	30%–40%	AD AD AD	Loss of function Gain of function (AP shortens) Gain of function (AP shortens)
KCNE1	21q22.1	MinKβ	LQT5 JLNS2 AF5	1%–3%	AD Recessive AD	Iks decrease Loss of function
KCNE2	21q22.1	MiRP1β	LQT6 AF2	1%–2% Rare	AD AD	Loss of function Gain of function (AP shortens)
KCNJ2	17q23	Kir2.1 α	SQT3 AF3 LQT7 CPVT3	Rare Rare Rare	AD AD AD	Gain of function Gain of function (AP shortens) Loss of function
KCNA5	12p13	Kv1.5 α	AF5			IKs ↓
ABCC9	12p12.1	SUR2A β	AF9 DCM			Ca2+ overload ↑ Ca2+ overload ↑
HCN4	15q24-q25	Potassium/sodium hyperpolarization-activated cyclic nucleotide-gated channel 4	SSS1		AD	
Na^+ Channel						
SCN5A	3p21	Nav1.5 α	LQT3, SIDS BrS1 SSS	5%–10% 20%–30% Rare	AD AD AR	Gain of function (INa ↑)
SCN4B	11q23	Nav1.5 β4	LQT10	Rare		INa↑
Ca^{++} Channel associated gene						
hRyR2	1q42	Ryanodine receptor 2	CPVT1	30%–50%	AD	SR Ca2+ leak ↑
CASQ2	1p13.3	Calsequestrin 2	CPVT2	<5%	AR	SR Ca2+ leak ↑
CACNA1C	12p13.3	Cav1.2α1c	LQT8, Timothy syndrome (TS1)	Rare	De novo mutation	Ica, L ↑
PLN	6q22.1	PLN β	DCM	?		Ca2+ overload ↑
Ion channel associated molecules						
ANK2	4q25	AnkyrinB	LQT4 AF7	Very rare	AD	Abnormal targeting of Ca2+ regulatory proteins
CAV3	3p25	Caveolin-3	LQT9 LQT10	Rare Rare		INa ↑
GPD1L	3p24	G3PD1L	BrS2	<1%	AD	
GJA5	1q21.1	Connexin 40	SSS (coinheritance with *SCN5A* mutation). AF4	Rare Rare	 Somatic	Connexin channel current↓ Connexin channel current↓

in congenital SSS (Benson et al. 2003). *SCN5A* missense mutation, D1275N, and a Cx40 promoter polymorphism were identified in a late-onset SSS case (Groenewegen et al. 2003).

Hypertrophic Cardiomyopathy

HCM is a common disease of the cardiac myocytes, with a population prevalence of 1 in 500, characterized by thickening of the left ventricular wall in the absence of increased external load. It can lead to heart failure and ventricular arrhythmias (Hughes and McKenna 2005) (see also Chapter 13) and causes 40%–50% of cases of SCD in young athletes in the United States (Maron et al. 1996).

To date, more than 450 different mutations have been identified within 13 myofilament-related genes (Table 16–3). The majority of HCM associated mutations occur in *MYH7* and *MYBPC3*, encoding the β-myosin heavy chain (β-MyHC) and myosin-binding protein C (MyBP-C) respectively. Mutations in cardiac troponin T (*TNNT2*), cardiac troponin I (*TNNI3*), essential myosin light chain (*MYL3*), regulatory myosin light chain (*MYL2*), a-tropomyosin (*TPM1*), and cardiac actin (*ACTC*) genes are rarer cause of HCM. About 50% of patients have no mutation in a sarcomeric or sarcomere-related genes.

Arrythmogenic Right Ventricular Dysplasia/Cardiomyopathy (ARVC)

ARVC is a genetic disorder of desmosomes, characterized by fibrofatty replacement of myocytes in the right ventricle and ventricular tachycardia. It can lead to syncope and young sudden death, often with only subtle histological changes identified, or to progressive cardiac failure. It is the commonest cause of sudden death in young athletes in Italy (Corrado et al. 2001). Congenital ARVC is predominantly an autosomal dominant disorder. To date, eight chromosomal loci and four definitive genes encoding desmosomal proteins have been identified (Table 16–3)—plakoglobin, desmoplakin, desmoglein 2, and plakophilin-2 (McKoy et al. 2000; Hodgkinson et al. 2005).

Table 16–3 Sarcomeric Disorders and Cardiomyopathies

Gene	Locus	Encoded Protein		Incidence of Cases (%)
HCM			Sarcomere Component	
MYH7	14q12	β-myosin heavy chain	Thick filament	44
MYBPC3	11p11.2	Myosin-binding protein C	Thick filament	35
TNNT2	1q32	Troponin T	Thin filament	7
TNNI3	19q13.4	Troponin I	Thin filament	5
TPM1	15q22.1	α-Tropomyosin	Thin filament	2.5
MYL2	12q24.3	Regulatory myosin light chain	Thick filament	2
MYL3	3p21	Essential myosin light chain	Thick filament	1
ACTC1	15q14	Actin	Thin filament	1
TTN	2q31	Titin	Thick filament/ Z-Disc	<1
CSRP3	11p15.1	Muscle LIM protein	Z-Disc	<1
TCAP	17q12	Telethonin	Z-Disc	<1
MYOZ2	4q26	Myozenin 2	Z-Disc	<1
VCL	10q22.1	Vinculin	Intercalated disc	<1
ARVC				
TGFβ-3	14q23–24	Transforming growth factor		
RYR-2	1q42–43	Cardiac ryanodine receptor		
_	14q12–22	_		
_	2q32.1–32.3	_		
_	3p23	_		
_	10p12–14	_		
_	10q22	_		
DSP	6p24	Desmoplakin		
PKP2	12p11	Plakophilin-2		
JUP	17q21	Plakoglobin		
WPW				
PRKAG2	7q36	AMPK		
		PRKAG2, LAMP2		

Biology of Channelopathy Arrhythmias

Potassium Channelopathies

Cardiac K^+ channels typically consist of a homomeric or heteromeric assembly of four voltage-gated, pore-forming α-subunits along with accessory β-subunits plus regulatory proteins. A typical cardiac K^+ α-subunit has six transmembrane domains (S1–S6), a voltage sensor (S4), and a pore loop containing a conserved K^+-selective signature sequence between S5 and S6A. Loss of function mutations in the cardiac K^+ channel genes is associated with the delayed repolarization, leading to LQTS, whereas gain of function mutations in *KCNQ1*, *KCNH2*, and *KCNJ2* are associated with SQTS (Priori et al. 2005; Schulze-Bahr 2005).

In vitro expression studies of mutant channels have been instrumental in the characterization of phenotypic consequences of LQTS-associated mutations and in identifying the physiological mechanisms by which the clinical phenotype is produced (Dumaine et al. 1996; Bianchi et al. 1999; Priori et al. 1999; Sanguinetti 1999; Lees-Miller et al. 2000; Huang et al. 2001; Roden 2001; Isbrandt et al. 2002; Tristani-Firouzi et al. 2002; Fodstad et al. 2004; Thomas et al. 2005). Expression studies have demonstrated that LQTS mutations of genes related with K^+ currents can produce loss of channel function by three mechanisms (Keating and Sanguinetti 2001; Aizawa et al. 2004; Wilson et al. 2005): (1) a net current reduction by altering the channel gating and kinetic properties (dominant negative effect); (2) prevention of assembly of functional channel protein (haploinsufficiency); and (3) an abnormal intracellular protein trafficking (dominant negative effect).

The cardiac slowly activating delayed rectifier current was induced when *KCNQ1* was coexpressed with *KCNE1*, a β-subunit of I_{Ks} channel. The I_{Ks} channel complex is composed of three different proteins in a specific ratio of *KCNQ1* isoform 1 (the channel pore), *KCNQ1* isoform 2 (an endogeneous N-terminal truncated *KCNQ1* splice variant), and *KCNE1* (Barhanin et al. 1996; Sanguinetti et al. 1996). The heterogeneity of I_{Ks} amplitude across the heart depends on the balance of expression of *KCNQ1* isoform 1 and 2 (Pereon et al. 2000). *KCNE1* appears to regulate the *KCNQ1* channel activity in a concentration-dependent manner (Romey et al. 1997). Hormones such as estrogens can alter the level of *KCNE1* expression and this may account for the gender differences in LQTS and vulnerability to torsades de pointes (Makkar et al. 1993; Kawasaki et al. 1995; Drici et al. 1996; Rodriguez et al. 2001; Moller and Netzer 2006).

The coexistence of deafness with JLNS is largely accounted for by the roles played by *KCNQ1/KCNE1* in the recycling circuit of K^+ ions in the cochlea and the affect on the sensitivity to auditory stimuli (Robbins 2001). However, patients with homozygous JLNS mutations of *KCNQ1* do not always present with coassociated deafness, reflecting the complexity of the mechanisms involved in K^+ channel-induced deafness (Priori et al. 1998).

Coexpression of the *KCNQ1* missense mutations with wild-type *KCNQ1* results in various degrees of I_{Ks} reduction (Chouabe et al. 1997; Donger et al. 1997). S4/S5 mutations modify coassembly with *KCNE1* (Li et al. 1998) and mutations in the pore regions and in the S5 regions are usually associated with the dominant-negative effects due to the disruption of the K^+ transport (Vatta et al. 2002). Mutations in the C- or N-termini and nonsense mutations seem to affect the subunits assembly and tetramerization of the channel (Wollnik et al. 1997; Dahimene et al. 2006; Wiener et al. 2008). Molecular modeling of gene variants is also available to researchers now that the partial crystal structure of *KCNQ1* is known (Smith et al. 2007) and examples of this are illustrated in Figure 16–3.

Heterozygous carriers of JLNS mutations generally have mild clinical effects, and two mutant alleles are required to cause the severe phenotype (Keating and Sanguinetti 2001). When JLNS mutations were expressed, the K^+ current was reduced to 50% most likely from haploinsufficiency (Chouabe et al. 1997; Wollnik et al. 1997; Mohammad-Panah et al. 1999). JLNS mutations appear to interfere with either the C-terminal or N-terminal assembly domains (Schmitt et al. 2000; Tyson et al. 2000), or may reduce protein expression due to nonsense-mediated mRNA decay (NMD) (Frischmeyer and Dietz 1999). However, it is difficult to predict phenotype and different effects of the mutation between individuals, as the functional effect of mutations differ by the relative amounts of mutant and wild-type protein (Huang et al. 2001).

The *KCNE1* C-terminal mutant, D76N, suppresses the I_{Ks} current in a dominant-negative manner (Splawski et al. 1997). This functional defect was rescued by the binding of activators of the I_{Ks} channel complex, such as 4,4'-diisothiocyanatostilbene-2,2'-disulfonic acid (DIDS) or mefenamic acid, to the extracellular N-terminal boundary of the *KCNE1* transmembrane segment, indicating that the C-terminal mutant produces loss of function by locking the cytoplasmic domain into inactive conformations (Abitbol et al. 1999). Trapping of *KCNE1* channels in the endoplasmic reticulum (ER) has also been reported, resulting in the prevention of *KCNQ1/KCNE1* association (Schulze-Bahr et al. 1997; Duggal et al. 1998). Studies have suggested that clinical manifestations of LQT5 mutations may be more complicated than expected

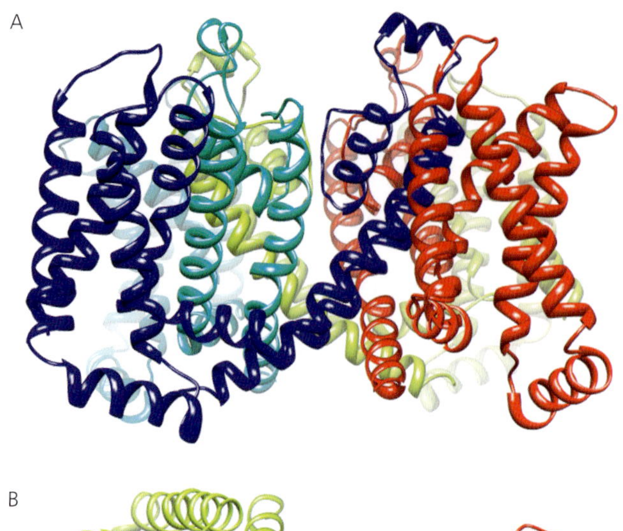

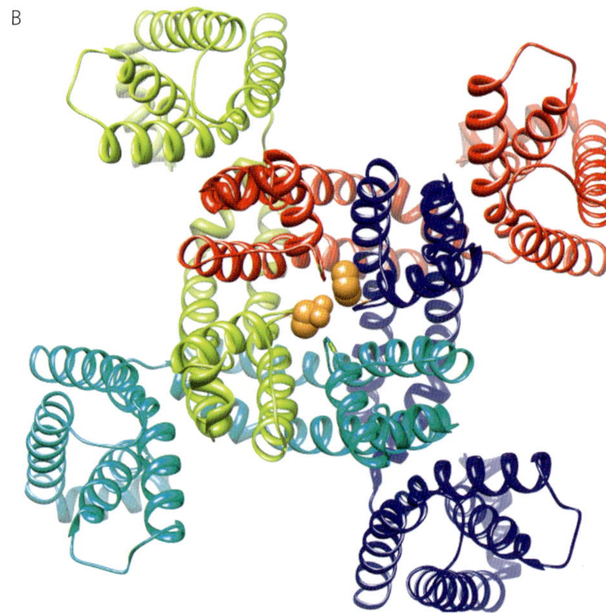

Figure 16–3 Examples of structural modeling of an ion channel. Tetrameric *KCNQ1* channel in open conformation. The chains of the receptor tetramer are shown in blue (A), green (B), lime (C), and red (D), visualized using the molecular graphics program Chimera (http://www.cgl.ucsf.edu/chimera/). **A.** The wild-type *KCNQ1* channel. **B.** *KCNQ1* with a G316E missense mutation. E316 on P loop is shown in orange for chains A and C, projected outward into the pore. For illustration, wild-type G316 shown in yellow on P loop of chains B and D, leaving the channel unobstructed. In this case, structural modeling of the ion channel can demonstrate that an introduction of a single mutation can disturb a pore region containing ion selectivity filter.

because *KCNE1* mutations exert differing effects on *KCNQ1* and *HERG* polypeptides (Bianchi et al. 1999; Ohyama et al. 2001; Priori et al. 2001). *HERG* interacts with *KCNE1*, when usual interactor *KCNE2* is not present (Bianchi et al. 1999; Ohyama et al. 2001; Priori et al. 2001).

Expression of some *HERG* mutant channels generate I_{Kr} current with altered gating or reduced amplitude, but there was no simple correlation between the position of the mutation and the functional consequences (Roden and Spooner 1999; Roden 2001). In cases of *HERG* mutants producing no I_{Kr} current, two mechanisms have been reported: (1) When the channel protein is not detected at the cell surface level, there may be defects in trafficking or protein stability (Zhou et al. 1998; Furutani et al. 1999; Petrecca et al. 1999). Mutated proteins are unglycosylated and retained in the ER, resulting in the reduction in the number of subunits for tertramerization. (2) A primary defect in gating is suggested when channel protein is detected at the cell surface (Furutani et al. 1999). The trafficking deficient subunits have also shown to tag tetrameric channel complexes for retention in the ER on coassembly (an acquired trafficking defect) (Ficker et al. 2000).

HERG mutations in the NBD region require *KCNE2* to produce the dominant negative effect (Cui et al. 2001). Heterozygous expression of *HERG* mutant and wild-type expressions showed no current suppression. However, when *KCNE2* was coexpressed K^+ current was partially reduced. *KCNE2* mutants reduce current due to the change in the gating of the channel, or faster deactivation kinetics (Abbott et al. 1999). *KCNE2* also transformed the voltage-dependant *KCNQ1* to a voltage-independent channel (Tinel et al. 2000).

Expression studies have provided evidence that acquired LQTS has a genetic predisposition, or at least a genetic risk factor. A mutation in *KCNE1* and a common polymorphism in *KCNE2* genes may affect the sensitivity to I_{Kr} blockers, leading to acquired LQTS (Abbott et al. 1999; Sesti et al. 2000). *HERG* and *KCNQ1* mutations, identified in patients with drug-associated LQTS reduce the K^+ current (Napolitano et al. 2000; Yang et al. 2002). A missense mutation identified in an individual with acquired LQTS exhibits a gain of function in the Na^+ channel features, persistent late Na^+ current, reduction in current density, and fast inactivation gating due to dispersed reopenings and prolonged channel activity (Bennett et al. 1995).

Sodium Channelopathies

The voltage-gated cardiac Na^+ channel (Nav1.5), encoded by *SCN5A* is expressed in human myocardium but not in skeletal muscle, liver, or uterus (Wang et al. 1995). Recently, an alternative *SCN5A* isoform was identified in the human central nervous system (Wang et al. 2008) and *SCN5A* is also expressed in limbic circuitry of rat brain (Hartmann et al. 1999). This may provide an explanation for LQTS patients presenting with suspected seizures—or phenocopies of seizures (Bezzina et al. 2001) although heart tissue remains the predominant site of expression. Nav1.5 is an important drug target for antiarrhythmic class Ia blockers (Lehnart et al. 2007) consistent with its importance in the depolarization dynamics of the cardiac action potential.

SCN5A mutations that cause even subtle defects in fast or slow gating in *SCN5A* receptors have profound effects on cardiac electrical activity, leading to significantly different cardiac phenotypes that have a high incidence of sudden death, usually at night or rest. The *SCN5A*-associated phenotypes include the following:

1. BrS.
2. Sudden unexplained nocturnal death syndrome (SUNDS), a disease allelic to BrS, is common in southeast Asia, and causes SCD (usually in males) during sleep (Vatta et al. 2002).
3. Isolated cardiac conduction disorder (ICCD), which is defined by isolated prolongation of the conduction parameter in the His-Purkinje conduction system but no ST segment elevation or QT prolongation (Tan et al. 2001).
4. SIDS and near SIDS cases (Schwartz et al. 2000a). Interestingly, Schwartz et al. (1998) found a prolonged QT interval in 50% of the 24 SIDS cases who died within the first year of life (SID cases), indicating the potential role of LQTS in SIDS. This suspicion has been confirmed in postmortem studies in young unexpected death syndrome cohorts and isolated retrospective diagnostic testing (Ackerman et al. 2001; Skinner et al. 2004).
5. SSS, also known as sinus node dysfunction. *SCN5A* mutations are associated with dominant form of SSS, whereas mutations in *HCN4* occur in recessive cases of SSS (Benson et al. 2003; Milanesi et al. 2006; Nof et al. 2007).

It is apparent, therefore that single *SCN5A* mutations may cause "overlap syndromes," that is, phenotypes that combine features of LQT3, BrS, and conduction disease (Tan et al. 2003) supported by model systems investigations that confirm that the interchangeable phenotypes can resonate from the same missense mutations (Abriel 2007). This raises the possibility that all *SCN5A*-associated diseases are allelic disorders or they may present the same syndrome, *SCN5A* syndrome, with different penetrance and severity.

Physiologically, *SCN5A* mutations result in defective I_{Na} and prolonged depolarization due to a delayed activation or incomplete inactivation of the Na^+ channel (Wehrens et al. 2000). Mutations in III-IV linker, the DI-DII linker, and the C-terminal demonstrate a prolonged Na^+ activity by altering the inactivation gating (Bennett et al. 1995; Dumaine et al. 1996; Wehrens et al. 2003). Heterologous expression of *SCN5A* mutations in III-IV linker exhibit a small, persistent Na^+ current during the AP plateau by allowing channel reopening, while a missense mutation in the S4 segment of the domain-IV region reduces channel activation by prolonging the channel opening with bursting behavior (Makita et al. 1998). A defect in the interaction between the *SCN5A* and β-subunits influences channel inactivation (An et al. 1998).

Interestingly, a *SCN5A* mutation, 1795insD in the C-terminus region, which is associated with both LQTS and BrS, produces opposite effects on the fast and slow components of inactivation (Bezzina et al. 1999; Veldkamp et al. 2000). At a slow heart rate, the sustained inward current was produced during AP plateau, whereas at fast heart rate, slow inactivation was enhanced by delaying recovery of channel availability between stimuli.

Calcium Receptors

HCM is a common cause of SCD in young individuals. The mechanisms underlying HCM-triggered arrhythmias are not yet determined. Although a few potential mechanisms including electrical instability and reentry cycles due to myocyte disarray have been suggested, few studies have been conducted to conclude a positive correlation between the degree of myofibrillar disarray and increased sudden death (Fineschi et al. 2005; Alcalai et al. 2008). Based on HCM-mutant mice models, alterations in Ca^{2+} homeostasis appear to be a probable cause for arrhythmias in HCM (Semsarian et al. 2002).

Alteration in Ca^{2+} level also accounts for several cardiac disorders such as CPVT, ARVD. *RYR-2* missense mutations in CPVT show a gain of function resulting in intracellular Ca^{2+} leak and delayed after depolarizations (Marks 2002; Paavola et al. 2007). Ryanodine receptors play an important role in regulating release of Ca^{2+} from the sarcoplasmic reticulum (SR). Mutations in *RYR-2* cause a decrease of calstabin2 (FKBP12.6) binding, which in turn phosphorylate RyR2-Ser2808 by protein kinase A. DCM-associated PLN mutation results in a gain of phospholamban function, which in turn inhibits SR Ca^{2+} reuptake by inactivating SERCA2a Ca^{2+} pumps and leading to intracellular Ca^{2+} overload and arrhythmia.

The Research and Diagnostic Pipeline

There are several challenges facing the molecular diagnostics of inherited cardiac disorders not least in correlating a specific genetic variant to the clinical phenotype. The clinical manifestations of arrhythmia syndromes are highly variable, even among the carriers of the same mutation (Schwartz et al. 2000b). In addition, model systems such as mouse models and cell culture lines often exhibit variable phenotypes that can be different in the human carrier. However, analysis of data on genotype-screened patients indicates that some gene-specific differences in some aspects of phenotype may exist, such as ECG pattern, the triggers for cardiac events, and age of onset.

The identification and characterization of genetic variants in arrhythmia syndromes is certainly enhancing our understanding of arrhythmogenesis, and this will ultimately result in better therapy strategies and management of patients. Issues remain around the identification of private missense mutations where the genetics requires functional platforms to add value to the diagnostic validity (Figure 16–1). Often large cohorts for population studies or specialized electrophysiology and primary cardiac cultures from animal models are outside the expertise envelope of a medical genetics diagnostic center. This makes it necessary that the diagnostic domain interacts with the research community before advising cardiologists on the pathogenicity status of gene variants that trigger downstream clinical interventions.

Lastly, it is important to keep investigating those cases in the various international cohorts, which remain gene negative. Recent descriptions of large deletions in LQTS, as revealed by MLPA (Eddy et al. 2008), show that returning to "cold-cases" have diagnostic value and that there is an ever-increasing capacity to find new genes through the various genomic platforms that are being developed. Despite the most common arrhythmia genes being linked to the cardiac action potential or sarcomeric function, there is also the possibility that arrhythmia in the wider population is a complex disorder where environment interacts with a polygenic susceptibility (Arking et al. 2006; Pfeufer 2007). The new candidate genes for arrhythmia will soon become apparent and are likely to involve genes that modulate ion channel function and genes that influence the quantitative multifactorial basis of the cardiac cycle intervals, the action potential kinetics, and myocardial dynamics.

References

Abbott GW, Sesti F, Splawski I, et al. MiRP1 forms I_{Kr} potassium channels with HERG and is associated with cardiac arrhythmia. *Cell.* 1999;97:175–187.

Abitbol I, Peretz A, Lerche C, Busch AE, Attali B. Stilbenes and fenamates rescue the loss of I_{Ks} channel function induced by an LQT5 mutation and other IsK mutants. *EMBO J.* 1999;18(15):4137–4148.

Abriel H. Roles and regulation of the cardiac sodium channel Na(v)1.5: recent insights from experimental studies. *Cardiovasc Res.* 2007;76(3):381–389.

Ackerman MJ, Siu BL, Sturner WQ, et al. Postmortem molecular analysis of SCN5A defects in sudden infant death syndrome. *JAMA.* 2001;286(18):2264–2269.

Aizawa Y, Ueda K, Wu LM, et al. Truncated KCNQ1 mutant, A178fs/105, forms hetero-multimer channel with wild-type causing a dominant-negative suppression due to trafficking defect. *FEBS Lett.* 2004;574(1–3):145–150.

Alcalai R, Seidman JG, Seidman CE. Genetic basis of hypertrophic cardiomyopathy: from bench to the clinics. *J Cardiovasc Electrophysiol.* 2008;19(1):104–110.

An RH, Wang XL, Kerem B, et al. Novel LQT-3 mutation affects Na+ channel activity through interactions between alpha- and beta 1-subunits. *Circ Res.* 1998;83(2):141–146.

Arking DE, Pfeufer A, Post W, et al. A common genetic variant in the NOS1 regulator NOS1AP modulates cardiac repolarization. *Nat Genet.* 2006;38(6):644–651.

Arnestad M, Crotti L, Rognum TO, et al. Prevalence of long-QT syndrome gene variants in sudden infant death syndrome. *Circulation.* 2007;115(3):361–367.

Barhanin J, Lesage F, Guillemare E, Fink M, Lazdunshki M, Romey G. KvLQT and Isk (minK) proteins associate to form the IKs cardiac potassium current. *Nature.* 1996;384:78–80.

Behr ER, Dalageorgou C, Christiansen M, et al. Sudden arrhythmic death syndrome: familial evaluation identifies inheritable heart disease in the majority of families. *Eur Heart J.* 2008;29(13):1670–1680.

Bellocq C, van Ginneken AC, Bezzina CR, et al. Mutation in the KCNQ1 gene leading to the short QT-interval syndrome. *Circulation.* 2004;109(20):2394–2397.

Bennett PB, Yazawa K, Makita N, George ALJ. Molecular mechanism for an inherited cardiac arrhythmia. *Nature.* 1995;376:683–685.

Benson DW, Wang DW, Dyment M, et al. Congenital sick sinus syndrome caused by recessive mutations in the cardiac sodium channel gene (SCN5A). *J Clin Invest.* 2003;112(7):1019–1028.

Bezzina C, Rook MB, Wilde AAM. Cardiac sodium channel and inherited arrhythmia syndromes. *Cardiovas Res.* 2001;49:257–217.

Bezzina C, Veldkamp MW, van den Berg MP, et al. A single Na+ channel mutation causing both long-QT and Brugada syndromes. *Circ Res.* 1999;85(12):1206–1213.

Bianchi L, Shen J, Dennis A, et al. Cellular dysfunction of LQT5-minK mutants: abnormalities of Iks, Ikr and trafficking in long QT syndrome. *Hum Mol Genet.* 1999;8(8):1499–1507.

Bjerregaard P, Gussak I. Short QT syndrome: mechanisms, diagnosis and treatment. *Nat Clin Pract Cardiovasc Med.* 2005;2(2):84–87.

Brugada P,Brugada J. Right bundle branch block, persistent ST elevation and sudden cardiac death: a distinct clinical and electrocardiographic syndrome. *J Am Coll Cardiol.* 1992;20(6):1391–1396.

Brugada R, Hong K, Dumaine R, et al. Sudden death associated with short-QT syndrome linked to mutations in HERG. *Circulation.* 2004;109(1):30–35.

Chen YH, Xu SJ, Bendahhou S, et al. KCNQ1 gain-of-function mutation in familial atrial fibrillation. *Science.* 2003;299(5604):251–254.

Chouabe C, Neyroud N, Guicheney P, Lazdunski M, Romey G, Barhanin J. Properties of KvLQT1 K+ channel mutations in Romano-Ward and Jervell and Lange-Nielsen inherited cardiac arrhythmias. *EMBO J.* 1997;16(17):5472–5479.

Corrado D, Basso C, Buja G, Nava A, Rossi L, Thiene G. Right bundle branch block, right precordial ST-segment elevation, and sudden death in young people. *Circulation.* 2001;103(5):710–717.

Cronk LB, Ye B, Kaku T, et al. Novel mechanism for sudden infant death syndrome: persistent late sodium current secondary to mutations in caveolin-3. *Heart Rhythm.* 2007;4(2):161–166.

Cui J, Kagan A, Qin D, Mathew J, Melmann YF, McDonald TV. Analysis of the cyclic nucleotide binding domain of the HERG potassium channel and interactions with KCNE2. *J Biol Chem.* 2001;276:17244–17251.

Dahimene S, Alcolea S, Naud P, et al. The N-terminal juxtamembranous domain of KCNQ1 is critical for channel surface expression: implications in the Romano-Ward LQT1 syndrome. *Circ Res.* 2006;99(10):1076–1083.

di Barletta MR, Viatchenko-Karpinski S, Nori A, et al. Clinical phenotype and functional characterization of CASQ2 mutations associated with catecholaminergic polymorphic ventricular tachycardia. *Circulation.* 2006;114(10):1012–1019.

Donger C, Denjoy I, Berthet M, et al. KVLQT1 C-terminal missense mutation causes a forme fruste long-QT syndrome. *Circulation.* 1997;96(9):2778–2781.

Doolan A, Langlois N, Semsarian C. Causes of sudden cardiac death in young Australians. *Med J Aust.* 2004;180(3):110–112.

Drici MD, Burklow TR, Haridasse V, Glazer RI, Woosley RL. Sex hormones prolong the QT interval and downregulate potassium channel expression in the rabbit heart. *Circulation.* 1996;94:1471–1474.

Duggal P, Vesely MR, Wattanasirichaigoon D, Villafane J, Kaushik V, Beggs AH. Mutation of the gene for IsK associated with both Jervell and Lange-Nielsen and Romano-Ward forms of long-QT syndrome. *Circulation.* 1998;97:142–146.

Dumaine R, Antzelevitch C. Molecular mechanisms underlying the long QT syndrome. *Curr Opin Cardiol.* 2002;17:36–42.

Dumaine R, Wang Q, Keating MT, et al. Multiple mechanisms of Na+ channel-linked long QT syndrome. *Circ Res.* 1996;78:916–924.

Eddy CA, MacCormick JM, Chung SK, et al. Identification of large gene deletions and duplications in KCNQ1 and KCNH2 in patients with long QT syndrome. *Heart Rhythm.* 2008;5(9):1275–1281.

Ficker E, Dennis A, Obejero-Paz CA, Castaldo P, Taglialatela M, Brown AM. Retention in the endoplasmic reticulum as a mechanism of dominant-negative current suppression in human long QT syndrome. *J Mol Cell Cardiol.* 2000;32:2327–2337.

Fineschi V, Silver MD, Karch SB, et al. Myocardial disarray: an architectural disorganization linked with adrenergic stress? *Int J Cardiol.* 2005;99(2):277–282.

Fodstad H, Swan H, Auberson M, et al. Loss-of-function mutations of the K+ channel gene KCNJ2 constitute a rare cause of long QT syndrome. *J Mol Cell Cardiol.* 2004;37(2):593–602.

Frischmeyer PA, Dietz HC. Nonsense-mediated mRNA decay in health and disease. *Hum Mol Genet.* 1999;8(10):1893–1900.

Furutani M, Trudeau MC, Hagiwara N, et al. Novel mechanism associated with an inherited cardiac arrhythmia. *Circulation.* 1999;99: 2290–2294.

Garcia-Touchard A, Somers VK, Kara T, et al. Ventricular ectopy during REM sleep: implications for nocturnal sudden cardiac death. *Nat Clin Pract Cardiovasc Med.* 2007;4(5):284–288.

Goldenberg I, Moss AJ, Peterson DR, et al. Risk factors for aborted cardiac arrest and sudden cardiac death in children with the congenital long-QT syndrome. *Circulation.* 2008;117(17):2184–2191.

Gollob MH, Green MS, Tang AS, et al. Identification of a gene responsible for familial Wolff-Parkinson-White syndrome. *N Engl J Med.* 2001;344(24):1823–1831.

Gollob MH, Jones DL, Krahn AD, et al. Somatic mutations in the connexin 40 gene (GJA5) in atrial fibrillation. *N Engl J Med.* 2006;354(25):2677–2688.

Groenewegen WA, Firouzi M, Bezzina CR, et al. A cardiac sodium channel mutation cosegregates with a rare connexin40 genotype in familial atrial standstill. *Circ Res.* 2003;92(1):14–22.

Harrison-Woolrych M, Clark DW, Hill GR, Rees MI, Skinner JR. QT interval prolongation associated with sibutramine treatment. *Br J Clin Pharmacol.* 2006;61(4):464–469.

Hartmann HA, Colom LV, Sutherland ML, Noebels JL. Selective localisation of cardiac SCN5A sodium channels in limbic regions of rat brain. *Nat Neurosci.* 1999;2(7):593–595.

Hobbs JB, Peterson DR, Moss AJ, et al. Risk of aborted cardiac arrest or sudden cardiac death during adolescence in the long-QT syndrome. *JAMA.* 2006;296(10):1249–1254.

Hodgkinson KA, Parfrey PS, Bassett AS, et al. The impact of implantable cardioverter-defibrillator therapy on survival in autosomal-dominant arrhythmogenic right ventricular cardiomyopathy (ARVD5). *J Am Coll Cardiol.* 2005;45(3):400–408.

Hong K, Piper DR, Diaz-Valdecantos A, et al. De novo KCNQ1 mutation responsible for atrial fibrillation and short QT syndrome in utero. *Cardiovasc Res.* 2005;68(3):433–440.

Huang L, Bitner-Glindzicz M, Tranebaerg L, Tinker A. A spectrum of functional effects for disease causing mutations in the Jervell and Lange-Nielsen syndrome. *Cardiovas Res.* 2001;51:670–680.

Hughes SE, McKenna WJ. New insights into the pathology of inherited cardiomyopathy. *Heart.* 2005;91(2):257–264.

Isbrandt D, Friederich P, Solth A, et al. Identification and functional characterization of a novel KCNE2 (MiRP1) mutation that alters HERG channel kinetics. *J Mol Med.* 2002;80(8):524–532.

Jervell A, Lange-Nielsen F. Congenital deaf-mutism, functional heart disease with prolongation of the Q-T interval, and sudden death. *Am Heart J.* 1957;54(1):59–68.

Kawasaki R, Machado C, Reinoehl J, et al. Increased propensity of women to develop torsades de pointes during complete heart block. *J Cardiovasc Electrophysiol.* 1995;6(11):1032–1038.

Keating MT, Sanguinetti MC. Molecular and cellular mechanisms of cardiac arrhythmias. *Cell.* 2001;104:569–580.

Knollmann BC, Roden DM. A genetic framework for improving arrhythmia therapy. *Nature.* 2008;451(7181):929–936.

Kobori A, Sarai N, Shimizu W, et al. Additional gene variants reduce effectiveness of beta-blockers in the LQT1 form of long QT syndrome. *J Cardiovasc Electrophysiol.* 2004;15(2):190–199.

Koopmann TT, Alders M, Jongbloed RJ, et al. Long QT syndrome caused by a large duplication in the KCNH2 (HERG) gene undetectable by current polymerase chain reaction-based exon-scanning methodologies. *Heart Rhythm.* 2006;3(1):52–55.

Kusano KF, Taniyama M, Nakamura K, et al. Atrial fibrillation in patients with Brugada syndrome relationships of gene mutation, electrophysiology, and clinical backgrounds. *J Am Coll Cardiol.* 2008;51(12): 1169–1175.

Lahat H, Pras E, Eldar M. A missense mutation in CASQ2 is associated with autosomal recessive catecholamine-induced polymorphic ventricular tachycardia in Bedouin families from Israel. *Ann Med.* 2004;36(suppl 1): 87–91.

Lahat H, Pras E, Olender T, et al. A missense mutation in a highly conserved region of CASQ2 is associated with autosomal recessive catecholamine-induced polymorphic ventricular tachycardia in Bedouin families from Israel. *Am J Hum Genet.* 2001;69(6):1378–1384.

Laitinen PJ, Brown KM, Piippo K, et al. Mutations of the cardiac ryanodine receptor (RyR2) gene in familial polymorphic ventricular tachycardia. *Circulation.* 2001;103(4):485–490.

Leenhardt A, Lucet V, Denjoy I, Grau F, Ngoc DD, Coumel P. Catecholaminergic polymorphic ventricular tachycardia in children: a 7-year follow-up of 21 patients. *Circulation.* 1995;91(5):1512–1519.

Lees-Miller JP, Duan Y, Teng GQ, Thorstad K, Duff HJ. Novel gain of function mechanism in K+ channel related long QT syndrome: altered gating and selectivity in the HERG N629D mutant. *Circ Res.* 2000;86:507–513.

Lehnart SE, Ackerman MJ, Benson DW Jr, et al. Inherited arrhythmias: a National Heart, Lung, and Blood Institute and Office of Rare Diseases workshop consensus report about the diagnosis, phenotyping, molecular mechanisms, and therapeutic approaches for primary cardiomyopathies of gene mutations affecting ion channel function. *Circulation.* 2007;116(20):2325–2345.

Li H, Chen Q, Moss AJ, et al. New mutations in the KVLQT1 potassium channel that cause long QT syndrome. *Circulation.* 1998;97:1264–1269.

Liu N, Colombi B, Raytcheva-Buono EV, Bloise R, Priori SG. Catecholaminergic polymorphic ventricular tachycardia. *Herz.* 2007;32(3):212–217.

Locati EH, Zareba W, Moss AJ, et al. Age- and sex-related differences in clinical manifestations in patients with congenital long-QT syndrome: findings from the International LQTS Registry. *Circulation.* 1998;97(22):2237–2244.

Lupoglazoff JM, Denjoy I, Villain E, et al. Long QT syndrome in neonates: conduction disorders associated with HERG mutations and sinus bradycardia with KCNQ1 mutations. *J Am Coll Cardiol.* 2004;43(5):826–830.

Makita N, Horie M, Nakamura T, et al. Drug-induced long-QT syndrome associated with a subclinical SCN5A mutation. *Circulation.* 2002;106:1269–1274.

Makita N, Shirai N, Nagashima M, et al. A de novo missense mutation of the human cardiac Na+ channel exhibiting novel molecular mechanisms of long QT syndrome. *FEBS Lett.* 1998;423:5–9.

Makkar RR, Fromm BS, Steinman RT, Meissner MD, Lehmann MH. Female gender as a risk factor for torsades de pointes associated with cardiovascular drugs. *JAMA.* 1993;270(21):2590–2597.

Marks AR, Priori S, Memmi M, Kontula K, Laitinen PJ. Involvement of the cardiac ryanodine receptor/calcium release channel in catecholaminergic polymorphic ventricular tachycardia. *J Cell Physiol.* 2002;190(1):1–6.

Maron BJ, Shirani J, Poliac LC, Mathenge R, Roberts WC, Mueller FO. Sudden death in young competitive athletes. Clinical, demographic, and pathological profiles. *JAMA.* 1996;276(3):199–204.

McKoy G, Protonotarios N, Crosby A, et al. Identification of a deletion in plakoglobin in arrhythmogenic right ventricular cardiomyopathy with palmoplantar keratoderma and woolly hair (Naxos disease). *Lancet.* 2000;355(9221):2119–2124.

Milanesi R, Baruscotti M, Gnecchi-Ruscone T, DiFrancesco D. Familial sinus bradycardia associated with a mutation in the cardiac pacemaker channel. *N Engl J Med.* 2006;354(2):151–157.

Mohamed U, Napolitano C, Priori SG. Molecular and electrophysiological bases of catecholaminergic polymorphic ventricular tachycardia. *J Cardiovasc Electrophysiol.* 2007;18(7):791–797.

Mohammad-Panah R, Demolombe S, Neyroud N, et al. Mutations in a dominant-negative isoform correlate with phenotype in inherited cardiac arrhythmias. *Am J Hum Genet.* 1999;64(4):1015–1023.

Moller C, Netzer R. Effects of estradiol on cardiac ion channel currents. *Eur J Pharmacol.* 2006;532(1–2):44–49.

Morita H, Wu J, Zipes DP. The QT syndromes: long and short. *Lancet.* 2008;372(9640):750–763.

Napolitano C, Schwartz PJ, Brown AM, et al. Evidence for a cardiac ion channel mutation underlying drug-induced QT prolongation and life-threatening arrhythmias. *J Cardiovasc Electrophysiol.* 2000;11:691–696.

Neyroud N, Tesson F, Denjoy I, et al. A novel mutation in the potassium channel gene KVLQT causes the Jervell and Lange-Nielson cardioauditory syndrome. *Nat Genet.* 1997;15:186–189.

Nof E, Luria D, Brass D, et al. Point mutation in the HCN4 cardiac ion channel pore affecting synthesis, trafficking, and functional expression is associated with familial asymptomatic sinus bradycardia. *Circulation.* 2007;116(5):463–470.

Ohyama H, Kajita H, Omori K, et al. Inhibition of cardiac delayed rectifier K+ currents by an antisense oligodeoxynucleotide against IsK (minK) and over-expression of IsK mutant D77N in neonatal mouse hearts. *Eur J Physiol.* 2001;442:329–335.

Paavola J, Viitasalo M, Laitinen-Forsblom PJ, et al. Mutant ryanodine receptors in catecholaminergic polymorphic ventricular tachycardia generate delayed after depolarizations due to increased propensity to Ca2+ waves. *Eur Heart J.* 2007;28(9):1135–1142.

Pereon Y, Demolombe S, Baro I, Drouin E, Charpentier F, Escande D. Differential expression of KvLQT1 isoforms across the human ventricular wall. *Am J Physiol.* 2000;278:H1908–H1915.

Petrecca K, Atanasiu R, Akhavan A, Shrier A. N-linked glycosylation sites determine HERG channel surface membrane expression. *J Physiol.* 1999;515(1):41–48.

Pfeufer A. Genetics of the ECG: QT or not QT a genetic analysis of a complex electrophysiological trait confirms several previously detected associations. *Eur J Hum Genet.* 2007;15(9):909–910.

Priori G, Bloise R, Crotti L. The long QT syndrome. *Europace.* 2001;3:16–27.

Priori SG, Barhanin J, Hauer RNW, et al. Genetic and molecular basis of cardiac arrhythmias: impact on clinical management parts I and II. *Circulation.* 1999;99:518–528.

Priori SG, Napolitano C, Tiso N, et al. Mutations in the cardiac ryanodine receptor gene (hRyR2) underlie catecholaminergic polymorphic ventricular tachycardia. *Circulation.* 2001;103(2):196–200.

Priori SG, Pandit SV, Rivolta I, et al. A novel form of short QT syndrome (SQT3) is caused by a mutation in the KCNJ2 gene. *Circ Res.* 2005;96(7):800–807.

Priori SG, Schwartz PJ, Napolitano C, et al. A recessive variant of the Romano-Ward long-QT syndrome? *Circulation.* 1998;97(24):2420–2425.

Puranik R, Chow CK, Duflou JA, Kilborn MJ, McGuire MA. Sudden death in the young. *Heart Rhythm.* 2005;2(12):1277–1282.

Robbins J. KCNQ potassium channels: physiology, pathophysiology, and pharmacology. *Pharmacol Ther.* 2001;90:1–19.

Roberts R. Genomics and cardiac arrhythmias. *J Am Coll Cardiol.* 2006;47(1):9–21.

Roden DM. Defective ion channel function in the long QT syndrome: multiple unexpected mechanisms. *J Mol Cell Cardiol.* 2001;33:185–187.

Roden DM. Clinical practice. Long-QT syndrome. *N Engl J Med.* 2008;358(2):169–176.

Roden DM, Lazzara R, Rosen M, Schwartz PJ, Towbin J. Vincent GM. Multiple mechanisms in the long-QT syndrome. *Circulation.* 1996;94:1996–2012.

Roden DM, Spooner PM. Inherited long QT syndromes: a paradigm for understanding arrhythmogenesis. *J Cardiovasc Electrophysiol.* 1999;10:1664–1683.

Rodriguez I, Kilborn MJ, Liu XK, Pezzullo JC, Woosley RL. Drug-induced QT prolongation in women during the menstrual cycle. *JAMA.* 2001;285(10):1322–1326.

Romano C, Gemme G, Pongiglione R. Aritmie cardiache rare dell'eta' pediatrica. *Clinica Pediatrica.* 1963;45:656–683.

Romey G, Attali B, Chouabe C, et al. Molecular mechanism and functional significance of the minK control of the KvLQT1 channel activity. *J Biol Chem.* 1997;272:16713–16716.

Sanguinetti MC. Dysfunction of delayed rectifier potassium channels in an inherited cardiac arrhythmia. *Ann N Y Acad Sci.* 1999;868:406–413.

Sanguinetti MC, Curran ME, Zou A, et al. Coassembly of KvLQT1 and minK (IsK) proteins to form cardiac IKs potassium channel. *Nature.* 1996;384:80–83.

Sauer AJ, Moss AJ, McNitt S, et al. Long QT syndrome in adults. *J Am Coll Cardiol.* 2007;49(3):329–337.

Schmitt N, Schwarz M, Peretz A, Abitbol I, Attali B, Pongs O. A recessive C-terminal Jervell and Lange-Nielsen mutation of the KCNQ1 channel impairs subunit assembly. *EMBO J.* 2000;19(3):332–340.

Schulze-Bahr E. Short QT syndrome or Andersen syndrome: Yin and Yang of Kir2.1 channel dysfunction. *Circ Res.* 2005;96(7):703–704.

Schulze-Bahr E, WangQ, Wedekind H, et al. KCNE1 mutations cause Jervell and Lange-Nielsen syndrome. *Nat Genet.* 1997;17:267–268.

Schwartz PJ, Priori SG, Bloise R, et al. Molecular diagnosis in a child with sudden infant death syndrome. *Lancet.* 2001;358(9290):1342–1343.

Schwartz PJ, Priori SG, Dumaine R, et al. A molecular link between the sudden infant death syndrome and the long QT syndrome. *N Eng J Med.* 2000a;343(4):262–267.

Schwartz PJ, Priori SG, Napolitano C. The long QT syndrome. In: Zipes DP, Jalife J. eds. *Cardiac Electrophysiology: From Cell to Bedside.* Philadelphia, USA, W.B. Saunders company; 2000b.

Schwartz PJ, Stramba-Badiale M, Segantini A, et al. Prolongation of the QT interval and the sudden infant death syndrome. *N Eng J Med.* 1998;338(24):1709–1714.

Semsarian C, Ahmad I, Giewat M, et al. The L-type calcium channel inhibitor diltiazem prevents cardiomyopathy in a mouse model. *J Clin Invest.* 2002;109(8):1013–1020.

Sesti F, Abbott GW, Wei J, et al. A common polymorphism associated with antibiotic-induced cardiac arrhythmia. *Proc Natl Acad Sci USA.* 2000;97(19):10613–10618.

Skinner JR, Chong B, Fawkner M, Webster DR, Hegde M. Use of the newborn screening card to define cause of death in a 12-year-old diagnosed with epilepsy. *J Paediatr Child Health.* 2004;40(11):651–653.

Smith JA, Vanoye CG, George AL Jr, Meiler J, Sanders CR. Structural models for the KCNQ1 voltage-gated potassium channel. *Biochemistry.* 2007;46(49):14141–14152.

Splawski I, Tristani-Firouzi M, Lehmann MH, Sanguinetti MC, Keating MT. Mutations in the hMink gene cause long QT syndrome and suppress IKs function. *Nat Genet.* 1997;17:338–340.

Tan HL, Bezzina CR, Smits JP, Verkerk AO, Wilde AA. Genetic control of sodium channel function. *Cardiovasc Res.* 2003;57(4):961–973.

Tan HL, Bink-Boelkens MTE, Bezzina C, et al. A sodium channel mutation causes isolated cardiac conduction disease. *Nature.* 2001;409:1043–1047.

Tan HL, Hofman N, van Langen IM, van der Wal AC, Wilde AA. Sudden unexplained death: heritability and diagnostic yield of cardiological and genetic examination in surviving relatives. *Circulation.* 2005;112(2):207–213.

Tester DJ, Ackerman MJ. Sudden infant death syndrome: how significant are the cardiac channelopathies? *Cardiovasc Res.* 2005;67(3):388–396.

Tester DJ, Ackerman MJ. Postmortem long QT syndrome genetic testing for sudden unexplained death in the young. *J Am Coll Cardiol.* 2007;49(2):240–246.

Tester DJ, Dura M, Carturan E, et al. A mechanism for sudden infant death syndrome (SIDS): stress-induced leak via ryanodine receptors. *Heart Rhythm.* 2007;4(6):733–739.

Tester DJ, Spoon DB, Valdivia HH, Makielski JC, Ackerman MJ. Targeted mutational analysis of the RyR2-encoded cardiac ryanodine receptor in sudden unexplained death: a molecular autopsy of 49 medical examiner/coroner's cases. *Mayo Clin Proc.* 2004;79(11):1380–1384.

Thomas D, Wimmer AB, Karle CA, et al. Dominant-negative I(Ks) suppression by KCNQ1-deltaF339 potassium channels linked to Romano-Ward syndrome. *Cardiovasc Res.* 2005;67(3):487–497.

Tinel N, Diochot S, Barsotto M, Lazdunski M, Barhanin J. KCNE2 confers background current characteristics to the cardiac KCNQ1 potassium channel. *EMBO J.* 2000;19(23):6326–6330.

Towbin J. Molecular genetic basis of sudden cardiac death. *Cardiovasc Pathol.* 2001;10:283–295.

Towbin JA, Vatta M. Molecular biology and the prolonged QT syndromes. *Am J Med.* 2001;110:385–398.

Tristani-Firouzi M, Jensen JL, Donaldson MR, et al. Functional and clinical characterization of KCNJ2 mutations associated with LQT7 (Andersen syndrome). *J Clin Invest.* 2002;110(3):381–388.

Tyson J, Tranebjaerg L, Bellman S, et al. IsK and KvLQT1: mutation in either of the two subunits of the slow component of the delayed rectifier potassium channel can cause Jervell and Lange-Nielsen syndrome. *Hum Mol Genet.* 1997;6(12):2179–2185.

Tyson J, Tranebjaerg L, McEntagart M, et al. Mutational spectrum in the cardioauditory syndrome of Jervell and Lange-Nielsen. *Hum Genet.* 2000;107:499–503.

Vatta M, Ackerman MJ, Ye B, et al. Mutant caveolin-3 induces persistent late sodium current and is associated with long-QT syndrome. *Circulation.* 2006;114(20):2104–2112.

Vatta M, Dumaine R, Varghese G, et al. Genetic and biophysical basis of sudden unexplained nocturnal death syndrome (SUNDS), a disease allelic to Brugada syndrome. *Hum Mol Genet.* 2002;11(3):337–345.

Veldkamp MW, Viswanathan PC, Bezzina C, Baartscheer A, Wilde AA, Balser JR. Two distinct congenital arrhythmias evoked by a multidysfunctional Na+ channel. *Circ Res.* 2000;86:E91–E97.

Wang J, Ou SW, Wang YJ, et al. New variants of Nav1.5/SCN5A encode Na+ channels in the brain. *J Neurogenet.* 2008;22(1):57–75.

Wang Q, Shen J, Splawski I, et al. SCN5A mutations associated with an inherited cardiac arrhythmia, long QT syndrome. *Cell.* 1995;80:805–811.

Wehrens XH, Rossenbacker T, Jongbloed R, et al. A novel mutation L619F in the cardiac Na+ channel SCN5A associated with long-QT syndrome (LQT3): a role for the I-II linker in inactivation gating. *Hum Mutat.* 2003;21(5):552–552.

Wehrens XHT, Abriel H, Cabo C, Benhorin J, Kass RS. Arrhythmogenic mechanism of an LQT-3 mutation of the human heart Na+ channel a-subunit. *Circulation.* 2000;102:584–590.

Wiener R, Haitin Y, Shamgar L, et al. The KCNQ1 (Kv7.1) COOH terminus, a multitiered scaffold for subunit assembly and protein interaction. *J Biol Chem.* 2008;283(9):5815–5830.

Wilson AJ, Quinn KV, Graves FM, Bitner-Glindzicz M, Tinker A. Abnormal KCNQ1 trafficking influences disease pathogenesis in hereditary long QT syndromes (LQT1). *Cardiovasc Res.* 2005;67(3):476–486.

Wollnik B, Schroeder BC, Kubisch C, Esperer HD, Wieacker P, Jentsch TJ. Pathophysiological mechanisms of dominant and recessive KVLQT1 K+ channel mutations found in inherited cardiac arrythmias. *Hum Mol Genet.* 1997;6(11):1943–1949.

Xia M, Jin Q, Bendahhou S, et al. A Kir2.1 gain-of-function mutation underlies familial atrial fibrillation. *Biochem Biophys Res Commun.* 2005;332(4):1012–1019.

Yamaguchi M, Shimizu M, Ino H, et al. Compound heterozygosity for mutations Asp611→Tyr in KCNQ1 and Asp609→Gly in KCNH2 associated with severe long QT syndrome. *Clin Sci.* 2005;108:143–150.

Yang P, Kanki H, Drolet B, et al. Allelic variants in long-QT disease genes in patients with drug-associated torsades de pointes. *Circulation.* 2002;105:1943–1948.

Yang Y, Xia M, Jin Q, et al. Identification of a KCNE2 gain-of-function mutation in patients with familial atrial fibrillation. *Am J Hum Genet.* 2004;75(5):899–905.

Zhou Z, Gong Q, Epstein ML, January CT. HERG channel dysfunction in human long QT syndrome. *J Biol Chem.* 1998;273(33):21061–21066.

17

The Long QT Syndrome and Catecholaminergic Polymorphic Ventricular Tachycardia

Tom Rossenbacker, Carlo Napolitano, and Silvia G Priori

Introduction

The two most important diseases associated with stress- or emotion-related cardiac arrhythmic events in young individuals with a structurally normal heart are long QT syndrome (LQTS) and catecholaminergic polymorphic ventricular tachycardia (CPVT). Both diseases are inherited cardiac arrhythmogenic disorders described in 1957 (Jervell and Lange-Nielsen 1957) and in 1975 (Reid et al. 1975), respectively. The origin of the syncope in this group of patients is often incorrectly attributed to neurological disorders. Such diagnostic lag should be avoided given the high mortality observed among untreated patients.

Although clinically recognized for many decades, it was only after the advent of molecular biology that a tremendous step forward was made in the understanding of the pathophysiology of LQTS and CPVT. The molecular bases of LQTS were revealed in the mid-1990s while the first causative CPVT mutations were only described in 2001: mutations in genes encoding ion channels or ion channels' controlling proteins emerged as the basis for the LQTS while mutations in calcium handling proteins have been shown to underlie CPVT. Besides the impact on the understanding of the mechanisms underlying both diseases, the identification of the molecular substrates has profoundly affected diagnostic methods. While genotyping was initially restricted to highly specialized research-oriented laboratories, nowadays genotyping of LQTS and CPVT patients has entered the clinical arena thanks to the close relationships between molecular genetics and clinical cardiology. The gaps in understanding the link between DNA defects and the clinical phenotype are progressively being filled and strategies are being developed to implement genotyping into clinical practice.

In this chapter we will focus on the description of the clinical profile of the two diseases and we will present an integrated view on the role of genetics in the management of LQTS and CPVT.

Clinical Phenotype of LQTS

LQTS is an inherited cardiac arrhythmogenic disease in which prolongation of cardiac repolarization alters electrical stability of the heart predisposing affected individuals to syncope and cardiac arrest (Schwartz et al. 2000a). The first arrhythmic manifestations occur mostly during adolescence (Zareba et al. 1995; Locati et al. 1998) and are usually triggered by increased sympathetic activity (Schwartz et al. 2001a).

The principal diagnostic and phenotypic hallmark of LQTS is an abnormally prolonged QT interval, although approximately 25%–30% of patients with a genetic mutation for LQTS have a *normal* QT interval (incomplete penetrance of mutations) (Priori et al. 1999; Zhang et al. 2000).

For diagnostic purposes, manual measurement of QT interval, preferentially in lead II, by an individual familiar with LQTS (Viskin et al. 2005) is preferred over automated techniques because of the difficulties in detecting the end of the T-wave that are commonly encountered in this disease. The Bazett's formula is generally used to correct the QT interval for heart rate. Historically, the diagnosis of LQTS has relied on point score systems that besides QTc duration incorporate other clinical aspects that are typical of LQTS. (Schwartz et al. 1993) Recently, the diagnostic accuracy of different diagnostic strategies and QT interval measurement solely has been compared in patients in whom genetic analysis has confirmed or dismissed the presence of the disease (Hofman et al. 2007). These data, together with a similar study (Napolitano et al. 2003), indicate that there is no benefit to introduce the use of the scores in the clinics and that therefore the QTc duration measurement remains the mainstay for clinical diagnosis (Rossenbacker and Priori 2007).

During the first visit of an individual with suspected LQTS it is critical to exclude the presence of clinical conditions or drugs that prolong QTc. It is therefore necessary to include in the first assessment a thorough clinical examination, echocardiography, history taking, and blood sample to uncover central nervous system disorders, structural heart diseases, electrolyte disturbances, and intake of drugs that can cause QT prolongation.

Arrhythmic events in LQTS patients are characterized by a distinguishing ventricular polymorphic tachyarrhythmia, called *torsades de pointes* (TdP), which can degenerate into ventricular fibrillation (Figure 17–1) (Viskin 1999). Symptoms caused by this tachyarrhythmia range from syncope (when TdP stops spontaneously) to cardiac arrest (when TdP deteriorates into ventricular fibrillation). Their occurrence is often precipitated by physical or emotional stress (Schwartz et al. 2001b). Syncopal episodes are

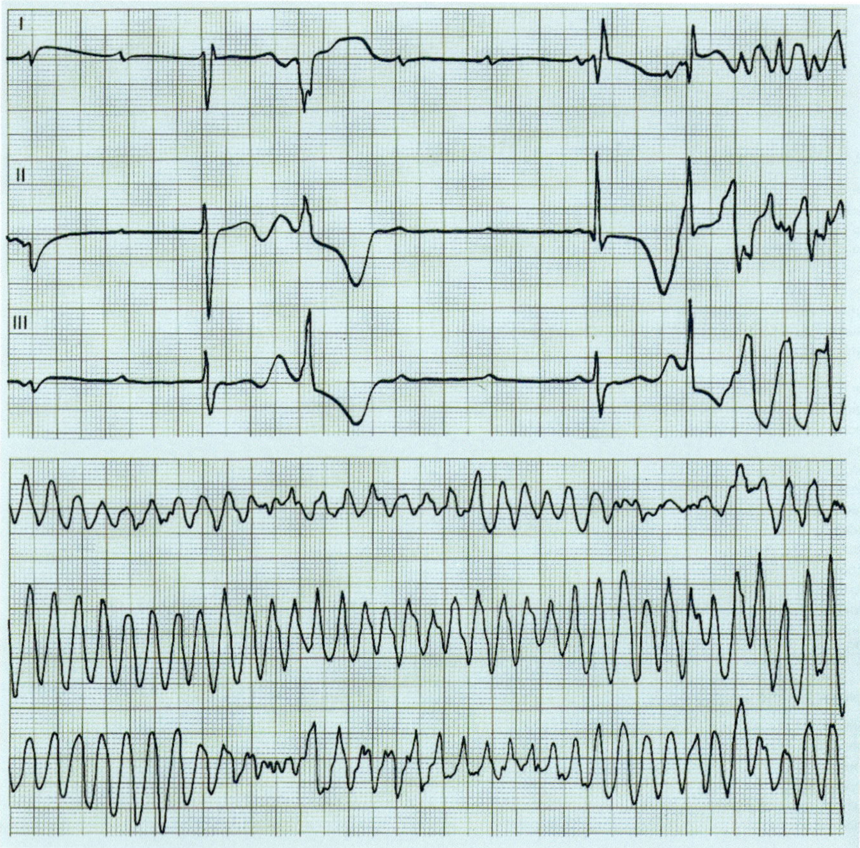

Figure 17–1 Tracing recorded during Holter monitoring in a LQTS patient showing torsades de pointes.

often mistaken for seizures as they can result in a loss of consciousness and tonic-clonic movements. Onset of symptoms is typically in the first two decades of life, including the neonatal period. The severity of the clinical manifestations of LQTS is highly variable, ranging from asymptomatic patients with a normal QTc interval to patients with sudden cardiac death (SCD) as first manifestation (Priori et al. 1999). In 12% of all patients, SCD occurs as first symptom; in 4% it may happen in the first year of life (Schwartz et al. 2000b). Up to 40% of LQTS patients are asymptomatic at the time of diagnosis (Ackerman 1998) and up to 25%–30% of all LQTS patients have a normal QTc interval (Zhang et al. 2000). Data collected in the 1980s, when it was ethically possible to compare symptomatic LQTS patients treated with antiadrenergic drugs to untreated patients showed that, in the absence of antiadrenergic therapy, symptomatic patients showed 20% mortality in the first year after the initial syncope and approximately 50% within 10 years (Schwartz 1985).

Accordingly, although the evidence comes from observational nonrandomized studies, β-blockers are considered the treatment of choice in LQTS patients (Moss 1998; Priori et al. 2001). Patients who have symptoms before β-blocker therapy have a high likelihood of experiencing recurrent cardiac events (32% within 5 years) despite being on β-blockers (Moss et al. 2000). Furthermore, 14% of patients with an aborted cardiac arrest before β-blocker therapy are expected to experience recurrent cardiac arrest or death within 5 years while on β-blockers (Moss et al. 2000). The only other effective treatment to abate mortality in LQTS is the implant of a cardioverter-defibrillator (ICD). Current guidelines advise the use of a defibrillator in LQTS patients who present with a cardiac arrest (Class I, level of evidence B), in patients presenting with sustained ventricular tachycardia (VT) (Class IIa, level of evidence B), in patients experiencing syncope while receiving β-blockers (Class IIa, level of evidence B) and, based on the observation of an excess of events among LQT2 and LQT3 patients despite β-blockers (Priori et al. 2004), the guidelines confer a Class IIb, level of evidence B recommendation for the implantation of an ICD as primary prevention of SCD in LQT2 and LQT3 patients, especially in patients with first event in early childhood (below age 7), which represents an additional risk factor for beta-blocker failure. (Zipes et al. 2006; Rossenbacker et al. 2007).

Genetics of LQTS

Genetic Basis and Molecular Correlates

The most common form of LQTS is autosomal dominant (Romano-Ward syndrome) (Romano et al. 1963; Ward 1964), although it has been reported that the Romano-Ward syndrome may also be transmitted as a recessive disorder (Priori et al. 1998; Larsen et al. 1999). LQTS in combination with deafness is inherited as an autosomal recessive trait (Jervell Lange-Nielsen [JLN] syndrome) (Jervell and Lange-Nielsen 1957). Autosomal dominant LQTS occurs with an estimated frequency of about 1 in 5,000 people in the general population (Kass and Moss 2003). The JLN syndrome is far less common with an estimated incidence of 1.6 to 6 cases per million (Splawski et al. 1997b). Recently, an interesting study demonstrated that in the Romano-Ward syndrome mutant

Table 17–1 Responsible Gene and Protein Function of LQTS and LQTS Spectrum Disorders

Disease	Gene	Protein Function
Romano-Ward syndrome		
LQT1	*KCNQ1*	I_{Ks}, α subunit
LQT2	*KCNH2*	I_{Kr}, α subunit
LQT3	*SCN5A*	I_{Na}, α subunit
LQT5	*KCNE1*	I_{Ks}, β subunit
LQT6	*KCNE2*	I_{Kr}, β subunit
Jervell Lange-Nielsen syndrome		
JLN1	*KCNQ1*	I_{Ks}, α subunit
Extremely rare LQTS variants		
LQT9	*CAV3*	Caveolin-3
LQT10	*SCN4B*	I_{Na}, β subunit
JLN2	*KCNE1*	I_{Ks}, β subunit
LQTS spectrum disorders		
Ankyrin-B syndrome	*ANK2*	Adaptor protein
Andersen-Tawil syndrome	*KCNJ2*	I_{K1}
Timothy syndrome	*CACNA1C*	$I_{Ca,L}$

alleles are transmitted more often to female offspring (Imboden et al. 2006).

In this section, we will focus on the Romano-Ward LQTS: LQT1, LQT2, LQT3, LQT5, and LQT6 and on the JLN LQTS: JLN1 and JLN2 (Table 17–1); LQT4, LQT7, and LQT8 will be discussed separately in the section on LQTS-spectrum diseases. According to the classification that we have elected to use in this chapter, the Romano-Ward syndrome depends on mutations affecting five genes, all encoding for subunits of cardiac sodium and potassium channels: *KCNQ1* (LQT1) (Wang et al. 1996), *KCNH2* (LQT2) (Curran et al. 1995), *SCN5A* (LQT3) (Wang et al. 1995), *KCNE1* (LQT5) (Splawski et al. 1997a), and *KCNE2* (LQT6) (Abbott et al. 1999). The JLN syndrome depends on homozygous or compound heterozygous mutations on either one of two genes: *KCNQ1* (JLN1) and *KCNE1* (JLN2) (Neyroud et al. 1997; Schulze-Bahr et al. 1997; Wang et al. 2002). It is not yet known if the simultaneous presence of a heterozygous defect in *KCNQ1* and in *KCNE1* would result in the JLN syndrome.

Very uncommon genetic variants such as LQT9 (mutation on caveolin gene) and LQT10 (mutation in the *SCN4B* gene) identified in a handful of patients worldwide remain anecdotal reports and it is impossible to tell whether they present distinguishing features and even if they should be considered part of the Romano-Ward syndrome or not—we have therefore listed them separately.

Finally, three LQTS-spectrum disorders have been identified in which specific cardiac and/or extracardiac manifestations are present and data available suggest keeping them separate from Romano-Ward syndrome.

Distribution of Mutations in Romano-Ward and Jervell Lange-Nielsen Syndromes

Based on the current knowledge about the molecular substrate of LQTS, 70% of Romano-Ward probands can be successfully genotyped by standard methods (Napolitano et al. 2005). Today, LQTS has been associated with hundreds of different mutations in the aforementioned genes (see http://www.fsm.it/cardmoc). The vast majority of mutations is found in *KCNQ1* and *KCNH2*, accounting for 84% of identified mutations in a study of Tester et al. in which a pool of 541 unrelated LQTS patients was tested for mutations in *KCNQ1*, *KCNH2*, *SCN5A*, *KCNE1*, and *KCNE2* (Tester et al. 2005). *SCN5A* counted for 15% of mutations (Tester et al. 2005). Only six *KCNE2* mutations have been linked so far with LQTS: three of the six patients with *KCNE2* mutations were asymptomatic and displayed only a mild QTc prolongation; among family members of these six probands, no clinically affected individuals were found and three silent gene carriers were identified.

Missense mutations are most common, followed by frameshift mutations, nonsense, splice-site mutations, and in-frame deletions (Tester et al. 2005). Of note, several mutations are private mutations even if the largest screening programs have been able to identify the presence of mutational hot spots (Napolitano et al. 1997, 2005; Murray et al. 1999).

The existence of a large number of private mutations on several genes mandates systematic screening of entire coding regions. To cope with this, the feasibility of an effective alternative strategy that may help bring genotyping closer to routine clinical practice has been reported (Napolitano et al. 2005). In a prospective study, it has been observed that 180 of 310 (58%) genotyped LQTS probands carried mutations on 64 nonprivate codons. These codons cover 3.5% of the *KCNQ1*, 2.2% of the *KCNH2*, and 0.4% of the *SCN5A* coding regions. Based on the evidence that in our study 88% of successfully genotyped patients carry mutations in the *KCNQ1* and *KCNH2* genes, it seems logical to propose that DNA of patients who test negative for the search for mutations in the 64 codons (first step) should be analyzed by sequencing the entire coding regions of *KCNQ1* and *KCNH2* genes (second step). Only patients who test negative to the first two steps would then move to the last level of this three-tier approach for LQTS genotyping and their DNA would be screened for mutations on *SCN5A*, *KCNE1*, and *KCNE2* genes.

Two or more coexisting mutations, both in the same gene and in different genes, are relatively common (Schwartz et al. 2003). Tester et al. identified 5% of their patient group as carriers of two pathogenic mutations (i.e., 10% of the genotype-positive group) (Tester et al. 2005). In another recent study, it was reported that 20 of 252 LQTS probands (7.9%) had two variants in the ion channel genes *KCNQ1*, *KCNH2*, *SCN5A*, or *KCNE1* (Westenskow et al. 2004). In the group with two mutations, QTc intervals were longer, the incidence of cardiac arrhythmia was higher and symptoms were more severe (Westenskow et al. 2004). These data favor a systematic screening of all LQTS genes, even when a first causal mutation is identified before completion of the entire screening.

Genotype–Phenotype Correlations in Romano-Ward and Jervell Lange-Nielsen Syndrome

Despite some overlap, the three major subtypes of LQTS (LQT1, LQT2, and LQT3) have their own clinical profile. Phenotypic differences in genetically distinct forms of LQTS may include each aspect of the clinical presentation: ECG characteristics (Moss et al. 1995), QT dynamics during exercise (Schwartz et al. 1995; Swan et al. 1999b), arrhythmia-related triggers (Schwartz et al. 2001), onset of arrhythmias (Tan et al. 2006), natural history (Priori et al. 2003), pregnancy-related cardiac events (Seth et al. 2007), and response to β-blocker therapy (Priori et al. 2004).

It has also been reported that LQT2 patients with mutations in the pore region of the *KCNH2* channel are at markedly increased risk for arrhythmia-related cardiac events compared to patients with nonpore mutations (Moss et al. 2002). Besides mutations in the pore, those in the PAS domain of the *KCNH2* channel may also have a deleterious impact (Rossenbacker et al. 2005a). Similarly, LQT1-associated mutations involving the transmembrane spanning domains of the *KCNQ1* channel are associated with higher cardiac event rates (Moss et al. 2007).

Patients with JLN syndrome have the most severe variant of LQTS, with a very early onset and major QTc prolongation. (Goldenberg et al. 2006) Subgroups have been identified in a study on 186 JLN patients: females, patients with a QTc ≤550 ms, those without events in the first year of life, and those with mutations on *KCNE1* are at relatively lower risk for aborted cardiac arrest and sudden cardiac death (Schwartz et al. 2006).

Uncommon LQTS Variants and LQTS "Spectrum Disorders"

1. Mutations on *CAV3* Gene and on *SCN4B* Gene

Caveolae are known membrane microdomains whose major component in the striated muscle is caveolin-3. Cardiac sodium channels localize in the caveolae. Recently, four novel mutations in *CAV3*-encoded caveolin-3 have been identified in 905 unrelated LQTS patients, suggesting that this new genetic form of LQTS (labeled LQT9) is extremely uncommon. Electrophysiological analysis of sodium current demonstrated that mutant *CAV-3* results in a two- to threefold increase in late sodium current compared to wild-type *CAV-3*, a pathophysiological mechanism well established to cause QT prolongation (Vatta et al. 2006).

Another susceptibility gene for LQTS is *SCN4B*, encoding for an auxiliary subunit to the pore-forming α-subunit *SCN5A*. Only one mutation in one LQTS patient has so far been found: the mutation leads to positive shift in inactivation of the sodium current, thus increasing sodium current (Medeiros-Domingo et al. 2007). Again, this form of LQTS (LQT10) is extremely rare and should not be targeted in the routine genetic screening of LQTS patients.

2. Ankyrin-B Disease

In 1995, shortly after the description of the subtypes LQT1, LQT2, and LQT3, a fourth LQTS locus was mapped to chromosome 4q25–26. The family, used in the linkage analysis, was assigned as suffering from LQT4 (Schott et al. 1995). Notably, the phenotype of a QTc prolongation in the family under study was associated with a number of atypical LQTS phenotypes: atrial fibrillation, a marked sinus bradycardia (leading to sinus node dysfunction), and uncommon polyphasic U waves. It took another 8 years before the responsible gene, *ANK2*, was isolated (Mohler et al. 2003). *ANK2* encodes for cardiac ankyrin-B, a structural protein that anchors ion channels to the cell membrane. In vitro studies indicated the pleiotropic effect of the responsible *ANK2* mutation (E1425G): a disruption in the cellular organization of the Na^+ pump, the Na^+/Ca^{2+} exchanger, and the inositol-1,4,5-trisphosphate receptors, leading to altered Ca^{2+} signaling (Mohler et al. 2003).

Since the initial description, a few more carriers of mutations in the *ANK2* gene have been described. In a large series, 3.3% of 269 patients, referred for LQTS genetic screening without mutations in *KCNQ1*, *KCNH2*, *SCN5A*, *KCNE1*, and *KCNE2*, hosted an *ANK2* variant; importantly, all patients had been diagnosed as atypical or borderline, most presenting with a normal QTc, non-exertional syncope, U waves, and/or sinus bradycardia (Sherman et al. 2005). Today, evidence is compelling that patients with *ANK2* mutations can display varying degrees of cardiac arrhythmias and that prolonged QTc intervals are *not* a consistent feature in *ANK2* mutation carriers. As also suggested in a study by Mohler et al. (2004), it seems logical to consider ankyrin-B dysfunction as a clinical entity, distinct from classic LQTS.

Interestingly, among the different cardiac arrhythmias described in *ANK2* mutation carriers is a catecholaminergic-triggered polymorphic VT, which may phenocopy catecholaminergic tachycardia (see below). However, the yield of *ANK2* mutations in patients with bidirectional VT (bVT) is unknown since a targeted mutation analysis of *ANK2* in patients with bVT and without *RYR2* and *CASQ2* mutations has not been performed yet.

3. Mutations in *KCNJ2*

Andersen-Tawil syndrome is a rare, clinically pleiotropic, disorder characterized by an abnormal repolarization (often marked prolongation of the *QUc* interval), ventricular arrhythmias (frequent premature ventricular contractions, bigeminy, and VT, typically nonsustained and bidirectional), hypokaliemic and/or hyperkaliemic periodic paralysis of skeletal muscle, and facial dysmorphic features (Plaster et al. 2001; Tristani-Firouzi et al. 2002). Characteristic dysmorphic features include low-set ears, micrognathia and clinodactyly. The syndrome is inherited in an autosomal dominant fashion, although several cases are sporadic. Mutations in the *KCNJ2*, gene encoding for the inward rectifier K^+ channel Kir2.1, have been associated with the syndrome (Plaster et al. 2001). *KCNJ2* mutations account for nearly two-thirds of reported cases (referred to as ATS1), with the molecular basis of the remaining one-third being still undefined. The full triad of clinical features (ventricular arrhythmias, periodic paralysis, and characteristic dysmorphic features) is present in only 58% to 78% of mutation-positive patients (Plaster et al. 2001), meaning that some patients present only the cardiac phenotype.

The observation that both a QTc prolongation and/or a bVT are part of the clinical spectrum of the KCNJ2-syndrome inspired some to screen the *KCNJ2* gene in patients referred for LQTS or CPVT genetic testing and to assign patients with *KCNJ2* mutations as LQTS subtype 7 or CPVT subtype 3 patients.

However, *KCNJ2* mutations were detected in nearly 2% (4 of 249) of patients referred for genetic arrhythmia testing who were negative for other known arrhythmia genes (Eckardt et al. 2007). Strikingly, these patients had a mean QTc of 418 ms (i.e., within the normal range), prominent U waves, marked ventricular ectopy, and polymorphic VT. Relevant differences exist between the phenotype linked to *KCNJ2* mutations and LQTS. A systematic assessment of the ECG features of 39 patients with *KCNJ2* mutations indicated that only 17% of patients had a QTc >460 ms and that the TU wave patterns were markedly abnormal (prolonged T wave downslope, wide TU junction and biphasic, enlarged U wave), both atypical characteristics of the LQTS phenotype (Zhang et al. 2005). Furthermore, ventricular ectopy is rather common in patients with *KCNJ2* mutations but very uncommon in LQTS patients. Based on these findings, a systematic screen for *KCNJ2* mutations in patients with a prolonged QTc time should not be encouraged.

In a small study, three of seven CPVT patients, without mutations in 23 exons of the RYR2 gene and without mutations in the *CASQ2* gene, carried *KCNJ2* mutations (Tester et al. 2006). Consistent with these observations, bVT has been reported to be part of the clinical spectrum of the Andersen-Tawil syndrome (Tristani-Firouzi et al. 2002; Zhang et al. 2005). The overlap between the arrhythymic phenotype of CPVT and ATS1 does not imply that there is a complete phenotypic mimicry. The adrenergic triggers for events and for (supra)ventricular arrhythmias are typical in CPVT1 and CPVT2 (see below), but not in patients with *KCNJ2* mutations. Additionally, sudden death is exceptional among *KCNJ2* mutation carriers (Sansone et al. 1997) but is a consistent feature of CPVT patients, and, finally, there are TU wave patterns characteristic for patients with *KCNJ2* mutations. These data prevent us from using the term CPVT3 for *KCNJ2* mutation carriers with bVT but encourage us to screen the *KCNJ2* gene in patients presenting with a bVT after exclusion of mutations in *RYR2* and *CASQ2* and after an expert investigation that includes neurological assessment and detection of facial dysmorphisms.

4. Timothy Syndrome

Timothy syndrome is a multiorgan dysfunction in which a prolonged QT interval (Figure 17–2), ventricular arrhythmias, and congenital heart disease are associated with extracardiac manifestations including webbing of fingers and toes, immune deficiency, intermittent hypoglycemia, cognitive abnormalities, and autism (Reichenbach et al. 1992; Marks et al. 1995; Splawski et al. 2004). The gene responsible for Timothy syndrome is *CACNA1C*, encoding for the calcium channel $Ca_v1.2$ (Splawski et al. 2004). The inheritance pattern of Timothy syndrome is sporadic in all but one family described so far. In the latter family, it was demonstrated that siblings were affected by the same mutation and that one unaffected parent was mosaic for the mutation (Splawski et al. 2004). To date only two mutations in *CACNA1C* have been identified in Timothy syndrome patients (Splawski et al. 2004; Splawski et al. 2005).

Genetic Modifiers

A plausible explanation for the clinical heterogeneity among LQTS patients sharing the same disease-causing mutation is the coexistence of modifier gene alleles, altering arrhythmia susceptibility. This concept has been demonstrated in a family segregating a novel, low-penetrant *KCNH2* mutation (A1116V) along with a common single nucleotide polymorphism (K897T) in *KCNH2*: family members who carried A1116V without K897T were asymptomatic, but in the proband, carrier of A1116V and K897T, the polymorphism exposed latent disease, as was also confirmed by biophysical analysis (Crotti et al. 2005).

Identification of the genetic modifiers, that will ultimately determine the final phenotype in LQTS patients, undoubtedly constitutes one of the current challenges for researchers in the field.

"Nongenotyped" LQTS Patients

Currently, investigators intensively hunt for other causal genes and even move to the noncoding regions of the LQTS genes in an attempt to genotype the remaining 30% of LQTS patients. In the approximately 30% of LQTS patients in whom conventional mutation screening fails to uncover a mutation, recent anecdotal studies report other genetic defects than the commonly found point mutations or small insertions and deletions in coding regions.

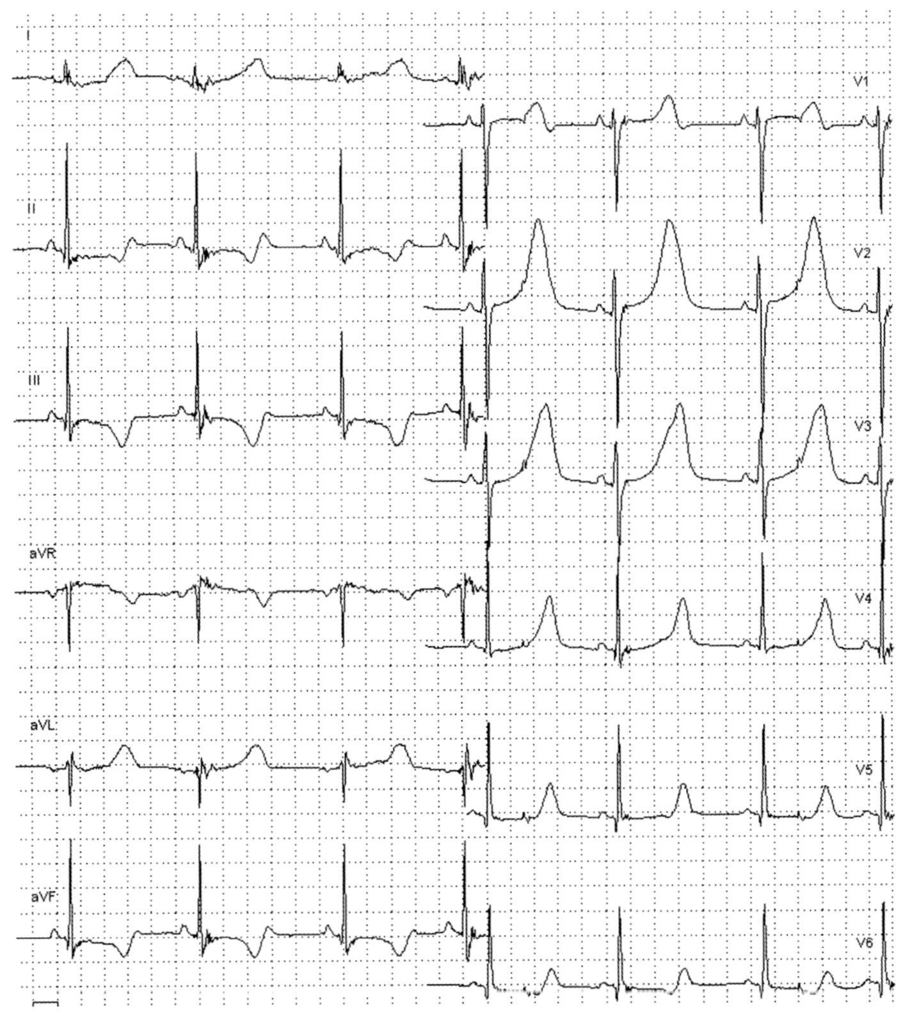

Figure 17–2 Twelve-lead ECG of a Timothy syndrome patient showing a markedly prolonged QT time with T-wave abnormalities (biphasic T-waves in inferior leads and giant T-waves in V2–V4).

Using a quantitative multiplex approach, a large gene rearrangement consisting of a tandem duplication of 3.7 kb in *KCNH2* has been found to be responsible for LQTS in a Dutch family (Koopmann et al. 2006). The rearrangement is undetectable by current polymerase-chain-reaction-based exon-scanning methodologies. It has to be determined in a larger series whether analysis for large gene alterations in routine genetic testing may provide a genetic diagnosis in a number of nongenotyped patients.

It is well known that base pairs around the exon–intron boundaries (donor and acceptor splice sites) are essential for normal splicing (Padgett et al. 1986). Sequence alterations at these locations are potentially disease causing by disruption of the splice site and, subsequently, exon skipping (Priori et al. 2002; Rossenbacker et al. 2005b). So far, it has been shown in two studies that disease-causing aberrations can be detected at less highly conserved nucleotide positions than either the obligatory GT or AG of the donor and acceptor splice sites. In one family, an intronic variant in *KCNH2*, T1945+6C, was identified. Splicing assay showed T1945+6C causing downstream intron retention. Complementary deoxyribonucleic acid with retained intron 7 failed to produce functional channels (Zhang et al. 2004). Another study described the pathophysiological role of an A to G branch point substitution in *KCNH2* in intron 9 at position -28 (IVS9–28A>G) (Crotti et al. 2007).

Clinical Phenotype of CPVT

CPVT is characterized by stress-induced ventricular tachyarrhythmias that often start manifesting during childhood (Napolitano and Priori 2004). The mean age of onset of symptoms is between 7 and 9 years (Leenhardt et al. 1995; Postma et al. 2005). The resting ECG of CPVT patients is normal, although some authors have reported lower-than-normal heart rates (Postma et al. 2005) and others have observed prominent U-waves (Leenhardt et al. 1995). Overall, these ECG features are not consistent and not sufficiently specific for diagnosis.

Ventricular arrhythmias in CPVT typically present with alternating QRS axis with 180° rotation on a beat-to-beat basis, the so-called bidirectional VT (bVT) (Figure 17–3). The onset of ectopic activity during exercise stress test is consistently observed at heart rates >110–120 bpm. The complexity and frequency of arrhythmias progressively worsens as workload increases. If exercise is not promptly discontinued, bVT may degenerate into polymorphic VT and ventricular fibrillation. Interestingly, supraventricular arrhythmias (isolated ectopic atrial beats, supraventricular tachycardia, short runs of atrial fibrillation) are part of the CPVT phenotype. A fast supraventricular rate caused by supraventricular arrhythmias may act as a trigger for the development of delayed afterdepolarizations, triggered activity, and onset of VT.

The most important step for diagnosis is the ability to reproduce the typical arrhythmic pattern of VT by exercise stress test or isoproterenol infusion. Holter monitoring also may be an important diagnostic tool for those patients in whom emotional stress is a major trigger.

CPVT should be regarded as a highly lethal disease; if left untreated, 80% of CPVT patients will develop symptoms (syncope, VT, or VF) by age 40 and overall mortality is 30%–50% (Cerrone et al. 2004). β-blockers are the first-line treatment. It is recommended that whenever the diagnosis of CPVT is established, β-blockers should be promptly initiated to prevent the occurrence of ventricular tachyarrhythmias (Priori et al. 2002). Unfortunately, up to 30% of patient on β-blockers require a defibrillator because of recurrence of symptoms and 50% of implanted patients receive appropriate shocks (Priori et al. 2002).

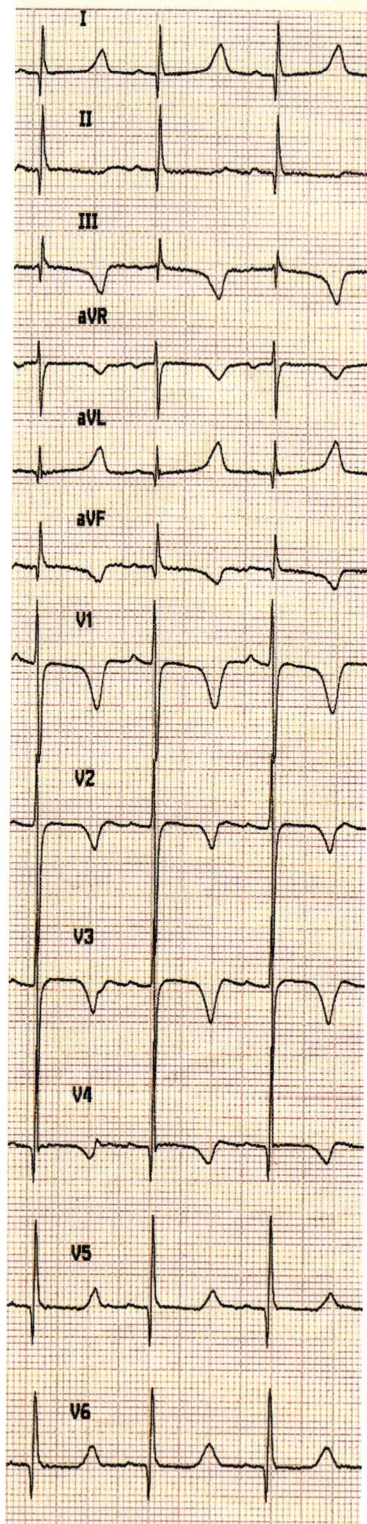

Figure 17–3 Tracing recorded during treadmill test in a CPVT patient showing a bidirectional ventricular tachycardia as a beat-to-beat alternation of the QRS axis.

Genetics of CPVT

Genetic Basis and Molecular Correlates

CPVT may have both an autosomal dominant and an autosomal recessive pattern of inheritance. The autosomal dominant variant is by far more frequent. It took several years and work of different groups to unveil the genetic substrate of the disease. The first advancement was made possible by linkage studies that were able to localize a CPVT locus to the long arm of chromosome 1 (Swan et al. 1999a). Subsequently, Priori et al., using the candidate gene approach, identified mutations in the cardiac ryanodine receptor (*RYR2*) in four CPVT probands (Priori et al. 2001). *RYR2* mutations cause uncontrolled Ca^{2+} release from the sarcoplasmic reticulum (SR) during electrical diastole (CPVT1). The gene encoding *RYR2* is one of the largest and most complex in the human genome (>800 kb, 105 exons): it encodes a large protein with a molecular weight of 565 kDA. The functional *RYR2* channel is a tetramer of four subunits. Each *RYR2* monomer is composed of the carboxy-terminal transmembrane Ca^{2+} pore-forming region, encompassing only 10% of the protein but with a critical role, as it is sufficient to form a functional Ca^{2+} release channel, and a large cytoplasmic domain, accounting for 90% of the protein that is responsible for regulatory functions.

The first autosomal recessive CPVT family was identified in a large Bedouin family; Lahat et al. linked the disease to the short arm of chromosome 1 and identified mutations in the cardiac calsequestrin gene (*CASQ2*) as the responsible gene for CPVT2 (Lahat et al. 2001a, 2001b). *CASQ2* is a SR Ca^{2+} buffering protein that plays an active role in the control of calcium release from SR to cytosol. Compound heterozygous carriership in nonconsanguineous families may occur (di Barletta et al. 2006).

Distribution of Mutations

The entire coding region of the *RYR2* gene contains 105 exons, rendering its full-length screening to be time consuming and expensive. Most laboratories target the genetic analysis to 25 exons, encoding for four discrete domains of the *RYR2* protein, in which all but one (E1724K) of the 69 *RYR2* mutations, identified so far, cluster: domain I (compressing amino acid (AA) 77–466), II (AA 2246–2534), III (AA 3778–4201), and IV (AA 4497–4959) (DI–DIV) (see http://www.fsm.it/cardmoc) (George et al. 2007). Mutation clustering in distinct *RyR2* domains is not linked to known genotype/phenotype characteristics. In contrast with the LQTS, all *RYR2* mutations, identified to date, are missense mutations.

One study showed that the yield of targeted screening was <40%, much lower than the expected 60% (Tester et al. 2006). It could be reasoned that confining genetic screens contributes to the disproportionate representation of mutation clustering into hot-spot regions and, therefore, a systematic analysis of the entire *RYR2* coding region is advisable.

Molecular Screening on LQTS- and CPVT-Related Genes in Selected Populations

Sudden Infant Death Syndrome

Approximately 5% of sudden infant death syndrome (SIDS) cases are believed to result from a cardiac channelopathy (Schwartz et al. 1998, 2000, 2001; Ackerman et al. 2001; Christiansen et al. 2005). A molecular study in 201 Norwegian SIDS victims showed that genetic variants in LQTS genes are present in 9.5% of SIDS victims (Arnestad et al. 2007). Another study implicated also *CAV3* mutations as a pathogenic basis of SIDS: 3 distinct *CAV3* mutations were identified in 3 of 50 black infants but no *CAV3* mutations were detected in 83 white infants (Cronk et al. 2007). Given the growing consistency of these and other (Tester and Ackerman 2005) molecular autopsy reports, the challenge is to find a cost-effective and efficient means for presymptomatic detection of LQTS to reduce the morbidity and mortality of the subset of SIDS etiologically related to LQTS genes and to determine whether newborn ECG screening is appropriate (Berul and Perry 2007).

The spectrum of channelopathies that can cause SIDS is even expanding as Tester et al. identified two *RYR2* mutations in 134 SIDS cases (Tester et al. 2007). Unfortunately, a clinical test to screen neonates for CPVT is currently not available.

Sudden Unexplained Death Syndrome

Another recent comprehensive postmortem study performed genetic testing in 49 sudden unexplained death (SUD) victims with an average age of death of 14 years (Tester and Ackerman 2007). Over one-third of decedents harbored a putative cardiac channel mutation: 7 hosted mutations in the *RyR2*-encoded calcium release channel and 10 carried LQTS susceptibility mutations (Tester and Ackerman 2007). Accordingly, postmortem cardiac channel genetic testing should be pursued in the evaluation of autopsy-negative SUD in order to provide reliable genetic counseling to the relatives of a SUD victim (see also Chapter 33).

Drowning Victims

Swimming is a relatively genotype-specific arrhythmogenic trigger for LQT1 (Schwartz et al. 2001). In a study by Choi et al. 43 of 388 index cases had a "positive-swimming-phenotype" of whom 33 and 10 had a high and low clinical probability of LQTS, respectively (Choi et al. 2004). In the former group, 28 (85%) patients carried a LQT1 mutation. Interestingly, in 9 of the 10 (90%) individuals of the latter group, a *RYR2* mutation was detected (Choi et al. 2004).

Clinical Applicability of Genetic Testing in LQTS and CPVT

Both the LQTS and CPVT present an excellent example of the stringent link between molecular genetics and clinical cardiology: the molecular information is directly applicable to the clinical care of LQTS and CPVT patients at the diagnostic and the therapeutic level.

Diagnosis

In patients with a definite clinical diagnosis of LQTS or CPVT, the identification of the mutant gene responsible for the disease confirms the clinically established diagnosis. More importantly, it offers the possibility for presymptomatic screening in patient's relatives and it may lead to specific modifications in the patient's management (see below). Therefore, a genetic diagnosis should be strived for in all patients with a definite clinical diagnosis of LQTS or CPVT.

In patients with a suspected clinical diagnosis, identification of a mutant gene turns a probable diagnosis into a certain diagnosis. The role for DNA diagnosis in these cases is substantial given, for example, the number of inherent difficulties that exist in identifying the phenotype solely from measurements of a 12-lead ECG. It should be stressed, however, that before costly and time-consuming genotyping is initiated, the diagnosis should be made as likely as possible: (1) lowering the cut-off value of a diagnostic QTc value will result in a substantial number of negative genetic results; (2) attempts should be made to examine first-degree relatives of patients with a suspected diagnosis to have more clues to a particular diagnosis.

In apparently asymptomatic relatives of a patient with LQTS or CPVT, genetic testing is highly informative for a variety of reasons. First, disease penetrance can be low; for example, in one large study, 36% of patients with a *KCNQ1* mutation were carriers with a normal QTc (Priori et al. 2003). However, asymptomatic mutation carriers are at risk for SCD. In case of the LQTS, silent gene carriers have a risk of 20% of having a syncope or cardiac arrest before age 40 years (Priori et al. 2003). These patients can be protected by avoiding precipitating factors for arrhythmias or by taking prophylactic medication. Second, silent gene carriers can generate affected offspring with possible overt phenotypes. Some patients may want to be aware of the probability to generated affected children. Third, prenatal diagnosis is emerging as an option for families affected by highly lethal forms of inherited arrhythmogenic diseases. Finally, presymptomatic genetic testing can identify noncarriers. This allows to reassure these persons and to discharge them from further medical follow-up. For all these reasons, it is recommended to perform molecular screening in all first-degree family members of positively genotyped patients. Moreover, once the disease-causing mutation has been identified in the proband, it is easy, fast, and cheap to screen for the culprit mutation among family members.

Therapy

Among the most important aspects that mark a departure from previous knowledge is the concept that the genetic substrate identifies distinct forms of LQTS that present specific characteristics and require different management.

Risk-stratification schemes have been proposed in the LQTS, based on two clinical features (gender and QTc) and the specific genetic locus (Priori et al. 2003). The incidence of a first cardiac event before the age of 40 years and before the initiation of any therapy is lower among LQT1 patients (30%) than among LQT2 (46%) and LQT3 (42%) patients (Priori et al. 2003). The risk of cardiac events among LQT1 patients is strongly dependent on the duration of the QTc interval: among patients with a QTc ≥ 500 ms, male patients are at high risk for a first cardiac event during childhood, whereas the risk for female patients is unchanged over time; among patients with a QTc < 500 ms, patients of either sex have a risk of a first cardiac event before the age of 40 years of less than 30% (Priori et al. 2003). Female LQT2 patients have a more severe prognosis irrespective of the duration of the QTc, whereas in LQT3 patients, prognosis is mainly influenced by sex: male patients have a higher probability of becoming symptomatic by the age of 40 years than female patients (Priori et al. 2003). Clinicians can use genetic data just like any other parameter that contributes to define the clinical profile of patients.

In the past, the concept is introduced that response to β-blocker therapy may be modulated by the genetic substrate. Given the high incidence of cardiac events during exercise in LQT1 patients, it is reasonable to hypothesize that β-blockers are particularly effective in the LQT1 subgroup (Schwartz et al. 2001). In a large β-blocker treated LQTS cohort, a gradient of risk from LQT1, LQT2 to LQT3 was reported: cardiac events occurred in 19 of 187 (10%) LQT1 patients, 27 of 120 (23%) LQT2 patients, and 9 of 28 (32%) LQT3 patients (Priori et al. 2004). These findings suggest that more aggressive therapy such as the prophylactic implant of an ICD may be warranted in LQT2 and LQT3 patients (Priori et al. 2004; Zipes et al. 2006).

The observation that arrhythmogenic triggers are, to a large extent, gene specific (Schwartz et al. 2001a) has led to specific gene-tailored management strategies in the LQTS. Competitive sports should not be allowed to LQT1 patients and they should avoid strenuous exercise, with special attention to swimming. Removal of telephones and alarm clocks from the bedroom of LQT2 patients should be strongly recommended given the specific auditory stimulus for events in LQTS subtype 2. Physical activity may not be restricted to LQT3 patients if an exercise test produces a significant shortening of the QT interval. An increase in extracellular concentration of K^+ may shorten the QT interval in LQT2 patients. In these patients, oral K^+ supplements may be beneficial. It has been demonstrated that mexiletine significantly shortens the QT interval in LQT3 patients: it is therefore reasonable to test the potential efficacy of Na^+ blockers in LQT3 patients.

Finally, the most ambitious step in the therapy of the cardiac inherited arrhythmogenic syndromes is to discover a novel therapy to correct the inborn defect by replacing the defective gene with gene therapy. This approach is currently in full development but can only be implemented if the diseased gene has been identified.

References

Abbott GW, Sesti F, Splawski I, et al. MiRP1 forms IKr potassium channels with HERG and is associated with cardiac arrhythmia. *Cell.* 1999;97(2):175–187.

Ackerman MJ. The long QT syndrome: ion channel diseases of the heart. *Mayo Clin Proc.* 1998;73(3):250–269.

Ackerman MJ, Siu BL, Sturner WQ, et al. Postmortem molecular analysis of SCN5A defects in sudden infant death syndrome. *J Am Med Assoc.* 2001;286(18):2264–2269.

Arnestad M, Crotti L, Rognum TO, et al. Prevalence of long-QT syndrome gene variants in sudden infant death syndrome. *Circulation.* 2007;115(3):361–367.

Berul CI, Perry JC. Contribution of long-QT syndrome genes to sudden infant death syndrome: is it time to consider newborn electrocardiographic screening? *Circulation.* 2007;115(3):294–296.

Cerrone M, Colombi B, Bloise R, et al. Clinical and molecular characterization of a large cohort of patients affected with CPVT (abstract). *Circulation.* 2004;110(suppl II):552.

Choi G, Kopplin LJ, Tester DJ, et al. Spectrum and frequency of cardiac channel defects in swimming-triggered arrhythmia syndromes. *Circulation.* 2004;110(15):2119–2124.

Christiansen M, Tonder N, Larsen LA, et al. Mutations in the HERG K(+)-ion channel: a novel link between long QT syndrome and sudden infant death syndrome. *Am J Cardiol.* 2005;95(3):433–434.

Cronk LB, Ye B, Kaku T, et al. Novel mechanism for sudden infant death syndrome: persistent late sodium current secondary to mutations in caveolin-3. *Heart Rhythm.* 2007;4(2):161–166.

Crotti L, Lundquist AL, Insolia R, et al. KCNH2-K897T is a genetic modifier of latent congenital long-QT syndrome. *Circulation.* 2005;112(9):1251–1258.

Crotti L, Marzena A, Lewandowska B, et al. Intronic branch point mutations may contribute to the current failure of identifying mutations in patients affected by the Long QT Syndrome (abstract). *Heart Rhythm Society Abstract Book.* 2007.

Curran ME, Splawski I, Timothy KW, et al. A molecular basis for cardiac arrhythmia: HERG mutations cause long QT syndrome. *Cell.* 1995;80(5):795–803.

di Barletta MR, Viatchenko-Karpinski S, Nori A, et al. Clinical phenotype and functional characterization of CASQ2 mutations associated with CPVT. *Circulation.* 2006;114(10):1012–1019.

Eckardt L, Farley AL, Rodriguez E, et al. KCNJ2 mutations in arrhythmia patients referred for LQT testing: a mutation T305A with novel effect on rectification properties. *Heart Rhythm.* 2007;4:323–329.

George CH, Jundi H, Thomas NL, et al. Ryanodine receptors and ventricular arrhythmias: emerging trends in mutations, mechanisms and therapies. *J Mol Cell Cardiol.* 2007;42(1):34–50.

Goldenberg I, Moss AJ, Zareba W, et al. Clinical course and risk stratification of patients affected with the Jervell and Lange-Nielsen syndrome. *J Cardiovasc Electrophysiol.* 2006;17(11):1161–1168.

Hofman N, Wilde AA, Kaab S, et al. Diagnostic criteria for congenital long QT syndrome in the era of molecular genetics: do we need a scoring system? *Eur Heart J.* 2007;28(5):575–580.

Imboden M, Swan H, Denjoy I, et al. Female predominance and transmission distortion in the long-QT syndrome. *N Engl J Med.* 2006;355(26):2744–2751.

Jervell A, Lange-Nielsen F. Congenital deaf mutism, functional heart disease with prolongation of the QT interval and sudden death. *Am Heart J.* 1957;54:59–68.

Kass RS, Moss AJ. Long QT syndrome: novel insights into the mechanisms of cardiac arrhythmias. *J Clin Invest.* 2003;112(6):810–815.

Koopmann TT, Alders M, Jongbloed RJ, et al. Long QT syndrome caused by a large duplication in the KCNH2 (HERG) gene undetectable by current polymerase chain reaction-based exon-scanning methodologies. *Heart Rhythm.* 2006;3(1):52–55.

Lahat H, Eldar M, Levy-Nissenbaum E, et al. Autosomal recessive catecholamine- or exercise-induced polymorphic ventricular tachycardia: clinical features and assignment of the disease gene to chromosome 1p13–21. *Circulation.* 2001a;103(23):2822–2827.

Lahat H, Pras E, Olender T, et al. A missense mutation in a highly conserved region of CASQ2 is associated with autosomal recessive catecholamine-induced polymorphic ventricular tachycardia in Bedouin families from Israel. *Am J Hum Genet.* 2001b;69(6):1378–1384.

Larsen LA, Fosdal I, Andersen PS, et al. Recessive Romano-Ward syndrome associated with compound heterozygosity for two mutations in the KVLQT1 gene. *Eur J Hum Genet.* 1999;7(6):724–728.

Leenhardt A, Lucet V, Denjoy I, et al. Catecholaminergic polymorphic ventricular tachycardia in children. A 7-year follow-up of 21 patients. *Circulation.* 1995;91(5):1512–1519.

Locati EH, Zareba W, Moss AJ, et al. Age- and sex-related differences in clinical manifestations in patients with congenital long-QT syndrome: findings from the International LQTS Registry. *Circulation.* 1998;97(22):2237–2244.

Marks ML, Whisler SL, Clericuzio C, et al. A new form of long QT syndrome associated with syndactyly. *J Am Coll Cardiol.* 1995;25(1):59–64.

Medeiros-Domingo A, Kaku T, Tester DJ, et al. SCN4B-encoded sodium channel beta4 subunit in congenital long-QT syndrome. *Circulation.* 2007;116(2):134–142.

Mohler PJ, Schott JJ, Gramolini AO, et al. Ankyrin-B mutation causes type 4 long-QT cardiac arrhythmia and sudden cardiac death. *Nature.* 2003;421(6923):634–639.

Mohler PJ, Splawski I, Napolitano C, et al. A cardiac arrhythmia syndrome caused by loss of ankyrin-B function. *Proc Natl Acad Sci USA.* 2004;101(24):9137–9142.

Moss AJ. Management of patients with the hereditary long QT syndrome. *J Cardiovasc Electrophysiol.* 1998;9(6):668–674.

Moss AJ, Shimizu W, Wilde AA, et al. Clinical aspects of type-1 long-QT syndrome by location, coding type, and biophysical function of mutations involving the KCNQ1 gene. *Circulation.* 2007;115(19):2481–2489.

Moss AJ, Zareba W, Benhorin J, et al. ECG T-wave patterns in genetically distinct forms of the hereditary long QT syndrome. *Circulation.* 1995;92(10):2929–2934.

Moss AJ, Zareba W, Hall WJ, et al. Effectiveness and limitations of beta-blocker therapy in congenital long-QT syndrome. *Circulation.* 2000;101(6):616–623.

Moss AJ, Zareba W, Kaufman ES, et al. Increased risk of arrhythmic events in long-QT syndrome with mutations in the pore region of the human ether-a-go-go-related gene potassium channel. *Circulation.* 2002;105(7):794–799.

Murray A, Donger C, Fenske C, et al. Splicing mutations in KCNQ1: a mutation hot spot at codon 344 that produces in frame transcripts. *Circulation.* 1999;100(10):1077–1084.

Napolitano C, Priori S, Schwartz PJ. Identification of a mutational hot spot in HERG-related long QT syndrome (LQT2): phenotypic implications. *Circulation.* 1997;96(Abstr Suppl I):212.

Napolitano C, Priori SG. Catecholaminergic polymorphic ventricular tachycardia. In Zipes DP, Jalife J eds. *Cardiac Electrphysiology.* Elsevier, Philadelphia, USA; 2004.

Napolitano C, Priori SG, Schwartz PJ, et al. Value and accuracy of clinical diagnostic criteria for the LQTS in the era of molecular diagnosis (abstract). *Circulation.* 2003;108(IV):363.

Napolitano C, Priori SG, Schwartz PJ, et al. Genetic testing in the long QT syndrome. *J Am Med Assoc.* 2005;294(23):2975–2980.

Neyroud N, Tesson F, Denjoy I, et al. A novel mutation in the potassium channel gene KVLQT1 causes the Jervell and Lange-Nielsen cardioauditory syndrome. *Nat Genet.* 1997;15(2):186–189.

Padgett RA, Grabowski PJ, Konarska MM, et al. Splicing of messenger RNA precursors. *Annu Rev Biochem.* 1986;55:1119–1150.

Plaster NM, Tawil R, Tristani-Firouzi M, et al. Mutations in Kir2.1 cause the developmental and episodic electrical phenotypes of Andersen's syndrome. *Cell.* 2001;105(4):511–519.

Postma AV, Denjoy I, Kamblock J, et al. Catecholaminergic polymorphic ventricular tachycardia: RYR2 mutations, bradycardia, and follow up of the patients. *J Med Genet.* 2005;42(11):863–870.

Priori SG, Aliot E, Blomstrom-Lundqvist C, et al. Task Force on Sudden Cardiac Death of the European Society of Cardiology. *Eur Heart J.* 2001;22(16):1374–1450.

Priori SG, Napolitano C, Memmi M, et al. Clinical and molecular characterization of patients with catecholaminergic polymorphic ventricular tachycardia. *Circulation.* 2002;106(1):69–74.

Priori SG, Napolitano C, Schwartz PJ. Low penetrance in the long-QT syndrome: clinical impact. *Circulation.* 1999;99(4):529–533.

Priori SG, Napolitano C, Schwartz PJ, et al. Association of long QT syndrome loci and cardiac events among patients treated with beta-blockers. *J Am Med Assoc.* 2004;292(11):1341–1344.

Priori SG, Napolitano C, Tiso N, et al. Mutations in the cardiac ryanodine receptor gene (hRyR2) underlie catecholaminergic polymorphic ventricular tachycardia. *Circulation.* 2001;103(2):196–200.

Priori SG, Schwartz PJ, Napolitano C, et al. A recessive variant of the Romano-Ward long-QT syndrome? *Circulation.* 1998;97(24):2420–2425.

Priori SG, Schwartz PJ, Napolitano C, et al. Risk stratification in the long-QT syndrome. *N Engl J Med.* 2003;348(19):1866–1874.

Reichenbach H, Meister EM, Theile H. The heart-hand syndrome. A new variant of disorders of heart conduction and syndactylia including osseous changes in hands and feet. *Kinderarztl Prax.* 1992;60(2):54–56.

Reid DS, Tynan M, Braidwood L, et al. Bidirectional tachycardia in a child. A study using His bundle electrography. *Br Heart J.* 1975;37(3):339–344.

Romano C, Gemme G, Pongiglione R. Aritmie cardiache rare dell'eta' pediatrica. *Clin Pediatr.* 1963;45:656–683.

Rossenbacker T, Mubagwa K, Jongbloed RJ, et al. Novel mutation in the Per-Arnt-Sim domain of KCNH2 causes a malignant form of long-QT syndrome. *Circulation.* 2005a;111(8):961–968.

Rossenbacker T, Priori SG. Clinical diagnosis of long QT syndrome: back to the caliper. *Eur Heart J.* 2007;28(5):527–528.

Rossenbacker T, Priori SG, Zipes D. The fight against sudden cardiac death: consensus guidelines as a reference. *Eur Heart J.* 2007; In press.

Rossenbacker T, Schollen E, Kuiperi C, et al. Unconventional intronic splice site mutation in SCN5A associates with cardiac sodium channelopathy. *J Med Genet.* 2005b;42(5):e29.

Sansone Sansone V, Griggs RC, Meola G, et al. Andersen's syndrome: a distinct periodic paralysis. *Ann Neurol.* 1997;42(3):305–312.

Schott JJ, Charpentier F, Peltier S, et al. Mapping of a gene for long QT syndrome to chromosome 4q25–27. *Am J Hum Genet.* 1995; 57(5):1114–1122.

Schulze-Bahr E, Wang Q, Wedekind H, et al. KCNE1 mutations cause Jervell and Lange-Nielsen syndrome. *Nat Genet.* 1997;17(3):267–268.

Schwartz PJ. Idiopathic long QT syndrome: progress and questions. *Am Heart J.* 1985;109(2):399–411.

Schwartz PJ, Moss AJ, Vincent GM, et al. Diagnostic criteria for the long QT syndrome. An update. *Circulation.* 1993;88(2):782–784.

Schwartz PJ, Priori SG, Bloise R, et al. Molecular diagnosis in a child with sudden infant death syndrome. *Lancet.* 2001b;358(9290):1342–1343.

Schwartz PJ, Priori SG, Dumaine R, et al. A molecular link between the sudden infant death syndrome and the long- QT syndrome. *N Engl J Med.* 2000b;343(4):262–267.

Schwartz PJ, Priori SG, Locati EH, et al. Long QT syndrome patients with mutations of the SCN5A and HERG genes have differential responses to Na+ channel blockade and to increases in heart rate. Implications for gene-specific therapy. *Circulation.* 1995;92(12):3381–3386.

Schwartz PJ, Priori SG, Napolitano C. The long QT syndrome. In Zipes DP, Jalife J. *Cardiac Electrophysiology.* W.B. Saunders, Philadelphia, USA; 2000a.

Schwartz PJ, Priori SG, Napolitano C. How really rare are rare diseases?: the intriguing case of independent compound mutations in the long QT syndrome. *J Cardiovasc Electrophysiol.* 2003;14(10):1120–1121.

Schwartz PJ, Priori SG, Spazzolini C, et al. Genotype-phenotype correlation in the long-QT syndrome: gene-specific triggers for life-threatening arrhythmias. *Circulation.* 2001a;103(1):89–95.

Schwartz PJ, Spazzolini C, Crotti L, et al. The Jervell and Lange-Nielsen syndrome: natural history, molecular basis, and clinical outcome. *Circulation.* 2006;113(6):783–790.

Schwartz PJ, Stramba-Badiale M, Segantini A, et al. Prolongation of the QT interval and the sudden infant death syndrome. *N Engl J Med.* 1998;338(24):1709–1714.

Seth R, Moss AJ, McNitt S, et al. Long QT syndrome and pregnancy. *J Am Coll Cardiol.* 2007;49(10):1092–1098.

Sherman J, Tester DJ, Ackerman MJ. Targeted mutational analysis of ankyrin-B in 541 consecutive, unrelated patients referred for long QT syndrome genetic testing and 200 healthy subjects. *Heart Rhythm.* 2005;2(11):1218–1223.

Splawski I, Timothy KW, Decher N, et al. Severe arrhythmia disorder caused by cardiac L-type calcium channel mutations. *Proc Natl Acad Sci USA.* 2005;102(23):8089–8096; discussion 8086–8088.

Splawski I, Timothy KW, Sharpe LM, et al. Ca(V)1.2 calcium channel dysfunction causes a multisystem disorder including arrhythmia and autism. *Cell.* 2004;119(1):19–31.

Splawski I, Timothy KW, Vincent GM, et al. Molecular basis of the long-QT syndrome associated with deafness. *N Engl J Med.* 1997b;336(22):1562–1567.

Splawski I, Tristani-Firouzi M, Lehmann MH, et al. Mutations in the hminK gene cause long QT syndrome and suppress IKs function. *Nat Genet.* 1997a;17(3):338–340.

Swan H, Piippo K, Viitasalo M, et al. Arrhythmic disorder mapped to chromosome 1q42-q43 causes malignant polymorphic ventricular tachycardia in structurally normal hearts. *J Am Coll Cardiol.* 1999a;34(7):2035–2042.

Swan H, Viitasalo M, Piippo K, et al. Sinus node function and ventricular repolarization during exercise stress test in long QT syndrome patients with KvLQT1 and HERG potassium channel defects. *J Am Coll Cardiol.* 1999b;34(3):823–829.

Tan HL, Bardai A, Shimizu W, et al. Genotype-specific onset of arrhythmias in congenital long-QT syndrome: possible therapy implications. *Circulation.* 2006;114(20):2096–2103.

Tester DJ, Ackerman MJ. Sudden infant death syndrome: how significant are the cardiac channelopathies? *Cardiovasc Res.* 2005;67(3):388–396.

Tester DJ, Ackerman MJ. Postmortem long QT syndrome genetic testing for sudden unexplained death in the young. *J Am Coll Cardiol.* 2007;49(2):240–246.

Tester DJ, Arya P, Will M, et al. Genotypic heterogeneity and phenotypic mimicry among unrelated patients referred for catecholaminergic polymorphic ventricular tachycardia genetic testing. *Heart Rhythm.* 2006;3(7):800–805.

Tester DJ, Dura M, Carturan E, et al. A mechanism for sudden infant death syndrome (SIDS): stress-induced leak via ryanodine receptors. *Heart Rhythm.* 2007;4(6):733–739.

Tester DJ, Will ML, Haglund CM, et al. Compendium of cardiac channel mutations in 541 consecutive unrelated patients referred for long QT syndrome genetic testing. *Heart Rhythm.* 2005;2(5):507–517.

Tristani-Firouzi M, Jensen JL, Donaldson MR, et al. Functional and clinical characterization of KCNJ2 mutations associated with LQT7 (Andersen syndrome). *J Clin Invest.* 2002;110(3):381–388.

Vatta M, Ackerman MJ, Ye B, et al. Mutant caveolin-3 induces persistent late sodium current and is associated with long-QT syndrome. *Circulation.* 2006;114(20):2104–2112.

Viskin S. Long QT syndromes and torsade de pointes. *Lancet.* 1999;354(9190):1625–1633.

Viskin S, Rosovski U, Sands AJ, et al. Inaccurate electrocardiographic interpretation of long QT: the majority of physicians cannot recognize a long QT when they see one. *Heart Rhythm.* 2005;2(6):569–574.

Wang Q, Curran ME, Splawski I, et al. Positional cloning of a novel potassium channel gene: KVLQT1 mutations cause cardiac arrhythmias. *Nat Genet.* 1996;12(1):17–23.

Wang Q, Shen J, Splawski I, et al. SCN5A mutations associated with an inherited cardiac arrhythmia, long QT syndrome. *Cell.* 1995;80(5):805–811.

Wang Z, Li H, Moss AJ, et al. Compound heterozygous mutations in KvLQT1 cause Jervell and Lange-Nielsen syndrome. *Mol Genet Metab.* 2002;75(4):308–316.

Ward O. A new familial cardiac syndrome in children. *J Iri Med Assoc.* 1964;54:103–106.

Westenskow P, Splawski I, Timothy KW, et al. Compound mutations: a common cause of severe long-QT syndrome. *Circulation.* 2004;109(15):1834–1841.

Zareba W, Moss AJ, le Cessie S, et al. Risk of cardiac events in family members of patients with long QT syndrome. *J Am Coll Cardiol.* 1995;26(7):1685–1691.

Zhang L, Benson DW, Tristani-Firouzi M, et al. Electrocardiographic features in Andersen-Tawil syndrome patients with KCNJ2 mutations: characteristic T-U-wave patterns predict the KCNJ2 genotype. *Circulation.* 2005;111(21):2720–2726.

Zhang L, Timothy KW, Vincent GM, et al. Spectrum of ST-T-wave patterns and repolarization parameters in congenital long-QT syndrome: ECG findings identify genotypes. *Circulation.* 2000;102(23):2849–2855.

Zhang L, Vincent GM, Baralle M, et al. An intronic mutation causes long QT syndrome. *J Am Coll Cardiol.* 2004;44(6):1283–1291.

Zipes DP, Camm AJ, Borggrefe M, et al. ACC/AHA/ESC 2006 Guidelines for Management of Patients With Ventricular Arrhythmias and the Prevention of Sudden Cardiac Death: a report of the American College of Cardiology/American Heart Association Task Force and the European Society of Cardiology Committee for Practice Guidelines (writing committee to develop Guidelines for Management of Patients With Ventricular Arrhythmias and the Prevention of Sudden Cardiac Death): developed in collaboration with the European Heart Rhythm Association and the Heart Rhythm Society. *Circulation.* 2006;114(10):e385–e484.

18

Acquired Repolarization Disorders

Elijah R Behr and John Camm

Introduction

There are four subgroups of congenital disorders of cardiac repolarization that have been described: the long and short QT syndromes, the Brugada syndrome, and catecholaminergic polymorphic ventricular tachycardia (Antzelevitch 2007). These conditions have been described in Chapters 17 and 19. The long QT syndrome (LQTS), and to a much lesser extent, the Brugada syndrome, have also been described in acquired forms, where the clinical features appear to have been precipitated by other factors, frequently medications, a phenomenon known as proarrhythmia (Ben-David et al. 1993). It has become evident, however, that there may be an underlying genetic predisposition to the development of proarrhythmia, particularly in the acquired long QT syndrome. This chapter will briefly describe the genetics of the congenital conditions, the clinical features of the acquired forms, and the relationship of genotype to the acquired phenotype, as it is currently understood. Future developments and the potential role for pharmacogenomics will be discussed.

The Acquired Long QT Syndrome

The Congenital Disorder

The LQTS is a cardiac disorder defined principally by the presence of abnormal prolongation of ventricular repolarization, which may manifest itself on the surface electrocardiogram (ECG) as QT interval prolongation and T-wave abnormalities. It may be associated with ventricular arrhythmias, specifically polymorphic ventricular tachycardia [Torsades de Pointes (TdP)] and ventricular fibrillation, causing syncope and/or sudden death (see Chapter 17). Its congenital form (Box 18–1) is associated with normal cardiac structure and function and was historically described in its autosomal dominant form as the Romano-Ward syndrome (Romano et al. 1963; Ward 1964), and in its more severe and autosomal recessive form with sensorineural deafness as the Jervell and Lang-Nielsen syndrome (Jervell et al. 1957). Its genetic basis has become more thoroughly understood over the past 15 years with the identification of disease-associated mutations in ten different genes linked to cardiac myocyte repolarization (Table 18–1).

> **Box 18–1**
>
> - Congenital LQTS has incomplete penetrance and is often clinically silent: the forme fruste.
> - The "repolarization reserve" is the result of the multiple inward and outward myocyte currents that influence repolarization and has an effective physiological redundancy of capacity.
> - The forme fruste represents a concealed reduction of repolarization reserve. When exposed to further insults to repolarization, the chance of developing acquired LQTS increases.

Overall these lead either to a net reduction or "loss of function" of outward potassium-rectifying currents or a net increase or "gain of function" in the inward sodium or calcium currents.

Both the Romano-Ward and Jervell and Lange-Nielsen syndromes have been linked to the potassium ion channel α and β subunits responsible for the slow rectifying current, IKs [respectively *KCNQ1* (Wang et al. 1996; Splawski et al. 1997a) and *KCNE1* (Splawski et al. 1997b; Schulze-Bahr et al. 1997b)]. In Jervell and Lang-Nielsen syndrome, homozygous or compound mutations occur in either gene (Schwartz et al. 2006). Romano-Ward has been associated with the potassium ion channel α and β subunits responsible for the rapid rectifying current, IKr [respectively *KCNH2/HERG* (Curran et al. 1995) and *KCNE2/MirP1* (Abbott et al. 1999)] and the sodium channel α and β subunits responsible for the inward sodium current [respectively *SCN5A* (Bennett et al. 1995; Wang et al. 1995) and *SCN4B* (Medeiros-Domingo et al. 2007)]. Mutations of the first five genes (excluding *SCN4B*) account for up to 70% of unrelated definite LQTS probands undergoing genetic testing, with *KCNQ1*- and *KCNH2*-associated LQTS (LQT1 and LQT2 respectively) accounting for approximately 40%–45% of genotyped patients each and *SCN5A*-associated disease (LQT3) being linked in 8%–15% (Splawski et al. 2000; Tester et al. 2005). Andersen (LQT7) and Timothy (LQT8) syndromes are both rare variants of LQTS associated with congenital multisystem disease. Andersen syndrome patients can present with dysmorphic features and hypokalemic periodic paralysis and the condition has been linked to mutations in *KCNJ2* encoding the inward rectifying potassium current, KIr2.1 (Plaster et al. 2001).

Table 18–1 The Congenital Long QT Syndrome: Subtypes, Their Genetic Basis, and Frequencies

Subtype	Chromosome	Gene	Product	Frequency in Overall Population
LQT1	11	*KCNQ1*	IKs α subunit	~30%
LQT2	7	*KCNH2*	IKr α subunit	~30%
LQT3	3	*SCN5A*	INa α subunit	~5%
LQT4	4	*ANKB*	Submembrane component	~2%
LQT5	21	*KNCE1*	IKs β subunit	~2%
LQT6	21	*KCNE2*	IKr β subunit	~2%
LQT7 (Andersen's)	23	*KCNJ2*	IK1	—
LQT8 (Timothy)	12	*CACNA1c*	Ca(V)1.2	—
LQT9	7	*CAV3*	Caveola component	~2%
LQT10	11	*SCN4B*	INa β subunit	—

Notes: Iks, slow rectifying current; Ikr, rapid rectifying current; Ina, inward sodium current; IK1, KIr 2.1 inward rectifying current; Ca(V)1.2, L-type calcium channel current.
Sources: Splawski et al. (2000), Tester et al. (2005), and Hofman et al. (2007).

Table 18–2 Risk Factors Associated with Acquired LQTS

Gender	Female
Electrolyte abnormalities	Hypokalemia, hypomagnesemia, hypocalcemia
Drugs	See Table 18–3 plus: Diuretic use, rapid intravenous infusion High drug concentrations (except quinidine) CYP2D6 and CYP3A inhibitors (grapefruit juice)
Cardiac disease	Bradycardia: sinus node disease, AV block Ischemic heart disease, cardiomyopathy Myocardial hypertrophy, myocarditis, valvular disease Shortly after conversion of atrial fibrillation.
Cerebrovascular disease	Intracranial hemorrhage, subarachnoid hemorrhage, stroke
Systemic conditions	Liver disease, renal disease, hypothyroidism, diabetes, obesity, anorexia nervosa
Genetic factors	Forme fruste and unrecognized congenital LQTS CYP3A and CYP2D6 slow metabolizer status LQTS gene polymorphism carriers

Sources: Makkar et al. (1993), Houltz et al. (1998), Yap et al. (1999), and Roden (2006).

Timothy syndrome can present with a severe form of LQTS, syndactyly, congenital heart disease, dysmorphic features, and developmental delay and has been associated with mutations of the Ca(V)1.2 calcium channel gene, *CACNA1c* (Splawski et al. 2004).

Mutations in Ankyrin B (ANKB) a submembrane protein that provides organizational support to membrane components including ion channels and pumps have been associated with LQTS in one pedigree (LQT4) (Mohler et al. 2003) as well as other arrhythmia syndromes less characteristic of LQTS (Mohler et al. 2004). Its frequency is difficult to assess due to the presence of single nucleotide polymorphisms (SNPs) in the general population but may be around 2% of the genotyped population (Sherman et al. 2005). A component of cardiac myocyte membrane caveolae, caveolin 3 (*CAV3*) (LQT10), has recently been demonstrated to associate with *SCN5A*, probably playing a regulatory role in sodium channel function such that nonconservative missense mutations have been identified in around 2% of LQTS patients causing a similar electrophysiological defect to *SCN5A*-linked LQT3 (Vatta et al. 2006).

Incomplete Penetrance and the Concept of "the Repolarization Reserve"

Long QT mutations vary dramatically in their effect and penetrance; indeed, individuals carrying mutations but with normal ECGs and phenotype have been identified: the "forme fruste" (Donger et al. 1997; Napolitano et al. 1997; Schulze-Bahr et al. 1997a; Priori et al. 1999). In fact, up to 80% of genetically proven LQTS fails to satisfy the criteria for "definite" LQTS proposed by Schwartz and Moss (Schwartz et al. 1993; Hofman et al. 2007) and penetrance can be as low as 25% (Priori et al. 1999). In addition, 5%–8% of successfully genotyped index cases carry more than one mutation, the digenic or compound state being associated with more severe disease and overt presentation than single mutation carriers (Schwartz et al. 2003; Westenskow et al. 2004). In around half the cases studied by Westenskow et al., the additional allele was identified as the nonsynonymous single nucleotide polymorphism (SNP) KCNE1-D85N. This exhibited cardiac electrophysiological manifestations of mild IKs loss-of-function and was prevalent in approximately 5% of the control and long QT samples in this study. It is therefore likely that there are many asymptomatic heterozygotes with relatively normal ECGs who carry single mutations or nonsynonymous SNPs that have only mild electrophysiological effects upon the individual.

The principle of multiple hits deleteriously affecting the ability of the myocardium to repolarize, eventually revealing the LQTS phenotype, had been conceptualized by Roden previously as a reduction of the repolarization reserve (Roden 1998). The repolarization reserve is the result of the multiple inward and outward myocyte currents that influence repolarization and has an effective physiological redundancy of capacity. This redundancy may already be impaired in the forme fruste individuals described above. The more severe, and the greater the number of additional lesions affecting repolarization, the greater the chance of further reduction of the repolarization reserve and phenotypic expression of LQTS. It has also been proposed that acquired lesions may have a role in causing such a reduction: acquired LQTS (Roden 1998).

The Acquired Disorder

The acquired LQTS is an uncommon condition that can occur in an unpredictable or idiosyncratic fashion despite the appreciation of acknowledged risk factors (Box 18–2). An individual's risk is increased by the presence of any combination of these potential predisposing factors (Table 18–2): female gender, certain drugs (Table 18–3), structural cardiac disease, metabolic abnormalities (hypokalemia, hypomagnesemia, and hypocalcemia), ECG abnormalities (bradycardia, conduction disease, and unrecognized congenital LQTS), and specific conditions (liver disease, diabetes mellitus, obesity, and anorexia nervosa) (Yap et al. 1999). In fact bradycardia and pauses appear acutely to be an important feature for the initiation of TdP in the acquired LQTS: the pause-dependent mechanism (Jackman et al. 1988; Figures 18–1 and 18–2).

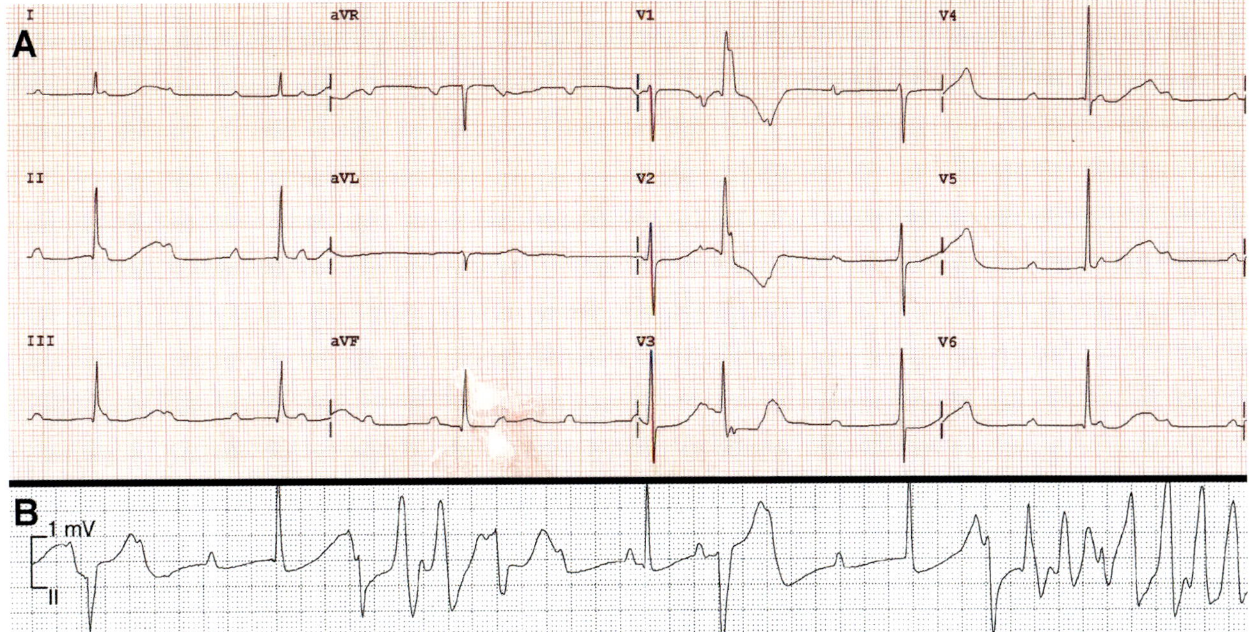

Figure 18–1 An example of acquired LQTS secondary to complete heart block: (A) 12-lead ECG demonstrating complete heart block, marked bradycardia, and QT prolongation with a late coupled ventricular ectopic generating a spontaneous beat with more severe QT and T-wave abnormality. (B) The same patient's rhythm strip is also shown demonstrating complete heart block with late-coupled ventricular ectopy, salvo, and TdP. The mechanism of initiation is known as pause-dependent initiation with a long-short-long pattern of spontaneous rhythm and ectopy resulting in exacerbation of repolarization.

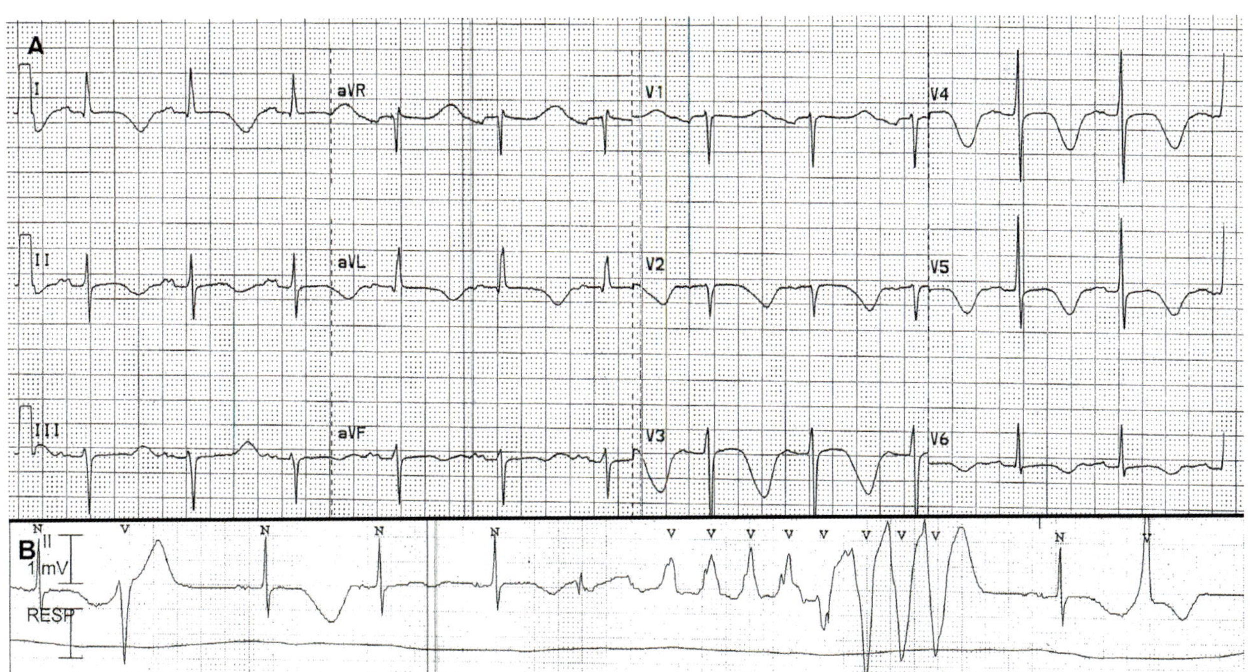

Figure 18–2 An example of acquired LQTS secondary to amiodarone in a patient with preexisting left ventricular hypertrophy secondary to hypertension: (A) 12-lead ECG demonstrating sinus rhythm with severe QT prolongation and widespread deep T-wave inversion. (B) A rhythm strip from the same patient showing typical long-short-long pattern resulting in deterioration in repolarization and eventually a short run of TdP.

Box 18–2

- The main cause of acquired LQTS is exposure to certain drugs.
- Over 100 medications have been described as causing acquired LQTS.
- It is an important public health issue for the medical profession, regulatory authorities, and the pharmaceutical industry.
- Recent research has focused on the understanding and prediction of risk in individuals and improving new drug design and development.
- A genetic and pharmacogenomic approach to risk evaluation has been taken.

Drug-Induced Long QT Syndrome

Acquired LQTS has been most commonly associated with exposure to certain over-the-counter and prescription drugs, both cardiac and noncardiac (Table 18–3). Its true incidence is unclear and varies depending on the markers, drugs, and populations being studied. The incidence of TdP in patients with cardiac disease receiving antiarrhythmics may be as high as 4%–5% (Soyka et al. 1990; Torp-Pedersen et al. 1999) while noncardiac drugs have been examined for their associated increase in risk of sudden unexplained death with dramatically lower event rates (Reilly et al. 2002; Ray et al. 2004). However low the true incidence of drug-induced TdP may be, it is clear that large numbers of patients are prescribed potential proarrhythmic agents, with an estimate of up to 3% of all prescriptions worldwide (De Ponti et al. 2000). The absolute numbers of individuals at potential risk are therefore significant.

The proarrhythmic drugs listed in Table 18–3 have been reported as associated with the acquired LQTS either alone, in combinations or, most commonly, in conjunction with the aforementioned predisposing factors. Over 100 medications have been described as prolonging the QT interval, although only a proportion has been associated with the development of TdP and may be described as torsadogenic (Brugada et al. 1988; Haverkamp et al. 2000; Figure 18–2). These are highlighted in the first column of Table 18–3. Some have been withdrawn or suspended due to the associated risk of sudden death: for example, terfenadine (Triludan) and cisapride (Prepulsid), prescribed for symptomatic but nonlife-threatening conditions (hayfever and gastroesophageal reflux, respectively). Unfortunately, there are torsadogenic drugs that are essential to medical practice and cannot be withdrawn: for example, halofantrine for drug-resistant malaria; macrolide antibiotics for penicillin-sensitive individuals; and neuroleptics for the treatment of psychotic illnesses (Figure 18–3).

The phenomenon of proarrhythmia has therefore become an important public health issue for the medical profession, regulatory authorities, and the pharmaceutical industry, in relation to existing torsadogenic agents and new drug development (De Ponti et al. 2000; Haverkamp et al. 2000; Yap et al. 2000). Most recent research has therefore focused on the understanding and prediction of risk in individuals and improving new drug design and development. With enhanced knowledge of congenital LQTS, a genetic and pharmacogenomic approach has been taken to investigate the predisposing risks that may underlie the acquired form (Roden 2006).

Pharmacokinetics and Pharmacodynamics of Drug-Induced Arrhythmia: Genetic Predisposition

In vitro functional studies using patch clamp technology have studied the exposure of wild-type HERG ion channels to known proarrhythmic agents such as cisapride, amitriptyline, and erythromycin and have demonstrated a loss of function in IKr (Antzelevitch et al. 1996; Rampe et al. 1997; Dumaine et al. 1998; Zhou et al. 1999; Jo et al. 2000; Kang et al. 2000). In fact it appears that virtually all nonantiarrhythmic torsadogens cause proarrhythmia by the direct blockade of HERG/IKr channels (Box 18–3).

Box 18–3

- The HERG/IKr channel is structurally vulnerable to the binding of drugs that cause QT prolongation.
- Most torsadogens cause proarrhythmia by the direct blockade of HERG/IKr channels.
- The disruption of HERG trafficking to the myocyte membrane is a more recently described mechanism of acquired LQTS.

The HERG channel is formed by coassembly of four identical α-subunits, coded for by *KCNH2*. Each subunit contains six α helical transmembrane domains, S1 to S6, which comprise two functionally distinct regions: the voltage sensor that is sensitive to transmembrane potential (S1–S4) and the potassium ion selective pore (S5–S6). The latter region forms the potassium ion selectivity filter at the extracellular side of the channel, below which the S6 domains form a wider central cavity. The cytoplasmic interface is obstructed by the S6 helices in the channel's closed state, which "open" when the channel is activated by a change in membrane potential (Sanguinetti et al. 2006).

Sanguinetti's group used alanine-scanning mutagenesis of the *KCNH2* gene and functional assessment of drug block of the cloned HERG channels by several different torsadogenic agents to determine the structural reason for the channel's vulnerability to drug blockade. The consistent binding site of all the drugs faced the cavity of the channel and consisted of amino acids with aromatic residues that are located in the S6 domain. These are unique to the HERG channel when compared to other potassium channels and one reason for HERG's susceptibility to high affinity drug block (Mitcheson et al. 2000) (Figure 18–4). In addition, while most potassium channels have a common Proline-Valine-Proline motif in the S6 domain forming part of the pore helix, this is absent in HERG. Introduction of this motif into the channel by mutagenic methods reduces its sensitivity to IKr blockade thus demonstrating a further mechanism for HERG's vulnerability (Fernandez et al. 2004).

More recently, an additional mechanism for diminished IKr function has been described: the disruption of HERG trafficking to the myocyte membrane by pentamidine, arsenic trioxide, probucol, or fluoxetine resulting in reduced expression of the IKr channel at the cell surface (Ficker et al. 2004; Cordes et al. 2005; Rajamani et al. 2006; Guo et al. 2007). This finding explained why pentamidine only blocks IKr at highly supratherapeutic levels yet chronic treatment at therapeutic levels can result in acquired LQTS, thus disrupting HERG channel expression at the cell surface (Kuryshev et al. 2005).

Other non-IKr mechanisms have occasionally been described. The diuretic indapamide has been recognized to cause QT prolongation and TdP by blockade of the IKs current (Turgeon et al. 1994). Activation of the inward sodium current has also been described as an additional possible torsadogenic effect of the class III antiarrhythmic and IKr blocker ibutilide and an investigational positive inotropic agent DPI-201 was found to cause TdP by this mechanism (Lee et al. 1998; Kuhlkamp et al. 2003).

The impact on cardiac electrophysiology of most torsadogenic agents depends on their plasma concentration at and their affinity

Table 18–3 Drugs Associated with Acquired LQTS

Drug Group	Definitely Torsadogenic	Possible Association with Acquired LQTS	Acquired LQTS Only Likely if Associated with Overdose or Concomitant Risk Factors (Table 17–2)
Antiarrhythmics			
Class I	Quinidine*, procainamide disopyramide ajmaline*, dihydroquinidine*	Flecainide propafenone pirmenol*, cibenzoline*	Mexiletine
Class III	Amiodarone sotalol d-sotalol*, dofetilide*, azimilide*, ibutilide*, sematilide*, ersentilide*, almokalant*, nifekalant*, terikalant*, dronedarone*		
Antianginals and vasodilators	Prenylamine*, terodiline*, lidoflazine*, bepridil*	Ardenafil	
Antihypertensives	Indapamide#	Nicardipine isradipine moexipril/hydrochlorthiazide	
Antihistamines	Terfenadine*, astemizole*	Ebastine*	Diphenhydramine
Serotonin agonists and antagonists	Cisapride*, ketanserin*, dolasetron	Ondansetron, granisetron	
Antimicrobials			
Macrolides	Erythromycin, clarithromycin, spiramycin	Azithromycin, roxithromycin*, telithromycin	
Fluoroquinolones	Sparfloxacin*, moxifloxacin	Gatifloxacin*, grepafloxacin*, levofloxacin, gemifloxacin*, ofloxacin	
Antifungals			Ketoconazole fluconazole itraconazole voriconazole
Antimalarials	Chloroquine halofantrine*, pentamidine#		Quinine
Others		Foscarnet amantadine	Cotrimoxazole trimethoprim sulfa
Psychiatric			
Tricyclic antidepressants			Amitriptyline nortriptyline desipramine*, clomipramine, imipramine, trimipramine, doxepin, trazodone, protriptyline*, amoxapine*
Serotonin reuptake inhibitors			Fluoxetine#, paroxetine, venlafaxine, sertraline, zimeldine*, citalopram
Phenothiazines	Thioridazine*, chlorpromazine	Trifluoperazine, prochlorperazine, fluphenazine	
Others	Haloperidol droperidol*, sertindole	Pimozide, mesoridazine, quetiapine, risperidone ziprasidone, maprotiline, lithium	Clozapine
Anticancer	Arsenic trioxide#	Tacrolimus tamoxifen geldanamycin#*, octreotide, sunitib	
Others	Probucol#, domperidone, levomethadyl*, methadone	Vasopressin, tizanidine, alfuzosin, amantidine, felbamate*, fosphenytoin, chloral hydrate, perflutren lipid microspheres (echocardiographic contrast)	Organophosphates*, galantamine, solifenacin, clobutinol*

Notes: * = unlicensed, withdrawn or suspended in the U.K. market; # = indirect IKr blockade or other mechanism of QT prolongation.

Source: Derived from Yap et al. (1999), reports from www.qtdrugs.org up to January 2008, case reports from www.pubmed.com up to January 2008, the British National Formulary edition 54 at www.bnf.org.

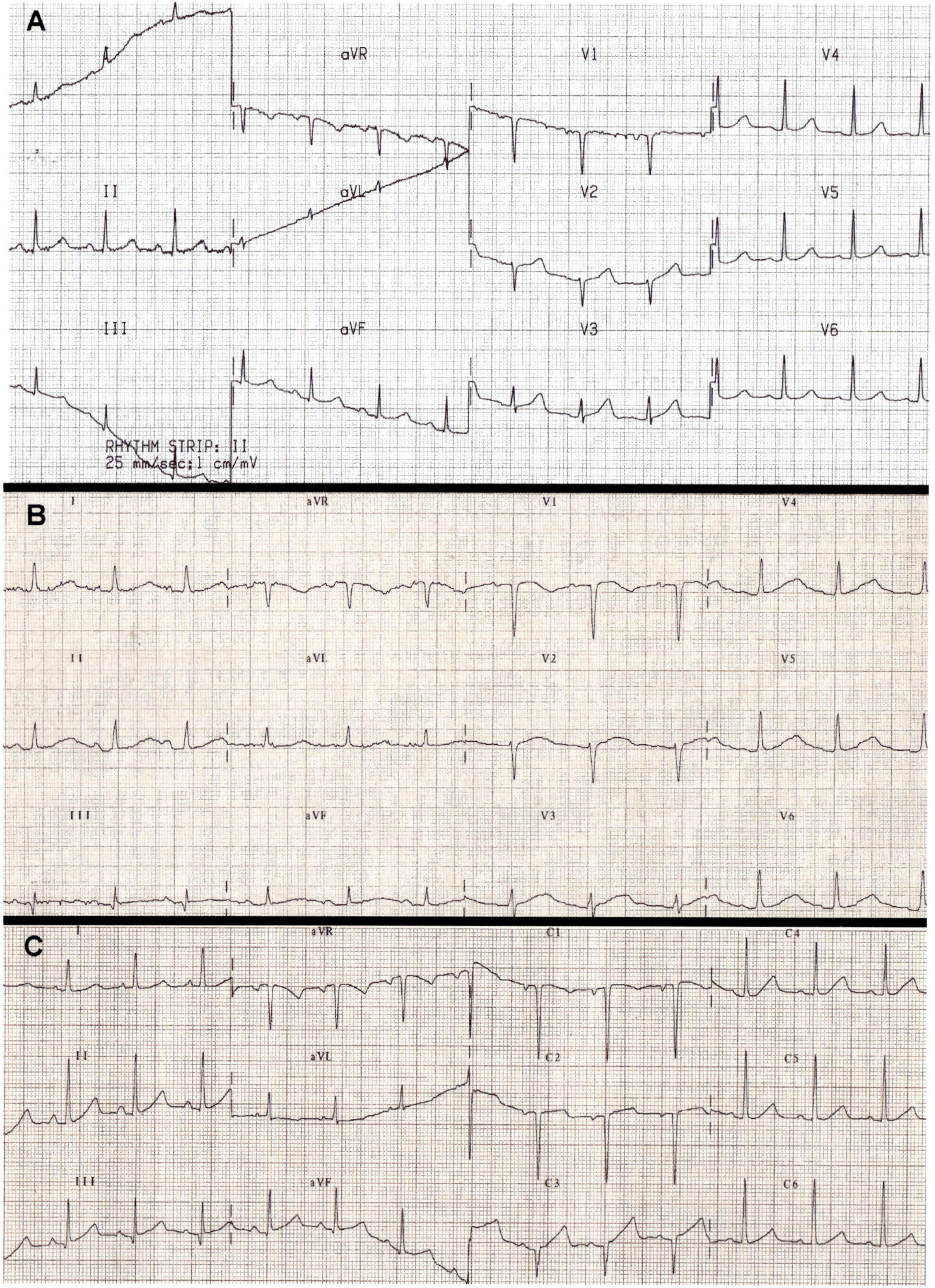

Figure 18–3 Three 12-lead ECGs from the same patient demonstrating: (a) a normal appearance in 1990 taken for incidental reasons when not on medication; (b) severe drug-induced QT prolongation and T-wave abnormalities while the patient receives thioridazine. The patient had suffered a syncopal episode and then a subsequent cardiac arrest; and (c) normalized QT prolongation and resolution of symptoms on trazodone but persistence of unusual peaked T-waves anterolaterally.

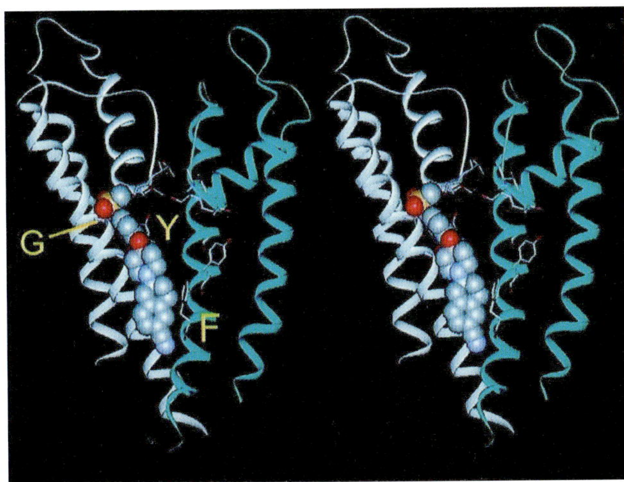

Figure 18–4 A stereoview of the S5-S6 domains of two HERG subunits with a docked molecule of MK-499 (IKr blocker) within the cavity of the homology model of the HERG K^+ channel. The aromatic residue amino acids G648, Y652, and F656 associated with the binding site are shown as stick models. Adapted from Mitcheson et al. 2000 with permission from *Proc Natl Acad Sci U S A.* published by the National Academy of Sciences.

Table 18–4 Some Common QT Prolonging Drugs Metabolized by Cytochrome P450 Enzymes and Common Inhibitors

	CYP2D6	CYP3A
Substrates	Haloperidol, thioridazine, propafenone, mexiletine	Amiodarone, disopyramide quinidine, propafenone, cisapride, erythromycin, pimozide, tamoxifen, terfenadine, astemizole, tricyclic antidepressants
Inhibitors	Amiodarone, cimetidine, quinidine, halofantrine	Amiodarone, cimetidine, clarithromycin, diltiazem, erythromycin, ketoconazole, itraconazole, verapamil, grapefruit juice

Source: Adapted from Aerssens et al. (2005).

for the HERG channel binding site and hence the potency of blockade (Yap et al. 1999). The only exception to this rule is quinidine that has been known to cause TdP at subtherapeutic concentrations (Roden et al. 1986). Drug concentration is increased either due to excess intake (overdose) and/or decreased elimination (e.g., renal and/or liver failure) (Yap et al. 1999). For many drugs this is an essential requirement for the development of acquired LQTS (see final column Table 18–3). Sometimes the delivery route of the drug is important. For example, intravenous erythromycin, given typically in intensive care and neonatal units, was found to have a much higher frequency of TdP when compared to the oral route (Tschida et al. 1996). This is thought to be due to the higher plasma levels achieved by the intravenous route.

When IKr blockers are coadministered their electrophysiological effect appears to be additive. If the additional agent interacts pharmacodynamically it may also have a synergistic effect. The presence of CYP2D6 and CYP3A cytochrome P450 enzyme inhibitors (see Table 18–4), some of which may block IKr in their own right (e.g., ketoconazole and erythromycin), decreases the metabolism of many QT-prolonging drugs and hence increases drug concentrations and the attendant risk of cardiac side effects (Zimmermann et al. 1992; Hoover et al. 1996; Michalets et al. 1998; Hayashi et al. 1999; Yap et al. 1999; Flockhart et al. 2000). Cisapride is metabolized by CYP3A and over a third of FDA reports of patients with cisapride induced TdP were found to have coadministration of CYP3A inhibitors (Aerssens et al. 2005). There is also genetic variation in the functionality of the cytochrome P450 enzymes with several known polymorphisms resulting in poor metabolizing states that are associated with higher drug concentrations and a potentially greater risk of TdP (Aerssens et al. 2005). For example, thioridazine and haloperidol are metabolized by CYP2D6. Around 10% of Caucasians carry a nonfunctional CYP2D6 polymorphism and they are the group at risk of TdP from elevated drug levels (von Bahr et al. 1991).

There are other drug properties that influence the impact of potential IKr blockers. These include any concomitant effects on other ion channels. Quinidine's ability to cause TdP at low concentrations reflects that its class I sodium channel and IKs blocking effects only occur at higher concentrations while IKr blockade occurs at much lower levels, particularly in the presence of hypokalemia (Yang et al. 1996). Other potent IKr blockers may not even cause QT prolongation due to their additional properties. Verapamil, for example, also blocks the inward calcium current, probably counteracting its IKr effects, while bepridil blocks both the inward calcium current, IKs and IKr and is torsadogenic (Chouabe et al. 2000). Amiodarone does prolong the QT interval by IKr blockade but is a relatively rare cause of TdP probably due to its concomitant sodium and calcium channel blocking effects (Mason et al. 1984).

The Impact of Gender and Hypokalemia

The female predisposition for drug-induced long QT results in up to three times more cases occurring amongst women when compared to men (Makkar et al. 1993). Women exhibit longer QT intervals than men with differing degrees of QT hysteresis that suggest a physiologically reduced repolarization reserve and increased vulnerability to proarrhythmia (Chauhan et al. 2002). While the understanding of this mechanism is incomplete in humans, studies in male and female rabbits and dogs have suggested differing mechanisms of prolongation of repolarization and risk for arrhythmias during exposure to IKr blockade: either the presence of testosterone was protective or the exposure to estrogens increased risk (Chen et al. 1999; Pham et al. 2001).

Intuitively, hypokalemia would be expected not to be deleterious to repolarization, but in fact prolongs the QT interval even causing TdP in itself (Kusano et al. 2001). It is a common finding in drug-induced LQTS, particularly with less potent torsadogenic agents (see final column of Table 18–3), and is often seen in association with diuretic usage. It is known to potentiate the effects of IKr blockade (Yang et al. 1996) and the mechanism may be due to enhanced IKr inactivation or enhanced channel block by extracellular sodium (Yang et al. 1997; Numaguchi et al. 2000).

Genetic Predisposition to Drug-Induced Long QT Syndrome: Mutations and Polymorphisms

Case reports have described individuals with drug-induced acquired LQTS who carry mutations of the genes implicated in the LQTS (Box 18–4). The carriers tended to be phenotypically normal once drug challenge was removed and therefore represented

Box 18–4

- Pharmacokinetic principles dictate the potency of IKr blocking effects of most torsadogenic drugs.
- Concomitant effects on other cardiac currents will alter the impact of IKr blockade on cardiac repolarization.
- The effect of torsadogens metabolized by cytochrome P450 enzymes may be increased by enzyme inhibitors.
- Polymorphisms of cytochrome P450 enzyme genes that cause loss of function may result in increased levels of torsadogenic agents.
- Female gender and hypokalemia are major predisposing factors for acquired LQTS.

the forme fruste end of the spectrum of incompletely penetrant LQTS with vulnerable repolarization reserve as described above. A first example was a clarithromycin induced TdP case that was heterozygous for the KCNE2-Q9E variant (Abbott et al. 1999). The HERG ion channel's sensitivity to the macrolide was actually increased by the presence of the mutated β subunit, with a greater binding affinity than for wild-type channels. It eventually became apparent, however, that Q9E is a polymorphism with a 3% allele frequency in the black population but is absent in the Caucasian population (Ackerman et al. 2003). This finding altered the potential importance of the variant significantly and serves as a cautionary note over interpretation of novel genetic results. A heterozygous carrier of the KCNH2-M124T mutation has been described as being aggravated by exposure to the cholesterol-lowering drug probucol (Hayashi et al. 2004). In both of these cases the preexisting heterozygous defect of the mutated HERG/Mirp1 IKr channel complexes therefore appears to be exacerbated by the IKr blocking/disrupting effects of the torsadogenic drug, causing a further reduction of repolarization reserve in these individuals.

Mutations in *KCNQ1* and *SCN5A* have also been identified in such cases: KCNQ1-Y315C pore mutation (Napolitano et al. 2000); KCNQ1-R555C C-terminal mutation (Donger et al. 1997); SCN5A-V1667I S5 region mutation (Piippo et al. 2001); and SCN5A-L1825P C-terminal mutation (Makita et al. 2002). As may be expected, carriers of unrecognized overt long QT syndrome mutations may also undergo acute exacerbations when exposed even to mild IKr blockers and should therefore avoid any such medications assiduously. For example, a young male carrier of KCNH2-A561P was exposed to a previously innocuous antitussive, clobutinol, and developed TdP. Patch clamping studies confirmed mild IKr blocking effects of the agent (Bellocq et al. 2004b).

In view of these case reports, larger series of patients with drug-induced TdP have also been studied for evidence of LQTS mutations (Wei et al. 1999; Sesti et al. 2000; Yang et al. 2002; Paulussen et al. 2004; Mank-Seymour et al. 2006). These findings are summarized in Table 18–5. A study of TdP secondary to dofetilide for the treatment of AF was the only series to examine the *ANKB* (LQT4) gene. It described a surprisingly high frequency of *ANKB* mutations as well as a significant overrepresentation of the common polymorphism SCN5A-H558R and a trend toward a higher proportion of KCNH2-R1047L (Mank-Seymour et al. 2006). These results were not replicated in the other studies.

Abbott et al.'s series of long QT patients, which described KCNE2-Q9E also, identified a heterozygous carrier of a mildly electrophysiologically active, or functional polymorphism, T8A, who when exposed to quinidine had developed TdP (Abbott et al. 1999). This was subsequently also described in the current largest of the series of drug-induced TdP cases after a patient was exposed to Bactrim (sulfamethoxazole and trimethoprim) (Sesti et al. 2000). Its allele frequency is 1%–2% in Caucasian populations and therefore was not overrepresented in these small numbers of TdP cases. Sesti et al. identified three other mutations of *KCNE2* as well: A116V, M54T, and I57T. The KCNE1-D85N polymorphism

Table 18–5 Numbers of Carriers of Mutations and Functional Polymorphisms with Associated Allele Frequencies Described in Three Series of Acquired Long QT Patients

Series Gene	Wei et al. 1999; Sesti et al. 2000; Yang et al. 2002	Paulussen et al. 2004	Mank-Seymour et al. 2006	Overall
KCNQ1: Mutations	1 (0.5%)	0	1 (1.5%)	2 (0.7%)
KCNE1: Polymorphism D85N	6 (3.5%) [1.1% controls]	3 (4.7%) [0 controls]	0	9 (3%)
KCNH2: Mutations Polymorphism R1047L	1 (0.5%) 0	1 (1.5%) 0	0 7.4% [2% controls p = 0.082]	2 (0.7%) 1.6%
KCNE2: Mutations Polymorphism T8A	3 (1.6%) 1 (0.5%)* [1.6% controls]	0 1 (2%) [0 controls]	0 0	3 (0.9%) 2 (1%)
SCN5A: Mutations Polymorphism H558R	3 (1.6%) 24%* [20% controls]	0 34%* [44% controls]	1 (1.5%) 37.5% [14.4% controls p = 0.004]	4 (1.3%) 29%
ANKB: Mutations	Not tested	Not tested	4 (5.8%)	4 (1.3%)
Total mutated alleles	8 (4.3%)	1 (1.5%)	6 (8.8%)	**15 (4.7%)**
Total cases	92	32	34	158

Notes: Square brackets indicate polymorphism frequencies in controls; * indicates no significant difference with polymorphism frequencies in controls. Where absolute numbers of alleles or cases are known these are included.

was found to be electrophysiologically active and associated with TdP in 7% of cases from the same series (3.5% allelic frequency) (Wei et al. 1999) and this has been subsequently confirmed in another series (Paulussen et al. 2004). It has a 2% minor allele frequency in Caucasian populations and thus was significantly overrepresented in TdP cases. Overall, it is apparent that there were low frequencies of forme fruste long QT mutations (9% of cases, 4.7% allele frequency) and there was a small but interesting group of electrophysiologically active, or functional, polymorphisms that were more frequent in different samples, only KCNE1-D85N demonstrating some consistency.

Three other studies have provided additional insights: (1) A large case-control study found the SCN5A-S1103Y polymorphism to be significantly overrepresented in black patients with apparently sporadic acquired arrhythmia (56% SS and SY) compared to a black control population where the minor allele frequency is 13% (OR 8.7 p = 0.000028). Thirty percent of these patients had drug-induced TdP and 13% had bradycardia-associated TDP (Splawski et al. 2002). (2) A Finnish study of 16 patients that only screened the four common Finnish founder mutations (KCNQ1-G589D and -IVS7–2A→G and KNCH2-L552S and -R176W) found that 3 (19%) were carriers (Lehtonen et al. 2007). (3) A polymorphism study of 7 dofetilide trial patients with TdP revealed that 2 (29%) carried the KCNH2-R1047L polymorphism compared to 5 out of 98 patients (5%) without TdP (Sun et al. 2004).

Genetic Predisposition in Other Forms of Acquired Long QT Syndrome: Complete Heart Block

In a proportion of patients with complete heart block, QT prolongation and TdP can occur and indicate a poor prognosis if unrecognized (see Figure 18–1). A French study examined a group of patients with permanent pacemakers for complete AV block and comparing those who presented with a QTc > 600 ms and TdP to those without such a phenotype. The acquired long QT group demonstrated 3/18 (17%) patients with mutations of *KCNH2* (R328C, R696C, and R1047L) that were all demonstrated to have functional effects causing IKr loss of function.

Hypokalemia

A genetic predisposition to TdP when exposed to hypokalemia without drug exposure has also been identified in a few reports. An apparently sporadic case of LQTS and TdP presented with a serum potassium of 2.6 mEq/L and a QTc of 620 ms. Genetic testing identified heterozygosity for a novel mutation, KCNQ1-R259C, causing a mild loss of function in IKs (Kubota et al. 2000). Hypokalemia, by its negative effect on HERG currents (Yang et al. 1997), had further reduced a genetically impaired repolarization reserve thus precipitating the acute deterioration. These findings have been replicated in a study of C-terminal *KCNQ1* mutations in two large families: S818L and V822M. The two probands in each pedigree presented with hypokalemia-associated TdP. Otherwise, the mutation was associated with a mild or forme fruste phenotype (Berthet et al. 1999). As with drug-induced disease, a polymorphism with low penetrance, KCNQ1-G643S, has been associated with hypokalemia- and bradycardia-induced LQTS. It has a 9% minor allele frequency in the Japanese population (Kubota et al. 2001).

Summary

Overall, many of the genetic findings in acquired LQTS appear to be specific to ethnic groups and the small populations that have been studied. While disease-causing mutations of the congenital LQTS may be more frequently detected as associated with drug-induced TdP in populations with founder gene effects their actual frequency appears low. If they are detected, however, it is reasonable to consider cascade evaluation and predictive testing in families provided they are counseled appropriately.

> **Box 18–5**
> - Mutations of the genes implicated in congenital LQTS are associated with the acquired condition in a small proportion of cases.
> - Polymorphisms of the same genes that have electrophysiologic consequences are also associated with the condition.
> - It appears likely that these variants might be of greater importance in specific ethnic populations.

There does appear, however, to be an increasing number of population-specific polymorphisms of the long QT genes that are carried by a higher proportion of the population but probably cause less severe reduction of repolarization reserve (Box 18–5). It is more reasonable to think of long QT mutations and polymorphisms not as distinct entities but as part of a spectrum of ion channel gene variants of varying electrophysiologic effects and differing frequencies depending on the population being examined. Their impact upon the repolarization reserve and subsequent interaction with environmental factors and other genes modulating repolarization and drug metabolism will determine their true significance as genetic tools for the prevention of sudden death. Currently their true clinical utility remains to be determined until studies are undertaken with larger sample sizes of different ethnicities and appropriately selected control groups.

The Brugada Syndrome

The Congenital Disorder

The Brugada syndrome is an inherited condition that is characterized by the presence of coved ST elevation and J point elevation of at least 2 mm in at least two of the right precordial ECG leads in the absence of cardiac structural disease (Brugada et al. 1992; Antzelevitch et al. 2005). It is also characterized by ventricular arrhythmias, atrial arrhythmias, syncope, and sudden death (see Chapter 19). The diagnosis in an individual requires the presence of the Brugada ECG pattern as described above (type 1) with at least one of the recognized diagnostic criteria: syncope, prior cardiac arrest, documented or inducible polymorphic ventricular tachycardia or ventricular fibrillation, a family history of sudden death <45 years old or type 1 Brugada pattern and/or nocturnal agonal respiration (Antzelevitch et al. 2005).

It has been associated with mutations in four genes: loss-of-function mutations affecting the sodium channel (*SCN5A*) also involved in LQT3 and found in approximately 20%–30% of cases (Chen et al. 1998; Antzelevitch et al. 2005); the glycerol-3-phosphate dehydrogenase 1-like (GPD1-L) gene found in one large pedigree and identified in around 1% of sudden infant death syndrome, causing reduced inward sodium currents (London et al. 2007; Van Norstrand et al. 2007); and loss-of-function mutations in *CACNA1C* and *CACNB2* encoding the α1- and β 2b-subunits of the L-type calcium channel in around 4% of consecutive probands and associated with a short QT interval (Antzelevitch et al. 2007).

As part of the diagnostic process, it is important to exclude other conditions that may mimic the Brugada ECG pattern. These include structural disease that may be hereditary (arrhythmogenic right ventricular cardiomyopathy) or acquired (e.g., acute myocardial infarction or ischemia of the right heart, pulmonary embolism, or cardiac compression) and similar ECG patterns in normal hearts (e.g., early repolarization syndrome, electrolyte imbalance, or hypothermia). They are separate clinical entities and have different pathophysiologies and prognoses (Antzelevitch et al. 2005).

The electrocardiographic marker for Brugada syndrome, the type 1 pattern, may be present continuously or intermittently. It is thought to be due to either one of two mechanisms: (1) The reduction of inward sodium current (and in some circumstances calcium current) leads to a loss of the action potential dome due to unopposed transient outward currents (Ito) in the subepicardial layer of the right ventricular outflow tract (RVOT) compared to the subendocardial layer where the dome is relatively preserved. This causes a transmural voltage gradient and phase 2 reentry, manifesting as ST elevation and T-wave inversion on the surface ECG, providing a substrate for triggered activity and reentry arrhythmia (Yan et al. 1999; Fish et al. 2004). (2) A slowing of conduction in the RVOT without a transmural voltage gradient has been demonstrated in an explanted Brugada syndrome carrier's heart. This was accompanied by localized fibrosis on histological examination (Coronel et al. 2005). Another study has confirmed the presence of subtle structural alterations on endomyocardial biopsy of the RVOT in Brugada syndrome carriers (Frustaci et al. 2005).

Whichever mechanism is accepted as a true reflection of the pathophysiology, it is clear that the ECG pattern can be dynamic and therefore intermittently present. It can also be incompletely expressed in a family. Known or suspected mutation carriers may display a normal ECG or a partial nondiagnostic Brugada pattern of a saddle-shaped ST segment with or without elevation: the type 2 and 3 ECG patterns respectively. In these cases a diagnostic challenge with a sodium channel blocker such as ajmaline, flecainide, or pilsicainide may induce the full-blown type 1 ECG pattern and support the diagnosis in a family member (Rolf et al. 2003; Antzelevitch et al. 2005).

It has become apparent subsequently that sporadic cases of the Brugada ECG pattern without a family history of the condition may be "unconcealed" by exposure to drugs with sodium channel blocking effects (Fujiki et al. 1999; Hermida et al. 2004). Theoretically, therefore, an acquired intervention that causes a sufficient imbalance of inward and outward currents in the RVOT may induce the surface ECG pattern in an individual although the likelihood of arrhythmias is unclear. Whether this requires an underlying genetic predisposition or represents latent Brugada syndrome has not been established (Box 18–6).

The Drug-Induced Brugada Syndrome

As alluded to, sporadic cases of drug-induced "acquired" Brugada ECG pattern have been described in the literature (see Table 18–6) most commonly secondary to potent sodium channel blockers such as the class I antiarrhythmics (Miyazaki et al. 1996; Fujiki et al. 1999). Other drugs with sodium channel blocking effects have also been described as causing the Brugada ECG pattern but usually only in overdose: the tricyclic and tetracyclic antidepressants, penothiazines, and selective serotonin reuptake inhibitors (Rouleau et al. 2001; Goldgran-Toledano et al. 2002; Copetti et al. 2005; Roberts-Thomson et al. 2007) as well as a recent report of phenytoin in overdose (Aloul et al. 2007).

Box 18–6

- Sporadic cases of the Brugada ECG pattern without a family history of the condition may be "unconcealed" by exposure to certain drugs.
- This is most commonly secondary to potent sodium channel blockers such as the class I antiarrhythmics.
- Other implicated sodium channel blockers include the tricyclic and tetracyclic antidepressants drugs.
- Calcium channel blockers, potassium channel openers, cocaine, and α-adrenergic agonists have also been implicated.

Table 18–6 Drugs Reported to Induce the Type 1 Brugada ECG Pattern

Antiarrhythmic drugs	
Sodium channel blockers	
Class IC drugs:	Flecainide, pilsicainide, propafenone
Class IA drugs:	Ajmaline*, procainamide, disopyramide, cibenzoline*
Calcium channel blockers	Verapamil
β-Blockers	Propranolol, atenolol, etc.
Antianginal drugs	
Calcium channel blockers	Nifedipine, diltiazem
Nitrate	Isosorbide dinitrate, nitroglycerine
Potassium channel openers	Nicorandil
Psychiatric drugs	
Tricyclic antidepressants	Amitriptyline, nortriptyline, desipramine, clomipramine
Tetracyclic antidepressants	Maprotiline
Phenothiazine	Perphenazine, cyamemazine*, thioridazine*
Selective serotonin reuptake inhibitors	Fluoxetine
Other drugs	Dimenhydrinate
	Cocaine intoxication
	Alcohol intoxication
	Bupivicaine
	α Adrenergic agonists
	Phenytoin

Source: Miyazaki et al. (1996); Antzelevitch et al. (2005); Copetti et al. (2005); Shimizu (2005); Aloul et al. (2007).

There are only limited cases of drugs causing the full-blown syndrome: the Brugada pattern in conjunction with ventricular arrhythmia (Tada et al. 2001; Goldgran-Toledano et al. 2002; Chow et al. 2005). One individual on therapeutic doses of desipramine developed new onset Brugada pattern with episodes of ventricular fibrillation, all of which resolved off the drug. He was found to be a heterozygous carrier for the common SCN5A-H558R polymorphism although its exact relationship to the development of the type 1 Brugada pattern is unclear (Chow et al. 2005). A series of 98 cases of cyclic antidepressant overdoses was reported in the *New England Journal* (Goldgran-Toledano et al. 2002). Twelve (12.3%) were associated with a type 1 ECG pattern. Three of these cases were in the same woman who presented three times with reproducible ECG changes giving an actual case frequency of 10/95 (10.5%). One of the patients presenting with the Brugada ECG died from recurrent ventricular fibrillation compared to one death in those without the Brugada ECG. While statistical significance was not demonstrated this did suggest a possible poor prognosis. In another retrospective French study of 65 cases, however, 15% demonstrated the type 1 ECG pattern but without any arrhythmia. The drugs involved were predominantly amitriptyline (66%) and clomipramine (29%) (Brahmi et al. 2007). Another larger series of around 400 cases of tricyclic overdoses found that only 2.3% developed the type 1 Brugada ECG pattern, again without any attendant increased risk of arrhythmia. Nortriptyline (4/52) and imipramine (3/49) appeared to be more effective than amitriptyline (0/177) in inducing the ECG pattern (Bebarta et al. 2007). The apparent discrepancy in these studies might relate to the differing binding affinities of the drugs involved for the sodium channel as well as different amounts of drug-ingested plasma concentrations and concomitant sodium channel blocking agents such as neuroleptics (Rouleau et al. 2001).

Reports of the neuroleptics causing the Brugada pattern are less common. Rouleau et al. described type 1 Brugada ECG patterns associated with a neuroleptic and tricyclic (cyamemazine and amitriptyline) overdose as well as a fluoxetine overdose. In addition, an individual taking therapeutic doses of trifluoperazine and loxapine presented with resuscitated sudden death associated with a type 1 ECG, which slowly resolved off medication. An electrophysiological study induced polymorphic ventricular tachycardia and an ICD was implanted. It is possible that this man represented a forme fruste case but genetic evaluation did not take place and there was no family history of note. Interestingly, flecainide challenge of the first two individuals failed to reinduce the type 1 ECG. Either the potency of sodium channel blockade was insufficient compared to the potency of the medications involved at supratherapeutic levels or additional mechanisms were at work (Rouleau et al. 2001).

β-blockers, nitrates, and verapamil have been described as exposing the Brugada ECG pattern by blockade of L-type calcium channels and reduction of the inward calcium current. Nicorandil has also been associated with induction of the pattern and this is probably due to augmentation of outward potassium currents (Shimizu 2005). Recreational cocaine usage is known to have induced Brugada syndrome acutely (Littmann et al. 2000). Although the mechanism is unclear it may involve sodium channel blockade or α-adrenergic receptor agonist actions. The individual described by Littmann et al. underwent a class I challenge that failed to induce the type I ECG, suggesting that the α-adrenergic action might be more important, at least in this case.

Electrophysiological and autonomic study of a small group of patients with Brugada syndrome has demonstrated an exacerbation of ST elevation after α-adrenergic stimulation with noradrenaline and methoxamine and cholinergic stimulation with edrophonium or intracoronary acetylcholine. Conversely, the pattern is ameliorated by β-adrenergic receptor stimulation with ispoprenaline and α antagonism with phentolamine and prazosin (Miyazaki et al. 1996). Hence autonomic modulation by drugs might induce the ECG pattern in latent cases of the Brugada syndrome, the common pathway probably being alteration of inward calcium currents.

Summary: What Does This Mean Currently?

The true significance of drug-induced Brugada is unclear. There has been little systematic study of such sporadic cases and the possibility of an underlying genetic predisposition has not been addressed as thoroughly as it has in acquired LQTS. This is probably due to the relative rarity of drug-induced Brugada compared to drug-induced long QT and the less complete understanding of the genetics and pathophysiology of the Brugada syndrome. Genetic testing has therefore featured little in these case reports.

There has, however, been one systematic study to determine the significance of the "acquired Brugada pattern." Hermida et al. studied 1,000 individuals who had occupational ECGs and detected a single spontaneous type 1 ECG and 5 ajmaline-induced type 1 ECGs (prevalence 0.5%). None of these individuals had *SCN5A* mutations or polymorphisms and all were asymptomatic without a family history.

The importance of acquired Brugada syndrome, its prognosis, and its relevance to the familial condition remains to be determined but it is reasonable to utilize existing risk stratification algorithms to guide management until more is understood about the condition (Box 18–7). Provided a normal resting ECG off drug is present and the patient is asymptomatic, the prognosis appears to be good once the provoking agent has been removed (Antzelevitch et al. 2005). One report does strike a cautionary note, however. It described a man with bipolar disorder who presented with the Brugada pattern and T-wave alternans secondary to amitriptyline overdose. His ECG normalized off drug but he unfortunately died suddenly before his investigations could be completed as they were delayed until his psychiatric state had improved (Roberts-Thomson et al. 2007).

The Short QT Syndrome

The short QT syndrome is a rare counterpart condition to the LQTS and, as its name suggests, its diagnosis depends on the presence of an inappropriately shortened QT interval. It is associated with ventricular arrhythmias and sudden death as well as a structurally normal heart (Gussak et al. 2000). It was found to

Box 18–7

- The frequency of ventricular arrhythmia appears low.
- Whether the drug-induced pattern indicates the presence of forme fruste Brugada syndrome is unknown.
- The true clinical significance is unclear at present.

be a familial condition (Gaita et al. 2003) and subsequently gain-of-function mutations have been described in *KCNQ1*, *KCNH2*, and *KCNJ2* (Brugada et al. 2004; Bellocq et al. 2004a; Hong et al. 2005; Priori et al. 2005). A crossover phenotype with Brugada syndrome has recently been described with loss-of-function mutations in *CACNA1C* and *CACNB2* (Antzelevitch et al. 2007). Arbitrary diagnostic QT interval cut-offs were set at <300 ms initially but as research has continued and the variable penetrance of the condition appreciated, upper limit QT values of 320–360 ms have been used (Gussak et al. 2002). It is apparent that there is substantial overlap with the normal end of the spectrum and the possibility of forme fruste disease that may place the individual at risk of acquired sudden death exists. Currently there have been no case reports of drug-induced arrhythmias but there are drugs in development that have been shown to shorten QT interval.

Conclusions

Genetic studies of the acquired LQTS support the view that while the risk attributable to mutations might be a small proportion of the total, there may be a much greater role played by functional polymorphisms in the genes implicated in the LQTS and other arrhythmia syndromes as well as hepatic drug metabolism. The search for other potential candidate genes has been cast wide utilizing novel methods for gene identification as well as high throughput and in silico technology. For example, using an in vivo worm-screening model (*Caenorhabditis elegans*), a polymorphism was identified in a HERG interacting protein, KCR1, which was of lower frequency in drug-induced TdP cases when compared to controls and hence might be a protective polymorphism (Petersen et al. 2004). In addition, a genome-wide association study has examined population QT interval variability and determined that specific variants of NOS1AP, a regulator of neuronal nitric oxidase, were associated with longer QT intervals (Arking et al. 2006). Provided these and similar findings can be explained in a biologically plausible way and proven experimentally, then unexpected targets beyond "arrhythmia" gene polymorphisms may be exposed.

Unfortunately many genome-wide association studies are fraught with difficulties due to the huge number of polymorphisms involved and the potential for throwing up false-positive results. Polymorphism haplotype studies may help to reduce the complexities of association studies due to the high linkage disequilibria seen with large haplotype blocks (Roden et al. 2005). In fact, recent data has linked haplotype blocks in the *SCN5A* promoter region and *KCNH2*, *KCNQ1*, and *KCNE1* to variation in cardiac conduction (QRS interval) and repolarization (QT interval) respectively (Pfeufer et al. 2005; Bezzina et al. 2006). International groups are now collecting larger groups of DNA samples from drug-induced TdP cases to undergo genome-wide study to identify novel candidate genes [the DARE study (www.dsru.org/gp_physician.html) and the Fondation leDucq Network (www.allianceagainstscd.org)]. A more selective approach is also being taken in order to assess more thoroughly potentially significant exons of the currently appreciated genetic targets for inherited arrhythmia syndromes. The results of these endeavors in pharmacogenomics will guide the understanding of genetic predisposition for acquired arrhythmic risk and potentially allow for preventive strategies based on risk stratification and risk reduction. The impact is likely to extend beyond just drug-induced arrhythmia but to other forms of acquired risk of sudden death.

There is also much more to understand about Brugada syndrome itself before the genetics of the acquired form will be appreciated. The same methods as described above may lead to novel genetic targets for evaluation. The acquired Brugada pattern may have a limited clinical relevance but given the overlap with the LQT3 form of LQTS and the increasing appreciation of the prevalence of the congenital condition (see Chapter 19), it is hopeful that its better understanding will also impact on the predisposition for acquired sudden death.

References

Abbott GW, Sesti F, Splawski I, et al. MiRP1 forms IKr potassium channels with HERG and is associated with cardiac arrhythmia. *Cell.* 1999;97(2):175–187.

Ackerman MJ, Tester DJ, Jones GS, Will ML, Burrow CR, Curran ME. Ethnic differences in cardiac potassium channel variants: implications for genetic susceptibility to sudden cardiac death and genetic testing for congenital long QT syndrome. *Mayo Clin Proc.* 2003;78(12):1479–1487.

Aerssens J, Paulussen AD. Pharmacogenomics and acquired long QT syndrome. *Pharmacogenomics.* 2005;6(3):259–270.

Aloul BA, Adabag AS, Houghland MA, Tholakanahalli V, et al. Brugada pattern electrocardiogram associated with supratherapeutic phenytoin levels and the risk of sudden death. *Pacing Clin Electrophysiol.* 2007;30(5):713–715.

Antzelevitch C. Role of spatial dispersion of repolarization in inherited and acquired sudden cardiac death syndromes. *Am J Physiol Heart Circ Physiol.* 2007;293(4):H2024–H2038.

Antzelevitch C, Brugada P, Borggrefe M, et al. Brugada syndrome: report of the Second Consensus Conference: endorsed by the Heart Rhythm Society and the European Heart Rhythm Association. *Circulation.* 2005;111(5):659–670.

Antzelevitch C, Pollevick GD, Cordeiro JM, et al. Loss-of-function mutations in the cardiac calcium channel underlie a new clinical entity characterized by ST-segment elevation, short QT intervals, and sudden cardiac death. *Circulation.* 2007;115(4):442–449.

Antzelevitch C, Sun ZQ, Zhang ZQ, Yan GX, et al. Cellular and ionic mechanisms underlying erythromycin-induced long QT intervals and torsade de pointes. *J Am Coll Cardiol.* 1996;28(7):1836–1848.

Arking DE, Pfeufer A, Post W, et al. A common genetic variant in the NOS1 regulator NOS1AP modulates cardiac repolarization. *Nat Genet.* 2006;38(6):644–651.

Bebarta VS, Phillips S, Eberhardt A, Calihan KJ, Waksman JC, Heard K. Incidence of Brugada electrocardiographic pattern and outcomes of these patients after intentional tricyclic antidepressant ingestion. *Am J Cardiol.* 2007;100(4):656–660.

Bellocq C, van Ginneken AC, Bezzina CR, et al. Mutation in the KCNQ1 gene leading to the short QT-interval syndrome. *Circulation.* 2004a;109(20):2394–2397.

Bellocq C, Wilders R, Schott JJ, et al. A common antitussive drug, clobutinol, precipitates the long QT syndrome 2. *Mol Pharmacol.* 2004b;66(5):1093–1102.

Ben-David J. Zipes DP. Torsades de pointes and proarrhythmia. *Lancet.* 1993;341(8860):1578–1582.

Bennett PB, Yazawa K, Makita N, George AL Jr. Molecular mechanism for an inherited cardiac arrhythmia. *Nature.* 1995;376(6542):683–685.

Berthet M, Denjoy I, Donger C, et al. C-terminal HERG mutations: the role of hypokalemia and a KCNQ1-associated mutation in cardiac event occurrence. *Circulation.* 1999;99(11):1464–1470.

Bezzina CR, Shimizu W, Yang P, et al. Common sodium channel promoter haplotype in Asian subjects underlies variability in cardiac conduction. *Circulation.* 2006;113(3):338–344.

Brahmi N, Thabet H, Kouraichi N, Driss I, Amamou M. Brugada syndrome and other cardiovascular abnormalities related to tricyclic antidepressants and related drugs intoxication. *Arch Mal Coeur Vaiss.* 2007;100(1):28–33.

Brugada P, Brugada J. Right bundle branch block, persistent ST segment elevation and sudden cardiac death: a distinct clinical and electrocardiographic syndrome. A multicenter report. *J Am Coll Cardiol.* 1992;20(6):1391–1396.

Brugada P, Wellens HJ. Arrhythmogenesis of antiarrhythmic drugs. *Am J Cardiol.* 1988;61(13):1108–1111.

Brugada R, Hong K, Dumaine R, et al. Sudden death associated with short-QT syndrome linked to mutations in HERG. *Circulation.* 2004;109(1):30–35.

Chauhan VS, Krahn AD, Walker BD, Klein GJ, Skanes AC, Yee R. Sex differences in QTc interval and QT dispersion: dynamics during exercise and recovery in healthy subjects. *Am Heart J.* 2002;144(5):858–864.

Chen Q, Kirsch GE, Zhang D, et al. Genetic basis and molecular mechanism for idiopathic ventricular fibrillation. *Nature.* 1998;392(6673):293–296.

Chen YJ, Lee SH, Hsieh MH, et al. Effects of 17 beta-estradiol on tachycardia-induced changes of atrial refractoriness and cisapride-induced ventricular arrhythmia. *J Cardiovasc Electrophysiol.* 1999;10(4):587–598.

Chouabe C, Drici MD, Romey G, Barhanin J. Effects of calcium channel blockers on cloned cardiac K+ channels IKr and Iks. *Therapie.* 2000;55(1):195–202.

Chow BJW, Gollob M, Birnie D. Brugada syndrome precipitated by a tricyclic antidepressant. *Heart.* 2005;91(5):651.

Copetti R, Proclemer A, Pillinini PP. Brugada-like ECG abnormalities during thioridazine overdose. *Br J Clin Pharmacol.* 2005;59(5):608.

Cordes JS, Sun Z, Lloyd DB, et al. Pentamidine reduces hERG expression to prolong the QT interval. *Br J Pharmacol.* 2005;145(1):15–23.

Coronel R, Casini S, Koopmann TT, et al. Right ventricular fibrosis and conduction delay in a patient with clinical signs of Brugada syndrome: a combined electrophysiological, genetic, histopathologic, and computational study. *Circulation.* 2005;112(18):2769–2777.

Curran ME, Splawski I, Timothy KW, Vincent GM, Green ED, Keating MT. A molecular basis for cardiac arrhythmia: HERG mutations cause long QT syndrome. *Cell.* 1995;80(5):795–803.

De Ponti F, Poluzzi E, Montanaro N, et al. QT-interval prolongation by non-cardiac drugs: lessons to be learned from recent experience. *Eur J Clin Pharmacol.* 2000;56(1):1–18.

Donger C, Denjoy I, Berthet M, et al. KVLQT1 C-terminal missense mutation causes a forme fruste long-QT syndrome. *Circulation.* 1997;96(9):2778–2781.

Dumaine R, Roy ML, Brown AM. Blockade of HERG and Kv1.5 by ketoconazole. *J Pharmacol Exp Ther.* 1998;286(2):727–735.

Fernandez D, Ghanta A, Kauffman GW, Sanguinetti MC. Physicochemical features of the hERG channel drug binding site. *J Biol Chem.* 2004;279(11):10120–10127.

Ficker E, Kuryshev YA, Dennis AT, et al. Mechanisms of arsenic-induced prolongation of cardiac repolarization. *Mol Pharmacol.* 2004;66(1):33–44.

Fish JM, Antzelevitch C. Role of sodium and calcium channel block in unmasking the Brugada syndrome. *Heart Rhythm.* 2004;1(2):210–217.

Flockhart DA, Drici MD, Kerbusch T, et al. Studies on the mechanism of a fatal clarithromycin-pimozide interaction in a patient with Tourette syndrome. *J Clin Psychopharmacol.* 2000;20(3):317–324.

Frustaci A, Priori SG, Pieroni M, et al. Cardiac histological substrate in patients with clinical phenotype of Brugada syndrome. *Circulation.* 2005;112(24):3680–3687.

Fujiki A, Usui M, Nagasawa H, Mizumaki K, Hayashi H, Inoue H. ST segment elevation in the right precordial leads induced with class IC antiarrhythmic drugs: insight into the mechanism of Brugada syndrome. *J Cardiovasc Electrophysiol.* 1999;10(2):214–218.

Gaita F, Giustetto C, Bianchi F, et al. Short QT syndrome: a familial cause of sudden death. *Circulation.* 2003;108(8):965–970.

Goldgran-Toledano D, Sideris G, Kevorkian JP. Overdose of cyclic antidepressants and the Brugada syndrome. *N Engl J Med.* 2002; 346(20):1591–1592.

Guo J, Massaeli H, Li W, et al. Identification of IKr and its trafficking disruption induced by probucol in cultured neonatal rat cardiomyocytes. *J Pharmacol Exp Ther.* 2007;321(3):911–920.

Gussak I, Brugada P, Brugada J, Antzelevitch C, Osbakken M, Bjerregaard P. ECG phenomenon of idiopathic and paradoxical short QT intervals. *Card Electrophysiol Rev.* 2002;6(1):49–53.

Gussak I, Brugada P, Brugada J, et al. Idiopathic short QT interval: a new clinical syndrome? *Cardiology.* 2000;94(2):99–102.

Haverkamp W, Breithardt G, Camm AJ, et al. The potential for QT prolongation and pro-arrhythmia by non-anti-arrhythmic drugs: clinical and regulatory implications. Report on a Policy Conference of the European Society of Cardiology. *Cardiovasc Res.* 2000;47(2):219–233.

Hayashi K, Shimizu M, Ino H, et al. Probucol aggravates long QT syndrome associated with a novel missense mutation M124T in the N-terminus of HERG. *Clin Sci.* 2004;107(2):175–182.

Hayashi Y, Ikeda U, Hashimoto T, Watanabe T, Mitsuhashi T, Shimada K. Torsades de pointes ventricular tachycardia induced by clarithromycin and disopyramide in the presence of hypokalemia. *Pacing Clin Electrophysiol.* 1999;22(4 Pt 1):672–674.

Hermida JS, Jandaud S, Lemoine JL, et al. Prevalence of drug-induced electrocardiographic pattern of the Brugada syndrome in a healthy population. *Am J Cardiol.* 2004;94(2):230–233.

Hofman N, Wilde AA, Tan HL. Diagnostic criteria for congenital long QT syndrome in the era of molecular genetics: do we need a scoring system? *Eur Heart J.* 2007;28(5):575–580.

Hong K, Bjerregaard P, Gussak I, Brugada R. Short QT syndrome and atrial fibrillation caused by mutation in KCNH2. *J Cardiovasc Electrophysiol.* 2005;16(4):394–396.

Hoover CA, Carmichael JK, Nolan PE Jr, Marcus FI. Cardiac arrest associated with combination cisapride and itraconazole therapy. *J Cardiovasc Pharmacol Ther.* 1996;1(3):255–258.

Houltz B, Darpö B, Edvardsson N et al. Electrocardiographic and clinical predictors of torsades de pointes induced by almokalant infusion in patients with chronic atrial fibrillation or flutter: a prospective study. *Pacing Clin Electrophysiol.* 1998:21(5):1044–1057.

Jackman WM, Friday KJ, Anderson JL, Aliot EM, Clark M, Lazzara R. The long QT syndromes: a critical review, new clinical observations and a unifying hypothesis. *Prog Cardiovasc Dis.* 1988;31(2):115–172.

Jervell A, Lange-Nielsen F. Congenital deaf-mutism, functional heart disease with prolongation of the Q-T interval and sudden death. *Am Heart J.* 1957;54(1):59–68.

Jo SH, Youm JB, Lee CO, Earm YE, Ho WK. Blockade of the HERG human cardiac K(+) channel by the antidepressant drug amitriptyline. *Br J Pharmacol.* 2000;129(7):1474–1480.

Kang J, Wang L, Cai F, Rampe D. High affinity blockade of the HERG cardiac K(+) channel by the neuroleptic pimozide. *Eur J Pharmacol.* 2000;392(3):137—140.

Kubota T, Horie M, Takano M, et al. Evidence for a single nucleotide polymorphism in the KCNQ1 potassium channel that underlies susceptibility to life-threatening arrhythmias. *J Cardiovasc Electrophysiol.* 2001;12(11):1223–1229.

Kubota T, Shimizu W, Kamakura S, Horie M. Hypokalemia-induced long QT syndrome with an underlying novel missense mutation in S4-S5 linker of KCNQ1 [In Process Citation]. *J Cardiovasc Electrophysiol.* 2000;11(9):1048–1054.

Kuhlkamp V, Mewis C, Bosch R, Seipel L. Delayed sodium channel inactivation mimics long QT syndrome 3. *J Cardiovasc Pharmacol.* 2003;42(1):113–117.

Kuryshev YA, Ficker E, Wang L, et al. Pentamidine-induced long QT syndrome and block of hERG trafficking. *J Pharmacol Exp Ther.* 2005;312(1):316–323.

Kusano KF, Hata Y, Yumoto A, Emori T, Sato T, Ohe T. Torsade de pointes with a normal QT interval associated with hypokalemia: a case report. *Jpn Circ J.* 2001;65(8):757–760.

Lee KS, Lee EW. Ionic mechanism of ibutilide in human atrium: evidence for a drug-induced Na+ current through a nifedipine inhibited inward channel. *J Pharmacol Exp Ther.* 1998;286(1):9–22.

Lehtonen A, Fodstad H, Laitinen-Forsblom P, Toivonen L, Kontula K, Swan H. Further evidence of inherited long QT syndrome gene mutations in antiarrhythmic drug-associated torsades de pointes. *Heart Rhythm.* 2007;4(5):603–607.

Littmann L, Monroe MH, Svenson RH. Brugada-type electrocardiographic pattern induced by cocaine. *Mayo Clin Proc.* 2000;75(8):845–849.

London B, Michalec M, Mehdi H, et al. Mutation in glycerol-3-phosphate dehydrogenase 1 like gene (GPD1-L) decreases cardiac Na+ current and causes inherited arrhythmias. *Circulation.* 2007;116(20):2260–2268.

Makita N, Horie M, Nakamura T, et al. Drug-induced long-QT syndrome associated with a subclinical SCN5A mutation. *Circulation.* 2002;106(10):1269–1274.

Makkar RR, Fromm BS, Steinman RT, Meissner MD, Lehmann MH. Female gender as a risk factor for torsades de pointes associated with cardiovascular drugs. *JAMA.* 1993;270(21):2590–2597.

Mank-Seymour AR, Richmond JL, Wood LS, et al. Association of torsades de pointes with novel and known single nucleotide polymorphisms in long QT syndrome genes *Am Heart J.* 2006;152(6):1116–1122.

Mason JW, Hondeghem LM, Katzung BG. Block of inactivated sodium channels and of depolarization-induced automaticity in guinea pig papillary muscle by amiodarone. *Circ Res.* 1984;55(3):278–285.

Medeiros-Domingo A, Kaku T, Tester DJ, et al. SCN4B-encoded sodium channel {beta}4 subunit in congenital long-QT syndrome. *Circulation.* 2007;116(2):134–142.

Michalets EL, Smith LK, Van Tassel ED. Torsade de pointes resulting from the addition of droperidol to an existing cytochrome P450 drug interaction. *Ann Pharmacother.* 1998;32(7–8):761–765.

Mitcheson JS, Chen J, Lin M, Culberson C, Sanguinetti MC. A structural basis for drug-induced long QT syndrome. *Proc Natl Acad Sci U S A.* 2000;97(22):12329–12333.

Miyazaki T, Mitamura H, Miyoshi S, Soejima K, Aizawa Y, Ogawa S. Autonomic and antiarrhythmic drug modulation of ST segment elevation in patients with Brugada syndrome. *J Am Coll Cardiol.* 1996;27(5):1061–1070.

Mohler PJ, Schott JJ, Gramolini AO, et al. Ankyrin-B mutation causes type 4 long-QT cardiac arrhythmia and sudden cardiac death. *Nature.* 2003;421(6923):634–639.

Mohler PJ, Splawski I, Napolitano C, et al. A cardiac arrhythmia syndrome caused by loss of ankyrin-B function. *Proc Natl Acad Sci U S A.* 2004;101(24):9137–9142.

Napolitano C, Priori SG, Schwartz PJ. Identification of a long QT syndrome molecular defect in drug-induced torsades de pointes (abstract). *Circulation.* 1997;96:I–211.

Napolitano C, Schwartz PJ, Brown AM, et al. Evidence for a cardiac ion channel mutation underlying drug-induced QT prolongation and life-threatening arrhythmias. *J Cardiovasc Electrophysiol.* 2000;11(6):691–696.

Numaguchi H, Johnson JP Jr, Petersen CI, Balser JR. A sensitive mechanism for cation modulation of potassium current. *Nat Neurosci.* 2000;3(5):429–430.

Paulussen AD, Gilissen RA, Armstrong M, et al. Genetic variations of KCNQ1, KCNH2, SCN5A, KCNE1, and KCNE2 in drug-induced long QT syndrome patients. *J Mol Med.* 2004;82(3):182–188.

Petersen CI, McFarland TR, Stepanovic SZ, et al. In vivo identification of genes that modify ether-a-go-go-related gene activity in Caenorhabditis elegans may also affect human cardiac arrhythmia. *Proc Natl Acad Sci U S A.* 2004;101(32):11773–11778.

Pfeufer A, Jalilzadeh S, Perz S, et al. Common variants in myocardial ion channel genes modify the QT interval in the general population. Results from the KORA study. *Circ Res.* 2005;96(6):693–701.

Pham TV, Sosunov EA, Gainullin RZ, Danilo P Jr, Rosen MR. Impact of sex and gonadal steroids on prolongation of ventricular repolarization and arrhythmias induced by I(K)-blocking drugs. *Circulation.* 2001;103(17):2207–2212.

Piippo K. Holmström S, Swan H, et al. Effect of the antimalarial drug halofantrine in the long QT syndrome due to a mutation of the cardiac sodium channel gene SCN5A. *Am J Cardiol.* 2001;87(7):909–911.

Plaster NM, Tawil R, Tristani-Firouzi M, et al. Mutations in Kir2.1 cause the developmental and episodic electrical phenotypes of Andersen's syndrome. *Cell.* 2001;105(4):511–519.

Priori SG, Napolitano C, Schwartz PJ. Low penetrance in the long-QT syndrome: clinical impact. *Circulation.* 1999;99(4):529–533.

Priori SG, Pandit SV, Rivolta I, et al. A novel form of short QT syndrome (SQT3) is caused by a mutation in the KCNJ2 gene. *Circ Res.* 2005;96(7):800–807.

Rajamani S, Eckhardt LL, Valdivia CR, et al. Drug-induced long QT syndrome: hERG K+ channel block and disruption of protein trafficking by fluoxetine and norfluoxetine. *Br J Pharmacol.* 2006;149(5):481–489.

Rampe D, Roy ML, Dennis A, Brown AM. A mechanism for the proarrhythmic effects of cisapride (Propulsid): high affinity blockade of the human cardiac potassium channel HERG. *FEBS Lett.* 1997;417(1):28–32.

Ray WA, Murray KT, Meredith S, Narasimhulu SS, Hall K, Stein CM. Oral erythromycin and the risk of sudden death from cardiac causes. *N Eng J Med.* 2004;351(11):1089–1096.

Reilly JG, Ayis SA, Ferrier IN, Jones SJ, Thomas SH. Thioridazine and sudden unexplained death in psychiatric in-patients. *Br J Psychiatry.* 2002;180(6):515–522.

Roberts-Thomson KC, Teo KS, Young GD. Drug-induced Brugada syndrome with ST-T wave alternans and long QT. *Int Med J.* 2007; 37(3):199–200.

Roden DM. Taking the idio out of idiosyncratic: predicting torsades de pointes. *Pacing Clin Electrophysiol.* 1998;21(5):1029–1034.

Roden DM. Long QT syndrome: reduced repolarization reserve and the genetic link. *J Int Med.* 2006;259(1):59–69.

Roden DM, Viswanathan PC. Genetics of acquired long QT syndrome. *J Clin Invest.* 2005;115(8):2025–2032.

Roden DM, Woosley RL, Primm RK. Incidence and clinical features of the quinidine-associated long QT syndrome: implications for patient care. *Am Heart J.* 1986;111(6):1088–1093.

Rolf S, Bruns HJ, Wichter T, et al. The ajmaline challenge in Brugada syndrome: diagnostic impact, safety, and recommended protocol. *Eur Heart J.* 2003;24(12):1104–1112.

Romano C, Gemme G, Pongiglione R. Aritmie cardiache rare in eta' pediatrica. *Clin Pediatr.* 1963;45:656–683.

Rouleau F, Asfar P, Boulet S, et al. Transient ST segment elevation in right precordial leads induced by psychotropic drugs: relationship to the Brugada syndrome. *J Cardiovasc Electrophysiol.* 2001;12(1):61–65.

Sanguinetti MC, Tristani-Firouzi M. hERG potassium channels and cardiac arrhythmia. *Nature.* 2006;440(7083):463–469.

Schulze-Bahr E, Wang Q, Wedekind H, Haverkamp W, Chen Q, Sun Y, Rubie C, Hördt M. Do mutations in cardiac ion channel genes predispose to drug-induced (acquired) long-QT syndrome? (abstract). *Circulation.* 1997a;96:I–211.

Schulze-Bahr E, Wang Q, Wedekind H, et al. KCNE1 mutations cause Jervell and Lange-Nielsen syndrome. *Nat Genet.* 1997b;17(3):267–268.

Schwartz PJ, Moss AJ, Vincent GM, Crampton RS. Diagnostic criteria for the long QT syndrome. An update. *Circulation.* 1993;88(2):782–784.

Schwartz PJ, Priori SG, Napolitano C. How really rare are rare diseases?: the intriguing case of independent compound mutations in the long QT syndrome. *J Cardiovasc Electrophysiol.* 2003;14(10):1120–1121.

Schwartz PJ, Spazzolini C, Crotti L, et al. The Jervell and Lange-Nielsen syndrome: natural history, molecular basis, and clinical outcome. *Circulation.* 2006;113(6):783–790.

Sesti F, Abbott GW, Wei J, et al. A common polymorphism associated with antibiotic-induced cardiac arrhythmia. *Proc Natl Acad Sci U S A.* 2000;97(19):10613–10618.

Sherman J, Tester DJ, Ackerman MJ. Targeted mutational analysis of ankyrin-B in 541 consecutive, unrelated patients referred for long QT syndrome genetic testing and 200 healthy subjects. *Heart Rhythm.* 2005;2(11):1218–1223.

Shimizu W. The Brugada syndrome: an update. *Int Med.* 2005;44(12):1224–1231.

Soyka LF, Wirtz C, Spangenberg RB. Clinical safety profile of sotalol in patients with arrhythmias. *Am J Cardiol.* 1990;65(2):74A–81A.

Splawski I, Shen J, Timothy KW, et al. Spectrum of mutations in long-QT syndrome genes: KVLQT1, HERG, SCN5A, KCNE1, and KCNE2. *Circulation.* 2000;102(10):1178–1185.

Splawski I, Timothy KW, Sharpe LM, et al. Ca(V)1.2 calcium channel dysfunction causes a multisystem disorder including arrhythmia and autism. *Cell.* 2004;119(1):19–31.

Splawski I, Timothy KW, Tateyama M, et al. Variant of SCN5A sodium channel implicated in risk of cardiac arrhythmia. *Science.* 2002;297(5585):1333–1336.

Splawski I, Timothy KW, Vincent GM, Atkinson DL, Keating MT. Molecular basis of the long-QT syndrome associated with deafness. *N Engl J Med.* 1997a;336(22):1562–1567.

Splawski I, Tristani-Firouzi M, Lehmann MH, Sanguinetti MC, Keating MT. Mutations in the hminK gene cause long QT syndrome and suppress IKs function. *Nat Genet.* 1997b;17(3):338–340.

Sun Z, Milos PM, Thompson JF, et al. Role of a KCNH2 polymorphism (R1047 L) in dofetilide-induced Torsades de Pointes. *J Mol Cell Cardiol.* 2004;37(5):1031–1039.

Tada H, Sticherling C, Oral H, Morady F. Brugada syndrome mimicked by tricyclic antidepressant overdose. *J Cardiovasc Electrophysiol.* 2001;12(2):275.

Tester DJ, Will ML, Haglund CM, Ackerman MJ. Compendium of cardiac channel mutations in 541 consecutive unrelated patients referred for long QT syndrome genetic testing. *Heart Rhythm.* 2005;2(5):507–517.

Torp-Pedersen C, Møller M, Bloch-Thomsen PE, et al. Dofetilide in patients with congestive heart failure and left ventricular dysfunction. *N Eng J Med.* 1999;341(12):857–865.

Tschida SJ, Guay DR, Straka RJ, Hoey LL, Johanning R, Vance-Bryan K. QTc-interval prolongation associated with slow intravenous erythromycin lactobionate infusions in critically ill patients: a prospective evaluation and review of the literature. *Pharmacotherapy.* 1996;16(4):663–674.

Turgeon J, Daleau P, Bennett PB, Wiggins SS, Selby L, Roden DM. Block of IKs, the slow component of the delayed rectifier K+ current, by the diuretic agent indapamide in guinea pig myocytes. *Circ Res.* 1994;75(5):879–886.

Van Norstrand DW, Valdivia CR, Tester DJ, et al. Molecular and functional characterization of novel glycerol-3-phosphate dehydrogenase 1 like gene (GPD1-L) mutations in sudden infant death syndrome. *Circulation.* 2007;116(20):2253–2259.

Vatta M, Ackerman MJ, Ye B, et al. Mutant caveolin-3 induces persistent late sodium current and is associated with long-QT syndrome. *Circulation.* 2006;114(20):2104–2112.

von Bahr C, Movin G, Nordin C, et al. Plasma levels of thioridazine and metabolites are influenced by the debrisoquin hydroxylation phenotype. *Clin Pharmacol Ther.* 1991;49(3):234–240.

Wang Q, Curran ME, Splawski I, et al. Positional cloning of a novel potassium channel gene: KVLQT1 mutations cause cardiac arrhythmias. *Nat Genet.* 1996;12(1):17–23.

Wang Q, Shen J, Splawski I, et al. SCN5A mutations associated with an inherited cardiac arrhythmia, long QT syndrome. *Cell.* 1995;80(5):805–811.

Ward OC. New familial cardiac syndrome in children. *J Irish Med Assoc.* 1964;54:103.

Wei J, Yang IC, Tapper AR, et al. KCNE1 polymorphism confers risk of drug-induced long QT syndrome by altering kinetic properties of I_{KS} potassium channels (abstract). *Circulation.* 1999;100(18(I):I–495.

Westenskow P, Splawski I, Timothy KW, Keating MT, Sanguinetti MC. Compound mutations: a common cause of severe long-QT syndrome. *Circulation.* 2004;109(15):1834–1841.

Yan GX, Antzelevitch C. Cellular basis for the brugada syndrome and other mechanisms of arrhythmogenesis associated with ST-segment elevation. *Circulation.* 1999;100(15):1660–1666.

Yang P, Kanki H, Drolet B, et al. Allelic variants in long-QT disease genes in patients with drug-associated torsades de pointes. *Circulation.* 2002;105(16):1943–1948.

Yang T, Roden DM. Extracellular potassium modulation of drug block of IKr: implications for torsade de pointes and reverse use-dependence. *Circulation.* 1996;93(3):407–411.

Yang T, Snyders DJ, Roden DM. Rapid inactivation determines the rectification and [K+]o dependence of the rapid component of the delayed rectifier K+ current in cardiac cells. *Circ Res.* 1997;80(6):782–789.

Yap YG, Camm AJ. Arrhythmogenic mechanisms of non-sedating antihistamines. *Clin Exp Allergy.* 1999;174–181.

Yap YG, Camm AJ. Risk of torsades de pointes with non-cardiac drugs. Doctors need to be aware that many drugs can cause QT prolongation. *BMJ.* 2000;320(7243):1158–1159.

Zhou Z, Vorperian VR, Gong Q, Zhang S, January CT. Block of HERG potassium channels by the antihistamine astemizole and its metabolites desmethylastemizole and norastemizole. *J Cardiovasc Electrophysiol.* 1999;10(6):836–843.

Zimmermann M, Duruz H, Guinand O. Torsades de Pointes after treatment with terfenadine and ketoconazole. *Eur Heart J.* 1992;13(7):1002–1003.

19

Brugada Syndrome

Pieter G Postema, Pascal FHM van Dessel, and Arthur AM Wilde

Introduction

The Brugada syndrome was described as a distinct clinical entity by the brothers Pedro and Josep Brugada in 1992. In their initial publication, they reported eight patients with a specific ECG pattern (Figure 19–1) and repeated episodes of aborted sudden cardiac death (Brugada and Brugada 1992). The contemporary concept of Brugada syndrome is a disorder characterized by sudden cardiac death at relatively young age, with familial segregation, an apparent absence of gross structural abnormalities or ischemic heart disease, and specific electrocardiographic characteristics (Wilde et al. 2002; Antzelevitch et al. 2005a). Sudden cardiac death is caused by fast polymorphic ventricular tachycardia (VT) and ventricular fibrillation (VF) that typically occur in situations associated with an increased vagal tone. In some patients with Brugada syndrome, the electrocardiographic characteristics and the life-threatening arrhythmias are provoked by fever or drugs. Brugada syndrome is characterized on the electrocardiogram (ECG) by ST segment elevation directly followed by a negative T-wave in the right precordial leads and in leads positioned one intercostal space higher (Figure 19–2), also referred to as a coved type Brugada ECG (Brugada et al. 1998; Shimizu et al. 2000; Sangwatanaroj et al. 2001) or type 1 Brugada ECG (Wilde et al. 2002). This specific ECG hallmark typically fluctuates over time, and in some patients it may only be elicited after provocation with class 1A or class 1C antiarrhythmic drugs (Miyazaki et al. 1996; Krishnan and Josephson 1998).

In retrospect, the type 1 Brugada ECG was described as early as 1953 in three otherwise healthy patients who presented with atypical substernal discomfort or for routine medical testing (Osher and Wolff 1953). One year later, ten more patients were described with ST elevation in the right precordial leads, including again clear-cut type 1 ECGs, without apparent heart disease and lack of events during follow-up (Edeiken 1954). Furthermore, only 3 years before the publication of Brugada and Brugada in 1992, the specific Brugada ECG has been described in one out of six cases of VF without apparent heart disease (Martini et al. 1989).

In the late 1970s and 1980s in the United States, unexplained nocturnal death was reported in many refugees from East and Southeast Asia, mainly men (Baron et al. 1983). This pattern of sudden death during sleep was already known for many centuries in Japan by the name *Pokkuri* (sudden unexpected death at night), and it was often prayed for as to end life without pain and suffering (Hattori et al. 2006). In the Philippines the same phenomenon is known as *Bangungut* (moaning and dying during sleep), in northeast Thailand as *laitai* (died during sleep), and in Laos as *non-laitai* (sleep death) (Otto et al. 1984; Nademanee et al. 1997). When studied, a considerable amount of these patients displayed a Brugada-type ECG (Nademanee et al. 1997).

Different genes have been associated with Brugada syndrome since its description. First, in the late 1990s, sodium channel mutations were documented in Brugada syndrome patients (Chen et al. 1998; Rook et al. 1999). Studies using heterologous expression in *Xenopus* oocytes demonstrated that sodium channels with the missense mutation recover more rapidly from inactivation than wild-type controls and that the frameshift mutation causes nonfunctional sodium channels. Over 90 *SCN5A* mutations associated with Brugada syndrome are described (Napolitano 2007), but *SCN5A* mutations are present in only 15%–30% of clinically diagnosed cases (Priori et al. 2000a; Smits et al. 2002). Second, the gene which encodes for the glycerol-3-phosphate dehydrogenase 1-like protein (GPD1L), was correlated with Brugada syndrome in a single large family (Weiss et al. 2002; London et al. 2007). In their preliminary report, London et al. report a reduction of sodium current in human embryonic kidney (HEK) cells expressing the mutated *GPD1L* gene versus wild-type controls, alike the *SCN5A* mutations linked with Brugada syndrome (Tan et al. 2003). Third, loss-of-function missense mutations in the genes encoding for the L-type calcium channel (*CACNA1C*, the α1 subunit, and the *CACNB2*, the β2b subunit) were reported in 9% of Brugada syndrome patients (Antzelevitch et al. 2007). Additionally, in a subset of these patients carrying a calcium channel mutation, the heart rate corrected QT interval appeared to be shorter than normal. Finally, loss-of-function mutations in *SCN1B* and *SCN3B* and gain-of-function mutations in *KCNE3* gene have been associated with Brugada syndrome (Watanabe et al. 2008; Hu et al. 2009; Delpon et al. 2008).

Notwithstanding the identification of as yet unknown genetic mutations and pathophysiologic mechanisms, clinical decision making in Brugada syndrome remains a daunting task. Implantation of an implantable cardioverter-defibrillator (ICD) is the only generally accepted therapy for the prevention of sudden

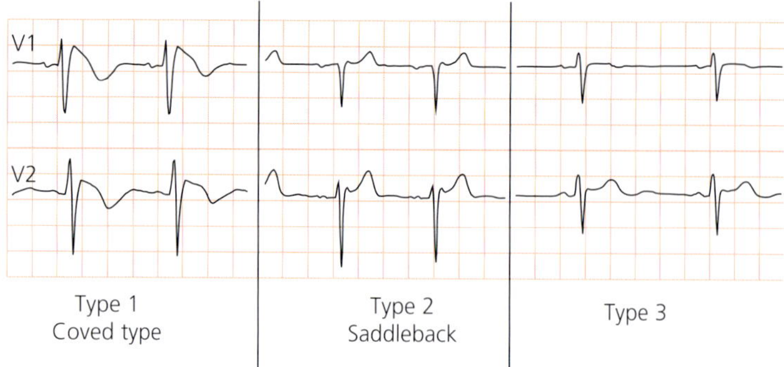

Figure 19–1 ST segment morphologies recognized in Brugada syndrome: type 1, 2, and 3.

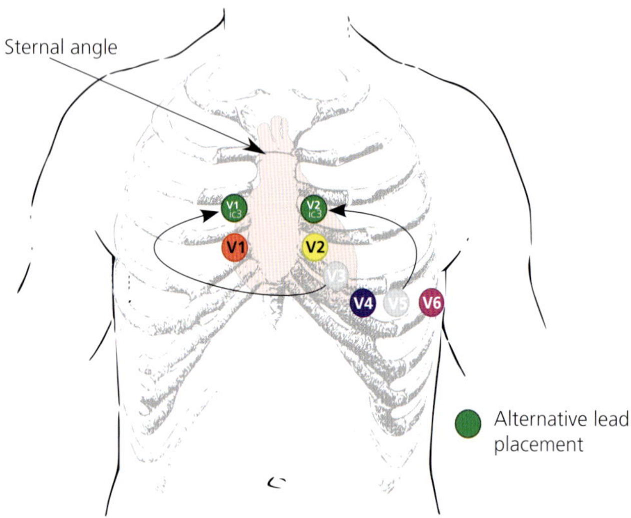

Figure 19–2 Placement of the ECG leads in Brugada syndrome. For use in practice, V3 and V5 are often relocated from their original positions to V1ic3 and V2ic3.

death in patients affected by Brugada syndrome (Brugada et al. 2002; Priori et al. 2002; Sacher et al. 2006; Kusmirek and Gold 2007). Oral therapy with quinidine may also prove valuable (Alings et al. 2001; Belhassen et al. 2004; Hermida et al. 2004; Mok et al. 2004b; Probst et al. 2007).

However, risk stratification in asymptomatic patients is heavily debated, as it is still unclear how to correctly identify the large number of patients who will not develop life-threatening arrhythmias.

Clinical Presentation

Epidemiology

The prevalence of the Brugada ECG is estimated at 1 per 2,000 (Antzelevitch et al. 2005a). This is quite similar to long QT syndrome with an estimated prevalence of 1 per 2,000 (Crotti et al. 2005), but less than hypertrophic cardiomyopathy with a prevalence of 1 per 500 (Maron et al. 1995). The exact prevalence of Brugada-like ECGs is difficult to estimate partly because the specific ECG pattern typically fluctuates over time and can be intermittently concealed. Furthermore, many patients with a spontaneous or inducible Brugada ECG are asymptomatic, and therefore remain without diagnosis. The prevalence of the spontaneous Brugada syndrome ECG seems to vary between different regions in the world (Figure 19–3). Brugada syndrome would be most prevalent in East and Southeast Asia, particularly Japan, Thailand, and the Philippines, where it is part of the sudden unexplained (nocturnal) death syndrome (SUDS or SUNDS), which is a leading cause of death among young men (Nademanee et al. 1997; Vatta et al. 2002; Gervacio-Domingo et al. 2007). In Europe, Brugada syndrome is quite extensively described (Priori et al. 2000a; Brugada et al. 2002; Eckardt et al. 2005). In the northern part of Europe as well as the United States (Greer and Glancy 2003) its prevalence seems to be lower (Junttila et al. 2004). The world wide prevalence of the spontaneous type 1 Brugada ECG from the current prevalence studies (Figure 19–3) is 0.06±0.14% and of the type 2–3 ECG this is 0.17±1.37% (n = 333685).

The Patient

Malignant arrhythmic events can occur at all ages, from childhood to the elderly (Brugada and Brugada 1992; Suzuki et al. 2000; Priori et al. 2000b) with a peak around the fourth decade (Antzelevitch et al. 2005a) of life. The youngest patient clinically diagnosed with Brugada syndrome was 2 days old, (Sanatani et al. 2005) and the oldest 85 years old (Huang and Marcus 2004). It is estimated that Brugada syndrome is responsible for 4%–12% of all sudden cardiac death and up to 20% of sudden cardiac deaths in patients without apparent structural heart disease (Antzelevitch et al. 2002). It may also be a cause of sudden infant death syndrome (SIDS) (Priori et al. 2000b; Skinner et al. 2005). Some patients present with palpitations or dizziness, but increasingly the clinical scenario is the detection of a Brugada ECG in an asymptomatic individual (Hermida et al. 2000; Atarashi et al. 2001; Eckardt et al. 2005). In a recent meta-analysis of 1,217 Brugada syndrome patients (defined by a spontaneous or inducible Brugada ECG and excluding case reports) the majority was asymptomatic (59%, range 0%–80%) (Paul et al. 2007).

When sudden death occurs, it is most likely the result of fast polymorphic VT originating from the right ventricle/right ventricular outflow tract (Morita et al. 2003), which subsequently degenerates into VF leading to cardiocirculatory arrest. The onset of these life-threatening arrhythmias typically occurs in situations with an augmented vagal tone (Kasanuki et al. 1997), during sleep (Matsuo et al. 1999), or after large meals (Ikeda et al. 2005; Mizumaki et al. 2007). Indeed, the latter gave rise to the suggestion of the use of a "full stomach test" as a diagnostic tool (Ikeda et al. 2006). Hyperthermia, for example fever, may also provoke the ECG or arrhythmias in a subset of affected patients (Gonzalez

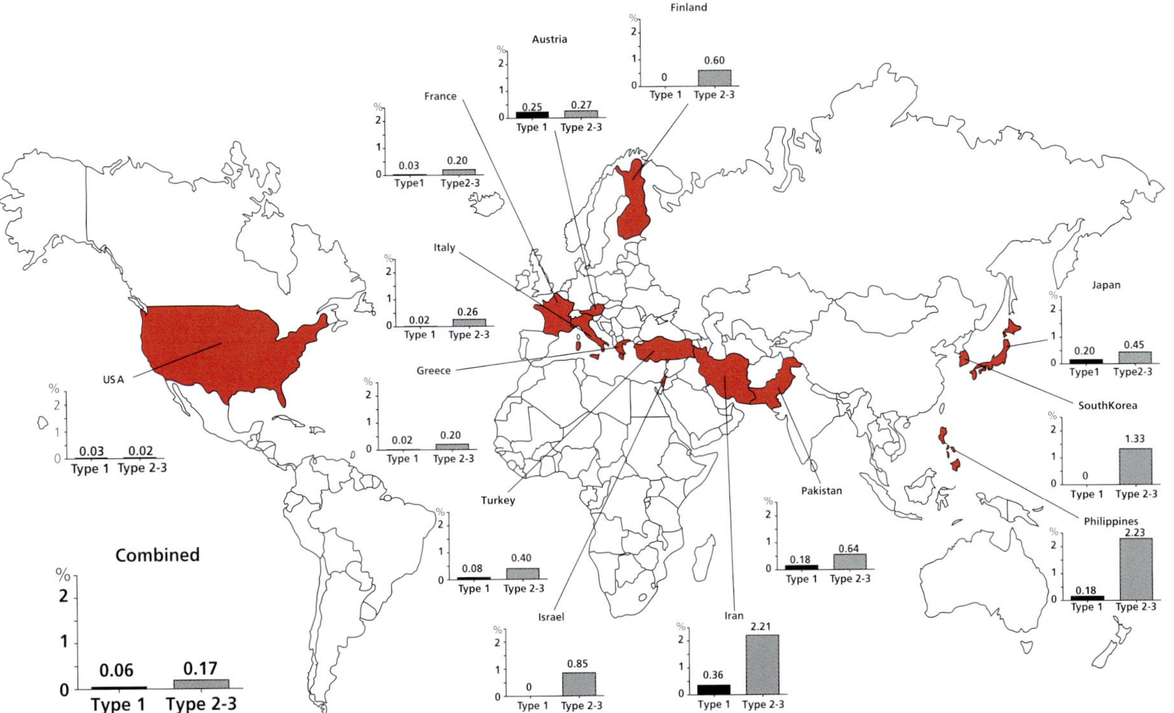

Figure 19–3 Combined prevalence data of the spontaneous Brugada syndrome ECG in different parts of the world from 2000 to 2009. Bars represent mean prevalence in percentages. Only reports in English were considered. Prevalence studies in adolescents or children (Yamakawa et al. 2004; Yoshinaga et al. 2004; Oe et al. 2005) were discarded for this figure. As the type 1 ECG was only recognized after the first consensus report (Wilde et al. 2002), prevalence in two studies was acknowledged as type 1 only (Monroe and Littmann 2000; Matsuo et al. 2001), a coved type ECG was acknowledged as type 1, a saddleback or suspicious ECG as type 2–3. It should be noted that the populations studied and the methods used vary importantly.

USA (Monroe and Littmann 2000; Greer and Glancy 2003; Ito et al. 2006; Donohue et al. 2008; Patel et al. 2009) n = 211272, type 1 0.03% (range 0–0.43), type 2–3 0.02% (range 0.01–0.15).

Finland (Junttila et al. 2004) n = 3021, type 1 0%, type 2–3 0.60% (one study).

Austria (Schukro et al. 2009) n = 4491, type 1 0.25%, type 2–3 0.27% (one study, note that this population is highly selected, another cohort revealed one type 1 out of 47606 ECGs: 0.002%).

France (Hermida et al. 2000; Blangy et al. 2005) n = 36309, type 1 0.03% (range 0.03–0.1), type 2–3 0.20% (range 0.04–6).

Italy (Gallagher et al. 2007) n = 12012, type 1 0.02%, type 2–3 0.26% (one study).

Greece (Letsas et al. 2007) n = 11488, type 1 0.02%, type 2–3 0.20% (one study).

Turkey (Bozkurt et al. 2006) n = 1238, type 1 0.08%, type 2–3 0.40% (one study).

Israel (Viskin et al. 2000) n = 592, type 1 0%, type 2–3 0.85% (one study).

Iran (Babaee Bigi et al. 2007) n = 3895, type 1 0.36%, type 2–3 2.21% (one study).

Pakistan (Wajed et al. 2008) n = 1100, type 1 0.18%, type 2–3 0.64% (one study).

Japan (Furuhashi et al. 2001; Matsuo et al. 2001; Miyasaka et al. 2001; Sakabe et al. 2003; Tsuji et al. 2008) n = 44135, type 1 0.20% (range 0.05–0.42), type 2–3 0.45% (range 0.09–0.93).

South Korea (Shin et al. 2005) n = 225, type 1 0%, type 2–3 1.33% (one study).

Philippines (Gervacio-Domingo et al. 2008) n = 3907, type 1 0.18%, type 2–3 2.23% (one study).

Combined prevalence; n = 333685, type 1 0.06% (range 0–0.43), type 2–3 0.17% (range 0.01–6).

Rebollo et al. 2000; Porres et al. 2002; Probst et al. 2007; Skinner et al. 2007; Tan and Meregalli 2007). Furthermore, a large number of drugs have been reported to induce Brugada syndrome, or Brugada syndrome-like ECG characteristics; for example antiarrhythmic drugs, antianginal drugs, psychotropic drugs, and also substances like cocaine and alcohol are included (Wilde et al. 2002; Antzelevitch et al. 2005a; Postema et al. 2009). Some Brugada syndrome patients experience agonal respiration at night, when arrhythmias are most prevalent (Nademanee et al. 1997; Matsuo et al. 1999). This may be explained by self-terminating VT, which can provoke (recurrent) syncope (Dubner et al. 1983; Patt et al. 1988; Kontny and Dale 1990; Bjerregaard et al. 1994). Clinical presentation with sustained monomorphic ventricular tachyarrhythmia, although quite uncommon, has also been described (Shimada et al. 1996; Boersma et al. 2001; Ogawa et al. 2001; Dinckal et al. 2003; Mok et al. 2004a).

In most patients premature ventricular complexes are scarce during 24-hour Holter monitoring, but premature ventricular complexes can occur very frequently, up to 500 per day (Bjerregaard et al. 1994) and may increase before the spontaneous onset of VF (Kakishita et al. 2000). The morphology of the preceding premature ventricular contractions appears to be identical to the first beat of VF. Repetitive episodes of VF may be initiated by premature ventricular contractions of similar morphology (Kakishita et al. 2000). Most premature ventricular contractions have a left bundle branch block morphology, indicating an origin in the right ventricle. There seems to be a predilection site of origin in the right ventricular outflow tract, but also extra systoles from the right ventricular free wall, septum and apex contribute and are capable of initiating VF (Morita et al. 2003). Further confirmation of the relationship between these right ventricular extra systoles and VF was derived from a study in three Brugada syndrome patients using endocardial catheter ablation of focal triggers of VF at different sites in the right ventricle (Haissaguerre et al. 2003). This therapy resulted in the absence of further episodes of tachyarrhythmias during short-term follow-up. Large studies using this strategy with long-term follow-up are lacking, however.

Although the most impressive ECG characteristics in Brugada syndrome are the changes in the right precordial leads, other ECG abnormalities are common. Supraventricular arrhythmias, for example, mainly atrial fibrillation, are very common with a prevalence between 10% and 39% (Eckardt et al. 2001; Morita et al. 2002; Naccarelli et al. 2002; Rossenbacker et al. 2004). Supraventricular arrhythmias were found to be more prevalent in patients who had an indication for ICD for either symptoms or inducible VT/VF during electrophysiological study (Bordachar et al. 2004; Bigi et al. 2007). Importantly, atrial arrhythmias may often lead to inappropriate ICD shocks (Bordachar et al. 2004; Sacher et al. 2006; Sarkozy et al. 2007).

For a syndrome that inherits an autosomal dominant trait with equal transmission to both genders, there is a striking male to female ratio of 4 to 1 (Gehi et al. 2006; Paul et al. 2007). Testosterone is probably a contributor to this gender disparity; surgical castration of two Brugada syndrome patients for prostate cancer normalized their ECGs (Matsuo et al. 2003), and testosterone levels in Brugada syndrome patients are higher when compared to controls (Shimizu et al. 2007). Sex hormones appear to modulate potassium and calcium currents during the repolarization phase of the action potential (Bidoggia et al. 2000). Where testosterone may shorten the action potential duration (Di Diego et al. 2002), estrogen may lengthen action potential duration (Pham et al. 2002). Furthermore, a different distribution of certain ion channels, particularly Ito, in males versus females may contribute (Di Diego et al. 2002).

Electrocardiography and Diagnosis

The Brugada ECG

Since its description in 1992, the signature sign of Brugada syndrome is its characteristic ECG (Brugada and Brugada 1992; Brugada et al. 2002). Patients with a spontaneous Brugada ECG and symptoms are at a high risk for sudden death secondary to VT/VF (Brugada et al. 2002; Priori et al. 2002; Eckardt et al. 2005; Gehi et al. 2006). The electrocardiographic manifestation of Brugada syndrome is typically dynamic and may often be concealed. The latter has important consequences for risk stratification and follow-up of these patients as patients with dynamic ECGs can still be at risk for future arrhythmic events (Ikeda et al. 2005; Tatsumi et al. 2006; Veltmann et al. 2006). Furthermore, the ECG may be influenced or elicited by hyperthermia and drugs.

The diagnosis of Brugada syndrome requires the demonstration of a "type 1" ECG pattern (Figure 19–1) (Wilde et al. 2002; Antzelevitch et al. 2005a). This type 1 Brugada ECG consists of ≥2 mm J point elevation in at least two of the three right precordial leads (V1 to V3), gradually descending into a negative T-wave (also known as a "coved type" morphology of the ST-T segment). The presence of a type 1 morphology in the third intercostal space above V1 and V2 (V1ic3 and V2ic3) accompanied by a type 1 morphology in V1 or V2 (Shimizu et al. 2000; Sangwatanaroj et al. 2001; Antzelevitch et al. 2005b) is by almost all authors also considered as diagnostic for a Brugada ECG. Furthermore, in some patients, Brugada syndrome is exclusively diagnosed on a type 1 ECG in the leads positioned in the third intercostal space (Shimizu et al. 2000; Sangwatanaroj et al. 2001; Meregalli et al. 2006). Importantly, with the placement of leads in the third intercostal space above V1 and V2 (Figure 19–2), sensitivity increases and there do not seem to be false-positive test results. Also the prognosis of patients with a spontaneous type 1 morphology exclusively in the leads positioned in the third intercostal seems to be similar to patients with a spontaneous type 1 morphology in V1 and V2 (Miyamoto et al. 2007). However, large prospective studies in the use of V1ic3 and V2ic3 are lacking. The type 1 ECG may be spontaneously present or provoked by drugs or hyperthermia. Furthermore, the definite diagnosis of Brugada syndrome requires, in addition to the type 1 ECG, either documented VT or VF, a family history of sudden cardiac death at <45 years old, coved-type ECGs in family members, syncope, inducibility of VT/VF with programmed electrical stimulation, or nocturnal agonal respiration (Wilde et al. 2002; Antzelevitch et al. 2005b).

There are two other ECG patterns recognized in Brugada syndrome, a type 2 and a type 3 ECG, although they are not specific and, importantly, not diagnostic (Figure 19–1). A type 2 Brugada ECG displays a "saddleback" appearance; it consists of ≥2 mm J elevation followed by a descending ST segment that does not reach the baseline and then gives rise to a positive or biphasic T-wave. A type 3 Brugada ECG has the morphology of a type 1 or type 2 ECG with ≥2 mm J elevation but is characterized by a smaller magnitude of the ST elevation (≤1 mm) (Wilde et al. 2002). Due to its typical dynamic nature, the type 1 ECG can change from and to a type 2, type 3, or normal ECG spontaneously or under influence of hyperthermia or drugs. Interestingly, the magnitude of ST elevation does not differ between Brugada syndrome patients with or without a *SCN5A* mutation (Smits et al. 2002). As discussed earlier in this chapter, many drugs and substances are capable of inducing a type 1 ECG in patients with Brugada syndrome. For clinical purposes this knowledge is used as a diagnostic tool to evoke a type 1 ECG in patients suspected of Brugada syndrome who do not display a spontaneous type 1 ECG, for example, in case of symptoms (syncope, aborted sudden cardiac death) or as part of familial screening for Brugada syndrome. For this purpose, sodium channel blockers such as ajmaline, flecainide, pilsicainide, or procainamide are mostly used (Table 19–1) (Wilde et al. 2002; Antzelevitch et al. 2005a). The diagnostic accuracy of drug challenge in patients suspected of Brugada syndrome is higher with the use of ajmaline over flecainide, while equally safe (Wolpert et al. 2005). Safety of drug challenges for Brugada syndrome is ensured when the test is performed using continuously 12-lead

Table 19–1 Drugs Used for Provocation of the Brugada ECG

Drug	Dosage and Administration
Ajmaline	IV 1 mg/kg over 5 minutes
Flecainide	IV 2 mg/kg over 10 minutes
Procainamide	IV 10 mg/kg over 10 minutes
Pilsicainide	IV 1 mg/kg over 10 minutes

Notes: IV denotes intravenously. Ajmaline administration particularly differs between studies (e.g., bolus every minute versus continuous administration, 5 minutes versus 10 minutes).
Source: Adapted from Antzelevitch et al. (2005a).

Table 19–2 Drugs Known to Induce Brugada or Brugada-like ECGs and Arrhythmias

	Drug Category
Antiarrhythmic Drugs	
1	To be avoided by Brugada syndrome patients
	Ajmaline, Flecainide, Pilsicainide, Procainamide, Propafenone
2	Preferably avoided by Brugada syndrome patients
	Amiodarone, Cibenzoline, Disopyramide, Lidocaine, Propranolol, Verapamil
Anesthetics	
1	To be avoided by Brugada syndrome patients
	Bupivacaine, Propofol
Psychotropic Drugs	
1	To be avoided by Brugada syndrome patients
	Amitriplyline, Clomipramine, Desipramine, Lithium, Loxapine, Nortriptyline, Trifluoperazine
2	Preferably avoided by Brugada syndrome patients
	Carbamazepine, Clonazepam, Cyamemazine, Delorazepam, Doxepin, Fluoxetine, Imipramine, Maprotiline, Perphenazine, Phenytoin, Thioridazine
Other Drugs and substances	
1	To be avoided by Brugada syndrome patients
	Acetylcholine, Alcohol (toxicity), Cocaine, Ergonovine
2	Preferably avoided by Brugada syndrome patients
	Demenhydrinate, Edrophonium, Indapamide

Source: Adapted from Postema et al. (2009), see also www.brugadadrugs.org.

Table 19–3 Differential Diagnosis for ST Segment Abnormalities in the Right Precordial ECG Leads

Differential Diagnosis
Right or left bundle branch block, left ventricular hypertrophy
Acute myocardial ischemia or infarction
Acute myocarditis
Right ventricular ischemia or infarction
Dissecting aortic aneurysm
Acute pulmonary thromboemboli
Various central and autonomic nervous system abnormalities
Heterocyclic antidepressant overdose
Duchenne muscular dystrophy
Friedreich's ataxia
Thiamine deficiency
Hypercalcemia
Hyperkalemia
Cocaine intoxication
Mediastinal tumor compressing right ventricular outflow tract
Arrhythmogenic right ventricular dysplasia/cardiomyopathy
Long QT syndrome type 3
Other Conditions
Early repolarization syndrome
Other normal variants (particularly in men)

Source: Adapted from Wilde et al. (2002).

ECG monitoring, with cardioverter defibrillators and advanced cardiac life support close at hand and discontinuation of the test when a type 1 ECG is obtained, when ventricular extra systoles or VT develops or when the QRS duration increases more than 30% (Wilde et al. 2002). As a type 1 ECG is associated with ventricular arrhythmias, drugs or substances associated with a type 1 ECG need to be avoided in patients diagnosed with Brugada syndrome (Table 19–2). Particular attention should also be given to general anesthesia in Brugada syndrome patients (Edge et al. 2002; Kim et al. 2004; Santambrogio et al. 2005; Cordery et al. 2006). The administration of isoproterenol, a β-receptor agonist, and/or quinidine may effectively be used to treat repetitive ventricular arrhythmias or electrical storms (Tanaka et al. 2001; Belhassen et al. 2004; Watanabe et al. 2006; Jongman et al. 2007; Ohgo et al. 2007).

As mentioned earlier, hyperthermia also evokes a type 1 ECG or ventricular arrhythmias in a subset of Brugada syndrome patients. Several reports revealed the presence of a type 1 ECG or episodes of arrhythmias during febrile illness, often in children (Saura et al. 2002; Dinckal et al. 2003; Todd et al. 2005; Probst et al. 2007; Skinner et al. 2007; Tan and Meregalli 2007). Elevation of the core body temperature as during hot baths may have a similar effect (Smith et al. 2003). Treating fever with antipyretic agents such as paracetamol (U.S.: Acetaminophen) and/or antibiotics may prove valuable in these cases. If hyperthermia persists and arrhythmias cannot be counteracted, cooling the patient by all means may be the ultimate rescue (personal communication Dr. Pedro Brugada, ESC congress 2006).

There is a wide differential diagnosis of clinical conditions accompanied by coved-like or elevated ST segments in the right precordial ECG leads, and these should be ruled out before a conclusive diagnosis of Brugada syndrome is made (Table 19–3) (Wilde et al. 2002). Relatively common causes include early repolarization (Gussak et al. 2000), myocardial infarction or ventricular aneurysms (Hermida et al. 2000; Kataoka 2000), vasospastic angina (Chinushi et al. 2001; Sasaki et al. 2006), electrolyte disturbances such as hyperkalemia or hypercalcemia (Douglas et al. 1984; Littmann et al. 2007; Wu et al. 2007), pericarditis or myocarditis (Buob et al. 2003; Kurisu et al. 2006; Hermida et al. 2007), left or right bundle branch block, and left ventricular hypertrophy (Zipes et al. 2005).

Other Electrocardiographic Characteristics

Other ECG characteristics associated with Brugada syndrome include conduction defects in the atria, conduction system, and ventricles. Frequently present are broad P-waves (Meregalli et al. 2006), long PQ interval (Smits et al. 2002), prolonged corrected sinus node recovery times, prolonged His-Ventricle intervals (HV), which may or may not be accompanied by prolonged Atrio-His (AH) intervals (Morita et al. 2002; Bordachar et al. 2004; Rossenbacker et al. 2004), sinus and AV node dysfunction (Morita et al. 2004), QRS axis deviation (Brugada and Brugada 1992), and broad QRS complexes (Meregalli et al. 2006). Conduction interval prolongation is frequently associated with the presence of *SCN5A* mutations (Smits et al. 2002). Furthermore, *SCN5A* mutations in Brugada syndrome patients may, as in Lev-Lenègres disease, worsen the phenotypic expression of the disease with aging and may lead to the necessity of pacemaker implantation (Kyndt et al. 2001; Rossenbacker et al. 2004; Probst et al. 2006). Although there is some variability of the heart rate corrected QT interval (QTc), it does not seem to prolong importantly when a type 1 Brugada ECG or VF develops (Brugada and Brugada 1992; Kakishita et al. 2000; Meregalli et al. 2006). This clearly distinguishes Brugada syndrome from long QT syndrome where excessive QTc prolongation is the hallmark of the disease (Schwartz et al. 1993). Overlap syndromes between Brugada syndrome and long QT syndrome (type 3) exist, based on a multidysfunctional sodium channel caused by specific *SCN5A* mutations (Bezzina et al. 1999; Veldkamp et al. 2000; Priori et al. 2000c; Grant et al. 2002). Interestingly, the phenotype of one of these mutations (SCN5A 1795insD) seems to be similar in a mouse model carrying the murine equivalent mutation (SCN5A 1798insD) with bradycardia, right ventricular conduction slowing, an increased vulnerability for arrhythmias and QTc prolongation (Remme et al. 2006). Conversely, shortened QTc intervals were noted in a subset of Brugada syndrome patients with calcium channel mutations (Antzelevitch et al. 2007). However, data regarding the calcium channel mutation and/or shortened QTc intervals are limited. Wide S-waves in the inferior leads are frequently observed before and after a type 1 ECG develops during drug challenge, which may reflect simultaneous slowing of right ventricular activation (Meregalli et al. 2006). Furthermore, S-waves ≥80 ms in V1 appear to be a good predictor for a history of VF (Atarashi and Ogawa 2003).

Signal-averaged ECGs show more variation in filtered QRS duration and late potentials in symptomatic patients (Kasanuki et al. 1997; Ikeda et al. 2001; Eckardt et al. 2002; Kanda et al. 2002; Nagase et al. 2002; Ikeda et al. 2005). Late potentials are generally regarded as delayed and disorganized ventricular activation and are related to ventricular tachyarrhythmias (Simson et al. 1983). In Brugada syndrome, however, other mechanisms have also been proposed: late potentials might for example represent a delayed second upstroke of the epicardial action potential, a local phase 2 reentry or an interventricular conduction delay (Antzelevitch 2002). These latter proposals have, however, not yet been validated as primary or cooperative pathophysiologic mechanisms of late potentials in Brugada syndrome.

In some case reports of patients who presented with VF, ST elevation in the inferior and/or lateral leads has been described in the absence of electrolyte disturbances, hypothermia, or myocardial ischemia (Kalla et al. 2000; Takagi et al. 2000; Ogawa et al. 2005; van den Berg and Wiesfeld 2006; Ueyama et al. 2007). In a French family, different *SCN5A* mutation carrying family members displayed either inferior or right precordial coved-type ST segment elevation (Potet et al. 2003). At present it is uncertain if these patients represent the same population as has been described by solely right precordial coved-type ST segments.

Pathophysiology and Genetics

Arrhythmia Mechanisms

Ventricular arrhythmias in Brugada syndrome often originate from ventricular extra systoles in the right ventricle, which subsequently initiate polymorphic VT or VF. The exact pathophysiology behind Brugada syndrome is, however, not clear and there might be different electrophysiological mechanisms involved. It seems that an increased vulnerability of the ventricles is present before the onset of VF. The coupling interval (i.e., the timing) of the premature ventricular complex, for example, may be important. In several electrophysiological studies, short coupled extra systoles (<200 ms) were necessary to induce VF while the coupling interval of the first premature ventricular complex of spontaneous VF is often (far) more than 300 ms (Kasanuki et al. 1997; Kakishita et al. 2000). There might furthermore be a relation between the vulnerability of the ventricle and the preceding RR interval following for example an extra systole, which may augment ST elevation and eventually degenerate into VF (Matsuo et al. 1998a). Notwithstanding the associated risk for sudden cardiac death of a type 1 ECG, it is not necessary for arrhythmias in Brugada syndrome, as was shown in Holter and ICD recordings documentation suggesting that there might be distinct—albeit possibly related—electrophysiological mechanisms involved. Moreover, a part of the patients with spontaneous type 1 ECGs will never have any symptoms (Osher and Wolff 1953; Edeiken 1954; Wilde and Duren 1999).

The Coved ST Segment

Ever since the first descriptions of Brugada syndrome, authors have been investigating possible mechanisms for this characteristic ECG feature (Edeiken 1954; Brugada and Brugada 1992; Corrado et al. 1996; Miyazaki et al. 1996; Brugada and Brugada 1997; Matsuo et al. 1998b; Antzelevitch 2001). Currently, there are two theories: the repolarization model and the depolarization model (Meregalli et al. 2005). The repolarization model has been developed by Yan and Antzelevitch in canine right ventricular wedge preparations (Yan et al. 1999). In this model, simultaneously measured epicardial and endocardial electrograms showed loss of action potential dome in the epicardium only when the wedge preparation was exposed to a potassium channel opener (pinacidil) or a combination of a sodium channel blocker (flecainide) and acetylcholine. This resulted in a transmural dispersion of repolarization with different lengths of action potentials across different cardiac layers, ST segment elevation on the ECG and it created a vulnerable window for (phase 2) reentry to occur between these layers and degenerate into ventricular tachyarrhythmias. Isoprotenerol, 4-aminopyridine, and quinidine were able to restore this loss of action potential dome, normalize the ST segments, and prevent the ventricular arrhythmias. This model resolves around a heterogeneous expression of the transient outward potassium current *I*to. This current seems to be expressed to a higher degree in the canine epicardium compared with the endocardium (Litovsky et al. 1988), in the right ventricle more than in the left ventricle (Di Diego et al. 1996), and in males more than in females (Di Diego et al. 2002), resulting in a higher susceptibility for *I*to augmentation over other currents and a consequential higher risk for ventricular tachyarrhythmias. Augmentation of *I*to would be enhanced by sodium current (*I*Na) reduction, either by a sodium channel mutation or sodium channel blockade. Furthermore, reduction of the calcium current (*I*Ca) and augmentation of the ATP-driven potassium current (*I*K-ATP) would give similar effects.

The second model explaining the coved-type morphology resolves around a depolarization disorder (Meregalli et al. 2005). In this model conduction slowing or conduction delay in the right ventricular outflow tract (RVOT) causes the type 1 morphology in the right precordial leads. Most evidence for this model is derived from clinical studies (Kasanuki et al. 1997; Fujiki et al. 1999; Ikeda et al. 2001; Kanda et al. 2002; Nagase et al. 2002; Takami et al. 2003; Izumida et al. 2004; Tukkie et al. 2004; Postema et al. 2008). Furthermore, conduction slowing may create the vulnerability for reentry of the right ventricle and give rise to ventricular extra systoles. The marked conduction slowing in atria and ventricles, which is seen during drug challenges with sodium channel blockers and in SCN5A mutation carriers particularly, further supports this model. However, neither the depolarization model nor the repolarization model currently fully explains the coved-type morphology, the vulnerability for ventricular arrhythmias, and the observed clinical and experimental data in Brugada syndrome. As with many diseases, it is likely that Brugada syndrome is not explained by one single mechanism (Meregalli et al. 2005; Aiba et al. 2006). The final common pathway of a spontaneous or inducible coved-type ECG and the vulnerability for ventricular arrhythmias may be started by distinct but cooperative mechanisms and may require tailored risk stratifications and treatment. Moreover, there might be other cooperative pathophysiological mechanisms such as structural myocardial abnormalities and gene–gene interactions.

Structural Changes

The most recent consensus criteria for Brugada syndrome recommend the exclusion of structural myocardial derangements in conjunction with the documentation of a type 1 ECG and the presence of at least one of the obligatory additional features (see section Electrocardiography and Diagnosis) before a conclusive diagnosis of Brugada syndrome can be made (Antzelevitch et al. 2005a). This reflects the hypothesis that Brugada syndrome is a pure electrical disease involving only myocardial channel abnormalities and thus the absence of structural changes. This issue has, however, been debated. A similarity between Brugada syndrome and arrhythmogenic right ventricular cardiomyopathy has been suggested (Martini et al. 1989; Tada et al. 1998; Martini and Nava 2004). Biventricular endomyocardial biopsies in 18 Brugada syndrome patients showed myocarditis, cardiomyopathy-like changes, or fatty infiltration in the right ventricle of all patients (without a control group) (Frustaci et al. 2005). Furthermore, in 8 out of these 18 patients (45%) there were similar findings in the left ventricle. Both magnetic resonance imaging (MRI) and echocardiography were negative in all patients. Interestingly, patients with fatty infiltration and cardiomyopathy-like changes all had a *SCN5A* mutation. In another case, right ventricular fibrosis and epicardial fatty infiltration was documented in the explanted heart of a *SCN5A* mutation carrying Brugada syndrome patient who experienced intolerable numbers of ICD discharges (up to 129 appropriate shocks in 5 months) (Coronel et al. 2005). This patient also had no clinically detected cardiac structural abnormalities before transplant. In a study using endocardial mapping it was noted that Brugada syndrome patients showed increased electrogram fractionation and abnormal conduction velocity restitution, both also related to structural changes (Postema et al. 2008). These reports suggest that there might be cooperative functional and structural derangements in Brugada syndrome, which may be enhanced by mutations in the sodium channel. In support of this hypothesis, mice and human data illustrate that *SCN5A* mutations may lead to impressive fibrosis accompanied by conduction disturbances, mainly in the right ventricle, which worsens with aging (Bezzina et al. 2003; Royer et al. 2005; van Veen et al. 2005; Remme et al. 2007). Fibrosis is probably missed in clinical practice as the clinical modalities to assess structural cardiac changes are incapable of detecting mild or diffuse abnormalities (Takagi et al. 2001; Takagi et al. 2003; Papavassiliu et al. 2004). Interestingly, a meta-analysis into risk stratification for ventricular tachyarrhythmias did not find an increased risk for patients carrying a *SCN5A* mutation (Gehi et al. 2006).

Genetics of Brugada Syndrome

Mutations have been identified in only 15%–30% of patients (Priori et al. 2000a; Smits et al. 2002). Although recent efforts in screening 16 putatively associated genes identified another ion channel (the calcium channel), this only resulted in a mutation diagnosis in 24% of patients (Antzelevitch et al. 2007).

The first mutation in Brugada syndrome patients was indentified in a collaborative effort of clinics in Europe and the United States in 1998 (Chen et al. 1998). A loss-of-function mutation in the *SCN5A* gene, encoding the pore-forming α-subunit of the human cardiac sodium channel protein (Nav1.5) was present in three out of six families with Brugada syndrome. Mutations leading to loss of sodium channel function can lead to a variety of disorders (Koopmann et al. 2006; McKusick 2007): Brugada syndrome (OMIM 601144), (progressive) cardiac conduction defects also known as Lev-Lenègres disease (OMIM 113900) (Schott et al. 1999), sick sinus syndrome (OMIM 608567) (Benson et al. 2003), Sudden infant death syndrome (OMIM 272120) (Priori et al. 2000b; Skinner et al. 2005), and dilated cardiomyopathy associated with conduction defects and arrhythmias (OMIM 601154) (McNair et al. 2004). In combination with other (atrial-specific modifier) genes, a loss-of-function defect may cause atrial standstill (Groenewegen et al. 2003). Mutations leading to a gain of function of the channel may cause long QT syndrome type 3 (OMIM 603830) (Wang et al. 1995) and also sudden infant death syndrome (OMIM 272120) (Ackerman et al. 2001; Wang et al. 2007). As mentioned earlier, certain mutations in the cardiac sodium channel gene may lead to combined phenotypes of loss-of-function and gain-of-function mutations, also referred to as an overlap syndrome (Bezzina et al. 1999; Priori et al. 2000c; Grant et al. 2002). *SCN5A* promoter polymorphisms in a haplotype variant may lead to variability in phenotypic expression as was shown recently in a study demonstrating slower cardiac conduction with a gene-dose effect in patients of Asian origin (Bezzina et al. 2006). The same holds for common *SCN5A* polymorphisms or the combination of different *SCN5A* mutations that may modulate the expression of the mutant gene(s) and disease (Baroudi et al. 2001; Hong et al. 2005; Rossenbacker et al. 2005; Poelzing et al. 2006).

Loss-of-function cardiac calcium channel mutations have recently been demonstrated in Brugada syndrome patients (Antzelevitch et al. 2007). These mutations involved the L-type calcium channel encoded by *CACNA1C* for the pore-forming Cav1.2 α1 subunit, and *CACNB2* for the Cavβ2b subunit involved in channel activation modulation of the α1 subunit. Mutations in the *GPD1L* gene have also been linked to Brugada syndrome in a single family (Weiss et al. 2002; London et al. 2007). The function of this gene is poorly understood at present but it may be involved in sodium channel trafficking and probably does not contribute more than 1% in Brugada syndrome (Koopmann et al. 2007; Rossenbacker and Priori 2007).

Exon mutations or duplications in the *SCN5A* gene and a large number of other candidate genes (*Caveolin-3*, *Irx-3*, *Irx-4*, *Irx-5*, *Irx-6*, *Plakoglobin*, *Plakophilin-2*, *SCN1B*, *SCN2B*, *SCN3B*, *SCN4B*, *KCNH2*, *KCNQ1*, *KCNJ2*, *KCNE1*, *KCNE2*, *KCNE3*, *KCND3*, *KCNIP2*, *KCNJ11*, and *CACNA2D1*) have been investigated in *SCN5A* mutation-negative Brugada syndrome patients with little success (Antzelevitch et al. 2007; Koopmann et al. 2007). Nevertheless, recently also mutations in several of these genes (*SCN1B*, *SCN3B* and *KCNE3*) have been associated with Brugada syndrome (Watanabe et al. 2008; Delpon et al. 2008; Hu et al. 2009). *SCN1B* and *SCN3B* encode for subunits of the cardiac sodium channel and these mutations cause a loss-of-function resulting in a Brugada Syndrome phenotype. *KCNE3* encodes for a subunit of MiRP2 which is involved in the transient outward current and a gain-of-function mutation resulted in the Brugada syndrome phenotype.

Interestingly, a recent study revealed common gene expression levels in Brugada syndrome patients irrespective of the culprit gene (Gaborit et al. 2009). This expression pattern involved not only cardiac sodium channel and its subunits, but also potassium channels and calcium channels.

Typically for Brugada syndrome, and other Mendelian disorders, is an incomplete penetrance and variable expression of the disease (Wilde and Bezzina 2005). Hence, not all mutation carriers are affected by the same degree and will thus not require the same treatment. Even so, the importance of diagnosing mutation carriers with little or no phenotypic expression of the disease is important because they still have a 50% chance of transmitting the genetic defect to their offspring, who in turn may be seriously symptomatic at young age. It is, however, not clear whether presymptomatic genetic testing in children of Brugada syndrome patients is to be advised (Viskin 2007). As symptomatic Brugada syndrome is rare in children, risk stratification is imperfect, and treatment may do more harm than good (see also the section on Clinical Decision Making), the consequences of a positive test result of presymptomatic genetic testing should be carefully considered.

Clinical Decision Making

Risk Stratification

After diagnosing Brugada syndrome, risk stratification for future ventricular arrhythmias is mandatory. The prognosis and risk stratification of Brugada syndrome patients is, however, debated. Risk for future ventricular arrhythmias is generally accepted to be high in patients who are known to have already experienced life-threatening ventricular arrhythmias, that is, patients with a history of aborted sudden cardiac death. Syncope, dizziness or nocturnal agonal respiration can also be caused by ventricular arrhythmias and are thus often regarded as high-risk features. However, this assumption can be erroneous and so other causes of these symptoms should also be sought.

A recent meta-analysis combined a history of sudden cardiac death and/or syncope as representative for a history of ventricular arrhythmias and found a relative risk (RR) of 3.34 [95% confidence interval (CI) 2.13–4.93] for the combined event of sudden cardiac death, syncope, or ICD shock during follow-up (Gehi et al. 2006). Also male gender, RR 3.47 (95% CI 1.58–7.63), and a spontaneous type 1 ECG versus a drug-induced type 1 ECG, RR 4.65 (95% CI 2.25–9.58), were positively associated with the occurrence of the combined events (sudden cardiac death and/or syncope) during follow-up. A family history of sudden cardiac death, a *SCN5A* mutation, or inducible ventricular arrhythmias during electrophysiological study were not associated with events during follow-up. Importantly, these risk factors are probably not independent.

As asymptomatic patients can experience ventricular arrhythmias, there is a dire need for reliable risk stratification in these patients. The role of the inducibility of ventricular arrhythmias during electrophysiological study in this matter has been debated in the recent years (Priori et al. 2002; Wilde et al. 2002; Brugada et al. 2003, 2005; Eckardt et al. 2005; Antzelevitch et al. 2005a). A recent meta-analysis to assess its prognostic role was not able to identify a significant role with regard to arrhythmic events during follow-up (Paul et al. 2007). In a combined effort of 14 centers in France and Japan, it was shown that 45% of the 220 studied Brugada syndrome patients received an ICD following inducibility of ventricular arrhythmias during electrophysiological study whilst being asymptomatic (Sacher et al. 2006). In this study there was an 8% rate of appropriate shocks for ventricular arrhythmias during >3 years follow-up, and a relatively low (2 to 5 times lower) rate of appropriate shocks in asymptomatic patients compared to the patients with syncope or aborted sudden cardiac death. There were no other factors (like a spontaneous type 1 ECG) apart from a clinical history of syncope or aborted sudden cardiac death predicting appropriate shocks. Of importance, approximately 20% of patients in each group suffered from inappropriate shocks during follow-up.

Noninvasive risk stratification has been attempted in relatively small cohorts of patients and yielded the strongest predictive value in spontaneous changes in the right precordial ST segments (Ikeda et al. 2005; Tatsumi et al. 2006; Veltmann et al. 2006). A standard cardiology workup including echocardiogram, 24-hour Holter, and an exercise test may be valuable to exclude differential diagnoses and to assess baseline conditions. Thorough cardiac imaging using MRI or CT does not seem to add significant clinical value at present, unless arrhythmogenic right ventricular cardiomyopathy needs to be excluded.

A summary of the current literature on risk stratification suggests that symptoms likely to be related to ventricular arrhythmias identify the patients at highest risk for future life-threatening arrhythmic events. Conversely, as asymptomatic patients have a very low risk of experiencing these arrhythmias, and the currently available treatment option (ICD implantation) may do more harm than good, they should be identified as low risk. A spontaneous type 1 ECG, whether or not accompanied by inducible arrhythmias during electrophysiological study, is seen by some as an indication for an ICD (see also section on Treatment). Naturally, risk stratification should be reevaluated in all patients during long-term follow-up using up-to-date consensus criteria.

Treatment

The most effective therapy to treat ventricular arrhythmias in Brugada syndrome is an ICD. Patients may, however, experience intolerable numbers of ICD shocks, up to 150 a day (Dinckal et al. 2003), as an ICD does not lower the vulnerability of the heart for ventricular arrhythmias. In some patients heart transplantation has been considered the only remaining option (Ayerza et al. 2002). Cardiologists should carefully weigh benefits versus possible harm, quality of life, and costs of ICDs as event rates are generally low and complications (in particular inappropriate shocks) are high in this population (Sacher et al. 2006). ICD implantation in the young specifically denotes several battery replacements, reimplantations over many decades, and increased morbidity. However, some Brugada syndrome patients may benefit from an ICD when they have lost a family member due to sudden cardiac death and intolerable anxiety diminishes their quality of life and impairs their daily activities.

Acute lowering of the vulnerability of the heart for ventricular arrhythmias may be accomplished by treating hyperthermia (e.g., cooling, antipyretics, antibiotics), correcting electrolyte disturbances, and the administration of quinidine and/or isoproterenol (Ohgo et al. 2007; Probst et al. 2007). Further chronic oral treatment with quinidine or several other agents may prove valuable (Belhassen et al. 2004; Ohgo et al. 2007). Excluding differential diagnoses in case of acute events is mandatory as VTs not due to Brugada syndrome may display a devastating response on isoproterenol (Francis et al. 2005).

All patients with Brugada syndrome should receive a list of avoidable drugs and substances, including a number of antiarrhythmic drugs (class Ia, Ic, and β-blockers), tricyclic antidepressants (with a relative contraindication for nontricyclic antidepressants), local anesthetics, opioid analgesics, propofol, potassium channel antagonists, lithium, α-adrenergic agonists, cocaine, and excessive use of alcohol (see www.brugadadrugs.org, Postema et al. 2009). Furthermore, patients should be instructed to obtain an ECG in case of fever at least once to assess whether their form of Brugada syndrome is hyperthermia sensitive. Long-term follow-up is mandatory in all Brugada syndrome patients. Symptomatic patients will have more frequent visits, but also asymptomatic patients should be seen with regular intervals for reassessment of the risk for arrhythmic events and genetic counselling in case of children. Genetic counselling should be advised for all adult patients.

Future Research

As Brugada syndrome is a relatively new entity, the knowledge and awareness of the disorder will continue to increase. In the first years after the description in 1992, many severely symptomatic patients were recognized, which led to the notion that Brugada syndrome is a malignant disease that is hard to manage (Brugada et al. 1992, 2002). More recently, many asymptomatic patients have been diagnosed and one of the great challenges for the future is to develop reliable risk stratification for arrhythmic events (Zipes et al. 2006). Risk stratification and treatment in the pediatric population affected with Brugada syndrome, although limited in numbers, should also receive greater attention. The pathophysiology of the ventricular arrhythmias and the coved-type ECG in the right precordial leads has been and will continue to be a major area of research. Although many animal and computer models are available, detailed descriptions of human data will continue to be important and will guide therapeutic interventions. Finally, further characterization of the genetic origin of Brugada syndrome will help to identify those silent carriers, and their offspring, who might be at risk and may clarify the complicated genotype–phenotype relationship in Brugada syndrome patients.

Acknowledgments

The authors wish to thank Paola G. Meregalli, MD, and Hanno L. Tan, MD, PhD for critical assessment of the manuscript and their suggestions.

References

Ackerman MJ, Siu BL, Sturner WQ, et al. Postmortem molecular analysis of SCN5A defects in sudden infant death syndrome. *JAMA.* 2001;286(18):2264–2269.

Aiba T, Shimizu W, Hidaka I, et al. Cellular basis for trigger and maintenance of ventricular fibrillation in the Brugada syndrome model high-resolution optical mapping study. *J Am Coll Cardiol.* 2006;47(10): 2074–2085.

Alings M, Dekker L, Sadee A, Wilde A. Quinidine induced electrocardiographic normalization in two patients with Brugada syndrome. *Pacing Clin Electrophysiol.* 2001;24(9 Pt 1):1420–1422.

Antzelevitch C. The Brugada syndrome: ionic basis and arrhythmia mechanisms. *J Cardiovasc Electrophysiol.* 2001;12(2):268–272.

Antzelevitch C. Late potentials and the Brugada syndrome. *J Am Coll Cardiol.* 2002;39(12):1996–1999.

Antzelevitch C, Brugada P, Borggrefe M, et al. Brugada syndrome: report of the second consensus conference. *Heart Rhythm.* 2005a;2(4):429–440.

Antzelevitch C, Brugada P, Borggrefe M, et al. Brugada syndrome: report of the second consensus conference: endorsed by the Heart Rhythm Society and the European Heart Rhythm Association. *Circulation.* 2005b;111(5):659–670.

Antzelevitch C, Brugada P, Brugada J, et al. Brugada syndrome: a decade of progress. *Circ Res.* 2002;91(12):1114–1118.

Antzelevitch C, Pollevick GD, Cordeiro JM, et al. Loss-of-function mutations in the cardiac calcium channel underlie a new clinical entity characterized by ST-segment elevation, short QT intervals, and sudden cardiac death. *Circulation.* 2007;115(4):442–449.

Atarashi H, Ogawa S. New ECG criteria for high-risk Brugada syndrome. *Circ J.* 2003;67(1):8–10.

Atarashi H, Ogawa S, Harumi K, et al. Three-year follow-up of patients with right bundle branch block and ST segment elevation in the right precordial leads: Japanese Registry of Brugada Syndrome. Idiopathic Ventricular Fibrillation Investigators. *J Am Coll Cardiol.* 2001;37(7):1916–1920.

Ayerza MR, de ZM, Goethals M, Wellens F, Geelen P, Brugada P. Heart transplantation as last resort against Brugada syndrome. *J Cardiovasc Electrophysiol.* 2002;13(9):943–944.

Babaee Bigi MA, Aslani A, Shahrzad S. Prevalence of Brugada sign in patients presenting with palpitation in southern Iran. *Europace.* 2007;9(4):252–255.

Baron RC, Thacker SB, Gorelkin L, Vernon AA, Taylor WR, Choi K. Sudden death among Southeast Asian refugees. An unexplained nocturnal phenomenon. *JAMA.* 1983;250(21):2947–2951.

Baroudi G, Pouliot V, Denjoy I, Guicheney P, Shrier A, Chahine M. Novel mechanism for Brugada syndrome: defective surface localization of an SCN5A mutant (R1432G). *Circ Res.* 2001;88(12):E78–E83.

Belhassen B, Glick A, Viskin S. Efficacy of quinidine in high-risk patients with Brugada syndrome. *Circulation.* 2004;110(13):1731–1737.

Benson DW, Wang DW, Dyment M, et al. Congenital sick sinus syndrome caused by recessive mutations in the cardiac sodium channel gene (SCN5A). *J Clin Invest.* 2003;112(7):1019–1028.

Bezzina C, Veldkamp MW, van den Berg MP, et al. A single Na(+) channel mutation causing both long-QT and Brugada syndromes. *Circ Res.* 1999;85(12):1206–1213.

Bezzina CR, Rook MB, Groenewegen WA, et al. Compound heterozygosity for mutations (W156X and R225W) in SCN5A associated with severe cardiac conduction disturbances and degenerative changes in the conduction system. *Circ Res.* 2003;92(2):159–168.

Bezzina CR, Shimizu W, Yang P, et al. Common sodium channel promoter haplotype in Asian subjects underlies variability in cardiac conduction. *Circulation.* 2006;113(3):338–344.

Bidoggia H, Maciel JP, Capalozza N, et al. Sex-dependent electrocardiographic pattern of cardiac repolarization. *Am Heart J.* 2000;140(3): 430–436.

Bigi MA, Aslani A, Shahrzad S. Clinical predictors of atrial fibrillation in Brugada syndrome. *Europace.* 2007;9(10):947–950.

Bjerregaard P, Gussak I, Kotar SL, Gessler JE, Janosik D. Recurrent syncope in a patient with prominent J wave. *Am Heart J.* 1994;127(5): 1426–1430.

Blangy H, Sadoul N, Coutelour JM, et al. Prevalence of Brugada syndrome among 35,309 inhabitants of Lorraine screened at a preventive medicine centre. *Arch Mal Coeur Vaiss.* 2005;98(3):175–180.

Boersma LV, Jaarsma W, Jessurun ER, Van Hemel NH, Wever EF. Brugada syndrome: a case report of monomorphic ventricular tachycardia. *Pacing Clin Electrophysiol.* 2001;24(1):112–115.

Bordachar P, Reuter S, Garrigue S, et al. Incidence, clinical implications and prognosis of atrial arrhythmias in Brugada syndrome. *Eur Heart J.* 2004;25(10):879–884.

Bozkurt A, Yas D, Seydaoglu G, Acarturk E. Frequency of Brugada-type ECG pattern (Brugada sign) in southern Turkey. *Int Heart J.* 2006;47(4):541–547.

Brugada J, Brugada P. Further characterization of the syndrome of right bundle branch block, ST segment elevation, and sudden cardiac death. *J Cardiovasc Electrophysiol.* 1997;8(3):325–331.

Brugada J, Brugada R, Antzelevitch C, Towbin J, Nademanee K, Brugada P. Long-term follow-up of individuals with the electrocardiographic pattern of right bundle-branch block and ST-segment elevation in precordial leads V1 to V3. *Circulation.* 2002;105(1):73–78.

Brugada J, Brugada R, Brugada P. Right bundle-branch block and ST-segment elevation in leads V1 through V3: a marker for sudden death in patients without demonstrable structural heart disease. *Circulation.* 1998;97(5):457–460.

Brugada P, Brugada J. Right bundle branch block, persistent ST segment elevation and sudden cardiac death: a distinct clinical and electrocardiographic syndrome. A multicenter report. *J Am Coll Cardiol.* 1992;20(6):1391–1396.

Brugada P, Brugada R, Brugada J. Should patients with an asymptomatic Brugada electrocardiogram undergo pharmacological and electrophysiological testing? *Circulation.* 2005;112(2):279–292.

Brugada P, Brugada R, Mont L, Rivero M, Geelen P, Brugada J. Natural history of Brugada syndrome: the prognostic value of programmed electrical stimulation of the heart. *J Cardiovasc Electrophysiol.* 2003;14(5):455–457.

Buob A, Siaplaouras S, Janzen I, et al. Focal parvovirus B19 myocarditis in a patient with Brugada syndrome. *Cardiol Rev.* 2003;11(1):45–49.

Chen Q, Kirsch GE, Zhang D, et al. Genetic basis and molecular mechanism for idiopathic ventricular fibrillation. *Nature.* 1998;392(6673):293–296.

Chinushi M, Kuroe Y, Ito E, Tagawa M, Aizawa Y. Vasospastic angina accompanied by Brugada-type electrocardiographic abnormalities. *J Cardiovasc Electrophysiol.* 2001;12(1):108–111.

Cordery R, Lambiase P, Lowe M, Ashley E. Brugada syndrome and anesthetic management. *J Cardiothorac Vasc Anesth.* 2006;20(3):407–413.

Coronel R, Casini S, Koopmann TT, et al. Right ventricular fibrosis and conduction delay in a patient with clinical signs of Brugada syndrome: a combined electrophysiological, genetic, histopathologic, and computational study. *Circulation.* 2005;112(18):2769–2777.

Corrado D, Nava A, Buja G, et al. Familial cardiomyopathy underlies syndrome of right bundle branch block, ST segment elevation and sudden death. *J Am Coll Cardiol.* 1996;27(2):443–448.

Crotti L, Stramba-Badiale M, Pedrazzini M, et al. Prevalence of the long QT syndrome [Abstract]. *Circulation.* 2005;112(17):U724.

Delpon E, Cordeiro JM, Nunez L, et al. Functional effects of KCNE3 mutation and its role in the development of Brugada Syndrome. *Circ Arrhythmia Electrophysiol.* 2008;1(3):209–218.

Di Diego JM, Cordeiro JM, Goodrow RJ, et al. Ionic and cellular basis for the predominance of the Brugada syndrome phenotype in males. *Circulation.* 2002;106(15):2004–2011.

Di Diego JM, Sun ZQ, Antzelevitch C. I(to) and action potential notch are smaller in left vs. right canine ventricular epicardium. *Am J Physiol.* 1996;271(2 Pt 2):H548–H561.

Dinckal MH, Davutoglu V, Akdemir I, Soydinc S, Kirilmaz A, Aksoy M. Incessant monomorphic ventricular tachycardia during febrile illness in a patient with Brugada syndrome: fatal electrical storm. *Europace.* 2003;5(3):257–261.

Donohue D, Tehrani F, Jamehdor R, Lam C, Movahed MR. The prevalence of Brugada ECG in adult patients in a large university hospital in the western United States. *Am Heart Hosp J.* 2008;6(1):48–50.

Douglas PS, Carmichael KA, Palevsky PM. Extreme hypercalcemia and electrocardiographic changes. *Am J Cardiol.* 1984;54(6):674–675.

Dubner SJ, Gimeno GM, Elencwajg B, Leguizamon J, Tronge JE, Quinteiro R. Ventricular fibrillation with spontaneous reversion on ambulatory ECG in the absence of heart disease. *Am Heart J.* 1983;105(4):691–693.

Eckardt L, Bruns HJ, Paul M, et al. Body surface area of ST elevation and the presence of late potentials correlate to the inducibility of ventricular tachyarrhythmias in Brugada syndrome. *J Cardiovasc Electrophysiol.* 2002;13(8):742–749.

Eckardt L, Kirchhof P, Loh P, et al. Brugada syndrome and supraventricular tachyarrhythmias: a novel association? *J Cardiovasc Electrophysiol.* 2001;12(6):680–685.

Eckardt L, Probst V, Smits JP, et al. Long-term prognosis of individuals with right precordial ST-segment-elevation Brugada syndrome. *Circulation.* 2005;111(3):257–263.

Edeiken J. Elevation of the RS-T segment, apparent or real, in the right precordial leads as a probable normal variant. *Am Heart J.* 1954;48(3):331–339.

Edge CJ, Blackman DJ, Gupta K, Sainsbury M. General anaesthesia in a patient with Brugada syndrome. *Br J Anaesth.* 2002;89(5):788–791.

Francis J, Sankar V, Nair VK, Priori SG. Catecholaminergic polymorphic ventricular tachycardia. *Heart Rhythm.* 2005;2(5):550–554.

Frustaci A, Priori SG, Pieroni M, et al. Cardiac histological substrate in patients with clinical phenotype of Brugada syndrome. *Circulation.* 2005;112(24):3680–3687.

Fujiki A, Usui M, Nagasawa H, Mizumaki K, Hayashi H, Inoue H. ST segment elevation in the right precordial leads induced with class IC antiarrhythmic drugs: insight into the mechanism of Brugada syndrome. *J Cardiovasc Electrophysiol.* 1999;10(2):214–218.

Furuhashi M, Uno K, Tsuchihashi K, et al. Prevalence of asymptomatic ST segment elevation in right precordial leads with right bundle branch block (Brugada-type ST shift) among the general Japanese population. *Heart.* 2001;86(2):161–166.

Gaborit N, Wichter T, Varro A, et al. Transcriptional profiling of ion channel genes in Brugada syndrome and other right ventricular arrhythmogenic diseases. *Eur Heart J.* 2009;30(4):487–496.

Gallagher MM, Forleo GB, Behr ER, et al. Prevalence and significance of Brugada-type ECG in 12,012 apparently healthy European subjects. *Int J Cardiol.* 2008;130(1):44–48.

Gehi AK, Duong TD, Metz LD, Gomes JA, Mehta D. Risk stratification of individuals with the Brugada electrocardiogram: a meta-analysis. *J Cardiovasc Electrophysiol.* 2006;17(6):577–583.

Gervacio-Domingo G, Isidro J, Tirona J, et al. The Brugada type 1 electrocardiographic pattern is common among Filipinos. *J Clin Epidemiol.* 2008;61(10):1067–1072.

Gervacio-Domingo G, Punzalan FE, Amarillo ML, Dans A. Sudden unexplained death during sleep occurred commonly in the general population in the Philippines: a sub study of the National Nutrition and Health Survey. *J Clin Epidemiol.* 2007;60(6):567–571.

Gonzalez Rebollo JM, Hernandez MA, Garcia A, Garcia de CA, Mejias A, Moro C. Recurrent ventricular fibrillation during a febrile illness in a patient with the Brugada syndrome. *Rev Esp Cardiol.* 2000;53(5):755–757.

Grant AO, Carboni MP, Neplioueva V, et al. Long QT syndrome, Brugada syndrome, and conduction system disease are linked to a single sodium channel mutation. *J Clin Invest.* 2002;110(8):1201–1209.

Greer RW, Glancy DL. Prevalence of the Brugada electrocardiographic pattern at the Medical Center of Louisiana in New Orleans. *J La State Med Soc.* 2003;155(5):242–246.

Groenewegen WA, Firouzi M, Bezzina CR, et al. A cardiac sodium channel mutation cosegregates with a rare connexin40 genotype in familial atrial standstill. *Circ Res.* 2003;92(1):14–22.

Gussak I, Antzelevitch C. Early repolarization syndrome: clinical characteristics and possible cellular and ionic mechanisms. *J Electrocardiol.* 2000;33(4):299–309.

Haissaguerre M, Extramiana F, Hocini M, et al. Mapping and ablation of ventricular fibrillation associated with long-QT and Brugada syndromes. *Circulation.* 2003;108(8):925–928.

Hattori K, McCubbin MA, Ishida DN. Concept analysis of good death in the Japanese community. *J Nurs Scholarsh.* 2006;38(2):165–170.

Hermida JS, Denjoy I, Clerc J, et al. Hydroquinidine therapy in Brugada syndrome. *J Am Coll Cardiol.* 2004;43(10):1853–1860.

Hermida JS, Lemoine JL, Aoun FB, Jarry G, Rey JL, Quiret JC. Prevalence of the Brugada syndrome in an apparently healthy population. *Am J Cardiol.* 2000;86(1):91–94.

Hermida JS, Six I, Jarry G. Drug-induced pericarditis mimicking Brugada syndrome. *Europace.* 2007;9(1):66–68.

Hong K, Guerchicoff A, Pollevick GD, et al. Cryptic 5' splice site activation in SCN5A associated with Brugada syndrome. *J Mol Cell Cardiol.* 2005;38(4):555–560.

Hu D, Barajas-Martinez H, Burashnikov E, et al. A mutation in the β3 subunit of the cardiac sodium channel associated with Brugada ECG phenotype. *Circ Cardiovasc Genet.* 2009;2(3):270–278.

Huang MH, Marcus FI. Idiopathic Brugada-type electrocardiographic pattern in an octogenarian. *J Electrocardiol.* 2004;37(2):109–111.

Ikeda T, Abe A, Yusu S, et al. The full stomach test as a novel diagnostic technique for identifying patients at risk of Brugada syndrome. *J Cardiovasc Electrophysiol.* 2006;17(6):602–607.

Ikeda T, Sakurada H, Sakabe K, et al. Assessment of noninvasive markers in identifying patients at risk in the Brugada syndrome: insight into risk stratification. *J Am Coll Cardiol.* 2001;37(6):1628–1634.

Ikeda T, Takami M, Sugi K, Mizusawa Y, Sakurada H, Yoshino H. Noninvasive risk stratification of subjects with a Brugada-type electrocardiogram and no history of cardiac arrest. *Ann Noninvasive Electrocardiol.* 2005;10(4):396–403.

Ito H, Yano K, Chen R, He Q, Curb JD. The prevalence and prognosis of a Brugada-type electrocardiogram in a population of middle-aged Japanese-American men with follow-up of three decades. *Am J Med Sci.* 2006;331(1):25–29.

Izumida N, Asano Y, Doi S, et al. Changes in body surface potential distributions induced by isoproterenol and Na channel blockers in patients with the Brugada syndrome. *Int J Cardiol.* 2004;95(2–3):261–268.

Jongman JK, Jepkes-Bruin N, Ramdat Misier AR, et al. Electrical storms in Brugada syndrome successfully treated with isoproterenol infusion and quinidine orally. *Neth Heart J.* 2007;15(4):151–154.

Junttila MJ, Raatikainen MJ, Karjalainen J, Kauma H, Kesaniemi YA, Huikuri HV. Prevalence and prognosis of subjects with Brugada-type ECG pattern in a young and middle-aged Finnish population. *Eur Heart J.* 2004;25(10):874–878.

Kakishita M, Kurita T, Matsuo K, et al. Mode of onset of ventricular fibrillation in patients with Brugada syndrome detected by implantable cardioverter defibrillator therapy. *J Am Coll Cardiol.* 2000;36(5):1646–1653.

Kalla H, Yan GX, Marinchak R. Ventricular fibrillation in a patient with prominent J (Osborn) waves and ST segment elevation in the inferior electrocardiographic leads: a Brugada syndrome variant? *J Cardiovasc Electrophysiol.* 2000;11(1):95–98.

Kanda M, Shimizu W, Matsuo K, et al. Electrophysiologic characteristics and implications of induced ventricular fibrillation in symptomatic patients with Brugada syndrome. *J Am Coll Cardiol.* 2002;39(11):1799–1805.

Kasanuki H, Ohnishi S, Ohtuka M, et al. Idiopathic ventricular fibrillation induced with vagal activity in patients without obvious heart disease. *Circulation.* 1997;95(9):2277–2285.

Kataoka H. Electrocardiographic patterns of the Brugada syndrome in right ventricular infarction/ischemia. *Am J Cardiol.* 2000;86(9):1056.

Kim JS, Park SY, Min SK, et al. Anaesthesia in patients with Brugada syndrome. *Acta Anaesthesiol Scand.* 2004;48(8):1058–1061.

Kontny F, Dale J. Self-terminating idiopathic ventricular fibrillation presenting as syncope: a 40-year follow-up report. *J Intern Med.* 1990;227(3):211–213.

Koopmann TT, Beekman L, Alders M, et al. Exclusion of multiple candidate genes and large genomic rearrangements in SCN5A in a Dutch Brugada syndrome cohort. *Heart Rhythm.* 2007;4(6):752–755.

Koopmann TT, Bezzina CR, Wilde AA. Voltage-gated sodium channels: action players with many faces. *Ann Med.* 2006;38(7):472–482.

Krishnan SC, Josephson ME. ST segment elevation induced by class IC antiarrhythmic agents: underlying electrophysiologic mechanisms and insights into drug-induced proarrhythmia. *J Cardiovasc Electrophysiol.* 1998;9(11):1167–1172.

Kurisu S, Inoue I, Kawagoe T, et al. Acute pericarditis uUnmasks ST-segment elevation in asymptomatic Brugada syndrome. *Pacing Clin Electrophysiol.* 2006;29(2):201–203.

Kusmirek SL, Gold MR. Sudden cardiac death: the role of risk stratification. *Am Heart J.* 2007;153(4 suppl):25–33.

Kyndt F, Probst V, Potet F, et al. Novel SCN5A mutation leading either to isolated cardiac conduction defect or Brugada syndrome in a large French family. *Circulation.* 2001;104(25):3081–3086.

Letsas KP, Gavrielatos G, Efremidis M, et al. Prevalence of Brugada sign in a Greek tertiary hospital population. *Europace.* 2007;9(11):1077–1180.

Litovsky SH, Antzelevitch C. Transient outward current prominent in canine ventricular epicardium but not endocardium. *Circ Res.* 1988;62(1):116–126.

Littmann L, Monroe MH, Taylor L III, Brearley WD Jr. The hyperkalemic Brugada sign. *J Electrocardiol.* 2007;40(1):53–59.

London B, Michalec M, Mehdi H, et al. Mutation in glycerol-3-phosphate dehydrogenase 1 like gene (GPD1-L) decreases cardiac Na+ current and causes inherited arrhythmias. *Circulation.* 2007;116(20):2260-2268.

Maron BJ, Gardin JM, Flack JM, Gidding SS, Kurosaki TT, Bild DE. Prevalence of hypertrophic cardiomyopathy in a general population of young adults. Echocardiographic analysis of 4111 subjects in the CARDIA Study. Coronary Artery Risk Development in (Young) Adults. *Circulation.* 1995;92(4):785–789.

Martini B, Nava A. 1988–2003. Fifteen years after the first Italian description by Nava-Martini-Thiene and colleagues of a new syndrome (different from the Brugada syndrome?) in the Giornale Italiano di Cardiologia: do we really know everything on this entity? *Ital Heart J.* 2004;5(1):53–60.

Martini B, Nava A, Thiene G, et al. Ventricular fibrillation without apparent heart disease: description of six cases. *Am Heart J.* 1989;118(6): 1203–1209.

Matsuo K, Akahoshi M, Nakashima E, et al. The prevalence, incidence and prognostic value of the Brugada-type electrocardiogram: a population-based study of four decades. *J Am Coll Cardiol.* 2001;38(3):765–770.

Matsuo K, Akahoshi M, Seto S, Yano K. Disappearance of the Brugada-type electrocardiogram after surgical castration: a role for testosterone and an explanation for the male preponderance. *Pacing Clin Electrophysiol.* 2003;26(7 Pt 1):1551–1553.

Matsuo K, Kurita T, Inagaki M, et al. The circadian pattern of the development of ventricular fibrillation in patients with Brugada syndrome. *Eur Heart J.* 1999;20(6):465–470.

Matsuo K, Shimizu W, Kurita T, et al. Increased dispersion of repolarization time determined by monophasic action potentials in two patients with familial idiopathic ventricular fibrillation. *J Cardiovasc Electrophysiol.* 1998b;9(1):74–83.

Matsuo K, Shimizu W, Kurita T, Inagaki M, Aihara N, Kamakura S. Dynamic changes of 12-lead electrocardiograms in a patient with Brugada syndrome. *J Cardiovasc Electrophysiol.* 1998a;9(5):508–512.

McKusick VA. OMIM—Online Mendelian Inheritance in Man. 2007. http://www.ncbi.nlm.nih.gov/sites/entrez?db=OMIM

McNair WP, Ku L, Taylor MR, et al. SCN5A mutation associated with dilated cardiomyopathy, conduction disorder, and arrhythmia. *Circulation.* 2004;110(15):2163–2167.

Meregalli PG, Ruijter JM, Hofman N, Bezzina CR, Wilde AA, Tan HL. Diagnostic value of flecainide testing in unmasking SCN5A-related Brugada syndrome. *J Cardiovasc Electrophysiol.* 2006;17(8):857–864.

Meregalli PG, Wilde AA, Tan HL. Pathophysiological mechanisms of Brugada syndrome: depolarization disorder, repolarization disorder, or more? *Cardiovasc Res.* 2005;67(3):367–378.

Miyamoto K, Yokokawa M, Tanaka K, et al. Diagnostic and prognostic value of a type 1 Brugada electrocardiogram at higher (third or second) V(1) to V(2) recording in men with Brugada syndrome. *Am J Cardiol.* 2007;99(1):53–57.

Miyasaka Y, Tsuji H, Yamada K, et al. Prevalence and mortality of the Brugada-type electrocardiogram in one city in Japan. *J Am Coll Cardiol.* 2001;38(3):771–774.

Miyazaki T, Mitamura H, Miyoshi S, Soejima K, Aizawa Y, Ogawa S. Autonomic and antiarrhythmic drug modulation of ST segment elevation in patients with Brugada syndrome. *J Am Coll Cardiol.* 1996;27(5): 1061–1070.

Mizumaki K, Fujiki A, Nishida K, et al. Postprandial augmentation of bradycardia-dependent ST elevation in patients with Brugada syndrome. *J Cardiovasc Electrophysiol.* 2007;18(8):839–844.

Mok NS, Chan NY. Brugada syndrome presenting with sustained monomorphic ventricular tachycardia. *Int J Cardiol.* 2004a;97(2):307–309.

Mok NS, Chan NY, Chiu AC. Successful use of quinidine in treatment of electrical storm in Brugada syndrome. *Pacing Clin Electrophysiol.* 2004b;27(6 Pt 1):821–823.

Monroe MH, Littmann L. Two-year case collection of the Brugada syndrome electrocardiogram pattern at a large teaching hospital. *Clin Cardiol.* 2000;23(11):849–851.

Morita H, Fukushima-Kusano K, Nagase S, et al. Site-specific arrhythmogenesis in patients with Brugada syndrome. *J Cardiovasc Electrophysiol.* 2003;14(4):373–379.

Morita H, Fukushima-Kusano K, Nagase S, et al. Sinus node function in patients with Brugada-type ECG. *Circ J.* 2004;68(5):473–476.

Morita H, Kusano-Fukushima K, Nagase S, et al. Atrial fibrillation and atrial vulnerability in patients with Brugada syndrome. *J Am Coll Cardiol.* 2002;40(8):1437–1444.

Naccarelli GV, Antzelevitch C, Wolbrette DL, Luck JC. The Brugada syndrome. *Curr Opin Cardiol.* 2002;17(1):19–23.

Nademanee K, Veerakul G, Nimmannit S, et al. Arrhythmogenic marker for the sudden unexplained death syndrome in Thai men. *Circulation.* 1997;96(8):2595–2600.

Nagase S, Kusano KF, Morita H, et al. Epicardial electrogram of the right ventricular outflow tract in patients with the Brugada syndrome: using the epicardial lead. *J Am Coll Cardiol.* 2002;39(12):1992–1995.

Napolitano C. Inherited arrhythmias database. 2007. http://www.fsm.it/cardmoc/.

Oe H, Takagi M, Tanaka A, et al. Prevalence and clinical course of the juveniles with Brugada-type ECG in Japanese population. *Pacing Clin Electrophysiol.* 2005;28(6):549–554.

Ogawa M, Kumagai K, Saku K. Spontaneous right ventricular outflow tract tachycardia in a patient with Brugada syndrome. *J Cardiovasc Electrophysiol.* 2001;12(7):838–840.

Ogawa M, Kumagai K, Yamanouchi Y, Saku K. Spontaneous onset of ventricular fibrillation in Brugada syndrome with J wave and ST-segment elevation in the inferior leads. *Heart Rhythm.* 2005;2(1):97–99.

Ohgo T, Okamura H, Noda T, et al. Acute and chronic management in patients with Brugada syndrome associated with electrical storm of ventricular fibrillation. *Heart Rhythm.* 2007;4(6):695–700.

Osher HL, Wollf L. Electrocardiographic pattern simulating acute myocardial injury. *Am J Med Sci.* 1953;226(5):541–545.

Otto CM, Tauxe RV, Cobb LA, et al. Ventricular fibrillation causes sudden death in Southeast Asian immigrants. *Ann Intern Med.* 1984;101(1): 45–47.

Papavassiliu T, Wolpert C, Fluchter S, et al. Magnetic resonance imaging findings in patients with Brugada syndrome. *J Cardiovasc Electrophysiol.* 2004;15(10):1133–1138.

Patel SS, Anees SS, Ferrick KJ. Prevalence of a Brugada pattern electrocardiogram in an urban population in the United States. Pacing Clin Electrophysiol. 2009;32(6):704–708.

Patt MV, Podrid PJ, Friedman PL, Lown B. Spontaneous reversion of ventricular fibrillation. *Am Heart J.* 1988;115(4):919–923.

Paul M, Gerss J, Schulze-Bahr E, et al. Role of programmed ventricular stimulation in patients with Brugada syndrome: a meta-analysis of worldwide published data. *Eur Heart J.* 2007;28(17):2126–2133.

Pham TV, Robinson RB, Danilo P Jr, Rosen MR. Effects of gonadal steroids on gender-related differences in transmural dispersion of L-type calcium current. *Cardiovasc Res.* 2002;53(3):752–762.

Poelzing S, Forleo C, Samodell M, et al. SCN5A polymorphism restores trafficking of a Brugada syndrome mutation on a separate gene. *Circulation.* 2006;114(5):368–376.

Porres JM, Brugada J, Urbistondo V, Garcia F, Reviejo K, Marco P. Fever unmasking the Brugada syndrome. *Pacing Clin Electrophysiol.* 2002;25(11):1646–1648.

Postema PG, Van Dessel PF, De Bakker JM, et al. Slow and Discontinuous Conduction Conspire in Brugada Syndrome: a Right Ventricular Mapping and Stimulation Study. *Circ Arrhythm Electrophysiol.* 2008;1(5):379–386.

Postema PG, Wolpert C, Amin AS, et al. Drugs and Brugada syndrome patients: review of the literature, recommendations and an up-to-date website (www.brugadadrugs.org), *Heart Rhythm.* 2009;6(9):1335–1341.

Potet F, Mabo P, Le Coq G, et al. Novel brugada SCN5A mutation leading to ST segment elevation in the inferior or the right precordial leads. *J Cardiovasc Electrophysiol.* 2003;14(2):200–203.

Priori SG, Napolitano C, Gasparini M, et al. Clinical and genetic heterogeneity of right bundle branch block and ST-segment elevation syndrome: a prospective evaluation of 52 families. *Circulation.* 2000a;102(20):2509–2515.

Priori SG, Napolitano C, Gasparini M, et al. Natural history of Brugada syndrome: insights for risk stratification and management. *Circulation.* 2002;105(11):1342–1347.

Priori SG, Napolitano C, Giordano U, Collisani G, Memmi M. Brugada syndrome and sudden cardiac death in children. *Lancet.* 2000b; 355(9206):808–809.

Priori SG, Napolitano C, Schwartz PJ, Bloise R, Crotti L, Ronchetti E. The elusive link between LQT3 and Brugada syndrome: the role of flecainide challenge. *Circulation.* 2000c;102(9):945–947.

Probst V, Allouis M, Sacher F, et al. Progressive cardiac conduction defect is the prevailing phenotype in carriers of a Brugada syndrome SCN5A mutation. *J Cardiovasc Electrophysiol.* 2006;17(3):270–275.

Probst V, Denjoy I, Meregalli PG, et al. Clinical aspects and prognosis of Brugada syndrome in children. *Circulation.* 2007;115(15): 2042–2048.

Remme CA, Engelen MA, van Brunschot S, et al. Severity of conduction disease and development of cardiac structural abnormalities in sodium channel disease depends on genetic background [Abstract]. *Heart Rhythm.* 2007;4(5 suppl):S60–S61.

Remme CA, Verkerk AO, Nuyens D, et al. Overlap syndrome of cardiac sodium channel disease in mice carrying the equivalent mutation of human SCN5A-1795insD. *Circulation.* 2006;114(24):2584–2594.

Rook MB, Bezzina AC, Groenewegen WA, et al. Human SCN5A gene mutations alter cardiac sodium channel kinetics and are associated with the Brugada syndrome. *Cardiovasc Res.* 1999;44(3):507–517.

Rossenbacker T, Carroll SJ, Liu H, et al. Novel pore mutation in SCN5A manifests as a spectrum of phenotypes ranging from atrial flutter, conduction disease, and Brugada syndrome to sudden cardiac death. *Heart Rhythm.* 2004;1(5):610–615.

Rossenbacker T, Priori SG. The Brugada syndrome. *Curr Opin Cardiol.* 2007;22(3):163–170.

Rossenbacker T, Schollen E, Kuiperi C, et al. Unconventional intronic splice site mutation in SCN5A associates with cardiac sodium channelopathy. *J Med Genet.* 2005;42(5):e29.

Royer A, van Veen TA, Le BS, et al. Mouse model of SCN5A-linked hereditary Lenegre's disease: age-related conduction slowing and myocardial fibrosis. *Circulation.* 2005;111(14):1738–1746.

Sacher F, Probst V, Iesaka Y, et al. Outcome after implantation of a cardioverter-defibrillator in patients with Brugada syndrome. A Multicenter Study. *Circulation.* 2006;114(22):2317–2324.

Sakabe M, Fujiki A, Tani M, Nishida K, Mizumaki K, Inoue H. Proportion and prognosis of healthy people with coved or saddle-back type ST segment elevation in the right precordial leads during 10 years follow-up. *Eur Heart J.* 2003;24(16):1488–1493.

Sanatani S, Mahkseed N, Vallance H, Brugada R. The Brugada ECG pattern in a neonate. *J Cardiovasc Electrophysiol.* 2005;16(3):342–344.

Sangwatanaroj S, Prechawat S, Sunsaneewitayakul B, Sitthisook S, Tosukhowong P, Tungsanga K. New electrocardiographic leads and the procainamide test for the detection of the Brugada sign in sudden unexplained death syndrome survivors and their relatives. *Eur Heart J.* 2001;22(24):2290–2296.

Santambrogio LG, Mencherini S, Fuardo M, Caramella F, Braschi A. The surgical patient with Brugada syndrome: a four-case clinical experience. *Anesth Analg.* 2005;100(5):1263–1266.

Sarkozy A, Boussy T, Kourgiannides G, et al. Long-term follow-up of primary prophylactic implantable cardioverter-defibrillator therapy in Brugada syndrome. *Eur Heart J.* 2007;28(3):334–344.

Sasaki T, Niwano S, Kitano Y, Izumi T. Two cases of Brugada syndrome associated with spontaneous clinical episodes of coronary vasospasm. *Intern Med.* 2006;45(2):77–80.

Saura D, Garcia-Alberola A, Carrillo P, Pascual D, Martinez-Sanchez J, Valdes M. Brugada-like electrocardiographic pattern induced by fever. *Pacing Clin Electrophysiol.* 2002;25(5):856–859.

Schott JJ, Alshinawi C, Kyndt F, et al. Cardiac conduction defects associate with mutations in SCN5A. *Nat Genet.* 1999;23(1):20–21.

Schukro C, Berger T, Stix G, et al. Regional prevalence and clinical benefit of implantable cardioverter defibrillators in Brugada syndrome. *Int J Cardiol.* 2009; doi:10.1016/j.ijcard.2009.03.136.

Schwartz PJ, Moss AJ, Vincent GM, Crampton RS. Diagnostic criteria for the long QT syndrome. An update. *Circulation.* 1993;88(2):782–784.

Shimada M, Miyazaki T, Miyoshi S, et al. Sustained monomorphic ventricular tachycardia in a patient with Brugada syndrome. *Jpn Circ J.* 1996;60(6):364–370.

Shimizu W, Matsuo K, Kokubo Y, et al. Sex hormone and gender difference--role of testosterone on male predominance in Brugada syndrome. *J Cardiovasc Electrophysiol.* 2007;18(4):415–421.

Shimizu W, Matsuo K, Takagi M, et al. Body surface distribution and response to drugs of ST segment elevation in Brugada syndrome: clinical implication of eighty-seven-lead body surface potential mapping and its application to twelve-lead electrocardiograms. *J Cardiovasc Electrophysiol.* 2000;11(4):396–404.

Shin SC, Ryu HM, Lee JH, et al. Prevalence of the Brugada-type ECG recorded from higher intercostal spaces in healthy Korean males. *Circ J.* 2005;69(9):1064–1067.

Simson MB, Untereker WJ, Spielman SR, et al. Relation between late potentials on the body surface and directly recorded fragmented electrograms in patients with ventricular tachycardia. *Am J Cardiol.* 1983;51(1):105–112.

Skinner JR, Chung SK, Montgomery D, et al. Near-miss SIDS due to Brugada syndrome. *Arch Dis Child.* 2005;90(5):528–529.

Skinner JR, Chung SK, Nel CA, et al. Brugada syndrome masquerading as febrile seizures. *Pediatrics.* 2007;119(5):e1206–e1211.

Smith J, Hannah A, Birnie DH. Effect of temperature on the Brugada ECG. *Heart.* 2003;89(3):272.

Smits JP, Eckardt L, Probst V, et al. Genotype-phenotype relationship in Brugada syndrome: electrocardiographic features differentiate SCN5A-related patients from non-SCN5A-related patients. *J Am Coll Cardiol.* 2002;40(2):350–356.

Suzuki H, Torigoe K, Numata O, Yazaki S. Infant case with a malignant form of Brugada syndrome. *J Cardiovasc Electrophysiol.* 2000;11(11):1277–1280.

Tada H, Aihara N, Ohe T, et al. Arrhythmogenic right ventricular cardiomyopathy underlies syndrome of right bundle branch block, ST-segment elevation, and sudden death. *Am J Cardiol.* 1998;81(4):519–522.

Takagi M, Aihara N, Kuribayashi S, et al. Localized right ventricular morphological abnormalities detected by electron-beam computed tomography represent arrhythmogenic substrates in patients with the Brugada syndrome. *Eur Heart J.* 2001;22(12):1032–1041.

Takagi M, Aihara N, Kuribayashi S, et al. Abnormal response to sodium channel blockers in patients with Brugada syndrome: augmented localised wall motion abnormalities in the right ventricular outflow tract region detected by electron beam computed tomography. *Heart.* 2003;89(2):169–174.

Takagi M, Aihara N, Takaki H, et al. Clinical characteristics of patients with spontaneous or inducible ventricular fibrillation without apparent heart disease presenting with J wave and ST segment elevation in inferior leads. *J Cardiovasc Electrophysiol.* 2000;11(8):844–848.

Takami M, Ikeda T, Enjoji Y, Sugi K. Relationship between ST-segment morphology and conduction disturbances detected by signal-averaged electrocardiography in Brugada syndrome. *Ann Noninvasive Electrocardiol.* 2003;8(1):30–36.

Tan HL, Bezzina CR, Smits JP, Verkerk AO, Wilde AA. Genetic control of sodium channel function. *Cardiovasc Res.* 2003;57(4):961–973.

Tan HL, Meregalli PG. Lethal ECG changes hidden by therapeutic hypothermia. *Lancet.* 2007;369(9555):78.

Tanaka H, Kinoshita O, Uchikawa S, et al. Successful prevention of recurrent ventricular fibrillation by intravenous isoproterenol in a patient with Brugada syndrome. *Pacing Clin Electrophysiol.* 2001;24(8 Pt 1):1293–1294.

Tatsumi H, Takagi M, Nakagawa E, Yamashita H, Yoshiyama M. Risk stratification in patients with Brugada syndrome: analysis of daily fluctuations in 12-lead electrocardiogram (ECG) and signal-averaged electrocardiogram (SAECG). *J Cardiovasc Electrophysiol.* 2006;17(7):705–711.

Todd SJ, Campbell MJ, Roden DM, Kannankeril PJ. Novel Brugada SCN5A mutation causing sudden death in children. *Heart Rhythm.* 2005;2(5):540–543.

Tsuji H, Sato T, Morisaki K, Iwasaka T. Prognosis of subjects with Brugada-type electrocardiogram in a population of middle-aged Japanese diagnosed during a health examination. *Am J Cardiol.* 2008;102(5):584–587.

Tukkie R, Sogaard P, Vleugels J, de GI, Wilde AA, Tan HL. Delay in right ventricular activation contributes to Brugada syndrome. *Circulation.* 2004;109(10):1272–1277.

Ueyama T, Shimizu A, Esato M, et al. A case of a concealed type of Brugada syndrome with a J wave and mild ST-segment elevation in the inferolateral leads. *J Electrocardiol.* 2007;40(1):39–42.

van den Berg MP, Wiesfeld AC. Brugada syndrome with ST-segment elevation in the lateral leads. *J Cardiovasc Electrophysiol.* 2006;17(9):1035.

van Veen TA, Stein M, Royer A, et al. Impaired impulse propagation in Scn5a-knockout mice: combined contribution of excitability, connexin expression, and tissue architecture in relation to aging. *Circulation.* 2005;112(13):1927–1935.

Vatta M, Dumaine R, Varghese G, et al. Genetic and biophysical basis of sudden unexplained nocturnal death syndrome (SUNDS), a disease allelic to Brugada syndrome. *Hum Mol Genet.* 2002;11(3):337–345.

Veldkamp MW, Viswanathan PC, Bezzina C, Baartscheer A, Wilde AA, Balser JR. Two distinct congenital arrhythmias evoked by a multidysfunctional Na(+) channel. *Circ Res.* 2000;86(9):E91–E97.

Veltmann C, Schimpf R, Echternach C, et al. A prospective study on spontaneous fluctuations between diagnostic and non-diagnostic ECGs in Brugada syndrome: implications for correct phenotyping and risk stratification. *Eur Heart J.* 2006;27(21):2544–2554.

Viskin S. Brugada syndrome in children: don't ask, don't tell? *Circulation.* 2007;115(15):1970–1972.

Viskin S, Fish R, Eldar M, et al. Prevalence of the Brugada sign in idiopathic ventricular fibrillation and healthy controls. *Heart.* 2000;84(1):31–36.

Wajed A, Aslam Z, Abbas SF, et al. Frequency of Brugada-type ECG pattern (Brugada sign) in an apparently healthy young population. *J Ayub Med Coll Abbottabad.* 2008;20(3):121–124.

Wang DW, Desai RR, Crotti L, et al. Cardiac sodium channel dysfunction in sudden infant death syndrome. *Circulation.* 2007;115(3):368–376.

Wang Q, Shen J, Li Z, et al. Cardiac sodium channel mutations in patients with long QT syndrome, an inherited cardiac arrhythmia. *Hum Mol Genet.* 1995;4(9):1603–1607.

Watanabe A, Kusano KF, Morita H, et al. Low-dose isoproterenol for repetitive ventricular arrhythmia in patients with Brugada syndrome. *Eur Heart J.* 2006;27(13):1579–1583.

Watanabe H, Koopmann TT, Le Scouarnec S, et al. Sodium channel beta1 subunit mutations associated with Brugada syndrome and cardiac conduction disease in humans. *J Clin Invest.* 2008;118(6):2260–2268.

Weiss R, Barmada MM, Nguyen T, et al. Clinical and molecular heterogeneity in the Brugada syndrome: a novel gene locus on chromosome 3. *Circulation.* 2002;105(6):707–713.

Wilde A, Duren D. Sudden cardiac death, RBBB, and right precordial ST-segment elevation. *Circulation.* 1999;99(5):722–723.

Wilde AA, Antzelevitch C, Borggrefe M, et al. Proposed diagnostic criteria for the Brugada syndrome. *Eur Heart J.* 2002;23(21):1648–1654.

Wilde AA, Bezzina CR. Genetics of cardiac arrhythmias. *Heart.* 2005;91(10):1352–1358.

Wolpert C, Echternach C, Veltmann C, et al. Intravenous drug challenge using flecainide and ajmaline in patients with Brugada syndrome. *Heart Rhythm.* 2005;2(3):254–260.

Wu LS, Wu CT, Hsu LA, Luqman N, Kuo CT. Brugada-like electrocardiographic pattern and ventricular fibrillation in a patient with primary hyperparathyroidism. *Europace.* 2007;9(3):172–174.

Yamakawa Y, Ishikawa T, Uchino K, et al. Prevalence of right bundle-branch block and right precordial ST-segment elevation (Brugada-type electrocardiogram) in Japanese children. *Circ J.* 2004;68(4):275–279.

Yan GX, Antzelevitch. Cellular basis for the Brugada syndrome and other mechanisms of arrhythmogenesis associated with ST-segment elevation. *Circulation.* 1999;100(15):1660–1666.

Yoshinaga M, Anan R, Nomura Y, et al. Prevalence and time of appearance of Brugada electrocardiographic pattern in young male adolescents from a three-year follow-up study. *Am J Cardiol.* 2004;94(9):1186–1189.

Zipes DP, Camm AJ, Borggrefe M, et al. ACC/AHA/ESC 2006 Guidelines for Management of Patients with Ventricular Arrhythmias and the Prevention of Sudden Cardiac Death: a report of the American College of Cardiology/American Heart Association Task Force and the European Society of Cardiology Committee for Practice Guidelines (writing committee to develop Guidelines for Management of Patients With Ventricular Arrhythmias and the Prevention of Sudden Cardiac Death): developed in collaboration with the European Heart Rhythm Association and the Heart Rhythm Society. *Circulation.* 2006;114(10):e385–e484.

Zipes DP, Libby P, Bonow RO, Braunwald E (eds). *Braunwald's Heart Disease: A Textbook of Cardiovascular Medicine*, 7th ed. Elsevier Saunders, Philadelphia; 2005.

20

Inherited Conduction Disease and Familial Atrial Fibrillation

Calum A MacRae

Introduction

Arrhythmias in general, and conduction disease and atrial fibrillation (AF) in particular, are common features in a broad range of heart diseases, both acquired and inherited. As a result of familiarity, these arrh0ythmias are often considered a consequence of final common pathways that are present in all forms of cardiac disease. However, diverse biological mechanisms are emerging as highly specific explanations for many arrhythmias, including conduction disease and AF. For example, AF is often conceived as a consequence of atrial distension, but in recent years roles for a host of other stimuli have emerged in the pathogenesis of this common arrhythmia. Inflammation, dehydration, and the renin-angiotensin system all have been implicated, and in many instances may coexist in an individual patient. Such diverse potential mechanisms have raised suggestions of innate complexity in the etiology of arrhythmias, with speculation on a proarrhythmic threshold that may be attained through many different pathways. A competing notion is that there are many forms of conduction disease or AF, each with a distinctive mechanism. It is likely that both hypotheses are valid. While in some individuals the concerted action of several pathways underlies the initiation of an arrhythmia, in others a single stimulus is sufficient. Genetic studies have proven remarkably powerful in the face of biological complexity, and in recent years inroads have begun to be made into the genetics of conduction disease and AF.

Inherited Conduction Disease

Multiple different disorders are included within the rubric of conduction disease, including perturbations of rhythm generation, atrioventricular (AV) conduction, and [intraventricular conduction]. There is considerable overlap among these syndromes, but also between classic conduction disease and many other cardiac disorders. As a result of the gestalt that such features represent generic effects of heart muscle damage, little effort has been focused on understanding the epidemiologic relationships between the various components of conduction disease and other cardiac phenotypes. Inherited forms of conduction disease offer a unique window into many syndromic associations (see Table 20–1) suggesting shared pathophysiologic mechanisms, but to date the responsible genes have proven largely inaccessible. For example, the relationship between AV conduction disease, ventricular preexcitation, and metabolic abnormalities extends across a number of conditions, but only as the genes for some of these disorders become known are the potential mechanistic links beginning to be understood.

Mechanisms of Conduction Disease

Inherited defects act at multiple time points throughout life. The patterning of cardiac form and function are closely intertwined, and subtle yet highly specific physiologic perturbations may lead to abnormal myocyte specification as well as macroscopic anatomic abnormalities.

Despite their phenotypic heterogeneity and highly specialized functions, peripheral conduction system cells and contractile myocytes are derived from common precursors. Although a significant proportion of AV conduction disease can be attributed to ischemic damage to the conduction tissues, the majority of conduction abnormalities are classified as degenerative. The underlying mechanism in these individuals is variously described as fibrosis or atrophy of the specialized conduction tissues. However, pathology studies are rather selected and almost all have failed to address the extent of coexisting ventricular disease. The disparate rates of progression in conduction disease suggest that other aspects of these disorders determine the final outcomes, and to some extent such differences are reflected in the patterns of conduction disease. The typical terminal events are sudden death or heart failure rather than bradycardia, suggesting that there is more to the pathophysiology than a simple failure of electrical conduction (Figure 20–1). Each syndrome may represent the distinctive involvement of a specific class of myocytes or a specific molecular pathway. For example, right bundle branch block with progressive leftward axis shift (classic bifascicular block) may represent a unique pattern of cell loss within the conduction system rather than the destruction of macroscopic fiber tracts that have proven histologically elusive. Similarly, particular metabolic defects may act on specific developmental events, in specific myocardial cell types, or through specific proarrhythmic pathways. These hypotheses are at least partly supported by the segregation of such conduction disease patterns through individual families.

Table 20–1 Genes and Loci Implicated in Conduction Disease

Specific Genes	Chromosome	Gene Name	Inheritance	Comments	Reference
	1q12–21	*LMNA*	AD	SA, AF, AV, DCM	Fatkin et al. 1999
	3p21–23	*SCN5A*	AD	SA, AF, AV, DCM	Schott et al. 1999
	7q36	*PRKAG2*	AD	AV, WPW, LVH	Arad et al. 2002
	15q23	*HCN4*	AD	SA	Milanesi et al. 2006
	19q13.32	Myotonin kinase	AD	AV, MD, Anticipation	Mahadevan et al. 1993
	Xq28	Emerin	XLD	SA, AV, MD	Bione et al. 1994
	Mitochondrial	Multiple genes	Maternal	SA, AF, AV	Anan et al. 2002
Genetic Loci	**Chromosome**	**Gene**	**Inheritance**		**Reference**
	19p13	Unknown	AD	AV	de Meeus et al. 1995

Notes: AD, autosomal dominant; XLD, X-linked; SA, sinoatrial conduction disease; AF, atrial fibrillation; AV, atrioventricular conduction disease; DCM, dilated cardiomyopathy; WPW, Wolff-Parkinson-White preexcitiation syndrome; LVH, left ventricular hypertrophy; MD, skeletal muscular dystrophy.

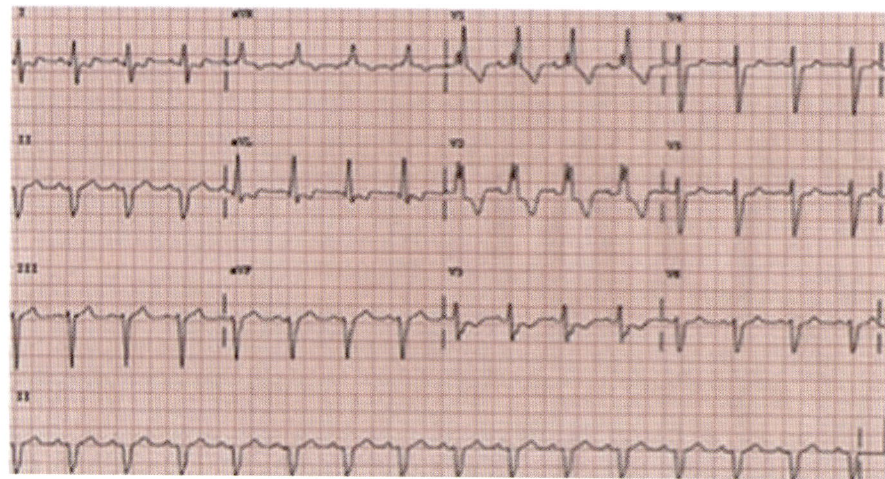

Figure 20–1 The classic ECG of advancing conduction disease often breeds true segregating through individual kindreds. While in some instances this may truly represent conduction disease involving the right bundle and one of the left-sided fascicles, the reproducibility of the progression in multiple individuals and the association with several diffuse myocardial diseases suggest the discrete involvement of a specific subset of myocytes or a specific pathway.

While to date the specific mechanisms responsible for most forms of human conduction disease remain obscure, some general insights have been gained from animal models and other experimental systems.

1. Sinoatrial Disease

Classic interpretation of sinoatrial disease as a focal degenerative disorder of the anatomic sinus node does not explain the distinctive associations of this syndrome with specific mutations causing structural human heart disease (Seidman and Seidman 2001). Precise genetic modeling of several human congenital structural anomalies or cardiomyopathies in the mouse also results in sinoatrial arrhythmias (Berul et al. 1997). These data suggest that either the primary disorder itself or a compensatory downstream response affects not only the fundamental structure or function of working myocytes, valve tissues, or vessels, but also specialized pacemaker and conduction tissue.

Mouse models of many different human disease alleles have unexpectedly caused sinus node disease, suggesting conduction system involvement in [different forms of] heart muscle disease. Some of these instances may represent the misinterpretation of secondary bradycardia and AV block resulting from preterminal hypoxia, acidosis, or other metabolic derangements (London 2001). A more general explanation is that many murine models are often imperfect transgenic overexpression models or harbor null alleles, and when specific knockin models of human mutant alleles are made phenotypes are much more faithfully reproduced without any associated pleiotropy. These findings suggest that the human disorders are the result of very specific perturbations of the pathway(s) in which the mutant proteins participate (Mohler et al. 2003; Casimiro et al. 2004).

2. AV Conduction Disease

Several knockout mice exhibit AV block, and further exploration in these models suggests that perturbations of action potential prolongation and cell–cell coupling play a mechanistic role in conduction disease. The transcription factor HF-1b is expressed in ventricular myocytes and the conduction system. Knockout of HF-1b results in sinus pauses, sinus bradycardia, and second- or third-degree AV block. These mice also develop spontaneous episodes of ventricular tachycardia. Analysis showed abnormal expression and distribution of *KCNE2*, connexin 40, and prolongation of the action potential duration that was at least in part due to diminished IK_s (Nguyen-Tran et al. 2000). Connexin 40 is expressed throughout the mouse atria and conduction system and is directly implicated in cell–cell coupling and impulse propagation. Therefore, it is not surprising that the connexin 40 knockout mouse has a prolonged PR interval with documented slowing of conduction in the AV node, and bundle branch system (VanderBrink et al. 2000). Several elegant papers have delineated the conduction deficits in these knockout models. There is evidence of tetralogy of Fallot and double outflow right ventricle on some genetic backgrounds (Gu et al. 2003), but concrete parallels with human disease are unclear. Some murine models have predicted human disease, such as the HCN4 null mice, but in general links with human disorders are [obscure], largely because of differences in the allelic structure of human disease. Few human disorders of conduction appear to result from true recessive null alleles, and the genes that cause human conduction disease may do so through gain of function that is difficult to predict.

The unique physiology of the cells within the conduction system is emphasized by the precise defects observed in several metabolic disorders including mitochondrial diseases, storage disorders, and inborn errors of metabolism. These [highly] specific [abnormalities] may partly reflect the role of calcium conductance and active transport in the conduction system, but many other molecular attributes including distinctive intercellular junctions, discrete membrane turnover, or unique sarcomeric protein isoforms may predispose the conduction system in these particular conditions. Differential sensitivity to metabolic defects also extends to other cell types, but may be more difficult to define anatomically. For example, ventricular myocytes appear particularly sensitive to defects in fatty acid oxidation. Passive storage itself may be quite localized, and many other intracellular processes are highly regionalized throughout the heart. Differential effects across apicobasal or endocardial-epicardial gradients result in [exaggerated] myocardial heterogeneity: a major substrate for reentrant arrhythmias.

Mouse modeling of the effects of cardiac sodium channel *SCN5A* gene dosage noted that haploinsufficient mice develop 2:1 AV block and display [slowed] myocardial conduction and myocardial fibrosis (Papadatos et al. 2002). In humans, [some] mutations in the *SCN5A* gene also result in isolated conduction system disease with AV block (Schott et al. 1999).

Types of Conduction Disease

The classical frameworks of conduction disease were defined in the 1950s [on a largely empirical basis] using the surface electrocardiogram. Rigorous anatomic correlation has long been a problem for several aspects of this framework, and many observations suggest that the relationships between structural and functional abnormalities are considerably less straightforward. Nevertheless, patterns of structure–function correlation have been observed, such as the extreme leftward axis deviation associated with ostium primum atrial septal defects. These observations suggest that there may be complex electrical pathways within the heart, which, by analogy to central nervous system nuclei, may be [electrically] coupled to the rest of the myocardium but play very specific [physiologic] roles. While there is essentially no postnatal cell division within the human heart, multiple cell types exist within the myocardial syncytium. Emerging data suggest that there are apicobasal and endocardial-epicardial gradients of electrical function within the adult ventricle, yet the precise factors responsible for the specification and maintenance of these gradients are unknown. Taken together these data suggest that the current classification of conduction disease may be further refined by human genetic studies.

Genetic Epidemiology of Conduction Disease

There have been few if any systematic studies of the heritability of conduction disease. The relatively advanced age of onset of most clinically significant AV block, and the widely held perception that the mechanisms of the syndrome are "degenerative" have undoubtedly contributed to this situation. Nevertheless, there is circumstantial evidence that a significant proportion of conduction disease at any age is likely inherited. There are multiple kindreds in the literature where conduction disorders cosegregate as apparently monogenic autosomal traits, both in isolation and in the context of other cardiac conditions.

The only well-studied subset of conduction disease is that occurring in association with dilated cardiomyopathy (DCM), where multiple kindreds have been described where the two disorders cosegregate as a single autosomal dominant trait (Graber et al. 1986). Cross-sectional studies of proband cohorts with idiopathic DCM find that approximately 30% of such cases have significant AV conduction disease (Schoeller et al. 1993). AV conduction disease is the only additional risk factor for mortality in these cohorts once left ventricular (LV) ejection fraction is accounted for. The AV block often precedes any detectable ventricular dysfunction, but this is not universal. In some families the evidence of ventricular disease is minimal. However, postmortem studies suggest that there is diffuse involvement of the atrial, nodal, and ventricular myocardium irrespective of the clinical picture.

Detailed studies are currently underway to unravel the details of the inherited contribution to conduction disease.

Mendelian Forms of Conduction Disease

Clinicians and geneticists share a search for new, more specific, more homogeneous phenotypes in an attempt to dissect syndromes, that is, collections of empiric symptoms, signs, and results into their component disorders. The study of extended families offers a unique opportunity to look for the subtle clues of such distinction. Clinical genetics can help to clarify the relationships between phenotypes, but ultimately the identification of the underlying primary genetic causes through molecular studies in such families will offer insights into these conditions. The genes have been cloned for several monogenic disorders in which conduction disease is prominent, and mechanistic understanding will hopefully aid in the genetic dissection of other Mendelian forms of conduction disease.

1. Sinoatrial Disease

I. HCN4 In vitro studies and murine modeling had identified the hyperpolarization-activated cyclic nucleotide-gated (HCN) channels as key components of the pacemaker current and predicted that these same channels might be a cause of familial sinoatrial disease. To date only isolated kindreds have been identified with mutations in the HCN4 channel gene, but these families exhibit highly penetrant sinus bradycardia. Interestingly, [such] kindreds do not display more complex arrhythmias, and affected individuals are essentially asymptomatic, further underlining the precision of many molecular defects.

II. Cardiac Sodium Channel There is some evidence that compound heterozyg[osity] for SCN5A alleles cause a rare congenital form of sick sinus syndrome, with sinus bradycardia or sinus arrest. The relationship to adult forms of this disorder is unknown. Heterozygous SCN5A mutations have also been implicated in occasional families with sinoatrial disease, AF, Brugada syndrome, AV block, and DCM. Resequencing of SCN5A in larger cohorts suggests that mutations in this gene are a rare cause of these phenotypes.

2. AV Conduction Disease with Dilated Cardiomyopathy

III. Myotonic Dystrophy Myotonic dystrophy is the most common form of muscular dystrophy and is due to an expansion of a trinucleotide repeat on human chromosome 19. Cardiac manifestations include varying degrees of AV block as well as sudden death. Occasional kindreds will display atrial arrhythmias, which may dominate the clinical picture. Dispute over the molecular mechanism of the cardiac defects has been addressed by the development of a mouse knockout model of the myotonic dystrophy protein kinase (DMPK). Mice deficient in DMPK display first-, second-, and third-degree AV block, while the haploinsufficient mice show first-degree AV block (Berul et al. 1999). By analogy with defects seen in the skeletal muscle of these mice, the mechanism of AV nodal pathology is thought to be due to alterations in the activation kinetics or amplitude of the ICa,L current.

IV. Emery Dreifuss Muscular Dystrophies The archetypal form of muscular dystrophy with prominent high-grade AV block was first described by Emery and Dreifuss (EDMD). Classically X-linked, but with autosomal dominant variants, the syndrome is characterized by onset in the first to third decade usually with tendon contractures. Progressive conduction disease is present in virtually all cases and leads to permanent pacing. Of note, when compared with the dystrophinopathies and myotonic dystrophy, atrial standstill is a hallmark of EDMD, but atrial arrhythmias and sudden death also are prominent in this syndrome. The extent of the associated cardiomyopathy is variable as is the humeroperoneal skeletal involvement. CPK is usually mildly elevated. Clinical genetics suggested that EDMD is a disorder of a distinct pathway and molecular studies confirmed this when mutations in a novel gene emerin, encoding a nuclear membrane protein, were identified as the cause of the X-linked form.

The major autosomal form of EDMD is caused by mutations in the lamin A/C gene, encoding another nuclear envelope protein. To date no unifying biological mechanism has been uncovered to explain the specific effects of mutations in emerin or lamin A/C on cardiac conduction system, myocardial contractility, and humeroperoneal muscle groups. Some animal models replicate clinical features of these disorders, but though effects on both transcription and nuclear integrity have been observed, the mechanism of restriction to particular tissues is obscure. The situation is further complicated by the marked pleiotropy observed with mutations in the lamin A/C gene. Mutations in this same gene have been implicated in a remarkable array of other clinical syndromes including Charcot-Marie-Tooth variants, isolated limb-girdle dystrophies, peripheral neuropathies, partial lipodystrophies, metabolic syndrome, and Hutchison-Gilford type progeria. Clearly, dissecting the mechanism by which mutations in a single gene can result in this degree of phenotypic complexity will be necessary if the fundamental biology of the disease is to be understood.

Interestingly, there may be subtle differences in the severity of the cardiac phenotypes seen in lamin A/C disease between genders. Many affected males will have significant cardiac disease, often with moderate or severe LV dysfunction, in the first two to three decades of life. Females bearing the same mutations are more likely to exhibit progressive conduction disease, less severe LV dysfunction, and will also develop skeletal symptoms later in life. These findings suggest that some of the apparent pleiotropy is a function of phenotypic resolution. It remains to be seen if a mechanistic interaction between lamin and emerin is the explanation for these genetic observations.

V. Dystrophinopathy Clinically, Duchenne and Becker muscular dystrophies are relatively well circumscribed. The trait is inherited as an X-linked recessive with onset in the first or second decade. Associated conduction disease is limited in that it rarely progresses to high-grade AV block but PR prolongation and a peculiar IVCD with a prominent R-wave in V1 are often seen. AF is unusual but typical DCM is often seen. Contractures are not observed, but skeletal muscle involvement is present although it may be subclinical as in the X-linked DCM families. Creatine phosphokinase is markedly elevated. The dystrophin gene is a large cytoskeletal protein with an actin-binding amino terminal domain, a central rod domain composed of spectrin repeats and a cysteine-rich domain as well as a unique carboxy terminal domain. It plays a central role in the dystrophin-glycoprotein complex, which also includes the sarcoglycans and the dystroglycans. [This complex] is thought to organize specific membrane domains, orchestrate signal transduction, and regulate sarcolemmal membrane cycling and membrane integrity. Interestingly, other members of the dystrophin-glycoprotein complex have been implicated in several recessive forms of muscular dystrophy where prominent cardiac phenotypes are not observed.

3. AV Conduction Disease with Hypertrophy

VI. PRKAG2 Disease Another form of inherited heart disease characterized by conduction system disease is caused by mutation of the gamma subunit of the AMP-activated protein kinase. This disorder is characterized by pseudohypertrophy of the left and right ventricles due to glycogen deposition in cardiac muscle, with both accessory pathways and conduction system disturbances (Arad et al. 2002). These families had previously been included under the rubric of hypertrophic cardiomyopathy on the basis of their inheritance patterns, adult onset, and echocardiographic features (MacRae et al. 1995). AF and atrial flutter are common, but high-grade AV block is the dominant clinical arrhythmia (MacRae et al. 1995). Clinical studies suggest that many asymptomatic individuals are maximally preexcited at rest, and so probably dependent on accessory AV connections from an early age. Syncope and sudden death are reported in PRKAG2 families, but the mechanism is not always clear.

Clinically the most prominent complaints are atypical chest pain, palpitations, and exertional limitation. The chest pain may arise from the chest wall, is usually postexertional rather than exertional, and is often accompanied by variable skeletal muscle pains or cramps after exertion similar to those seen in classic McArdle's syndrome. Exertional limitation appears to correlate with exercise hypotension, and also may reflect peripheral muscle metabolic signals rather than any specific cardiac abnormality. The index of suspicion for PRKAG2 disease is raised by massive LV wall thickening (>30 mm) and by the presence of high-grade AV block, as these features are rare in hypertrophic heart disease caused by sarcomere gene mutations.

A mouse model carrying a mutation responsible for the human disease has been generated that faithfully reproduces the three characteristic phenotypes found in the human disease (Arad et al. 2003). In this model the annulus fibrosis that normally insulates the atria and ventricles is penetrated by glycogen-filled cardiomyocytes that appear to be responsible for ventricular preexcitation.

Of note, there is significant phenotypic overlap between PRKAG2 disease and Danon disease, which previously had been classified as a glycogen storage disorder, despite the inconsistent presence of glycogen on biopsy (Arad et al. 2005). The identification of mutations in the lysosomal-associated membrane protein LAMP2 confirmed this as a vacuolar myopathy. The clinical course is malignant, complicated by ventricular arrhythmias and intractable heart failure, and this may explain the failure to observe AV block in this syndrome.

VII. Other Rare Storage Disorders Many of the classic metabolic storage disorders are associated with cardiac involvement (Guertl et al. 2000). Neurologic or respiratory failure is often the cause of early death. Cardiac manifestations, including massive LV wall thickening (a combination of deposition and true hypertrophy) and valvular involvement, though present to some degrees in all cases, may emerge as a problem only later in life in those who survive as a result of therapeutic intervention or less penetrant alleles (Kelly and Strauss 1994; Guertl et al. 2000). Prominent evidence of AV conduction disease, often with ventricular preexcitation, is seen in all of these diseases, while atrial arrhythmias are also a frequent problem.

Pompe's disease typically results in massive thickening of the ventricular wall in childhood, sometimes with endocardial fibroelastosis (Kelly and Strauss 1994; Guertl et al. 2000). There is usually evidence of ventricular preexcitation as well as bizarre fractionation of the entire surface electrogram (Moses et al. 1989). While ectopy is commonly seen, arrhythmias do not dominate the clinical course and death is usually from cardiorespiratory failure. Defects in glycogen phosporylase (McArdle's disease), brancher or debrancher enzymes, all are reported to cause AV conduction system disease and DCM with disproportionate wall thickening (Guertl et al. 2000). In these disorders, heart failure and sudden death are seen occasionally.

Anderson-Fabry disease is an X-linked storage disorder characterized by angiokeratomata, acroparesthiae, abdominal pain, renal, and cardiac disease (Guertl et al. 2000). Female heterozygotes often exhibit much less penetrant forms of the disease and late-onset variants with predominant cardiac involvement exist (Chimenti et al. 2004). In general, the incidence of cardiovascular symptoms in males and females is similar. Ventricular thickening is common especially in males, and correlates with the risk of nonsustained ventricular tachycardia (Shah et al. 2005). AF is the most frequent arrhythmia. AV conduction system disease and preexcitation are less common than in many other storage disorders.

Cardiac involvement is the rule rather than the exception in a host of other rare storage disorders including mucopolysaccharidoses, mucolipidoses, gangliosidoses, and neuronal ceroid lipofuscinosis (Guertl et al. 2000). The majority of these conditions are recessive and lethal in childhood. Reports of arrhythmias are rare, but are dominated by AV block.

VIII. Disorders of Lipid Metabolism At rest, free fatty acids constitute the predominant myocardial substrate; so it is not surprising that several inherited disorders of fatty acid oxidation present with early-onset cardiomyopathy and arrhythmias. Abnormal carnitine transport into cells or into mitochondria as well as defects in several mitochondrial enzymes required for fatty acid oxidation can result in cardiomyopathies (Bonnet et al. 1999; Longo et al. 2006). Overt cardiac involvement is present in over 50% of those with fatty acid oxidation defects. Presentation is usually precipitated by fasting, depletion of glycogen stores, and consequent dependence on fatty acid as an energy substrate. In typical acute metabolic crises, characterized by hypoglycemia, lactic acidosis, hepatic dysfunction, blunted ketone formation, and hypotonia, arrhythmias are a common feature (Bonnet et al. 1999). Arrhythmias may be prominent in a substantial minority of cases, irrespective of overt evidence of cardiomyopathy. Sinus node dysfunction, paroxysmal supraventricular arrhythmias, AV block, and intraventricular conduction abnormalities all are reported (Bonnet et al. 1999). It is difficult to make definitive correlations in such rare disorders, but there may be a propensity to specific arrhythmias with different defects. While the majority of fatty acid oxidation disorders are recognized in the first 2 to 3 years of life, there are well-documented cases that have presented in adulthood (Feillet et al. 2003).

4. AV Conduction Disease with Structural Congenital Heart Disease

IX. Holt-Oram Syndrome (TBX5) Conduction disease is a feature of [the] Holt-Oram hand-heart syndrome caused by mutations in the transcription factor TBX5. First-degree AV block is often present even when anatomical septal defects are not found. The role of TBX5 in the specification and maintenance of the proximal conduction system is emerging from elegant studies in the mouse.

X. NKX2.5 Mutations in the NKX2.5 gene, an ortholog of the Drosophila homeobox gene tinman that is required for cardiac development, result in atrial septal defects and conduction system disease. More complex congenital heart defects have also been associated with this gene, but precise genotype–phenotype correlations with respect to associated conduction disease have not emerged.

Specific Loci for Which the Disease Genes are not Yet Known

There are several disorders where conduction disease is a prominent feature and genetic analyses have identified a unique genomic locus, but to date the causal gene has not been identified. These include the progressive familial heart blocks, forms of isolated AV conduction disease, and conduction disease found in association with several forms of congenital heart disease.

There are also additional loci yet to be discovered for many forms of conduction disease. Families exist with sick sinus syndrome, AV conduction disease, isolated bundle branch blocks, and autosomal dominant EDMD, which do not map to any of the known loci for each of these conditions. The tremendous genetic heterogeneity seen in other inherited cardiac disorders is likely to be present in conduction disease, and a concerted effort in clinical and molecular investigation will be required to unravel the genetic contribution to conduction disease.

Candidate Genes

To date the candidates that have been studied in conduction disease reflect the causal genes already outlined above. As there have been few systematic attempts to collect proband-based cohorts with conduction disease large candidate screening efforts have not been published. As such cohorts emerge, and as resequencing technologies improve, the genes encoding other cardiac isoforms of ion channels and many interacting proteins will likely emerge as candidates. Similarly, other nuclear membrane protein genes will likely be screened in AV conduction disease with DCM.

Somatic Mutations

1. Mitochondrial Disorders

Specific mitochondrial DNA defects have quite variable effects as a result of differences in the extent of tissue heteroplasmy for mutant mitochondria. However, cardiac involvement is a central feature of several of the classic mitochondrial syndromes (Kelly and Strauss 1994). Cardiac expression of these defects is usually in the form of cardiomyopathy. AV conduction disease is a common feature of Kearns-Sayre syndrome and accessory AV connections are also reported (Anan et al. 1995). Importantly, the mutated gene in myotonic dystrophy (see above) recently has been implicated in mitochondrial function.

Common Forms of Conduction Disease

In the vast majority of human conduction disease there is no obvious inherited contribution. Sinoatrial disease and some degree of AV conduction disease are common in aging populations, and in most instances it is assumed that this is a reflection, as has been noted, of long-term degenerative processes. These features do not exclude an inherited component to the etiology, and the absence of symptoms in all but the latest stages of conduction disease may lead to significant difficulties in the detection of heritability should it exist. There is sufficient evidence from isolated families and population studies of heart rate, QRS duration, and other forms of conduction disease that systematic approaches to the genetic architecture of conduction disease are warranted. Some insights may be gained from ongoing genome-wide association studies for a range of electrocardiographic parameters including heart rate, [PR interval] and QRS duration.

Endophenotypes

Ultimately, understanding the genetic basis of conduction defects will likely require higher resolution phenotypes, causally related to the underlying diseases. The exploration of efficient noninvasive techniques to identify homogeneous subsets of conduction disease will improve the resolution of any genetic approaches. Potential subclinical phenotypes primarily involved in the underlying syndromes (so called endophenotypes) may include signal-averaged ECG, improved techniques for the detection of cardiomyopathy, and a host of extracardiac phenotypes. For example, the detection of subclinical limb-girdle skeletal myopathy has helped dissect the role of lamin mutations in AV block. Resolving phenotypic complexity in this way will be the key to advancing our understanding of the genetic basis of conduction disease, or indeed any other heritable disorder, and will require an intensive clinical investigation effort.

Current Clinical Implications

Our current understanding of the genetic contribution to conduction disease is rather limited, and the major clinical utility of these insights at present is to inform diagnosis and to aid in the identification of subsets that may benefit from additional therapy and prognosis. Thus, in those kindreds in which AV block and DCM cosegregate, the early presence of conduction disease may allow [cascade] screening efforts to be focused on individuals who are likely to develop subclinical LV dysfunction and benefit from the introduction of afterload reduction using angiotensin-converting enzyme inhibitors or angiotensin receptor blockers. Clearly, subtle conduction system disease may also be a marker for cardiac manifestations in a host of primary myocardial disorders, and so may aid in management under specific circumstances, such as anesthesia in subjects with mitochondrial disease.

Ultimately, the lack of systematic data on prognosis and the absence of specific therapies preclude the use of genetic insights over traditional clinical parameters, for example, standard electrocardiographic indications for permanent pacing. At present, there is no clear role for genetic testing in most forms of conduction system disease. The prevalence of lamin A/C mutations in AV block segregating with DCM or PRKAG2 mutations when such block is associated with increased wall thickness has led to commercial efforts to introduce genetic testing. Until predictive utility is compared with standard clinical criteria or there are specific therapies, it is difficult to justify testing outside of stringent research protocols.

Outstanding Questions and Future Directions

A host of questions remain in the genetics of inherited conduction disease. The role of major gene effects in late-onset forms of conduction disease will require extensive clinical studies and family collections, as will approaches to the genetic architecture of conduction disease. Study designs such as the kin-cohort strategy will ultimately be able to dissect gene–gene and gene–environment interactions. The identification of discrete subsets using biomarkers or other endophenotypes will aid clinical practice even if the inherited contribution to conduction disease is relatively small. Understanding the genetic basis and pathophysiology of inherited forms of conduction disease will [eventually] enable [improved] prediction of the need for pacing or anticoagulation, as well as allowing insights into the role of electrical stimuli in cardiac physiology and the development of novel therapies for conduction disease and its associated phenotypes.

Familial Atrial Fibrillation

AF, a disorder characterized by rapid, irregular electrical activation of the atrium, affects over 2 million Americans and is a major risk factor for heart failure and stroke (Chugh et al. 2001; Go et al. 2001) Despite the substantial morbidity associated with this arrhythmia, the etiology of AF remains poorly understood (Nattel 2002; Coyne et al. 2006).

AF is seen in virtually every form of structural heart disease, but also may exist in isolated forms (Kopecky et al. 1987; Chugh et al. 2001). The broad range of associations may suggest a complex final common pathway, although by analogy with other human syndromes, it is likely that AF represents an aggregation of unresolved, discrete phenotypes (Keating and Sanguinetti 2001; Seidman and Seidman 2001). Even in the face of apparent heterogeneity, there is evidence of a heritable etiologic contribution to some forms of AF, and in particular idiopathic, or lone AF (Darbar et al. 2003; Fox et al. 2004; Ellinor et al. 2005; Arnar et al. 2006). These findings suggest that there may be a genetically determined threshold for vulnerability to the arrhythmia.

Mechanistic Framework

As for conduction disease, the primary etiology of most forms of AF is unknown, and mechanistic insights rely on data from large animal models correlated with clinical observations in humans. Electrophysiologic studies using multiple electrodes or optical mapping have led to the emergence of overlapping conceptual models (Nattel 2002; Waldo 2003). Early canine studies suggested that increased automaticity could generate AF, but later work implicated single reentry circuits of very short cycle length as rapid "drivers" of AF. More recent optical mapping data has introduced the concept of focal reentry circuits rapidly stimulating the atria (Waldo 2003), while clinical observations demonstrating ectopic foci, most commonly in the pulmonary veins, have consolidated the role of spontaneous activity in the initiation of AF (Haissaguerre et al. 1998). These automatic foci have been reported not just in pulmonary veins, but also in other venous structures. These regions of increased automaticity are physically close to extensive nervous plexi, and there are already data that this innervation may play a role in promoting pulmonary vein ectopy (Katritsis and Ellenbogen 2004). A consensus is emerging that autonomous foci, single local reentrant circuits, and multiple reentrant circuits all may play a role in AF.

It has proven difficult to identify the primary molecular abnormalities in AF as the arrhythmia itself distorts the substrate, thus confounding the relationship between causal factors and epiphenomena (Allessie et al. 2002; Brundel et al. 2002). AF induces electrical, contractile, and molecular changes in the atrial myocytes that arise within minutes and may persist for a considerable time (Ausma et al. 2001). These changes include shortening of the atrial effective refractory period and loss of rate adaptation. The expression levels and subcellular compartmentalization of numerous ion channels, connexins, and calcium handling proteins are altered by AF, in part reactivating the fetal transcription program (Brundel et al. 2002; Nattel 2002). The remodeling process appears to be largely triggered by increased intracellular calcium, but other mechanisms also may be involved. Pretreatment with calcium channel blockers abrogates some components of remodeling, but may have a net proarrhythmic effect (Nattel 2002). The ultimate outcome of atrial remodeling is sarcomere loss, patchy apoptosis, focal inflammation, and fibrosis in the atria (Frustaci et al. 1997; Allessie et al. 2002; Nattel 2002).

One hint at the underlying biologic basis of a reduced threshold for AF is the beneficial effect of angiotensin-converting enzyme inhibition on the incidence of the arrhythmia in populations with subclinical LV dysfunction (Vermes et al. 2003). These data suggest that the inhibition of this pathway [may] prevent or delay the onset of AF possibly through effects on progression of an underlying myopathy, a hypothesis further supported by similar effects on AF in heart failure cohorts (Mann 1999; Li, Czernuszewicz et al. 2001; Madrid et al. 2002).

Types of Atrial Fibrillation

Clinical studies have suggested that there are discrete triggers for AF in many patients. Thus, several series have identified individuals where vagal stimuli, exercise, or inflammation appear to be the relevant precipitants. It remains to be seen if these various triggers will breed true in familial forms of AF, but to date this does not appear to be the case. These preliminary data further support the proposal that the fundamental diathesis in inherited forms of AF is a reduced threshold for the arrhythmia, though this may occur through many distinct pathways.

Genetic Epidemiology

A genetic predisposition to AF has only recently been appreciated. AF develops in individuals within some families at a relatively young age in the absence of any evidence of structural

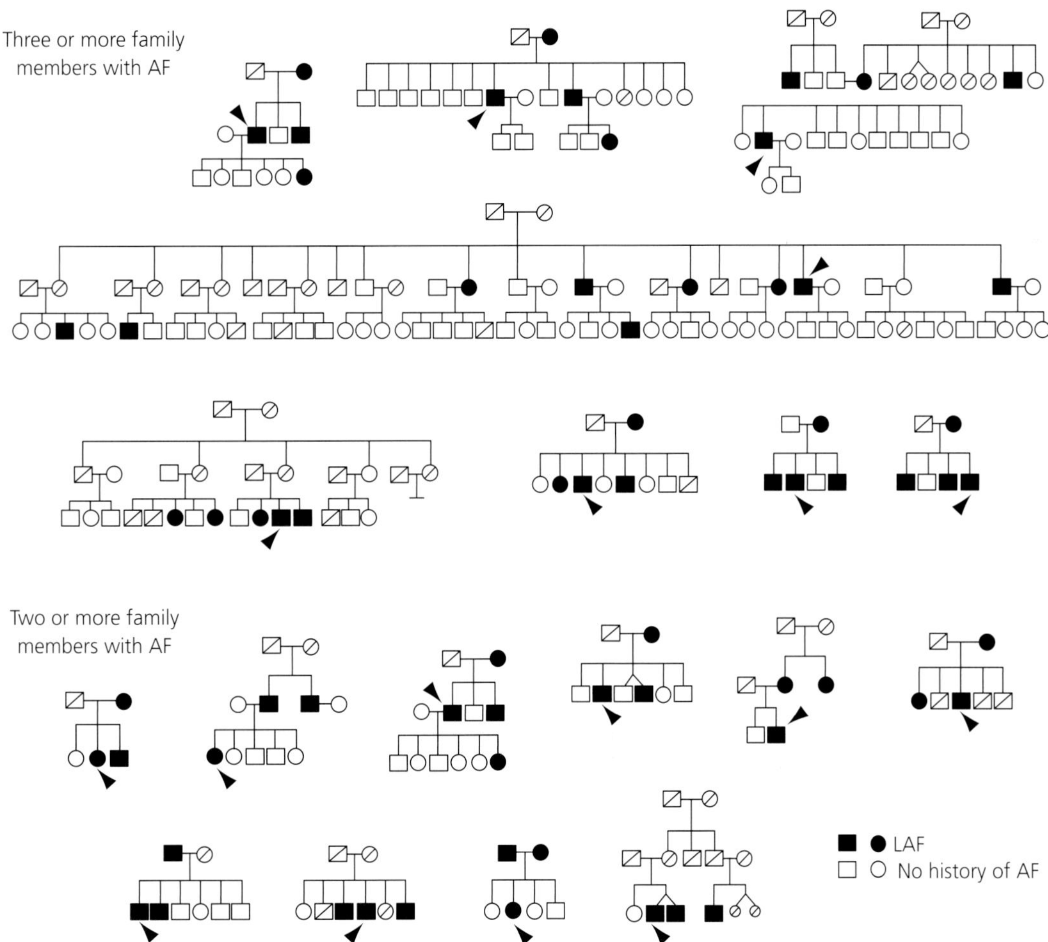

Figure 20–2 Families with 'Lone AF' (LAF). Lone AF kindreds are most often consistent with an autosomal dominant inheritance with markedly reduced penetrance. This is not unexpected for a phenotype that is paroxysmal and often asymptomatic, but constrains efforts to map and clone the responsible genes. Novel [and] persistent endophenotypes will be necessary to improve our understanding of the genetics of such traits.

heart disease and without any apparent etiology, but these families were typically considered rare (Wolff 1943; Figure 20–2). Work from the Framingham Heart Study looking at subjects over a 19-year period identified an association between AF in offspring and parental occurrence of the arrhythmia, particularly in those under the age of 75 years and in those without antecedent heart disease. Parental AF approximately doubled the 4-year risk of developing AF even after adjustment for risk factors such as hypertension, diabetes mellitus, or myocardial infarction (Fox et al. 2004). A genetic predisposition for AF in the general population was further supported by a study of AF in a large Icelandic population (Arnar et al. 2006). First-degree relatives of those with AF had a 1.77 higher relative risk for the arrhythmia compared with the general population. The relative risk was as high as 4–5-fold greater when patients under 60 years old were studied.

Even higher levels of heritability have been observed in more selected populations with AF. A retrospective review of over 2,000 subjects with AF referred to the Mayo Clinic found that 5% (or 15% in those with lone AF) had a family history of the same arrhythmia (Darbar et al. 2003). In prospective studies of a cohort with lone AF almost 40% had at least one relative with the arrhythmia, and a substantial number reported having multiple affected relatives (Ellinor et al. 2005). The arrhythmia could be verified in the vast majority of relatives, and when simple sibling recurrence risks were estimated as an index of heritability, a substantially increased relative risk of approximately 70-fold was observed in male siblings.

AF also is associated with many inherited forms of human heart disease for which the molecular defects have been cloned (Keating and Sanguinetti 2001; Seidman and Seidman 2001; see Table 20–2). Although these conclusions are based on small numbers of families, it appears that AF is a prominent feature only in specific families, rather than across all the mutant alleles from a single gene (Gruver et al. 1999; Chen et al. 2003; Mohler et al. 2003). It will take considerable work, including comprehensive animal modeling, to dissect the complex relationships between individual genes and AF.

Mendelian Forms of Atrial Fibrillation

Genetic studies have proven a powerful means of dissecting complex biological phenomena, often revealing previously unsuspected etiologic pathways. In many cases, studies of rare families have uncovered mechanisms applicable to all forms of a disease.

Mendelian forms of AF do occur, and their existence suggests that perturbation of single genes is sufficient to cause the arrhythmia.

1. KCNQ1

In one large family of Chinese descent, investigators identified a mutation in KCNQ1, a potassium channel that underlies the slow repolarizing current in cardiomyocytes known as I_{Ks}. The disease locus was mapped to the region on the short arm of chromosome 11 containing the *KCNQ1* gene (Chen et al. 2003). Sequencing revealed a serine to glycine missense mutation at position 140 (S140G) in affected family members. Unlike the mutations in *KCNQ1* associated with the long QT syndrome, which typically result in a loss of channel function, the S140G mutation resulted in a gain of channel function. In cultured cells, expression of the S140G mutant channel resulted in dramatically enhanced potassium channel currents and markedly altered potassium channel gating kinetics, changes that would be predicted to increase I_{Ks}. Such an increase would be expected to lead to a shortening of the action potential duration and thus make atrial myocytes vulnerable to reentry and subsequent AF.

While the identification of this mutation provided an initial inroad into the pathogenesis of AF, this family also illustrates our limited understanding of the role of the *KCNQ1* channel in repolarization. Specifically, it remains unclear why with a mutation that results in a gain of function in *KCNQ1* (albeit in vitro), is associated with delayed ventricular repolarization (as manifested by a prolonged QT interval on their electrocardiograms) in more than half of the individuals with the S140G mutation.

Other *KCNQ1* mutations have been described in single families with AF, One such mutation R14C had no significant effect on *KCNQ1/KCNE1* current amplitudes in cultured cells at baseline; however, upon exposure to hypotonic solution, mutant channels exhibited a marked increase in currents compared to wild-type channels. Interestingly, of those who carried the R14C mutation, only those with left atrial dilatation had AF leading the authors to propose a "two-hit" hypothesis of AF. They also identified a mutation in *KCNE2* in two of the kindreds. Like the S140G mutation in *KCNQ1*, the mutation in *KCNE2* (R27C) also increased the amplitude of I_{Ks} (Yang et al. 2004).

Other "gain-of-function" mutations in *KCNQ1* have been associated with the short QT syndrome and AF (Bellocq et al. 2004). Based on this association, they sequenced the *KCNQ1* gene and found a valine to methionine mutation in position 141. Like the S140G mutation, V141M mutant channels when expressed in vitro displayed enhanced current density and altered gating kinetics.

Table 20–2 [Mendelian] Genes and Loci Implicated in Atrial Fibrillation

Specific Genes	Chromosome	Gene Name	Inheritance	Comments	Reference
	11p15.5	KCNQ1/KvLQT1	AD	Disparate effects on QT	Chen et al. 2003
	21q22.1	KCNE2/MiRP1	AD	Limited data	Yang et al. 2004
	17q23.1–24.2	KCNJ2	AD	Limited data	Xia et al. 2005
	12p13	KCNA5	AD	Limited data	Olson et al. 2006
	1q21.1	GJA5/Connexin 40	Presumed somatic	Limited data	Gollob et al. 2006
Genetic loci	Chromosome	Gene	Inheritance		Reference
	5p13	Unknown	AR		Oberti et al. 2004
	6q14-q16	Unknown	AD	Overlaps with DCM locus	Ellinor et al. 2003a
	10q22-q24	Unknown	AD	Overlaps with DCM locus	Brugada et al. 1997
	10p11-q21	Unknown	AD		Volders et al. 2007

Notes: AD, autosomal dominant; AR, autosomal recessive; DCM, dilated cardiomyopathy.

Specific Loci for Which the Disease Genes Are Not Yet Known

To date five independent loci for AF have been described. At three of these loci the disease is quite typical of the lone AF seen in clinical practice (Brugada et al. 1997; Darbar et al. 2003; Ellinor et al. 2003b). At the remaining locus, which is recessive, the disease has unusual features including fetal or neonatal onset (Oberti et al. 2004). There is evidence of considerable genetic heterogeneity, as other families do not map to any of the loci described. Even in the large families used to identify these genetic loci, AF is incompletely penetrant. The very nature of the arrhythmia (paroxysmal and often asymptomatic) may have resulted in the genetic contribution being underestimated.

Candidate Genes

Since the initial report of mutations in *KCNQ1* in families with AF, multiple reports of associating sequence variants in a variety of ion channels with AF have emerged. Missense variants in several potassium channels and in the sodium channel have been identified in individual subjects, [and] occasionally [with more rigorous genetic support] in larger extended kindreds.

Despite these data, the role of ion channel mutations in AF remains uncertain. For the vast majority of the sequence variants identified to date, there are few genetic data to substantiate a causal role in the arrhythmia. Even for the reported gain of function mutations in *KCNQ1* where the genetic data are more robust, there is discordance between the available in vitro data and observed effects on atrial and ventricular electrophysiology. Understanding the allele-specific and regional expression of this imprinted gene, and modeling the specific disease alleles in vivo may shed light on these discrepancies, but to date the precise mechanism by which AF and QT prolongation coexist is unclear. In vitro data for other ion channel variants have failed to identify a unifying physiologic mechanism, which may not be unexpected for a phenotype so common as AF, but in the presence of other limitations raises serious concerns about the pathophysiologic role of ion channel variants in the arrhythmia.

The data obtained in heterologous expression systems may not reflect in vivo physiology where many other accessory proteins, local membrane composition, and significant redundancy all may modify the final phenotype. In addition, apparent mutations may have no effect in the context of the powerful homeostatic influences of other biologic pathways. Human genetic studies reveal many examples of profound in vitro effects that fail to translate into an in vivo phenotype. The absence of robust genetic support in humans or in animal models is only compounded by other circumstantial evidence. Ion channel gene mutations, if causal in AF, certainly are responsible for only a very small fraction of disease. Resequencing studies of each of the ion channel genes implicated to date have identified only a handful of putative mutations, which even if they were all causal would represent less than 1% of all AF. Importantly, in most such studies the control populations have not been subjected to parallel resequencing, so that similar rare variants with modest functional consequences that may well exist in normal individuals would not have been revealed. It should also be noted that there are no functional data available for the majority of sequence variants purported to cause AF.

Somatic Mutations

The genes encoding the connexins have also been examined as potential candidates for AF. Prior work has shown that mice with null alleles of *GJA5*, the gene for connexin 40, exhibit atrial reentrant arrhythmias (Hagendorff et al. 1999). From this work, Gollob and coworkers considered this gene as a potential candidate in individuals with idiopathic AF who underwent pulmonary vein isolation surgery (Gollob et al. 2006). An analysis of DNA isolated from their cardiac tissue showed that 4 of the 15 subjects had mutations in *GJA5* that markedly interfered with the electrical coupling between cells. In 3 of the patients, DNA isolated from their lymphocytes lacked the same mutation in *GJA5* suggesting that the connexin40 mutations arose after fertilization, possibly during cardiac organogenesis. One of the four individuals carried the mutation in both cardiac tissue and in their lymphocytes arguing that, in this instance, the mutation was transmitted in the germline; however, more information about the transmission of AF in relatives of this individual was not available.

Common Forms of Atrial Fibrillation

Although traditional methods such as linkage analysis can be applied to families where the phenotype and pattern of inheritance are consistent with a monogenic disorder, the genetic contribution to AF in the general population is less clear. In order to identify smaller genetic effects active across the population, investigators have undertaken genetic association studies. These studies have typically tested a small number of variants and have been directed at candidate genes previously believed to be involved in AF. Examples include genes in the renin-angiotensin system (Tsai et al. 2004), interleukins, signaling molecules (Schreieck et al. 2004), gap junction proteins, and ion channels. Such studies are necessarily limited by the low prior probability of any polymorphism truly being associated with AF. Further complicating these analyses are the small sample sizes, a lack of replication in distinct populations, as well as phenotypic and genetic heterogeneity.

In recent years, genome-wide association studies (GWAS) have been made possible by advancements in genotyping technology that allow investigators to assay hundreds of thousands of polymorphisms in parallel (Risch 2000). While GWAS have the potential to identify new pathways for disease, they also have a number of limitations. In particular, with hundreds of thousands of individual associations being tested, these studies have a high likelihood of producing a false-positive result. False positives can also emerge from ethnicity, or population stratification. Ultimately, replication of the results in other populations may be the best test of whether a result is a true positive (Risch 2000).

Recently, the results of a GWA study for AF were reported and a locus on the long arm of chromosome 4 (4q25) was identified that demonstrated a highly significant association ($p = 3.3x10^{-41}$) with AF (Gudbjartsson et al. 2007). The investigators were able to replicate their original findings in other populations. At present, the mechanism of action of the associated genetic variants is unclear. Interestingly, the markers lie upstream from a gene that plays a role in the development of the left atrium: the paired-like homeodomain transcription factor 2, *PITX2* (Franco and Campione 2003). This gene has been shown to suppress the emergence of pacemaker cells outside the sinus node in early development. Further work should help clarify the mechanism underlying the association of these markers with AF, and identify other loci associated with the arrhythmia.

Outstanding Questions

Largely due to the lack of any known major proximate cause for AF, the conceptual framework used to understand the arrhythmia has changed little in the past 50 years. A comparison with other episodic electrical disorders such as epilepsy may be helpful. AF parallels the global disorganized electrical activity of a generalized seizure, which may represent the common endpoint of a range of distinct focal arrhythmias. In epilepsy the discovery of discrete mechanisms led to reevaluation of the entire classification of seizures, and [to] the advent of targeted and thus more successful therapies. By analogy the potential mechanisms for AF will likely include disorders of ion channels, developmental patterning defects affecting structure or function, and metabolic abnormalities, among others. The challenge for cardiologists is to identify these primary pathways and to merge them with the classic concepts of the arrhythmia building on the therapeutic successes of the past five decades. Ultimately, improving our understanding of the proximal causes in each subtype of AF may lead to more effective therapies.

Endophenotypes

The completion of the human genome project, and insights gained from the study of major Mendelian disorders have led to a reappraisal of the role of phenotype in understanding human disease (Freimer and Sabatti 2003). Syndromes that previously were treated as homogeneous entities from the standpoint of therapy or clinical trials have begun to be revealed as aggregates of multiple discrete diseases. For example, the long QT syndrome now is known to represent several discrete disorders, each with distinctive electrocardiographic features that were not described until after the causal genes had been cloned (Moss et al. 1995). In more common clinical entities there may be unrecognized, phenotypically distinct subsets accessible only through high-resolution investigation. By changing the resolution of clinical investigation we may encounter components of the underlying arrhythmogenic substrate that are causally related to AF but that occur earlier in the disease process or are not paroxysmal in nature (Leboyer et al. 1998). Such endophenotypes might be uncovered through reappraisal of classic clinical findings, or through existing investigative tools including signal averaged EKG, Holter, CT scan, MRI, and known biomarkers. However, the discovery of novel aspects of the AF substrate undoubtedly will involve the use of unbiased approaches including proteomics, metabolomics, and cellular profiling. It will be interesting to see if classic associations between AF and other phenomena such as thromboembolism or heart failure are general features of all forms of the arrhythmia, or are restricted to specific subsets, for example, those with dysregulated endothelial function.

Several groups have identified perturbations of atrial endocrine pathways during AF or in cohorts with previous AF. No consensus has emerged, but findings to date suggest that some AF subgroups have a biomarker profile similar to that seen in congestive heart failure. These data, if confirmed, would define a clear mechanism for the known epidemiologic links between AF and heart failure, and immediately enable the identification of those at risk for either phenotype (Wang et al. 2003). Importantly, while of immediate clinical utility, refined phenotypes also can be used to define cohorts with increased clinical and etiological homogeneity for long-term investigation. In family studies endophenotypes allow the robust extension of nuclear families and would accelerate the discovery of the causal genes.

Ultimately, faithful animal models of human disease, precisely recapitulating the molecular defects through homologous recombination or "knockin" methods will be generated. Parallels with other murine models suggest that the specific phenotypes associated with mutations in a given gene may actually be the result of distinct perturbations of particular signaling pathways, and may not be modeled by the simple disruption of the function of that gene (Casimiro et al. 2004).

Current Clinical Implications

As for conduction disease, the major clinical utility of these insights at present is to inform diagnosis and to aid in the identification of subsets that may benefit from additional therapy and prognosis. A careful family history will play a major role in the management of those presenting with AF as it may facilitate screening and also suggest the early introduction of prognostically useful therapies such as angiotensin-converting enzyme inhibitors or angiotensin receptor blockers. Perhaps the most useful information at present is simply the realization that the condition is often inherited, as this may stimulate additional clinical genetic insights and furnish the material for new molecular studies.

Future Directions

In order to improve the utility of genetic studies for AF we will need to overcome a number of obstacles. A critical step in any genetic study is the ability to correctly assign the diagnosis. While on first pass this may seem straightforward; it can be challenging in AF, a condition that can be asymptomatic, paroxysmal, and have an onset later in life. Further complicating studies of AF are the genotypic and phenotypic heterogeneity. AF may represent the final common, rather than a single pathway for a number of distinct pathogenic insults such as heart failure, hypertension, or thyroid abnormalities.

Several different strategies will converge to help resolve the [genetic basis of] AF. Novel third-generation sequencing technologies will allow large-scale studies in subjects and controls. GWAS will define the common small effect alleles contributing to atrial arrhythmias. In vivo modeling of some of the putative AF alleles may resolve questions on the net effects on atrial and ventricular electrophysiology, though this will likely require the use of organisms other than the mouse. Emerging technologies will uncover subclinical endophenotypes for AF, facilitating genetic studies of informative families with Mendelian AF. The identification of the causal genes at several Mendelian loci and the evaluation of these genes in large series of less selected AF subjects will define new pathways predisposing to the arrhythmia. Importantly the known loci do not contain any obvious ion channel genes, suggesting that distinctive mechanisms are responsible for such AF. Overlap with known loci for cardiomyopathy exists, and the relationship between AF and heart failure is likely to be much more fundamental than simple elevations of atrial pressure. As investigators explore the links between these novel AF genes and emerging macromolecular complexes regulating ion channel conductance and downstream signaling, the mechanistic role of ion channels in AF will be established.

In order to address these challenges, we will have to continue to improve upon the characterization and classification of AF. The identification of endophenotypes or subtle, heritable traits that cosegregate with AF may help to refine ongoing genetic studies. For AF, endophenotypes such as specific P-wave morphologies, pulmonary venous anatomy as assessed by computed tomography or magnetic resonance imaging, or biomarkers that are heritable and easily detectable may be helpful.

Conclusions

Like the arrhythmias themselves, advances in our understanding of conduction disease and AF have been slowly progressive or even episodic. The next challenge in discerning the etiology of these arrhythmias will require distillation of heterogeneous syndromes into distinct biological entities. An emphasis is needed on the identification of primary pathways through novel genetic techniques or other unbiased approaches. The ultimate goal of investigators is refinement, which will permit the development of discrete preventative therapies targeted to the proximate cause of each form of arrhythmia, rather than against a final common outcome.

References

Allessie M, Ausma J, Schotten U. Electrical, contractile and structural remodeling during atrial fibrillation. *Cardiovasc Res.* 2002;54(2): 230–246.

Anan R, Nakagawa M, Miyata M, et al. Cardiac involvement in mitochondrial diseases. A study on 17 patients with documented mitochondrial DNA defects. *Circulation.* 1995;91(4):955–961.

Arad M, Benson DW, Perez-Atayde AR, et al. Constitutively active AMP kinase mutations cause glycogen storage disease mimicking hypertrophic cardiomyopathy. *J Clin Invest.* 2002;109(3):357–362.

Arad M, Maron BJ, Gorham JM, et al. Glycogen storage diseases presenting as hypertrophic cardiomyopathy. *N Engl J Med.* 2005;352(4):362–372.

Arad M, Moskowitz IP, Patel VV, et al. Transgenic mice overexpressing mutant PRKAG2 define the cause of Wolff-Parkinson-White syndrome in glycogen storage cardiomyopathy. *Circulation.* 2003;107(22): 2850–2856.

Arnar DO, Thorvaldsson S, Manolio TA, et al. Familial aggregation of atrial fibrillation in Iceland. *Eur Heart J.* 2006;27(6):708–712.

Ausma J, Litjens N, Lenders MH, et al. Time course of atrial fibrillation-induced cellular structural remodeling in atria of the goat. *J Mol Cell Cardiol.* 2001;33(12):2083–2094.

Bellocq C, van Ginneken AC, Bezzina CR, et al. Mutation in the KCNQ1 gene leading to the short QT-interval syndrome. *Circulation.* 2004;109(20): 2394–2397.

Berul CI, Christe ME, Aronovitz MJ, Seidman CE, Seidman JG, Mendelsohn ME. Electrophysiological abnormalities and arrhythmias in alpha MHC mutant familial hypertrophic cardiomyopathy mice. *J Clin Invest.* 1997;99(4):570–576.

Berul CI, Maguire CT, Aronovitz MJ, et al. DMPK dosage alterations result in atrioventricular conduction abnormalities in a mouse myotonic dystrophy model. *J Clin Invest.* 1999;103(4):R1–R7.

Bione S, Maestrini E, Rivella S, Mancini M, Regis S, Romeo G, Toniolo D.1. Identification of a novel X-linked gene responsible for Emery-Dreifuss muscular dystrophy. *Nat Genet.* 1994;8(4):323–323.

Bonnet D, Martin D, Pascale De Lonlay, et al. Arrhythmias and conduction defects as presenting symptoms of fatty acid oxidation disorders in children. *Circulation.* 1999;100(22):2248–2253.

Brugada R, Tapscott T, Czernuszewicz GZ, et al. Identification of a genetic locus for familial atrial fibrillation. *N Engl J Med.* 1997;336(13):905–911.

Brundel BJ, Henning RH, Kampinga HH, Van Gelder IC, Crijns HJ. Molecular mechanisms of remodeling in human atrial fibrillation. *Cardiovasc Res.* 2002;54(2):315–324.

Casimiro MC, Knollmann BC, Yamoah EN, et al. Targeted point mutagenesis of mouse Kcnq1: phenotypic analysis of mice with point mutations that cause Romano-Ward syndrome in humans. *Genomics.* 2004;84(3):555–564.

Chen YH, Xu SJ, Bendahhou S, et al. KCNQ1 gain-of-function mutation in familial atrial fibrillation. *Science.* 2003;299(5604):251–254.

Chimenti C, Pieroni M, Morgante E, et al. Prevalence of Fabry disease in female patients with late-onset hypertrophic cardiomyopathy. *Circulation.* 2004;110(9):1047–1053.

Chugh SS, Blackshear JL, Shen WK, Hammill SC, Gersh BJ. Epidemiology and natural history of atrial fibrillation: clinical implications. *J Am Coll Cardiol.* 2001;37(2):371–378.

Coyne KS, Paramore C, Grandy S, Mercader M, Reynolds M, Zimetbaum P. Assessing the direct costs of treating nonvalvular atrial fibrillation in the United States. *Value Health.* 2006;9(5):348–356.

Darbar D, Herron KJ, Ballew JD, et al. Familial atrial fibrillation is a genetically heterogeneous disorder. *J Am Coll Cardiol.* 2003;41(12):2185–2192.

de Meeus A, Stephan E, Debrus S, Jean MK, Loiselet J, Weissenbach J, Demaille J, Bouvagnet P. An isolated cardiac conduction disease maps to chromosome 19q. *Circ Res.* 1995;77(4):735–740.

Ellinor PT, Shin JT, Moore RK, Yoerger DM, Macrae CA. A genetic locus for atrial fibrillation maps to Chromosome 6q12–21. *Circulation.* 2003a;107:2880.

Ellinor PT, Shin JT, Moore RK, Yoerger DM, MacRae CA. Locus for atrial fibrillation maps to chromosome 6q14–16. *Circulation.* 2003b;107(23): 2880–2883.

Ellinor PT, Yoerger DM, Ruskin JN, MacRae CA. Familial aggregation in lone atrial fibrillation. *Hum Genet.* 2005;118(2):179–184.

Fatkin D, MacRae C, Sasaki T, Wolff MR, Porcu M, Frenneaux M, et al. Missense mutations in the rod domain of the lamin A/C gene as causes of dilated cardiomyopathy and conduction-system disease. *N Engl J Med.* 1999;341(23):1715–1724.

Feillet F, Steinmann G, Vianey-Saban C, et al. Adult presentation of MCAD deficiency revealed by coma and severe arrythmias. *Intensive Care Med.* 2003;29(9):1594–1597.

Fox CS, Parise H, D'Agostino RB Sr, et al. Parental atrial fibrillation as a risk factor for atrial fibrillation in offspring. *JAMA.* 2004;291(23):2851–2855.

Franco D, Campione M. The role of Pitx2 during cardiac development. Linking left-right signaling and congenital heart diseases. *Trends Cardiovasc Med.* 2003;13(4):157–163.

Freimer N, Sabatti C. The human phenome project. *Nat Genet.* 2003;34(1): 15–21.

Frustaci A, Chimenti C, Bellocci F, Morgante E, Russo MA, Maseri A. Histological substrate of atrial biopsies in patients with lone atrial fibrillation. *Circulation.* 1997;96(4):1180–1184.

Go AS, Hylek EM, Phillips KA, et al. Prevalence of diagnosed atrial fibrillation in adults: national implications for rhythm management and stroke prevention: the Anticoagulation and Risk Factors in Atrial Fibrillation (ATRIA) Study. *JAMA.* 2001;285(18):2370–2375.

Gollob MH, Jones DL, Krahn AD, et al. Somatic mutations in the connexin 40 gene (GJA5) in atrial fibrillation. *N Engl J Med.* 2006;354(25): 2677–2688.

Graber HL, Unverferth DV, Baker PB, Ryan JM, Baba N, Wooley CF. Evolution of a hereditary cardiac conduction and muscle disorder: a study involving a family with six generations affected. *Circulation.* 1986;74(1):21–35.

Gruver EJ, Fatkin D, Dodds GA, et al. Familial hypertrophic cardiomyopathy and atrial fibrillation caused by Arg663His beta-cardiac myosin heavy chain mutation. *Am J Cardiol.* 1999;83(12A):13H–18H.

Gu H, Smith FC, Taffet SM, Delmar M. High incidence of cardiac malformations in connexin40-deficient mice. *Circ Res.* 2003;93(3):201–206.

Gudbjartsson DF, Arnar DO, Helgadottir A, et al. Variants conferring risk of atrial fibrillation on chromosome 4q25. *Nature.* 2007;448(7151):353–357.

Guertl B, Noehammer C, Hoefler G. Metabolic cardiomyopathies. *Int J Exp Pathol.* 2000;81(6):349–372.

Hagendorff A, Schumacher B, Kirchhoff S, Lüderitz B, Willecke K. Conduction disturbances and increased atrial vulnerability in Connexin40-deficient mice analyzed by transesophageal stimulation. *Circulation.* 1999;99(11):1508–1515.

Haissaguerre M, Jais P, Shah DC, et al. Spontaneous initiation of atrial fibrillation by ectopic beats originating in the pulmonary veins. *N Engl J Med.* 1998;339(10):659–666.

Katritsis DG, Ellenbogen KA. Is isolation of all four pulmonary veins necessary in patients with paroxysmal atrial fibrillation? *Pacing Clin Electrophysiol.* 2004;27(7):938–940.

Keating MT, Sanguinetti MC. Molecular and cellular mechanisms of cardiac arrhythmias. *Cell.* 2001;104(4):569–580.

Kelly DP, Strauss AW. Inherited cardiomyopathies. *N Engl J Med.* 1994;330(13):913–919.

Kopecky SL, Gersh BJ, McGoon MD, et al. The natural history of lone atrial fibrillation. A population-based study over three decades. *N Engl J Med.* 1987;317(11):669–674.

Leboyer M, Bellivier F, Nosten-Bertrand M, Jouvent R, Pauls D, Mallet J. Psychiatric genetics: search for phenotypes. *Trends Neurosci.* 1998;21(3): 102–105.

Li D, Czernuszewicz GZ, Gonzalez O, et al. Novel cardiac troponin T mutation as a cause of familial dilated cardiomyopathy. *Circulation.* 2001;104(18):2188–2193.

London B. Cardiac arrhythmias: from (transgenic) mice to men. *J Cardiovasc Electrophysiol.* 2001;12:1089–1991.

Longo N, Amat di San Filippo C, Pasquali M. Disorders of carnitine transport and the carnitine cycle. *Am J Med Genet C Semin Med Genet.* 2006;142(2): 77–85.

MacRae CA, Ghaisas N, Kass S, et al. Familial hypertrophic cardiomyopathy with Wolff-Parkinson-White syndrome maps to a locus on chromosome 7q3. *J Clin Invest.* 1995;96(3):1216–1220.

Madrid AH, Bueno MG, Rebollo JM, et al. Use of irbesartan to maintain sinus rhythm in patients with long-lasting persistent atrial fibrillation: a prospective and randomized study. *Circulation.* 2002;106(3):331–336.

Mahadevan D, Thanki N, McPhie P, Beeler JF, Yu JC, Wlodawer A, Heidaran MA. Comparison of calcium-dependent conformational changes in the N-terminal SH2 domains of p85 and GAP defines distinct properties for SH2 domains. *Biochemistry.* 1994;33(3):746–754.

Mann DL. Mechanisms and models in heart failure: a combinatorial approach. *Circulation.* 1999;100(9):999–1008.

Milanesi R, Baruscotti M, Gnecchi-Ruscone T, DiFrancesco D. Familial sinus bradycardia associated with a mutation in the cardiac pacemaker channel. *N Engl J Med.* 2006;354(2):151–157.

Mohler PJ, Schott JJ, Gramolini AO, et al. Ankyrin-B mutation causes type 4 long-QT cardiac arrhythmia and sudden cardiac death. *Nature.* 2003;421(6923):634–639.

Moses SW, Wanderman KL, Myroz A, Frydman M. Cardiac involvement in glycogen storage disease type III. *Eur J Pediatr.* 1989;148(8):764–766.

Moss AJ, Zareba W, Benhorin J, et al. ECG T-wave patterns in genetically distinct forms of the hereditary long QT syndrome. *Circulation.* 1995;92(10):2929–2934.

Nattel S. New ideas about atrial fibrillation 50 years on. *Nature.* 2002;415(6868):219–226.

Nguyên-Trân VT, Kubalak SW, Minamisawa S, et al. A novel genetic pathway for sudden cardiac death via defects in the transition between ventricular and conduction system cell lineages. *Cell.* 2000;102(5):671–682.

Oberti C, Wang L, Li L, et al. Genome-wide linkage scan identifies a novel genetic locus on chromosome 5p13 for neonatal atrial fibrillation associated with sudden death and variable cardiomyopathy. *Circulation.* 2004;110(25):3753–3759.

Olson TM, Alekseev AE, Liu XK, et al. Kv1.5 channelopathy due to KCNA5 loss-of-function mutation causes human atrial fibrillation. *Hum Mol Genet.* 2006;15(14):2185–2191.

Papadatos GA, Wallerstein PM, Head CE, et al. Slowed conduction and ventricular tachycardia after targeted disruption of the cardiac sodium channel gene Scn5a. *Proc Natl Acad Sci USA.* 2002;99(9):6210–6215.

Risch NJ. Searching for genetic determinants in the new millennium. *Nature.* 2000;405(6788):847–856.

Schoeller R, Andresen D, Büttner P, Oezcelik K, Vey G, Schröder R. First- or second-degree atrioventricular block as a risk factor in idiopathic dilated cardiomyopathy. *Am J Cardiol.*1993;71(8):720–726.

Schott JJ, Alshinawi C, Kyndt F, et al. Cardiac conduction defects associate with mutations in SCN5A. *Nat Genet.* 1999;23(1):20–21.

Schreieck J, Dostal S, von Beckerath N, et al. C825T polymorphism of the G-protein beta3 subunit gene and atrial fibrillation: association of the TT genotype with a reduced risk for atrial fibrillation. *Am Heart J.* 2004;148(3):545–550.

Seidman JG, Seidman C. The genetic basis for cardiomyopathy: from mutation identification to mechanistic paradigms. *Cell.* 2001;104(4): 557–567.

Shah JS, Hughes DA, Sachdev B, et al. Prevalence and clinical significance of cardiac arrhythmia in Anderson-Fabry disease. *Am J Cardiol.* 2005;96(6):842–846.

Tsai CT, Lai LP, Lin JL, et al. Renin-angiotensin system gene polymorphisms and atrial fibrillation. *Circulation.* 2004;109(13):1640–1646.

VanderBrink BA, Sellitto C, Saba S, et al. Connexin40-deficient mice exhibit atrioventricular nodal and infra-Hisian conduction abnormalities. *J Cardiovasc Electrophysiol.* 2000;11(11):1270–1276.

Vermes E, Tardif JC, Bourassa MG, et al. Enalapril decreases the incidence of atrial fibrillation in patients with left ventricular dysfunction: insight from the Studies of Left Ventricular Dysfunction (SOLVD) trials. *Circulation.* 2003;107(23):2926–2931.

Volders PG, Zhu Q, Timmermans C, et al. Mapping a novel locus for familial atrial fibrillation on chromosome 10p11-q21. *Heart Rhythm.* 2007;4(4):469–475.

Waldo AL. Mechanisms of atrial fibrillation. *J Cardiovasc Electrophysiol.* 2003;14(12 suppl):S267–S274.

Wang TJ, Larson MG, Levy D, et al. Temporal relations of atrial fibrillation and congestive heart failure and their joint influence on mortality: the Framingham Heart Study. *Circulation.* 2003;107(23):2920–2925.

Wolff L. Familial auricular fibrillation. *N Engl J Med.* 1943;229:396–398.

Xia M, Jin Q, Bendahhou S, et al. A Kir2.1 gain-of-function mutation underlies familial atrial fibrillation. *Biochem Biophys Res Commun.* 2005;332(4):1012–1019.

Yang Y, Xia M, Jin Q, et al. Identification of a KCNE2 gain-of-function mutation in patients with familial atrial fibrillation. *Am J Hum Genet.* 2004;75(5):899–905.

21

Familial Hypercholesterolemia

Ian FW McDowell, S Gaye Hadfield, and Steve E Humphries

Introduction

Familial hypercholesterolemia (FH) is one of the commonest identified genetic disorders to cause premature heart disease. It is an inborn error of metabolism affecting the clearance of low-density lipoprotein cholesterol (LDL-C) that leads to early onset coronary artery atherosclerosis, which can be prevented by medication to lower LDL-C. Despite this, many clinicians remain relatively unaware of how to diagnose and manage FH, such that less than 15% of all individuals in the United Kingdom predicted to have the condition are adequately diagnosed or treated. This chapter concentrates on the genetic basis of FH and issues relating to cascade testing. The key issues relating to clinical diagnosis and treatment are also discussed.

Background

Prevalence

The prevalence of heterozygous FH is widely quoted as 1 in 500 of the population for those of European descent. However, this figure is a general estimate and there are limited hard data to substantiate it. In the Netherlands, where there is a national program for FH (Umans-Eckenhausen et al. 2001), it has been found that the frequency is closer to 1 in 400, in regions where there is a high awareness of the condition. There are several defined communities with higher prevalence rates (Austin et al. 2004) such as the French Canadian population in Quebec (1 in 120), Norway (1 in 300), and the white Afrikaner population in South Africa (1 in 70), all attributable to a founder gene effect. In the United Kingdom, one report (Neil et al. 2000) estimated the overall prevalence in one geographical region (Oxfordshire) as being 1 in 2,000, but noted that prevalence was particularly low in subjects under 35 years (due to underdiagnosis) and reached 1 in 625 in middle-aged men and women, which is therefore the likely true estimate in the region. The incidence of FH in the Middle East is relatively high and some of the early descriptions were based on extended kindreds from Lebanon. Although there is little hard data and no comprehensive surveys have been published, the prevalence of FH in individuals of black and Asian origin appears to be lower (Austin et al. 2004), though it is thought that this may in part be due to underdiagnosis. The prevalence of individuals with a clinical diagnosis of homozygous FH is about 1 in 10^6 of the population.

Current State of Clinical Services for FH

Clinical services for FH vary widely between different countries and different health care systems. In some countries, most notably the Netherlands, there is a coordinated national approach, particularly for cascade testing (Umans-Eckenhausen et al. 2001). Through this program there is heightened awareness of the diagnosis and a national service for DNA testing. Physicians are encouraged to apply diagnostic criteria in possible cases and send samples for DNA analysis. If the diagnosis is confirmed by DNA testing then family cascade testing is carried out as part of a national public health program. Individuals for whom a diagnosis of FH is made are treated by local physicians often in conjunction with hospital lipid clinics. In Netherlands it is estimated that from the prevalence of 1 in 400, there are likely to be approximately 24,000 individuals with FH of whom 13,000 (by 2007) have been diagnosed by molecular testing and cascading. Cascade testing is being actively pursued in several other countries including Norway (Leren 2004a), Denmark (Damgaard et al. 2005), and Spain (Pocovi et al. 2004).

In the United Kingdom, the diagnosis and management of FH is largely based around hospital lipid clinics. However, these clinics operate independently and there is no formal collaboration between different centers; a survey in 2004 suggested that <15% of the predicted number of U.K. FH patients had been identified and were being treated (Marks et al. 2004). The lipid clinics are led by physicians with varying training including chemical pathologists, metabolic physicians, and cardiologists. In most parts of the United Kingdom, FH is not regarded as part of the remit of clinical geneticists. Although there are several centers in the United Kingdom where DNA testing has been carried out as part of research projects, it has not been widely used for diagnosis and there is no formal process for cascade testing within families, though pilot studies have demonstrated that it is feasible (Hadfield and Humphries 2005). A DNA diagnostic service for FH is available although funding for these tests is not yet routinely available through the NHS (Heath et al. 1999), an exception to this applies in Northern Ireland where lipid clinics actively collaborate and have access to DNA testing to support family cascade testing (Graham et al. 1999).

Metabolic Basis of FH

The key components of cholesterol and lipid metabolism are shown in Figure 21–1. FH is an inborn error of LDL metabolism leading to accumulation of LDL-C particles in the blood. In most cases this is due to defects in the LDL-receptor (LDL-R), and the lower number of functional receptors on the surface of the liver results in a reduced clearance of LDL-C and thus its accumulation in the plasma. In heterozygous FH serum LDL-C (and total cholesterol) values are approximately double the usual values. The slower clearance of LDL-C particles leads to a reduction in LDL particle triglyceride content. Hence, serum total triglyceride values for individuals with FH are usually within the "normal range." Elevation of serum triglyceride suggests that there may be another coexisting condition (e.g., diabetes) or else calls the diagnosis of FH into doubt (see section 7). Elevated LDL-C concentrations promote atherosclerosis, particularly in the coronary arteries, and the study of FH has led to much of the current understanding of the role of cholesterol and LDL-C in the pathogenesis of atherosclerosis.

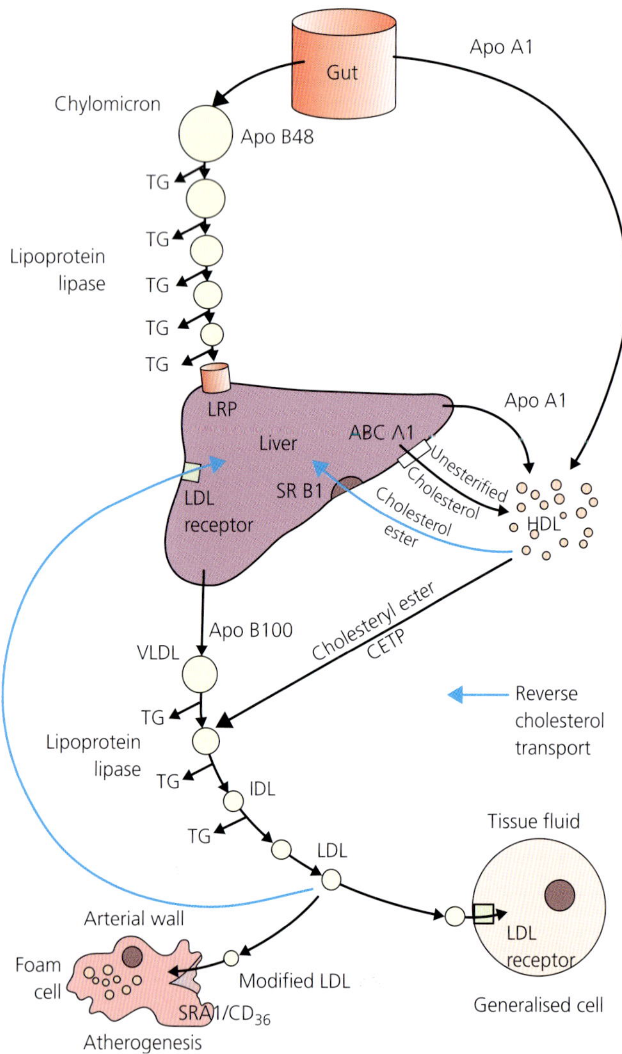

Figure 21–1 The role of cholesterol in the metabolism of lipoprotein. Adapted from Charlton-Menys and Durrington 2008 with permission.

Genetic Basis of FH

FH is an autosomal dominant condition, with most cases being caused by one of the many different mutations in the *LDLR* gene, which encodes the LDL-receptor. The *LDLR* gene is located at 19p13.2, and is composed of 18 exons spanning 45 kb (Soutar and Naoumova 2007). The transcript is 5.3 kb long and encodes a peptide of 860 residues. Functional domains of the peptide correspond with the exons as follows: signal sequence—exon 1, ligand binding domain—exons 2–6, epidermal growth factor precursor-like domain—exons 7–14, O-linked carbohydrate domain—exon 15, transmembrane domain—exon 16, and cytoplasmic domain—exons 17 and 18. As shown in Figure 21–2, *LDLR* is expressed ubiquitously under the control of sterol-regulated negative feedback, mediated by three 16 bp imperfect repeats (sterol regulatory elements) and a TATA-like sequence in the promoter.

To date over 1,000 different mutations have been reported worldwide with more than 100 so far identified in patients in the United Kingdom (Leigh et al. 2008). Sixty-five percent of the variants are DNA substitutions, 24% (n = 260) small DNA rearrangements (<100 bp) and 11% large DNA rearrangements (>100 bp). The DNA substitutions and small rearrangements occur along the length of the gene, with 24 in the promoter region, 86 in intronic sequences, and 839 in the exons (93 nonsense variants, 499 missense variants, and 204 frame-shift rearrangements). Reported variants occur in all exons, with the highest number in exon 4 (186/839); this exon is the largest and codes for the critical ligand binding region, where any missense variant is likely to be pathogenic. Using the function-prediction computer programs, 87% of the missense variants are predicted to have a deleterious effect on LDL-R activity, and it is probable that at least half of the remaining 13% are also pathogenic, but their role in FH causation requires confirmation by in vitro and/or family studies.

In 3% to 5% of U.K. FH patients, the hypercholesterolemia is caused by a single mutation in the *APOB* gene on chromosome 2p that encodes apolipoprotein B, which is the major protein of the LDL-C particle and the ligand for the LDL-R. While formally being given the name Familial Defective ApoB (FDB), this disorder is, however, phenotypically almost indistinguishable from FH. The mutation, which alters a single amino acid (previously R3500Q, now designated p.R3527Q), has been shown to reduce the affinity of the LDL-C particle (Myant 1993), leading to slower clearance and thus LDL-C accumulation. The defect is not as severe as FH (Myant 1993), since the normal number of LDL-Rs present on the liver can clear lipoprotein particles containing apoE normally. The defect is known to be expressed as hyperlipidemia in childhood (Myant 1993); FDB may present with the classical FH phenotype (high LDL, tendon xanthomata, and premature CHD), but typically the phenotype is less pronounced with less expression of clinical features.

In 2003, defects in a third gene causing monogenic hypercholesterolemia was identified (Abifadel et al. 2003). The gene called protein convertase subtilisin/kexin type 9 (*PCSK9*), codes for an enzyme that has also been called "neural apoptosis regulated convertase 1" (NARC-1), which has been found to be involved in degrading the LDL-R protein in the lysosome of the cell and preventing it recycling (Kwon et al. 2008). Gain-of-function mutations in the *PCSK9* gene will therefore cause increased degradation

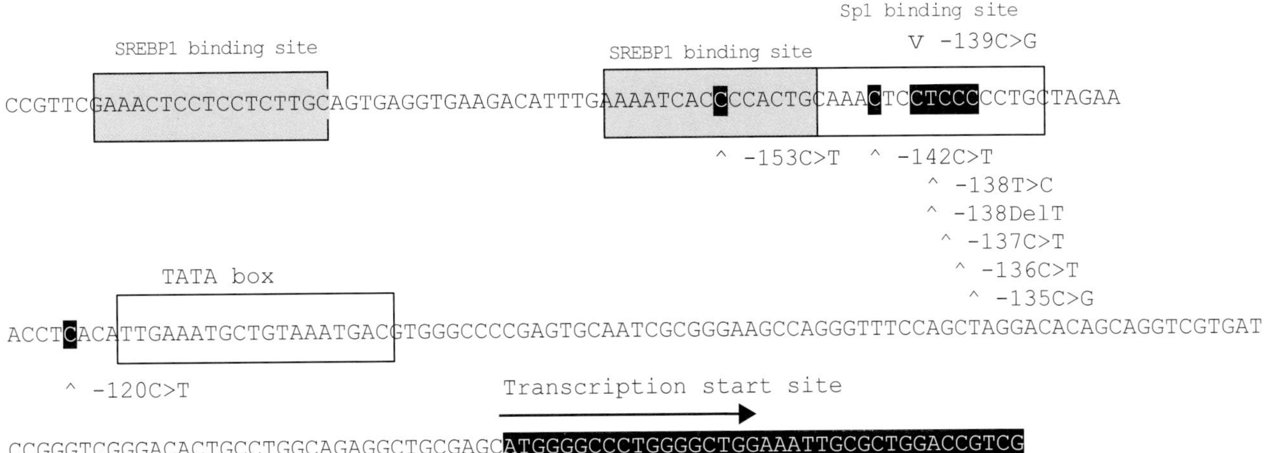

Figure 21–2 *LDLR* promoter and reported FH-causing sequence changes. Reprinted from Smith AJ, Ahmed F, Nair D, et al. A functional mutation in the *LDLR* promoter (-139C>G) in a patient with familial hypercholesterolemia. *Eur J Hum Genet.* 2007;15(11):1186–1189, with permission.

of LDL-Rs, reduced numbers of receptors on the surface of the cell and monogenic hypercholesterolemia. To date, 11 likely causative mutations have been reported in the *PCSK9* gene in autosomal dominant hypercholesterolemia patients (Lambert 2007), but only one of these appears to be common in the United Kingdom. This mutation, D374Y, has been reported in several independent families (Timms et al. 2004; Leren 2004b; Naoumova 2005; Sun et al. 2005) and is present in roughly 2% of U.K. DFH patients (Humphries et al. 2006a, 2006b). In contrast to FDB, this mutation usually presents with clinical features at the more severe end of the FH spectrum. Finally, there is some evidence to suggest that at least one, and possibly two, other gene loci may also cause the disorder (Varret et al. 2008) but their identity is not yet established.

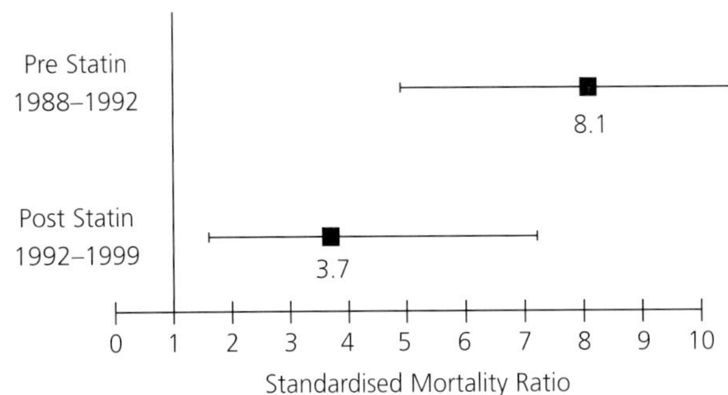

Figure 21–3 Standardized mortality ratio for DFH and PFH men and women aged 20–59 years before and after the introduction of statins. Reprinted from Betteridge DJ, Broome K, Durrington PN et al. Mortality in treated heterozygous familial hypercholesterolaemia: implications for clinical management. *Atherosclerosis.* 1999;142: 105–112, with permission.

Clinical Implications of FH

Vascular Disease

The main clinical consequence of FH is premature coronary heart disease (CHD). In homozygous FH, aortic stenosis can also occur due to lipid deposition; this can sometimes occur in heterozygotes but even if detected is usually not clinically significant. Early studies of FH documented the natural history of the condition. These studies showed that men with heterozygous FH who are not treated have a 50% incidence of clinically evident CHD by the age of 50 years and women a 30% incidence (Slack 1969; Stone et al. 1974). FH can therefore be regarded as accelerating the process of CHD by approximately 20 years on average. In homozygous FH, CHD is very markedly accelerated, often causing symptoms in childhood.

The atherosclerosis in FH has a particular predilection for the coronary arteries. Although carotid intimal thickening does occur in FH, there appears to be little or no increase in the incidence of stroke or peripheral vascular disease in FH. It is widely assumed that the risk of accelerated CHD in FH is directly related to both the concentration of LDL-C and the duration of exposure. It is also influenced by other cardiovascular risk factors particularly male gender and smoking, and factors such as low levels of HDL (Neil et al. 2004b) and elevated levels of Lp(a) (Durrington 2007).

Impact of Treatments on Disease

The natural history of FH has been significantly improved by medical interventions particularly statin therapy to lower LDL-cholesterol. Placebo-controlled trials of LDL-C-lowering therapy in FH would be unethical. Therefore much of the evidence for this comes from observational data from the Simon Broome register. The register was established in 1980 and now contains data on over 4,000 patients aged 18 years or more with treated heterozygous FH. All patients are "flagged" with the Office of National Statistics (ONS) allowing accurate follow-up data on frequency and causes of mortality. Over the course of this observation treatment of FH was transformed by the introduction of statins in the early 1990s. The relative coronary risk in 20–50 year olds prior to the introduction of statins was eightfold (The Simon Broome Register Group 1991), equivalent roughly to a 23-year reduction in life expectancy. As shown in Figure 21–3, in the statin era this has been reduced to threefold (Betteridge et al. 1999), equivalent to a roughly 9-year improvement in life expectancy, raising the possibility that with early identification and the availability of the new more potent statins, life expectancy for FH patients may not be significantly reduced at all. This is supported by more recent analysis of Simon Broome data, which shows that the overall standardized mortality rate for individuals with FH is indistinguishable from the general population, due to major reductions in CHD plus additional reductions in cancers associated with smoking (Neil et al. 2005). This has been interpreted as indicating that the lifestyle interventions in FH (smoking cessation and healthy diet) have a secondary benefit of also reducing the incidence of these conditions.

Treatment of FH

The aim of treatment in FH is directed toward preventing the development and/or progression of CHD. This is achieved by a combination of LDL lowering and general enhancement of cardiovascular protection.

"Lifestyle" Factors

Smoking has a major potentiating action on the development of coronary atheroma and its complications in FH. Therefore it is particularly important that individuals with FH do not smoke and this is a key aspect for health care intervention in children and young people diagnosed with FH. Other general lifestyle factors are also likely to be important, in a similar way as for individuals in the general population. The importance of diet in FH is to provide a general cardioprotective effect rather than to achieve a clinically important lowering of LDL-C. Dietary measures have a relatively small (less than 10%) effect on serum cholesterol values and some individuals (particularly children) need to be advised against excessively restrictive diets. The nutriceutical products, stanols and sterols, which inhibit cholesterol absorption, can reduce serum LDL-C by approximately 10%. These agents may therefore be of some benefit in FH, particularly in combination with statin therapy although large trials to confirm this are lacking. Stanols and sterols appear to be safe and well tolerated, though there is no evidence on their effect of cardiovascular outcomes.

Medication

Although dietary advice is important in counseling for FH patients, all will require lifelong lipid-lowering medication to achieve and maintain a clinically useful reduction in plasma LDL-C levels.

Statins

Statin therapy has revolutionized the treatment of FH. The statin class of lipid-lowering drugs acts by inhibiting HMG-CoA reductase. This is the rate-limiting step for endogenous cholesterol synthesis. In hyperlipidemic patients including those with heterozygous FH, this leads to an upregulation of LDL-R expression on the cell surface leading to increased internalization of LDL-C from the blood. As shown in Figure 21–4, LDL-C concentrations are consistently lowered by 30%–55% depending on the agent and dosage. In homozygous FH patients statins are generally less effective due to the lack (or very low level) of functioning LDL-receptors.

The statins are taken as a single tablet per day. They are generally well tolerated and very extensive postmarketing surveillance has proven their excellent overall safety record. Physicians have become very confident in prescribing these drugs and they now are the third most widely used class of prescription drug in the United Kingdom. Several of the widely used statins (simvastatin and atorvasatin) have either come off patent or are shortly to do so with subsequent reductions in cost with the introduction of generic products. The recent NICE Guideline for FH has shown that treatment of FH patients with the more potent statins is cost-effective, and recommends titration to achieve a greater than 50% reduction of LDL-C from baseline levels.

Cholesterol Absorption Inhibitors (Ezetimibe)

Ezetimibe is a specific inhibitor of cholesterol absorption in the brush border of the small intestine. This inhibits the absorption of dietary cholesterol and more importantly blocks the reuptake of cholesterol secreted in the bile. Consequently, there is a net flux of cholesterol from the liver and upregulation of cell surface LDL-receptors to compensate. Ezetimibe has a modest LDL-C-lowering action when used as monotherapy, but is particularly effective when combined with a statin when it increases the LDL-C-lowering effect by 15%–20% (John et al. 2008). Ezetimibe is generally well tolerated. The use of ezetimibe in combination with a statin has become a widely used treatment approach in FH. This is based on the efficacy of LDL-C lowering combined with excellent tolerability and safety data. However, there is as yet no outcome studies to demonstrate benefit in terms of cardiovascular outcome. A study of ezetimibe in combination with simvastatin compared to simvastatin alone in FH did not demonstrate any additional benefit from ezetimibe in terms of reducing carotid intimal medial thickness (IMT). However, it has been argued that the study did not have sufficient power to demonstrate a significant benefit (Brown and Taylor 2008), especially in this group of well-treated FH patients where starting IMT was already low. Currently the NICE guidelines recommend use of ezetimibe for FH patients as an adjunct to statins or where statins are not tolerated or are contraindicated.

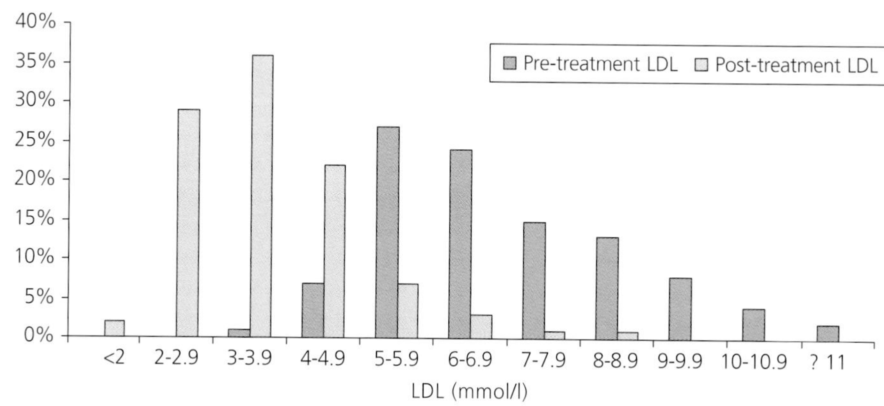

Figure 21–4 Histogram showing distribution of recorded LDL-cholesterol pre- and post-treatment in FH patients. P value difference pre-LDL-cholesterol and post-LDL-cholesterol = <0.001. Reprinted from Hadfield SG, Horara S, Starr BJ et al. Are patients with familial hypercholesterolaemia well managed in lipid clinics? An audit of eleven clinics from the Department of Health Familial Hypercholesterolaemia Cascade Testing project. *Ann Clin Biochem.* 2008;45(Pt 2):199–205, with permission.

Other Lipid-Lowering Medications

Several other drugs do have a role in FH mainly as third-line agents. These are bile acid sequestrants, nicotinic acid derivatives, and fibrates but will not be discussed further in this chapter.

LDL Apheresis

LDL apheresis is a technique that removes LDL from the blood by absorption onto a column as part of an extra corporeal circulation. This is the treatment of choice for individuals with homozygous FH because of the aggressive and early nature of cardiovascular disease, and the relative ineffectiveness of statins in these individuals who lack any functional LDL-receptors. It usually requires creation of an arteriovenous fistula similar to that for hemodialysis and treatments are undertaken at two weekly intervals. In the United Kingdom treatment is currently provided for 0.6 individuals/million of the population and as such is classified as an "orphan treatment." The use of LDL apheresis may occasionally be an option in some heterozygous FH patients for whom medication is ineffective or not tolerated if there is severe and progressive coronary artery disease despite all other treatment measures. The indications for LDL apheresis have recently been considered by a U.K. working group (Thompson et al. 2008) and also by the NICE clinical guideline development group on FH (NICE 2008, www.nice.org.uk/cg071).

Antisense Oligonucleotides

This a novel form of therapy that is being pioneered for patients with homozygous FH. It is based on the principle that oligonucleotides directed against messenger RNA for apolipoprotein B will inhibit hepatic apoB synthesis and hence LDL production. The oligonucleotides are given as subcutaneous injections. Phase I and phase II studies have demonstrated a significant reduction in plasma LDL-C concentrations (30%–50%) with weekly subcutaneous injections and appear to be well tolerated (Kastelein et al. 2006; Akdim et al. 2007).

Drug Treatment of Children

In homozygous FH treatment of children is clearly indicated because of the very early onset of cardiovascular disease. In heterozygous FH there remains debate as to the age at which drug treatment (principally statins) should be started. Vascular studies in children with FH have demonstrated endothelial dysfunction by the age of 10 years (Celermajer et al. 1992). However, for most individuals with FH, clinically evident vascular disease does not become evident until middle age. There is often a reluctance to prescribe lifelong medication in a child who is outwardly healthy, particularly if the lipid concentrations are not particularly high in adult terms, as well as concern that statins might interfere with growth and development. It has been common practice in the United Kingdom to defer statin therapy until after the age of 16 years in individuals with FH. However, this is not in keeping with the clinical evidence available. Controlled trials of statins in children and adolescents with FH have not shown any adverse effects on growth and development (Arambepola et al. 2007), and have also shown that carotid intimal medial thickening can be prevented in children with statin treatment (Koeijvoets et al. 2005; Bhatnagar 2006). Clinical experience would also indicate that initiation of medication is often more acceptable to a 10-year-old than a rebellious teenager, thereby running the risk of missing out altogether on statin treatment. Combined with increasing confidence on the overall safety and efficacy of statins, there is now a strong case for actively considering statin therapy in children with FH from the age of 10 years onward, especially in families with a history of early onset coronary disease (NICE 2008 clinical guideline).

Drug Treatment of Girls and Women of Childbearing Potential

Case reports indicate a small increase in the incidence of congenital fetal abnormalities in pregnancies where the mother has taken statins in the three months preceding conception or in the early stages of pregnancy (Edison and Muenke 2004). Therefore, it is important that women of childbearing age who are being recommended for statin therapy should also be given clear contraceptive advice. This then raises the issue as to when statin therapy should be initiated in girls with FH, particularly given that, in general, women have a degree of atheroprotection until after the menopause. One possible course of action would be to withhold statins completely until there is no further prospect of pregnancy. Given the current trend to delay having a family till the late twenties or later this would seem an unjustifiable risk. Current practice therefore would be that treatment of girls from the age of 10 years is indicated, provided there are clear plans with relation to family planning. This will minimize the time they spend with high LDL-C and this will reduce their long-term coronary risk. As with boys, the decision as to when statin therapy should be initiated is strongly based on clinical judgment and patient preference and will differ for different individuals and different families.

Diagnosis of FH

Clinical Diagnosis

Diagnosis of FH is based on a combination of clinical features, family history, lipid measurements, and DNA analysis. In the United Kingdom the diagnosis of FH is usually based on criteria developed by the Simon Broome (SB) FH register (1991) (Table 21–1), which more recently have been adapted to include the provision for a DNA analysis. Alternative approaches are the Dutch scoring system (Umans-Eckenhausen et al. 2001) and the MedPed criteria. The U.S. MedPed Program (Williams et al. 1993) uses criteria that take account of the prior probability of having FH, which will vary for first-, second-, and third-degree relatives and the general population. Different cut points are then provided for each of these categories for four age groups. However, a comparison of the different

Table 21–1 The Simon Broome Diagnostic Criteria for FH (Simon Broome 1991)

In Adults, total cholesterol above 7.5mmol/L or LDL above 4.9 mmol/L.

For children (<16 years of age) total cholesterol above 6.7 mmol/L or LDL above 4.0 mmol/L.

Plus for a diagnosis of **Definite FH**

Tendon xanthomas in patient or 1st- or 2nd-degree relative **OR** DNA-based evidence of FH.

Plus for a diagnosis of **Possible FH**

Family history of myocardial infarction below age 50 in 2nd-degree relative, below age 60 in 1st-degree relative, OR a Family history of raised cholesterol levels, above 7.5mmol/L in adult 1st- or 2nd-degree relative; above 6.7 mmol/L in child or sibling under 16 years.

methods of clinical diagnosis compared to the "Gold-Standard" of the presence of a DNA mutation suggests that there is little to choose between the approaches in terms of specificity or sensitivity, and in the United Kingdom the Simon Broome criteria are recommended.

The Simon Broome criteria distinguishes individuals as those with a clinical diagnosis of "definite" or "possible" FH, based on the presence of absence of tendon xanthomas (TX), as a sign of the presence of long-term elevation of plasma cholesterol levels. However, TX do not usually develop until the third decade of life, and are not present in all affected members of a family, so while the presence of TX is useful their absence is not definitive, especially in young individuals. In clinical practice "possible" diagnoses outnumber definite diagnoses by approximately two to one, which means that in most cases the diagnosis remains uncertain (Hadfield et al. 2008).

It is important to try to distinguish between acquired polygenic hypercholesterolemia and FH. Patients with FH have sustained elevation of LDL-cholesterol from birth and are at a higher risk of coronary disease for any given LDL concentration. As a consequence of this pattern, as shown in Figure 21–5 the LDL-C years score calculated as the accumulated "exposure" of LDL-C over time, rose at a much greater rate in mutation carriers than in noncarriers. By the age of 50 years, the (gender-averaged) LDL-C score of a mutation carrier was the equivalent of a noncarrier of roughly 75 years of age, explaining the roughly 20 years earlier age of onset of CHD in such patients (Slack 1969; Stone et al. 1974). Consequently, they warrant more intensive cholesterol-lowering therapy than suggested by published risk charts based on their age, sex, LDL levels, and other coronary risk factors.

Clinical Utility of a DNA Diagnosis

Genetic testing for FH is available in the United Kingdom but has not been extensively used to date, in contrast to some other European countries such as the Netherlands and Spain. A DNA-based approach may impact on the clinical assessment and treatment of the patient and family in several ways.

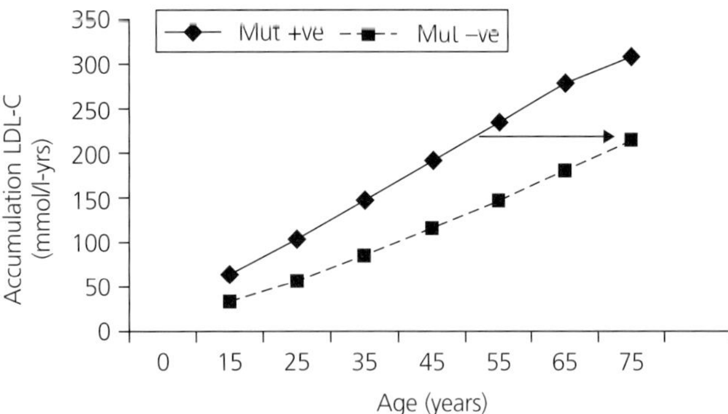

Figure 21–5 Graph showing accumulation of LDL-C "burden" in mutation carriers and non- carriers. The LDL-C years score in mutation carriers and non-carriers was calculated (Umans-Eckenhausen, 2001)as the median of the observed LDL-C level multiplied by the number of years.That is for the 15-year time point it was calculated as the median LDL-C of the 0-14 years subjects (adjusted for gender) multiplied by 15, and for all other time points shown multiplied by 10 years, and summed over time.Reprinted from Starr B, Hadfield SG, Hutten BA, Landsberg P, Leren TP, Damgaard D , Neil HAW and Humphries SE Development of sensitive and specific age- and gender-specific Low Density Lipoprotein cholesterol cut-offs for diagnosis of relatives with Familial Hypercholesterolaemia in cascade testing. *Clin Chem Lab Med* 2008, with permission.

1. Diagnostic Certainty in Probands

In case series of patients with a "clinical diagnosis of FH" the detection rates for identifying a causal mutation range from 30% to 90% (Heath et al. 2001; Graham et al. 2005). The differences in detection rates for particular case series can be explained partially by the variable stringency of criteria applied to clinical diagnosis and the steadily improving capability of DNA methodology to detect a wider range of mutations. It is likely that current methodology can detect a mutation in "true" FH in approximately 85% of cases (McDowell et al. 2007). It also compares favorably with the detection rate in other complex diseases such as breast cancer, where BRAC1/2 screening achieves an overall detection rate of <30% (Bergman et al. 2005; Capalbo et al. 2006).

2. Diagnostic Certainty for Family Members

Once the causative mutation in the patient has been found, molecular testing in relatives is possible in all family members and this allows unequivocal diagnosis. The diagnostic uncertainty caused by the overlap in cholesterol levels between the general population and FH subjects can be eradicated, eliminating false-negative diagnosis. This test is age independent unlike cholesterol, which varies significantly according to age. A single test, once in the lifetime, will be able to ascertain FH status, and early diagnosis in children would also be possible. A DNA versus cholesterol diagnostic study of an extended Irish family showed that 15%–20% of family members would have been incorrectly diagnosed based on cholesterol testing alone (Ward et al. 1996), and in a Finnish study, 10%–20% of relatives would have been misdiagnosed (Koivisto et al. 1992). Recent data from the DNA-based family tracing study in the Netherlands indicates that over 25% of people may have been misdiagnosed if cholesterol testing alone was done (van Aalst-Cohen et al. 2006).

3. Personalizing Diagnosis and Treatment

Several studies suggest that individuals with a DNA diagnosis of FH have a greater risk of developing CHD than those where no mutation can be found (Humphries 2005). In this U.K. study of 409 DFH patients, after adjusting for age, sex, smoking, and systolic blood pressure, compared to those with no detectable mutation, the odds ratio of having CHD in those with an *LDLR* mutation was 1.84-fold higher, for *APOB* 3.40-fold higher, and for *PCSK9* almost 20-fold higher (p = 0.0003 overall). The high risk in *LDLR* and *PCSK9* p.Y374-carrying subjects was partly but not completely explained by their higher pretreatment cholesterol levels (*LDLR, PCSK9,* no mutation, 10.29mmol/L vs. 13.12mmol/L, vs. 9.85mmol/L, p = 0.0002). Thus knowledge of the mutation may be useful in identifying those families where earlier or more aggressive treatment with statins is warranted.

In addition, several studies have shown that particular "severe" *LDLR* mutations have higher lipid levels and CHD risk (Kotze et al. 1993; Graham et al. 1999), as do patients with "null" mutations (Alonso et al. 2008). In genetically heterogeneous populations such as in the United Kingdom, such comparisons are difficult due to the relatively low frequency of any single mutation. In the U.K. cohort, the most common mutation was in intron3 (c.313 + 1G>A), which has been demonstrated to disrupt correct splicing, and result in a functionally "null" allele since the predicted mRNA is in frame with exon 3 deleted (Sun et al. 1995). In the U.K. cohort, carriers of this mutation had mean untreated cholesterol levels 1.35 mmol/L higher, and LDL-C levels 0.62 mmol/L higher than those with no mutation, and a 51% higher risk of having CHD (after taking into account age, gender, and smoking history). By contrast, one of the common mutations in the Netherlands, N543H, appears to have a mild phenotype (Souverein et al. 2007).

From a clinical point of view, the important issue is whether patients carrying different types of mutations respond differently to statin therapy. Since the LDL-lowering effect is mainly due to the upregulation of the patient's normal *LDLR* gene, a priori, the type of defect in the mutated *LDLR* gene is unlikely to have a large effect, and this is essentially borne out by the available data (Sun et al. 1998; Heath et al. 1999). Patients carrying the *APOB* mutation, who have two normal *LDLR* genes, usually show a good response to modest doses of statins (Myant 1993; Heath et al. 1999). In part this is because a large proportion of the triglyceride-rich lipoprotein precursors to circulating LDL are removed by the upregulated LDL-Rs, using apoE as the ligand (Myant 1993). Conversely, in patients carrying the common *PCSK9* p.D374Y mutation, untreated LDL-C levels are often extremely high, and may find it hard to achieve ideal LDL-cholesterol levels, even on high doses of a potent statin (Naoumova 2005; Humphries 2006a, 2006b). This explains their reported higher CHD risk.

1. Adherence to Treatment

Several studies have shown that a DNA diagnosis leads to higher levels of adherence to treatment (Leren et al. 2004).

Determining the Pathogenesis of DNA Mutations

Mutation screening for FH is potentially complicated by the fact that many *LDLR* mutations are family specific and by the presence of numerous polymorphisms that are not pathologically significant. Once the specific base change has been detected in the DNA of an FH patient, the potential functional significance of the change must be evaluated, using defined criteria (see www.cmgs.org—Bell et al. 2007). All possible classes of sequence changes in the *LDLR* have been reported (Leigh et al. 2008). In general, mutations causing a premature stop codon, or a frame-shift mutation or a large deletion or rearrangement of the gene, are all likely to result in the generation of a truncated protein, which in almost all cases will be dysfunctional. If such a mutation is detected, it is almost undoubtedly the cause of FH in this patient.

For missense mutations two types must be distinguished. The first are those that alter a critical amino acid, for example, one that changes or adds a residue such as cysteine, or substitutes a large bulky amino acid such as tryptophan for a small one such as glycine. Mutations causing such substitutions are very likely to result in a defective LDL-receptor and therefore to be the cause of FH in the patient. The second are those missense mutations that cause a conservative amino acid change, or that occur in a noncritical region of the protein, and these may not be FH-causing and their effect must be interpreted with caution. Ideally, the deleterious effect of such mutations needs to be confirmed by expression in vitro, and where they cause either a major defect in binding or in the number of LDL-receptor molecules on the surface of the cell, they can be designated as FH-causing. Unfortunately, such assays are time consuming and technically demanding and the majority of detected missense mutations have not been tested in this way. However, where a mutation alters an amino acid that is conserved across species, or the same mutation has been detected in more than one unrelated patient with heterozygous FH, or in a patient with homozygous FH, and where the mutation occurs on different haplotypes (i.e., is an independent mutation), such a mutation could safely be designated as definite FH.

The final class of mutations may also require in vitro testing to confirm their deleterious effect, and these are mutations in splice junctions, at intron–exon boundaries, within the promoter or upstream region, within introns, within the wobble position of amino acids, or within the 3' untranslated region. Formally, all such mutations must be treated as only possible FH-causing until expressed, but a mutation in the conserved AG sequence that occurs within the intron side of the exon/intron boundary is extremely likely to be causing a splice defect, although it may not be possible to predict the exact effect on messenger RNA splicing and therefore LDL-receptor function. By contrast, changes occurring in the wobble position of a codon that do not alter the predicted amino acid residue at the position are extremely unlikely to be of functional significance, although there are reported examples in other genes of such apparently "silent" changes altering RNA splicing and thus disrupting protein function (Kimchi-Sarfaty et al. 2007).

Laboratory Approaches to DNA Diagnostics

Clinical genetics laboratories currently use one of several different rapid screening methods such as SSCP (Heath et al. 1999) or dHPLC (Graham et al. 1999) that check exon by exon for any sequence differences from normal and then only sequence these. A commercially available kit for screening for deletions and rearrangements of the *LDLR* gene is also now available, and it is known that up to 5% of U.K. FH patients may have such a deletion (Sun et al. 1992). In an attempt to provide a more cost-effective and rapid means of mutation screening an amplification refractory mutation system (ARMS) (Newton et al. 1989) has been designed to detect 11 mutations in the *LDLR* gene, the common mutation (p.R3527Q) in the *APOB* gene and one (p.D374Y) mutation in the *PCSK9* gene. These were selected for inclusion on the basis of their frequency in a cohort of 409 U.K. FH patients (Humphries 2006a, 2006b) where these 13 mutations would have identified the defect in 34% of the whole cohort, explaining 54% of the mutations detected by a full *LDLR* gene screen. These estimates have been confirmed in a subsequent U.K.-wide study of 400 patients attending ten U.K. lipid clinics (Taylor et al. 2007). Results can be obtained within a week of sample receipt, and the high detection rate and good specificity make this a useful initial DNA diagnostic test for U.K. patients.

Currently the cost for a complete screen of the *LDLR* gene and a test for the single common *APOB* and *PCSK9* mutations is about £400 with the cost of a single mutation test in a relative of a patient with a known mutation being about £150. Although this is substantially higher than the cost of a full plasma lipid profile at approximately £12, a DNA diagnosis provides an unequivocal result and need never be repeated. Over the next few years its cost is likely to fall significantly as new, automated, higher throughput methods are developed, including more rapid methods to sequence the whole of the gene.

Cascade Testing

Modeling has shown that "cascade testing," that is, contacting first-degree relatives of FH probands (index cases) and identifying affected relatives by their elevated cholesterol levels, is a cost-effective method of finding additional patients (Marks et al. 2002). This has been used successfully in Manchester (Bhatnagar et al. 2000) and Oxfordshire (Marks et al. 2006) in the United Kingdom and extensively in other countries in Europe, most notably in Holland (Umans-Eckenhausen et al. 2001). To examine how applicable this is in the United Kingdom, the Department of Health has recently funded five pilot sites within England to determine the efficiency of cascade testing within the current social structure and the framework of the National Health Service. Experience from the national cascade screening program in the Netherlands from 1994 onward (Umans-Eckenhausen et al. 2001) demonstrates that 90% of relatives respond to a direct approach and similarly 97% of parents in Oxfordshire agreed to their children being tested (Marks et al. 2006).

However, there is an overlap between the frequency distribution for LDL-C in children with FH and their unaffected brothers and sisters (Kwiterovich et al. 1974; Leonard et al. 1977), which leads to false-positive and false-negative rates of between 8% and 18%. The plasma total and LDL-C levels that are used as diagnostic criteria for FH probands in the general population are too stringent for use in relatives, given the higher prior probability of a first-degree relative being FH (50% vs. 1/500). This problem has been addressed in the "MedPed" cut-offs (Williams et al. 1993) that used a priori probabilities and odds ratios, calculated from published U.S. cholesterol and LDL-C data, to develop cholesterol and LDL-C cut-offs that would give a specificity of 98% for first-, second-, and third-degree relatives also taking into account their age, since cholesterol levels in the general population rise with age. Starr et al. (2008) have used a Bayesian approach with a large, anonymized sample of genetically tested first-degree relatives of Netherlands FH probands (mutation carriers/noncarriers $n = 825/2,469$), to develop age- and gender-specific LDL-C diagnostic cut-offs for first-degree relatives. In children (<15 years) the overlap is approximately 20% but as levels rise with age the overlap increases to the point where there is an unacceptable high degree of false-negative and false-positive diagnosis based on the use of the intersection value (Figure 21–6). This clearly limits the utility of LDL-C cut-offs for an unambiguous diagnosis in this age group. The authors developed cut-off charts: (1) individuals with levels greater than 50% probability of FH (based on age and gender) were given the diagnosis of FH; (2) those with levels less than a 20% probability were given the diagnosis of not-FH; and (3) for the remainder of relatives, where an unambiguous diagnosis could not be given, the subjects were recommended for further testing before a definite diagnosis on lipid levels would be made. These cut-offs have a balanced specificity and sensitivity, which is more appropriate for cascade testing purposes. The authors suggest that country-specific LDL-C cut-offs may lead to greater accuracy for identifying FH patients but should be used with caution and only when a DNA-based diagnosis is not available, since any false-positive results will lead to non-FH subjects becoming probands for further cascade screening, which by definition cannot result in any new FH subjects being detected. This can only be effectively avoided by the use of DNA diagnostic tests.

To achieve maximum efficiency for cascade testing, the optimum method is, once permission has been obtained from the index case, for a direct approach to be made to first-degree relatives by the genetic nurse. This ensures accurate transmission of information, and thus fewer relatives are lost to follow-up by the failure of the index case to contact for any of several personal reasons, including often simply being too busy. Although the ethics of directly approaching family members has been contested, an examination of the ethical arguments against it has shown these to be unsubstantiated for a treatable disease like FH (Newson and Humphries 2005), provided permission to approach relatives is obtained from the index case. While a direct approach may cause a possible breach of confidentiality, if consent from the patient to discuss their condition with a relative were withheld, this would deny relatives the opportunity of risk-reducing treatment. In a systematic literature review of FH cascade testing approaches (Newson and Humphries 2005), little or no evidence was found for adverse effects of direct contact in seven reported studies where direct contact with permission has been used without adverse effects. Criteria were proposed that would allow an appropriate balance to be struck between maximizing the efficiency of family tracing and respecting the interests of probands and their relatives.

Family (Genetic) Counseling

The success of genetic testing for FH will depend, in part, on how learning of a genetic vulnerability affects an individual's motivation to reduce risks. Given the common perception that genetic risks are immutable (Marteau and Lerman 2001), assessing risk using genetic as opposed to nongenetic tests may decrease motivation to engage in risk-reducing behaviors by strengthening beliefs that the disease is neither preventable nor controllable. In addition, it is unknown whether there are any long-term detrimental psychological effects associated with a DNA-based diagnosis of FH, although identification of FH by non-DNA methods has been shown to be of low emotional impact (Tonstad 1996; Tonstad et al. 1996). Data from a detailed evaluation of the psychological impact of DNA-based and non-DNA-based diagnosis of FH in a randomized controlled trial found that mean anxiety and depression levels were in the normal range for both the DNA-based and the non-DNA testing arm (Marteau et al. 2004). Interestingly, a diagnosis based on DNA was perceived as more accurate and seemed to weaken belief in the effectiveness of behavior change, namely, altering diet, in reducing cholesterol, with a trend toward reinforcing belief in biologically based ways of reducing cholesterol, namely, taking medication. In support of this, those who attributed more importance to genes in causing a heart attack reported greater adherence to their cholesterol-lowering medication (Marteau et al. 2004). Thus we predict that confirming a diagnosis or identifying increased risk of disease using DNA could increase perceptions of control in those already aware of their risks for a condition for which biologically based treatments are perceived to be effective. While more studies need to be carried out in this field, these data give no strong concern about any adverse psychological impact of the use of DNA testing in families with FH.

Worry has also been expressed about whether a DNA-based diagnosis of FH may lead to employment discrimination or reduce an individual's ability to obtain life insurance, although again there is little evidence to support either of these concerns. There is currently a moratorium on the use of DNA information for insurance underwriting (recently extended to 2014), and the insurance industry appears to be taking a helpful view of the situation with FH. A survey of insurance companies (Neil et al. 2004a) reported that while patients with FH are (appropriately) seen to be at higher risk than the general population, and would be quoted a higher premium because of their higher risk, companies are prepared to reduce this premium where patients have their LDL-C levels reduced by statin therapy.

Recommendations and Future Perspectives

The genetic and metabolic basis of FH is well understood and highly effective treatments are now available. These treatments (particularly statin medication) prevent the development and

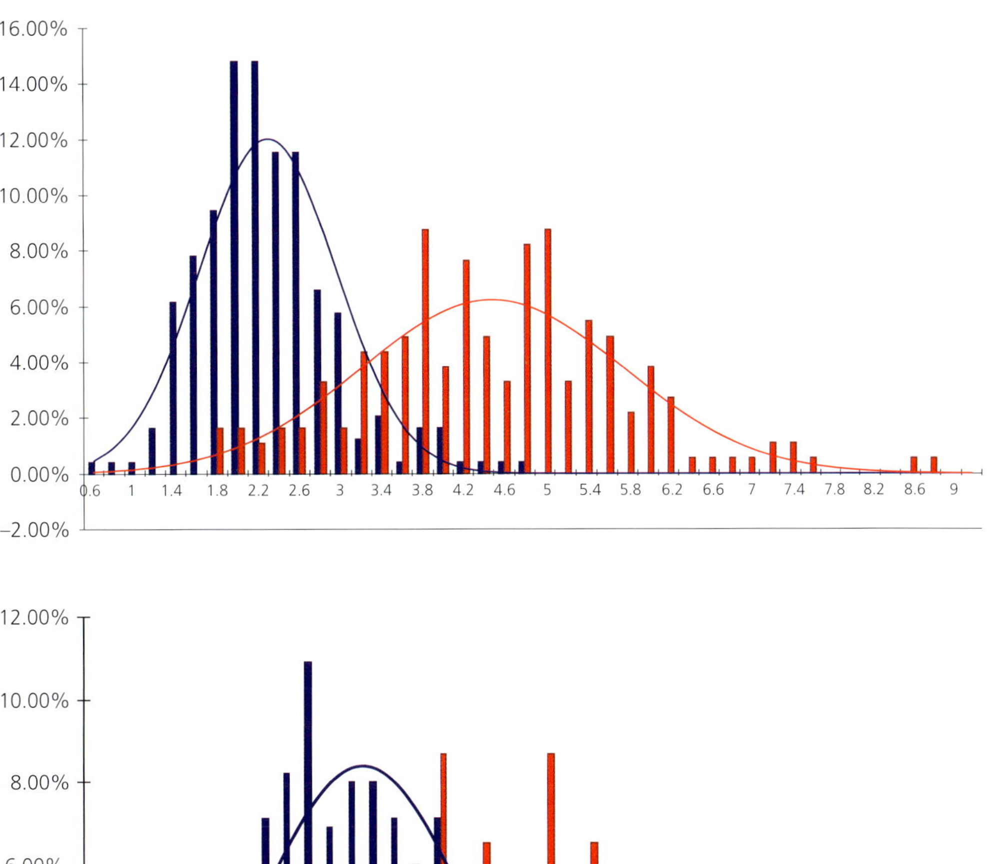

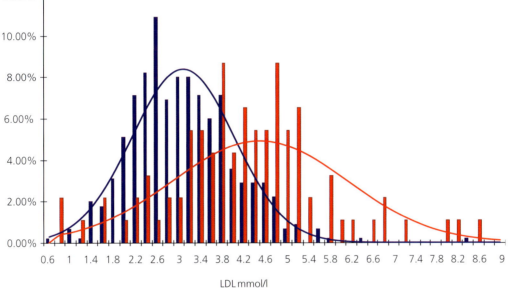

Figure 21–6 Histogram of the observed frequency of LDL-cholesterol levels in mutation carriers (red) and noncarriers (blue), for males (a) aged <15 (b) aged 45–54. Reprinted from Starr B, Hadfield SG, Hutten BA et al. Development of sensitive and specific age- and gender-specific Low Density Lipoprotein cholesterol cut-offs for diagnosis of relatives with Familial Hypercholesterolaemia in cascade testing. *Clin Chem Lab Med.* 2008, with permission.

progression of CHD, such that the standardized mortality rate for individuals identified and appropriately treated with high potency statins, appears now to be similar to the general population. FH can be diagnosed by a combination of clinical features, biochemical (cholesterol) testing, and DNA testing (Neil et al. 2008). Recent developments in DNA technology have made such testing much faster and sensitive and of relatively low cost. Cascade testing has been shown to be an efficient mechanism for family tracing to identify individuals who warrant treatment. In some countries, particularly the Netherlands, national programs, based on systematic cascade testing from mutation-positive individuals have been introduced, and this is now recommended in the United Kingdom. Although the clinical utility of DNA testing in the diagnosis of FH patients has been reported by many groups, its utility in patient management and its cost-effectiveness has yet to be determined unequivocally. More information will need to be collected regarding the negative and positive predictive values of DNA testing and a detailed cost–benefit analysis, to support its widespread introduction to complement diagnosis of FH by lipid levels alone.

Acknowledgments

SEH acknowledges BHF support (RG 2005/014) and SGH acknowledges support by a grant from the Department of Health to the London *IDEAS* Genetics Knowledge Park. IMCD acknowledges support for the Wales FH project from the Wales Gene

Park, Chief Medical Officer for Wales, HEART U.K., British Heart Foundation, Astra Zeneca, MSD, and Pfizer Ltd.

References

Abifadel M, Varret M, Rabes JP, et al. Mutations in PCSK9 cause autosomal dominant hypercholesterolemia. *Nat Genet.* 2003;34:154–156.

Akdim F, Stroes ES, Kastelein JJ. Antisense apolipoprotein B therapy: where do we stand? *Curr Opin Lipidol.* 2007;18:397–400, Review.

Alonso R, Mata N, Castillo S, et al. Cardiovascular disease in familial hypercholesterolaemia: influence of low-density lipoprotein receptor mutation type and classic risk factors. *Atherosclerosis.* 2008;200(2):315–321.

Arambepola C, Farmer AJ, Perera R, Neil HA. Statin treatment for children and adolescents with heterozygous familial hypercholesterolaemia: a systematic review and meta-analysis. *Atherosclerosis.* 2007;195(2):339–347.

Austin MA, Hutter CM, Zimmern RL, Humphries SE. Genetic causes of monogenic heterozygous familial hypercholesterolemia: a HuGE prevalence review. *Am J Epidemiol.* 2004;160(5):407–420.

Bergman A, Flodin A, Engwall Y, et al. A high frequency of germline BRCA1/2 mutations in western Sweden detected with complementary screening techniques. *Fam Cancer.* 2005;4:89–96.

Betteridge DJ, Broome K, Durrington PN, et al. Scientific Steering Committee on behalf of the Simon Broome Register Group—Mortality in treated heterozygous familial hypercholesterolaemia: implications for clinical management. *Atherosclerosis.* 1999;142:105–112.

Bhatnagar D. Diagnosis and screening for familial hypercholesterolaemia: finding the patients, finding the genes. *Ann Clin Biochem.* 2006;43:441–456.

Bhatnagar D, Morgan J, Siddiq S, Mackness MI, Miller JP, Durrington PN. Outcome of case finding among relatives of patients with known heterozygous familial hypercholesterolaemia. *BMJ.* 2000;321:1497–1500.

Brown BG, Taylor AJ. Does ENHANCE diminish confidence in lowering LDL or in ezetimibe? *N Eng J Med.* 2008;358:1504–1507.

Capalbo C, Ricevuto E, Vestri A, et al. BRCA1 and BRCA2 genetic testing in Italian breast and/or ovarian cancer families: mutation spectrum and prevalence and analysis of mutation prediction models. *Ann Oncol.* 2006;7(suppl 7):734–740.

Celermajer DS, Sorensen KE, Gooch VM, et al. Non-invasive detection of endothelial dysfunction in children and adults at risk of atherosclerosis. *Lancet.* 1992;340(8828):1111–1115.

Damgaard D, Larsen ML, Nissen PH, et al. The relationship of molecular genetic to clinical diagnosis of familial hypercholesterolemia in a Danish population. *Atherosclerosis.* 2005;180:155–160.

DeMott K, Nherera L, Shaw EJ, et al. Clinical Guidelines and Evidence Review for Familial hypercholesterolaemia: the identification and management of adults and children with familial hypercholesterolaemia. London: National Collaborating Centre for Primary Care and Royal College of General Practitioners; 2008. Available at: http://www.nice.org.uk/nicemedia/pdf/CG071FullGuideline.pdf.

Durrington PN. *Hyperlipidaemia. Diagnosis and Management.* 3rd ed. London: Hodder Arnold; 2007.

Edison RJ, Muenke M. Central nervous system and limb anomalies in case reports of first-trimester statin exposure. *N Engl J Med.* 2004;350(15):1579–1582.

Graham CA, McClean E, Ward AJ, et al. Mutation screening and genotype:phenotype correlation in familial hypercholesterolaemia. *Atherosclerosis.* 1999;147(2):309–316.

Graham CA, McIlhatton BP, Kirk CW, et al. Genetic screening protocol for familial hypercholesterolemia which includes splicing defects gives an improved mutation detection rate. *Atherosclerosis.* 2005;182(2):331–340.

Hadfield SG, Horara S, Starr BJ, et al. Are patients with familial hypercholesterolaemia well managed in lipid clinics? An audit of eleven clinics from the Department of Health Familial Hypercholesterolaemia Cascade Testing project. *Ann Clin Biochem.* 2008;45(Pt 2):199–205.

Hadfield SG, Humphries SE. Implementation of cascade testing for the detection of familial hypercholesterolaemia. *Curr Opin Lipidol.* 2005;16:428–433.

Heath KE, Gudnason V, Humphries SE, Seed M. The type of mutation in the low density lipoprotein receptor gene influences the cholesterol-lowering response of the HMG-CoA reductase inhibitor simvastatin in patients with heterozygous familial hypercholesterolaemia. *Atherosclerosis.* 1999;143(1):41–54.

Heath KE, Humphries SE, Middleton-Price H, Boxer M. A molecular genetic service for diagnosing individuals with familial hypercholesterolaemia (FH). *Eur J Hum Gen.* 2001;9:244–252.

Humphries SE, Cranston T, Allen M, et al. Mutational analysis in UK patients with a clinical diagnosis of familial hypercholesterolaemia: relationship with plasma lipid traits, heart disease risk and utility in relative tracing. *J Mol Med.* 2006a;84:203–214.

Humphries SE, Whittall RA, Hubbart CS, et al. Genetic causes of familial hypercholesterolaemia in patients in the UK: relation to plasma lipid levels and coronary heart disease risk. *J Med Genet.* 2006b;43:943–949.

John JP, Fatima Akdim K, Erik SG, et al. Simvastatin with or without ezetimibe in familial hypercholesterolemia. *N Eng J Med.* 2008;358:1431–1443.

Kastelein JJ, Wedel MK, Baker BF, et al. Potent reduction of apolipoprotein B and low-density lipoprotein cholesterol by short-term administration of an antisense inhibitor of apolipoprotein B. *Circulation.* 2006;114:1729–1735.

Kimchi-Sarfaty C, Oh JM, Kim I-W, et al. A "silent" polymorphism in the MDR1 gene changes substrate specificity. *Science.* 2007;315:525–528.

Koeijvoets KC, Rodenburg J, Hutten BA, Wiegman A, Kastelein JJ, Sijbrands EJ. Low-density lipoprotein receptor genotype and response to pravastatin in children with familial hypercholesterolemia: substudy of an intima-media thickness trial. *Circulation.* 2005;112(20):3168–3173.

Koivisto PVI, Koivisto U-M, Miettinen TA, Kontula K. Diagnosis of heterozygous familial hypercholesterolaemia. DNA analysis complements clinical examination and analysis of serum lipid levels. *Arterioscler & Thromb.* 1992;12:584–592.

Kotze MJ, De Villiers WJ, Steyn K, et al. Phenotypic variation among familial hypercholesterolemics heterozygous for either one of two Afrikaner founder LDL receptor mutations. *Arterioscler & Thromb.* 1993;13(10):1460–1468.

Kwiterovich PO Jr, Fredrickson DS, Levy RI. Familial hypercholesterolemia (one form of familial type II hyperlipoproteinemia). A study of its biochemical, genetic and clinical presentation in childhood. *J Clin Invest.* 1974;53:1237–1249.

Kwon HJ, Lagace TA, McNutt MC, Horton JD, Deisenhofer J. Molecular basis for LDL receptor recognition by PCSK9. *Proc Natl Acad Sci USA.* 2008;105(6):1820–1825.

Lambert G. Unravelling the functional significance of PCSK9. *Curr Opin Lipidol.* 2007;18(3):304–309.

Leigh SE, Foster AH, Whittall RA, Hubbart CS, Humphries SE. Update and analysis of the University College London low density lipoprotein receptor familial hypercholesterolemia database. *Ann Hum Genet.* 2008;72(Pt 4):485–498.

Leonard JV, Whitelaw AG, Wolff OH, Lloyd JK, Slack J. Diagnosing familial hypercholesterolaemia in childhood by measuring serum cholesterol. *Br Med J.* 1977;1:1566–1568.

Leren TP. Cascade genetic screening for familial hypercholesterolemia. *Clin Genet.* 2004a;66:483–487.

Leren TP. Mutations in the PCSK9 gene in Norwegian subjects with autosomal dominant hypercholesterolemia. *Clin Genet.* 2004b;65(5):419–422.

Leren TP, Manshaus T, Skovholt U, et al. Application of molecular genetics for diagnosing familial hypercholesterolemia in Norway: results from a family-based screening program. *Semin Vasc Med.* 2004;4:75–85.

Marks D, Thorogood M, Farrer JM, et al. Census of clinics providing specialist lipid services in the UK. *J Pub Health.* 2004;26:353–354.

Marks D, Thorogood M, Neil SM, Humphries SE, Neil HA. Cascade screening for familial hypercholesterolaemia: implications of a pilot study for national screening programmes. *J Med Screen.* 2006;13(3):156–159.

Marks D, Wonderling D, Thorogood M, Lambert H, Humphries SE, Neil HA. Cost effectiveness analysis of different approaches of screening for familial hypercholesterolaemia. *BMJ.* 2002;324:1303.

Marteau T, Senior V, Humphries SE, et al. Psychological impact of genetic testing for familial hypercholesterolemia within a previously aware population: a randomized controlled trial. *Am J Med Genet.* 2004;128A(3):285–293.

Marteau TM, Lerman C. Genetic risk and behavior change. *Br Med J.* 2001;322:1056–1059.

McDowell I, Watson M, Townsend D, Featherstone K, Parham K, Whatley S. An evaluation of DNA diagnostics for familial hypercholesterolaemia including a study of personal and family implications (Abstract). *Atherosclerosis.* 2007;194:282.

Myant NB. Familial defective apolipoprotein B-100: a review, including some comparisons with familial hypercholesterolaemia. *Atherosclerosis.* 1993;104(1–2):1–18.

Naoumova RP, Tosi I, Patel D, et al. Severe hypercholesterolemia in four British families with the D374Y mutation in the PCSK9 gene: long-term follow-up and treatment response. *Arterioscler Thromb Vasc Biol.* 2005;25:2654–2660.

Neil HA, Hammond T, Mant D, Humphries SE. Effect of statin treatment for familial hypercholesterolaemia on life assurance: results of consecutive surveys in 1990 and 2002. *BMJ.* 2004a;328:500–501.

Neil HA, Hawkins MM, Durrington PN, et al. Non-coronary heart disease mortality and risk of fatal cancer in patients with treated heterozygous familial hypercholesterolaemia: a prospective registry study. *Atherosclerosis.* 2005;179(2):293–297.

Neil HAW, Cooper J, Betteridge DJ, et al. Reductions in all-cause, cancer and coronary mortality in statin-treated patients with heterozygous familial hypercholesterolaemia: a prospective registry study. *Eur Heart J.* 2008;29(21):2625–2633. Epub Oct 7, 2008.

Neil HAW, Hammond T, Huxley R, et al. The extent of under-diagnosis of familial hypercholesterolaemia in routine practice: results of a prospective register study. *BMJ.* 2000;321:148.

Neil HAW, Seagroatt V, Betteridge DJ, et al. Established and emerging coronary risk factors in patients with heterozygous familial hypercholesterolaemia. *Heart.* 2004b;90:1431–1437.

Newson AJ, Humphries SE. Cascade testing in familial hypercholesterolaemia: how should family members be contacted? *Eur J Hum Genet.* 2005;13:401–408.

Newton CR, Graham A, Heptinstall LE, et al. Analysis of any point mutation in DNA. The Amplification Refractory Mutation System (ARMS). *Nucleic Acids Res.* 1989;17:2503–2516.

Pocovi M, Civeira F, Alonso R, Mata P. Familial hypercholesterolemia in Spain: case-finding program, clinical and genetic aspects. *Semin Vasc Med.* 2004;4:67–74.

Scientific Steering Committee on behalf of The Simon Broome Register Group: the risk of fatal coronary heart disease in familial hypercholesterolaemia. *BMJ.* 1991;303:893–896.

Slack J. Risks of ischaemic heart-disease in familial hyperlipoproteinaemic states. *Lancet.* 1969;2:1380–1382.

Smith AJ, Ahmed F, Nair D, et al. A functional mutation in the LDLR promoter (-139C>G) in a patient with familial hypercholesterolemia. *Eur J Hum Genet.* 2007;15(11):1186–1189.

Soutar AK, Naoumova RP. Mechanisms of disease: genetic causes of familial hypercholesterolemia. *Nat Clin Pract Cardiovasc Med.* 2007;4(4):214–225.

Souverein OW, Defesche JC, Zwinderman AH, Kastelein JJP, Tanck MWT. Influence of LDL-receptor mutation type on age at first cardiovascular event in patients with familial hypercholesterolaemia. *Eur Heart J.* 2007;28(3):299–304.

Starr B, Hadfield SG, Hutten BA, et al. Development of sensitive and specific age- and gender-specific low density lipoprotein cholesterol cut-offs for diagnosis of relatives with familial hypercholesterolaemia in cascade testing. *Clin Chem Lab Med.* 2008;46(6):791–803.

Stone NJ, Levy RI, Fredrickson DS, Verter J. Coronary artery disease in 116 kindred with familial type II hyperlipoproteinemia. *Circulation.* 1974;49:476–488.

Sun X-M, Eden ER, Tosi I, et al. Evidence for effect of mutant PCSK9 on apolipoprotein B secretion as the cause of unusually severe dominant hypercholesterolaemia. *Hum Mol Genet.* 2005;14(9):1161–1169.

Sun X-M, Patel DD, Bhatnagar D, Knight BL, Soutar AK. Characterization of a splice-site mutation in the gene for the LDL receptor associated with an unpredictably severe clinical phenotype in English patients with heterozygous FH. *Arterioscler Thromb Vasc Biol.* 1995;15(2):219–227.

Sun X-M, Patel DD, Knight BL, Soutar AK. Influence of genotype at the low density lipoprotein (LDL) receptor gene locus on the clinical phenotype and response to lipid-lowering drug therapy in heterozygous familial hypercholesterolaemia. The Familial Hypercholesterolaemia Regression Study Group. *Atherosclerosis.* 1998;136(1):175–185.

Sun X-M, Webb JC, Gudnason V, et al. Characterization of deletions in the LDL receptor gene in patients with familial hypercholesterolemia in the United Kingdom. *Arterioscler Thromb.* 1992;12:762–770.

Taylor A, Tabrah S, Wang D, et al. Multiplex ARMS analysis to detect 13 common mutations in familial hypercholesterolaemia. *Clin Genet.* 2007;71(6):561–568.

Thompson GR, Heart UK. LDL Apheresis working group recommendations for the use of LDL apheresis *Atherosclerosis.* 2008;198(2):247–255.

Timms KM, Wagner S, Samuels ME, et al. A mutation in PCSK9 causing autosomal-dominant hypercholesterolemia in a Utah pedigree. *Hum Genet.* 2004;114:349–353.

Tonstad S. Familial hypercholesterolaemia: a pilot study of parents and children's concerns. *Acta Pediatr.* 1996;85:1307–1313.

Tonstad S, Novik TS, Vandvik IH. Psychosocial function during treatment for familial hypercholesterolaemia. *Pediatrics.* 1996;98:249–255.

Umans-Eckenhausen MAW, Defesche JC, Sijbrands EJG, Scheerder RLJM, Kastelein JJP. Review of first 5 years of screening for familial hypercholesterolaemia in the Netherlands. *Lancet.* 2001;357:165–168.

van Aalst-Cohen ES, Jansen AC, Tanck MW, et al. Diagnosing familial hypercholesterolaemia: the relevance of genetic testing. *Eur Heart J.* 2006;27(18):2240–2246.

Varret M, Abifadel M, Rabès JP, Boileau C. Genetic heterogeneity of autosomal dominant hypercholesterolemia. *Clin Genet.* 2008;73(1):1–13.

Ward AJ, O'Kane M, Nicholls DP, Young IS, Nevin N, Graham CA. A novel single base deletion in the LDLR gene (211 del G). Effect on serum lipid profiles and the influence of other genetic polymorphisms in the ACE, APOE and APOB genes. *Atherosclerosis.* 1996;120:83–91.

Williams RR, Hunt SC, Schumacher MC, et al. Diagnosing heterozygous familial hypercholesterolemia using new practical criteria validated by molecular genetics. *Am J Cardiol.* 1993;72:171–176.

www.cmgs.org—Bell J, Bodmer D, Sistermans E, Ramsden SC. Practice guidelines for the Interpretation and Reporting of Unclassified Variants (UVs) in Clinical Molecular Genetics. 2007.

22

Genetics of Coronary Artery Disease

Yoshiji Yamada, Sahoko Ichihara, and Tamotsu Nishida

Introduction

Recent progress in human genetics and genomics research, highlighted by completion of the nucleotide sequence of the human genome by the Human Genome Project (International Human Genome Sequencing Consortium 2004), has provided substantial benefits to clinical medicine, including facilitation of the characterization of disease pathogenesis at the molecular level and the development of panels of genetic markers for assessment of disease risk. In particular, determination of single nucleotide polymorphisms (SNPs) and haplotype blocks and the specification of tag SNPs in each haplotype block for four ethnic groups by the International HapMap Project (The International HapMap Consortium 2007) have led to increasingly effective approaches to the identification of genetic variation associated with various multifactorial diseases, providing new insight into the pathogenesis of these conditions. Furthermore, technological developments such as cDNA microarrays and SNP chips that provide huge amounts of genetic information have made possible the detection of genetic differences among individuals at the whole-genome level.

Selection of the most appropriate strategies for disease prevention or therapy on the basis of genetic information for a given individual is referred to as personalized or individualized medicine. In conventional medicine, medications are prescribed on the basis of the diagnosis and severity of the disease. However, the efficacy of drugs and the incidence of side effects vary among individuals. The goal of treatment based on genetic or genomic information is to be able to predict therapeutic outcome or side effects in an individual, thereby increasing the effectiveness and safety of therapy. In addition, the clarification of disease etiologies at the molecular level and the identification of genetic variants that confer disease susceptibility are likely to contribute both to disease prevention and to the development of new medicines.

Myocardial infarction (MI) is an important clinical problem because of its large contribution to mortality. In the United States, the total number of individuals affected by coronary artery disease (CAD) was 15.8 million in 2004, with nearly 450,000 patients dying annually from this condition (Rosamond et al. 2007). The annual incidence of MI was 565,000 new attacks and 300,000 recurrent attacks, with an annual mortality of 157,000 (Rosamond et al. 2007). As in the United States, coronary heart disease (CHD) is the most common cause of death in the United Kingdom, where it is responsible for around 101,000 deaths each year (British Heart Foundation; http://www.heartstats.org/homepage.asp). In Japan, the total number of individuals affected by CAD was 910,000 in 2005 and approximately 50,000 people die annually from MI (Ministry of Health, Labor, and Welfare of Japan).

The main causal and treatable risk factors for MI include hypertension, hypercholesterolemia or dyslipidemia, diabetes mellitus, and smoking. In addition to these risk factors, recent studies have shown the importance of genetic factors and of interactions between multiple genes and environmental factors in this condition (Topol et al. 2006; Arnett et al. 2007; Kullo and Ding 2007). The common forms of CAD and MI are thus thought to be multifactorial and to be determined by many genes, each with a relatively small effect, working alone or in combination with modifier genes or environmental factors (or both). The "common disease, common variants" hypothesis proposes that genetic variants present in many normal individuals contribute to overall CAD risk. In addition, susceptibility to some common diseases may be conferred, in part, by rarer variants (Arnett et al. 2007).

Despite recent advances in therapy, such as drug-eluting stents (Marroquin et al. 2008), for acute coronary syndrome (ACS), CAD remains the leading cause of death in the United States and United Kingdom and the second leading cause of death in Japan. Disease prevention is an important strategy for reducing the overall burden of CAD and MI, and the identification of biomarkers for disease risk is key both for risk prediction and for potential intervention to reduce the chance of future events.

Familial Aggregation of CAD

Twin and family studies have established that CAD aggregates in families, with a family history of early onset CAD having long been considered a risk factor for the disease (Scheuner 2003). The familial clustering of CAD might be explained in part by heritable quantitative variation in known CAD risk factors. However, evidence suggests that family history contributes to an increased risk of CAD independently of the known risk factors (Yusuf et al. 2004; Murabito et al. 2005). High-risk families account for a substantial proportion of early onset CAD cases in the general population.

In one study, families with a history of early onset CAD represented only 14% of the general population but accounted for 72% of early onset CAD cases (men aged <55 years, women aged <65 years) and 48% of CAD at all ages (Williams et al. 2001). A history of early onset CAD in a first-degree relative approximately doubles a person's risk of CAD, although the reported relative risk ranges from 1.3 to 11.3 (Myers et al. 1990; Roncaglioni et al. 1992; Friedlander et al. 1998; Lloyd-Jones et al. 2004; Yusuf et al. 2004; Kaikkonen et al. 2006). The highest relative hazard of CAD-related death is seen in monozygotic twins, when one twin dies of early onset CAD (Yusuf et al. 2004). Furthermore, sibling history of MI seems to be a greater risk factor than parental history of early onset CAD (Nasir et al. 2004). A family risk score for CAD has been proposed to evaluate the ratio of observed CAD events to expected events in an individual's first-degree relatives, with adjustment for age and sex at the onset of the first event (Li et al. 2000). A higher family risk score is associated with greater CAD risk (Kullo and Ding 2007).

Mendelian Disorders Associated with CAD and MI

Genes responsible for familial hypercholesterolemia and Tangier disease are the prototypical examples of causal genes for Mendelian disorders associated with CAD and MI. Familial hypercholesterolemia is an autosomal dominant disorder characterized by pronounced increases in the serum concentrations of total cholesterol and low-density lipoprotein (LDL)-cholesterol. Cholesterol deposition accounts for the associated findings, which include tendon xanthomas and markedly increases the risk for CAD and MI. One of the underlying causes of familial hypercholesterolemia is a defect in the LDL receptor, which is responsible for the uptake of most circulating LDL-cholesterol by the liver. Familial hypercholesterolemia is an uncommon disorder, and homozygosity for an associated mutation results in exceptionally high LDL-cholesterol levels that lead to progressive CAD and MI in the first decade of life. In addition to mutations of the LDL receptor gene (*LDLR*), familial hypercholesterolemia can be caused by mutations in the apolipoprotein B100 gene (*APOB*), proprotein convertase subtilisin/kexin type 9 gene (*PCSK9*), cytochrome P450, family 7, subfamily A, polypeptide 1 gene (*CYP7A1*), and LDL-receptor adaptor protein 1 gene (*ARH*). Studies of the molecular basis of familial hypercholesterolemia led to identification of the pathways of LDL-cholesterol metabolism and the subsequent development of statins (Goldstein and Brown 1973; Rader et al. 2003; Arnett et al. 2007; Kullo and Ding 2007; Robin et al. 2007; Soutar and Naoumova 2007).

Rare allelic variants of genes thought to influence high-density lipoprotein (HDL)-cholesterol metabolism, including those for ATP-binding cassette, subfamily A, member 1 (*ABCA1*), apolipoprotein A-I (*APOA1*), and lecithin-cholesterol acyltransferase (*LCAT*), are associated with syndromes characterized by a low plasma concentration of HDL-cholesterol but are also found in individuals from the general population with low HDL-cholesterol levels (Cohen et al. 2004; Frikke-Schmidt et al. 2004). Tangier disease is a rare autosomal recessive disorder characterized by diffuse deposition of cholesterol esters throughout the reticuloendothelial system and by the classic manifestation of enlarged yellow tonsils. Affected individuals have low plasma HDL-cholesterol levels as a result of loss-of-function mutations in *ABCA1* (Bodzioch et al. 1999; Brooks-Wilson et al. 1999; Rust et al. 1999). In families affected by Tangier disease, the onset of CAD occurs substantially earlier in mutation carriers than in noncarriers (Clee et al. 2000; van Dam et al. 2002). The increased incidence of early onset CAD in *ABCA1* mutation carriers is likely attributable to the accumulation of lipid-laden macrophage foam cells in the vascular wall and the consequent development and progression of atherosclerosis (Oram and Heinecke 2005).

The genes for familial hypercholesterolemia and Tangier disease were identified by linkage analysis, given that each condition segregates in a Mendelian pattern with a clear marker for the presence of the mutant gene. Clinical genetic testing is available for both of these disorders. The efficacy of testing is limited, however, to confirmation of the clinical diagnosis in an individual with an abnormal lipid profile or to prenatal diagnosis. The real power of genetic testing is to identify at-risk individuals who cannot otherwise be identified because they lack other clinical or laboratory markers (Robin et al. 2007). Several Mendelian disorders of lipid metabolism associated with increased CAD risk have yielded new insight into the mechanisms of CAD. The examination of disease pathogenesis and gene function in such Mendelian disorders may increase our understanding of the etiology of complex traits (Antonarakis and Beckmann 2006). In addition, common variation in genes implicated in Mendelian disorders might be used to determine disease susceptibility in the general population (Kullo and Ding 2007).

Linkage Analysis of MI, ACS, or CAD

Several genome-wide linkage analyses of families or sib pairs have identified chromosomal loci linked to or genetic variations that confer susceptibility to MI, ACS, or CAD (Pajukanta et al. 2000; Francke et al. 2001; Broeckel et al. 2002; Harrap et al. 2002; Wang et al. 2003, 2004; Hauser et al. 2004; Helgadottir et al. 2004; The BHF Family Heart Study Research Group 2005; Farrall et al. 2006). The published results of genome-wide linkage analyses for these conditions are summarized in Table 22–1. Genomic regions identified in the published linkage studies as being correlated with MI or CAD are largely nonoverlapping, suggestive of genetic complexity in which multiple genes are responsible for the development of these conditions, although phenotypic heterogeneity could also have contributed to the nonreplicability of results.

The deCODE Genetics group (Helgadottir et al. 2004) performed linkage analysis with 1,068 microsatellite markers and found a linkage peak (LOD score of 2.86) at chromosomal region 13q12-q13 for 296 Icelandic families (713 individuals) enrolled on the basis of a history of MI. The researchers then genotyped an additional 120 microsatellite markers in this interval in 802 individuals with MI and 837 controls, and they found that a four-marker SNP haplotype spanning the arachidonate 5-lipoxygenase–activating protein gene (*ALOX5AP*) was associated with MI (odds ratio, 1.8) and stroke (odds ratio, 1.7). A subsequent study found that *ALOX5AP* was associated with CAD in British individuals and with stroke in Icelandic and Scottish populations (Helgadottir et al. 2005).

On the basis of the results of the same genome-wide scan, the deCODE Genetics group (Helgadottir et al. 2006) performed fine mapping to determine that a five- to seven-marker SNP haplotype of the leukotriene A4 hydrolase gene (*LTA4H*) accounted for a linkage peak at 12q22. Of particular interest with this haplotype was its ancestry-specific association with the incidence and risk of MI. In European-Americans, the relative risk for MI was only 1.2, with a population attributable risk of 4.6%, whereas among

Table 22–1 Genome-Wide Linkage Analyses of Myocardial Infarction (MI), Acute Coronary Syndrome (ACS), or Coronary Heart Disease (CHD)

Chromosomal Locus	Marker/Gene Symbol	Phenotype	Reference
1p34-p36	D1S1597	MI	Wang et al. 2004
1q25	D1S518	ACS	Hauser et al. 2004
2p12-q23.3	D2S2271	CHD	The BHF Family Heart Study Research Group 2005
2p12-q23.3	D2S2216	MI	The BHF Family Heart Study Research Group 2005
2q21.1-q22	D2S129, D2S2313	CHD	Pajukanta et al. 2000
2q36-q37.3	D2S125	ACS	Harrap et al. 2002
3q13	D3S2460	CHD	Hauser et al. 2004
3q27	D3S1262, D3S1580	CHD, MI	Francke et al. 2001
10q23	D10S185	CHD	Francke et al. 2001
13q12	D13S289/*ALOX5AP*	MI	Helgadottir et al. 2004
14q	D14S1426	MI	Broeckel et al. 2002
15q26	D15S120/*MEF2A*	CHD, MI	Wang et al. 2003
16p13-pter	D16S423	CHD	Francke et al. 2001
17p11.2-q21	D17S921, D17S787	CHD	Farrall et al. 2006
Xq23-q26	DXS1072, DXS1212	CHD	Pajukanta et al. 2000

individuals of African ancestry the relative risk was 3.5 and the population attributable risk was 14% (Helgadottir et al. 2006). Two different genes (*ALOX5AP* and *LTA4H*) in the same inflammation-related pathway of leukotriene B4 production were thus found to be associated with disease in a single genome-wide scan. This pathway had already been implicated in studies of murine experimental atherosclerosis as well as in human epidemiological and pathological studies (Mehrabian et al. 2002; Spanbroek et al. 2003; Dwyer et al. 2004). In addition, a small-molecule inhibitor of ALOX5AP was shown to reduce both leukotriene production and the plasma concentration of C-reactive protein (CRP), an important biomarker for CAD, in a pilot, placebo-controlled, randomized trial with individuals harboring the risk *ALOX5AP* or *LTA4H* haplotype (Hakonarson et al. 2005). Of note, *LTA4H* was the first MI-linked gene to show an ancestry-specific risk (Topol et al. 2006; Damani and Topol 2007).

Association Studies of MI or CAD

Various association studies of unrelated individuals have identified genetic variations that confer susceptibility to MI or CAD (Box 22–1). The published results for genes associated with these conditions are summarized in Table 22–2. Numerous candidate genes have been implicated, but those that show reproducible associations between risk alleles and CAD or MI in replication studies are few. The candidate gene approach has been widely applied to analysis of the possible association between genetic variants and disease, with genes selected on the basis of a priori hypotheses regarding their potential etiologic role. It is characterized as a hypothesis-testing approach because of the biological observation supporting a role for the proposed candidate gene. The candidate gene approach is not able, however, to identify disease-associated polymorphisms in unknown genes. The recent development of high-density genotyping arrays has improved the resolution of unbiased genome-wide scans for common variants associated with multifactorial diseases. Currently, the genome-wide association study (GWAS) makes use of high-throughput genotyping technologies that include about 1 million probes for SNPs and 1 million probes for copy number variations to examine their relation to clinical conditions or measurable traits. Since 2005, nearly 100 loci for as many as 40 common diseases or traits have been identified by GWAS, many in genes not previously suspected of having a role in the condition studied, and some in genomic regions containing no known genes. Although GWAS represent a substantial advance in the search for genetic variants that influence disease, they also have important limitations, including the potential for generating false-positive or false-negative results and for biases related to the selection of study participants and genotyping errors (Pearson and Manolio 2008).

Mendelian Randomization

Mendelian randomization analysis is a relatively recent development in genetic epidemiology based on Mendel's second law, which states that the inheritance of one trait is independent of that of other traits (Keavney 2002; Davey Smith and Ebrahim 2003). It relies on common genetic polymorphisms that are known to influence exposure patterns (such as the propensity to drink alcohol) or to have effects equivalent to those produced by modifiable exposures (such as an increased serum cholesterol concentration). Associations between genetic variants and outcomes are not generally confounded by behavioral or environmental exposures, with the result that observational studies of genetic variants have similar properties to intention to treat analyses in randomized controlled trials. The simplest way of appreciating the potential of Mendelian randomization analysis is to consider applications of the underlying principles. The inferences that can be drawn from Mendelian randomization studies depend on the different ways in which genetic variants can serve as a proxy for environmentally modifiable exposures (Davey Smith and Ebrahim 2005).

The relations of polymorphisms of the CRP gene (*CRP*) to circulating CRP concentrations and the prevalence of CAD or

Table 22–2 Genes Shown to be Related to the Prevalence of Myocardial Infarction or Coronary Artery Disease

Chromosomal Locus	Gene Name	Gene Symbol	Reference
1p36.3	5,10-Methylenetetrahydrofolate reductase	*MTHFR*	Gallagher et al. 1996; Yamada et al. 2006
1p36.2	Natriuretic peptide precursor A	*NPPA*	Gruchala et al. 2003
1p35.1	Gap junction protein, α-4	*GJA4*	Yamada et al. 2002
1p34.1-p32	Proprotein convertase, subtilisin/kexin-type, 9	*PCSK9*	Cohen et al. 2006
1p34	Low-density lipoprotein receptor-related protein 8, apolipoprotein E receptor	*LRP8*	Shen et al. 2007
1p31.3-p31.2	Cytochrome P450, subfamily IIJ, polypeptide 2	*CYP2J2*	Liu et al. 2007
1p22-p21	Coagulation factor III	*F3*	Ott et al. 2004
1p22.1	Glutamate-cysteine ligase, modifier subunit	*GCLM*	Nakamura et al. 2002
1q21-q23	C-reactive protein, pentraxin-related	*CRP*	Lange et al. 2006
1q23-q25	Selectin E	*SELE*	Yoshida et al. 2003
1q23-q25	Selectin P	*SELP*	Tregouet et al. 2002
1q25	Tumor necrosis factor ligand superfamily, member 4	*TNFSF4*	Wang et al. 2005
1q25.2-q25.3	Prostaglandin-endoperoxide synthase 2	*PTGS2*	Cipollone et al. 2004
1q32	Complement factor H	*CFH*	Kardys et al. 2006
1q42-q43	Angiotensinogen	*AGT*	Katsuya et al. 1995
1q44	Olfactory receptor, family 13, subfamily G, member 1	*OR13G1*	Shiffman et al. 2005
2p24	Apolipoprotein B	*APOB*	Hegele et al. 1986
2p12-p11.2	Vesicle-associated membrane protein 8	*VAMP8*	Shiffman et al. 2006
2q14	Interleukin 1-β	*IL1B*	Iacoviello et al. 2005
2q31	Collagen, type III, α-1	*COL3A1*	Muckian et al. 2002
3pter-p21	Chemokine, CX3C motif, receptor 1	*CX3CR1*	Lavergne et al. 2005
3p25	Peroxisome proliferator-activated receptor-gamma	*PPARG*	Ridker et al. 2003
3p21	Chemokine, CC motif, receptor 2	*CCR2*	Ortlepp et al. 2003
3p21	Chemokine, CC motif, receptor 5	*CCR5*	Gonzalez et al. 2001
3q13.3-q21	Calcium-sensing receptor	*CASR*	Marz et al. 2007
3q21-q25	Angiotensin-receptor 1	*AGTR1*	Tiret et al. 1994
3q26.3-q27	Thrombopoietin	*THPO*	Webb et al. 2001
3q27	Adipocyte, C1Q, and collagen domain containing	*ADIPOQ*	Ohashi et al. 2004
4q22-q24	Microsomal triglyceride transfer protein, 88-kD	*MTP*	Ledmyr et al. 2004
4q26-q28	Annexin A5	*ANXA5*	Gonzalez-Conejero et al. 2002
4q28	Fibrinogen, B β polypeptide	*FGB*	Behague et al. 1996
4q28-q31	Fatty acid binding protein 2	*FABP2*	Georgopoulos et al. 2007
4q32.3	Palladin, cytoskeletal associated protein	*PALLD*	Shiffman et al. 2005
5q13	Thrombospondin IV	*THBS4*	Topol et al. 2001
5q23-q31	Integrin, α-2	*ITGA2*	Moshfegh et al. 1999
5q31.1	Monocyte differentiation antigen CD14	*CD14*	Hubacek et al. 1999
5q32-q34	β -2-adrenergic receptor	*ADRB2*	Sala et al. 2001
5q33-qter	Factor XII	*F12*	Endler et al. 2001
5q34	Potassium channel, calcium-activated, large conductance, subfamily M, β member 1	*KCNMB1*	Senti et al. 2005
6p25-p24	Factor XIII, A1 subunit	*F13A1*	Kohler et al. 1998
6p21.3	Lymphotoxin-α	*LTA*	Ozaki et al. 2002
6p21.3	Tumor necrosis factor	*TNF*	Vendrell et al. 2003
6p21.2	Kinesin family member 6	*KIF6*	Iakoubova et al. 2008
6p21.2-p12	Phospholipase A2, group VII	*PLA2G7*	Yamada et al. 1998
6p12	Glutamate-cysteine ligase, catalytic subunit	*GCLC*	Koide et al. 2003
6p12	Vascular endothelial growth factor	*VEGF*	Howell et al. 2005
6q22	c-Ros oncogene 1, receptor tyrosine kinase	*ROS1*	Shiffman et al. 2005
6q22-q23	Ectonucleotide pyrophosphatase/phosphodiesterase 1	*ENPP1*	Bacci et al. 2005

Table 22–2 (Continued)

Chromosomal Locus	Gene Name	Gene Symbol	Reference
6q23	Arginase, liver	*ARG1*	Dumont et al. 2007
6q25.1	Estrogen receptor 1	*ESR1*	Shearman et al. 2003
6q25.3	Superoxide dismutase 2, mitochondrial	*SOD2*	Fujimoto et al. 2008
6q26	Lipoprotein(a)	*LPA*	Holmer et al. 2003
6q27	Thrombospondin II	*THBS2*	Topol et al. 2001
7p21	Interleukin 6	*IL6*	Georges et al. 2001
7q21.3	Paraoxonase 1	*PON1*	Serrato and Marian 1995
7q21.3-q22	Plasminogen activator inhibitor 1	*PAI1*	Eriksson et al. 1995; Yamada et al. 2002
7q36	Nitric oxide synthase 3	*NOS3*	Shimasaki et al. 1998
8p22	Lipoprotein lipase	*LPL*	Jemaa et al. 1995; Yamada et al. 2006
8p12	Plasminogen activator, tissue	*PLAT*	Ladenvall et al. 2002
9p21.3	Cyclin-dependent kinase inhibitor 2A/B	*CDKN2A/B* (?)	Helgadottir et al. 2007; McPherson et al. 2007; Samani et al. 2007; Wellcome Trust Case Control Consortium 2007
9q22-q31	ATP-binding cassette, subfamily A, member 1	*ABCA1*	Tregouet et al. 2004
9q32-q33	Toll-like receptor 4	*TLR4*	Edfeldt et al. 2004
10q24-q26	β -1-adrenergic receptor	*ADRB1*	Iwai et al. 2003
11q22-q23	Matrix metalloproteinase 1	*MMP1*	Pearce et al. 2005
11q23	Apolipoprotein A-V	*APOA5*	Talmud et al. 2004
11q23	Apolipoprotein C-III	*APOC3*	Olivieri et al. 2002
11q23	Matrix metalloproteinase 3	*MMP3*	Ye et al. 1995; Yamada et al. 2002
12p13.2	Taste receptor, type 2, member 50	*TAS2R50*	Shiffman et al. 2008
12p13	Guanine nucleotide-binding protein, β-3	*GNB3*	Naber et al. 2000
12p13-p12	Low-density lipoprotein, oxidized, receptor 1	*OLR1*	Mango et al. 2005
12q22	Leukotriene A4 hydrolase	*LTA4H*	Helgadottir et al. 2006
13q12	Arachidonate 5-lipoxygenase-activating protein	*ALOX5AP*	Helgadottir et al. 2004
13q12.1	Insulin promoter factor 1	*IPF1*	Yamada et al. 2006
13q14.11	Carboxypeptidase B2, plasma	*CPB2*	Juhan-Vague et al. 2002
13q34	Factor VII	*F7*	Iacoviello et al. 1998
13q34	Collagen, type IV, α 1	*COL4A1*	Yamada et al. 2008
14q13	Proteasome subunit, α-type, 6	*PSMA6*	Ozaki et al. 2006
15q15	Thrombospondin I	*THBS1*	Zwicker et al. 2006
15q21-q23	Lipase, hepatic	*LIPC*	Dugi et al. 2001
16p13.3	Deoxyribonuclease I	*DNASE1*	Kumamoto et al. 2006
16p13	Major histocompatibility complex, class II, transactivator	*MHC2TA*	Swanberg et al. 2005
16p11.2	Vitamin K epoxide reductase complex, subunit 1	*VKORC1*	Wang et al. 2006
16q13	Matrix metalloproteinase 2	*MMP2*	Vasku et al. 2004
16q21	Cholesteryl ester transfer protein, plasma	*CETP*	Kuivenhoven et al. 1998
16q24	Cytochrome b(-245), α subunit	*CYBA*	Inoue et al. 1998
17pter-p12	Glycoprotein Ib, platelet, α polypeptide	*GP1BA*	Murata et al. 1997
17p13	Chemokine, CXC motif, ligand 16	*CXCL16*	Lundberg et al. 2005
17q11.1-q12	Solute carrier family 6, member 4	*SLC6A4*	Fumeron et al. 2002
17q11.2-q12	Chemokine, CC motif, ligand 2	*CCL2*	McDermott et al. 2005
17q21.1-q21.2	Chemokine, CC motif, ligand 11	*CCL11*	Zee et al. 2004
17q21.32	Integrin, β-3	*ITGB3*	Weiss et al. 1996
17q23	Angiotensin I-converting enzyme	*ACE*	Cambien et al. 1992
17q23	Platelet-endothelial cell adhesion molecule 1	*PECAM1*	Elrayess et al. 2004
19p13	Purinergic receptor P2Y, G protein-coupled, 11	*P2RY11*	Amisten et al. 2007
19p13.3-p13.2	Intercellular adhesion molecule 1	*ICAM1*	Podgoreanu et al. 2006
19p13.2	Zinc finger protein 627	*ZNF627*	Shiffman et al. 2005; Yamada et al. 2008

(Continued)

Table 22–2 (Continued)

Chromosomal Locus	Gene Name	Gene Symbol	Reference
19q13.1	Transforming growth factor, β 1	*TGFB1*	Yokota et al. 2000
19q13.2	Apolipoprotein E	*APOE*	Wilson et al. 1994
19q13.2	Heterogeneous nuclear ribonucleoprotein U-like 1	*HNRPUL1*	Shiffman et al. 2006
19q13.4	Glycoprotein VI, platelet	*GP6*	Croft et al. 2001
19q13.4	Fc fragment of IgA, receptor for	*FCAR*	Iakoubova et al. 2006
20p11.2	Thrombomodulin	*THBD*	Wu et al. 2001
20q11.2-q13.1	Matrix metalloproteinase 9	*MMP9*	Zhang et al. 1999
20q13.11-q13.13	Prostaglandin I2 synthase	*PTGIS*	Nakayama et al. 2002
21q21.2	ADAM metallopeptidase with thrombospondin type 1 motif, 1	*ADAMTS1*	Sabatine et al. 2008
22q11.2	Catechol-O-methyltransferase	*COMT*	Eriksson et al. 2004
22q12	Heme oxygenase 1	*HMOX1*	Ono et al. 2004
22q12-q13	Lectin, galactoside-binding, soluble, 2	*LGALS2*	Ozaki et al. 2004

Box 22–1 Key Points

- Twin and family studies have established that CAD aggregates in families, with a family history of early onset CAD being considered a risk factor for the disease (Chapter 4).
- Genes responsible for familial hypercholesterolemia and Tangier disease are the prototypical examples of causal genes for Mendelian disorders associated with CAD and MI (Chapter 3 and 21).
- Several genome-wide linkage analyses of families or sib pairs have identified chromosomal loci linked, or genetic variations that confer susceptibility, to MI, ACS, or CAD (Chapter 4).
- Various association studies of unrelated individuals have identified genetic variations that confer susceptibility to MI or CAD. Numerous candidate genes have been implicated, but those that show reproducible associations between risk alleles and CAD or MI in replication studies are few (Chapter 4).
- Mendelian randomization analysis is a relatively recent development in genetic epidemiology and is based on Mendel's second law, which states that the inheritance of one trait is independent of that of other traits.

Box 22–2 Key Points

- A meta-analysis has indicated that the 677C→T (Ala222Val) polymorphism of *MTHFR* is associated with CAD in the Middle East and Asia, but not in Europe, North America, or Australia, with this geographic variability possibly reflecting higher folate intake in the latter regions (Chapter 4).
- The *G* (Stop) allele of the 1595C→G (Ser447Stop) polymorphism of *LPL* has been shown to be related to decreased plasma triglyceride or increased HDL-cholesterol levels, or both, and was found to be associated with a reduced risk of CAD or MI (Chapter 4).
- A meta-analysis of association between *APOE* genotype and CAD revealed that, compared with individuals with the ε3/ε3 genotype, carriers of the ε4 allele had a higher risk for CHD, whereas the ε2 allele was not associated with CAD risk (Chapter 4).

MI have been examined by Mendelian randomization analysis. Pooled data from 4,659 Caucasian men in six studies revealed that individuals homozygous for the *T* allele of the 1444C→T polymorphism of *CRP* had a higher circulating CRP concentration than carriers of the *C* allele. However, men with the *TT* genotype were not at increased risk of nonfatal MI (Casas et al. 2006). This unbiased and nonconfounded estimate of the effect of *CRP* genotype on coronary events was smaller than estimates provided by previous studies. In two independent prospective cohort studies of 32,826 women and 18,225 men in the United States, the minor alleles of 1919A→T and 4741G→C polymorphisms of *CRP* were associated with higher plasma CRP levels and those of 2667G→C and 3872C→T polymorphisms of *CRP* were associated with lower plasma CRP levels. Two of the five common haplotypes of *CRP* were associated with lower CRP levels. However, neither the individual SNPs nor the common haplotypes were associated with risk of CAD in the direction that would be predicted by their association with CRP levels (Pai et al. 2008). These data suggest that the underlying inflammatory processes that predict coronary events cannot be captured solely by variation in *CRP*. The CRP CAD Genetics Collaboration is a consortium of investigators generating and pooling analyses of data on genetic determinants of circulating CRP levels and CAD. These data should help to clarify the likelihood and magnitude of any causal association between circulating CRP concentration and CAD. The collaboration is likely to advance understanding of the relevance of low-grade inflammation to CAD and indicate whether or not CRP itself should be prioritized as a therapeutic target for long-term prevention strategies (CRP CAD Genetics Collaboration 2008).

Candidate Gene Association Studies for MI or CAD

Association studies based on the candidate gene approach have revealed many polymorphisms to be associated with the prevalence of MI or CAD (Table 22–2). In this section, we discuss the association of polymorphisms in *MTHFR*, *LPL*, and *APOE* with MI or CAD (Box 22–2).

5,10-Methylenetetrahydrofolate Reductase

Homocysteine is a sulfur-containing amino acid that plays a pivotal role in methionine metabolism. 5,10-Methylenetetrahydrofolate reductase (MTHFR) catalyzes the reduction of

5,10-methylenetetrahydrofolate to 5-methylenetetrahydrofolate, a reaction that provides a substrate for the methylation of homocysteine to methionine catalyzed by methionine synthase. Individuals with the 677C→T (Ala222Val) substitution of *MTHFR* manifest reduced MTHFR activity and higher plasma homocysteine levels compared with those without it (Deloughery et al. 1996; Ma et al. 1996; Schwartz et al. 1997). Association of the 677C→T (Ala222Val) polymorphism of *MTHFR* with CAD or MI has been described by several groups, with the *TT* genotype being a risk factor for these conditions (Gallagher et al. 1996; Kluijtmans et al. 1996; Morita et al. 1997; Mager et al. 1999; Yamada et al. 2006). Other studies, however, did not support such an association (Schwartz et al. 1997; Folsom et al. 1998). These apparently contradictory results are attributable, at least in part, to differences in intake of folate and other B vitamins (Verhoef et al. 1998). A meta-analysis of the association of the 677C→T (Ala222Val) polymorphism of *MTHFR* with the risk of CAD in 11,162 cases and 12,758 controls from 40 studies revealed that individuals with the *TT* genotype had an odds ratio of 1.16 for CAD compared with those with the *CC* genotype (Klerk et al. 2002). These observations suggest that impaired folate metabolism, resulting in high homocysteine concentrations, is an important determinant of CAD. Another meta-analysis of the association of the 677C→T (Ala222Val) polymorphism of *MTHFR* with CAD in 26,000 cases and 31,183 controls from 80 studies yielded an overall odds ratio of 1.14 for the *TT* genotype versus the *CC* genotype; odds ratios for Europe, Australia, and North America were about 1.0, whereas those for the Middle East and Asia were 2.61 and 1.23, respectively (Lewis et al. 2005). These results indicate that the 677C→T (Ala222Val) polymorphism of *MTHFR* is associated with CAD in the Middle East and Asia, but not in Europe, North America, or Australia, with this geographic variability possibly reflecting higher folate intake in the latter regions (Lewis et al. 2005).

Lipoprotein Lipase

Lipoprotein lipase (LPL) is the rate-limiting enzyme in lipolysis of triglyceride-rich lipoproteins in the circulation. It is synthesized in parenchymal cells of adipose tissue as well as in skeletal and cardiac muscle, and it is then transferred to heparan sulfate binding sites of the vascular endothelium (Kastelein et al. 2000). The hydrolytic function of LPL is important for the processing of triglyceride-rich chylomicrons and very low-density lipoproteins to remnant particles as well as for the transfer of phospholipids and apolipoproteins to HDL. LPL also plays an important role in the receptor-mediated removal of lipoproteins from the circulation (Groenemeijer et al. 1997). *LPL* is polymorphic, with amino acid substitutions of the encoded protein affecting triglyceride and HDL-cholesterol levels, which are implicated in atherosclerosis risk (Wittrup et al. 1999). The 1595C→G (Ser447Stop) substitution of *LPL* results in carboxyl-terminal truncation of LPL by two amino acids. This change is thought to increase the binding affinity of the protein for receptors or to facilitate or otherwise affect its formation of dimers (Wittrup et al. 1999). The *G* (Stop) allele of the 1595C→G (Ser447Stop) polymorphism has also been shown to be related to decreased plasma triglyceride or increased HDL-cholesterol levels, or both (Jemaa et al. 1995; Groenemeijer et al. 1997; Kuivenhoven et al. 1997; Wittrup et al. 1999). In addition, the *G* (Stop) allele of this polymorphism was found to be associated with a reduced risk of CAD or MI (Wittrup et al. 1999; Yang et al. 2004; Yamada et al. 2006). Evidence suggests that the catalytic activity and stability of the truncated variant of LPL may be largely normal, but that it may be present at higher concentrations in the circulation, resulting in a higher level of LPL activity (Zhang et al. 1996; Groenemeijer et al. 1997; Humphries et al. 1998; Henderson et al. 1999).

Apolipoprotein E

Apolipoprotein E (ApoE) plays an important role in lipid transport and metabolism. Three common alleles (ε2, ε3, and ε4) of *APOE* encode the three major isoforms (E2, E3, and E4) of ApoE, which differ at amino acid positions 112 and 158. Allelic variation of *APOE* accounts for interindividual variability in total cholesterol and LDL-cholesterol concentrations, with studies in human populations demonstrating associations of the ε4 and ε2 alleles with increased and decreased LDL-cholesterol levels, respectively (Sing and Davignon 1985; Ehnholm et al. 1986; Xhignesse et al. 1991). The various ApoE isoforms interact differently with specific lipoprotein receptors, ultimately affecting circulating levels of cholesterol (Eichner et al. 2002). ApoE from very low-density lipoprotein, chylomicrons, and chylomicron remnants binds to specific receptors on cells in the liver. Carriers of the ε2 allele of *APOE* are less efficient than carriers of the ε3 or ε4 alleles at synthesizing very low-density lipoprotein and chylomicrons and at transferring them from plasma to the liver as a result of the binding properties of the ApoE2 isoform. Thus, compared to carriers of the ε3 or ε4 alleles, carriers of the ε2 allele are slower to clear dietary fat from their blood (Weintraub et al. 1987). The difference in uptake of postprandial lipoprotein particles results in differences in regulation of hepatic LDL receptors, which in turn contribute to genotypic differences in total and LDL-cholesterol levels (Davignon et al. 1988; Hallman et al. 1991; Schaefer et al. 1994).

The relation of *APOE* polymorphisms to CAD or MI has been extensively investigated in the last two decades. In many studies, the ε4 allele has been associated with CAD or MI (van Bokxmeer and Mamotte 1992; Wilson et al. 1994; Lahoz et al. 2001). A meta-analysis of 15,492 subjects with CAD and 32,965 controls pooled from 48 studies revealed that, compared with individuals with the ε3/ε3 genotype, carriers of the ε4 allele had a higher risk for CAD (odds ratio, 1.42), whereas the ε2 allele was not associated with CAD risk (Song et al. 2004). The ε4 allele of *APOE* is thus an important risk factor for CAD.

The –219G→T SNP of *APOE* has been associated with MI for men in France and Northern Ireland, with the *T* allele representing a risk factor for this condition (Lambert et al. 2000). Consistent with its location in the promoter region of *APOE*, the –219G→T SNP was shown to be associated with the plasma concentration of ApoE, with the *T* allele conferring a reduced ApoE concentration (Lambert et al. 2000). The deleterious influence of the *T* allele on MI therefore cannot be explained by its effect on the circulating level of ApoE. The *T* allele of this SNP was also shown to be a risk factor for CAD in low-risk Japanese men (Hirashiki et al. 2003).

Genome-Wide Association Studies of MI or CAD

GWAS have identified susceptibility genes for various multifactorial diseases including CAD and MI (Table 22–3).

Lymphotoxin-α

Screening of 65,671 SNPs revealed that two polymorphisms of the lymphotoxin-α gene (*LTA*) were associated with susceptibility to MI in a study with 1133 MI patients and 1878 controls

Table 22–3 Genome-Wide Association Studies of Myocardial Infarction (MI) or Coronary Heart Disease (CHD)

Chromosomal Locus	Gene Symbol	Phenotype	SNP Array	Reference
6p21.3	*LTA*	MI	Japanese SNP database	Ozaki et al. 2002
9p21.3	*CDKN2A/B* (?)	CHD	100K custom array	McPherson et al. 2007
9p21.3	*CDKN2A/B* (?)	MI	Hap 300K array (Illumina)	Helgadottir et al. 2007
9p21.3	*CDKN2A/B* (?)	CHD	GeneChip 500K array (Affymetrix)	Wellcome Trust Case Control Consortium 2007
9p21.3	*CDKN2A/B* (?)	CHD	GeneChip 500K array (Affymetrix)	Samani et al. 2007

(Ozaki et al. 2002). Functional analysis in vitro indicated that the *G* allele of one of these two polymorphisms, 252A→G in intron 1 (rs909253), was associated with an increase in the transcriptional activity of *LTA*, and that the *A* (Asn) allele of the second SNP, 804C→A (Thr26Asn) in exon 3 (rs1041981), was associated with increased expression of the genes for vascular cell adhesion molecule 1 and selectin E. Ozaki et al. (2002) thus suggested that variants of *LTA* are risk factors for MI and that they influence the vascular inflammation that underlies this condition. These researchers subsequently showed that the 3279C→T polymorphism in intron 1 of the lectin, galactoside-binding, soluble, 2 gene (*LGALS2*) was associated with the prevalence of MI (Ozaki et al. 2004). LGALS2 plays a role in the secretion of LTA from smooth muscle cells and macrophages, and the identified polymorphism affects the transcriptional activity of *LGALS2*. These results suggested that an LGALS2–LTA axis is important in the pathophysiology of coronary atherosclerosis and thrombosis.

The relation of seven SNPs (rs2071590, rs1800683, rs909253, rs746868, rs2857713, rs3093543, rs1041981) distributed throughout *LTA* and of their corresponding haplotypes to risk of MI was examined in the International Study of Infarct Survival (ISIS) case-control study involving 6,928 cases of nonfatal MI and 2,712 unrelated controls (Clarke et al. 2006). The seven SNPs were in strong linkage disequilibrium with each other and formed six common haplotypes. None of the SNPs or haplotypes was associated with risk of MI. A meta-analysis of rs909253 or rs1041981 in six previously published studies and the ISIS study (Clarke et al. 2006) found no association with CAD risk in a recessive model (odds ratio, 1.07) and only a moderate association in a dominant model (odds ratio, 1.09). Overall, these studies suggest that these common polymorphisms of *LTA* are not associated with susceptibility to CAD or MI. Given that the effect of *LTA* variants on the development of MI might differ among ethnic groups or among individuals exposed to different environmental factors such as smoking, further investigation is warranted with large independent subject panels of different ethnic groups.

1. Chromosome 9p21.3

In 2007, independent GWAS based on the use of SNP chips identified four SNPs on chromosome 9p21.3 that were associated with CAD or MI in several white cohorts (Helgadottir et al. 2007; McPherson et al. 2007; Samani et al. 2007; Wellcome Trust Case Control Consortium 2007). McPherson et al. (2007) identified two susceptibility SNPs (rs10757274 and rs2383206) that were located within 20 kbp of each other on chromosome 9p21.3 and were associated with CAD in a Canadian population and five other white cohorts. Helgadottir et al. (2007) described an association between MI and two SNPs (rs2383207 and rs10757278) located in the same 9p21.3 region in an Icelandic population, and they replicated the finding in four white cohorts. The same genetic locus was also identified by a GWAS performed with 1,926 CAD cases and 3,000 controls from a British population (Wellcome Trust Case Control Consortium 2007), and the finding was replicated in a German population (Samani et al. 2007). Association of SNPs on chromosome 9p21.3 was also replicated for MI in an Italian population (Shen et al. 2008b) and for CAD in a Korean population (Shen et al. 2008a). Interestingly, the independent population-based case-control studies also identified several SNPs at 9p21.3 that were significantly associated with type 2 diabetes mellitus in white populations in England (Zeggini et al. 2007), Finland (Scott et al. 2007), and Sweden (Saxena et al. 2007). In addition to MI, SNP rs10757278 at this locus was found to be associated with abdominal aortic aneurysm and intracranial aneurysm (Helgadottir et al. 2008). Schunkert et al. (2008) genotyped a SNP (rs1333049) representing the 9p21.3 locus in seven case-control studies including a total of 4,645 subjects with MI or CAD and 5,177 controls. The risk allele (*C*) of this SNP was uniformly associated with MI or CAD in each study, with pooled analysis revealing the odds ratio per copy of the risk allele to be 1.29. Meta-analysis of rs1333049 in 12,004 cases and 28,949 controls provided further evidence for association of this SNP with MI or CAD, yielding an odds ratio of 1.24 per risk allele (Box 22–3).

The prospective Northwick Park Heart Study II analyzed complete trait and genotype information available for 2,057 men (183 CAD events over 10.8 years). For a panel of selected genotypes for *UCP2*, *APOE*, *LPL*, *APOA4*, *IL6*, and *PECAM1*, CAD risk estimates incorporating conventional risk factors (age, triglyceride and cholesterol levels, systolic blood pressure, and smoking) and genetic risk interactions were more effective than those based on conventional risk factors alone (Humphries et al. 2007). In a study of the same cohort involving 2,742 men (270 CAD events over 15 years), although rs10757274 at 9p21.3 was associated with CAD, it did not add substantially to the usefulness of the Framingham risk score based on conventional risk factors alone for predicting future CAD events. However, it did improve reclassification of CAD risk and thus may be of clinical utility (Talmud et al. 2008).

Although this broad replication of the association with chromosome 9p21.3 provides important new information on the molecular genetics of CAD and MI, the underlying mechanism is as yet elusive. The region is defined by two flanking recombination hot spots and contains the coding sequences of genes for two cyclin-dependent kinase inhibitors, *CDKN2A* and *CDKN2B*. These genes play an important role in regulation of the cell cycle and belong to a family of genes that have been implicated in the pathogenesis of atherosclerosis as a result of their contribution to inhibition of cell growth by transforming growth factor–β1. However, the SNPs associated most strongly with MI or CAD lie considerably upstream of these genes, with the nearest being located 10 kbp upstream of *CDKN2B*. Although an effect mediated through one or both of these genes is possible, other explanations

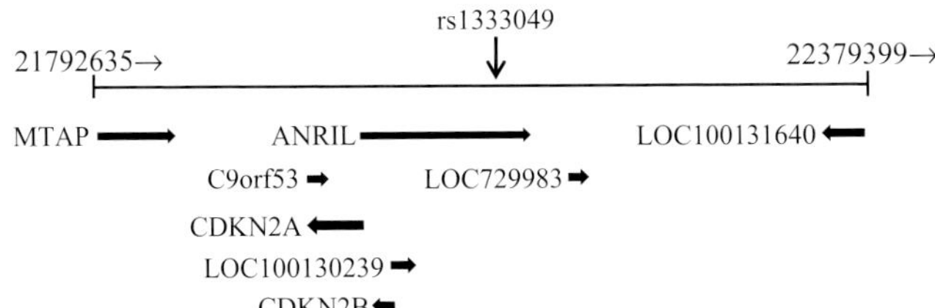

Figure 22–1 Genomic region at chromosome 9p21.3. The schema shows genomic context at chromosome 9p21.3 related to MI and CAD by genome-wide association studies.

for the association of the 9p21.3 region with MI or CAD need to be considered (Schunkert et al. 2008).

The high-risk CAD haplotype at 9p21.3 [T (rs10116277)–T (rs6475606)–G (rs10738607)–T (rs10757272)–G (rs10757274)–G (4977574)–G (2891168)–G (1333042)–G (2383206)–G (2383207)–C (1333045)–G (10757278)–C (1333048)–C (1333049)] was recently shown to overlap with exons 13 to 19 of *ANRIL* (Broadbent et al. 2008; Figure 22–1), a newly annotated gene for a large antisense noncoding RNA that was identified by deletion analysis of an extended French family with hereditary melanoma–neural system tumors (Pasmant et al. 2007). Reverse transcription and polymerase chain reaction analysis showed that *ANRIL* is expressed in atheromatous human vessels (specimens of abdominal aortic aneurysm or carotid endarterectomy), which manifest a cell type profile similar to that of atherosclerotic coronary arteries. *ANRIL* was found to be expressed in vascular endothelial cells, monocyte-derived macrophages, and coronary smooth muscle cells (Broadbent et al. 2008), all of which contribute to atherosclerosis. Little is known of the function of *ANRIL*, as is typical of most genes for noncoding RNAs, which in general are thought to participate in transcriptional control (Mattick and Makunin 2006). A survey of the dbSNP database revealed no SNPs that map within the exons of *ANRIL* that colocalize with the risk haplotype. However, multiple SNPs coupled to the high-risk haplotype map to intronic or downstream sequences of this gene; these variants are plausible candidates for determinants of the level of *ANRIL* expression. The targets of *ANRIL* action remain to be discovered as do any interactions with neighboring genes (Broadbent et al. 2008). Clarification of the functional relevance of SNPs at 9p21.3 to CAD and MI may provide insight into the pathogenesis of these conditions as well as into the role of genetic factors in their development.

Box 22–3 Key Points

- A GWAS and subsequent analysis have suggested that an LGALS2-LTA axis is important in the pathophysiology of coronary atherosclerosis and thrombosis (Chapter 3).
- Independent GWAS based on the use of SNP chips have identified four SNPs on chromosome 9p21.3 that were associated with CAD or MI in several white cohorts. Meta-analysis of rs1333049 provided further evidence for association of this SNP with MI or CAD, yielding an odds ratio of 1.24 per risk allele (Chapter 4).
- Although broad replication of the association with chromosome 9p21.3 provides important new information on the molecular genetics of CAD and MI, the underlying mechanism is as yet elusive. Clarification of the functional relevance of SNPs at 9p21.3 to CAD and MI may provide insight into the pathogenesis of these conditions as well as into the role of genetic factors in their development.

Conclusion

There has been a growing effort to find genetic variants that confer risk for CAD and MI as a means to understand the underlying biological events of these conditions. Such studies may ultimately lead to the personalized prevention of MI (Yamada 2006). It may thus become possible to predict the future risk for MI in each individual on the basis of conventional laboratory examinations and genetic analyses. It should also be possible to assess how the risk level of an individual will decrease if treatable risk factors, including hypertension, diabetes mellitus, hypercholesterolemia or dyslipidemia, and smoking, are ameliorated or eliminated. Furthermore, it may be possible to prevent an individual from undergoing MI by medical intervention based on his or her genotype for specific polymorphisms. In the future, we may have the ability to use specific therapeutic agents individualized on the basis of certain genetic susceptibility factors, thereby increasing the efficacy and limiting the toxicity of treatment (Damani and Topol 2007). Identification of disease susceptibility genes will thus contribute to the prevention, early diagnosis, and treatment of CAD and MI.

References

Amisten S, Melander O, Wihlborg AK, Berglund G, Erlinge D. Increased risk of acute myocardial infarction and elevated levels of C-reactive protein in carriers of the Thr-87 variant of the ATP receptor P2Y11. *Eur Heart J.* 2007;28:13–18.

Antonarakis SE, Beckmann JS. Mendelian disorders deserve more attention. *Nat Rev Genet.* 2006;7:277–282.

Arnett DK, Baird AE, Barkley RA, et al. Relevance of genetics and genomics for prevention and treatment of cardiovascular disease: a scientific statement from the American Heart Association Council on Epidemiology and Prevention, the Stroke Council, and the Functional Genomics and Translational Biology Interdisciplinary Working Group. *Circulation.* 2007;115:2878–2901.

Bacci S, Ludovico O, Prudente S, et al. The K121Q polymorphism of the ENPP1/PC-1 gene is associated with insulin resistance/atherogenic phenotypes, including earlier onset of type 2 diabetes and myocardial infarction. *Diabetes.* 2005;54:3021–3025.

Behague I, Poirier O, Nicaud V, et al. β Fibrinogen gene polymorphisms are associated with plasma fibrinogen and coronary artery disease in patients with myocardial infarction. The ECTIM Study. Etude Cas-Temoins sur l'Infarctus du Myocarde. *Circulation.* 1996;93:440–449.

Bodzioch M, Orso E, Klucken J, et al. The gene encoding ATP-binding cassette transporter 1 is mutated in Tangier disease. *Nat Genet.*1999; 22:347–351.

Broadbent HM, Peden JF, Lorkowski S, et al. Susceptibility to coronary artery disease and diabetes is encoded by distinct, tightly linked SNPs in the ANRIL locus on chromosome 9p. *Hum Mol Genet.* 2008;17:806–814.

Broeckel U, Hengstenberg C, Mayer B, et al. A comprehensive linkage analysis for myocardial infarction and its related risk factors. *Nat Genet.* 2002;30:210–214.

Brooks-Wilson A, Marcil M, Clee SM, et al. Mutations in ABC1 in Tangier disease and familial high-density lipoprotein deficiency. *Nat Genet.* 1999;22:336–345.

Cambien F, Poirier O, Lecerf L, et al. Deletion polymorphism in the gene for angiotensin-converting enzyme is a potent risk factor for myocardial infarction. *Nature.* 1992;359:641–644.

Casas JP, Shah T, Cooper J, et al. Insight into the nature of the CRP-coronary event association using Mendelian randomization. *Int J Epidemiol.* 2006;35:922–931.

Cipollone F, Toniato E, Martinotti S, et al. A polymorphism in the cyclooxygenase 2 gene as an inherited protective factor against myocardial infarction and stroke. *JAMA*. 2004;291:2221–2228.

Clarke R, Xu P, Bennett D, et al. Lymphotoxin-alpha gene and risk of myocardial infarction in 6,928 cases and 2,712 controls in the ISIS case-control study. *PLoS Genet*. 2006;2:e107.

Clee SM, Kastelein JJ, van Dam M, et al. Age and residual cholesterol efflux affect HDL cholesterol levels and coronary artery disease in ABCA1 heterozygotes. *J Clin Invest*. 2000;106:1263–1270.

Cohen JC, Boerwinkle E, Mosley TH Jr, Hobbs HH. Sequence variations in PCSK9, low LDL, and protection against coronary heart disease. *N Engl J Med*. 2006;354:1264–1272.

Cohen JC, Kiss RS, Pertsemlidis A, Marcel YL, McPherson R, Hobbs HH. Multiple rare alleles contribute to low plasma levels of HDL cholesterol. *Science*. 2004;305:869–872.

Croft SA, Samani NJ, Teare MD, et al. Novel platelet membrane glycoprotein VI dimorphism is a risk factor for myocardial infarction. *Circulation*. 2001;104:1459–1463.

CRP CHD Genetics Collaboration. Collaborative pooled analysis of data on C-reactive protein gene variants and coronary disease: judging causality by Mendelian randomisation. *Eur J Epidemiol*. 2008;23:531–540.

Damani SB, Topol EJ. Future use of genomics in coronary artery disease. *J Am Coll Cardiol*. 2007;50:1933–1940.

Davey Smith G, Ebrahim S. "Mendelian randomization": can genetic epidemiology contribute to understanding environmental causes of disease? *Int J Epidemiol*. 2003;32:1–22.

Davey Smith G, Ebrahim S. What can Mendelian randomization tell us about modifiable behavioural and environmental exposures? *Br Med J*. 2005;330:1076–1079.

Davignon J, Gregg RE, Sing CF. Apolipoprotein E polymorphism and atherosclerosis. *Arteriosclerosis*. 1988;8:1–21.

Deloughery TG, Evans A, Sadeghi A, et al. Common mutation in methylenetetrahydrofolate reductase. Correlation with homocysteine metabolism and late-onset vascular disease. *Circulation*. 1996;94:3074–3078.

Dugi KA, Brandauer K, Schmidt N, et al. Low hepatic lipase activity is a novel risk factor for coronary artery disease. *Circulation*. 2001;104:3057–3062.

Dumont J, Zureik M, Cottel D, et al. Association of arginase 1 gene polymorphisms with the risk of myocardial infarction and common carotid intima-media thickness. *J Med Genet*. 2007;44:526–553.

Dwyer JH, Allayee H, Dwyer KM, et al. Arachidonate 5-lipoxygenase promoter genotype, dietary arachidonic acid, and atherosclerosis. *N Engl J Med*. 2004;350:29–37.

Edfeldt K, Bennet AM, Eriksson P, et al. Association of hypo-responsive toll-like receptor 4 variants with risk of myocardial infarction. *Eur Heart J*. 2004;25:1447–1453.

Ehnholm C, Lukka M, Kuusi T, Nikkilä E, Utermann G. Apolipoprotein E polymorphism in the Finnish population: gene frequencies and relation to lipoprotein concentrations. *J Lipid Res*. 1986;27:227–235.

Eichner JE, Dunn ST, Perveen G, Thompson DM, Stewart KE, Stroehla BC. Apolipoprotein E polymorphism and cardiovascular disease: a HuGE review. *Am J Epidemiol*. 2002;155:487–495.

Elrayess MA, Webb KE, Bellingan GJ, et al. R643G polymorphism in PECAM-1 influences transendothelial migration of monocytes and is associated with progression of CHD and CHD events. *Atherosclerosis*. 2004;177:127–135.

Endler G, Mannhalter C, Sunder-Plassmann H, et al. Homozygosity for the C→T polymorphism at nucleotide 46 in the 5' untranslated region of the factor XII gene protects from development of acute coronary syndrome. *Br J Haematol*. 2001;115:1007–1009.

Eriksson AL, Skrtic S, Niklason A, et al. Association between the low activity genotype of catechol-O-methyltransferase and myocardial infarction in a hypertensive population. *Eur Heart J*. 2004;25:386–391.

Eriksson P, Kallin B, van't Hooft FM, Bavenholm P, Hamsten A. Allele-specific increase in basal transcription of the plasminogen-activator inhibitor 1 gene is associated with myocardial infarction. *Proc Natl Acad Sci USA*. 1995;92:1851–1855.

Farrall M, Green FR, Peden JF, et al. Genome-wide mapping of susceptibility to coronary artery disease identifies a novel replicated locus on chromosome 17. *PLoS Genet*. 2006;2:755–761.

Folsom AR, Nieto FJ, McGovern PG, et al. Prospective study of coronary heart disease incidence in relation to fasting total homocysteine, related genetic polymorphisms, and B vitamins: the Atherosclerosis Risk in Communities (ARIC) Study. *Circulation*. 1998;98:204–210.

Francke S, Manraj M, Lacquemant C, et al. A genome-wide scan for coronary heart disease suggests in Indo-Mauritians a susceptibility locus on chromosome 16p13 and replicates linkage with the metabolic syndrome on 3q27. *Hum Mol Genet*. 2001;10:2751–2765.

Friedlander Y, Siscovick DS, Weinmann S, et al. Family history as a risk factor for primary cardiac arrest. *Circulation*. 1998;97:155–160.

Frikke-Schmidt R, Nordestgaard BG, Jensen GB, Tybjaerg-Hansen A. Genetic variation in ABC transporter A1 contributes to HDL cholesterol in the general population. *J Clin Invest*. 2004;114:1343–1353.

Fujimoto H, Taguchi JI, Imai Y, et al. Manganese superoxide dismutase polymorphism affects the oxidized low-density lipoprotein-induced apoptosis of macrophages and coronary artery disease. *Eur Heart J*. 2008;29:1267–1274.

Fumeron F, Betoulle D, Nicaud V, et al. Serotonin transporter gene polymorphism and myocardial infarction: etude Cas-Temoins de l'Infarctus du Myocarde (ECTIM). *Circulation*. 2002;105:2943–2945.

Gallagher PM, Meleady R, Shields DC, et al. Homocysteine and risk of premature coronary heart disease. Evidence for a common gene mutation. *Circulation*. 1996;94:2154–2158.

Georges JL, Loukaci V, Poirier O, et al. Interleukin-6 gene polymorphisms and susceptibility to myocardial infarction: the ECTIM study. *J Mol Med*. 2001;79:300–305.

Georgopoulos A, Bloomfield H, Collins D, et al. Codon 54 polymorphism of the fatty acid binding protein (FABP) 2 gene is associated with increased cardiovascular risk in the dyslipidemic diabetic participants of the Veterans Affairs HDL Intervention Trial (VA-HIT). *Atherosclerosis*. 2007;194:169–174.

Goldstein JL, Brown MS. Familial hypercholesterolemia: identification of a defect in the regulation of 3-hydroxy-3-methylglutaryl coenzyme A reductase activity associated with overproduction of cholesterol. *Proc Natl Acad Sci USA*. 1973;70:2804–2808.

Gonzalez P, Alvarez R, Batalla A, et al. Genetic variation at the chemokine receptors CCR5/CCR2 in myocardial infarction. *Genes Immun*. 2001;2:191–195.

Gonzalez-Conejero R, Corral J, Roldan V, et al. A common polymorphism in the annexin V Kozak sequence (–1C>T) increases translation efficiency and plasma levels of annexin V, and decreases the risk of myocardial infarction in young patients. *Blood*. 2002;100:2081–2086.

Groenemeijer BE, Hallman MD, Reymer PW, et al. Genetic variant showing a positive interaction with β-blocking agents with a beneficial influence on lipoprotein lipase activity, HDL cholesterol, and triglyceride levels in coronary artery disease patients. The Ser447-stop substitution in the lipoprotein lipase gene. *Circulation*. 1997;95:2628–2635.

Gruchala M, Ciecwierz D, Wasag B, et al. Association of the ScaI atrial natriuretic peptide gene polymorphism with nonfatal myocardial infarction and extent of coronary artery disease. *Am Heart J*. 2003;145:125–131.

Hakonarson H, Thorvaldsson S, Helgadottir A, et al. Effects of a 5-lipoxygenase-activating protein inhibitor on biomarkers associated with risk of myocardial infarction. *JAMA*. 2005;293:2245–2256.

Hallman DM, Boerwinkle E, Saha N, et al. The apolipoprotein E polymorphism: a comparison of allele frequencies and effects in nine populations. *Am J Hum Genet*. 1991;49:338–349.

Harrap SB, Zammit KS, Wong ZY, et al. Genome-wide linkage analysis of the acute coronary syndrome suggests a locus on chromosome 2. *Arterioscler Thromb Vasc Biol*. 2002;22:874–878.

Hauser ER, Crossman DC, Granger CB, et al. A genomewide scan for early-onset coronary artery disease in 438 families: the GENECARD Study. *Am J Hum Genet*. 2004;75:436–447.

Hegele RA, Huang LS, Herbert PN, et al. Apolipoprotein B-gene DNA polymorphisms associated with myocardial infarction. *N Engl J Med*. 1986;315:1509–1515.

Helgadottir A, Gretarsdottir S, St Clair D, et al. Association between the gene encoding 5-lipoxygenase-activating protein and stroke replicated in a Scottish population. *Am J Hum Genet*. 2005;76:505–509.

Helgadottir A, Manolescu A, Helgason A, et al. A variant of the gene encoding leukotriene A4 hydrolase confers ethnicity-specific risk of myocardial infarction. *Nat Genet.* 2006;38:68–74.

Helgadottir A, Manolescu A, Thorleifsson G, et al. The gene encoding 5-lipoxygenase activating protein confers risk of myocardial infarction and stroke. *Nat Genet.* 2004;36:233–239.

Helgadottir A, Thorleifsson G, Magnusson KP, et al. The same sequence variant on 9p21 associates with myocardial infarction, abdominal aortic aneurysm and intracranial aneurysm. *Nat Genet.* 2008;40:217–224.

Helgadottir A, Thorleifsson G, Manolescu A, et al. A common variant on chromosome 9p21 affects the risk of myocardial infarction. *Science.* 2007;316:1491–1493.

Henderson HE, Kastelein JJ, Zwinderman AH, et al. Lipoprotein lipase activity is decreased in a large cohort of patients with coronary artery disease and is associated with changes in lipids and lipoproteins. *J Lipid Res.* 1999;40:735–743.

Hirashiki A, Yamada Y, Murase Y, et al. Association of gene polymorphisms with coronary artery disease in low- or high-risk subjects defined by conventional risk factors. *J Am Coll Cardiol.* 2003;42:1429–1437.

Holmer SR, Hengstenberg C, Kraft HG, et al. Association of polymorphisms of the apolipoprotein(a) gene with lipoprotein(a) levels and myocardial infarction. *Circulation.* 2003;107:696–701.

Howell WM, Ali S, Rose-Zerilli MJ, Ye S. VEGF polymorphisms and severity of atherosclerosis. *J Med Genet.* 2005;42:485–490.

Hubacek JA, Rothe G, Pit'ha J, et al. C(−260)→T polymorphism in the promoter of the CD14 monocyte receptor gene as a risk factor for myocardial infarction. *Circulation.* 1999;99:3218–3220.

Humphries SE, Cooper JA, Talmud PJ, Miller GJ. Candidate gene genotypes, along with conventional risk factor assessment, improve estimation of coronary heart disease risk in healthy UK men. *Clin Chem.* 2007;53:8–16.

Humphries SE, Nicaud V, Margalef J, Tiret L, Talmud PJ. Lipoprotein lipase gene variation is associated with a paternal history of premature coronary artery disease and fasting and postprandial plasma triglycerides: the European Atherosclerosis Research Study (EARS). *Arterioscler Thromb Vasc Biol.* 1998;18:526–534.

Iacoviello L, Di Castelnuovo A, De Knijff P, et al. Polymorphisms in the coagulation factor VII gene and the risk of myocardial infarction. *N Engl J Med.* 1998;338:79–85.

Iacoviello L, Di Castelnuovo A, Gattone M, et al. Polymorphisms of the interleukin-1β gene affect the risk of myocardial infarction and ischemic stroke at young age and the response of mononuclear cells to stimulation in vitro. *Arterioscler Thromb Vasc Biol.* 2005;25:222–227.

Iakoubova OA, Tong CH, Chokkalingam AP, et al. Asp92Asn polymorphism in the myeloid IgA Fc receptor is associated with myocardial infarction in two disparate populations: CARE and WOSCOPS. *Arterioscler Thromb Vasc Biol.* 2006;26:2763–2768.

Iakoubova OA, Tong CH, Rowland CM, et al. Association of the Trp719Arg polymorphism in kinesin-like protein 6 with myocardial infarction and coronary heart disease in 2 prospective trials: the CARE and WOSCOPS trials. *J Am Coll Cardiol.* 2008;51:435–443.

Inoue N, Kawashima S, Kanazawa K, Yamada S, Akita H, Yokoyama M. Polymorphism of the NADH/NADPH oxidase p22 phox gene in patients with coronary artery disease. *Circulation.* 1998;97:135–137.

International Human Genome Sequencing Consortium. Finishing the euchromatic sequence of the human genome. *Nature.* 2004;431:931–945.

Iwai C, Akita H, Kanazawa K, et al. Arg389Gly polymorphism of the human β1-adrenergic receptor in patients with nonfatal acute myocardial infarction. *Am Heart J.* 2003;146:106–109.

Jemaa R, Fumeron F, Poirier O, et al. Lipoprotein lipase gene polymorphisms: associations with myocardial infarction and lipoprotein levels, the ECTIM study. Etude Cas Temoins sur l'Infarctus du Myocarde. *J Lipid Res.* 1995;36:2141–2146.

Juhan-Vague I, Morange PE, Aubert H, et al. Plasma thrombin-activatable fibrinolysis inhibitor antigen concentration and genotype in relation to myocardial infarction in the north and south of Europe. *Arterioscler Thromb Vasc Biol.* 2002;22:867–873.

Kaikkonen KS, Kortelainen ML, Linna E, Huikuri HV. Family history and the risk of sudden cardiac death as a manifestation of an acute coronary event. *Circulation.* 2006;114:1462–1467.

Kardys I, Klaver CC, Despriet DD, et al. A common polymorphism in the complement factor H gene is associated with increased risk of myocardial infarction: the Rotterdam Study. *J Am Coll Cardiol.* 2006;47:1568–1575.

Kastelein JJ, Jukema JW, Zwinderman AH, et al. Lipoprotein lipase activity is associated with severity of angina pectoris. *Circulation.* 2000;102:1629–1633.

Katsuya T, Koike G, Yee TW, et al. Association of angiotensinogen gene T235 variant with increased risk of coronary heart disease. *Lancet.* 1995;345:1600–1603.

Keavney B. Genetic epidemiological studies of coronary heart disease. *Int J Epidemiol.* 2002;31:730–736.

Klerk M, Verhoef P, Clarke R, et al. MTHFR 677C→T polymorphism and risk of coronary heart disease: a meta-analysis. *JAMA.* 2002;288:2023–2031.

Kluijtmans LA, van den Heuvel LP, Boers GH, et al. Molecular genetic analysis in mild hyperhomocysteinemia: a common mutation in the methylenetetrahydrofolate reductase gene is a genetic risk factor for cardiovascular disease. *Am J Hum Genet.* 1996;58:35–41.

Kohler HP, Stickland MH, Ossei-Gerning N, Carter A, Mikkola H, Grant PJ. Association of a common polymorphism in the factor XIII gene with myocardial infarction. *Thromb Haemost.* 1998;79:8–13.

Koide S, Kugiyama K, Sugiyama S, et al. Association of polymorphism in glutamate-cysteine ligase catalytic subunit gene with coronary vasomotor dysfunction and myocardial infarction. *J Am Coll Cardiol.* 2003;41:539–545.

Kuivenhoven JA, Groenemeyer BE, Boer JM, et al. Ser447stop mutation in lipoprotein lipase is associated with elevated HDL cholesterol levels in normolipidemic males. *Arterioscler Thromb Vasc Biol.* 1997;17:595–599.

Kuivenhoven JA, Jukema JW, Zwinderman AH, et al. The role of a common variant of the cholesterol ester transfer protein gene in the progression of coronary atherosclerosis. *N Engl J Med.* 1998;338:86–93.

Kullo IJ, Ding K. Mechanisms of disease: the genetic basis of coronary heart disease. *Nat Clin Pract Cardiovasc Med.* 2007;4:558–569.

Kumamoto T, Kawai Y, Arakawa K, et al. Association of Gln222Arg polymorphism in the deoxyribonuclease I (DNase I) gene with myocardial infarction in Japanese patients. *Eur Heart J.* 2006;27:2081–2087.

Ladenvall P, Johansson L, Jansson JH, et al. Tissue-type plasminogen activator −7,351C/T enhancer polymorphism is associated with a first myocardial infarction. *Thromb Haemost.* 2002;87:105–109.

Lahoz C, Schaefer EJ, Cupples LA, et al. Apolipoprotein E genotype and cardiovascular disease in the Framingham Heart Study. *Atherosclerosis.* 2001;154:529–537.

Lambert JC, Brousseau T, Defosse V, et al. Independent association of an APOE gene promoter polymorphism with increased risk of myocardial infarction and decreased APOE plasma concentrations—the ECTIM study. *Hum Mol Genet.* 2000;9:57–61.

Lange LA, Carlson CS, Hindorff LA, et al. Association of polymorphisms in the CRP gene with circulating C-reactive protein levels and cardiovascular events. *JAMA.* 2006;296:2703–2711.

Lavergne E, Labreuche J, Daoudi M, et al. Adverse associations between CX3CR1 polymorphisms and risk of cardiovascular or cerebrovascular disease. *Arterioscler Thromb Vasc Biol.* 2005;25:847–853.

Ledmyr H, McMahon AD, Ehrenborg E, et al. The microsomal triglyceride transfer protein gene −493T variant lowers cholesterol but increases the risk of coronary heart disease. *Circulation.* 2004;109:2279–2284.

Lewis SJ, Ebrahim S, Davy Smith G. Meta-analysis of MTHFR 677C→T polymorphism and coronary heart disease: does totality of evidence support causal role for homocysteine and preventive potential of folate? *Br Med J.* 2005;331:1053–1056.

Li R, Bensen JT, Hutchinson RG, et al. Family risk score of coronary heart disease (CHD) as a predictor of CHD: the Atherosclerosis Risk in Communities (ARIC) study and the NHLBI family heart study. *Genet Epidemiol.* 2000;18:236–250.

Liu PY, Li YH, Chao TH, et al. Synergistic effect of cytochrome P450 epoxygenase CYP2J2*7 polymorphism with smoking on the onset of premature myocardial infarction. *Atherosclerosis.* 2007;195:199–206.

Lloyd-Jones DM, Nam BH, D'Agostino RB Sr, et al. Parental cardiovascular disease as a risk factor for cardiovascular disease in middle-aged adults: a prospective study of parents and offspring. *JAMA.* 2004;291:2204–2211.

Lundberg GA, Kellin A, Samnegard A, et al. Severity of coronary artery stenosis is associated with a polymorphism in the CXCL16/SR-PSOX gene. *J Intern Med.* 2005;257:415–422.

Ma J, Stampfer MJ, Hennekens CH, et al. Methylenetetrahydrofolate reductase polymorphism, plasma folate, homocysteine, and risk of myocardial infarction in US physicians. *Circulation.* 1996;94:2410–2416.

Mager A, Lalezari S, Shohat T, et al. Methylenetetrahydrofolate reductase genotypes and early-onset coronary artery disease. *Circulation.* 1999;100:2406–2410.

Mango R, Biocca S, del Vecchio F, et al. In vivo and in vitro studies support that a new splicing isoform of OLR1 gene is protective against acute myocardial infarction. *Circ Res.* 2005;97:152–158.

Marroquin OC, Selzer F, Mulukutla SR, et al. A comparison of bare-metal and drug-eluting stents for off-label indications. *N Engl J Med.* 2008;358:342–352.

Marz W, Seelhorst U, Wellnitz B, et al. Alanine to serine polymorphism at position 986 of the calcium-sensing receptor associated with coronary heart disease, myocardial infarction, all-cause and cardiovascular mortality. *J Clin Endocrinol Metab.* 2007;92:2363–2369.

Mattick JS, Makunin IV. Non-coding RNA. *Hum Mol Genet.* 2006; 15:R17–R29.

McDermott DH, Yang Q, Kathiresan S, et al. CCL2 polymorphisms are associated with serum monocyte chemoattractant protein-1 levels and myocardial infarction in the Framingham Heart Study. *Circulation.* 2005;112:1113–1120.

McPherson R, Pertsemlidis A, Kavaslar N, et al. A common allele on chromosome 9 associated with coronary heart disease. *Science.* 2007; 316:1488–1491.

Mehrabian M, Allayee H, Wong J, et al. Identification of 5-lipoxygenase as a major gene contributing to atherosclerosis susceptibility in mice. *Circ Res.* 2002;91:120–126.

Morita H, Taguchi J, Kurihara H, et al. Genetic polymorphism of 5,10-methylenetetrahydrofolate reductase (MTHFR) as a risk factor for coronary artery disease. *Circulation.* 1997;95:2032–2036.

Moshfegh K, Wuillemin WA, Redondo M, et al. Association of two silent polymorphisms of platelet glycoprotein Ia/IIa receptor with risk of myocardial infarction: a case-control study. *Lancet.* 1999;353:351–354.

Muckian C, Fitzgerald A, O'Neill A, O'Byrne A, Fitzgerald DJ, Shields DC. Genetic variability in the extracellular matrix as a determinant of cardiovascular risk: association of type III collagen COL3A1 polymorphisms with coronary artery disease. *Blood.* 2002;100:1220–1223.

Murabito JM, Pencina MJ, Nam BH, et al. Sibling cardiovascular disease as a risk factor for cardiovascular disease in middle-aged adults. *JAMA.* 2005;294:3117–3123.

Murata M, Matsubara Y, Kawano K, et al. Coronary artery disease and polymorphisms in a receptor mediating shear stress-dependent platelet activation. *Circulation.* 1997;96:3281–3286.

Myers RH, Kiely DK, Cupples LA, Kannel WB. Parental history is an independent risk factor for coronary artery disease: the Framingham Study. *Am Heart J.* 1990;120:963–969.

Naber CK, Husing J, Wolfhard U, Erbel R, Siffert W. Interaction of the ACE D allele and the GNB3 825T allele in myocardial infarction. *Hypertension.* 2000;36:986–989.

Nakamura S, Kugiyama K, Sugiyama S, et al. Polymorphism in the 5'-flanking region of human glutamate-cysteine ligase modifier subunit gene is associated with myocardial infarction. *Circulation.* 2002;105:2968–2973.

Nakayama T, Soma M, Saito S, et al. Association of a novel single nucleotide polymorphism of the prostacyclin synthase gene with myocardial infarction. *Am Heart J.* 2002;143:797–801.

Nasir K, Michos ED, Rumberger JA, et al. Coronary artery calcification and family history of premature coronary heart disease: sibling history is more strongly associated than parental history. *Circulation.* 2004;110:2150–2156.

Ohashi K, Ouchi N, Kihara S, et al. Adiponectin I164T mutation is associated with the metabolic syndrome and coronary artery disease. *J Am Coll Cardiol.* 2004;43:1195–1200.

Olivieri O, Stranieri C, Bassi A, et al. ApoC-III gene polymorphisms and risk of coronary artery disease. *J Lipid Res.* 2002;43:1450–1457.

Ono K, Goto Y, Takagi S, et al. A promoter variant of the heme oxygenase-1 gene may reduce the incidence of ischemic heart disease in Japanese. *Atherosclerosis.* 2004;173:315–319.

Oram JF, Heinecke JW. ATP-binding cassette transporter A1: a cell cholesterol exporter that protects against cardiovascular disease. *Physiol Rev.* 2005;85:1343–1372.

Ortlepp JR, Vesper K, Mevissen V, et al. Chemokine receptor (CCR2) genotype is associated with myocardial infarction and heart failure in patients under 65 years of age. *J Mol Med.* 2003;81:363–367.

Ott I, Koch W, von Beckerath N, et al. Tissue factor promotor polymorphism—603 A/G is associated with myocardial infarction. *Atherosclerosis.* 2004;177:189–191.

Ozaki K, Inoue K, Sato H, et al. Functional variation in LGALS2 confers risk of myocardial infarction and regulates lymphotoxin-α secretion in vitro. *Nature.* 2004;429:72–75.

Ozaki K, Ohnishi Y, Iida A, et al. Functional SNPs in the lymphotoxin-α gene that are associated with susceptibility to myocardial infarction. *Nat Genet.* 2002;32:650–654.

Ozaki K, Sato H, Iida A, et al. A functional SNP in PSMA6 confers risk of myocardial infarction in the Japanese population. *Nat Genet.* 2006;38:921–925.

Pai JK, Mukamal KJ, Rexrode KM, Rimm EB. C-reactive protein (CRP) gene polymorphisms, CRP levels, and risk of incident coronary heart disease in two nested case-control studies. *PLoS ONE.* 2008;3:e1395.

Pajukanta P, Cargill M, Viitanen L, et al. Two loci on chromosomes 2 and X for premature coronary heart disease identified in early- and late-settlement populations of Finland. *Am J Hum Genet.* 2000;67:1481–1493.

Pasmant E, Laurendeau I, Heron D, Vidaud M, Vidaud D, Bieche I. Characterization of a germ-line deletion, including the entire INK4/ARF locus, in a melanoma-neural system tumor family: identification of ANRIL, an antisense noncoding RNA whose expression coclusters with ARF. *Cancer Res.* 2007;67:3963–3969.

Pearce E, Tregouet DA, Samnegard A, et al. Haplotype effect of the matrix metalloproteinase-1 gene on risk of myocardial infarction. *Circ Res.* 2005;97:1070–1076.

Pearson TA, Manolio TA. How to interpret a genome-wide association study. *JAMA.* 2008;299:1335–1344.

Podgoreanu MV, White WD, Morris RW, et al. Inflammatory gene polymorphisms and risk of postoperative myocardial infarction after cardiac surgery. *Circulation.* 2006;114:I275–I281.

Rader DJ, Cohen J, Hobbs HH. Monogenic hypercholesterolemia: new insights in pathogenesis and treatment. J Clin Invest. 2003;111:1795–1803.

Ridker PM, Cook NR, Cheng S, et al. Alanine for proline substitution in the peroxisome proliferator-activated receptor gamma-2 (PPARG2) gene and the risk of incident myocardial infarction. *Arterioscler Thromb Vasc Biol.* 2003;23:859–863.

Robin NH, Tabereaux PB, Benza R, Korf BR. Genetic testing in cardiovascular disease. *J Am Coll Cardiol.* 2007;50:727–737.

Roncaglioni MC, Santoro L, D'Avanzo B, et al. Role of family history in patients with myocardial infarction: an Italian case-control study. GISSI-EFRIM Investigators. *Circulation.* 1992;85:2065–2072.

Rosamond W, Flegal K, Friday G, et al. Heart disease and stroke statistics—2007 update: a report from the American Heart Association Statistics Committee and Stroke Statistics Subcommittee. *Circulation.* 2007;115:e69–e171.

Rust S, Rosier M, Funke H, et al. Tangier disease is caused by mutations in the gene encoding ATP-binding cassette transporter 1. *Nat Genet.* 1999;22:352–355.

Sabatine MS, Ploughman L, Simonsen KL, et al. Association between ADAMTS1 matrix metalloproteinase gene variation, coronary heart disease, and benefit of statin therapy. *Arterioscler Thromb Vasc Biol.* 2008;28:562–567.

Sala G, Di Castelnuovo A, Cuomo L, et al. The E27 β2-adrenergic receptor polymorphism reduces the risk of myocardial infarction in dyslipidemic young males. *Thromb Haemost.* 2001;85:231–233.

Samani NJ, Erdmann J, Hall AS, et al. Genomewide association analysis of coronary artery disease. *N Engl J Med.* 2007;357:443–453.

Saxena R, Voight BF, Lyssenko V, et al. Genome-wide association analysis identifies loci for type 2 diabetes and triglyceride levels. *Science.* 2007;316:1331–1336.

Schaefer EJ, Lamon-Fava S, Johnson S, et al. Effects of gender and menopausal status on the association of apolipoprotein E phenotype with plasma lipoprotein levels: results from the Framingham Offspring Study. *Arterioscler Thromb Vasc Biol.* 1994;14:1105–1113.

Scheuner MT. Genetic evaluation for coronary artery disease. *Genet Med.* 2003;5:269–285.

Schunkert H, Götz A, Braund P, et al. Repeated replication and a prospective meta-analysis of the association between chromosome 9p21.3 and coronary artery disease. *Circulation.* 2008;117:1675–1684.

Schwartz SM, Siscovick DS, Malinow MR, et al. Myocardial infarction in young women in relation to plasma total homocysteine, folate, and a common variant in the methylenetetrahydrofolate reductase gene. *Circulation.* 1997;96:412–417.

Scott LJ, Mohlke KL, Bonnycastle LL, et al. A genome-wide association study of type 2 diabetes in Finns detects multiple susceptibility variants. *Science.* 2007;316:1341–1345.

Senti M, Fernandez-Fernandez JM, Tomas M, et al. Protective effect of the KCNMB1 E65K genetic polymorphism against diastolic hypertension in aging women and its relevance to cardiovascular risk. *Circ Res.* 2005;97:1360–1365.

Serrato M, Marian AJ. A variant of human paraoxonase/arylesterase (HUMPONA) gene is a risk factor for coronary artery disease. *J Clin Invest.* 1995;96:3005–3008.

Shearman AM, Cupples LA, Demissie S, et al. Association between estrogen receptor α gene variation and cardiovascular disease. *JAMA.* 2003;290:2263–2270.

Shen GQ, Li L, Girelli D, et al. An LRP8 variant is associated with familial and premature coronary artery disease and myocardial infarction. *Am J Hum Genet.* 2007;81:780–791.

Shen GQ, Li L, Rao S, et al. Four SNPs on chromosome 9p21 in a South Korean population implicate a genetic locus that confers high cross-race risk for development of coronary artery disease. *Arterioscler Thromb Vasc Biol.* 2008a;28:360–365.

Shen GQ, Rao S, Martinelli N, et al. Association between four SNPs on chromosome 9p21 and myocardial infarction is replicated in an Italian population. *J Hum Genet.* 2008b;53:144–150.

Shiffman D, Ellis SG, Rowland CM, et al. Identification of four gene variants associated with myocardial infarction. *Am J Hum Genet.* 2005;77:596–605.

Shiffman D, O'Meara ES, Bare LA, et al. Association of gene variants with incident myocardial infarction in the Cardiovascular Health Study. *Arterioscler Thromb Vasc Biol.* 2008;28:173–179.

Shiffman D, Rowland CM, Louie JZ, et al. Gene variants of VAMP8 and HNRPUL1 are associated with early-onset myocardial infarction. *Arterioscler Thromb Vasc Biol.* 2006;26:1613–1618.

Shimasaki Y, Yasue H, Yoshimura M, et al. Association of the missense Glu298Asp variant of the endothelial nitric oxide synthase gene with myocardial infarction. *J Am Coll Cardiol.* 1998;31:1506–1510.

Sing CF, Davignon J. Role of apolipoprotein E genetic polymorphism in determining normal plasma lipid and lipoprotein variation. *Am J Hum Genet.* 1985;37:268–285.

Song Y, Stampfer MJ, Liu S. Meta-analysis: apolipoprotein E genotypes and risk for coronary heart disease. *Ann Intern Med.* 2004;141:137–147.

Soutar AK, Naoumova RP. Mechanism of disease: genetic causes of familial hypercholesterolemia. *Nat Clin Pract Cardiovasc Med.* 2007;4:214–225.

Spanbroek R, Grabner R, Lotzer K, et al. Expanding expression of the 5-lipoxygenase pathway within the arterial wall during human atherogenesis. *Proc Natl Acad Sci USA.* 2003;100:1238–1243.

Swanberg M, Lidman O, Padyukov L, et al. MHC2TA is associated with differential MHC molecule expression and susceptibility to rheumatoid arthritis, multiple sclerosis and myocardial infarction. *Nat Genet.* 2005;37:486–494.

Talmud PJ, Cooper JA, Palmen J, et al. Chromosome 9p21.3 coronary heart disease locus genotype and prospective risk of CHD in healthy middle-aged men. *Clin Chem.* 2008;54:467–474.

Talmud PJ, Martin S, Taskinen MR, et al. APOA5 gene variants, lipoprotein particle distribution, and progression of coronary heart disease: results from the LOCAT study. *J Lipid Res.* 2004;45:750–756.

The BHF Family Heart Study Research Group. A genomewide linkage study of 1,933 families affected by premature coronary artery disease: The British Heart Foundation (BHF) Family Heart Study. *Am J Hum Genet.* 2005;77:1011–1020.

The International HapMap Consortium. A second generation human haplotype map of over 3.1 million SNPs. *Nature.* 2007;449:851–861.

Tiret L, Bonnardeaux A, Poirier O, et al. Synergistic effects of angiotensin-converting enzyme and angiotensin-II type 1 receptor gene polymorphisms on risk of myocardial infarction. *Lancet.* 1994;344:910–913.

Topol EJ, McCarthy J, Gabriel S, et al. Single nucleotide polymorphisms in multiple novel thrombospondin genes may be associated with familial premature myocardial infarction. *Circulation.* 2001;104:2641–2644.

Topol EJ, Smith J, Plow EF, Wang QK. Genetic susceptibility to myocardial infarction and coronary artery disease. *Hum Mol Genet.* 2006;15:R117–R123.

Tregouet DA, Barbaux S, Escolano S, et al. Specific haplotypes of the P-selectin gene are associated with myocardial infarction. *Hum Mol Genet.* 2002;11:2015–2023.

Tregouet DA, Ricard S, Nicaud V, et al. In-depth haplotype analysis of ABCA1 gene polymorphisms in relation to plasma ApoA1 levels and myocardial infarction. *Arterioscler Thromb Vasc Biol.* 2004;24:775–781.

van Bokxmeer FM, Mamotte CDS. Apolipoprotein ε4 homozygosity in young men with coronary heart disease. *Lancet.* 1992;340:879–880.

van Dam MJ, de Groot GE, Clee SM, et al. Association between increased arterial-wall thickness and impairment in ABCA1-driven cholesterol efflux: an observational study. *Lancet.* 2002;359:37–42.

Vasku A, Goldbergova M, Izakovicova Holla L, et al. A haplotype constituted of four MMP-2 promoter polymorphisms (–1575G/A, –1306C/T, –790T/G and –735C/T) is associated with coronary triple-vessel disease. *Matrix Biol.* 2004;22:585–591.

Vendrell J, Fernandez-Real JM, Gutierrez C, et al. A polymorphism in the promoter of the tumor necrosis factor-α gene (–308) is associated with coronary heart disease in type 2 diabetic patients. *Atherosclerosis.* 2003;167:257–264.

Verhoef P, Rimm EB, Hunter DJ, et al. A common mutation in the methylenetetrahydrofolate reductase gene and risk of coronary heart disease: results among U.S. men. *J Am Coll Cardiol.* 1998;32:353–359.

Wang L, Fan C, Topol SE, Topol EJ, Wang Q. Mutation of *MEF2A* in an inherited disorder with features of coronary artery disease. *Science.* 2003;302:1578–1581.

Wang Q, Rao S, Shen GQ, et al. Premature myocardial infarction novel susceptibility locus on chromosome 1p34–36 identified by genomewide linkage analysis. *Am J Hum Genet.* 2004;74:262–271.

Wang X, Ria M, Kelmenson PM, et al. Positional identification of *TNFSF4*, encoding OX40 ligand, as a gene that influences atherosclerosis susceptibility. *Nat Genet.* 2005;37:365–372.

Wang Y, Zhang W, Zhang Y, et al. VKORC1 haplotypes are associated with arterial vascular diseases (stroke, coronary heart disease, and aortic dissection; *Circulation.* 2006;113:1615–1621.

Webb KE, Martin JF, Hamsten A, et al. Polymorphisms in the thrombopoietin gene are associated with risk of myocardial infarction at a young age. *Atherosclerosis.* 2001;154:703–711.

Weintraub MS, Eisenberg S, Breslow JL. Dietary fat clearance in normal subjects is regulated by genetic variation in apolipoprotein E. *J Clin Invest.* 1987;80:1571–1577.

Weiss EJ, Bray PF, Tayback M, et al. A polymorphism of a platelet glycoprotein receptor as an inherited risk factor for coronary thrombosis. *N Engl J Med.* 1996;334:1090–1094.

Wellcome Trust Case Control Consortium. Genome-wide association study of 14,000 cases of seven common diseases and 3,000 shared controls. *Nature.* 2007;447:661–678.

Williams RR, Hunt SC, Heiss G, et al. Usefulness of cardiovascular family history data for population-based preventive medicine and medical research (the Health Family Tree Study and the NHLBI Family Heart Study). *Am J Cardiol.* 2001;87:129–135.

Wilson PW, Myers RH, Larson MG, Ordovas JM, Wolf PA, Schaefer EJ. Apolipoprotein E alleles, dyslipidemia, and coronary heart disease. The Framingham Offspring Study. *JAMA.* 1994;272:1666–1671.

Wittrup HH, Tybjærg-Hansen A, Nordestgaard BG. Lipoprotein lipase mutations, plasma lipids and lipoproteins, and risk of ischemic heart disease. A meta-analysis. *Circulation.* 1999;99:2901–2907.

Wu KK, Aleksic N, Ahn C, et al. Thrombomodulin Ala455Val polymorphism and risk of coronary heart disease. *Circulation.* 2001;103:1386–1389.

Xhignesse M, Lussier-Cacan S, Sing CF, Kessling AM, Davignon J. Influences of common variants of apolipoprotein E on measures of lipid metabolism in a sample selected for health. *Arterioscler Thromb.* 1991;11:1100–1110.

Yamada Y. Identification of genetic factors and development of genetic risk diagnosis systems for cardiovascular diseases and stroke. *Circ J.* 2006;70:1240–1248.

Yamada Y, Ichihara S, Fujimura T, Yokota M. Identification of the G994→T missense mutation in exon 9 of the plasma platelet-activating factor acetylhydrolase gene as an independent risk factor for coronary artery disease in Japanese men. *Metabolism.* 1998;47:177–181.

Yamada Y, Izawa H, Ichihara S, et al. Prediction of the risk of myocardial infarction from polymorphisms in candidate genes. *N Engl J Med.* 2002;347:1916–1923.

Yamada Y, Kato K, Oguri M, et al. Genetic risk for myocardial infarction determined by polymorphisms of candidate genes in Japanese individuals. *J Med Genet.* 2008;45:216–221.

Yamada Y, Matsuo H, Segawa T, et al. Assessment of genetic risk for myocardial infarction. *Thromb Haemost.* 2006;96:220–227.

Yang Y, Ruiz-Narvaez E, Niu T, Xu X, Campos H. Genetic variants of the lipoprotein lipase gene and myocardial infarction in the Central Valley of Costa Rica. *J Lipid Res.* 2004;45:2106–2109.

Ye S, Watts GF, Mandalia S, Humphries SE, Henney AM. Preliminary report: genetic variation in the human stromelysin promoter is associated with progression of coronary atherosclerosis. *Br Heart J.* 1995;73:209–215.

Yokota M, Ichihara S, Lin TL, Nakashima N, Yamada Y. Association of a T29→C polymorphism of the transforming growth factor-β1 gene with genetic susceptibility to myocardial infarction in Japanese. *Circulation.* 2000;101:2783–2787.

Yoshida M, Takano Y, Sasaoka T, Izumi T, Kimura A. E-selectin polymorphism associated with myocardial infarction causes enhanced leukocyte-endothelial interactions under flow conditions. *Arterioscler Thromb Vasc Biol.* 2003;23:783–788.

Yusuf S, Hawken S, Ounpuu S, et al. Effect of potentially modifiable risk factors associated with myocardial infarction in 52 countries (the INTERHEART study): case-control study. *Lancet.* 2004;364:937–952.

Zee RY, Cook NR, Cheng S, et al. Threonine for alanine substitution in the eotaxin (CCL11) gene and the risk of incident myocardial infarction. *Atherosclerosis.* 2004;175:91–94.

Zeggini E, Weedon MN, Lindgren CM, et al. Replication of genome-wide association signals in UK samples reveals risk loci for type 2 diabetes. *Science.* 2007;316:1336–1341.

Zhang B, Ye S, Herrmann SM, et al. Functional polymorphism in the regulatory region of gelatinase B gene in relation to severity of coronary atherosclerosis. *Circulation.* 1999;99:1788–1794.

Zhang H, Henderson H, Gagne SE, et al. Common sequence variants of lipoprotein lipase: standardized studies of in vitro expression and catalytic function. *Biochim Biophys Acta.* 1996;1302:159–166.

Zwicker JI, Peyvandi F, Palla R, et al. The thrombospondin-1 N700S polymorphism is associated with early myocardial infarction without altering von Willebrand factor multimer size. *Blood.* 2006;108:1280–1283.

23

Genetics of Essential Hypertension

Mark Caulfield, Stephen J Newhouse, and Patricia B Munroe

Introduction

The global public health significance of hypertension can be judged by the simple fact that there are over 1 billion people with high blood pressure worldwide. The World Health Organisation (WHO) suggests that this will rise to 1.5 billion by 2020 (Murray et al. 2002). It is estimated that blood pressure played an important part in 50% of the 16.7 million cardiovascular deaths worldwide (Lewington et al. 2002; Murray et al. 2002; Petersen et al. 2005).

It is only during the 1950s that treatments that effectively reduce blood pressure began to emerge. Before that, various approaches were tried as treatments for hypertension including full dental clearance and colonic lavage, with no success (Pickering 1995). A particularly poignant reminder of how little could be done to lower blood pressure arises from the records kept by Franklin D. Roosevelt's personal physician, who diligently recorded the inexorable rise of the president's blood pressure, eventually causing a fatal stroke in April 1945 (Calhoun and Oparil 1995).

Since the 1940s multiple new therapies have been developed that have been shown to effectively reduce stroke and heart attack. In spite of the availability of multiple different therapeutic strategies, public health data from Western economies show that hypertension remains poorly controlled. Indeed, only 10% achieve current targets and up to 20% of subjects are resistant to current treatments (Primatesta et al. 2001; Petersen et al. 2005). This is partly because of the need for a broader range of more effective therapies, but it is also true that the discovery pipeline for new blood pressure treatments is relatively thin. Therefore it is possible that an understanding of the genetic factors elevating blood pressure might lead to new pathways for therapy (Dominiczak 2004).

In this chapter the lessons from genetic studies of simple Mendelian forms of hypertension, family-based linkage studies, and early genome-wide association studies are described.

The Complexity of Hypertension and Evidence of Heritability

Epidemiological studies indicate that hypertension arises from a complex interplay of lifestyle factors, such as sodium intake, alcohol and weight, and genetic factors, with genes contributing up to 30% toward blood pressure variation (Dominiczak 2004; Mein 2004). Family studies have estimated that the recurrence risk to a sibling (λs) for hypertension lies between 2.5 and 3.5 (Mein et al. 2004; WTCCC 2007). This has led to large-scale national and international collaborations, such as the British Genetics of Hypertension (BRIGHT) Study in the United Kingdom (www.brightstudy.ac.uk). The BRIGHT study contributed to the first phase of the Wellcome Trust Case Control Consortium (WTCCC) genome-wide association scans in a paper identifying new genes for several common diseases (WTCCC 2007).

Pharmacogenomics of Antihypertensive Response

It is possible that the pharmacodynamic response to antihypertensives may also be influenced by genetic variation. Investigation in this area would be valuable because it is estimated that the United Kingdom spent £864 million on this therapeutic area in the past year (www.nice.org.uk). There are no published heritability studies on blood pressure response to antihypertensives. However, genetic variation is known to determine response to other pharmaceutical treatments, and response to blood pressure lowering treatment varies between individuals of different ethnic backgrounds. This suggests that at least part of the variation in response may relate to genetic background. As trials to determine heritability of blood pressure response would be difficult (requiring treatment and monitoring of many related individuals), large-scale genetic association studies may be the simplest method to determine whether and to what extent treatment response is genetic (Arnett et al. 2005; Davis et al. 2005). To date, pharmacogenetic responses to antihypertensives have largely been investigated in underpowered studies and there has been no large-scale genome scans published from a major blood pressure outcome trial (Dominiczak 2004; www.nice.org.uk).

Lessons from Mendelian Forms of Human Hypertension

There are several rare Mendelian forms of hypertension with distinctive co-phenotypes, such as the hypertension and hypokalemia seen in Liddle's syndrome and glucorticoid suppressible

Table 23–1 Mendelian Disorders with Systemic Hypertension

Disorder	Protein	Inheritance	MIM#	Map	Gene
GRA	CYP11B2	AD	103900	8q21	*CYP11B2, CYP11B1-hybrid*
Liddle Syndrome	SCNN1B SCNN1G	AD	177200	16p13-p12	*β or γ EnaC*
Hypertension in pregnancy	Mineralocorticoid receptor binding	AD	605115	4q31.1	*MR*
PHA2	WNK1, WNK4	AD	145260	17q21-q22 1q31-q42	*WNK1, WNK4*
FH2	Unknown	AD	605635	7p22	Unknown
Mineralocorticoid excess syndrome	11β-HSD2	AR	207765	16q22	*11β-HSD2*
11-β hydroxylase deficiency	11-β hydroxylase	AR	202010	8q21	*CYP11B1*
17-α hydroxylase deficiency	17-α hydroxylase	AR	202110	10q24.3	*CYP17A1*

Notes: MIM, Victor McKusick's Mendelian Inheritance in Man; AD, autosomal dominant; AR, autosomal recessive; GRA, glucocorticid remediable aldosteronism; PHA2, pseudohypoaldosteronism type 2, Gordon's syndrome; FH2, familial hyperaldosteronism type 2 is a syndrome with hyperplastic adrenals (recently described by Geller et al. 2008).

hyperaldosteronism (Dominiczak 2004). The elucidation of the genetic basis of these simple Mendelian forms of hypertension has offered the greatest progress in hypertension genomics (Table 23–1) (Dominiczak 2004). As in other common complex disorders, for example, type 2 diabetes, it is possible that genes identified as leading to these more dramatic, but rare forms of hypertension, could also harbor more subtle common, or rare variants, contributing to essential hypertension.

There are several common features that emerge from the study of these Mendelian forms of human hypertension:

1. It may be possible to possess the gene defect causing the Mendelian syndrome but not manifest the phenotype (Dominiczak 2004; Mein et al. 2004). This implies there may be other susceptibility factors, either modifier genes or lifestyle influences at work.
2. Even when the disorder has been localized to a particular chromosomal segment identification of causative defect may still be very challenging.
3. To date all the known mechanisms for these rare disorders influence sodium homeostasis (Dominiczak 2004; Mein et al. 2004).

Pseudohypoaldosteronism Type II (Gordon's Syndrome)

This autosomal dominant form of hypertension, known as pseudohypoaldosteronism type II, shares several features with the commoner form of essential hypertension. These include onset in middle age and responsiveness to thiazide diuretics (Dominiczak 2004). The syndrome had originally been mapped to three different chromosomes in different families, which illustrates some of the genetic heterogeneity even within these rare disorders (Mansfield et al. 1997). Subsequently, a new kindred with the features of this trait allowed identification of a gain-of-function deletion in the gene encoding the serine threonine kinase, *WNK1* (with no lysine serine threonine kinase) on chromosome 12 (Mansfield et al. 1997; Wilson et al. 2001). By chance, bioinformatic interrogation of public domain databases identified another serine threonine

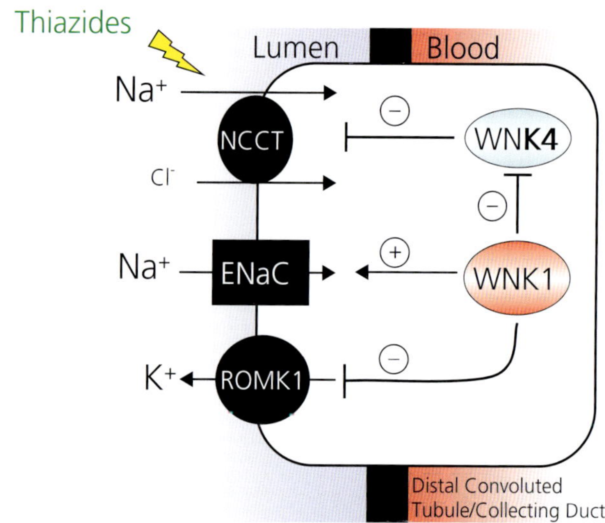

Figure 23–1 Schematic showing interactions of serine threonine kinases *WNK1* and *WNK4* in the distal convoluted tubule. A schematic showing a distal convoluted tubular epithelial cells and the interactions of the serine threonine kinases, *WNK1* and *WNK4*, which act as molecular switches upon the sodium chloride cotransporter (NCCT) which is the target for thiazide diuretics. The diagram also indicates interaction of *WNK1* with the inwardly rectifying potassium channel (ROMK) and the epithelial sodium channel (ENAC) located in the collecting ducts.

kinase, known as *WNK4*, with strong homology to *WNK1* and located within the chromosome 17 region previously linked to pseudohypoaldosteronism type II (Wilson et al. 2001). The identification of mutations within *WNK4* that could cause loss of enzymatic function-fueled functional studies that have begun to shed light on this important regulatory system for sodium in the distal nephron (Wilson et al. 2001). These studies reveal that *WNK* kinases are molecular switches in a cascade, which regulates sodium reabsorption via the sodium chloride cotransporter

(NCCT) and, to some extent, the epithelial sodium channel in the collecting ducts (Kahle et al. 2008) (see Figure 23–1). In the context of the phenotypic response to therapy it is interesting that the sodium chloride cotransporter is the target for thiazide diuretics in the distal nephron. The findings in this rare Mendelian form of hypertension raise the possibility that subtler suceptibility variants might be implicated in essential hypertension.

Variations with Serine Threonine Kinase and Blood Pressure

To explore the relationship of these serine theronine kinases to essential hypertension, common genetic variation within the *WNK1* and *WNK4* genes has been studied in 700 parent–offspring trios from the BRIGHT study, using family-based association testing (Newhouse et al. 2005). The *WNK4* gene showed no evidence of association. However, an association with blood pressure and essential hypertension was detected using an initial set of eight single nucleotide polymorphisms (SNPs) within the *WNK1* gene (Newhouse et al. 2005). This was rapidly followed up in 500 nuclear families, unselected for blood pressure level, within the Genetic Regulation of Arterial Pressure in Communities Study where an association with ambulatory blood pressure parameters was demonstrated (Tobin et al. 2005). These encouraging findings have been developed further into large-scale case-control and population-based analyses in cohorts that are currently ongoing. This gene appears to be one of the first to have translated from a Mendelian hypertensive phenotype, where it has a large effect on blood pressure, into a more subtle but nevertheless important role in blood pressure regulation (Newhouse et al. 2005; Tobin et al. 2005). These findings may also present a novel drug target or pathway for target discovery in the treatment of hypertension.

Common Variants in Mendelian Trait Genes and Blood Pressure Regulation

A recent investigation of common variation in genes responsible for several monogenic hypertensive and hypotensive disorders suggests that the findings with pseudohypoaldosteronism type II will not be unique (Tobin et al. 2008). In 520 nuclear families with 24-hour ambulatory blood pressure and related cardiovascular traits, 298 tagging and putative functional SNPs offering 82% coverage across 11 candidate loci were genotyped (Tobin et al. 2008). Within the *KCNJ1* gene, coding for the inwardly rectifying potassium channel known as ROMK, five SNPs were associated with mean 24-hour systolic or diastolic blood pressure (Tobin et al. 2008). There were weaker associations with mean 24-hour systolic, or diastolic blood pressure, for variants in the calcium sensing receptor gene, the mineralocorticoid receptor (NR3C2), and the β and γ subunits of the epithelial sodium channel genes (*SCNN1B* and *SCNN1G*) (Tobin et al. 2008). Alongside findings described above, this indicates that common variants in genes responsible for some Mendelian disorders of hypertension and hypotension do affect blood pressure in the general population.

Rare Variation in Mendelian Traits and Blood Pressure

It is important to consider the possibility that rare variants in genes encoding Mendelian blood pressure syndromes could contribute to common complex diseases, such as hypertension (Dominiczak 2004; Tobin et al. 2008). This has recently been explored in the Framingham Heart Study (FHS) where the effect of rare mutations that might influence blood pressure was tested in each of the sodium chloride cotransporter (*SLC12A3* or *NCCT*), *SLC12A1* (NKCC2), and the inwardly rectifying potassium channel, ROMK (*KCNJ1*) genes (Ji et al. 2008). These genes cause rare recessive disorders with substantial effects on blood pressure. It is therefore of considerable interest to discover that rare mutations, in these same genes that alter renal salt handling, associate with significant blood pressure reductions in the population (Ji et al. 2008). These findings have important implications for the genetic architecture of hypertension and it remains possible that multiple rare variants will be important contributors to this phenotype.

Linkage Analysis to Identify Genes for Hypertension

In the 1990s large-scale family resources based on affected sibling pairs were identified for linkage based genome scans (www.bright-study.ac.uk; Caulfield et al. 2003; Munroe et al. 2006; Rice et al. 2006; Wu et al. 2006). This approach typically tested for excess sharing of alleles at 400 microsatellite markers spread evenly across the genome and expressed this as a likelihood of linkage divided by a likelihood of nonlinkage that gave a LOD score. It rapidly became clear that conventional significance thresholds for LOD scores of 3.0, or greater, would not be attainable in common complex traits (Caulfield et al. 2003; Munroe et al. 2006; Rice et al. 2006; Wu et al. 2006). In hypertension, the BRIGHT study and a U.S. competitor study, the Family Blood Pressure Program, undertook large-scale linkage-based genome scans (www.bright-study.ac.uk; Caulfield et al. 2003; Rice et al. 2006; Wu et al. 2006) The BRIGHT study identified modest support for four loci on chromosome 2, 5q, 6q, 8p in 2,010 affected sibling pairs. These were followed up with a denser grid of additional microsatellites, which reduced support for linkage to chromosomes 2, 6, and 8 loci (Caulfield et al. 2003; Munroe et al. 2006). However, this process did find increased support for linkage of the chromosome 5q locus, in both affected sibling pairs and in 700 parent–offspring trios (Munroe et al. 2006). This chromosome 5 locus spans 22 mega bases (mb) but contains a 2 mb repetitive region right in the middle of the interval. This has been poorly mapped to date and as yet no gene has been identified for hypertension on chromosome 5q (Munroe et al. 2006). This disappointing experience in hypertension has been mirrored in linkage analysis of many common disorders (Caulfield et al. 2003; Mein et al. 2004; Munroe et al. 2006). The lack of findings from these family-based linkage scans created the impetus for genome-wide association studies as a route to access smaller gene effect sizes than could be identified by conventional linkage analysis.

The Advances Enabling Genome-Wide Association Scanning

A series of major international initiatives began with the Human Genome Mapping Project and developed in the SNP consortium created an inventory of more than 12 million SNPs spread across the genome (Manolio et al. 2008). This enabled the International Haplotype Mapping Project (HAPMAP) to correlate the positions of these SNPs allowing us to economize on genotyping effort by employing SNPs that tag genetic variation that is not directly typed (www.hapmap.org). Genome-wide association studies are greatly facilitated by high-throughput technological advances using chip technology that permit genotyping of up to 1 million SNPs covering 80% of genetic variation across the genome.

As the genotyping chip technologies began to emerge, simulations were run to test the coverage of these tools using data from HAPMAP and the Seattle Resequencing Project on a subset of cardiovascular and inflammatory genes (Wallace et al. 2007; Manolio et al. 2008; www.hapmap.org/). The findings suggested that sequence variations known as short interspersed elements (SINES) and long interspersed elements (LINES) based on repetitive sequences that are common around inflammatory genes could reduce tag SNP coverage and thereby risk missing associations within, or close by these variations (Wallace et al. 2007). These data need further corroboration as the range of genes with deep resequencing increases with the new generation of long-range clonal sequencers, such as Solexa or 454.

Genome-Wide Association Scan of Seven Common Diseases

The WTCCC published a trail blazing genome-wide association study (GWAS) study in 2,000 cases from each of seven common diseases in June 2007 (WTCCC 2007). As a control group, 3,000 common controls (1,500 National Blood Service donors and 1,500 1958 birth cohort participants) drawn from across the United Kingdom were used as the comparator for each disease (Figure 23–2) (WTCCC 2007).

In the Wellcome study, generation of the highest fidelity data set necessitated the development or adaptation of multiple quality assurance steps, to minimize the risk of erroneous data contained in the 9 billion genotypes (WTCCC 2007). Initial quality control samples with <95% of SNPs scored were eliminated as this implied a DNA problem. In addition, markers were removed if they were found to be unreliable or had an unknown map assignment, or if they had less than 95% genotype capture, or exhibited strong deviation from Hardy-Weinberg equilibrium. Furthermore, checks were run for cryptic or undeclared relationships and to verify gender assignment (WTCCC 2007).

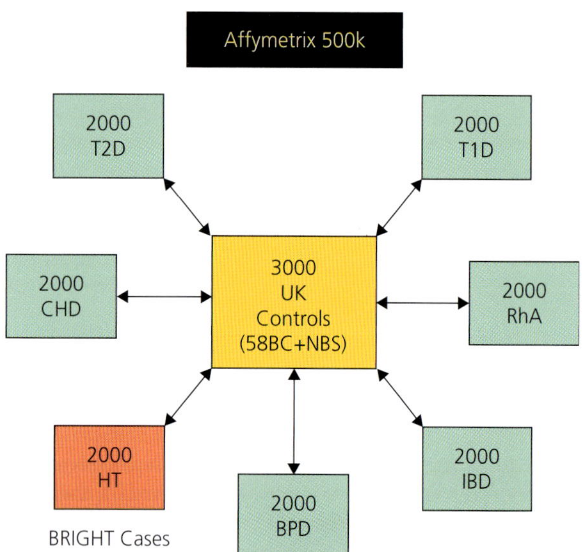

Figure 23–2 The design of the WTCCC. GWAS of seven common complex disorders compared with common controls (Adapted with permission of Prof. Mark McCarthy, Oxford).

A particular area of concern that has previously been raised is that there may be hidden population substructure or regional variation in allelic frequencies. This could distort any subsequent analysis and create outliers that are not well matched in the case and control groups. In the WTCCC, this was approached by dividing Britain into 12 geographic regions, and comparing allele frequencies across 400,000 markers that passed our quality control steps (WTCCC 2007). This detected a mere 13 markers with allelic differences on a northwest- southeast diagonal line. These frequencies resemble those seen in Scandinavia and it is tempting to speculate they may represent the influence of Viking invasions in the middle of the first millennium.

The HAPMAP allows researchers to use our wet bench typed SNPs to tag, and therefore impute, untyped SNPs using various methodologies (Marchini 2007). This imputation step can allow us to take up to 2.5 million real or imputed SNPs forward into statistical analysis. In the analysis of genome-wide association studies it is absolutely vital to correct for multiple statistical comparisons and select a stringent p-value to accept genome-wide significance. The most broadly accepted approach to date is to adopt a p-value threshold of less than 5×10^{-7} (WTCCC 2007).

Results from the Hypertension Genome-Wide Association Scan

In the first phase of WTCCC, 2,000 hypertensives from the BRIGHT Study were subjected to a genome-wide scan using the Affymetrix 500 chip and compared with 3,000 common controls (WTCCC 2007). A comparable number and distribution of suggestive association signals in the range $p < 10^{-4}$ to 10^{-7} were found when compared with the six other diseases investigated. Unlike most of these disorders there were no signals attaining the experiment-wide significance threshold of $p < 5 \times 10^{-7}$ (WTCCC 2007). To satisfy replication criteria the p-value for statistical significance must become smaller and ideally below 5×10^{-8} to take account of up to 1 million independent statistical tests (see section on Diabetes Meta-analysis) (see Figure 23–3).

There are several potential reasons for these findings; first, the use of common controls without phenotyping for a highly prevalent disorder may have imposed a penalty on power because of "caseness" amongst the controls. As part of the experiment we estimated that if 5% of the controls were cases this would be equivalent to a 10% reduction in the size of the control group (WTCCC 2007). As the U.K. prevalence of hypertension is circa 30% there could have been a substantial penalty on power for this genome-wide association scan. Second, some of the strongest candidate genes for hypertension were poorly tagged by the Affymetrix chip, for example, the serine threonine kinase *WNK1* (Newhouse et al. 2005; Tobin et al. 2005; WTCCC 2007). Third, the WTCCC experiment was a pathfinder experiment powered to detect effect sizes of 1.5 or greater for common alleles as illustrated in the table. It is highly plausible that very common, complex disorders, such as hypertension, arise from odds ratios (OR) or genotype effect sizes between 1.2 and 1.5, which will only be detectable in large data sets. This observation resonates with the

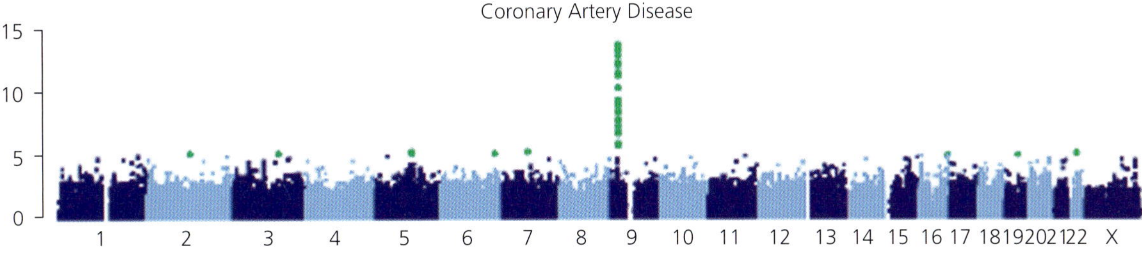

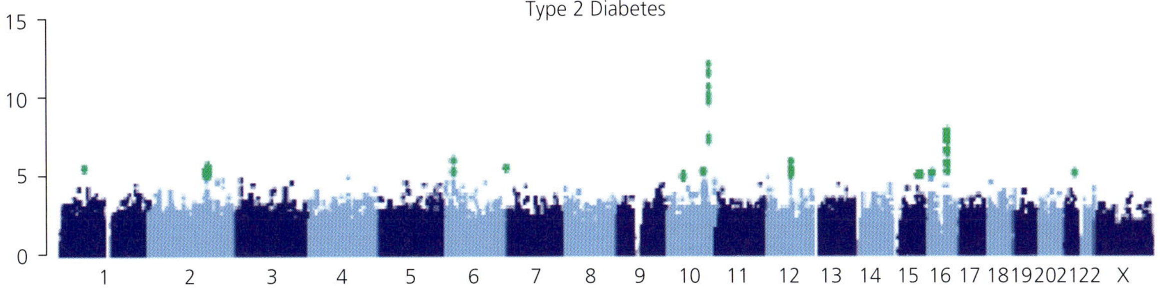

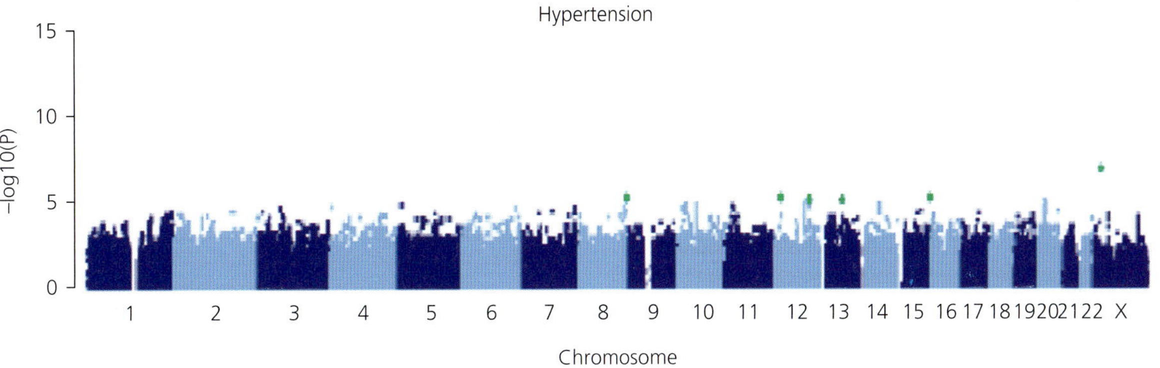

Figure 23–3 Manhattan plots from type 2 diabetes, CHD, and hypertension. Manhattan plots for genome-wide association scan data from the WTCCC contrasting results for the common cardiovascular disorders of coronary disease, type 2 diabetes with hypertension. Here *p*-value is on the vertical axis and the chromosome is on the horizontal axis. This shows clear signals for coronary disease and diabetes but nothing of genome-wide significance for hypertension. The Wellcome Trust Case Control Consortium. *Nature.* 2007;447:661–678, with permission of Nature Publishing Group.

lower recurrence risk ratio of between 2.0 and 3.5 for hypertension compared to most of the other diseases under test in the Wellcome Trust study.

Lessons from Case

Lessons from Control Collaborations on GWAS

The benefit of extra numbers in enabling access to lower genotype effect sizes is nicely illustrated in the coronary artery disease meta-analysis of WTCCC 2,000 cases compared with a smaller number of German scans (Samani et al. 2007). This identified novel loci and confirmed known loci. This theme has been developed further in the type 2 diabetes consortium known as Diagram. The expanded case-control meta-analysis allowed further new genes to be identified and then replicated in a staged design (Zegginni et al. 2008). This staged design offers the value of an initial combined meta-analysis, in this case including 4,549 cases and 5,579 controls, with follow-up of 69 independent signals in a second stage involving 10,000 cases and 12,000 controls. The results of this second stage enabled economic focusing of wet bench SNP genotyping on 11 of the 69 signals, which were taken into a further 14,000 cases and 43,000 controls. From this study, a total of six new loci for type 2 diabetes were identified with $p < 5 \times 10^{-8}$, which illustrates the potential of both enlarged sample size and the economy of a staged design (Zegginni et al. 2008).

Lessons for Further Hypertension Case-Control Analyses

The power simulations shown in Table 23–2 illustrate the limitations of the WTCCC experiment for hypertension. The key message from all case-control analyses in other traits is that expanding the numbers with high-fidelity phenotyping is likely to improve the prospect of identifying new loci (Samani et al. 2007;

Table 23–2 The percentage power of the hypertension 2,000 cases (drawn from the top 10% of BP distribution) versus 3,000 common controls, unselected for blood pressure, where the letter *q* denotes the column with allele frequencies and the top row is the genotype relative risk. This shows that the study had limited power to detect association in a discrete allelic frequency range for an effect size of 1.5 in original the WTCCC experiment (WTCCC 2007)

Q	1.2	1.3	1.4	1.5
0.1	0.000	0.002	0.010	0.030
0.2	0.002	0.018	0.093	0.256
0.4	0.011	0.122	0.444	**0.797**
0.6	0.015	0.176	0.599	**0.915**
0.8	0.005	0.068	0.345	0.750
0.9	0.001	0.011	0.077	0.222

Zegginni et al. 2008). To that end we are concluding an 8,000 hypertensive case versus 8,500 control (many selected to be normotensive) genome scan analysis (Table 23–2). The power simulations conducted prior to this experiment indicate that a study of this size can begin to access effect sizes ranging from 1.2 to 1.5 dramatically enhancing the likelihood of gene detection in more recalcitrant complex traits, such as hypertension (Table 23–2).

Lessons from GWAS on Quantitative Anthropometric Phenotypes

The Genetic Investigation of Anthropometric Traits (GIANT) consortium has now published separate papers based on meta-analyses of height and body mass index as quantitative traits, which may serve future blood pressure based GWAS (Frayling et al. 2007; Weedon et al. 2008).

The experience gained in the genome scan meta-analysis for height is encouraging for blood pressure because up to 20 novel genes were identified from the first phase of the GIANT collaboration (Weedon et al. 2008). However, it must be noted that there are important distinctions between height and blood pressure phenotypes:

1. Although some loss of height occurs with aging and in post-menopausal women a person's height is relatively fixed after puberty and is therefore not a dynamic variable like blood pressure.
2. Height is relatively robustly and simply measured. Typically, individuals have relatively high recall for their height and will query values that vary from expectation.

A trait that is rather closer to blood pressure as a phenotype is body mass index (height in meters squared divided by the weight in kilograms) (Frayling et al. 2007). Since the initial discovery of the fused toes gene (FTO) as a gene for body mass index (BMI) this has proved to be a challenging trait for gene identification (Frayling et al. 2007). In a separate meta-analysis led by the GIANT consortium, following the approaches used above, common variation at the melanocortin-4 receptor gene locus was found to influence fat mass and BMI (Loos et al. 2008). This necessitated meta-analysis of GWAS of 16,876 subjects and follow-up in replication resources of over 60,352 subjects (Loos et al. 2008). The BMI phenotype has some common features with blood pressure, which may serve to inform future study:

1. BMI like blood pressure is a dynamic variable and may change over the course of a day.
2. Weight change may be independent of fat mass and can be influenced by fluid homeostasis or hydration.
3. Measurement although relatively simple may vary between equipment.

Lessons from Quantitative Traits for Genome-Wide Scans in Blood Pressure

The implication from studies on gene discovery for BMI is that when effect sizes are small in a challenging dynamic phenotype, then high-quality measurements and large numbers of subjects are necessary for successful gene detection. For blood pressure analyses, the BRIGHT consortium have formed collaborations with other complementary European and U.S. quantitative blood pressure GWAS population-based analyses with high-fidelity blood pressure measurements. This has prompted large-scale blood pressure meta-analysis of 26,800 subjects led by a consortium known as GLOBAL BP Gen.

Replication Studies and Minimizing the "Winners Curse"

Association from genome-wide studies requires validation in appropriately powered replication studies (NCI-NHGRI 2007). The participants will ideally be drawn from the same population background and ideally have similarly detailed phenotyping. The replication resources should be genotyped for the originally associated SNP or a proxy in complete linkage disequilibrium. The expectation is that stochastic variation, or genetic heterogeneity will mean that a sample size of approximately double that seen in the initial study will often be needed to detect smaller *p*-values than that observed in the original study, for example, $<5 \times 10^{-8}$. This is especially likely to be true for blood pressure and hypertension signals where "winners curse" is likely to operate as *p*-values will very likely be close to the genome-wide significance threshold. Recently, very useful consensus guidance on standards for replication has been published (NCI-NHGRI 2007).

Investigating Hypertensive Biochemical Cophenotypes

Serum and urine biochemistry measurements are regularly used in clinical investigation of hypertension to identify abnormal lipid profiles and target organ damage (e.g., renal function). It is conceivable that these traits may be under tighter genetic control than disorders, such as hypertension. Such heritable quantitative traits may permit identification of novel pathways, or explain coexistent risk factors for cardiovascular disease. To test this hypothesis, we recently published a genome-wide quantitative trait analysis of 25 biochemical intermediate traits from serum and urine samples from hypertensive participants in the BRIGHT study (Wallace et al. 2008). This analysis identified novel gene signals for urate and lipid parameters that we validated in silico in secondary data sets, or by de novo genotyping.

The SLC2A9 Gene Influences Serum Urate

The Framingham study suggests urate levels are markedly heritable and there are many strands of evidence that show a correlation between increased serum urate, blood pressure, and hypertension (Li et al. 2007; Wallace et al. 2008) and a link between raised urate

Table 23–3 The Power for GWAS of 8,000 Cases versus 8,500 Controls

Q	1.2	1.3	1.4	1.5
0.1	0.094	0.504	**0.86**	**0.979**
0.2	0.440	**0.953**	**1.00**	**1.000**
0.4	**0.894**	**1.000**	**1.00**	**1.000**
0.6	**0.941**	**1.000**	**1.00**	**1.000**
0.8	0.735	**0.999**	**1.00**	**1.000**
0.9	0.253	**0.917**	**1.00**	**1.000**

Notes: Simulations of power for the comparison of GWAS of 8,000 cases drawn from the top 10% of blood pressure distribution compared with 1,500 population controls with no blood pressure information plus 7,000 population controls with blood pressure data enabling selection of normotensive controls.

and other cardiovascular disorders. Two studies have identified a common allele which is present in 79% of the White European population in the glucose transporter gene *SLC2A9*, that increases serum urate levels by 0.02 mmol/L for each allelic copy—this explains approximately 3.5% of urate variance (Li et al. 2007; Wallace et al. 2008). The *SLC2A9* gene is most strongly expressed in the kidney and liver, but interestingly it is also expressed at low levels in chondrocytes and has since been associated with gout, which affects 3.9 million Americans (Vitart et al. 2008; Döring et al. 2008). Additional studies are underway to assess if *SLC2A9* may explain the association between serum urate, blood pressure, and cardiovascular disease.

The Identification of Novel Genes Influencing Low Density Lipoprotein Levels

Dyslipidemia is commonly identified in the routine investigation of hypertensive patients. Associations between lipid parameters and various genes were identified in GWAS followed by in silico replication using publicly available data (see Table 23–4 for summary of findings) (Wallace et al. 2008).

The main novel finding is association of serum LDL, total cholesterol, and SNPs in gene regions containing *PSRC1* and *CELSR2*. There is very little known about the function of the *PSRC1* (proline/serine-rich coiled-coil 1) gene product beyond a role within the WNT/β-catenin signaling pathway, which has been implicated in LDL processing in the liver. The second gene in that block *CELSR2* (cadherin, EGF LAG seven-pass G-type receptor 2) has not yet had a specific function determined (Wallace et al. 2008).

In the coronary artery disease meta-analysis, this gene cluster was identified as associated with ischemic heart disease but due to routine statin use in these patients no connection was made to LDL (Samani et al. 2007). Therefore, this genome scan in hypertension was able to define the potential mechanism for coronary artery disease etiology through LDL level because of the absence of statin consumption in the hypertensive subjects (Wallace et al. 2008). In addition to our own replication shown in Table 23–4 of several lipid parameters, these findings (especially *PSRC1* and *CELSR2)* have since been replicated in other studies on lipid parameters (Samani et al. 2008; Sandhu et al. 2008; Willer et al. 2008).

Genome-wide Approaches—Copy Number Variants

Genome structural variation involves DNA segments of up to several mega bases and comprises deletions, insertions, inversions, and translocations (Estivill and Armengol 2007). The most

Table 23–4 Quantitative Influences of Genes on Lipid Levels Identified from a GWAS of Hypertensives Showing Gene Identifier and Chromosome

Trait	Chromosome	Gene	Hypertension	Diabetic	Combined
LDL	1	*PSCR1, CELSR2*	1×10^{-7}	4×10^{-8}	3×10^{-14}
LDL	19	*APOE*	2×10^{-2}	3×10^{-14}	8×10^{-14}
LDL	2	*APOB*	3×10^{-5}	5×10^{-9}	8×10^{-14}
HDL	8	*LPL*	2×10^{-5}	1×10^{-6}	1×10^{-10}
HDL	16	*CETP*	6×10^{-3}	1×10^{-9}	1×10^{-10}
TRIG	1	*ANGPTL3*	3×10^{-4}	2×10^{-4}	3×10^{-7}
TRIG	2	*GCKR*	4×10^{-7}	3×10^{-8}	8×10^{-14}
TRIG	8	*LPL*	1×10^{-9}	3×10^{-7}	5×10^{-15}
TRIG	11	*APOA5*	1×10^{-11}	1×10^{-4}	3×10^{-12}

Notes: Column 5 shows confirmation in a second population of publicly available diabetes and combined *p*-values. LDL, low-density lipoprotein; HDL, high-density lipoprotein; Trig, triglycerides (Wallace et al. 2008).

common structural variations are copy number variants (CNV) due to extra segments or deletions of DNA. There were initial thoughts that these might be tagged using SNPs as proxies for different alleles of these structural changes. Although this could work for simple biallelic CNVs, the more abundant polymorphic CNVs appear to have more complex inheritance pattern and importantly may not follow patterns of Mendelian inheritance (Estivill and Armengol 2007). It is highly plausible that many existing GWAS have failed to capture adequately the contribution of some CNVs to common disease because the current chips are populated with readily typable common variants. This is being addressed by commercial providers with allocation of features to identify CNV on SNP gene chips and the development of array-based comparative genomic hybridization products (Nimblegen and Agilent) (Estivill and Armengol 2007). These latter technologies could explore the complete genome, and may offer greater CNV typing accuracy. Recently, the WTCCC has selected the Agilent comparative genomic hybridization array for a genome-wide study of CNV in the same seven diseases studied by genome-wide association including hypertension.

The Challenge of Finding Genes for Human Hypertension

The genetic architecture of human hypertension still remains to be elucidated but there is evidence of progress. It is clear that there were no signals identified in the WTCCC greater than 1.5 but it is equally clear that the Affymetrix gene chip did not tag some known candidates well, for example, *WNK1* (WTCCC 2007). In addition, observations in rare Mendelian forms of hypertension have translated into common and rare variation affecting blood pressure. Although these need further corroboration in other populations and functional studies this represents real progress. It is also true that some signals that are not confirmed reside in genomic areas of CNV and may be resolved by ongoing WTCCC work. The large-scale collaborative initiatives in both case-control and population-based cohorts described herein offer real prospects of accessing the level of genotype relative risk that will be associated with a very common disorder such as hypertension with very strong lifestyle influence. The main reasons for pursuing these low genotype effect sizes are to gain a better understanding of the molecular physiology of blood pressure regulation and to identify new points of pharmacological intervention. The ultimate goal is to reduce further the burgeoning global epidemic of cardiovascular disease (Murray et al. 2002).

References

Arnett DK, Baird AE, Barkley RA, et al. Relevance of genetics and genomics for prevention and treatment of cardiovascular disease: a scientific statement from the American Heart Association Council on Epidemiology and Prevention, the Stroke Council, and the Functional Genomics and Translational Biology Interdisciplinary Working Group. *Circulation.* 2007;115(22):2878–2901.

Arnett DK, Davis BR, Ford CE, et al. Pharmacogenetic association of the angiotensin-converting enzyme insertion/deletion polymorphism on blood pressure and cardiovascular risk in relation to antihypertensive treatment: the Genetics of Hypertension-Associated Treatment (GenHAT) study. *Circulation.* 2005;111(25):3374–3383.

Calhoun DA, Oparil S. Hypertensive crisis since FDR—a partial victory. *N Engl J Med.* 1995;332(15):1029–1030.

Caulfield M, Munroe P, Pembroke J, et al. Genome-wide mapping of human loci for essential hypertension. *Lancet.* 2003;361(9375):2118–2123.

Dominiczak AF, Brain N, Charchar F, McBride M, Hanlon N, Lee WK. Genetics of hypertension: lessons learnt from mendelian and polygenic syndromes. *Clin Exp Hypertens.* 2004;26(7–8):611–620. Review.

Döring A, Gieger C, Mehta D, et al. SLC2A9 influences uric acid concentrations with pronounced sex-specific effects. *Nat Genet.* 2008;40(4):430–436. Epub 2008 Mar 9.

Estivill X, Armengol L. Copy number variants and common disorders: filling the gaps and exploring complexity in genome-wide association studies. *PLoS Genet.* 2007;3(10):1787–1799.

Frayling TM, Timpson NJ, Weedon MN, et al. A common variant in the FTO gene is associated with body mass index and predisposes to childhood and adult obesity. *Science.* 2007;316(5826):889–894. Epub 2007 Apr 12.

Geller DS, Zhang J, Wisgerhof MV, Shackleton C, Kashgarian M, Lifton RP. A novel form of human mendelian hypertension featuring nonglucocorticoid-remediable aldosteronism. *J Clin Endocrinol Metab.* 2008;93(8):3117–3123.

http://www.brightstudy.ac.uk/

http://www.hapmap.org/

http://www.nice.org.uk/download.aspx?o=442062

Ji W, Foo JN, O'Roak BJ, et al. Rare independent mutations in renal salt handling genes contribute to blood pressure variation. *Nat Genet.* 2008;40(5):592–599. Epub 2008 Apr 6.

Kahle KT, Ring AM, Lifton RP. Molecular physiology of the WNK kinases. *Annu Rev Physiol.* 2008;70:329–355. Review.

Lewington S, Clarke R, Qizilbash N, Peto R, Collins R. Prospective Studies Collaboration. Age-specific relevance of usual blood pressure to vascular mortality: a meta-analysis of individual data for one million adults in 61 prospective studies. *Lancet.* 2002;360(9349):1903–1913.

Li S, Sanna S, Maschio A, et al. The GLUT9 gene is associated with serum uric acid levels in Sardinia and Chianti cohorts. *PLoS Genet.* 2007;3(11):e194.

Loos RJ, Lindgren CM, Li S, et al. Common variants near MC4R are associated with fat mass, weight and risk of obesity. *Nat Genet.* 2008;40(6):768–775. Epub 2008 May 4.

Manolio TA, Brooks LD, Collins FS. A HapMap harvest of insights into the genetics of common disease. *J Clin Invest.* 2008;118(5):1590–1605.

Mansfield TA, Simon DB, Farfel Z, et al. Multilocus linkage of familial hyperkalaemia and hypertension, pseudohypoaldosteronism type II, to chromosomes 1q31–42 and 17p11-q21. *Nat Genet.* 1997;16(2):202–205.

Marchini J, Howie B, Myers S, McVean G, Donnelly P. A new multipoint method for genome-wide association studies by imputation of genotypes. *Nat Genet.* 2007;39(7):906–913. Epub 2007 Jun 17.

Mein CA, Caulfield MJ, Dobson RJ, Munroe PB. Genetics of essential hypertension. *Hum Mol Genet.* 2004;13(Spec No 1):R169–R175. Epub 2004 Feb 5. Review.

Munroe PB, Wallace C, Xue MZ, et al. Increased support for linkage of a novel locus on chromosome 5q13 for essential hypertension in the British Genetics of Hypertension Study. *Hypertension.* 2006;48(1):105–111. Epub 2006 Jun 5.

Murray C, Lopez A, Rodgers A, Vaughan P. World Health Organisation Report 2002. *Reducing Risks, Promoting Healthy Life.* World Heath Organisation; 2002.

NCI-NHGRI Working Group on Replication in Association Studies, Chanock SJ, Manolio T, et al. Replicating genotype-phenotype associations. *Nature.* 2007;447(7145):655–660.

Newhouse SJ, Wallace C, Dobson R, et al. Haplotypes of the WNK1 gene associate with blood pressure variation in a severely hypertensive population from the British Genetics of Hypertension study. *Hum Mol Genet.* 2005;14(13):1805–1814.

Petersen S, Peto V, Rayner M, Leal J, Luengo-Fernandez R, Gray A. *European Cardiovascular Disease Statistics.* London, British Heart Foundation; 2005.

Pickering GW. *High Blood Pressure.* London, Churchill; 1955:314–315, Chapter 9, pages 184–203.

Primatesta P, Brookes M, Poulter NR. Improved hypertension management and control: results from the health survey for England 1998. *Hypertension.* 2001;38(4):827–832.

Rice T, Cooper RS, Wu X, et al. Meta-analysis of genome-wide scans for blood pressure in African American and Nigerian samples. The National Heart, Lung, and Blood Institute GeneLink Project. *Am J Hypertens.* 2006;19(3):270–274.

Samani NJ, Braund PS, Erdmann J, et al. The novel genetic variant predisposing to coronary artery disease in the region of the PSRC1 and CELSR2 genes on chromosome 1 associates with serum cholesterol. *J Mol Med.* 2008;86(11):1233–1241 Epub ahead of print.

Samani NJ, Erdmann J, Hall AS, et al. Genomewide association analysis of coronary artery disease. *N Engl J Med.* 2007;357(5):443–453. Epub 2007 Jul 18.

Sandhu MS, Waterworth DM, Debenham SL, et al. LDL-cholesterol concentrations: a genome-wide association study. *Lancet.* 2008;371(9611):483–491.

The Wellcome Trust Case Control Consortium. Genome-wide association study of 14,000 cases of seven common diseases and 3,000 shared controls. *Nature.* 2007;447:661–678.

Tobin MD, Raleigh SM, Newhouse S, et al. Association of WNK1 gene polymorphisms and haplotypes with ambulatory blood pressure in the general population. *Circulation.* 2005;112(22):3423–3429.

Tobin MD, Tomaszewski M, Braund PS, et al. Common variants in genes underlying monogenic hypertension and hypotension and blood pressure in the general population. *Hypertension.* 2008;51(6):1658–1664. Epub 2008 Apr 28.

Vitart V, Rudan I, Hayward C, et al. SLC2A9 is a newly identified urate transporter influencing serum urate concentration, urate excretion and gout. *Nat Genet.* 2008;40(4):437–442. Epub 2008 Mar 9.

Wallace C, Dobson RJ, Munroe PB, Caulfield MJ. Information capture using SNPs from HapMap and whole-genome chips differs in a sample of inflammatory and cardiovascular gene-centric regions from genome-wide estimates. *Genome Res.* 2007;17(11):1596–1602. Epub 2007 Sep 25.

Wallace C, Newhouse SJ, Braund P, et al. Genome-wide association study identifies genes for biomarkers of cardiovascular disease: serum urate and dyslipidemia. *Am J Hum Genet.* 2008;82(1):139–149.

Weedon MN, Lango H, Lindgren CM, et al. Genome-wide association analysis identifies 20 loci that influence adult height. *Nat Genet.* 2008;40(5):575–583. Epub 2008 Apr 6.

Willer CJ, Sanna S, Jackson AU, et al. Newly identified loci that influence lipid concentrations and risk of coronary artery disease. *Nat Genet.* 2008;40(2):161–169. Epub 2008 Jan 13.

Wilson FH, Disse-Nicodème S, Choate KA, et al. Human hypertension caused by mutations in WNK kinases. *Science.* 2001;293(5532):1107–1112.

Wu X, Kan D, Province M, et al. An updated meta-analysis of genome scans for hypertension and blood pressure in the NHLBI Family Blood Pressure Program (FBPP). *Am J Hypertens.* 2006;19(1):122–127. www.brightstudy.ac.uk

Zeggini E, Scott LJ, Saxena R, et al. Meta-analysis of genome-wide association data and large-scale replication identifies additional susceptibility loci for type 2 diabetes. *Nat Genet.* 2008;40(5):638–645. Epub 2008 Mar 30.

24

Stroke

Yoshiji Yamada, Sahoko Ichihara, and Tamotsu Nishida

Introduction

Recent progress in human genetics and genomics research, highlighted by the completion of the nucleotide sequence of the human genome by the Human Genome Project (Lander et al. 2001), has provided substantial benefits to clinical medicine, including facilitation of the characterization of disease pathophysiology at the molecular level and the development of panels of genetic markers for assessment of disease risk. In particular, determination of single nucleotide polymorphisms (SNPs) and haplotype blocks and the specification of tag SNPs in each haplotype block for four ethnic groups by the International HapMap Project (The International HapMap Consortium 2005) have led to increasingly effective approaches to the identification of genetic variation associated with various multifactorial diseases, providing new insight into the pathogenesis of these conditions. Furthermore, the development of technologies such as DNA microarrays and SNP chips that provide huge amounts of genetic information has made possible the detection of genetic differences among individuals at the whole-genome level. Selection of the most appropriate strategies for disease prevention and therapy on the basis of genetic information for a given individual is referred to as personalized or individualized medicine. In conventional medicine, medications are prescribed on the basis of the diagnosis and severity of the disease. However, the efficacy of drugs and the incidence of side effects vary among individuals. The goal of treatment based on genetic or genomic information is to be able to predict therapeutic outcome or side effects in an individual, thereby increasing the effectiveness and safety of treatment. In addition, the clarification of disease etiologies at the molecular level and the identification of genes that confer disease susceptibility, with genetic factors being thought to account for 20%–70% of such susceptibility to common complex diseases, are likely to contribute both to disease prevention and to the development of new medicines.

Stroke is a complex multifactorial disorder that is thought to result from an interaction between a person's genetic background and various environmental factors. It is a common and serious condition, with about 700,000 individuals experiencing a new or recurrent stroke and nearly 150,000 deaths from stroke-related causes in 2004 in the United States. The prevalence of stroke in the United States is 5.7 million. Of all such events, 88% are ischemic stroke, 9% are intracerebral hemorrhage, and 3% are subarachnoid hemorrhage (Rosamond et al. 2007). In the United Kingdom, 133,000 individuals have a first or recurrent stroke and there are 60,000 deaths from stroke-related causes each year. The prevalence of stroke is 0.9 million, with 69% of such events being ischemic stroke, 13% intracerebral hemorrhage, and 6% subarachnoid hemorrhage (The Stroke Association, United Kingdom, 2006). In Japan, the prevalence of stroke is 1.4 million (61% ischemic stroke, 25% intracerebral hemorrhage, 11% subarachnoid hemorrhage), with nearly 132,000 deaths from this condition each year (Ministry of Health, Labor, and Welfare of Japan, 2005). Despite recent advances in acute stroke therapy, stroke remains the leading cause of severe disability and the third leading cause of death, after heart disease and cancer, in Western countries and Japan (Warlow et al. 2003). The identification of biomarkers of stroke risk is important both for risk prediction and for intervention to avert future events.

Genetics of Stroke

Ischemic and hemorrhagic stroke may have both shared and different determinants, although the genetic variants that influence these clinical conditions are probably different. Studies with twins, siblings, and families have provided substantial evidence for heritability of common forms of stroke (Bak et al. 2002), but the genetic determinants remain largely unknown. Specific mutations in several monogenic stroke disorders have been identified (Meschia and Worrall 2003). Although these observations provide insight into the pathophysiological processes of stroke, these mutations are rare and do not contribute substantially to stroke risk in the general population.

A family history of stroke is regarded as an important risk factor for this disease (Williams et al. 2001). A positive family history might be the result of shared genes, a shared environment, or both. Despite the identification of rare Mendelian stroke syndromes in humans (Tournier-Lasserve et al. 1991; Hassan and Markus 2000), many candidate gene association studies for common forms of stroke have produced no consistent results and data on the genetic epidemiology of stroke are conflicting (Hassan and Markus 2000; Hademenos et al. 2001). The incidence of ischemic stroke, intracerebral hemorrhage, or subarachnoid hemorrhage differs among ethnic groups, which may be attributable to differences in the distribution and frequency of genetic polymorphisms as well as in environmental factors such as diet, exercise, and other lifestyle aspects. Given that some gene polymorphisms characteristic of specific ethnic groups may be related to stroke, it is necessary to examine the relations of gene polymorphisms to stroke in each ethnic group.

Single-Gene Disorders Associated with Stroke

Several conditions in which stroke occur are inherited in a classical Mendelian pattern as autosomal dominant, autosomal recessive, or X-linked disorders (Natowicz and Kelley 1987; Hassan and Markus 2000; Tournier-Lasserve 2002). In most of these conditions, stroke is just one component of the disease phenotype, but in others it is the prominent or sole clinical manifestation (Tournier-Lasserve 2002). Studies of some Mendelian forms of stroke have identified the genes responsible (Carr et al. 2002). In particular, an autosomal dominant form of stroke—cerebral arteriopathy, autosomal dominant, with subcortical infarcts and leukoencephalopathy (CADASIL)—has been well characterized genetically and shown to be attributable to mutation of the notch, drosophila, homolog of, 3 gene (*NOTCH3*) (Box 24–1). Linkage analysis thus mapped the responsible gene to a defined region of human chromosome 19q12 (Tournier-Lasserve et al. 1993; Chabriat et al. 1995); the gene was then isolated by positional cloning, and the mutation was identified and its functional role confirmed (Joutel et al. 1996, 1997).

Two deadly forms of inherited intracerebral hemorrhage have been described in the Dutch and Icelandic populations (Hademenos et al. 2001). Hereditary cerebral hemorrhage with amyloidosis, Dutch type (HCHWA-D) is due to a mutation in the amyloid β A4 precursor protein gene (*APP*) (Levy et al. 1990). The Icelandic form of this condition (HCHWA-I) is due to mutations in the gene coding for cystatin 3 (*CST3*), a serine protease inhibitor (Jensson et al. 1987; Palsdottir et al. 1988). These disorders are characterized by the development of cerebral hemorrhage at an age of 40–50 years for HCHWA-D and 20–30 years for HCHWA-I. Both are associated with amyloid deposition in cortical and leptomeningeal arterioles (Hademenos et al. 2001). Mutations of the integral membrane protein 2B gene (*ITM2B*) have also been shown to result in autosomal dominant amyloid angiopathies, which lead to cerebral hemorrhage, vascular dementia, or both (Vidal et al. 1999). The krev interaction trapped 1 gene (*KRIT1*) has also been identified as one of the genes responsible for cavernous angiomas (Laberge-le Couteulx et al. 1999).

Another Mendelian condition associated with stroke is mitochondrial myopathy, encephalopathy, lactic acidosis, and strokelike episodes (MELAS), a genetically heterogeneous mitochondrial disorder with a variable clinical phenotype. It is accompanied by features of central nervous system involvement, including seizures, hemiparesis, hemianopsia, cortical blindness, and episodic vomiting (Pavlakis et al. 1984; Montagna et al. 1988). This syndrome has been attributed to single nucleotide mutations in mitochondrial DNA. The mutations are usually, but not exclusively, missense and lie within the $tRNA^{Leu(UUR)}$ gene, with an A→G transition at position 3243 (Enter et al. 1991) and a T→C transition at position 3271 (Sakuta et al. 1993) being most frequently reported. Individuals who have inherited one (Ciafaloni et al. 1992; Macmillan et al. 1993) or both (Pulkes et al. 2000) of these mutations have a greater predisposition to stroke (Carr et al. 2002).

> **Box 24–1 Key Point**
>
> - Several genes responsible for Mendelian forms of stroke have been identified. One of the best characterized examples is the role of mutations of the notch, drosophila, homolog of, 3 gene (*NOTCH3*) in cerebral arteriopathy, autosomal dominant, with subcortical infarcts and leukoencephalopathy (CADASIL), a condition that leads to lacunar infarcts and vascular dementia (Chapter 3).

Ischemic stroke is occasionally attributable to an underlying connective tissue disorder that results in arterial dissection (Carr et al. 2002). In Marfan syndrome, extension of aortic dissection into the common carotid artery can occur and result in stroke (Spittell et al. 1993). Defects in collagen synthesis in Ehlers-Danlos syndrome type IV can predispose affected individuals to spontaneous dissection of the extracranial carotid and vertebral arteries (Schievink et al. 1990). Fabry disease is an X-linked disorder caused by a deficiency of α-galactosidase A and is associated with a high risk of both stroke and coronary heart disease (Crutchfield et al. 1998).

Identification of the genes responsible for Mendelian forms of stroke by reverse genetics has provided new insights into the pathophysiology of stroke (Tournier-Lasserve 2002). These observations constitute the basis for clinically useful molecular diagnostic tests. Despite their low prevalence, monogenic conditions should always be considered in young patients who present with stroke or in patients of any age with no evidence of vascular risk factors, especially when there is a family history. Indeed, the risk of stroke both in individuals known to have the mutated gene and in their relatives is high. For example, in the case of an autosomal dominant disorder with complete penetrance, all persons who carry the mutated gene will have a stroke, as will half of their first-degree relatives (Tournier-Lasserve 2002).

Genetic Epidemiology of Common Forms of Stroke

The etiology of common forms of stroke is multifactorial and includes both genetic and environmental factors. Studies with families have estimated that the relative risk of stroke in a first-degree relative of an individual who has a stroke is between 1.5 and 2.5. Such a risk is low at the individual level and does not have practical clinical implications. However, this slight increase in the risk of stroke is important at the population level, because of the high incidence of stroke (Tournier-Lasserve 2002). Identification of genetic variants that contribute to the increased risk of stroke is therefore clinically important.

Common stroke is extremely heterogeneous and most likely results in part from the additive or multiplicative effects of a wide spectrum of pathogenic alleles, each of which confers a small degree of risk. Some of these alleles may predispose individuals to specific types or subtypes of stroke by affecting certain intermediate factors that either lead to stroke, such as the intimal-medial thickness of the carotid artery, or have a direct independent effect on the risk of stroke. In addition, gene variants may also modulate the severity of stroke (Tournier-Lasserve 2002).

In spite of the large number of studies that have identified genes or polymorphisms associated with stroke, only a small number of the findings of these studies have been confirmed by independent replication or in other ethnic groups. One reason for this inconsistency is that many studies have combined ischemic and hemorrhagic stroke and it is unlikely that these different pathological conditions are under the same genetic influences (Floßmann et al. 2004). Another reason is that, although ischemic stroke is a highly complex trait, few studies have assessed subtypes of ischemic stroke or have had sufficient statistical power to do so (Floßmann et al. 2004). Many studies have thus analyzed atherosclerotic cerebral infarction and cardiogenic cerebral embolism collectively as ischemic stroke; the former results from the development of atherosclerotic stenosis in carotid or vertebral arteries, whereas the latter is attributable to the obstruction of cerebral arteries by thrombi that are generated in the cardiac atrium or ventricle as a result of arrhythmia such as atrial fibrillation or of valvular or ischemic heart disease. However, it can be argued that atherosclerosis is also responsible for most cardiogenic embolic strokes, given that many such events are the consequence of thrombus formation on the damaged endocardial surface in acute myocardial infarction or within a ventricular aneurysm caused by damage to cardiac muscle secondary to previous myocardial infarction (Gulcher et al. 2005). Most cardiogenic strokes used to be caused by atrial fibrillation secondary to mitral stenosis associated with rheumatic heart disease, but the incidence of childhood rheumatic fever has decreased markedly in the era of penicillin (Wilhelmsen et al. 2001a, 2001b). Most cases of atrial fibrillation are now caused by cardiac damage secondary to coronary heart disease. A substantial proportion of cardiogenic embolic strokes is therefore related to atherosclerosis of coronary arteries (Gulcher et al. 2005). The etiology of intracardiac thrombi is diverse, however, including lone atrial fibrillation and other arrhythmias, valvular heart disease, cardiomyopathies, as well as coronary heart disease. Atherothrombotic cerebral infarction and cardiogenic embolic stroke are thus different disorders. Given that the effects of gene polymorphisms or haplotypes on the development of common forms of stroke are likely to be small, it is necessary to examine these disorders separately in order to identify associated genetic variants.

Molecular Genetics of Ischemic Stroke

Stroke can be divided into two major varieties, ischemic and hemorrhagic stroke, with most (~80%) cases being ischemic (Humphries and Morgan 2004). Ischemic stroke is characterized by a sudden decrease in blood flow to one or more central nervous system territories (Gulcher et al. 2005) and is a heterogeneous disease caused by different pathogenic mechanisms that include both environmental and genetic factors (Box 24–2).

Box 24–2 Key Points

- Ischemic stroke, which accounts for approximately 80% of all stroke cases, is a complex and heterogeneous disorder.
- Principal subtypes of ischemic stroke include large-vessel occlusive disease, small-vessel occlusive disease, and cardiogenic embolic stroke.
- The pathological basis for most cases of ischemic stroke is atherosclerosis, with plaque rupture and subsequent overriding thrombosis being the final precipitating event in many instances.
- Several important studies have identified candidate genes, including *PDE4D*, *ALOX5AP*, and *IL6*, which confer susceptibility to ischemic stroke (Chapter 4).

Studies with twins, siblings, and families have provided substantial evidence for stroke heritability (Bak et al. 2002). A mechanistic approach to the study of ischemic stroke, as advocated in the Trial of ORG 10172 in Acute Stroke Treatment (TOAST) study (Adams et al. 1993), is the best suited to genetic research (Morgan and Humphries 2005). This approach classifies ischemic stroke into five subtypes: (1) large-artery atherosclerosis; (2) small-vessel occlusion; (3) cardiogenic embolism; (4) stroke of other determined etiology; and (5) stroke of undetermined etiology. It was applied in a family history study of 1,000 individuals with ischemic stroke and 800 controls (Jerrard-Dunne et al. 2003). This study found that a family history of vascular disease was a risk factor for both small-vessel occlusion and large-vessel atherosclerosis, but not for cardiogenic embolic stroke or stroke of undetermined etiology. These findings suggest that genetic research may be most fruitful when focused on the former two subtypes of ischemic stroke (Morgan and Humphries 2005).

Accurate phenotyping and performance of separate analyses according to stroke subtypes are thus essential. Focusing on particular stroke subtypes will likely make a study more efficient and markedly reduce the necessary sample sizes (Jerrard-Dunne et al. 2003). Another way of increasing the statistical power of a study may be to focus on early onset cases, as is in any genetic predisposition. Family history studies, such as prospective twin studies (Brass et al. 1992), suggest that the genetic component of stroke is stronger in such individuals.

The main cause of ischemic stroke is atherothrombosis, with the principal and treatable risk factors including hypertension, hypercholesterolemia, and diabetes mellitus (Goldstein et al. 2001). In addition to these conventional risk factors, genetic variants are important in the pathogenesis of ischemic stroke (Hassan and Markus 2000, 2004). Prediction of the risk for ischemic stroke beyond the usual clinical risk factors on the basis of genetic variants would be useful for deciding how aggressively to target the risk factors currently amenable to treatment. Furthermore, it might prompt earlier carotid imaging of patients at risk in order to detect asymptomatic carotid stenosis (Humphries and Morgan 2004).

A whole-genome linkage analysis of families or sibling pairs showed that chromosomal region 5q12 was linked to ischemic stroke (Gretarsdottir et al. 2002). A large number of genetic epidemiological studies of unrelated individuals has identified many genes that are related to the prevalence of ischemic stroke (Table 24–1), including those for apolipoprotein E (Kessler et al. 1997), 5,10-methylenetetrahydrofolate reductase (Morita et al. 1998; Kohara et al. 2003), paraoxonase 1 (Voetsch et al. 2002), interleukin 6 (Pola et al. 2003; Flex et al. 2004; Yamada et al. 2006), vitamin K epoxide reductase complex, subunit 1 (Wang et al. 2006), nitric oxide synthase 3 (Elbaz et al. 2000b), and cyclooxygenase 2 (Cipollone et al. 2004).

The Icelandic deCODE group identified two genes associated with ischemic stroke, the phosphodiesterase 4D, cAMP-specific gene (*PDE4D*) (Gretarsdottir et al. 2003), and arachidonate 5-lipoxygenase-activating protein gene (*ALOX5AP*) (Helgadottir et al. 2004). These associations were with specific haplotypes of each gene, but no disease-specific mutations in either gene have been identified (Markus and Alberts 2006). The deCODE researchers grouped together all subtypes of ischemic stroke, including thrombotic, embolic, large vessel, and small vessel. Although the end result of all these strokes is the same, blood vessels tend to be affected in different ways. It will be of interest to see whether the

Table 24–1 Genes Shown to be Related to the Prevalence of Ischemic Stroke

Chromosomal Locus	Gene Name	Gene Symbol	Reference
1p36.3	5,10-Methylenetetrahydrofolate reductase	*MTHFR*	Morita et al. 1998
1p36.2	Natriuretic peptide precursor A	*NPPA*	Rubattu et al. 2004
1q21-q23	C-reactive protein, pentraxin-related	*CRP*	Morita et al. 2006
1q23-q25	Selectin P	*SELP*	Zee et al. 2004
1q25.2-q25.3	Prostaglandin-endoperoxide synthase 2	*PTGS2*	Cipollone et al. 2004
2q14	Interleukin 1-β	*IL1B*	Iacoviello et al. 2005
2q14.2	Interleukin 1 receptor antagonist	*IL1RN*	Worrall et al. 2007
3pter-p21	Chemokine, CX3C motif, receptor 1	*CX3CR1*	Lavergne et al. 2005
3p25	Peroxisome proliferator-activated receptor-γ	*PPARG*	Lee et al. 2006
4p16.3	Adducin 1	*ADD1*	Morrison et al. 2001
4q28	Fibrinogen, B β polypeptide	*FGB*	Kessler et al. 1997
4q28-q31	Fatty acid-binding protein 2	*FABP2*	Carlsson et al. 2000
5q12	Phosphodiesterase 4D, cAMP-specific	*PDE4D*	Gretarsdottir et al. 2003
5q23-q31	Integrin, α-2	*ITGA2*	Carlsson et al. 1999
5q31.1	Interleukin 4	*IL4*	Zee et al. 2004
5q32-q33.1	Glutathione peroxidase 3	*GPX3*	Voetsch et al. 2007
5q33-qter	Coagulation factor XII	*F12*	Santamaria et al. 2004
6p25-p24	Factor XIII, A1 subunit	*F13A1*	Elbaz et al. 2000a
6p21.3	Lymphotoxin-α	*LTA*	Szolnoki et al. 2005
6q25.1	Estrogen receptor 1	*ESR1*	Shearman et al. 2005
6q27	Apolipoprotein (a)	*LPA*	Sun et al. 2003
7p21	Interleukin 6	*IL6*	Pola et al. 2003; Yamada et al. 2006
7q21.3	Paraoxonase 1	*PON1*	Voetsch et al. 2002
7q21.3-q22	Plasminogen activator inhibitor 1	*PAI1*	Wiklund et al. 2005
7q36	Nitric oxide synthase 3	*NOS3*	Elbaz et al. 2000b
8p22	Lipoprotein lipase	*LPL*	Shimo-Nakanishi et al. 2001
8p21-p12	Epoxide hydrolase 2, cytosolic	*EPHX2*	Fornage et al. 2005
8p12	Plasminogen activator, tissue	*PLAT*	Saito et al. 2006
11p11	Coagulation factor II	*F2*	De Stefano et al. 1998
11q12	Angiotensin-receptor-like 1	*AGTRL1*	Hata et al. 2007
11q23	Apolipoprotein A-V	*APOA5*	Havasi et al. 2006
12p13	Guanine nucleotide-binding protein, β-3	*GNB3*	Morrison et al. 2001
12p13	Sodium channel, nonvoltage-gated 1, α subunit	*SCNN1A*	Hsieh et al. 2005
13q12	Arachidonate 5-lipoxygenase-activating protein	*ALOX5AP*	Helgadottir et al. 2004
14q11.2	Cathepsin G	*CTSG*	Herrmann et al. 2001
14q22	Prostaglandin E receptor 2, EP2 subtype	*PTGER2*	Hegener et al. 2006
14q22-q23	Protein kinase C, eta	*PRKCH*	Kubo et al. 2007
16p11.2	Vitamin K epoxide reductase complex, subunit 1	*VKORC1*	Wang et al. 2006
16q24	Cytochrome b(-245), α subunit	*CYBA*	Ito et al. 2000
17pter-p12	Glycoprotein Ib, platelet, α polypeptide	*GPIBA*	Baker et al. 2001
17q21.32	Integrin, β-3	*ITGB3*	Ridker et al. 1997
17q23	Angiotensin I-converting enzyme	*ACE*	Margaglione et al. 1996
19p13.3	Thromboxane A2 receptor, platelet	*TBXA2R*	Kaneko et al. 2006
19p13.3-p13.2	Intercellular adhesion molecule 1	*ICAM1*	Pola et al. 2003
19p13.2	Low-density lipoprotein receptor	*LDLR*	Frikke-Schmidt et al. 2004
19q13.1	Transforming growth factor, β-1	*TGFB1*	Kim and Lee 2006
19q13.2	Apolipoprotein E	*APOE*	Kessler et al. 1997

Box 24–3 Key Points

- The Icelandic deCODE group identified *PDE4D* as a gene associated with ischemic stroke.
- Both risk-raising and risk-lowering haplotypes of *PDE4D* were identified, but no disease-specific mutations of the gene have been detected.
- The association was demonstrated only for large-artery and cardiogenic embolic strokes, not with small-vessel disease stroke.
- Reduced intracellular levels of cAMP promote smooth muscle cell proliferation and migration, key events in atherosclerosis, making an association of PDE4D, which selectively degrades cAMP, with stroke etiology plausible.
- The regulation of intracellular cAMP concentration by PDE4D in vascular smooth muscle cells or endothelial cells, or even in macrophages, may be a key determinant of stroke risk (Chapter 4).

genes identified by the deCODE group are related to all of these diverse mechanisms (Alberts 2003).

In the following section, candidate genes of particular interest (*PDE4D*, *ALOX5AP*, and *IL6*) for common forms of ischemic stroke are reviewed (Box 24–3).

Candidate Genes for Ischemic Stroke

Phosphodiesterase 4D, cAMP-Specific Gene (*PDE4D*)

A genome-wide linkage study indicated that a gene on chromosome 5q might contribute to the risk of stroke (Gretarsdottir et al. 2002). A case-control study was performed to determine which linkage disequilibrium block within the linkage peak showed the strongest association with ischemic stroke. Markers in the alternative promoter region corresponding to one of the eight isoforms of PDE4D showed the strongest association (Gretarsdottir et al. 2003). The subtypes of ischemic stroke with the highest risk ratios were large-vessel occlusive disease and cardiogenic stroke; there was no association with small-vessel occlusive disease. The frequency of the most significant haplotype in each of these two patient subgroups was approximately 30%, and the relative risk was 1.98 for the two subgroups combined. A mutually exclusive haplotype that conferred protection and was present in 28% of control individuals and associated with a relative risk of 0.68 was also identified. *PDE4D* variants thus conferred substantial risk for two forms of ischemic stroke related to atherosclerosis (Gulcher et al. 2005). Neither the risk nor protective haplotypes were associated with underlying missense or nonsense mutations, but they did correlate with the expression of *PDE4D* (Gretarsdottir et al. 2003).

PDE4D degrades the second messenger cAMP (Fukumoto et al. 1999), which is a key signaling molecule in cell types that are important in the pathogenesis of atherosclerosis (Gulcher et al. 2005). A decrease in cAMP levels in vascular smooth muscle cells in vitro promoted the proliferation and migration of these cells, processes that are characteristic of atherosclerosis (Pan et al. 1994; Palmer et al. 1998; Fukumoto et al. 1999; Houslay and Adams 2003). Inhibitors of PDE4 were found to block smooth muscle proliferation induced in the rat carotid artery by balloon injury (Indolfi et al. 1997, 2000). *PDE4D* is also expressed in activated macrophages and may therefore play a role in inflammation within atherosclerotic plaques, possibly contributing to atherogenesis or plaque instability, or both (Lusis 2000; Libby 2002; Naghavi et al. 2003). Increased activity of one or more isoforms of PDE4D resulting from dysregulation of transcript splicing or translation may thus increase the risk for ischemic stroke, with the decreased risk conferred by the identified protective haplotype possibly being due to a reduced activity of PDE4D (Gulcher et al. 2005).

Studies that have attempted to replicate this association of *PDE4D* with stroke have yielded diverse results (Markus and Alberts 2006). In a U.K. population, no overall association was found with ischemic stroke, but possible associations were identified with cardiogenic embolic stroke and large-artery stroke (Bevan et al. 2005). A U.S. study reported an association of *PDE4D* with ischemic stroke, especially with large-artery stroke (Meschia et al. 2005). In contrast, no association was found in a German stroke cohort (Lohmussaar et al. 2005) or a Swedish stroke cohort of individuals aged <75 years (Nilsson-Ardnor et al. 2005). A linkage study with a second Swedish population confirmed linkage of ischemic stroke to 5q12 (Nilsson-Ardnor et al. 2005), but no linkage was detected in an American population (Meschia et al. 2005). No association of *PDE4D* was found with carotid intimal-medial thickness (Bevan et al. 2005), suggesting that the gene does not exert its effects by accelerating early atherosclerosis (Markus and Alberts 2006).

Arachidonate 5-Lipoxygenase-Activating Protein Gene (*ALOX5AP*)

A linkage and association study in Iceland demonstrated that the gene encoding arachidonate 5-lipoxygenase-activating protein (*ALOX5AP*) confers risk for both myocardial infarction and ischemic stroke (Helgadottir et al. 2004). The locus associated with myocardial infarction was initially mapped to chromosome 13q through a genome-wide linkage scan conducted on 296 families with this condition (Helgadottir et al. 2004). An independent linkage study of Icelandic stroke patients without myocardial infarction identified the same locus (Helgadottir et al. 2004). The haplotype defined by microsatellite markers that showed the strongest association with myocardial infarction covered a region containing *ALOX5AP* (Gulcher et al. 2005). A haplotype that spans *ALOX5AP* (HapA) and is defined by four SNPs was subsequently shown to be associated with myocardial infarction, with a relative risk of 1.8. The same haplotype was then found to confer risk for stroke in the Icelandic population with a relative risk of 1.7 (Gulcher et al. 2005). HapA is relatively common and is carried by 27% of Icelandic patients with stroke. Another haplotype within *ALOX5AP*, HapB, showed a significant association with myocardial infarction in British cohorts, with a relative risk of 2.0 (Helgadottir et al. 2004). The association of both haplotypes with stroke in Scottish individuals was subsequently demonstrated (Helgadottir et al. 2005).

ALOX5AP participates in the initial steps of leukotriene synthesis. Arachidonic acid is thus converted to leukotriene A4 by the action of 5-lipoxygenase and its activating protein, ALOX5AP. Inflammatory lipid mediators, including leukotrienes B4, C4, D4, and E4 (Dixon et al. 1990), are then produced from leukotriene A4 by the action of leukotriene A4 hydrolase and leukotriene C4 synthase. The amount of leukotriene B4 synthesized by ionomycin-stimulated neutrophils from individuals with myocardial infarction was greater than that produced by those from control individuals (Helgadottir et al. 2004), supporting the notion that increased activity of the leukotriene pathway plays a role in the pathogenesis of myocardial infarction (Gulcher et al. 2005). Moreover, the observed difference in the release of leukotriene B4 was largely accounted for by carriers of HapA, whose cells produced more leukotriene B4 than did those from noncarriers. Although leukotriene B4 production was not measured in cells from patients with stroke, a similar increase would be expected, given that the HapA variant of *ALOX5AP* shows similar associations with ischemic stroke and myocardial infarction. Elevated levels of leukotriene B4 might contribute to atherogenesis or plaque instability by promoting inflammation at atherosclerotic plaques (Gulcher et al. 2005).

A role for upregulation of the leukotriene pathway in atherosclerosis is further supported by the observation that expression of enzymes of the 5-lipoxygenase pathway is increased in human atheromas, with the number of 5-lipoxygenase-positive cells (macrophages, dendritic cells, mast cells, and neutrophils) being markedly increased in advanced lesions (Spanbroek et al. 2003). Furthermore, the arachidonate 5-lipoxygenase gene (*ALOX5*) has been implicated in the development of atherosclerosis in mice by the finding that the loss of only one *ALOX5* allele confers protection against atherosclerosis in animals deficient in the low-density lipoprotein (LDL) receptor (Mehrabian et al. 2002). An increased activity of the leukotriene biosynthetic pathway associated with specific *ALOX5AP* variants might thus promote the processes of atherogenesis and subsequent plaque instability, increasing the chance of ischemic stroke on the background of atherosclerosis (Box 24–4) (Gulcher et al. 2005).

Several groups have attempted to replicate the association of ischemic stroke with *ALOX5AP* (Markus and Alberts 2006). Whereas the deCODE group replicated the association in a Scottish stroke population (Helgadottir et al. 2005), a case-control study in Germany reported a weak association with an *ALOX5AP* polymorphism (Lohmussaar et al. 2005), and no association in a case-control study and no linkage to this chromosomal region in a sibling-pair study were found in American populations (Bevan et al. 2005). Several explanations are possible for such disparate results (Markus and Alberts 2006). There might be substantial genetic heterogeneity for ischemic stroke, leading to different results in different study populations. Other population-specific genetic differences also might account for divergent results among patients in different countries. Lastly, random chance might produce spurious positive associations in some populations and studies, but not in others.

Interleukin 6 Gene (*IL6*)

Interleukin 6 plays a key role in promotion of the acute inflammatory response and in regulation of the production of acute phase proteins such as C-reactive protein (Heinrich et al. 1990). It contributes to the inflammatory response by activating endothelial cells (Romano et al. 1997) and stimulating the synthesis of fibrinogen (Dalmon et al. 1993). This cytokine is thus likely important in the pathogenesis of vascular inflammation. A –174G→C polymorphism of *IL6* was shown to be associated both with intimal-medial thickness of the carotid artery (Rauramaa et al. 2000; Rundek et al. 2002), an important predictor of new myocardial infarction and stroke (O'Leary et al. 1999), and with coronary heart disease (Humphries et al. 2001). This polymorphism was also found to be associated with a history of ischemic stroke (Pola et al. 2003; Flex et al. 2004) and with the severity of ischemic stroke in young patients (Greisenegger et al. 2003), with the *G* allele being a risk factor for this condition. However, this polymorphism has not been detected in the Japanese population (Yamada, unpublished data). The –572G→C polymorphism of *IL6* was also shown to be significantly associated with the prevalence of atherothrombotic cerebral infarction, with the *C* allele representing a risk factor for this condition (Yamada et al. 2006).

Cerebral ischemia induces the expression of IL6 in neurons and astrocytes (Maeda et al. 1994; Suzuki et al. 1999). The serum concentration of IL6 also increases within several days after ischemic stroke. Indeed, the ischemic brain appears to be a major source of IL6, given that the serum concentration of this cytokine correlates with infarct size and that its concentration in cerebrospinal fluid is greater than that in serum (Tarkowski et al. 1995). These various observations suggest that variants of *IL6* play an important role in the development and outcome of ischemic stroke.

Molecular Genetics of Intracerebral Hemorrhage

Intracerebral hemorrhage is responsible for approximately 10% of all strokes, including a large proportion of fatal or severe cases. Advancing age and hypertension are the most important risk factors for intracerebral hemorrhage. Familial aggregation of cases of intracerebral hemorrhage was demonstrated in a prospective study in North Carolina in the United States, which found that 10% of affected individuals had a family history of intracerebral hemorrhage (Alberts et al. 2002). No significant clinical demographic differences separated affected individuals with or without a family history of intracerebral hemorrhage. Genetic factors may influence not only the development of intracerebral hemorrhage but also the prevalence of certain risk factors for this condition, such as hypertension. Furthermore, such genetic factors may interact with environmental factors such as diet and cigarette smoking. The etiology of intracerebral hemorrhage is complex and the genetic determinants of this condition are still largely unknown (Box 24–5).

Box 24–4 Key Points

- The Icelandic deCODE group identified *ALOX5AP* as a susceptibility gene for ischemic stroke (Chapter 4).
  - This association was made with specific haplotypes of the gene, but no disease-specific mutations in *ALOX5AP* have been identified.
  - ALOX5AP is required for the conversion of arachidonic acid to leukotriene A4 by 5-lipoxygenase.
  - Leukotriene A4 is converted to leukotriene B4, which plays an important role in leukocyte chemotaxis and inflammatory responses, key processes in atherosclerosis.

Box 24–5 Key Points

- The occurrence of intracerebral hemorrhage in a first-degree relative is a risk factor for this condition.
- Intracerebral hemorrhage is usually attributed to hypertensive small-vessel disease, with the most common sites of hemorrhage being the basal ganglia, cerebellum, and pons.
- In some patients, the hemorrhage is lobar in location, and such patients often do not have hypertension. This category of hemorrhage is referred to as lobar intracerebral hemorrhage.
- The ε2 and ε4 alleles of *APOE* have been identified as risk factors for lobar intracerebral hemorrhage, likely due to their association with cerebral amyloid angiopathy (Chapter 4).

Table 24–2 Genes Shown to be Associated with Intracerebral Hemorrhage

Chromosomal Locus	Gene Name	Gene Symbol	Reference
6p25-p24	Factor XIII, A1 subunit	*F13A1*	Reiner et al. 2001
6q27	Apolipoprotein (a)	*LPA*	Sun et al. 2003
7p21	Interleukin 6	*IL6*	Yamada et al. 2006
9q34.1	Endoglin	*ENG*	Alberts et al. 1997
13q34	Collagen, type IV, α-1	*COL4A1*	Gould et al. 2006
14q32.1	α-1-antichymotrypsin	*AACT*	Vila et al. 2000
16p11.2	Vitamin K epoxide reductase complex, subunit 1	*VKORC1*	Wang et al. 2006
17q23	Angiotensin I-converting enzyme	*ACE*	Slowik et al. 2004b
17q23-qter	Apolipoprotein H	*APOH*	Xia et al. 2004
19q13.2	Apolipoprotein E	*APOE*	O'Donnell et al. 2000

Intracerebral hemorrhage is usually attributed to hypertensive small-vessel disease, with the most common sites of hemorrhage being the basal ganglia, cerebellum, and pons. In some individuals with intracerebral hemorrhage, however, the hemorrhage is lobar in location, such as in the frontal, parietal, temporal, or occipital cortex, and such patients often do not have hypertension (Massaro et al. 1991). This category of hemorrhage, referred to as lobar intracerebral hemorrhage, may represent a distinct pathogenetic subgroup (Sacco 2000). The occurrence of lobar intracerebral hemorrhage was shown to be associated with the ε2 and ε4 alleles of the apolipoprotein E gene (*APOE*) (O'Donnell et al. 2000; Woo et al. 2005). These associations, in particular with ε4, are presumably due to the association of *APOE* with cerebral amyloid angiopathy (Greenberg et al. 1996).

Various association studies of unrelated individuals have identified genes that are related to intracerebral hemorrhage (Table24–2), but the role of genetic predisposition to this condition has not been determined definitively. In the following sections, candidate genes for intracerebral hemorrhage that are of particular interest (*APOE*, *COL4A1*, and *IL6*) are reviewed.

Candidate Genes for Intracerebral Hemorrhage

Apolipoprotein E Gene (*APOE*)

Cerebral amyloid angiopathy is a frequent cause of lobar intracerebral hemorrhage (Sacco 2000). The main pathological feature of this condition is the infiltration of cortical vessels by β-amyloid, a homogeneous eosinophilic substance found in the brain of elderly individuals and an important component of the senile plaques in patients with Alzheimer's disease. The incidence of lobar intracerebral hemorrhage due to cerebral amyloid angiopathy increases markedly with age, with most affected individuals being over the age of 60 years and many having antecedent memory loss. Patients with cerebral amyloid angiopathy and intracerebral hemorrhage have a lower mortality rate and a greater risk of recurrence than do those with other types of intracerebral hemorrhage (Sacco 2000).

The ε4 and ε2 alleles of *APOE* were identified as predictors of recurrent lobar intracerebral hemorrhage in patients with cerebral amyloid angiopathy (O'Donnell et al. 2000). The risk of recurrence at 2 years was 28% for carriers of the ε2 or ε4 alleles, compared with 10% for patients with the ε3 allele. The presence of the ε2 or ε4 alleles is thus considered a potent risk factor for recurrence (Sacco 2000).

Other studies have shown that the frequency of the ε4 allele of *APOE* is increased in patients with cerebral amyloid angiopathy, whereas the ε2 allele may be associated with an increased risk of intracerebral hemorrhage in individuals with this condition (Greenberg et al. 1995, 1998; Nicoll et al. 1997; O'Donnell et al. 2000). These observations may be partially explained by the association of the ε4 allele with Alzheimer's disease, which is present in up to 50% of patients with cerebral amyloid angiopathy. In addition, the age of onset of intracerebral hemorrhage in individuals with cerebral amyloid angiopathy was found to be earlier in carriers of the ε4 allele of *APOE* than in carriers of other alleles of this gene (Greenberg et al. 1996).

Collagen, Type IV, α-1 Gene (*COL4A1*)

Mutations in *COL4A1* have been detected in families with cerebral small-vessel disease (Gould et al. 2005, 2006). *COL4A1* was initially identified as the causative gene in a mouse mutant with perinatal cerebral hemorrhage and porencephaly (Gould et al. 2005). Mice heterozygous for the responsible mutation develop recurrent hemorrhage in the basal ganglia, a typical site of intracerebral hemorrhage in hypertensive patients. Subsequent analysis of families with porencephaly and cerebral small-vessel disease revealed several mutations of human *COL4A1* in affected individuals (Gould et al. 2005, 2006; van der Knaap et al. 2006).

Type IV collagens are an integral component of the vascular basement membrane. COL4A1 and COL4A2, the most abundant type IV collagens, form heterotrimers. Repeated Gly-Pro-X motifs of these collagen molecules are required for formation of a triple helix during collagen assembly, and most mutations identified in *COL4A1* affect Gly residues within these motifs. It was therefore hypothesized that *COL4A1* mutations interfere with triple-helix formation or heterotrimer secretion. Indeed, analysis of heterozygous embryonic tissue has suggested that the mutations inhibit collagen secretion into the basement membrane. Ultrastructural abnormalities in capillaries of carriers of *COL4A1* mutations are indicative of disordered assembly of the basement membrane (Dichgans and Hegele 2007).

The phenotypic spectrum associated with *COL4A1* mutations is broad and strongly related to small-vessel disease. Key features include leukoencephalopathy, microhemorrhages, and clinically overt hemorrhage. The structural compromise of small blood vessels is reflected by the observations that birth trauma, brain trauma, or oral anticoagulants may trigger intracerebral hemorrhage in carriers of *COL4A1* mutations (Gould et al. 2005, 2006). Genes that encode proteins associated with the vascular basement membrane are thus potential candidates for causative agents of intracerebral hemorrhage and leukoencephalopathy (Dichgans and Hegele 2007).

Interleukin 6 Gene (*IL6*)

The −174G→C polymorphism of *IL6* has been associated with intracerebral hemorrhage at brain arteriovenous malformations (Pawlikowska et al. 2004). Furthermore, a high plasma level of IL6 was shown to be an independent predictor of early hematoma growth associated with intracerebral hemorrhage (Silva et al. 2005). These observations suggest that IL6 plays a role in the onset and progression of intracerebral hemorrhage. The −572G→C polymorphism of *IL6* was significantly associated with the prevalence of intracerebral hemorrhage as well as atherothrombotic cerebral infarction, with the *C* allele representing a risk factor for these conditions (Yamada et al. 2006).

The association of polymorphisms of *IL6* with intracerebral hemorrhage implicates inflammatory processes in the pathophysiology of this condition. Cytokines induce the production of matrix metalloproteinases, which degrade the extracellular matrix around blood vessels and may damage the vascular wall (Rosenberg 2002). Local release of IL6 by endothelial cells may therefore contribute to vascular wall instability by stimulating the release and activation of matrix metalloproteinases (Dasu et al. 2003). The association of polymorphisms of *IL6* with intracerebral hemorrhage might thus be attributable to matrix metalloproteinase-mediated weakening of vessel walls already compromised by hemodynamic stress.

Molecular Genetics of Subarachnoid Hemorrhage

Subarachnoid hemorrhage is most commonly caused by rupture of an aneurysm on an intracranial artery (Ruigrok et al. 2005a). About 2% of the general population has an intracranial aneurysm (Rinkel et al. 1998). Rupture of an aneurysm is most common between 40 and 60 years of age and prognosis after rupture is poor, with half of affected individuals dying within 1 month and 20% remaining dependent on support for activities of daily life (Longstreth et al. 1993; Inagawa et al. 1995; Hop et al. 1997). The incidence of aneurysmal subarachnoid hemorrhage in the general population is low (about 8 per 100,000 person-years) (Linn et al. 1996), but the young age at onset and the poor prognosis mean that the loss of productive life-years is similar to that associated with ischemic stroke (Johnston et al. 1998) (Box 24–6).

Subarachnoid hemorrhage is 1.6 times more common in women than in men (Rinkel et al. 1998). Hormonal factors probably explain this sex-specific risk, given that it is higher in postmenopausal women than in premenopausal women (Longstreth et al. 1994). Smoking, alcohol consumption, and hypertension are also common risk factors for aneurysmal subarachnoid hemorrhage (Teunissen et al. 1996; Ruigrok et al. 2001). In addition to these environmental risk factors, genetic factors play an important role in the pathogenesis of subarachnoid hemorrhage associated with intracranial aneurysms. First-degree relatives of affected individuals are thus at up to seven times greater risk than is the general population (Bromberg et al. 1995; Schievink et al. 1995; Braekeleer et al. 1996; Ronkainen et al. 1997; Gaist et al. 2000), and approximately 10% of patients with aneurysmal subarachnoid hemorrhage have first- or second-degree relatives with subarachnoid hemorrhage or unruptured intracranial aneurysms (Norrgard et al. 1987; Ronkainen et al. 1993; Bromberg et al. 1995; Schievink et al. 1995; Wang et al. 1995; Braekeleer et al. 1996).

> **Box 24–6 Key Points**
>
> - Intracranial aneurysm, which accounts for the vast majority of cases of subarachnoid hemorrhage, has a multifactorial etiology, with cigarette smoking, female sex, hypertension, and alcohol consumption being major risk factors.
> - Genetic factors likely contribute to the development of intracranial aneurysm because familial predisposition is the strongest risk factor for aneurysmal subarachnoid hemorrhage.
> - Familial clustering is apparent in approximately 10% of patients with subarachnoid hemorrhage, and first-degree relatives of affected individuals have a three- to sevenfold greater risk of developing subarachnoid hemorrhage than does the general population.
> - Intracranial aneurysm is associated with certain heritable disorders, including polycystic kidney disease and Ehlers-Danlos syndrome (Chpater 28).

Several additional lines of evidence further support a role for genetic factors in the etiology of intracranial aneurysm. First, several genetic diseases, such as adult polycystic kidney disease (Chapman et al. 1992), Marfan syndrome (ter Berg et al. 1986), glucocorticoid-remediable aldosteronism (Litchfield et al. 1998), and Ehlers-Danlos syndrome type IV (de Paepe et al. 1988), increase the risk of the formation of intracranial aneurysm. Second, familial recurrence of nonsyndromic intracranial aneurysm has been described (Fox and Ko 1980; Morooka and Waga 1983; Maroun et al. 1986; Elshunnar and Whittle 1990). Indeed, there is a three- to fivefold increase in the risk for this condition in first-degree relatives of affected individuals compared with the general population (Stehbens 1998; Ronkainen et al. 1999). Recent genetic linkage analyses have mapped loci for intracranial aneurysm to chromosomal regions 1p34.3-p36.13 (Nahed et al. 2005), 2p13 (Roos et al. 2004), 5q22-q31 (Onda et al. 2001), 7q11 (Onda et al. 2001), 11q24-q25 (Ozturk et al. 2006), 14q22 (Onda et al. 2001), 14q23-q31 (Ozturk et al. 2006), 17cen (Yamada et al. 2004), 19q13 (Yamada et al. 2004), 19q13.3 (Van der Voet et al. 2004), and Xp22 (Yamada et al. 2004).

The pathogenesis of subarachnoid hemorrhage from a ruptured aneurysm is poorly understood. Hemodynamic factors and structural properties of the arterial wall may contribute to the development of intracranial aneurysms, but the trigger factors remain unknown. Disruption of the extracellular matrix is likely to be a factor in the pathophysiology given that intracranial aneurysms are associated with heritable disorders of connective tissue and the extracellular matrix (Chapman et al. 1992; Schievink et al. 1994; Ruigrok et al. 2005a). Moreover, the amount of structural proteins of the extracellular matrix has been found to be reduced in the intracranial arterial wall of many ruptured intracranial aneurysms as well as in skin biopsies and intracranial and extracranial arteries of patients with aneurysms (Neil-Dwyer et al. 1983; Hegedus 1984; Ostergaard and Oxlund 1987; Ostergaard et al. 1987; Chyatte et al. 1990; Skirgaudas et al. 1996; van den Berg et al. 1997).

Magnetic resonance angiography is not sufficiently effective for screening the first-degree relatives of individuals with sporadic subarachnoid hemorrhage for intracranial aneurysms (The Magnetic Resonance Angiography in Relatives of Patients with Subarachnoid Hemorrhage Study Group 1999), and repeated screening is necessary to identify newly developed aneurysms in familial subarachnoid hemorrhage (Raaymakers et al. 1998). Given that a familial predisposition is the strongest risk factor for the development of intracranial aneurysms (Rinkel et al. 1998; Ruigrok et al. 2001), the identification of genetic risk factors might provide further diagnostic capability. In the future, genotype assessment might thus help to identify first-degree relatives of individuals with subarachnoid hemorrhage who are at high risk of developing one or more intracranial aneurysms (Ruigrok et al. 2005a). Furthermore, identification of these genetic factors should provide insight into the pathophysiology of intracranial aneurysms (Ruigrok et al. 2005a). The identification of disease susceptibility genes and increased understanding of the disease pathophysiology may lead to new therapeutic interventions to prevent the development, growth, or rupture of intracranial aneurysms (Ruigrok et al. 2005a).

Various association studies of unrelated individuals have identified genes that are related to subarachnoid hemorrhage or intracranial aneurysm (Table 24–3). However, the genes that confer susceptibility to these conditions have not been determined definitively. Candidate genes for subarachnoid hemorrhage or intracranial aneurysm that are of particular interest (*ELN*, *LIMK1*, *TNFRSF13B*, and *TNF*) are reviewed in the following section.

Candidate Genes for Subarachnoid Hemorrhage and Intracranial Aneurysm

Elastin Gene (*ELN*) and LIM Domain Kinase 1 Gene (*LIMK1*)

A recent study showed that a functional haplotype spanning *ELN* and *LIMK1* confers susceptibility to intracranial aneurysm (Akagawa et al. 2006). *ELN* is located within the chromosome 7q11 linkage region and was recognized earlier to be a positional and functional candidate gene for intracranial aneurysm (Onda et al. 2001). However, allelic association studies yielded variable results (Hofer et al. 2003; Ruigrok et al. 2004). A systematic analysis of 166 SNPs and haplotypes that reside within the chromosome 7q linkage peak identified a highly significant association between intracranial aneurysm and a distinct linkage disequilibrium block containing the 3' untranslated region of *ELN* and the promoter region of *LIMK1* (Akagawa et al. 2006). The strongest association was found with the *ELN* +695G→C tag SNP for a risk haplotype composed of the functional *ELN* + 502A insertion and the *LIMK1* –187C→T SNP. Both the genotype and haplotype associations were replicated in an independent cohort. Functional studies revealed that the *ELN* +502A insertion reduces the rate of *ELN* transcription, whereas the *LIMK1* –187C→T SNP reduces promoter activity (Dichgans and Hegele 2007). Synergism between genetic variants of *ELN* and *LIMK1* in their effects on vascular stability and distensibility seems plausible because (1) elastin is a major structural component of the internal elastic lamina in cerebral arteries; (2) *ELN* plays a key role in vascular development and remodeling; (3) secreted elastin

Table 24–3 Genes Associated with Subarachnoid Hemorrhage

Chromosomal Locus	Gene Name	Gene Symbol	Reference
1p36.1	Heparan sulfate proteoglycan of basement membrane	*HSPG2*	Ruigrok et al. 2006a
1p34.2	Polycystic kidney disease 1-like	*PKD1-like*	Yamada et al. 2006
5q12-q14	Chondroitin sulfate proteoglycan 2	*CSPG2*	Ruigrok et al. 2006b
5q23-q31	Fibrillin 2	*FBN2*	Ruigrok et al. 2006a
6p21.3	Tumor necrosis factor	*TNF*	Yamada et al. 2006
7p21	Interleukin 6	*IL6*	Morgan et al. 2006
7q11.2	Elastin	*ELN*	Akagawa et al. 2006
7q11.23	Lim domain kinase 1	*LIMK1*	Akagawa et al. 2006
7q21.3-q22	Plasminogen activator inhibitor 1	*PAI1*	Ruigrok et al. 2006a
7q22.1	Collagen, type I, α-2	*COL1A2*	Yoneyama et al. 2004
7q36	Nitric oxide synthase 3	*NOS3*	Khurana et al. 2004
9q34.1	Endoglin	*ENG*	Takenaka et al. 1999
11q13	Uncoupling protein 3	*UCP3*	Yamada et al. 2006
13q34	Collagen, type IV, α-1	*COL4A1*	Ruigrok et al. 2006a
14q32.1	α-1-antichymotrypsin	*AACT*	Slowik et al. 2005
16p13.3-p13.12	Polycystic kidney disease 1	*PKD1*	Watnick et al. 1999
17p11.2	Tumor necrosis factor receptor superfamily, member 13B	*TNFRSF13B*	Inoue et al. 2006
17q21.32	Integrin, β-3	*ITGB3*	Iniesta et al. 2004
17q23	Angiotensin I-converting enzyme	*ACE*	Slowik et al. 2004a
20q11.2-q13.1	Matrix metalloproteinase 9	*MMP9*	Peters et al. 1999
22q12	Heme oxygenase 1	*HMOX1*	Morgan et al. 2005

activates a G protein-coupled signaling pathway that stimulates organization of actin stress fibers; and (4) LIMK1 is a regulator of the actin cytoskeleton (Dichgans and Hegele 2007).

Tumor Necrosis Factor Receptor Superfamily, Member 13b (TNFRSF13B)

Sequence variation in *TNFRSF13B* was shown to contribute to risk for intracranial aneurysm (Inoue et al. 2006). Sequence analysis of genes in a linkage peak on chromosome 17p revealed several potentially deleterious changes in *TNFRSF13B* that segregated with intracranial aneurysm in pedigrees. Sequencing of a portion of *TNFRSF13B* in a large case-control sample showed that several potentially functional rare variants were more frequent in cases than in controls. Finally, association analyses suggested that one of the *TNFRSF13B* haplotypes was protective. Interactions of genetic factors such as *TNFRSF13B* with known risk factors for aneurysm formation, such as smoking and hypertension, remain an important area of research (Dichgans and Hegele 2007).

Tumor Necrosis Factor Gene (TNF)

The amounts of TNF mRNA and protein as well as that of a proapoptotic downstream target, Fas-associated death domain protein, were found to be increased in human intracranial aneurysms (Jayaraman et al. 2005). TNF and Fas-associated death domain protein may adversely affect cerebral arteries by promoting inflammation and subsequent apoptosis in vascular and immune cells, thereby weakening the vessel wall (Jayaraman et al. 2005). TNF induces apoptosis in cultured cerebral endothelial cells by activating the protease caspase 3 (Kimura et al. 2003). Furthermore, the concentration of TNF in the hemorrhagic cerebrospinal fluid of individuals who had experienced subarachnoid hemorrhage was greater for those with an unfavorable outcome than for those with a good outcome (Mathiesen et al. 1997). The −863C→A polymorphism of *TNF* was shown to be significantly associated with the prevalence of subarachnoid hemorrhage, with the *A* allele representing a risk factor for this condition (Yamada et al. 2006). In addition, individuals with the *A* allele of this polymorphism of *TNF* have a higher risk of a poor outcome after subarachnoid hemorrhage (Ruigrok et al. 2005b). The −308G→A polymorphism of *TNF* has also been associated with aneurysmal subarachnoid hemorrhage (Fontanella et al. 2007). These observations suggest that *TNF* may play important roles in the development of intracranial aneurysm and outcome after subarachnoid hemorrhage.

Conclusions

There has been a growing effort to find genetic variants that confer risk for common forms of stroke as a means to understand the underlying biological events. Such studies may ultimately lead to the personalized prevention of stroke (Yamada 2006). It may thus become possible to predict the future risk for each type of stroke in each individual on the basis of conventional laboratory analyses and genetic evaluation. It should also be possible to assess how the risk level of an individual will decrease if treatable risk factors, including hypertension, diabetes mellitus, hyperlipidemia, and smoking, are ameliorated or eliminated. Furthermore, it may be possible to prevent an individual from having a stroke by medical intervention based on his or her genotype for specific polymorphisms. For example, it would be beneficial to prescribe an antiplatelet drug if an individual at risk has a glycoprotein Ib, platelet, α polypeptide gene (*GP1BA*) variant that results in an increase in platelet function. Prescription of folic acid would also be effective if an individual at risk has a 5,10-methylenetetrahydrofolate reductase gene (*MTHFR*) polymorphism that results in an increase in the plasma homocysteine concentration and consequent acceleration of the development of atherosclerosis. Identification of disease susceptibility genes will thus contribute to the prevention, early diagnosis, and treatment of stroke.

References

Adams HP Jr, Bendixen BH, Kappelle LJ, et al. Classification of subtype of acute ischemic stroke. Definitions for use in a multicenter clinical trial. TOAST. Trial of Org 10172 in Acute Stroke Treatment. *Stroke.* 1993;24:35–41.

Akagawa H, Tajima A, Sakamoto Y, et al. A haplotype spanning two genes, ELN and LIMK1, decreases their transcripts and confers susceptibility to intracranial aneurysms. *Hum Mol Genet.* 2006;15:1722–1734.

Alberts MJ. Stroke genetics update. *Stroke.* 2003;34:342–344.

Alberts MJ, Davis JP, Graffagnino C, et al. Endoglin gene polymorphism as a risk factor for sporadic intracerebral hemorrhage. *Ann Neurol.* 1997;41:683–686.

Alberts MJ, McCarron MO, Hoffmann KL, Graffagnino C. Familial clustering of intracerebral hemorrhage: a prospective study in North Carolina. *Neuroepidemiology.* 2002;21:18–21.

Bak S, Gaist D, Sindrup SH, Skytthe A, Christensen K. Genetic liability in stroke: a long-term follow-up study of Danish twins. *Stroke.* 2002;33:769–774.

Baker RI, Eikelboom J, Lofthouse E, et al. Platelet glycoprotein Ibα Kozak polymorphism is associated with an increased risk of ischemic stroke. *Blood.* 2001;98:36–40.

Bevan S, Porteous L, Sitzer M, Markus HS. Phosphodiesterase 4D gene, ischemic stroke, and asymptomatic carotid atherosclerosis. *Stroke.* 2005;36:949–953.

Braekeleer DM, Pérussee L, Cantin L, Bouchard JM, Mathieu J. A study of inbreeding and kinship in intracranial aneurysms in the Saguenay Lac-Saint-Jean region (Quebec, Canada). *Ann Hum Genet.* 1996;60:99–104.

Brass LM, Isaacsohn JL, Merikangas KR, Robinette CD. A study of twins and stroke. *Stroke.* 1992;23:221–223.

Bromberg JE, Rinkel GJ, Algra A, et al. Subarachnoid haemorrhage in first and second degree relatives of patients with subarachnoid haemorrhage. *BMJ.* 1995;311:288–289.

Carlsson LE, Santoso S, Spitzer C, Kessler C, Greinacher A. The α_2 gene coding sequence T807/A873 of the platelet collagen receptor integrin $\alpha_2\beta_1$ might be a genetic risk factor for the development of stroke in younger patients. *Blood.* 1999;93:3583–3586.

Carlsson M, Orho-Melander M, Hedenbro J, Almgren P, Groop LC. The T 54 allele of the intestinal fatty acid-binding protein 2 is associated with a parental history of stroke. *J Clin Endocrinol Metab.* 2000;85:2801–2804.

Carr FJ, McBride MW, Carswell HV, et al. Genetic aspects of stroke: human and experimental studies. *J Cerebr Blood Flow Metab.* 2002;22:767–773.

Chabriat H, Vahedi K, Iba-Zizen MT, et al. Clinical spectrum of CADASIL: a study of 7 families. Cerebral autosomal dominant arteriopathy with subcortical infarcts and leukoencephalopathy. *Lancet.* 1995;346:934–939.

Chapman AB, Rubinstein D, Hughes, R, et al. Intracranial aneurysms in autosomal dominant polycystic kidney disease. *N Engl J Med.* 1992;327:916–920.

Chyatte D, Reilly J, Tilson MD. Morphometric analysis of reticular and elastin fibers in the cerebral arteries of patients with intracranial aneurysms, *Neurosurgery.* 1990;26:939–943.

Ciafaloni E, Ricci E, Shanske S, et al. MELAS: clinical features, biochemistry, and molecular genetics. *Ann Neurol.* 1992;31:391–398.

Cipollone F, Toniato E, Martinotti S, et al. A polymorphism in the cyclooxygenase 2 gene as an inherited protective factor against myocardial infarction and stroke. *JAMA.* 2004;291:2221–2228.

Crutchfield KE, Patronas NJ, Dambrosia JM, et al. Quantitative analysis of cerebral vasculopathy in patients with Fabry disease. *Neurology.* 1998;50:1746–1749.

Dalmon J, Laurent M, Courtois G. The human β fibrinogen promoter contains a hepatocyte nuclear factor 1-dependent interleukin-6-responsive element. *Mol Cell Biol.* 1993;13:1183–1193.

Dasu MR, Barrow RE, Spies M, Herndon DN. Matrix metalloproteinase expression in cytokine stimulated human dermal fibroblasts. *Burns.* 2003;29:527–531.

de Paepe A, van Landegem W, de Keyser F, de Reuck J. Association of multiple intracranial aneurysms and collagen type III deficiency. *Clin Neurol Neurosurg.* 1988;90:53–56.

De Stefano V, Chiusolo P, Paciaroni K, et al. Prothrombin G20210A mutant genotype is a risk factor for cerebrovascular ischemic disease in young patients. *Blood.* 1998;91:3562–3565.

Dichgans M, Hegele RA. Update on the genetics of stroke and cerebrovascular disease 2006. *Stroke.* 2007;38:216–218.

Dixon RA, Diehl RE, Opas E, et al. Requirement of a 5-lipoxygenase-activating protein for leukotriene synthesis. *Nature.* 1990;343:282–284.

Elbaz A, Poirier O, Canaple S, Chedru F, Cambien F, Amarenco P. The association between the Val34Leu polymorphism in the factor XIII gene and brain infarction. *Blood.* 2000a;95:586–591.

Elbaz A, Poirier O, Moulin T, Chedru F, Cambien F, Amarenco P. Association between the Glu298Asp polymorphism in the endothelial constitutive nitric oxide synthase gene and brain infarction. The GENIC Investigators. *Stroke.* 2000b;31:1634–1639.

Elshunnar KS, Whittle IR. Familial intracranial aneurysms: report of five families. *Br J Neurosurg.* 1990;4:181–186.

Enter C, Muller-Hocker J, Zierz S, et al. A specific point mutation in the mitochondrial genome of Caucasians with MELAS. *Hum Genet.* 1991;88:233–236.

Flex A, Gaetani E, Papaleo P, et al. Proinflammatory genetic profiles in subjects with history of ischemic stroke. *Stroke.* 2004;35:2270–2275.

Floßmann E, Schulz UGR, Rothwell PM. Systematic review of methods and results of studies of the genetic epidemiology of ischemic stroke. *Stroke.* 2004;35:212–227.

Fontanella M, Rainero I, Gallone S, et al. Tumor necrosis factor-α gene and cerebral aneurysms. *Neurosurgery.* 2007;60:668–672.

Fornage M, Lee CR, Doris PA, et al. The soluble epoxide hydrolase gene harbors sequence variation associated with susceptibility to and protection from incident ischemic stroke. *Hum Mol Genet.* 2005;14:2829–2837.

Fox JL, Ko JP. Familial intracranial aneurysms. Six cases among 13 siblings. *J Neurosurg.* 1980;52:501–503.

Frikke-Schmidt R, Nordestgaard BG, Schnohr P, Tybjaerg-Hansen A. Single nucleotide polymorphism in the low-density lipoprotein receptor is associated with a threefold risk of stroke. A case-control and prospective study. *Eur Heart J.* 2004;25:943–951.

Fukumoto S, Koyama H, Hosoi M, et al. Distinct role of cAMP and cGMP in the cell cycle control of vascular smooth muscle cells: cGMP delays cell cycle transition through suppression of cyclin D1 and cyclin-dependent kinase 4 activation. *Circ Res.* 1999;85:985–991.

Gaist D, Vaeth M, Tsiropulos I, et al. Risk of subarachnoid haemorrhage in first degree relatives of patients with subarachnoid haemorrhage: follow up study based on national registries in Denmark. *BMJ.* 2000;320:141–145.

Goldstein LB, Adams R, Becker K, et al. Primary prevention of ischemic stroke: a statement for healthcare professionals from the Stroke Council of the American Heart Association. *Stroke.* 2001;32:280–299.

Gould DB, Phalan FC, Breedveld GJ, et al. Mutations in Col4a1 cause perinatal cerebral hemorrhage and porencephaly. *Science.* 2005;308:1167–1171.

Gould DB, Phalan FC, van Mil SE, et al. Role of COL4A1 in small-vessel disease and hemorrhagic stroke. *N Engl J Med.* 2006;354:1489–1496.

Greenberg SM, Briggs ME, Hyman BT, et al. Apolipoprotein E epsilon 4 is associated with the presence and earlier onset of hemorrhage in cerebral amyloid angiopathy. *Stroke.* 1996;27:1333–1337.

Greenberg SM, Rebeck GW, Vonsattel JP, Gomez-Isla T, Hyman BT. Apolipoprotein E epsilon 4 and cerebral hemorrhage associated with amyloid angiopathy. *Ann Neurol.* 1995;38:254–259.

Greenberg SM, Vonsattel JP, Segal AZ, et al. Association of apolipoprotein E epsilon 2 and vasculopathy in cerebral amyloid angiopathy. *Neurology.* 1998;50:961–965.

Greisenegger S, Endler G, Haering D, et al. The (–174) G/C polymorphism in the interleukin-6 gene is associated with the severity of acute cerebrovascular events. *Thromb Res.* 2003;110:181–186.

Gretarsdottir S, Sveinbjornsdottir S, Jonsson HH, et al. Localization of a susceptibility gene for common forms of stroke to 5q12. *Am J Hum Genet.* 2002;70:593–603.

Gretarsdottir S, Thorleifsson G, Reynisdottir ST, et al. The gene encoding phosphodiesterase 4D confers risk of ischemic stroke. *Nat Genet.* 2003;35:131–138.

Gulcher JR, Gretarsdottir S, Helgadottir A, Stefansson K. Genes contributing to risk for common forms of stroke. *Trends Mol Med.* 2005;11:217–224.

Hademenos GJ, Alberts MJ, Awad I, et al. Advances in the genetics of cerebrovascular disease and stroke. *Neurology.* 2001;56:997–1008.

Hassan A, Markus HS. Genetics and ischaemic stroke. *Brain.* 2000; 123:1784–1812.

Hata J, Matsuda K, Ninomiya T, et al. Functional SNP in an Sp1-binding site of AGTRL1 gene is associated with susceptibility to brain infarction. *Hum Mol Genet.* 2007;16:630–639.

Havasi V, Szolnoki Z, Talian G, et al. Apolipoprotein A5 gene promoter region T-1131C polymorphism associates with elevated circulating triglyceride levels and confers susceptibility for development of ischemic stroke. *J Mol Neurosci.* 2006;29:177–183.

Hegedus K. Some observations on reticular fibers in the media of the major cerebral arteries: a comparative study of patients without vascular diseases and those with ruptured berry aneurysms. *Surg Neurol.* 1984;22:301–307.

Hegener HH, Diehl KA, Kurth T, Gaziano JM, Ridker PM, Zee RY. Polymorphisms of prostaglandin-endoperoxide synthase 2 gene, and prostaglandin-E receptor 2 gene, C-reactive protein concentrations and risk of atherothrombosis: a nested case-control approach. *J Thromb Haemost.* 2006;4:1718–1722.

Heinrich PC, Castell JV, Andus T. Interleukin-6 and the acute phase response. *Biochem J.* 1990;265:621–636.

Helgadottir A, Gretarsdottir S, St Clair D, et al. Association between the gene encoding 5-lipoxygenase-activating protein and stroke replicated in a Scottish population. *Am J Hum Genet.* 2005;76:505–509.

Helgadottir A, Manolescu A, Thorleifsson G, et al. The gene encoding 5-lipoxygenase activating protein confers risk of myocardial infarction and stroke. *Nat Genet.* 2004;36:233–239.

Herrmann SM, Funke-Kaiser H, Schmidt-Petersen K, et al. Characterization of polymorphic structure of cathepsin G gene: role in cardiovascular and cerebrovascular diseases. *Arterioscler Thromb Vasc Biol.* 2001;21:1538–1543.

Hofer A, Hermans M, Kubassek N, et al. Elastin polymorphism haplotype and intracranial aneurysms are not associated in Central Europe. *Stroke.* 2003;34:1207–1211.

Hop JW, Rinkel GJE, Algra A, van Gijn J. Case fatality rates and functional outcome after subarachnoid haemorrhage: a systematic review. *Stroke.* 1997;28:660–664.

Houslay MD, Adams DR. PDE4 cAMP phosphodiesterases: modular enzymes that orchestrate signalling cross-talk, desensitization and compartmentalization. *Biochem J.* 2003;370:1–18.

Hsieh K, Lalouschek W, Schillinger M, et al. Impact of αENaC polymorphisms on the risk of ischemic cerebrovascular events: a multicenter case-control study. *Clin Chem.* 2005;51:952–956.

Humphries SE, Luong LA, Ogg MS, Hawe E, Miller GJ. The interleukin-6—174 G/C promoter polymorphism is associated with risk of coronary heart disease and systolic blood pressure in healthy men. *Eur Heart J.* 2001;22:2243–2252.

Humphries SE, Morgan L. Genetic risk factors for stroke and carotid atherosclerosis: insights into pathophysiology from candidate gene approaches. *Lancet Neurol.* 2004;3:227–235.

Iacoviello L, Di Castelnuovo A, Gattone M, et al. Polymorphisms of the interleukin-1β gene affect the risk of myocardial infarction and ischemic stroke at young age and the response of mononuclear cells to stimulation in vitro. *Arterioscler Thromb Vasc Biol.* 2005;25: 222–227.

Inagawa T, Tokuda Y, Ohbayashi N, Takaya M, Moritake K. Study of aneurysmal subarachnoid hemorrhage in Izumo City, Japan. *Stroke.* 1995;26:761–766.

Indolfi C, Avvedimento EV, Di Lorenzo E, et al. Activation of cAMP–PKA signaling *in vivo* inhibits smooth muscle cell proliferation induced by vascular injury. *Nat Med.* 1997;3:775–779.

Indolfi C, Di Lorenzo E, Rapacciuolo A, et al. 8-Chloro-cAMP inhibits smooth muscle cell proliferation *in vitro* and neointima formation induced by balloon injury *in vivo*. *J Am Coll Cardiol.* 2000;36:288–293.

Iniesta JA, Gonzalez-Conejero R, Piqueras C, Vicente V, Corral J. Platelet GP IIIa polymorphism HPA-1 (PlA) protects against subarachnoid hemorrhage. *Stroke.* 2004;35:2282–2286.

Inoue K, Mineharu Y, Inoue S, Yamada S, et al. Search on chromosome 17 centromere reveals TNFRSF13B as a susceptibility gene for intracranial aneurysm: a preliminary study. *Circulation.* 2006;113:2002–2010.

Ito D, Murata M, Watanabe K, et al. C242T polymorphism of NADPH oxidase p22 PHOX gene and ischemic cerebrovascular disease in the Japanese population. *Stroke.* 2000;31:936–939.

Jayaraman T, Berenstein V, Li X, et al. Tumor necrosis factor α is a key modulator of inflammation in cerebral aneurysms. *Neurosurgery.* 2005;57:558–564.

Jensson O, Gudmundsson G, Arnason A, et al. Hereditary cystatin C (gamma-trace) amyloid angiopathy of the CNS causing cerebral hemorrhage. *Acta Neurol Scand.* 1987;76:102–114.

Jerrard-Dunne P, Cloud G, Hassan A, Markus HS. Evaluating the genetic component of ischemic stroke subtypes: a family history study. *Stroke.* 2003;34:1364–1369.

Johnston SC, Selvin S, Gress DR. The burden, trends, and demographics of mortality from subarachnoid hemorrhage. *Neurology.* 1998;50:1413–1418.

Joutel A, Corpechot C, Ducros A, et al. Notch3 mutations in CADASIL, a hereditary adult-onset condition causing stroke and dementia. *Nature.* 1996;383:707–710.

Joutel A, Corpechot C, Ducros A, et al. Notch3 mutations in cerebral autosomal dominant arteriopathy with subcortical infarcts and leukoencephalopathy (CADASIL), a mendelian condition causing stroke and vascular dementia. *Ann NY Acad Sci.* 1997;826:213–217.

Kaneko Y, Nakayama T, Saito K, et al. Relationship between the thromboxane A2 receptor gene and susceptibility to cerebral infarction. *Hypertens Res.* 2006;29:665–671.

Kessler C, Spitzer C, Stauske D, et al. The apolipoprotein E and β-fibrinogen G/A–455 gene polymorphisms are associated with ischemic stroke involving large-vessel disease. *Arterioscler Thromb Vasc Biol.* 1997;17:2880–2884.

Khurana VG, Sohni YR, Mangrum WI, et al. Endothelial nitric oxide synthase gene polymorphisms predict susceptibility to aneurysmal subarachnoid hemorrhage and cerebral vasospasm. *J Cerebr Blood Flow Metab.* 2004;24:291–297.

Kim Y, Lee C. The gene encoding transforming growth factor β1 confers risk of ischemic stroke and vascular dementia. *Stroke.* 2006;37:2843–2845.

Kimura H, Gules I, Meguro T, Zhang JH. Cytotoxicity of cytokines in cerebral microvascular endothelial cell. *Brain Res.* 2003;990:148–156.

Kohara K, Fujisawa M, Ando F, et al. MTHFR gene polymorphism as a risk factor for silent brain infarcts and white matter lesions in the Japanese general population: The NILS-LSA Study. *Stroke.* 2003;34:1130–1135.

Kubo M, Hata J, Ninomiya T, et al. A nonsynonymous SNP in PRKCH (protein kinase C-eta) increases the risk of cerebral infarction. *Nat Genet.* 2007;39:212–217.

Laberge-le Couteulx S, Jung HH, Labauge P, et al. Truncating mutations in CCM1, encoding KRIT1, cause hereditary cavernous angiomas. *Nat Genet.* 1999;23:189–193.

Lander ES, Linton LM, Birren B, et al. Initial sequencing and analysis of the human genome. *Nature.* 2001;409:860–921.

Lavergne E, Labreuche J, Daoudi M, et al. Adverse associations between CX3CR1 polymorphisms and risk of cardiovascular or cerebrovascular disease. *Arterioscler Thromb Vasc Biol.* 2005;25:847–853.

Lee BC, Lee HJ, Chung JH. Peroxisome proliferator-activated receptor-γ2 Pro12Ala polymorphism is associated with reduced risk for ischemic stroke with type 2 diabetes. *Neurosci Lett.* 2006;410:141–145.

Levy E, Carman MD, Fernandez-Madrid IJ, et al. Mutation of the Alzheimer's disease amyloid gene in hereditary cerebral hemorrhage, Dutch type. *Science.* 1990;248:1124–1126.

Libby P. Inflammation in atherosclerosis. *Nature.* 2002;420:868–874.

Linn FHH, Rinkel GJE, Algra A, van Gijn J. Incidence of subarachnoid hemorrhage: role of region, year and rate of computed tomography: a meta-analysis. *Stroke.* 1996;27:625–629.

Litchfield WR, Anderson BF, Weiss RJ, Lifton RP, Dluhy RG. Intracranial aneurysm and hemorrhagic stroke in glucocorticoid-remediable aldosteronism. *Hypertension.* 1998;31:445–450.

Lohmussaar E, Gschwendtner A, Mueller JC, et al. ALOX5AP gene and the PDE4D gene in a central European population of stroke patients. *Stroke.* 2005;36:731–736.

Longstreth WT, Nelson LM, Koepsell TD, van Belle G. Clinical course of spontaneous subarachnoid hemorrhage: a population-based study in King County, Washington. *Neurology.* 1993;43:712–718.

Longstreth WT, Nelson LM, Koepsell TD, van Belle G. Subarachnoid hemorrhage and hormonal factors in women. A population-based case-control study. *Ann Intern Med.* 1994;121:168–173.

Lusis AJ. Atherosclerosis. *Nature.* 2000;407:233–241.

Macmillan C, Lach B, Shoubridge EA. Variable distribution of mutant mitochondrial DNAs (tRNA(Leu[3243])) in tissues of symptomatic relatives with MELAS: the role of mitotic segregation. *Neurology.* 1993;43:1586–1590.

Maeda Y, Matsumoto M, Hori O, et al. Hypoxia/reoxygenation-mediated induction of astrocyte interleukin 6: a paracrine mechanism potentially enhancing neuron survival. *J Exp Med.* 1994;180:2297–2308.

Margaglione M, Celentano E, Grandone E, et al. Deletion polymorphism in the angiotensin-converting enzyme gene in patients with a history of ischemic stroke. *Arterioscler Thromb Vasc Biol.* 1996;16:304–309.

Markus HS, Alberts MJ. Update on genetics of stroke and cerebrovascular disease 2005. *Stroke.* 2006;37:288–290.

Maroun FB, Murray GP, Jacob JC, Mangan MA, Faridi M. Familial intracranial aneurysms: report of three families. *Surg Neurol.* 1986;25:85–88.

Massaro AR, Sacco RL, Mohr JP, et al. Clinical discriminators of lobar and deep hemorrhages: the Stroke Data Bank. *Neurology.* 1991;41:1881–1885.

Mathiesen T, Edner G, Ulfarsson E, Andersson B. Cerebrospinal fluid interleukin-1 receptor antagonist and tumor necrosis factor-α following subarachnoid hemorrhage. *J Neurosurg.* 1997;87:215–220.

Mehrabian M, Allayee H, Wong J, et al. Identification of 5-lipoxygenase as a major gene contributing to atherosclerosis susceptibility in mice. *Circ Res.* 2002;91:120–126.

Meschia JF, Brott TG, Brown RD Jr, et al. Phosphodiesterase 4D and 5-lipoxygenase activating protein in ischemic stroke. *Ann Neurol.* 2005;58:351–361.

Meschia JF, Worrall BB. New advances in identifying genetic anomalies in stroke-prone probands. *Curr Atheroscler Rep.* 2003;5:317–323.

Ministry of Health, Labor, and Welfare of Japan, 2005. Available at: http://www.mhlw.go.jp/toukei/saikin/hw/jinkou/geppo/nengai08/index.html.

Montagna P, Gallassi R, Medori R, et al. MELAS syndrome: characteristic migrainous and epileptic features and maternal transmission. *Neurology.* 1988;38:751–754.

Morgan L, Cooper J, Montgomery H, Kitchen N, Humphries SE. The interleukin-6 gene −174G→C and −572G→C promoter polymorphisms are related to cerebral aneurysms. *J Neurol Neurosurg Psychiatry.* 2006;77:915–917.

Morgan L, Hawe E, Palmen J, Montgomery H, Humphries SE, Kitchen N. Polymorphism of the heme oxygenase-1 gene and cerebral aneurysms. *Br J Neurosurg.* 2005;19:317–321.

Morgan L, Humphries SE. The genetics of stroke. *Curr Opin Lipidol.* 2005;16:193–199.

Morita A, Nakayama T, Soma M. Association study between C-reactive protein genes and ischemic stroke in Japanese subjects. *Am J Hypertens.* 2006;19:593–600.

Morita H, Kurihara H, Tsubaki S, et al. Methylenetetrahydrofolate reductase gene polymorphism and ischemic stroke in Japanese. *Arterioscler Thromb Vasc Biol.* 1998;18:1465–1469.

Morooka Y, Waga S. Familial intracranial aneurysms: report of four families. *Surg Neurol.* 1983;19:260–262.

Morrison AC, Doris PA, Folsom AR, Nieto FJ, Boerwinkle E; Atherosclerosis Risk in Communities Study. G-protein β3 subunit and α-adducin polymorphisms and risk of subclinical and clinical stroke. *Stroke.* 2001;32:822–829.

Naghavi M, Libby P, Falk E, et al. From vulnerable plaque to vulnerable patient: a call for new definitions and risk assessment strategies: part I. *Circulation.* 2003;108:1664–1672.

Nahed BV, Seker A, Guclu B, et al. Mapping a Mendelian form of intracranial aneurysm to 1p34.3–p36.13. *Am J Hum Genet.* 2005;76:172–179.

Natowicz M, Kelley RI. Mendelian etiologies of stroke. *Ann Neurol.* 1987;22:175–192.

Neil-Dwyer G, Bartlett JR, Nicholls AC, Narcisi P, Pope FM. Collagen deficiency and ruptured cerebral aneurysms: a clinical and biochemical study. *J Neurosurg.* 1983;59:16–20.

Nicoll JA, Burnett C, Love S, et al. High frequency of apolipoprotein E epsilon 2 allele in hemorrhage due to cerebral amyloid angiopathy. *Ann Neurol.* 1997;41:716–721.

Nilsson-Ardnor S, Wiklund PG, Lindgren P, et al. Linkage of ischemic stroke to the PDE4D region on 5q in a Swedish population. *Stroke.* 2005;36:1666–1671.

Norrgard O, Angquist KA, Fodstad H, Forsell A, Lindberg M. Intracranial aneurysms and heredity. *Neurosurgery.* 1987;20:236–239.

O'Donnell HC, Rosand J, Knudsen KA, et al. Apolipoprotein E genotype and the risk of recurrent lobar intracerebral hemorrhage. *N Engl J Med.* 2000;342:240–245.

O'Leary DH, Polak JF, Kronmal RA, Manolio TA, Burke GL, Wolfson SK Jr. Carotid artery intima and media thickness as a risk factor for myocardial infarction and stroke in older adults. Cardiovascular Health Study Collaborative Research Group. *N Eng J Med.* 1999;340:14–22.

Onda H, Kasuya H, Yoneyama T, et al. Genomewide-linkage and haplotype-association studies map intracranial aneurysm to chromosome 7q11. *Am J Hum Genet.* 2001;69:804–819.

Ostergaard JR, Oxlund H. Collagen type III deficiency in patients with rupture of intracranial saccular aneurysms. *J Neurosurg.* 1987;67:690–696.

Ostergaard JR, Reske-Nielsen E, Oxlund H. Histological and morphometric observations on the reticular fibers in the arterial beds of patients with ruptured intracranial saccular aneurysms. *Neurosurgery.* 1987;20:554–558.

Ozturk AK, Nahed BV, Bydon M, et al. Molecular genetic analysis of two large kindreds with intracranial aneurysms demonstrates linkage to 11q24–25 and 14q23–31. *Stroke.* 2006;37:1021–1027.

Palmer D, Tsoi K, Maurice DH. Synergistic inhibition of vascular smooth muscle cell migration by phosphodiesterase 3 and phosphodiesterase 4 inhibitors. *Circ Res.* 1998;82:852–861.

Palsdottir A, Abrahamson M, Thorsteinsson L, et al. Mutation in cystatin C gene causes hereditary brain haemorrhage. *Lancet.* 1988;2:603–604.

Pan X, Arauz E, Krzanowski JJ, Fitzpatrick DF, Polson JB. Synergistic interactions between selective pharmacological inhibitors of phosphodiesterase isozyme families PDE III and PDE IV to attenuate proliferation of rat vascular smooth muscle cells. *Biochem Pharmacol.* 1994;48:827–835.

Pavlakis SG, Phillips PC, DiMauro S, De Vivo DC, Rowland LP. Mitochondrial myopathy, encephalopathy, lactic acidosis, and strokelike episodes: a distinctive clinical syndrome. *Ann Neurol.* 1984;16:481–488.

Pawlikowska L, Tran MN, Achrol AS, et al. Polymorphisms in genes involved in inflammatory and angiogenic pathways and the risk of hemorrhagic presentation of brain arteriovenous malformations. *Stroke.* 2004;35:2294–2300.

Peters DG, Kassam A, St Jean PL, Yonas H, Ferrell RE. Functional polymorphism in the matrix metalloproteinase-9 promoter as a potential risk factor for intracranial aneurysm. *Stroke.* 1999;30:2612–2616.

Pola R, Flex A, Gaetani E, Flore R, Serricchio M, Pola P. Synergistic effect of –174 G/C polymorphism of the interleukin-6 gene promoter and 469 E/K polymorphism of the intercellular adhesion molecule-1 gene in Italian patients with history of ischemic stroke. *Stroke.* 2003;34:881–885.

Pulkes T, Sweeney MG, Hanna MG. Increased risk of stroke in patients with the A12308G polymorphism in mitochondria. *Lancet.* 2000;356:2068–2069.

Raaymakers TWM, Rinkel GJE, Ramos LMP. Initial and follow up screening for aneurysms in familial subarachnoid hemorrhage. *Neurology.* 1998;51:1125–1130.

Rauramaa R, Vaisanen SB, Luong LA, et al. Stromelysin-1 and interleukin-6 gene promoter polymorphisms are determinants of asymptomatic carotid artery atherosclerosis. *Arterioscler Thromb Vasc Biol.* 2000;20:2657–2662.

Reiner AP, Schwartz SM, Frank MB, et al. Polymorphisms of coagulation factor XIII subunit A and risk of nonfatal hemorrhagic stroke in young white women. *Stroke.* 2001;32:2580–2586.

Ridker PM, Hennekens CH, Schmitz C, Stampfer MJ, Lindpaintner K. PIA1/A2 polymorphism of platelet glycoprotein IIIa and risks of myocardial infarction, stroke, and venous thrombosis. *Lancet.* 1997;349:385–388.

Rinkel GJE, Djibuti M, Algra A, van Gijn J. Prevalence and risk of rupture of intracranial aneurysms. *Stroke.* 1998;29:251–256.

Romano M, Sironi M, Toniatti C, et al. Role of IL-6 and its soluble receptor in induction of chemokines and leukocyte recruitment. *Immunity.* 1997;6:315–325.

Ronkainen A, Hernesniemi J, Puranen M, et al. Familial intracranial aneurysms. *Lancet.* 1997;349:380–384.

Ronkainen A, Hernesniemi J, Ryynanen M. Familial subarachnoid hemorrhage in east Finland, 1977–1990. *Neurosurgery.* 1993;33:787–796.

Ronkainen A, Niskanen M, Piironen R, Hernesniemi J. Familial subarachnoid hemorrhage. Outcome study. *Stroke.* 1999;30:1099–1102.

Roos YB, Pals G, Struycken PM, et al. Genome-wide linkage in a large Dutch consanguineous family maps a locus for intracranial aneurysms to chromosome 2p13. *Stroke.* 2004;35:2276–2281.

Rosamond W, Flegal K, Friday G, et al. Heart disease and stroke statistics—2007 update: a report from the American Heart Association Statistics Committee and Stroke Statistics Subcommittee. *Circulation.* 2007;115:e69–e171.

Rosenberg GA. Matrix metalloproteinases in neuroinflammation. *Glia.* 2002;39:279–291.

Rubattu S, Stanzione R, Di Angelantonio E, et al. Atrial natriuretic peptide gene polymorphisms and risk of ischemic stroke in humans. *Stroke.* 2004;35:814–818.

Ruigrok YM, Buskens E, Rinkel GJE. Attributable risk of common and rare determinants of subarachnoid hemorrhage. *Stroke.* 2001;32:1173–1175.

Ruigrok YM, Rinkel GJ, van't Slot R, Wolfs M, Tang S, Wijmenga C. Evidence in favor of the contribution of genes involved in the maintenance of the extracellular matrix of the arterial wall to the development of intracranial aneurysms. *Hum Mol Genet.* 2006a;15:3361–3368.

Ruigrok YM, Rinkel GJ, Wijmenga C. Genetics of intracranial aneurysms. *Lancet Neurol.* 2005a;4:179–189.

Ruigrok YM, Rinkel GJ, Wijmenga C. The versican gene and the risk of intracranial aneurysms. *Stroke.* 2006b;37:2372–2374.

Ruigrok YM, Seitz U, Wolterink S, Rinkel GJ, Wijmenga C, Urban Z. Association of polymorphisms and haplotypes in the elastin gene in Dutch patients with sporadic aneurysmal subarachnoid hemorrhage. *Stroke.* 2004;35:2064–2068.

Ruigrok YM, Slooter AJ, Bardoel A, Frijns CJ, Rinkel GJ, Wijmenga C. Genes and outcome after aneurysmal subarachnoid haemorrhage. *J Neurol.* 2005b;252:417–422.

Rundek T, Elkind MS, Pittman J, et al. Carotid intima-media thickness is associated with allelic variants of stromelysin-1, interleukin-6, and hepatic lipase genes: the Northern Manhattan Prospective Cohort Study. *Stroke.* 2002;33:1420–1423.

Sacco RL. Lobar intracerebral hemorrhage. *N Engl J Med.* 2000;342:276–279.

Saito K, Nakayama T, Sato N, et al. Haplotypes of the plasminogen activator gene associated with ischemic stroke. *Thromb Haemost.* 2006;96:331–336.

Sakuta R, Goto Y, Horai S, Nonaka I. Mitochondrial DNA mutations at nucleotide positions 3243 and 3271 in mitochondrial myopathy, encephalopathy, lactic acidosis, and stroke-like episodes: a comparative study. *J Neurol Sci.* 1993;115:158–160.

Santamaria A, Mateo J, Tirado I, et al. Homozygosity of the T allele of the 46 C→T polymorphism in the F12 gene is a risk factor for ischemic stroke in the Spanish population. *Stroke.* 2004;35:1795–1799.

Schievink WI, Limburg M, Oorthuys JWE, Fleury P, Pope FM. Cerebrovascular disease in Ehlers-Danlos syndrome type IV. *Stroke.* 1990;21:626–632.

Schievink WI, Michels VV, Piepgras DG. Neurovascular manifestations of heritable connective tissue disorders: a review. *Stroke.* 1994;25:889–903.

Schievink WI, Schaid DJ, Michels VV, Piepgras DG. Familial aneurysmal subarachnoid hemorrhage: a community based study. *J Neurosurg.* 1995;83:426–429.

Shearman AM, Cooper JA, Kotwinski PJ, et al. Estrogen receptor α gene variation and the risk of stroke. *Stroke.* 2005;36:2281–2282.

Shimo-Nakanishi Y, Urabe T, Hattori N, et al. Polymorphism of the lipoprotein lipase gene and risk of atherothrombotic cerebral infarction in the Japanese. *Stroke.* 2001;32:1481–1486.

Silva Y, Leira R, Tejada J, et al. Molecular signatures of vascular injury are associated with early growth of intracerebral hemorrhage. *Stroke.* 2005;36:86–91.

Skirgaudas M, Awad IA, Kim J, Rothbart D, Criscuolo G. Expression of angiogenesis factors and selected vascular wall matrix proteins in intracranial saccular aneurysms. *Neurosurgery.* 1996;39:537–545.

Slowik A, Borratynska A, Pera J, et al. II Genotype of the angiotensin-converting enzyme gene increases the risk for subarachnoid hemorrhage from ruptured aneurysm. *Stroke.* 2004a;35:1594–1597.

Slowik A, Borratynska A, Turaj W, et al. α_1-Antichymotrypsin gene (SERPINA3) A/T polymorphism as a risk factor for aneurysmal subarachnoid hemorrhage. *Stroke.* 2005;36:737–740.

Slowik A, Turaj W, Dziedzic T, et al. DD genotype of ACE gene is a risk factor for intracerebral hemorrhage. *Neurology.* 2004b;63:359–361.

Spanbroek R, Grabner R, Lotzer K, et al. Expanding expression of the 5-lipoxygenase pathway within the arterial wall during human atherogenesis. *Proc Natl Acad Sci USA.* 2003;100:1238–1243.

Spittell PC, Spittell JA Jr, Joyce JW, et al. Clinical features and differential diagnosis of aortic dissection: experience with 236 cases (1980 through 1990). *Mayo Clin Proc.* 1993;68:642–651.

Stehbens WE. Familial intracranial aneurysms: an autopsy study. *Neurosurgery.* 1998;43:1258–1259.

Sun L, Li Z, Zhang H, et al. Pentanucleotide TTTTA repeat polymorphism of apolipoprotein(a) gene and plasma lipoprotein(a) are associated with ischemic and hemorrhagic stroke in Chinese: a multicenter case-control study in China. *Stroke.* 2003;34:1617–1622.

Suzuki S, Tanaka K, Nogawa S, et al. Temporal profile and cellular localization of interleukin-6 protein after focal cerebral ischemia in rats. *J Cerebr Blood Flow Metab.* 1999;19:1256–1262.

Szolnoki Z, Havasi V, Talian G, et al. Lymphotoxin-α gene 252G allelic variant is a risk factor for large-vessel-associated ischemic stroke. *J Mol Neurosci.* 2005;27:205–211.

Takenaka K, Sakai H, Yamakawa H, et al. Polymorphism of the endoglin gene in patients with intracranial saccular aneurysms. *J Neurosurg.* 1999;90:935–938.

Tarkowski E, Rosengren L, Blomstrand C, et al. Early intrathecal production of interleukin-6 predicts the size of brain lesion in stroke. *Stroke.* 1995;26:1393–1398.

ter Berg HW, Bijlsma JB, Veiga Pires JA, et al. Familial association of intracranial aneurysms and multiple congenital anomalies. *Arch Neurol.* 1986;43:30–33.

Teunissen LL, Rinkel GJE, Algra A, van Gijn J. Risk factors for subarachnoid hemorrhage: a systematic review. *Stroke.* 1996;27:544–549.

The International HapMap Consortium. A haplotype map of the human genome. *Nature.* 2005;437:1299–1320.

The Magnetic Resonance Angiography in Relatives of Patients with Subarachnoid Hemorrhage Study Group. Risks and benefits of screening of intracranial aneurysms in first-degree relatives of patients with sporadic subarachnoid hemorrhage. *N Engl J Med.* 1999;341:1344–1350.

The Stroke Association. United Kingdom; 2006. Available at: http://www.stroke.org.uk.

Tournier-Lasserve E. New players in the genetics of stroke. *N Engl J Med.* 2002;347:1711–1712.

Tournier-Lasserve E, Iba-Zizen MT, Romero N, Bousser MG. Autosomal dominant syndrome with strokelike episodes and leukoencephalopathy. *Stroke.* 1991;22:1297–1302.

Tournier-Lasserve E, Joutel A, Melki J. Cerebral autosomal dominant arteriopathy with subcortical infarcts and leukoencephalopathy maps to chromosome 19q12. *Nat Genet.* 1993;3:256–259.

van den Berg JS, Limburg M, Pals G, et al. Some patients with intracranial aneurysms have a reduced type III/type I collagen ratio. A case-control study. *Neurology.* 1997;49:1546–1551.

van der Knaap MS, Smit LM, Barkhof F, et al. Neonatal porencephaly and adult stroke related to mutations in collagen IV A1. *Ann Neurol.* 2006;59:504–511.

Van der Voet M, Olson JM, Kuivaniemi H, et al. Intracranial aneurysms in Finnish families: confirmation of linkage and refinement of the interval to chromosome 19q13.3. *Am J Hum Genet.* 2004;74:564–571.

Vidal R, Frangione B, Rostagno A, et al. A stop-codon mutation in the BRI gene associated with familial British dementia. *Nature.* 1999;399:776–781.

Vila N, Obach V, Revilla M, Oliva R, Chamorro A. α_1-Antichymotrypsin gene polymorphism in patients with stroke. *Stroke.* 2000;31:2103–2105.

Voetsch B, Benke KS, Damasceno BP, Siqueira LH, Loscalzo J. Paraoxonase 192 Gln→Arg polymorphism: an independent risk factor for nonfatal arterial ischemic stroke among young adults. *Stroke.* 2002;33:1459–1464.

Voetsch B, Jin RC, Bierl C, et al. Promoter polymorphisms in the plasma glutathione peroxidase (GPx-3) gene: a novel risk factor for arterial ischemic stroke among young adults and children. *Stroke.* 2007;38:41–49.

Wang PS, Longstreth WT Jr, Koepsell TD. Subarachnoid hemorrhage and family history: a population-based case-control study. *Arch Neurol.* 1995;52:202–204.

Wang Y, Zhang W, Zhang Y, et al. VKORC1 haplotypes are associated with arterial vascular diseases (stroke, coronary heart disease, and aortic dissection). *Circulation.* 2006;113:1615–1621.

Warlow C, Sudlow C, Dennis M, Wardlaw J, Sandercock P. Stroke. *Lancet.* 2003;362:1211–1224.

Watnick T, Phakdeekitcharoen B, Johnson A, et al. Mutation detection of PKD1 identifies a novel mutation common to three families with aneurysms and/or very-early-onset disease. *Am J Hum Genet.* 1999;65:1561–1571.

Wiklund PG, Nilsson L, Ardnor SN, et al. Plasminogen activator inhibitor-1 4G/5G polymorphism and risk of stroke: replicated findings in two nested case-control studies based on independent cohorts. *Stroke.* 2005;36:1661–1665.

Wilhelmsen L, Rosengren A, Eriksson H, Lappas G. Heart failure in the general population of men—morbidity, risk factors and prognosis. *J Intern Med.* 2001a;249:253–261.

Wilhelmsen L, Rosengren A, Lappas G. Hospitalizations for atrial fibrillation in the general male population: morbidity and risk factors. *J Intern Med.* 2001b;250:382–389.

Williams RR, Hunt SC, Heiss G, et al. Usefulness of cardiovascular family history data for population-based preventive medicine and medical research (the Health Family Tree Study and the NHLBI Family Heart Study). *Am J Cardiol.* 2001;87:129–135.

Woo D, Kaushal R, Chakraborty R, et al. Association of apolipoprotein E4 and haplotypes of the apolipoprotein E gene with lobar intracerebral hemorrhage. *Stroke.* 2005;36:1874–1879.

Worrall BB, Brott TG, Brown RD Jr, et al. IL1RN VNTR polymorphism in ischemic stroke. Analysis in 3 populations. *Stroke.* 2007;38:1189–1196.

Xia J, Yang QD, Yang QM, et al. Apolipoprotein H gene polymorphisms and risk of primary cerebral hemorrhage in a Chinese population. *Cerebrovasc Dis.* 2004;17:197–203.

Yamada S, Utsunomiya M, Inoue K, et al. Genome-wide scan for Japanese familial intracranial aneurysms: linkage to several chromosomal regions. *Circulation.* 2004;14:3727–3733.

Yamada Y. Identification of genetic factors and development of genetic risk diagnosis systems for cardiovascular diseases and stroke. *Circ J.* 2006;70:1240–1248.

Yamada Y, Metoki N, Yoshida H, et al. Genetic risk for ischemic and hemorrhangic stroke. *Arterioscler Thromb Vasc Biol.* 2006;26:1920–1925.

Yoneyama T, Kasuya H, Onda H, et al. Collagen type I α2 (COL1A2) is the susceptible gene for intracranial aneurysms. *Stroke.* 2004;35:443–448.

Zee RY, Cook NR, Cheng S, et al. Polymorphism in the P-selectin and interleukin-4 genes as determinants of stroke: a population-based, prospective genetic analysis. *Hum Mol Genet.* 2004;13:389–396.

25

Pulmonary Arterial Hypertension

Jennifer Thomson and Richard C Trembath

Introduction

Pulmonary arterial hypertension (PAH) is defined clinically by the presence of pulmonary hypertension (mean pulmonary artery pressure greater than 25 mmHg at rest or greater than 30 mmHg during exercise) *and* a normal pulmonary artery wedge pressure (less than or equal to 12 mmHg at rest) (Harris and Heath 1962). Idiopathic PAH is the presence of PAH in the absence of known causes and without a family history of the disease (Table 25–1; Launay 2003). When two or more relatives have idiopathic disease, this is termed familial PAH (Launay 2003).

The pulmonary circulation is a high-flow, low-resistance system that recruits normally closed vessels during increased cardiac outputs, thus maintaining pulmonary artery pressures at 30 mmHg or below (Hughes et al. 1997). The pulmonary vascular bed differs from the systemic circulation, exhibiting minimal resting tone and vasoconstriction in response to hypoxia (von Euler and Liljestrand 1946). In idiopathic PAH, an anatomic decrease in cross-sectional area of peripheral pulmonary arteries occurs through neointimal formation, vascular remodeling, and in situ thrombus. In addition, there is reduced vasoconstriction and distensibility, leading to increased pulmonary vascular resistance. By the time a patient is symptomatic, the structural changes of PAH are well developed. Initially cardiac output remains normal at rest but does not appropriately increase with exercise. As the disease progresses, cardiac output becomes decreased at rest and right ventricular failure ensues (Rubin 1997).

The History of Idiopathic PAH and Terminology

In 1891, Ernst Romberg described "pulmonary arteriosclerosis" in a 24-year-old man with unexplained right heart failure (Romberg 1891). Although this is likely to delineate the first histological description of idiopathic PAH, the case of a 59-year-old gentleman with right ventricular failure in the absence of gross cardiopulmonary disease in 1865 may represent the earliest clinical report (Klob 1865).

The concept of "primary pulmonary arteriosclerosis" reached the English literature in 1909 with numerous case reports to follow, including two sisters with the condition (Sanders 1909). However, of these, very few fulfilled Brenner's 1935 clinical criteria that "before the diagnosis is made, all the factors commonly thought to cause secondary pulmonary vascular sclerosis must be absent and there must be marked hypertrophy of the right ventricle" (Brenner 1935). The hypothesis that pulmonary hypertension caused right ventricular hypertrophy remained unproven until the evolution of right heart catheterization in 1941 and the ability to measure pulmonary capillary pressure in 1949 (Cournand and Ranges 1941; Hellems et al. 1949; Wood 1950). The development of this technique allowed antemortem diagnosis of idiopathic PAH and the quantitative evaluation of therapeutic measures (Brill and Krygier 1941). For the first time, reports of familial PAH could be confirmed.

In 1973, the World Health Organisation held a symposium in Geneva in response to the increased incidence of PAH relating to the appetite suppressant aminorex (Gurtner et al. 1968; Hatano and Strasser 1973). "Primary pulmonary hypertension" was agreed as a description of the clinical diagnosis in the absence of known causes, whereas the term "plexogenic pulmonary arteriopathy" was created for the histopathological appearances of intimal fibrosis, necrotizing arteritis, and plexiform lesions seen in the absence of lung or heart disease. The term "primary pulmonary hypertension" has now been superseded by "idiopathic pulmonary arterial hypertension" (Table 25–1).

Epidemiology of Idiopathic PAH

Idiopathic PAH has an estimated incidence of one to two per million population per year (Rich et al. 1987; Rubin 1993). However, the prevalence from autopsy studies ranges from 83 to 1,302 per million in unselected cases (MacCallum 1931; Goodale and Thomas 1954; McDonnell et al. 1983). In a more recent report in the United States, the average annual age-adjusted mortality from idiopathic PAH during the period 1979–1996 was three per million population (Lilienfeld and Rubin 2000). Lilienfeld and Rubin particularly comment on the paucity of data regarding incidence and prevalence of this disease. Idiopathic PAH is reported in many countries, including North America, in Europe, Asia, and Australasia. In the 1981–1985 National Institutes of Health idiopathic PAH study (NIH study), the distribution of patients by nationality was similar to that of the general population in the United States (Rich et al. 1987). At the time of entry into the NIH study the age range of patients was 1–81 years with a mean of 36.4 years (Rich et al. 1987). Females more often presented in the third

Table 25–1 International Symposium Classification of Pulmonary Hypertension, Venice 2003

1. Pulmonary arterial hypertension
Idiopathic
Hereditary (at least two affected individuals in one family or causative gene mutation identified)
Related to collagen vascular disease, congenital heart disease, portal hypertension, human immunodeficiency virus, drugs, and toxins
With significant venous and/or capillary involvement
Persistent pulmonary hypertension of the newborn
2. Pulmonary hypertension with left heart disease
Atrial or ventricular disease
Valvular heart disease
3. Pulmonary hypertension with lung disease and/or hypoxemia
Chronic obstructive pulmonary disease
Interstitial lung disease
Sleep disorders; alveolar hypoventilation; chronic exposure to high altitude
Developmental abnormalities
4. Pulmonary hypertension due to chronic thrombotic and/or embolic disease
Thromboembolic obstruction of proximal pulmonary arteries
Thromboembolic obstruction of distal pulmonary arteries
Pulmonary embolism (tumor, parasites, foreign material)
5. Others
Sarcoidosis, histiocytosis X, lymphangiomatosis, pulmonary vessel compression (adenopathies, tumors, fibrosing mediastinitis)

Note: Modified at the California World Health Organisation Symposium in 2008.
Source: Launay 2003.

decade and males in the fourth decade of life. In a National idiopathic PAH survey in Israel, 44 patients were enrolled between 1988 and 1997 with a mean age of diagnosis of 42.8 years, ranging from 16 to 63 years (Appelbaum et al. 2001). However, in neither report is information available regarding age of onset of symptoms. A greater number of females than males develop idiopathic PAH. Exact ratios vary between studies as cohort size and inclusion criteria differ but ranges from 1.7:1 to 4.2:1 (females to males) (Wagenvoort et al. 1970; Rich et al. 1987; Oakley 1994; Appelbaum 2001).

Risk Factors for PAH

At the World Health Organisation meeting in 1998, a risk factor for PAH was defined as "any factor or condition that is suspected to play a causal or facilitating role in the development of the disease" (Table 25–2; Rich 1998a). However, a family history of PAH is an important omission from this list.

Pregnancy and Estrogens

From 1978 until 1996, there were 27 case reports of PAH in pregnancy with a maternal mortality of 30%, all deaths occurring within 35 days of delivery (Weiss et al. 1998). Maternal prognosis depended on early diagnosis of the disease, individually tailored treatment during pregnancy and particular focus on the postpartum period. There was 12% fetal mortality. The most likely reason for PAH to occur in labor, delivery, or postpartum is the significant alteration in cardiac output and blood volume at this time. In the normal situation, cardiac output is 18% greater immediately after delivery than upon completion of the first stage and is maintained until day four postpartum (Adams and Alexander 1958). Thus, pulmonary blood flow increases by 20% postdelivery. Therefore, a large volume shift could lead to acute right ventricular failure in a PAH patient. Alternatively, the sudden decrease in volume of the uterus could decrease venous return to the right atrium and therefore cardiac output (Nielsen and Fabricius 1961). Furthermore, the hypercoagulable state in pregnancy may lead to thromboembolism or increased in situ thrombus formation in small pulmonary arteries (Pechet and Pechet 1961).

Female reproductive steroids have been associated with hyperplasia in a variety of organs in humans and animals. In a series of 16 women either taking oral contraceptives, pregnant or postpartum, all had evidence of intimal thickening in systemic or pulmonary blood vessels (Irey and Norris 1973). Pulmonary vascular obstruction by intimal fibrosis was found in one of three women with congenital septal defects who deteriorated whilst taking oral contraceptives (Oakley and Sommerville 1968). During the NIH prospective study of PAH patients, oral contraceptive use was analyzed. Fifty-four percent of females had taken such hormones, similar to the rate in the general population (Rich et al. 1987). Of the variables assessed, only age for users of these contraceptives compared with nonusers showed a difference (30.0 +/– 8.4 years compared with 39.9 +/–17.3 years, $p<0.002$). Estrogen therapy is listed as an unlikely risk factor for pulmonary hypertension. However, the case of a postmenopausal lady with a family history of PAH who developed the condition 6 months after commencing hormone replacement therapy, having been asymptomatic with a normal ECG, CXR, and ECHO 2 months prior to therapy, highlights the need for reexamining this issue (Morse et al. 1999).

PAH in Associated Studies

As listed in Table 25–1, there is a heterogeneous group of disorders associated with PAH, including collagen vascular disease, congenital heart disease, portal hypertension, HIV infection, drugs, and toxins, for example, appetite suppressants and adulterated rapeseed oil. The clinical, hemodynamic, histopathological, and prognostic features of the pulmonary vasculopathy in these conditions are similar to idiopathic PAH. However, only a minority of individuals with these related disorders develop idiopathic-type PAH. Therefore, these individuals may have a genetic susceptibility for the development of PAH, which is triggered by an injurious agent or other pathologic process.

Clinical Features of Idiopathic PAH

The most common initial symptoms in adults and older children are nonspecific breathlessness (60%), fatigue (19%), and fainting (8%) (Table 25–3) (Rich et al. 1987). Infants and young children may present with similar symptoms and are commonly misdiagnosed with asthma (Haworth 2008). With progression of disease, patients may also experience chest pain, palpitations, and other symptoms of right heart failure. Ten percent of patients report features of Raynaud's phenomenon. Hemoptysis and hoarseness (from left recurrent laryngeal nerve compression by an enlarged pulmonary artery known as Ortner syndrome) are uncommon. Sudden death may occur.

The physical findings depend on the severity of the pulmonary hypertension. Central cyanosis is apparent in 20% and peripheral edema in 32% of affected individuals (Rich et al. 1987). There is a raised jugular venous pressure with prominent *a* and *v*

Table 25–2 World Health Organisation Classification of PAH Risk, 1998 (Evian)

Categories	Definite[a]	Very likely[b]	Possible[c]	Unlikely[d]
Demographic and medical conditions	Gender		Pregnancy, systemic hypertension	Obesity
Drugs and toxins	Aminorex, fenfluramine, toxic, rapeseed oil	Amphetamines, L-tryptophan	Meta-amphetamine, cocaine, chemotherapeutic agents	Antidepressants, oral contraceptive pill, estrogen therapy, cigarette smoking
Diseases	HIV infection	Portal hypertension, collagen vascular disease, congenital systemic-pulmonary shunts	Thyroid disorders	

Source: Rich 1998a.
[a]An association based on several different observations and often including a major controlled study or clear epidemic.
[b]Several concordant observations or a general consensus amongst experts.
[c]An association based on case reports, registries such as the NIH and expert opinions.
[d]Risk factors that have been proposed but for which no additional evidence has been forthcoming.

Table 25–3 Clinical Features of Idiopathic PAH in the National Institutes of Health Study 1981–1985

Symptom	At Onset of Disease (Percentage of Persons)	At Time of Enrolment in Study (Percentage of Persons)
Breathlessness	60	98
Fatigue	19	73
Syncope	8	36
Chest pain	7	47
Near syncope	5	41
Palpitations	5	33
Leg edema	3	37

Source: Rich et al. 1987.

waves. Right ventricular heave may occur. There is an increased pulmonary component of the second heart sound (P2) in 93% of patients and right-sided third and fourth heart sounds. Tricuspid and pulmonary regurgitation is audible in 40% and 13% of subjects respectively (Rich et al. 1987). Additional physical signs may be indicative of an underlying cause of disease but there are none known to be specific to idiopathic PAH.

Investigations

Recognition of idiopathic PAH can be lengthy due to its nonspecific presentation, few clinical signs, and the numerous investigations required to exclude known etiologies of pulmonary hypertension. The "gold standard" investigation for determining pulmonary artery pressure is cardiac catheterization. A Swan-Ganz triple lumen thermodynamic cardiac catheter study is best performed in specialist centers for interpretation of results, acute drug trials, and management of complications. In PAH, right atrial pressure and pulmonary artery pressure are increased, pulmonary artery wedge pressure is normal, and cardiac output is normal or reduced (Rubin 1997). Pulmonary vasoreactivity is currently defined as a decrease in mean PAP of at least 10 mmHg to a level ≤40 mmHg with either no change or an increase in cardiac output. Recent studies have shown that 22% of patients (n = 67) demonstrate pulmonary vasoreactivity following administration of epoprostenol, adenosine, nitric oxide, or high dose nifedipine (Elliott et al. 2006). The reason for vasoresponsiveness in these patients and not others is unknown but may reflect early pathology or possibly a specific subset of the disorder. Of note, previous analyses of pulmonary reactivity have been based on an alternative definition and therefore are not comparable to current studies.

Cardiac catheterization is an invasive procedure that may cause cardiorespiratory arrest in a compromised patient. Hence, a number of other tests are often undertaken prior to catheterization to determine (1) an indirect measure of pulmonary hypertension such as echocardiography (ECHO), (2) the consequences of pulmonary hypertension such as hypoxia and right heart strain using arterial blood gas measurements, the electrocardiogram (ECG), and chest radiography, and (3) assessment of possible underlying causes (Table 25–1).

Features of pulmonary hypertension demonstrated by ECHO include impaired left ventricular filling, paradoxical septal motion, right atrial and ventricular enlargement, and pulmonary and tricuspid regurgitation (Goodman et al. 1974). Doppler studies can be used to measure the tricuspid regurgitant jet velocity and the relationship of acceleration time in the pulmonary outflow tract, indicative of pulmonary artery systolic flow and pressure. The ECG commonly demonstrates features of right heart overload such as right axis deviation, right ventricular hypertrophy, and right ventricular strain (Rich et al. 1987). Sinus rhythm is usually present although life-threatening arrhythmias may occur. Chest radiography (CXR) may portray prominence of the main pulmonary artery, enlarged hilar vessels, decreased peripheral vessels, and right ventricular hypertrophy. However, in 6% the CXR is relatively normal despite significant pulmonary hypertension, emphasizing the lack of sensitivity of this investigation (Rich et al. 1987).

Respiratory function tests may display a mild restrictive defect and a reduced diffusing capacity for carbon monoxide (Rich et al. 1987). Arterial blood gases invariably depict hypoxia with a chronic respiratory alkalosis. Lung perfusion scanning is often normal although patchy defects may be observed (Rich et al. 1987). Magnetic resonance imaging may be used to evaluate right ventricular function (Tardivon et al. 1994). Pulmonary angiography shows characteristic pruning of distal vessels in patients with idiopathic PAH. Positive antinuclear antibodies at titres of 1:80 dilutions or greater are found in 40% of individuals with PAH compared to 6% of individuals with pulmonary hypertension of known causes and the general population (Rich et al. 1986). However, this does not necessarily imply an associated collagen vascular disease. Although histological analysis of explant or autopsy material cannot identify hypertension per se, the presence of characteristic changes in the pulmonary arteries, in the absence of known causes, supports a diagnosis of idiopathic PAH, as discussed later.

Treatment of Idiopathic PAH

Until relatively recently, treatment options were limited to avoidance of circumstances that may aggravate the disease (e.g., hypoxic conditions such as high altitude, pregnancy, oral contraceptives, and hormone replacement therapy), oxygen supplementation, diuretics, and heart-lung transplantation. There are now an increasing number of therapeutic interventions and an American College of Chest Physicians consensus panel has developed and updated guidelines for diagnosis and treatment of PAH (Badesch et al. 2004, 2007). Referral of patients with PAH to specialized pulmonary vascular units is strongly recommended for optimum diagnostic evaluation and treatment.

Deep vein thrombosis (secondary to right heart failure and impaired mobility) and pulmonary in situ thrombus formation (caused by sluggish flow, dysfunctional pulmonary vascular endothelium, abnormal fibrinolysis, enhanced procoagulant activity, and/or platelet abnormalities) are potential complications of PAH. Hence, the administration of oral anticoagulants alone can improve survival (Fuster et al. 1984).

High oral doses of calcium channel blockers, such as nifedipine and diltiazem, produce a sustained improvement in 25% of PAH patients who respond to an acute vasodilator trial. Hence, approximately 10% of patients benefit from this form of vasodilator treatment (Rich et al. 1992). Endothelium-derived vasodilators and vasoconstrictors modulate pulmonary vascular tone. In PAH patients, circulating levels of the vasodilator prostacyclin (PGI2) are reduced with increased urinary excretion of metabolites (Christman et al. 1992). In addition, pulmonary arterial endothelial cells have reduced expression of prostacyclin synthase (Tuder et al. 1999). Continuous intravenous prostacyclin (sodium epoprostenol; Flolan) improves hemodynamics and exercise tolerance and prolongs survival in severe PAH (Barst et al. 1996). In some patients, pulmonary artery pressure decreases despite lack of acute vasodilator response (McLaughlin et al. 1998). Properties of the drug other than its vasodilator activity, including the inhibition of platelet aggregation and effects on vascular remodeling, may be responsible for these long-term effects and improved survival. However, major drawbacks include its expense, short half-life, side effects, and the requirement of an indwelling Hickman line susceptible to sepsis. The success of prostacyclin therapy led to trials of more stable analogs via other routes of administration. The use of treprostinil (subcutaneous or intravenous), iloprost (inhalation), and beraprost (oral) have shown significant improvements in pulmonary hemodynamics and exercise capacity (Galie et al. 2002; Olschewski et al. 2002). Clinical trials continue with alternative drugs based on observations of other vasoactive mediators.

Phosphodiesterase type 5, responsible for cyclic 3'-5'-guanosine monophosphate (cGMP) metabolism in the lung, is thought to influence pulmonary vascular tone and structure (Cohen et al. 1996; Fukumoto et al. 1999). In support of these observations, sildenafil, a phosphodiesterase type 5 inhibitor, reduces pulmonary artery pressure in PAH patients (Prasad et al. 2000; Sastry et al. 2002). Endothelin-1 is a powerful vasoconstrictor, mitogen and profibrotic agent thought to play a role in intimal proliferation and vasoconstriction. PAH patients have enhanced expression and increased concentrations of endothelin (Stewart et al. 1991; Giaid et al. 1993). Initial trials of bosentan, an oral dual receptor antagonist of endothelin-1, show some improvement in exercise capacity and pulmonary hemodynamics but has been discontinued in a proportion of patients due to raised aminotransferases (Channick et al. 2001; Rubin et al. 2002; Humbert et al. 2007).

Surgical interventions remain an option for PAH patients in whom medical therapy has been unsuccessful (Doyle et al. 2004). Blade balloon atrial septostomy creates a right to left shunt in the atria allowing decompression of the right heart and improved filling of the left-sided chambers. This technique may be used as palliative therapy in selected PAH patients with recurrent syncope or refractory right heart failure (Kerstein et al. 1995; Rich et al. 1997). A patient failing on medical therapy may be referred for a heart and/or lung transplant (Reitz et al. 1982; Pasque et al. 1995). However, drawbacks include lack of donor organs, the need for long-term immunosuppression, and organ rejection. Interestingly, disease recurrence has never been reported following a heart and/or lung transplant, emphasizing that local pulmonary factors are crucial in the pathogenesis of idiopathic PAH.

Prognosis in Idiopathic PAH

The two most frequent mechanisms of death in PAH are progressive right ventricular failure (47%) and sudden unexpected death (26%) (Dresdale et al. 1951; D'Alonzo et al. 1991). Outlook is directly proportional to cardiopulmonary hemodynamics, particularly raised right atrial and pulmonary artery pressures and decreased cardiac index (cardiac output divided by body surface area) (D'Alonzo et al. 1991). Age of onset, duration of symptoms, gender, and family history do not affect prognosis (D'Alonzo et al. 1991; Loyd et al. 1995). Cardiopulmonary exercise testing by means of a "6-minute" walk can be used to monitor disease progression. Exercise capacity, oxygen consumption, and ventilatory responses correlate well with pulmonary hemodynamics and long-term survival (D'Alonzo et al. 1987; Barst et al. 1996).

In the 1980s, the median survival was 2.8 years from diagnosis (D'Alonzo et al. 1991). However, prognosis has improved recently with increasing knowledge and availability of therapies. First, the introduction of anticoagulants enhanced prospects and, in the 10% of patients who respond to calcium antagonists, there is a 90% 5-year survival rate (Rich et al. 1992). The use of continuous intravenous prostacyclin has increased 3-year survival rates from 40.6% to 63.3% and is comparable to lung transplantation (50%–60%) (Glanville et al. 1987; Barst et al. 1994).

In a series of 137 idiopathic PAH patients from the United Kingdom, Oakley describes the onset of symptoms to death ranging from 2 months to 42 years (Oakley 1994). There are additional idiopathic PAH case reports of unusually long duration between 15 and 40 years in length (Nielsen and Fabricius 1961; Charters et al. 1970; Wagenvoort et al. 1970; Trell 1973; Suarez 1979). The natural history of pathological changes within the pulmonary vasculature in idiopathic PAH is unclear. Although the majority of individuals have progressive disease, the cases described with long duration highlight the variability observed and serve to question the possible elements that modify the course of the condition.

Vascular Remodeling in Idiopathic PAH

In large elastic pulmonary arteries the media contains smooth muscle cells and collagen fibers between concentric elastic layers. In contrast, the media of smaller muscular pulmonary arteries (external diameter 100–1,000 μm) is predominantly composed of concentric smooth muscle fibers (Hatano and Strasser 1973). Precapillary pulmonary arteries of less than 80 μm in diameter are normally devoid of smooth muscle and have a single internal elastic lamina.

Some or all of the histopathological features listed below may be present and are characteristic, but not pathognomic, of idiopathic PAH (Figures 25–1 and 25–2). Identical changes can also occur in PAH associated with congenital heart disease, portal hypertension, human immunodeficiency virus, collagen vascular disease, appetite suppressants, and shistosomiasis (Gordon et al. 1954; Naye 1968; Wagenvoort et al. 1970; Moser and Bloor 1993; Tuder et al. 1994)

Intimal fibrosis and fibroelastosis develop in a characteristic concentric "onion skin" configuration (Wagenvoort et al. 1964). The elastic pulmonary arteries often reveal patchy atheromatosis and rupture of the intima and/or media with potential aneurysm formation (Heath and Edwards 1958; Nienaber et al. 1986; Masuda et al. 1996; Wekerle et al. 1998; Wunderbaldinger et al. 2000; Cherwek and Amundson 2003). Smooth muscle cell hypertrophy is observed in pulmonary arteries between 100 and 1,000 μm in external diameter (Hatano and Strasser 1973). There is muscularization of arteries less than 80 μm in diameter with formation of distinct internal and external elastic laminae and increased extracellular matrix (Hatano and Strasser 1973; Pietra 1994). In some instances, fibrinoid vascular necrosis and arteritis is present in the walls of muscular pulmonary arteries (Wagenvoort et al. 1970). There is fibroblast proliferation and differentiation within the adventitia and an increase in matrix proteins (Chazova et al. 1995). Plexiform lesions resemble disorganized vessels and are composed of proliferating endothelial cells, smooth muscle cells, myofibroblasts, and macrophages (Figure 25–3; Smith et al. 1990; Tuder et al. 1994; Atkinson et al. 2002). These lesions usually arise from a hypertrophied muscular pulmonary artery, approximately 100–200 μm in diameter, which has just branched from its parent artery. Plexiform lesions are thought to be the result of an angiogenic response to local ischemia or hypoxia, occurring distal to vascular obstructive lesions (Wagenvoort 1959; Eddahibi et al. 2002). In one study, 70% of PAH patients (n = 110) had plexiform lesions (Wagenvoort et al. 1970). Clusters of markedly dilated thin-walled vessels or angiomatoid lesions may occur in up to 62% of PAH patients (n = 110) (Wagenvoort et al. 1970). In situ thrombus may develop in the lumen of small pulmonary arteries.

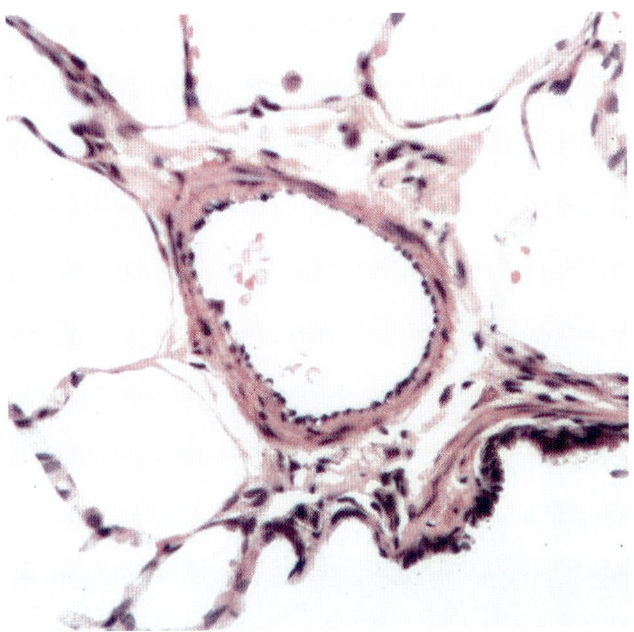

Figure 25–1 Cross-section of a normal small pulmonary artery (Trembath et al. 2001).

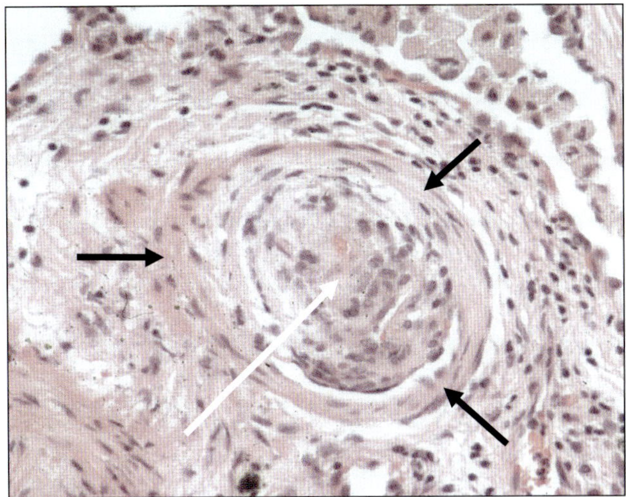

Figure 25–2 Cross-section demonstrating a thick-walled peripheral pulmonary artery (black arrow) occluded by a cellular intimal proliferation (white arrow) in idiopathic PAH (Trembath et al. 2001).

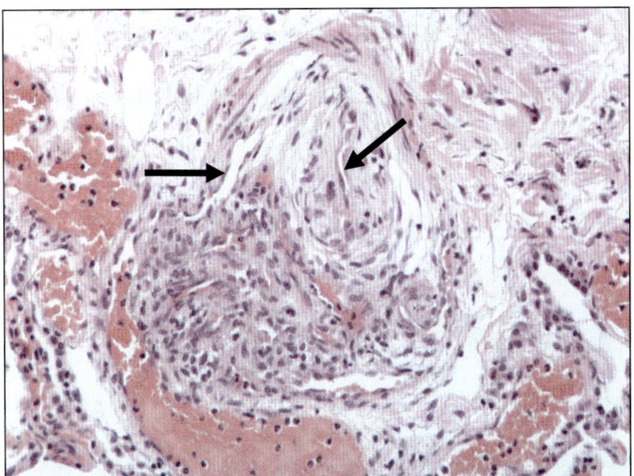

Figure 25–3 Cross-section showing a plexiform lesion with thin-walled capillary channels (arrowed) (Trembath et al. 2001).

Familial Pulmonary Arterial Hypertension

In 1927, two sisters with gross right ventricular dilatation, pulmonary artery atheroma, and endothelial proliferation were presented to the Association of Physicians, United Kingdom

(Clarke et al. 1927). The meeting concluded that "there is some inherited influence at work in the persons of this family, the nature of which is entirely hidden from us." In 1954, Dresdale was able to confirm for the first time the hemodynamic findings of PAH in two sisters and one son subsequent to the development of cardiac catheterization (Cournand and Ranges 1941; Dresdale et al. 1954). Since that time, over 200 families have been documented in North America and many others in Europe, Australasia, and Asia.

Mode of Inheritance and Gene Penetrance

Having met a family with two affected males and three affected females in three generations, Melmon and Braunwald proposed that genetic transmission of familial PAH was autosomal dominant with variable penetrance (Melmon and Braunwald 1963). In addition to this pedigree, there were other cases of male to male transmission, thus excluding X-linked inheritance (Kingdon et al. 1966; Loyd et al. 1984).

From the National Institute of Health (NIH) study of 187 PAH patients, 6% had at least one first-degree relative with PAH (Rich et al. 1987). The occurrence of inherited PAH appears to be low for a number of reasons: (1) a full family history is often not obtained; (2) incomplete gene penetrance may mask a family history of the condition; (3) loss of contact between relatives; and (4) misdiagnosis may also hamper acknowledgment of an inherited condition (Newman et al. 2001).

In familial PAH, the gene penetrance is variable and not all individuals inheriting the disease gene will develop PAH in their lifetime, for example, a kindred in which two affected relatives were identified with six intervening asymptomatic obligate gene carriers (Elliott et al. 1995). Gene penetrance appears to depend on a number of factors, including age, gender, and as yet unidentified variables. In one study of 24 PAH families, there were 99 symptomatic (72 females, 27 males) and 25 asymptomatic obligate gene carriers (12 females, 13 males) (Loyd et al. 1995). Hence 86% of females assumed to have the altered gene, from pedigree analysis alone, had developed PAH compared to 68% of males. In these families, the age correction for penetrance was calculated as 10% by 10 years of age and 92% by 70 years of age. In one large family, 18 individuals developed PAH out of a total of 41 gene carriers equating to an overall gene penetrance of 44% (Newman et al. 2001). However, no studies to date have calculated the disease gene penetrance using both clinical and molecular data, to overcome bias from exclusion of nonobligate gene carriers.

Age of Onset and Anticipation

In the NIH study there was no difference in age at time of enrolment between those with and without a family history of PAH (Rich et al. 1987). However, Kingdon noted the apparent tendency of familial PAH to occur at an earlier age in successive generations, raising the possibility of anticipation (Penrose 1948; Kingdon et al. 1966; Crow 1991). Loyd et al. analyzed 24 families with 124 affected or obligate carriers for evidence of anticipation (Loyd et al. 1995). The mean age at death in each generation decreased from 45.6 +/– 11.2 years (n = 13) in the first generation to 36.3 +/– 12.6 years (n = 41) in the second generation to 24.2 +/– 11.0 years (n = 42) in the third generation ($p<0.05$). Loyd's group hypothesized that the apparent anticipation observed in their familial PAH cohort was due to the presence of trinucleotide repeat expansion in genomic DNA. They utilized the repeat expansion detection (RED) assay but demonstrated the presence of many expanded triplets in control subjects as well as familial PAH patients (Loyd et al. 1997). To date, there has been no evidence of trinucleotide repeat expansion as the underlying biological mechanism for anticipation in familial PAH.

Clinical Features of Familial PAH

The clinical, histopathological, and prognostic features of familial PAH are indistinguishable from those of idiopathic PAH cases with no known family history, as previously described in this chapter.

Clinical Screening for Relatives at Risk of PAH

Idiopathic PAH is thought to pass from a reversible vasoconstrictive to an irreversible proliferative stage, a process that may occur before the onset of symptoms and signs. Treatment at an early stage of disease maybe easier, more effective, and less costly than later more intensive therapy, although no prospective trials have been undertaken to date (Rich et al. 1992; Barst et al. 1996; Higenbottam et al. 1998). Therefore, screening is recommended for this condition (Rich 1998a). For relatives of idiopathic PAH patients, screening should include a thorough history and examination followed by a transthoracic ECHO, the preferred screening test for pulmonary hypertension, being sensitive, simple, safe, and relatively inexpensive (Rich 1998a). One drawback of using ECHO as a screening test at rest is that at least 70% of the pulmonary circulation must be obstructed before pulmonary artery pressure rises. Performing ECHO during exercise is more likely to detect evidence of pulmonary artery occlusion, although this is a difficult technique (Grunig et al. 2000). A CXR and ECG may also be undertaken as part of screening investigations. Suggested frequency of testing is at the time of diagnosis of the index case, if symptomatic or every 3 years in asymptomatic individuals. If estimated pulmonary artery pressure is greater than 40 mmHg, cardiac catheterization is recommended (Rich 1998a).

Identification of a Gene Predisposing to Pulmonary Arterial Hypertension

Familial PAH Linkage Studies

In 1997, two research groups independently mapped a PAH susceptibility gene to a locus on chromosome 2q31–33, designated *PPH1* (MIM 178600) (Morse et al. 1997; Nichols et al. 1997). Based on recombination events in affected families, the candidate region was narrowed to 4.8cM between markers *D2S115* and *D2S1384* (Figure 25–4; Machado et al. 2000). All families appeared linked, suggesting genetic homogeneity, and there was no evidence of a founder haplotype.

The PPH1 Critical Interval and Construction of a Physical Map

To assist in positional cloning of the gene, Machado et al. verified and extended a published YAC map at chromosome 2q33 to anchor a BAC/PAC contig, including genomic sequences available at GenBank (Hadano et al. 1999; Machado et al. 2000). By means of database and PCR screening, 79 potential transcriptional units were positioned within a 5.8 Mb interval between *D2S115* and *D2S1384*, including 15 partially or completely characterized genes (Machado et al. 2000).

The Bone Morphogenetic Protein Receptor Type 2 Gene

One of the 15 known genes in the interval, the bone morphogenetic protein receptor type 2 (*BMPR2*) gene represented a strong biological candidate. The gene encodes for the 1,038 amino acid

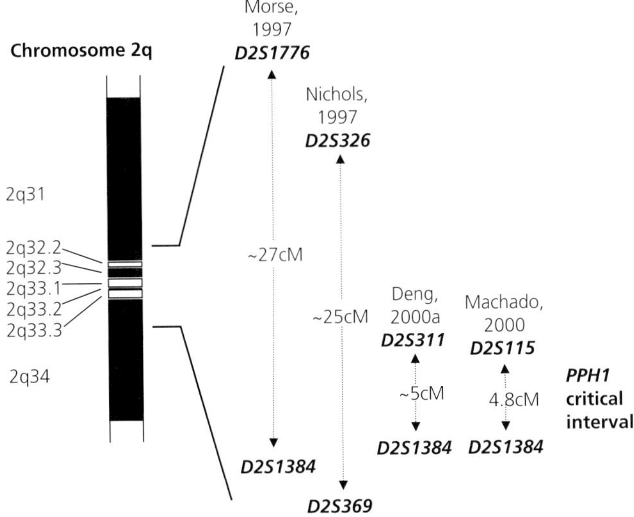

Figure 25–4 Ideogram of chromosome 2q and reduction of the *PPH1* critical interval.

bone morphogenetic protein type II receptor (BMPR-II), a transmembrane serine/threonine kinase receptor member of the transforming growth factor β (TGFβ) superfamily. The TGFβ signaling pathway is involved in many cellular mechanisms, including vascular differentiation and proliferation (Schulick et al. 1998). DNA sequencing subsequently identified pathological sequence variants in the *BMPR2* gene to underlie familial PAH (International PPH Consortium et al. 2000; Deng et al. 2000b).

BMPR2 Gene Structure

The *BMPR2* gene was originally identified in 1995 through a yeast two-hybrid screen using TGFβ family type I receptors as bait (Kawabata et al. 1995; Liu et al. 1995; Rosenzweig et al. 1995). The genomic structure of the mouse *bmpr2* gene was determined in 1997 and the human *BMPR2* gene localized to 2q33–34 in 1999 (Beppu et al. 1997; Astrom et al. 1999). The gene has 13 exons spanning over 80 kilobases (kb) (Figure 25–5). Two large introns (one and three) contribute to a majority of the gene size.

BMPR-II Protein Structure

Forty-nine of 51 nucleotides of the signal peptide are encoded in exon 1. The major part of the extracellular (ligand-binding) region is encoded by exons 2 and 3 (Figure 25–5). Crystal structure of the activin A receptor type II extracellular domain, a related type II receptor of the TGFβ superfamily, reveals a typical pattern of four disulfide bridges and three β-pleated sheets conferring a three-finger fold similar to snake toxin (Greenwald et al. 1999). The cysteine residues that form the disulphide bridges are conserved in both type I and II receptors of the TGFβ superfamily (Massague et al. 1998). Exon 4 encodes the entire transmembrane region and exons 5–11 the serine/threonine kinase region (Figure 25–5). Exons 12 and 13 encode the long cytoplasmic carboxy-terminus tail, unique to BMPR-II. Alternative splicing can yield a shortened form of BMPR-II of 530 amino acids, lacking the region encoded by exon 12 (Kawabata et al. 1995; Liu et al. 1995).

There is 96.6% homology of the human and mouse BMPR-II amino acid sequence. The receptor is also distantly related to DAF4, a BMP type II receptor in *Caenorhabditis elegans* (Beppu et al. 1997). Using Northern blot and reverse transcriptase polymerase chain reaction (RT-PCR) analysis, long and short forms of BMPR-II are ubiquitously expressed in fetal and adult tissue, including lung (Nohno et al. 1995; Rosenzweig et al. 1995). More specifically, BMPR-II localizes immunohistologically to endothelial cells and myofibroblasts within PAH obliterative lesions (Morrell et al. 2001). In addition, BMPR-II expression is markedly reduced in the peripheral lung of familial and idiopathic PAH patients compared to less marked reduction in pulmonary hypertension of known cause, possibly representing reduced expression from not only the mutant but also the wild-type allele (Atkinson et al. 2002).

PAH and *BMPR2* Gene Mutations

To date, using direct sequencing, denaturing high-performance liquid chromatography (DHPLC), Southern blotting, and multiplex ligation-dependent probe amplification (MLPA) a total of 298 heterozygous *BMPR2* mutations have been identified, 88 of which are novel (Machado et al. 2006). Using these methods, over 70% of PAH patients with at least one affected relative and 10%–40% with no known family history have identifiable *BMPR2* gene

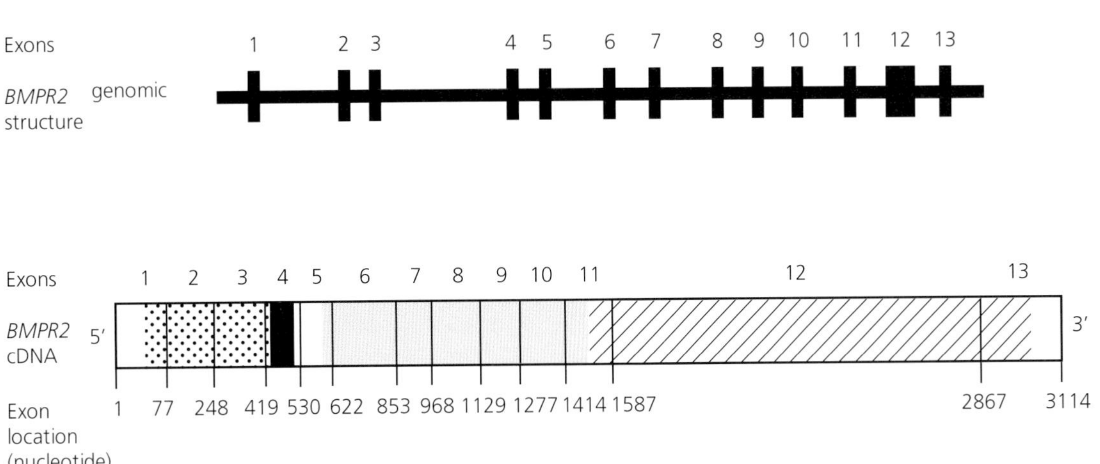

Figure 25–5 BMPR2 genomic structure, complimentary DNA (cDNA) and encoded domains. The locations of the exons are indicated by the nucleotide start position, below the cDNA. The stippled area denotes the sequence encoding the ligand binding domain, the black area the transmembrane domain, the grey area the kinase domain and the striped area the cytoplasmic tail.

mutations of similar type (Thomson et al. 2000; Aldred et al. 2006; Morisaki et al. 2004; Machado et al. 2006). Sixty-eight percent of mutations predict premature protein truncation, including 29% nonsense, 24% frame-shift, 9% splice-site, and 6% gene duplications/deletions (Machado et al. 2006). Thus, haploinsufficiency is the predominant molecular mechanism underlying *BMPR2* gene predisposition to PAH (Machado et al. 2001).

BMPR2 missense mutations in PAH tend to cluster in regions of the gene encoding receptor domains and are confined to exons 2, 3, 6–9, 11, and 12 (Machado et al. 2006). The extracellular ligand-binding domain of BMPR-II is dependent on the formation of five disulfide bridges by ten cysteine residues in exons 2 and 3 (Greenwald et al. 1999). Amino acid substitutions in this domain are common. Analysis of cysteine mutant constructs demonstrates cytosolic retention, probably due to loss of protein conformation (Rudarakanchana et al. 2002). In the BMPR-II catalytic domain, missense mutations are typically restricted to regions crucial to kinase activity and display a near complete abolition of signaling through the Smad pathway (Rudarakanchana et al. 2002). Amino acid substitutions are infrequently detected in the BMPR-II cytoplasmic domain and, in contrast, appear to activate Smad-independent pathways, notably p38MAPK (Rudarakanchana et al. 2002).

A proportion of families remain in which *BMPR2* gene mutations have not yet been identified. Parts of the *BMPR2* gene are unsequenced in these kindreds, such as intronic sequences. Genetic heterogeneity must be considered where linkage has not been established due to insufficient DNA samples from relevant family members, although there has been no firm evidence to suggest this. Finally, the possibility of phenocopies cannot be totally excluded.

Studying DNA of asymptomatic parents from idiopathic PAH patients determined that these *BMPR2* gene mutations can be inherited or de novo (Thomson et al. 2000). As the number of patient–parent trios reported for *BMPR2* gene analysis is currently small in idiopathic PAH, testing of further individuals is required to determine more accurately the proportion of inherited versus spontaneous mutations.

Genotype/Phenotype Correlations of PAH and *BMPR2* Gene Mutations

Interestingly only a few patients with *BMPR2* gene mutations have evidence of pulmonary vasoreactivity following an acute vasodilator challenge. In contrast, a much greater number of cases of PAH without identifiable *BMPR2* gene mutations respond to an acute vasodilator challenge. Fifty percent of males (n = 5) and 27.5% of females (n = 11) amongst 50 idiopathic PAH patients had identifiable *BMPR2* gene mutations (Thomson et al. 2000). One of nine patients with a mutation was known to be responsive to vasodilators on acute challenge during right heart catheterization compared to 10 of 21 without mutations (unpublished data). Published studies are consistent with this observation. Vasoreactivity was identified in 3.7%–4% of patients with *BMPR2* gene mutations compared to 33%–35% of patients without mutations ($p = 0.003$) (Elliott et al. 2006; Rosenzweig et al. 2008). Hence, determination of *BMPR2* mutations appears to help identify individuals who are unlikely to respond to acute vasodilator testing and, thus, unlikely to benefit from calcium channel blockers.

Other clinical features, prognosis, pulmonary artery pressure, and histological examination of pulmonary arteries, do not distinguish between those with and without a *BMPR2* gene mutation. Marked differences in the age of onset are noted both within and between families with *BMPR2* gene mutations, for example, age of onset varied from 1 to 42 years in one documented family and 14 to 60 years in another kindred (Machado et al. 2001). Such variance may reflect a genotype–phenotype relationship or independent genetic and environmental modifiers.

BMPR2 Gene Mutations Identified in Associated PAH Conditions

The incidence of PAH escalated in Switzerland, Austria, and Germany in the late 1960s subsequent to the availability of the appetite suppressant aminorex fumarate (2-amino-5-phenyl-2-oxazoline) (Gurtner 1969, 1985). In the early 1990s Brenot reported a group of patients with PAH who had used derivatives of the appetite suppressant fenfluramine, particularly dexfenfluramine (Brenot et al. 1993). A case-control study of 95 European PAH patients showed that use of appetite suppressant drugs, particularly fenfluramine, dexfenfluramine, and amphetamine-like compounds for more than 3 months, is associated with a 23.1-fold increased risk of developing a disorder clinically and histologically indistinguishable from idiopathic PAH (Abenhaim et al. 1996). The effect of appetite suppressants is independent of body mass index, thus obesity per se is not responsible for the increased risk of PAH.

BMPR2 gene mutations have since been detected in a minority of individuals who have developed pulmonary hypertension after the ingestion of appetite suppressants. In 33 French PAH patients who had taken fenfluramine and/or dexfenfluramine, 4 heterozygous *BMPR2* gene mutations were identified (Humbert et al. 2002). In addition, novel missense *BMPR2* gene mutations have been detected in 6 of 106 subjects with congenital heart disease and PAH (Roberts et al. 2004). The cardiac abnormalities in the mutation-positive cases included complete atrioventricular canals, atrial septal defects, patent ductus arteriosus, partial anomalous pulmonary venous return, and one ventricular septal defect. However, the mutation spectrum in PAH associated with both appetite suppressants and congenital heart disease is different to that of familial and idiopathic disease (Machado et al. 2006). The relationship of these *BMPR2* gene variants is unknown but may represent rare susceptibility alleles that only cause PAH in association with additional genetic or environmental factors. Thirty patients with HIV-associated PAH (19 French and 11 American) have been analyzed for *BMPR2* gene mutations but none found to date (Morse 2002). *BMPR2* mutations have not been identified in one case of chronic thromboembolic disease and a number of patients with connective tissue disease (Atkinson et al. 2002; Tew et al. 2002).

Implications of Genetic Analysis in the Management of Inherited PAH

Identification of underlying pathogenic mechanisms has important implications for patient diagnosis, genetic counseling, and clinical screening in PAH gene mutation carriers. The absence of specific clinical features and noninvasive investigative tools frequently contributes to a delay in securing the diagnosis of idiopathic PAH. Molecular genetic analysis should now be considered as a potential diagnostic aid for this group of patients. The identification of a gene mutation in a proband is highly significant for relatives, whether it be for the offspring of an individual with a de novo mutation or a larger number of family members where the gene variant has clearly been inherited. While clinical methods of screening in PAH aim to detect evidence of disease in an asymptomatic individual, predictive genetic testing identifies susceptibility to the pathogenic process.

Ideally, the identification of a PAH gene carrier would prompt lifestyle modifications and therapeutic measures that could prevent the onset of the disease. However, there have been no prospective trials to date determining the effect of such measures. Furthermore, knowledge of disease gene status may cause undue anxiety in an individual who never actually develops PAH and there is the possibility of being prejudiced by insurance agencies in the future. Conversely, those found not to be PAH gene mutation carriers would no longer have the worry of manifesting the disease or transmitting the disease gene to offspring. In addition, they would not require long-term clinical screening and females could commence a pregnancy in safety with respect to PAH. Due to these important issues, predictive genetic testing should only be undertaken with appropriate genetic counseling.

Bone Morphogenetic Proteins and the TGFβ Signaling Pathway

Bone morphogenetic proteins (BMPs) were originally identified as proteins capable of inducing bone formation at extraskeletal sites in vivo (Wozney et al. 1988). BMPs belong to the TGFβ superfamily of ligands and are regulated through reversible interactions with extracellular antagonists, including noggin, chordin, and DAN (Piek et al. 1999; Reddi 2001). BMPs and other TGFβ superfamily ligands transduce their signals through formation of heteromeric complexes of two different types of serine/threonine kinase receptors, type I and type II (Figure 25–6; ten Dijke et al. 1994). The constitutively active cytoplasmic kinase domain of the type II receptor phosphorylates a glycine-serine rich domain (GS loop) on the proximal intracellular portion of the type I receptor. This activates the type I receptor kinase domain initiating phosphorylation of cytoplasmic signaling proteins called SMADs (Figure 25–6; Raftery and Sutherland 1999). BMPs signal via activation of SMAD1, SMAD5, and SMAD8 (Receptor or R-SMADs), complexing with SMAD4 (Comediator or CoSMAD) and translocating to the nucleus to regulate gene transcription (Figure 25–6; Kawabata et al. 1998; Shi and Massague 2003). The specificity of the TGFβ signaling pathway is dependent on a number of positive and negative regulatory elements in different cell types at multiple levels of the cascade, including ligand binding, receptor interaction, SMAD activation, and transcription augmentation (Ring and Cho 1999; Nohe 2002). Interruption of any stage of this process may result in a pathological process (Blobe et al. 2000).

Pathogenesis of idiopathic PAH

Evidence suggests that the combination of vascular injury and changes in hemodynamics may direct the neointimal response (Voelkel and Tuder 1995; Stenmark et al. 1997). Endothelial cell damage also transforms the pulmonary vascular bed to a procoagulant state (Ryan 1986). Idiopathic PAH patients have enhanced platelet activity with increased circulating serotonin, plasminogen activator inhibitor and fibrinopeptide A, and decreased levels of thrombomodulin (Eisenberg et al. 1990; Herve et al. 1995; Welsh et al. 1996). Thrombotic lesions are present in one-third of patients and anticoagulant therapy improves survival (Wagenvoort et al. 1970; Pietra et al. 1989). Thus, hypercoagulability and in situ thrombus contribute to progression of disease. The imbalance in the growth inhibitory vasodilators (prostacyclin and nitric oxide) and the growth-promoting vasoconstrictors (endothelin-1, thromboxane A2, and serotonin) is thought to be a consequence of endothelial dysfunction and an important factor in the vascular remodeling that occurs in idiopathic PAH (Palmer et al. 1987; Christman et al. 1992). In cell culture, loss of BMPR-II leads to apoptosis susceptibility in pulmonary artery endothelial cells and proliferation of pulmonary artery smooth muscle cells (Morrell et al. 2001; Teichert-Kuliszewska et al. 2006).

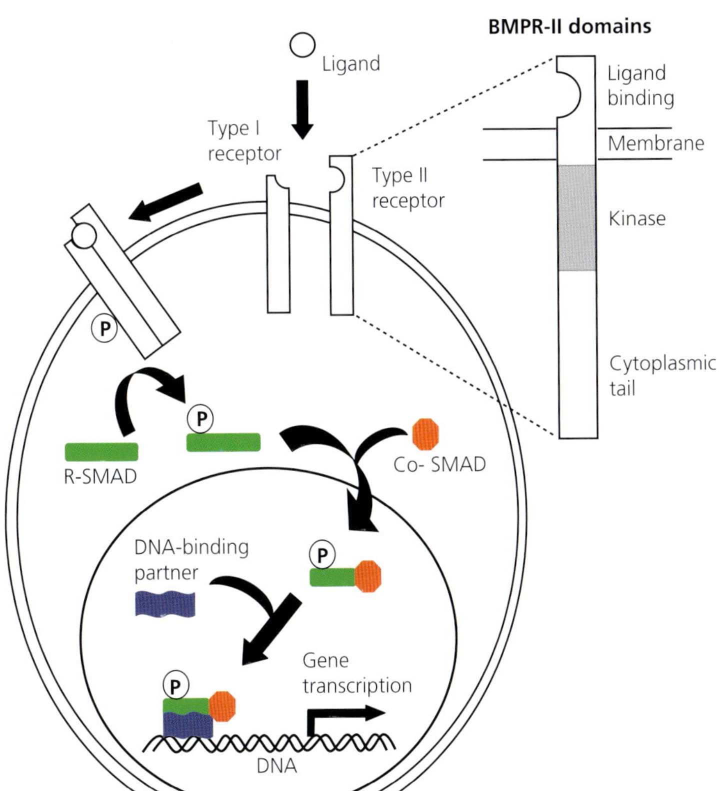

Figure 25–6 BMPR-II domains and the SMAD-dependent TGFβ signaling pathway (Thomson et al. 2000). Following ligand binding, BMPR-II forms a heteromeric complex with a type I receptor, resulting in activation of the type I receptor kinase domain. This activates phosphorylation (P) of SMADs leading to signal transduction.

Interestingly, conditional heterozygous or homozygous bmpr2 deletions specifically in pulmonary endothelial cells predisposes mice to develop PAH (Hong et al. 2008). Homozygous *bmpr2* mutant (bmpr2$^{-/-}$) mice die in utero before mesoderm formation (Beppu et al. 2000). Heterozygous *bmpr2* mutant mice (bmpr2$^{+/-}$) are morphologically normal and fertile but under inflammatory stress are more susceptible to increased right ventricular systolic pressure and vascular remodeling than wild type (Beppu et al. 2004; Song et al. 2005). Transgenic mice expressing a dominant negative *bmpr2* gene expressed postnatally in smooth muscle results in increased right ventricular systolic pressure but only modest vascular remodeling (West et al. 2004), suggesting that other genetic and environmental factors play an important role in the development of PAH.

One of the fundamental structural changes in the pulmonary vasculature in idiopathic PAH is the abnormal synthesis and deposition of connective tissue proteins, particularly elastin and collagen, within different layers of the vessel wall (Todorovich-Hunter et al. 1988). Using the rat model of pulmonary hypertension induced by monocrotaline injection, an endogenous vascular elastase has been identified in serum that promotes proliferation and migration of vascular smooth muscle (Zhu et al. 1994). Experiments in these rats show that elastase inhibitors can prevent or retard proliferative and migratory responses (Cowan et al. 2000).

Many idiopathic PAH patients have evidence of autoimmunity and/or active inflammation, including circulating antinuclear antibodies, elevated serum interleukin 1 (IL-1) and interleukin 6 (IL-6), and increased pulmonary expression of platelet-derived growth factor or macrophage inflammatory protein 1α (Humbert et al. 1995). Perivascular inflammatory infiltrates with T- and B-lymphocytes and macrophages occur in association with plexiform lesions (Tuder et al. 1994). IL-1 and IL-6 promote thrombosis and are potent mitogens, hence inflammatory responses may alter pulmonary vascular reactivity and contribute to vessel wall remodeling and in situ thrombus (Nawroth et al. 1986).

The pathogenesis of idiopathic PAH remains unclear despite the identification of BMPR-II defects as a major predisposing factor and countless studies of varying pulmonary vascular cellular and molecular mechanisms. The identification of modifier genes of the BMP/TGFβ signaling pathways will help determine the pathogenesis of PAH in susceptible individuals.

Pulmonary Arterial Hypertension and Hereditary Hemorrhagic Telangiectasia (HHT)

The association between repeated epistaxis and small mucocutaneous "angiomas" was first reported by Rendu in 1896, followed by Osler observing this as heritable and Weber characterizing a triad of features, defining the disease that became known as the Osler-Rendu-Weber syndrome (Rendu 1896; Osler 1901; Weber 1907). Now more widely referred to as hereditary hemorrhagic telangiectasia (HHT), this autosomal dominant condition consisting of telangiectasia and arteriovenous malformations of both systemic and pulmonary circulations is diagnosed clinically using the Curaçao consensus criteria (Shovlin et al. 2000).

HHT has been described in all racial groups. The prevalence is estimated at 1 per 10,000 population, occurring more frequently in the Dutch Antilles, parts of France, and the Danish island of Funen and Fyn (Vase et al. 1985; Vase and Grove 1986; Bideau et al. 1989; Plauchu et al. 1989; Porteous et al. 1992; Jessurun et al. 1993). HHT is equally frequent in males and females (Peery 1987).

Clinical Features of HHT

Epistaxis is present in up to 96% of patients and is usually the earliest clinical symptom of HHT (Plauchu et al. 1989). Other features of HHT include facial and buccal telangiectasia, arteriovenous malformations (AVMs), and gastrointestinal hemorrhage. AVMs consist of thin-walled vascular spaces between arteries and veins, which may reach several centimeters in diameter. There may be single or multiple feeding arteries but no intervening capillaries are present. In HHT, AVMs occur particularly in the brain, liver, and lungs. An estimated 10% of patients will die from HHT-related complications, particularly from the consequences of paradoxical emboli due to pulmonary AVMs.

Pulmonary Manifestations of HHT

AVMs in the lungs occur between the pulmonary arterial and venous systems (PAVMs) (Bosher et al. 1959; White et al. 1983). They either consist of microscopic telangiectatic vessels or complex macroscopic structures, up to 50 mm in diameter. Eighty percent of PAVMs are associated with HHT and 14%–30% of individuals with HHT develop PAVMs (Haitjema et al. 1996b; Shovlin et al. 1997a). They tend to present in early adulthood and more often in females (ratio 1.9 female: 1 male) (Dutton et al. 1995; Shovlin et al. 1995). Approximately half of all HHT patients with PAVMs are asymptomatic despite clinical signs (Dines et al. 1983). A major complication is the free passage of emboli from the venous system to the cerebral circulation causing transient ischemic attacks, cerebrovascular accidents (30%–40%), and cerebral abscesses (5%–20%), accounting for the majority of the 4%–22% mortality rate in symptomatic but untreated patients with PAVMs (Sluiter-Eringa et al. 1969; Dines et al. 1974). Massive pulmonary hemorrhage may occur from spontaneous rupture (Shovlin et al. 1995).

Pulmonary hypertension is infrequently recognized in the presence of HHT and may be attributed to other facets of the disease or its treatment. Systemic AVMs may produce an increased workload on the heart causing high output cardiac failure. The resultant increase in left atrial pressure can lead to raised pulmonary artery wedge pressure and PAH (Holman 1962; Childers et al. 1967; Haitjema et al. 1996a). Another potential mechanism for the development of pulmonary hypertension in HHT is in situ thrombus formation in PAVMs or thromboembolism from deep veins or systemic AVMs (Pritchard and Llewelyn 1987; White et al. 1994; Clouston et al. 1995). One of the treatments for epistaxis and gastrointestinal bleeding in HHT is estrogen, a well-established cause of increased coagulability (Poller 1978). Finally, pulmonary hypertension in association with a personal or family history of HHT can be due to a primary abnormality of the pulmonary vasculature that is clinically, hemodynamically, and histologically similar to idiopathic PAH associated with *BMPR2* gene mutations (Sapru et al. 1969; Trell et al. 1972b; Trembath et al. 2001). Pulmonary artery pressure is not frequently measured in patients with HHT and the lack of hemodynamic data may conceal a true incidence of associated PAH.

Genotype/Phenotype Correlations of HHT and Pulmonary Vascular Disease

Mutations in four genes, *endoglin, ALK1, SMAD4,* and *BMPR2,* have been described in patients with HHT. However, only *ALK1* and *BMPR2* pathogenic variants have been detected in individuals with idiopathic-type PAH in association with HHT.

The coding region of *ALK1* contains 9 exons, numbered 2–10, with exon 1 containing the 5' untranslated region, spanning greater than 15 kb of genomic DNA (ten Dijke et al. 1993; Berg et al. 1997). The *ALK1* gene encodes a 503 amino acid TGFβ type I cell surface receptor. *ALK1* is homologous to other TGFβ type I receptors, with an extracellular domain containing 10 cysteine residues and an intracellular domain consisting of a serine/threonine kinase domain, GS loop, and a short C-terminal tail (Hanks et al. 1988; Attisano et al. 1993; ten Dijke et al. 1993, 1994; Hanks and Hunter 1995). *ALK1* gene mutations have been identified as underlying idiopathic-type PAH in over 20 cases of HHT (Trembath et al. 2001; Harrison et al. 2003; Abdalla et al. 2004). Experiments using 15 different GFP or myc-tagged *ALK1* mutant constructs show that all but three are retained in the endoplasmic reticulum, supporting haploinsufficiency as the predominant molecular mechanism in PAH associated with HHT (Harrison et al. 2003). In total, six *ALK1* gene mutations predisposing to PAH are postulated to affect activity of the highly conserved GS loop domain that contains sites phosphorylated by type II receptors. Furthermore, four mutations, all identified in subjects with HHT-associated PAH, arise within the NANDOR BOX (Huse et al. 1999; Harrison et al. 2003; Abdalla et al. 2004). The NANDOR BOX is a highly conserved COOH domain of ALK1 from codons 479 to 489, that regulates GS domain phosphorylation and subsequent activation of the TGFβ receptor complex (Garamszegi et al. 2001; Harrison et al. 2003). In HHT only families, there have been no *ALK1* gene mutations identified in exons 5 or 10 that encode the GS loop and NANDOR BOX respectively. Hence, ALK1 variants that affect normal activity of the GS loop domain may be particularly important in the maintenance of normal pulmonary vasculature.

The high level of expression of ALK1 in endothelial cells, vascular smooth muscle cells, and placenta parallels that of endoglin (ten Dijke et al. 1993; Attisano et al. 1993; Caniggia et al. 1997; Roelen et al. 1997). However, in rats, the expression of ALK1 is greatest in pulmonary blood vessels (Panchenko et al. 1996). Mice lacking ALK1 die by midgestation with severe arteriovenous malformations resulting from fusion of major arteries and veins, indicating that ALK1 is required for developing distinct arterial and venous vascular beds (Urness et al. 2000). These vascular defects are associated with enhanced expression of angiogenic factors and proteases and are characterized by deficient differentiation and recruitment of vascular smooth muscle cells, demonstrating that ALK1 is essential for structural, functional, and molecular distinctions between arteries and veins (Oh et al. 2000; Urness et al. 2000). Mice heterozygous for loss-of-function mutations in ALK1 developed vascular lesions in the skin, extremities, oral cavity, lung, liver, intestine, spleen, and brain, similar to those seen in HHT2 patients (Srinivasan et al. 2003).

Recently, a 36-year-old woman with PAH, PAVMs, epistaxis, and telangiectasia was reported harboring a *BMPR2* nonsense gene mutation (Rigelsky et al. 2008). Hence, a similar PAH phenotype may arise from abnormalities of two different receptor members of the TGFβ superfamily, ALK1 and BMPR-II.

In direct contrast to PAH, PAVMs classically give rise to decreased pulmonary vascular resistance, increased cardiac output, and normal to low pulmonary artery pressure due to the presence of a low-resistance shunt (Moyer et al. 1962; Waldhausen and Abel 1966; Gomes et al. 1969). The suggestion has been made that PAVMs may cause PAH through hypoxia-induced vasospasm (Hasleton et al. 1968). However, there are few reports of PAVMs associated with PAH, despite their presence in 14%–30% of HHT patients (Haitjema et al. 1996b; Le Roux et al. 1970; Sperling et al. 1977; Rodan et al. 1981; Yoshida et al. 1995; Shovlin et al. 1997a). Interestingly, there are cases of PAH developing in patients following embolization or resection of pulmonary arteriovenous fistulae both in the presence and absence of HHT (Le Roux et al. 1970; Rodan et al. 1981; Haitjema et al. 1996b). Hence, the notion that PAVMs may well mask the presence of an obliterative pulmonary artery disorder in HHT, by way of a low-resistance shunt, is not inconceivable. As such, a diagnosis of PAH may be made less frequently in individuals with *ENG* mutations who have a higher degree of PAVMs (Berg et al. 1996, 2003). Indeed, no *ENG* gene mutations have yet been found in relation to idiopathic-type PAH disease. However, this study and others show PAVMs can occur in association with *ALK1* mutations, demonstrating the need to screen for pulmonary as well as systemic vascular malformations in all patients with HHT, irrespective of genotype (Berg et al. 1996; McDonald et al. 2000; Kjeldsen et al. 2001; Harrison et al. 2003; Abdalla et al. 2003b).

The presence of two seemingly diverse pathogenic processes, dilated vascular malformations and obliterative small pulmonary vessel disease, is intriguing. However, a similar paradox is well described in the systemic circulation in which arterial wall disease, such as atheroma, can lead to narrowing or dilatation of the vessel lumen in the same individual (Burn and Young 1992). Likewise, in idiopathic PAH, obliterative lesions can simultaneously occur in the small pulmonary arteries with atheroma and even aneurysms described in the larger pulmonary arteries (Wagenvoort et al. 1970; Nienaber et al. 1986; Cherwek and Amundson 2003). TGFβ signaling affects both vascular differentiation and proliferation, and overexpression of the TGFβ1 ligand promotes intimal growth and apoptosis simultaneously in vascular endothelium (Schulick et al. 1998). The pleiotropic nature of TGFβ as a growth factor offers a potential explanation for the variable complications of HHT. The net effect of ALK1 dysfunction may depend on local vascular interactions and other environmental or genetic factors.

Expansion of the HHT phenotype to include idiopathic-type PAH is clinically important for a number of reasons. Assessment of all pulmonary hypertensive patients should include a family history and HHT should form part of the differential diagnosis. Clinically, symptoms of breathlessness and syncope in an HHT patient are usually secondary to chronic hemorrhage and anemia from telangiectasia. However, these symptoms are also common in PAH and this diagnosis should be considered particularly in individuals who do not respond to iron therapy or blood transfusions. The potential occurrence of an obliterative process in the pulmonary vasculature should provide a better understanding of physiological and hemodynamic changes in HHT patients, important when considering embolization or ligation of a PAVM, which may be hazardous following closure of low-resistance channels.

Conclusions

Pathogenic variants in the *BMPR2* gene have been identified as the major predisposing factor in at least 70% of familial PAH and 10%–40% of patients with no known family history of the disease. In contrast, *ALK1* gene mutations are predominantly associated with PAH in association with HHT. However, both genes encode receptor members of the TGFβ signaling pathway and, as such, have identified the importance of this cascade in the maintenance of normal pulmonary vascular integrity. The identification of substantial numbers of genetically at-risk individuals, through international collaborative efforts, will enable assessment of the natural history of PAH and identification of disease biomarkers and modifiers. Greater understanding of underlying pathogenic mechanisms will ultimately allow for the development of novel and safer therapies.

References

Abdalla SA, Gallione CJ, Barst RJ, et al. Primary pulmonary hypertension in families with hereditary haemorrhagic telangiectasia. *Eur Respir J.* 2004;23:373–377.

Abdalla SA, Geisthoff UW, Bonneau D, et al. Visceral manifestations in hereditary haemorrhagic telangiectasia type 2. *J Med Genet.* 2003b; 40:494–502.

Abenhaim L, Moride Y, Brenot F, et al. Appetite-suppressant drugs and the risk of primary pulmonary hypertension. International Primary Pulmonary Hypertension Study Group. *N Engl J Med.* 1996;335:609–616.

Adams J, Alexander AM. Alterations in cardiovascular physiology during labor. *Obstet Gynecol.* 1958;12:542–549.

Aldred MA, Vijayakrishnan J, James V, et al. BMPR2 gene rearrangements account for a significant proportion of mutations in familial and idiopathic pulmonary arterial hypertension. *Hum Mutat.* 2006;27:212–213.

Appelbaum L, Yigla M, Bendayan D, et al. Primary pulmonary hypertension in Israel: a national survey. *Chest.* 2001;119:1801–1806.

Astrom A-K, Jin D, Imamura T, et al. Chromosomal localization of three human genes encoding bone morphogenetic protein receptors. *Mamm Genome.* 1999;10:299–302.

Atkinson C, Stewart S, Upton PD, et al. Primary pulmonary hypertension is associated with reduced pulmonary vascular expression of type II bone morphogenetic protein receptor. *Circulation.* 2002;105:1672–1678.

Attisano L, Carcamo J, Ventura F, Weis FM, Massague J, Wrana JL. Identification of human activin and TGF beta type I receptors that form heteromeric kinase complexes with type II receptors. *Cell.* 1993; 75:671–680.

Badesch DB, Abman SH, Ahearn GS, et al. Medical therapy for pulmonary arterial hypertension: ACCP evidence-based clinical practice guidelines. *Chest.* 2004;126:35S–62S.

Badesch DB, Abman SH, Simmoneau G, Rubin LJ, McLaughlin VV. Medical therapy for pulmonary arterial hypertension: updated ACCP evidence-based clinical practice guidelines. *Chest.* 2007;131:1917–1928.

Barst RJ, Rubin LJ, Long WA, et al. A comparison of continuous intravenous epoprostenol (prostacyclin) with conventional therapy for primary pulmonary hypertension. The Primary Pulmonary Hypertension Study Group. *N Engl J Med.* 1996;334:296–302.

Barst RJ, Rubin LJ, McGoon MD, Caldwell EJ, Long WA, Levy PS. Survival in primary pulmonary hypertension with long-term continuous intravenous prostacyclin. *Ann Intern Med.* 1994;121:409–415.

Beppu H, Ichinose F, Kawai N, et al. BMPR-II heterozygous mice have mild pulmonary hypertension and an impaired pulmonary vascular remodeling response to prolonged hypoxia. *Am J Physiol Lung Cell Mol Physiol.* 2004;287:L1241–1247.

Beppu H, Kawabata M, Hamamoto T, et al. BMP type II receptor is required for gastrulation and early development of mouse embryos. *Dev Biol.* 2000;221:249–258.

Beppu H, Minowa O, Miyazano K, Kawabata M. cDNA cloning and genomic organization of the mouse BMP type II receptor. *Biochem Biophys Res Commun.* 1997;27:499–504.

Berg JN, Gallione CJ, Stenzel TT, et al. The activin receptor-like kinase 1 gene: genomic structure and mutations in hereditary hemorrhagic telangiectasia. *Am J Hum Genet.* 1997;61:60–76.

Berg J, Porteous M, Reinhardt D, et al. Hereditary haemorrhagic telangiectasia: a questionnaire based study to delineate the different phenotypes caused by endoglin and ALK1 mutations. *J Med Genet.* 2003;40:585–590.

Berg JN, Guttmacher AE, Marchuk DA, Porteous ME. Clinical heterogeneity in hereditary hemorrhagic telangiectasia: are pulmonary arteriovenous malformations more common in families linked to endoglin? *J Med Genet.* 1996;33:256–257.

Bideau A, Plauchu H, Brunet G, Robert J-M. Etude epidemiologique de la maladie de Rendu-Osler en France. *Population.* 1989;1:9–28.

Blobe GC, Schiemann WP, Lodish HF. Role of transforming growth factor beta in human disease. *N Engl J Med.* 2000;342:1350–1358.

Bosher LHJ, Blake DA, Byrd BR. An analysis of the pathologic anatomy of pulmonary arteriovenous aneurysms with particular reference to the applicability of local excision. *Surgery.* 1959;45:91–104.

Brenner O. Pathology of the vessels of the pulmonary circulation. *Arch Intern Med.* 1935;56:976–1014.

Brenot F, Herve P, Petitpretz P, Parent F, Duroux P, Simonneau G. Primary pulmonary hypertension and fenfluramine use. *Br Heart J.* 1993;70:537–541.

Brill I, Krygier J. Primary pulmonary vascular sclerosis. *Arch Intern Med.* 1941;68:560.

Burnand KG, Young AE. (eds.) *The New Aird's Companion in Surgical Studies.* Churchill Livingstone, New York; 1992.

Caniggia I, Taylor CV, Ritchie JW, Lye SJ, Letarte M. Endoglin regulates trophoblast differentiation along the invasive pathway in human placental villous explants. *Endocrinology.* 1997;138:4977–4988.

Channick R, Badesch DB, Tapson VF, et al. Effects of the dual endothelin receptor antagonist bosentan in patients with pulmonary hypertension: a placebo-controlled study. *J Heart Lung Transplant.* 2001;20:262–263.

Charters AD, Baker W, de C. Primary pulmonary hypertension of unusually long duration. *Br Heart J.* 1970;32:130–133.

Chazova I, Loyd JE, Zhdanov VS, Newman JH, Belenkov Y, Meyrick B. Pulmonary artery adventitial changes and venous involvement in primary pulmonary hypertension. *Am J Pathol.* 1995;146:389–397.

Cherwek H, Amundson S. Pulmonary artery aneurysm. *N Engl J Med.* 2003;348:e1.

Childers RW, Ranniger K, Rabinowitz M. Intrahepatic arteriovenous fistula with pulmonary vascular obstruction in Osler-Rendu-Weber disease. *Am J Med.* 1967;43:304–312.

Christman BW, McPherson CD, Newman JH, et al. An imbalance between the excretion of thromboxane and prostacyclin metabolites in pulmonary hypertension. *N Engl J Med.* 1992;327:70–75.

Clarke RC, Coombs C, Hadfield G, Todd A. On certain abnormalities, congenital and acquired, of the pulmonary artery. *QJM.* 1927;21:51–70.

Clouston JE, Pais SO, White CS, Dempsey JE, Templeton PA. Pulmonary arteriovenous malformation: diagnosis and treatment of spontaneous thrombosis and recanalization. *J Vasc Interv Radiol.* 1995;6:143–145.

Cohen AH, Hanson K, Morris K, et al. Inhibition of cyclic 3'-5'-guanosine monophosphate-specific phosphodiesterase selectively vasodilates the pulmonary circulation in chronically hypoxic rats. *J Clin Invest.* 1996;97:172–179.

Cournand A, Ranges H. Catheterisation of the right auricle in man. *Proc Soc Exper Biol and Med.* 1941;46:462.

Cowan KN, Heilbut A, Humpl T, Lam C, Ito S, Rabinovitch M. Complete reversal of fatal pulmonary hypertension in rats by a serine elastase inhibitor. *Nat Med.* 2000;6:698–702.

Crow TJ. A note on Survey of cases of familial mental illness by L.S. Penrose. *Eur Arch Psychiatry Clin Neurosci.* 1991;240:314–324.

D'Alonzo GE, Barst RJ, Ayres SM, et al. Survival in patients with primary pulmonary hypertension. Results from a national prospective registry. *Ann Intern Med.* 1991;115:343–349.

D'Alonzo GE, Gianotti LA, Pohil RL, et al. Comparison of progressive exercise performance of normal subjects and patients with primary pulmonary hypertension. *Chest.* 1987;92:57–62.

Deng Z, Haghighi F, Helleby L, et al. Fine mapping of PPH1, a gene for familial primary pulmonary hypertension, to a 3-cM region on chromosome 2q33. *Am J Respir Crit Care Med.* 2000a;161:1055–1059.

Deng Z, Morse JH, Slager SL, et al. Familial primary pulmonary hypertension (gene PPH1) is caused by mutations in the bone morphogenetic protein receptor-II gene. *Am J Hum Genet.* 2000b;67:737–744.

Dines DE, Arms RA, Bernatz PE, Gomes MR. Pulmonary arteriovenous fistulas. *Mayo Clin Proc.* 1974;49:460–465.

Dines DE, Seward JB, Bernatz PE. Pulmonary arteriovenous fistulas. *Mayo Clin Proc.* 1983;58:176–181.

Doyle RL, McCrory D, Channick RN, Simmoneau G, Conte R. Surgical Treatments/Interventions for Pulmonary Arterial Hypertension.

ACCP Evidence-based Clinical Practice Guidelines. *Chest.* 2004;126:63S–71S.

Dresdale DT, Michtom R, Schultz M. Recent studies in primary pumonary hypertension. *Bull NY Acad Med.* 1954;30:195–207.

Dresdale DT, Schultz M, Michtom R. Primary pulmonary hypertension. I. Clinical and haemodynamic study. *Am J Med.* 1951;11:686–705.

Dutton J, Jackson JE, Hughes JM, et al. Pulmonary arteriovenous malformations: results of treatment with coil embolization in 53 patients. *Am J Roentgenol.* 1995;165:1119–1125.

Eddahibi S, Morrell NW, d'Ortho MP, Naeije R. Pathobiology of pulmonary arterial hypertension. *Eur Respir J.* 2002;20:1559–1572.

Eisenberg PR, Lucore C, Kaufman L, Sobel BE, Jaffe AS, Rich S. Fibrinopeptide A levels indicative of pulmonary vascular thrombosis in patients with primary pulmonary hypertension. *Circulation.* 1990;82:841–847.

Elliott G, Alexander G, Leppert M, Yeates S, Kerber R. Coancestry in apparently sporadic primary pulmonary hypertension. *Chest.* 1995;108:973–977.

Elliott G, Glissmeyer EW, Havlena GT, et al. Relationship of BMPR2 mutations to vasoreactivity in pulmonary arterial hypertension. *Circulation.* 2006;113:2509–2515.

Fukumoto S, Koyama H, Hosoi M, et al. Distinct role of cAMP and cGMP in the cell cycle control of vascular smooth muscle cells: cGMP delays cell cycle transition through suppression of cyclin D1 and cyclin-dependent kinse 4 activation. *Circ Res.* 1999;85:985–991.

Fuster V, Steele PM, Edwards WD, Gersh BJ, McGoon MD, Frye RL. Primary pulmonary hypertension: natural history and the importance of thrombosis. *Circulation.* 1984;70:580–587.

Galie N, Humbert M, Vachiery F, et al. Effects of beraprost sodium, an oral prostacyclin analogue, in patients with pulmonary arterial hypertension: a randomized, double-blind, placebo-controlled trial. *J Am Coll Cardiol.* 2002;39:1496–1502.

Garamszegi N, Dore JJ Jr, Penheiter SG, Edens M, Yao D, Leof EB. Transforming growth factor beta receptor signaling and endocytosis are linked through a COOH terminal activation motif in the type I receptor. *Mol Biol Cell.* 2001;12:2881–2893.

Giaid A, Yanagisawa M, Langleben D, et al. Expression of endothelin-1 in the lungs of patients with pulmonary hypertension. *N Engl J Med.* 1993;328:1732–1739.

Glanville AR, Burke CM, Theodore J, Robin ED. Primary pulmonary hypertension. Length of survival in patients referred for heart-lung transplantation. *Chest.* 1987;91:675–681.

Gomes MR, Bernatz PE, Dines DE. Pulmonary arteriovenous fistulas. *Ann Thorac Surg.* 1969;C7:582–593.

Goodale FJ, Thomas W. Primary pulmonary arterial disease, observation with special reference to medial thickening of small arteries and arterioles. *Arch Pathol.* 1954;58:568.

Goodman DJ, Harrison DC, Popp RL. Echocardiographic features of primary pulmonary hypertension. *Am J Cardiol.* 1974;33:438–443.

Gordon AJ, Donoso E, Kuhn LA, Ravitch MM, Himmelstein A. Patent ductus arteriosus with reversal of flow. *N Engl J Med.* 1954;251:923–927.

Greenwald J, Fischer WH, Vale WW, Choe S. Three-finger toxin fold for the extracellular ligand-binding domain of the type II activin receptor serine kinase. *Nat Struct Biol.* 1999;6:18–22.

Grunig E, Janssen B, Mereles D, et al. Abnormal pulmonary artery pressure response in asymptomatic carriers of primary pulmonary hypertension gene. *Circulation.* 2000;102:1145–1150.

Gurtner HP. Pulmonary hypertension produced by ingestion of substances. *Bull Physio-Path Resp.* 1969;5:435.

Gurtner HP. Aminorex and pulmonary hypertension. A review. *Cor Vasa.* 1985;27:160–171.

Gurtner HP, Gertsch M, Salzmann C, Scherrer M, Stucki P, Wyss F. Haufen sich die primer vascularen forman des chronischen cor pulmonale? (Are the primary vascular forms of chronic pulmonary heart disease becoming more common?) *Schweiz Med Wochenschr.* 1968;98:1579–1589.

Hadano S, Nichol K, Brinkman RR, et al. A yeast artifical chromosome-based physical map of the juvenile amyotrophic lateral sclerosis (ALS2) critical region on human chromosome 2q33-q34. *Genomics.* 1999;55:106–112.

Haitjema T, tenBerg JM, Overtoom TT, Ernst JM, Westermann CJ. Unusual complications after embolization of a pulmonary arteriovenous malformation. *Chest.* 1996a;109:1401–1404.

Haitjema T, Westermann CJ, Overtoom TT, et al. Hereditary hemorrhagic telangiectasia (Osler-Weber-Rendu disease): new insights in pathogenesis, complications, and treatment. *Arch Intern Med.* 1996b;156:714–719.

Hanks SK, Hunter T. Protein kinases 6. The eukaryotic protein kinase superfamily: kinase (catalytic) domain structure and classification. *FASEB J.* 1995;9:576–596.

Hanks SK, Quinn AM, Hunter T. The protein kinase family: conserved features and deduced phylogeny of the catalytic domains. *Science.* 1988;241:42–52.

Harris P, Heath D. *The Human Pulmonary Circulation.* Livingstone, Edinburgh; 1962.

Harrison RE, Flanagan JA, Sankelo M, et al. Molecular and functional analysis identifies ALK-1 as the predominant cause of pulmonary hypertension related to hereditary haemorrhagic telangiectasia. *J Med Genet.* 2003;40:865–871.

Hasleton PS, Heath D, Brewer DB. Hypertensive pulmonary vascular disease in states of chronic hypoxia. *J Path & Bact.* 1968;95:431–440.

Hatano S, Strasser T. Primary pulmonary hypertension. Report on a WHO meeting. Geneva. World Health Organisation. 1973;7–45.

Haworth SG. The management of pulmonary hypertension in children. *Arch Dis Child.* 2008;93:620–625.

Heath D, Edwards JE. A description of six grades of structural changes in the pulmonary arteries with special reference to congenital cardiac septal defects. *Circulation.* 1958;18:533–547.

Hellems H, Haynes F, Dexter L. Pumonary 'capillary' pressure in man. *J Appl Physiol.* 1949;2:24–29.

Herve P, Launay JM, Scrobohaci ML, et al. Increased plasma serotonin in primary pulmonary hypertension. *Am J Med.* 1995;99:249–254.

Higenbottam T, Butt AY, McMahon A, Westerbeck R, Sharples L. Long-term intravenous prostaglandin (epoprostenol or iloprost) for treatment of severe pulmonary hypertension. *Heart.* 1998;80:151–155.

Holman E. Contribution to cardiovascular physiology gleaned from clinical and experimental observations of abnormal arteriovenous communications. *J Cardiovasc Surg.* 1962;3:48–63.

Hong KH, Lee YJ, Lee E, et al. Genetic ablation of the BMPR2 gene in pulmonary endothelium is sufficient to predispose to pulmonary arterial hypertension. *Circulation.* 2008;118:722–730.

Hughes JMB. In: Crystal RG, West JB, Weibel ER, Barnes PJ, (eds.) *The Lung: Scientific Foundations.* Lippincott-Raven. Philadelphia; 1997.

Humbert M, Deng Z, Simonneau G, et al. BMPR2 germline mutations in pulmonary hypertension associated with fenfluramine derivatives. *Eur Respir J.* 2002;20:518–523.

Humbert M, Monti G, Brenot F, et al. Increased interleukin-1 and interleukin-6 serum concentrations in severe primary pulmonary hypertension. *Am J Respir Crit Care Med.* 1995;151:1628–1631.

Humbert M, Segal ES, Kiely DG, Carlsen J, Schwierin B, Hoeper MM. Results of European post-marketing surveillance of bosentan in pulmonary hypertension. *Eur Respir J.* 30:2007;338–344.

Huse M, Chen YG, Massague J, Kuriyan J. Crystal structure of the cytoplasmic domain of the type I TGF receptor in complex with FKBP12. *Cell.* 1999;96:425–436.

International PPH Consortium, Lane KB, Machado RD, et al. Heterozygous germline mutations in BMPR2, encoding a TGF-beta receptor, cause familial primary pulmonary hypertension. The International PPH Consortium. *Nat Genet.* 2000;26:81–84.

Irey NS, Norris HJ. Intimal vascular lesions associated with female reproductive steroids. *Arch Pathol.* 1973;96:227–234.

Jessurun GA, Kamphuis DJ, van der Zande FH, Nossent JC. Cerebral arteriovenous malformations in The Netherlands Antilles. High prevalence of hereditary hemorrhagic telangiectasia-related single and multiple cerebral arteriovenous malformations. *Clin Neurol Neurosurg.* 1993; 95:193–198.

Kawabata M, Chytil A, Moses HL. Cloning of a novel type II serine/threonine kinase receptor through interaction with the type I transforming growth factor-beta receptor. *J Biol Chem.* 1995;270:5625–5630.

Kawabata M, Imamura T, Miyazano K. Signal transduction by bone morphogenetic proteins. *Cytokine Growth Factor Rev.* 1998;9:49–61.

Kerstein D, Levy PS, Hsu DT, Hordof AJ, Gersony WM, Barst RJ. Blade balloon atrial septostomy in patients with severe primary pulmonary hypertension. *Circulation.* 1995;91:2028–2035.

Kingdon HS, Cohen LS, Roberts WC, Braunwald E. Familial occurrence of primary pulmonary hypertension. *Arch Intern Med.* 1966;118:422–426.

Kjeldsen AD, Brusgaard K, Poulsen L, et al. Mutations in the ALK-1 gene and the phenotype of hereditary hemorrhagic telangiectasia in two large Danish families. *Am J Med Genet.* 2001;98:298–302.

Klob J. *Wiener Wochenbatt,* 1865;XXI, 45.

Launay D. Third International Symposium on Pulmonary Hypertension. Venezia, Italia, 23–25 June 2003. *Rev Med Interne.* 2003;24:853–856.

Le Roux BT, Gibb BH, Wainwright J. Pulmonary arteriovenous fistula with bilharzial pulmonary hypertension. *Br Heart J.* 1970;32:571–574.

Lilienfeld DE, Rubin LJ. Mortality from primary pulmonary hypertension in the United States, 1979–1996. *Chest.* 2000;117:796–800.

Liu F, Ventura F, Doody J, Massague J. Human type II receptor for bone morphogenetic proteins (BMPs): extension of the two-kinase receptor model to the BMPs. *Mol Cell Biol.* 1995;15:3479–3486.

Loyd JE, Butler MG, Foroud TM, Conneally PM, Phillips JA III, Newman JH. Genetic anticipation and abnormal gender ratio at birth in familial primary pulmonary hypertension. *Am J Respir Crit Care Med.* 1995;152:93–97.

Loyd JE, Primm RK, Newman JH. Familial primary pulmonary hypertension: clinical patterns. *Am Rev Respir Dis.* 1984;129:194–197.

Loyd JE, Slovis B, Phillips JA III, et al. The presence of genetic anticipation suggests that the molecular basis of familial primary pulmonary hypertension may be trinucleotide repeat expansion. *Chest.* 1997;111: 82S–83S.

MacCallum W. Obliterative pumonary arteriosclerosis. *Bull Johns Hopkins Hosp.* 1931;49:37–48.

Machado RD, Aldred MA, James V, et al. Mutations of the TGF-beta type II receptor BMPR2 in pulmonary arterial hypertension. *Hum Mutat.* 2006;27:121–132.

Machado RD, Pauciulo MW, Fretwell N, et al. A physical and transcript map based upon refinement of the critical interval for PPH1, a gene for familial primary pulmonary hypertension. *Genomics.* 2000;68:220–228.

Machado RD, Pauciulo MW, Thomson JR, et al. BMPR2 haploinsufficiency as the inherited molecular mechanism for primary pulmonary hypertension. *Am J Hum Genet.* 2001;68:92–102.

Massague J. TGF-beta signal trasnduction. *Annu Rev Biochem.* 1998;67:753–791.

Masuda S, Ishii T, Asuwa N, Ishikawa Y, Kiguchi H, Uchiyama T. Concurrent pulmonary arterial dissection and saccular aneurysm associated with primary pulmonary hypertension. *Arch Pathol Lab Med.* 1996;120:309–312.

McDonald JE, Miller FJ, Hallam SE, Nelson L, Marchuk D, Ward KJ. Clinical manifestations in a large hereditary hemorrhagic telangiectasia (HHT) type 2 kindred. *Am J Med Genet.* 2000;93:320–327.

McDonnell PJ, Toye PA, Hutchins GM. Primary pulmonary hypertension and cirrhosis: are they related? *Am Rev Respir Dis.* 1983;127:437–441.

McLaughlin VV, Genthner DE, Panella MM, Rich S. Reduction in pulmonary vascular resistance with long-term epoprostenol (prostacyclin) therapy in primary pulmonary hypertension. *N Engl J Med.* 1998;338:273–277.

Melmon K, Braunwald E. Familial pulmonary hypertension. *N Engl J Med.* 1963;26:770–775.

Morisaki H, Nakanishi N, Kyotani S, Takashima A, Tomoike H, Morisaki T. BMPR2 mutations found in Japanese patients with familial and sporadic primary pulmonary hypertension. *Hum Mutat.* 2004;23:632.

Morrell NW, Yang X, Upton PD, et al. Altered growth responses of pulmonary artery smooth muscle cells from patients with primary pulmonary hypertension to transforming growth factor-beta(1) and bone morphogenetic proteins. *Circulation.* 2001;104:790–795.

Morse JH. Bone morphogenetic protein receptor 2 mutations in pulmonary hypertension. *Chest.* 2002;121(3 Suppl):50S–53S.

Morse JH, Horn EM, Barst RJ. Hormone replacement therapy: a possible risk factor in carriers of familial primary pulmonary hypertension. *Chest.* 1999;116:847.

Morse JH, Jones AC, Barst RJ, Hodge SE, Wilhelmsen KC, Nygaard TG. Mapping of familial primary pulmonary hypertension locus (PPH1) to chromosome 2q31-q32. *Circulation.* 1997;95:2603–2606.

Moser KM, Bloor CM. Pulmonary vascular lesions occurring in patients with chronic major vessel thromboembolic pulmonary hypertension. *Chest.* 1993;103:685–692.

Moyer JH, Glantz G, Brest AN. Pulmonary arteriovenous fistulas; physiologic and clinical considerations. *Am J Med.* 1962;32:417–435.

Nawroth PP, Handley DA, Esmon CT, Stern DM. Interleukin 1 induces endothelial cell procoagulant while suppressing cell-surface anticoagulant activity. *Proc Natl Acad Sci USA.* 1986;83:3460–3464.

Naye RL. Primary pulmonary hypertension with coexisting portal hypertension: a retrospective study of six cases. *Circulation.* 1968;22:376–384.

Newman JH, Wheeler L, Lane KB, et al. Mutation in the gene for bone morphogenetic protein receptor II as a cause of primary pulmonary hypertension in a large kindred. *N Engl J Med.* 2001;345:319–324.

Nichols WC, Koller DL, Slovis B, et al. Localization of the gene for familial primary pulmonary hypertension to chromosome 2q31–32. *Nat Genet.* 1997;15:277–280.

Nielsen NC, Fabricius J. Primary pulmonary hypertension with special reference to prognosis. *Acta Med Scand.* 1961;170:731.

Nienaber CA, Spielmann RP, Montz R, Bleifeld W, Mathey DG. Development of pulmonary aneurysm in primary pulmonary hypertension: a case report. *Angiology.* 1986;37:319–324.

Nohe A, Hassel S, Ehrlich M, et al. The mode of bone morphogenetic protein (BMP) receptor oligomerization determines different BMP-2 signaling pathways. *J Biol Chem.* 2002;277:5330–5338.

Nohno T, Ishikawa T, Saito T, et al. Identification of a human type II receptor for bone morphogenetic protein-4 that forms differential heteromeric complexes with bone morphogenetic protein type I receptors. *J Biol Chem.* 1995;270:22522–22526.

Oakley C, Sommerville J. Oral contraceptives and progressive pulmonary vascular disease. *Lancet.* 1968;1:890–983.

Oakley CW. Primary pulmonary hypertension. Case series from the United Kingdom. *Chest.* 1994;105:29S–32S.

Oh SP, Seki T, Goss KA, et al. Activin receptor-like kinase 1 modulates transforming growth factor-beta 1 signaling in the regulation of angiogenesis. *Proc Natl Acad Sci USA.* 2000;97:2626–2631.

Olschewski H, Simonneau G, Galie N, et al. Inhaled iloprost for severe pulmonary hypertension. *N Engl J Med.* 2002;347:322–329.

Osler W. A family form of recurring epistaxis associated with multiple telangiectases of the skin and mucous membranes. *Bull Johns Hopkins Hosp.* 1901;12:333–337.

Palmer RM, Ferrige AG, Moncada S. Nitric oxide release accounts for the biologic activity of endothelium-derived relaxing factor. *Nature.* 1987;327:524–526.

Panchenko MP, Williams MC, Brody JS, Yu Q. Type I receptor serine-threonine kinase preferentially expressed in pulmonary blood vessels. *Am J Physiol.* 1996;270:L547–L558.

Pasque MK, Trulock EP, Cooper JD, et al. Single lung transplantation for pulmonary hypertension. Single institution experience in 34 patients. *Circulation.* 1995;92:2252–2258.

Pechet L, Alexander B. Increased clotting factors in pregnancy. *N Engl J Med.* 1961;265:1093–1097.

Peery WH. Clinical spectrum of hereditary hemorrhagic telangiectasia (Osler-Weber-Rendu disease). *Am J Med.* 1987;82:989–997.

Penrose LS. The problem of anticipation in pedigrees of dystrophica myotonica. *Ann Eugen.* 1948;14:125–132.

Piek E, Heldin CH, ten Dijke P. Specificity, diversity, and regulation in TGF-beta superfamily signaling. *FASEB J.* 1999;13:2105–2124.

Pietra GG. Histopathology of primary pulmonary hypertension. *Chest.* 1994;105:2S–6S.

Pietra GG, Edwards WD, Kay JM, et al. Histopathology of primary pulmonary hypertension. A qualitative and quantitative study of pulmonary blood vessels from 58 patients in the National Heart, Lung, and Blood Institute, Primary Pulmonary Hypertension Registry. *Circulation.* 1989;80:1198–1206.

Plauchu H, de Chadarevian JP, Bideau A, Robert JM. Age-related clinical profile of hereditary hemorrhagic telangiectasia in an epidemiologically recruited population. *Am J Med Genet.* 1989;32:291–297.

Poller L. Oral contraceptives, blood clotting and thrombosis. *Br Med Bull.* 1978;34:151–156.

Porteous ME, Burn J, Proctor SJ. Genetic heterogeneity in hereditary haemorrhagic telangiectasia. *J Med Genet.* 1992;31:527–530.

Prasad S, Wilkinson J, Gatzoulis MA. Sildenafil in primary pulmonary hypertension. *N Engl J Med.* 2000;343:1342.

Pritchard GA, Llewelyn MB. Mesenteric vein thrombosis as a complication of hereditary haemorrhagic telangiectasia. *J R Coll Surg Edinb.* 1987;5:325–326.

Raftery LA, Sutherland DJ. TGF-beta family signal transduction in Drosophila development: from Mad to Smads. *Dev Biol.* 1999;210:251–268.

Reddi AH. Interplay between bone morphogenetic proteins and cognate binding proteins in bone and cartilage development: noggin, chordin and DAN. *Arthritis Res.* 2001;3:1–5.

Reitz BA, Wallwork JL, Hunt SA, et al. Heart-lung transplantation: successful therapy for patients with pulmonary vascular disease. *N Engl J Med.* 1982;306:557–564.

Rendu M. Epistaxis repetees chez un sujet porteur de petits angiomes cutanes et muqueux. *Gaz Hop (Paris).* 1896;135:132–133.

Rich S. Executive summary from the world symposium on primary pulmonary hypertension, Evian, France, September 6–10, 1998a, cosponsored by the World Health Organization. http://www.who.int/entity/cardiovascular_diseases/resources/publications /en.

Rich S, Dantzker DR, Ayres SM, et al. Primary pulmonary hypertension. A national prospective study. *Ann Intern Med.* 1987;107:216–223.

Rich S, Dodin E, McLaughlin VV. Usefulness of atrial septostomy as a treatment for primary pulmonary hypertension and guidelines for its application. *Am J Cardiol.* 1997;80:369–371.

Rich S, Kaufmann E, Levy PS. The effect of high doses of calcium-channel blockers on survival in primary pulmonary hypertension. *N Engl J Med.* 1992;327:76–81.

Rich S, Kieras K, Hart K, Groves BM, Stobo JD, Brundage BH. Antinuclear antibodies in primary pulmonary hypertension. *J Am Coll Cardiol.* 1986;8:1307–1311.

Rigelsky CM, Jennings C, Lehtonen R, Minai OA, Eng C, Aldred MA. BMPR2 mutation in a patient with pulmonary arterial hypertension and suspected hereditary hemorrhagic telangiectasia. *Am J Med Genet A.* 2008;146A, 2551–2556.

Ring CJ, Cho KWY. Specificity in transforming growth factor-beta signalling pathways. *Am J Hum Genet.* 1999;64:691–697.

Roberts KE, McElroy JJ, Wong WP, et al. BMPR2 mutations in pulmonary arterial hypertension with congenital heart disease. *Eur Respir J.* 2004;24:371–374.

Rodan BA, Goodwin JD, Chen JT, Ravin CE. Worsening pulmonary hypertension after resection of arteriovenous fistula. *Am J Roentgenol.* 1981;137:864–866.

Roelen BA, van Rooijen MA, Mummery CL. Expression of ALK-1, a type 1 serine/threonine kinase receptor, coincides with sites of vasculogenesis and angiogenesis in early mouse development. *Dev Dyn.* 1997;209:418–430.

Romberg E. Ueber sklerose der lungenarterie. *Deutsch Arch f klin Med.* 1891;48:197–206.

Rosenzweig BL, Imamura T, Okadome T, et al. Cloning and characterization of a human type II receptor for bone morphogenetic proteins. *Proc Natl Acad Sci USA.* 1995;92:7632–7636.

Rosenzweig EB, Morse JH, Knowles JA, et al. Clinical implications of determining BMPR2 mutation status in a large cohort of children and adults with pulmonary arterial hypertension. *J. Heart Lung Transpl.* 2008;27:668–674.

Rubin LJ. Primary pulmonary hypertension. *Chest.* 1993;104:236–250.

Rubin LJ. Primary pulmonary hypertension. *N Engl J Med.* 1997;336:111–117.

Rubin LJ, Badesch D, Barst RJ, et al. Bosentan therapy for pulmonary arterial hypertension. *N Engl J Med.* 2002;346:896–903.

Rudarakanchana N, Flanagan J, Chen H, et al. Functional analysis of bone morphogenetic protein type II receptor mutations underlying primary pulmonary hypertension. *Hum Mol Genet.* 2002;11:1517–1525.

Ryan US. The endothelial surface and responses to injury. *Fed Proc.* 1986;45:101–108.

Sanders WE. Primary pulmonary arteriosclerosis with hypertrophy of the right ventricle. *Arch Intern Med.* 1909;3:257–262.

Sapru RP, Hutchinson DC, Hall JI. Pulmonary hypertension in patients with pulmonary arteriovenous fistulae. *Br Heart J.* 1969;31:559–569.

Sastry BK, Narasimhan C, Reddy NK, et al. A study of clinical efficacy of sildenfil in patients with primary pulmonary hypertension. *Indian Heart J.* 2002;54:410–414.

Schulick AH, Taylor AJ, Zuo W, et al. Overexpression of transforming growth factor beta 1 in arterial endothelium causes hyperplasia, apoptosis, and cartilaginous metaplasia. *Proc Natl Acad Sci USA.* 1998;95:6983–6988.

Shi Y, Massague J. Mechanisms of TGF-beta signaling from cell membrane to the nucleus. *Cell.* 2003;113:685–700.

Shovlin CL. Molecular defects in rare bleeding disorders: hereditary haemorrhagic telangiectasia. *Thromb Haemost.* 1997a;78:145–150.

Shovlin CL, Guttmacher AE, Buscarini E, et al. Diagnostic criteria for hereditary hemorrhagic telangiectasia. *Am J Med Genet.* 2000;91:66–67.

Shovlin CL, Hughes JM, Scott J, Seidman CE, Seidman JG. Characterization of endoglin and identification of novel mutations in hereditary hemorrhagic telangiectasia. *Am J Hum Genet.* 1997b;61:68–79.

Shovlin CL, Winstock AR, Peters AM, Jackson JE, Hughes JM. Medical complications of pregnancy in hereditary haemorrhagic telangiectasia. *QJM.* 1995;88:879–887.

Sluiter-Eringa H, Orie NG, Sluiter HJ. Pulmonary arteriovenous fistula. Diagnosis and prognosis in noncomplainant patients. *Am Rev Respir Dis.* 1969;100:177–188.

Smith P, Heath D, Yacoub M, Madden B, Caslin A, Gosney J. The ultrastructure of plexogenic pulmonary arteriopathy. *J Pathol.* 1990; 160:111–121.

Song Y, Jones JE, Beppu H, Keaney JF, Loscalzo J, Zhang Y-Y. Increased susceptibility to pulmonary hypertension in heterozygous BMPR2-mutant mice. *Circulation.* 2005;112:553–562.

Sperling DC, Cheitlin M, Sullivan RW, Smith A. Pulmonary arteriovenous fistulas with pulmonary hypertension. *Chest.* 1977;71:753–757.

Srinivasan S, Hanes MA, Dickens T, et al. A mouse model for hereditary hemorrhagic telangiectasia (HHT) type 2. *Hum Mol Genet.* 2003;12:473–482.

Stenmark KR, Mecham RP. Cellular and molecular mechanisms of pulmonary vascular remodelling. *Annu Rev Physiol.* 1997;59:89–144.

Stewart DJ, Levy RD, Cernacek P, Langleben D. Increased plasma endothelin-1 in pulmonary hypertension: marker or mediator of disease? *Ann Intern Med.* 1991;114:464–469.

Suarez LD, Sciandro EE, Llera JJ, Perosio AM. Long-term follow-up in primary pulmonary hypertension. *Br Heart J.* 1979;41:702–708.

Tardivon AA, Mousseaux E, Brenot F, et al. Quantification of hemodynamics in primary pulmonary hypertension with magnetic resonance imaging. *Am J Respir Crit Care Med.* 1994;150:1075–1080.

Teichert-Kuliszewska K, Kutryk MJ, Kuliszewski MA, et al. Bone morphogenetic protein receptor-2 signalling promotes pulmonary arterial endothelial cell survival: complications for loss-of-function mutations in the pathogenesis of pulmonary hypertension. *Cir Res.* 2006;98:209–217.

ten Dijke P, Franzen P, Yamashita H, Ichijo H, Heldin CH, Miyazono K. Serine/threonine kinase receptors. *Prog Growth Factor Res.* 1994;5:55–72.

ten Dijke P, Ichijo H, Franzen P, et al. Activin receptor-like kinases: a novel subclass of cell-surface receptors with predicted serine/threonine kinase activity. *Oncogene.* 1993;8:2879–2887.

Tew MB, Arnett FC, Reveille JD, Tan FK. Mutations of bone morphogenetic protein receptor type II are not found in patients with pulmonary hypertension and underlying connective tissue diseases. *Arthritis Rheum.* 2002;46:2829–2830.

Thomson JR, Machado RD, Pauciulo MW, et al. Sporadic primary pulmonary hypertension is associated with germline mutations of the gene encoding BMPR-II, a receptor member of the TGF- beta family. *J Med Genet.* 2000;37:741–745.

Todorovich-Hunter L, Johnson DJ, Ranger P, Keeley FW, Rabinovitch M. Altered elastin and collagen synthesis associated with progressive pulmonary hypertension induced by monocrotaline: a biochemical and ultrastructural study. *Lab Invest.* 1988;58:184–195.

Trell E. Benign, idiopathic pulmonary hypertension? Two further cases of unusually long duration. *Acta Med Scand.* 1973;193:137–143.

Trell E, Johansson BW, Linell F, Ripa J. Familial pulmonary hypertension and multiple abnormalities of large systemic arteries in Osler's disease. *Am J Med.* 1972b;53:50–63.

Trembath RC, Thomson JR, Machado RD, et al. Clinical and molecular genetic features of pulmonary hypertension in patients with hereditary hemorrhagic telangiectasia. *N Engl J Med.* 2001;345:325–334.

Tuder RM, Cool CD, Geraci MW, et al. Prostacyclin synthase expression is decreased in lungs from patients with severe pulmonary hypertension. *Am J Respir Crit Care Med.* 1999;159:1925–1932.

Tuder RM, Groves B, Badesch DB, Voelkel NF. Exuberant endothelial cell growth and elements of inflammation are present in plexiform lesions of pulmonary hypertension. *Am J Pathol.* 1994;144:275–285.

Urness D, Sorensen LK, Li DY. Arteriovenous malformations in mice lacking activin receptor-like kinase-1. *Nat Genet.* 2000;26:328–331.

Vase P, Grove O. Gastrointestinal lesions in hereditary hemorrhagic telangiectasia. *Gastroenterology.* 1986;91:1079–1083.

Vase P, Holm M, Arendrup H. Pulmonary arteriovenous fistulas in hereditary hemorrhagic telangiectasia. *Acta Med Scand.* 1985;218:105–109.

Voelkel NF, Tuder RM. Cellular and molecular mechanisms in the pathogenesis of severe pulmonary hypertension. *Eur Respir J.* 1995;8:2129–2138.

von Euler US, Liljestrand G. Observations on the pulmonary arterial blood pressure in the cat. *Acta Physiol Scand.* 1946;12:301–320.

Wagenvoort CA. The morphology of certain vascular lesions in pulmonary hypertension. *J Path & Bact.* 1959;78:503.

Wagenvoort CA, Heath D, Edwards JE. *The Pathology of the Pulmonary Vasculature.* Springfield. Illinois. Charles C Thomas Publisher; 1964:172.

Wagenvoort CA, Wagenvoort N. Primary pulmonary hypertension: a pathologic study of the lung vessels in 156 clinically diagnosed cases. *Circulation.* 1970;42:1163–1184.

Waldhausen JA, Abel FL. The circulatory effects of pulmonary arteriovenous fistulas. *Surgery.* 1966;59:76–80.

Weber FP. Multiple hereditary developmental angiomata (telangiectases) of the skin and mucous membranes associated with recurring haemorrhages. *Lancet.* 1907;2:160–162.

Weiss BM, Zemp L, Seifert B, Hess OM. Outcome of pulmonary vascular disease in pregnancy: a systematic overview from 1978 through 1996. *J Am Coll Cardiol.* 1998;31:1650–1657.

Wekerle T, Klepetko W, Taghavi S, Birsan T. Lung transplantation for primary pulmonary hypertension and giant pulmonary artery aneurysm. *Ann Thorac Surg.* 1998;65:825–827.

Welsh CH, Hassell KL, Badesch DB, Kressin DC, Marlar RA. Coagulation and fibrinolytic profiles in patients with severe pulmonary hypertension. *Chest.* 1996;110:710–717.

West J, Fagan K, Steudel W, et al. Pulmonary hypertension in transgenic mice expressing a dominant-negative BMPRII gene in smooth muscle. *Circ Res.* 2004;94:1109–1114.

White CS, Templeton PA, Pais SO, Clouston J. MR angiographic diagnosis of recanalization in a thrombosed pulmonary arteriovenous malformation. *J Thorac Imaging.* 1994;9:105–107.

White RI Jr, Mitchell SE, Barth KH, et al. Angioarchitecture of pulmonary arteriovenous malformations: an important consideration before embolotherapy. *Am J Roentgenol.* 1983;140:681–686.

Wood P. Congenital heart diseases. A review of its clinical aspects in the light of experience gained by means of modern techniques. *Br Med J.* 1950;2:693–698.

Wozney JM, Rosen V, Celeste AJ, et al. Novel regulators of bone formation: molecular clones and activities. *Science.* 1988;242:1528–1534.

Wunderbaldinger P, Bernhard C, Uffmann M, Kurkciyan I, Senbaklavaci O, Herold CJ. Acute pulmonary trunk dissection in a patient with primary pulmonary hypertension. *J Comput Assist Tomogr.* 2000;24:92–95.

Yoshida F, Terasawa A, Hosoe M, Mishima N, Suzuki M, Goshima K. Long-term observation of a case of pulmonary arteriovenous fistula with pulmonary hypertension. *Intern Med.* 1995;34:574–576.

Zhu L, Wigle D, Hinek A, et al. The endogenous vascular elastase that governs development and progression of monocrotaline-induced pulmonary hypertension in rats is a novel enzyme related to the serine proteinase adipsin. *J Clin Invest.* 1994;94:1163–1171.

26

The Heart and Inherited Metabolic Disease

Mike Champion and Maureen Cleary

Introduction

The heart is a metabolically active organ and therefore inborn errors of metabolism (IEMs) inevitably present with cardiac manifestations as their primary symptom. The heart has a large energy requirement derived from a number of different sources including glucose, free fatty acids, pyruvate and ketone bodies. In utero, a major source of energy is from pyruvate via glycolysis. Postdelivery, fatty acids are the major source of energy production via fat oxidation (Strauss and Johnson 1996). Blocks in energy metabolism or the provision of substrate for energy production may therefore present with cardiac dysfunction. Examples include mitochondrial cytopathies and fat oxidation defects. Mitochondrial disorders are covered in detail in Chapter 31. However, IEMs that result in failure to make or break complex molecules may result in disordered embryogenesis and structural cardiac defects, for example, congenital disorders of glycosylation or progressive storage that interferes with the mechanics of the heart such as Fabry disease and the mucopolysaccharidoses. For some disorders such as Pompe disease (glycogen storage disease type II), fat oxidation defects and mitochondrial cytopathies, cardiac involvement may be the presenting feature for which the patient is investigated, whereas for many IEMs heart involvement is just one element of their condition and other noncardiac features are more prominent such as is seen in the mucopolysaccharidoses, organic acidemias, and some glycogen storage disorders (types III and IV).

IEMs that involve the heart tend to present in one of five ways: cardiomyopathy, arrhythmia, valve dysfunction, structural heart disease, or cardiovascular disease. Cardiomyopathy and arrhythmias will be discussed in more detail below. Valve involvement is usually secondary to storage disorders that result in valve deformity leading to incompetence, stenosis, or a mixture of both. Structural lesions are seen in dysmorphic syndromes, typically cholesterol biosynthesis defects and maternal phenylketonuria (PKU). Disorders with associated hypercoagulability may result in cardiac or pulmonary thrombosis of which homocystinuria (β cystathionine synthase deficiency) is the most important. Inherited lipid disorders (Chapter 21) and coronary artery disease (Chapter 22) are discussed separately.

Cardiomyopathy

Many IEMs that present with cardiac involvement present with cardiomyopathy. In one Australian study an underlying syndrome or genetic cause was identified in 58% of cases of pediatric hypertrophic cardiomyopathy but only 3 out of 80 subjects (4%) had an identified IEM (Nugent et al. 2005). For many patients, the clinical characteristics of the cardiomyopathy are nonspecific and therefore a metabolic work-up becomes essential if an IEM is to be identified. Diagnostic clues in the history include consanguinity as most IEMs are inherited in an autosomal recessive fashion. Exceptions include Barth syndrome which is an X-linked cardioskeletal myopathy with neutropenia secondary to a defect in cardiolipin metabolism secondary to mutations in the TAZ gene (Barth et al. 2004). Fabry disease and Danon disease are also X-linked conditions. Matrilineal inheritance is seen in mitochondrial cytopathies (see Chapter 31).

Clinical Presentation

Further clues may be gained from the obstetric history. Fetal long chain fat oxidation disorders are associated with maternal hepatic symptoms during pregnancy including acute fatty liver of pregnancy (AFLP) and the HELLP (hemolysis, elevated liver enzymes, and low platelets) syndrome. Although carrier status is usually sufficient for healthy living in the mother, the additional metabolic burden of pregnancy in conjunction with an affected fetus producing larger amounts of the metabolite is sufficient to cause liver impairment in the mother. Fetal long chain fat oxidation defects are the cause of AFLP or HELLP syndrome in only a minority of cases, but it remains essential that the diagnosis is excluded in the infant at birth as these are treatable conditions, which if not detected early have poorer and even fatal outcomes (Ibdah et al. 2000). Diagnosis requires plasma acylcarnitines in the neonate as urinary organic acid profiles may be inappropriately reassuring in a fed neonate.

Hypoglycemia is a common feature of fat oxidation defects, glycogen storage disorders, and mitochondrial cytopathies and therefore symptoms suggestive of this should be actively sought whilst taking the history. Examination is usually unrewarding with most IEMs having no dysmorphic features. Exceptions

Table 26–1. Metabolic Investigations in Cardiac Disease

Investigation	Finding	Disorder
Echocardiography	Dilated or hypertrophic cardiomyopathy Pericardial effusion	Barth syndrome, fat oxidation defects, storage disorders including Pompe, mitochondrial disorders, GSD III CDG
ECG	Giant complexes, short PR interval	Pompe
Full blood count + differential	Neutropenia Megaloblastic anemia	Barth syndrome, organic acidemias B_1/B_{12} defects
Vacuolated lymphocytes		Pompe, MPS, mucolipidoses
Transferrin glycoforms		CDG
Lactate	Elevated lactate	Mitochondrial disorders, fat oxidation defects, organic acidemias NB also seen in poor perfusion, hypoxia, etc.
Acylcarnitine profile and free carnitine	Very low carnitine Abnormal profile	Carnitine transporter defect Fat oxidation defects
Cardiolipins	Abnormal profile	Barth Syndrome
CK	Elevated CK	Pompe, GSD III, Fat oxidation defects
Ammonia	Elevated ammonia	Organic Acidaemias Fat oxidation
Urinary organic acids	Abnormal profile Dicarboxylic aciduria Methylglutaconate	Organic acidemias, mitochondrial disorders Fat oxidation defects Barth syndrome
Urinary glycosaaminoglycans		Mucopolysaccharidoses
Urinary oligosaccharides		Mucolipidoses
Second-line tests		
White cell enzymes		Storage disorders
Muscle biopsy		Mitochondrial disorders
Skin biopsy		Fat oxidation studies
Mitochondrial DNA	Point mutations, deletion	Mitochondrial disorders
DNA, selenium and thiamine ± red cell transketolase		
7-dehydrocholesterol	Structural heart defect	Smith Lemli Opitz

Notes: CDG, congenital disorders of glycosylation; GSD, glycogen storage disease; MPS, mucopolysaccharidoses.

to this include storage disorders such as Hurler syndrome with coarse facies, corneal clouding, and dysostosis multiplex and children with congenital disorders of glycosylation (CDGs) that can have dysmorphic features with abnormal fat distribution, inverted nipples, and edema. Patients with Fabry disease have angiokeratomas, typically within the bathing-trunk distribution and corneal dystrophy (cornea verticillata). Skeletal myopathy is often associated with inborn errors presenting with cardiomyopathy; however, hypotonia is a common finding in patients with severe cardiac failure. The paucity of physical signs to indicate an underlying IEM means that a metabolic screen is needed to detect most cases (see Table 26–1).

Investigations

The presence of massive hypertrophy of the myocardium on ECG and echocardiography in a neonate is suggestive of Pompe disease. The presence of a pericardial effusion may suggest the presence of CDG. There is often associated hypoalbuminemia in conjunction with pleural effusions and abdominal ascites. Dilated cardiomyopathy in a male infant may indicate Barth syndrome. Further supportive evidence includes neutropenia and the presence of methylglutaconate in the urine. As the neutropenia is highly variable even within the same patient, ranging from normal neutrophil count to complete absence, serial sampling is necessary.

Examination of peripheral blood film may detect vacuolated lymphocytes suggestive of storage disease but should be performed by a hematologist or pathologist with experience in this area (Anderson et al. 2005). Electron microscopy may help identify the likely storage material and hence the diagnosis.

Transferrin isoelectric focusing is the screening test for CDGs, however, this can give a false-negative result in the early weeks of life (Clayton et al. 1993). This is thought to be secondary to fetal isoforms with the mature isoelectric focusing pattern not being established until after the first few months of life and therefore prenatal testing biochemically has proven unreliable. An early abnormal result would confirm the diagnosis, but a normal result should be assessed again at a later stage if CDG remains a possibility.

Measuring plasma lactate is an important key metabolic test but this has to be taken under scrupulous conditions as a squeezed sample will result in spurious elevation, which is the commonest cause of an elevated result. If a free-flowing venous sample proves impossible, an arterial sample should be taken to assess the lactate concentration. An elevated lactate is seen in mitochondrial disorders, organic acidemias, and fat oxidation defects but it must be remembered that the commonest reason for an elevated lactate is a secondary rather than primary cause including poor perfusion and hypoxia, which are not uncommon in the severely sick child with heart failure.

Plasma acylcarnitines and free carnitine levels are the investigation of choice for fat oxidation and carnitine defects. Carnitine depletion is not uncommon in acute decompensation; however, very low levels less than 5 μmol/L are highly suggestive of a carnitine transporter defect (CTD). Further evidence for the condition can be gained examining urinary carnitine excretion, which will show low tubular reabsorption.

Urinary organic acid analysis examines over 350 metabolic compounds and the specific signature may suggest or indicate a specific metabolic diagnosis. Measurement of urinary glycosaminoglycans and oligosaccharides help exclude storage disorders.

Second-line tests include white cell enzymes specifically looking for storage disorders such as Fabry disease. Muscle biopsy is often required to establish a mitochondrial diagnosis, particularly in children where nuclear DNA (nDNA) mutations are more frequent compared to adult mitochondrial disease and relatively few genes have been identified. Diagnosis therefore relies on respiratory chain enzymology. Skin biopsy and fibroblast culture can be used for confirmatory tests both in fat oxidation defects looking at fat oxidation flux studies and further investigation of mitochondrial disorders to confirm a generalized defect looking at respiratory chain enzymology in fibroblasts. Fibroblasts can also be used as a source of DNA and banked for future investigation should further potential diagnoses come to light. Similarly, a blood sample for DNA should be taken at the time for storage.

Selenium assay is often performed as part of the cardiomyopathy screen as selenium deficiency is a treatable cause of cardiomyopathy. Selenium deficiency is very rare, except in a few geographic regions where the soil has very little selenium. Outside these regions, selenium deficiency is more likely in malnourished patients, including those receiving total parenteral nutrition (TPN) (Johnson et al. 1981). Selenium is absorbed in the small intestine and has been described in patients with Crohn's disease and cystic fibrosis.

Treatment

When considering the initial management of patients with cardiomyopathy where a metabolic cause has been questioned, there is usually no specific management to be undertaken until a diagnosis has been secured. Fat restriction may be considered in the patient with a suspected long chain fat oxidation defect; however, this can be rapidly confirmed or excluded on acylcarnitine assay. It is important to ensure an adequate intake of carbohydrate, particularly where a fat oxidation defect or glycogen storage disorder is considered. This, however, may be contraindicated in the patient with a congenital lactic acidosis as high carbohydrate intakes may exacerbate lactate production. In these patients, carbohydrate may need to be controlled if increasing concentrations are associated with higher lactate levels. The use of empiric carnitine is much debated and remains controversial (Stanley 1995). It is the treatment of choice in CTD with improvement in both cardiac and skeletal function, but its role in fat oxidation disorders with secondary carnitine deficiency is unclear. When carnitine is low it would appear logical to supplement with carnitine in the hope that it might help remove accumulating metabolites, though there is concern that carnitine will promote fatty acid uptake within the mitochondria leading to greater accumulation (Lieu et al. 1997). It has therefore been suggested that the secondary carnitine deficiency might be a protective adaptation to prevent long chain acylcarnitine accumulation and their toxic effect.

Box 26–1 Kearns-Sayre Syndrome Diagnostic Criteria

- Onset before age 20 years
- Pigmentary retinopathy
- Progressive external ophthalmoplegia plus one of the following
  - cardiac conduction block
  - cerebrospinal fluid protein >100 mg/dL
  - cerebellar ataxia

In patients with intractable lactic acidosis, a thiamine bolus may be given as this is a rare reversible cause of cardiomyopathy. Similar to selenium deficiency, this is rare and is more common with artificial diets such as TPN where vitamin supplementation may have been inadvertently deficient. Reversal of the acidosis and elevated lactate occurs within hours if this is the underlying cause.

Arrhythmias

Arrhythmias are not an uncommon accompaniment to cardiomyopathy, especially dilated cardiomyopathy. Disturbances in the conduction system with associated dysrhythmias are seen in a number of IEMs including fat oxidation defects, mitochondrial cytopathies, and Fabry disease. Kearns-Sayre syndrome is associated with heart block and is one of the diagnostic criteria (Rowland et al. 1983; see Box 26–1).

Kearns-Sayre syndrome is a mitochondrial cytopathy with large-scale deletions of mitochondrial DNA found in over 90% of patients. The conduction defects seen include prolonged intraventricular conduction time, bundle branch block, and atrioventricular block and insertion of a pacemaker may be life saving. Conduction defects are also seen in Barth syndrome, especially in cases with noncompaction of the left ventricle where the ECG is normally abnormal with right or left axis deviation, left or right bundle branch block, and on occasion nonspecific ST segment changes. Associated arrhythmias include atrial fibrillation, paroxysmal supraventricular tachycardia, ventricular arrhythmias, and sudden death (Gilbert-Barness and Barness 2006).

Fat oxidation disorders and disorders of the carnitine cycle are associated with tachyarrhythmias including supraventricular or ventricular tachycardia. The toxic effects of accumulating long chain acylcarnitines have been proposed as a potential mechanism. Accumulation of glycosphingolipid in the myocardium and conduction system in Fabry disease results in arrhythmias including intermittent supraventricular tachycardias and shortening of the PR interval.

Fat Oxidation Disorders

Fatty acid oxidation in mitochondria is an important source of energy production. The commonest presentation within disorders of fat oxidation is hypoketotic hypoglycemia and encephalopathy. Muscle involvement is a feature in many of the disorders as is cardiac involvement, particularly cardiomyopathy but also arrhythmias (see Figure 26–1).

The fat oxidation pathway comprises four key components: the carnitine cycle—essential for the entry of long chain free fatty acids into the mitochondrion, the β oxidation cycle whereby the activated fatty acylcarnitines are progressively shortened by two carbon atoms each turn of the cycle to produce acetyl-CoA, electron

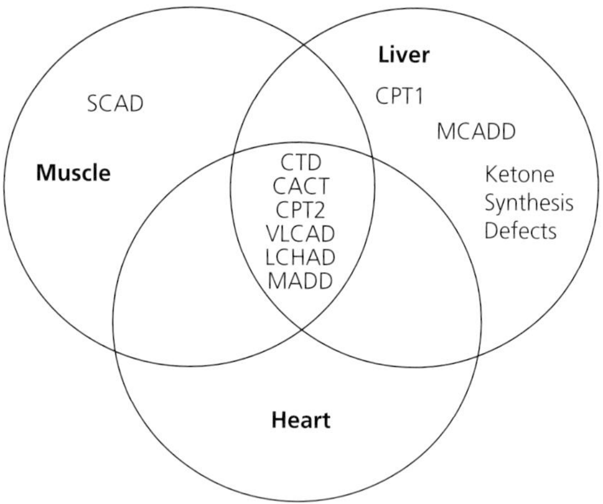

Figure 26–1 Clinical presentations of fat oxidation defects. CACT, carnitine acylcarnitine translocase deficiency; CPT, carnitine palmitoyl transferase; CTD, carnitine transporter defect; LCHAD, long chain hydoxyacyl-CoA dehydrogenase deficiency; MADD, multiple acyl-CoA dehydrogenase deficiency; MCADD, medium chain acyl-CoA dehydrogenase deficiency; SCAD, short chain acyl-CoA dehydrogenase deficiency; VLCAD, very long chain acyl-CoA dehydrogenase deficiency.

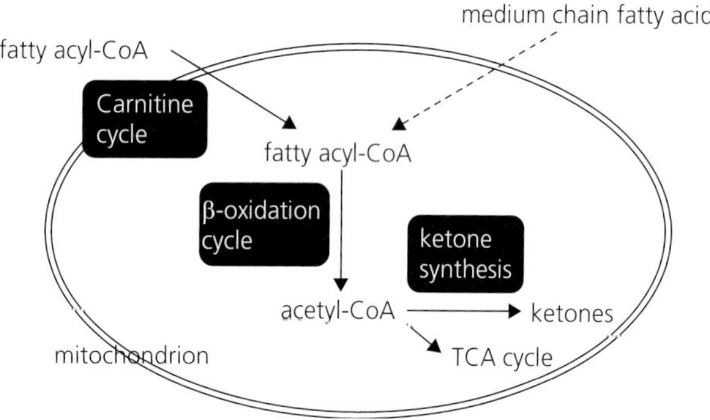

Figure 26–2 Fat oxidation pathway.

transfer from the β oxidation cycle to the respiratory chain for ATP synthesis, and ketone synthesis converting the acetyl-coA to ketone bodies for export to be utilized as an energy source within the body, particularly the brain. Fat cannot be used directly by the brain and therefore needs to be converted first in the liver to ketone bodies before the brain can utilize it as an energy source (see Figure 26–2).

Fat oxidation disorders should always be considered in patients with cardiomyopathy, especially hypertrophic cardiomyopathy, but also arrhythmias, particularly the long chain fat oxidation defects. Acylcarnitines is the key investigation as a block in fat oxidation is revealed by a build up of the acylcarnitines at that particular chain length, for example, MCADD (medium chain acyl-coA dehydrogenase deficiency) C8–10 and VLCAD (very long chain acyl-coA dehydrogenase deficiency) C14:1. The acylcarnitine profile in plasma, or on a blood spot, can prove very useful in diagnosing the specific metabolic defect. The utilization of blood spots on filter paper forms the basis of the U.K. Newborn Screening Programme for MCADD. In other European countries, United States, and Australia extended newborn screening includes other fat oxidation disorders; however, presentation and indeed death can occur prior to the screening result being available in a number of these conditions (Schulze et al. 2003; Waisbren et al. 2003). Acylcarnitine analysis in bile may prove diagnostically useful in postmortem investigation, particularly where there has been sudden death with hepatic, muscle, or myocardial lipid accumulation (Rashed et al. 1995).

Specific acylcarnitine profiles occur in SCAD (short chain acyl-CoA dehydrogenase deficiency), SCHAD (short chain hydroxy acyl-CoA dehydrogenase deficiency), MCADD, VLCAD, LCHAD (long chain hydroxy acyl-CoA dehydrogenase deficiency), trifunctional protein deficiency, and MADD (multiple acyl-CoA dehydrogenase deficiency also known as glutaric aciduria type II). The free carnitine concentration may also prove helpful. In most fat oxidation disorders, the free carnitine is reduced secondary to carnitine depletion resulting from the increased excretion of the specific acylcarnitines in the urine. In CTD, free carnitine levels are very low due to a failure of entry of carnitine into the cells and increased urinary excretion. Very high levels of carnitine (150%–200% of normal) are associated with CPT1 (carnitine palmitoyl transferase 1) deficiency; however, this condition is associated with the hepatic fat oxidation presentation, that is, hypoketotic hypoglycemia and liver dysfunction. Prior to acylcarnitine analysis and better diagnostic techniques, many of these conditions were diagnosed as Reye's syndrome (Saudubray et al. 1999).

Acylcarnitine analysis is complemented by urinary organic acid analysis, particularly during times of intercurrent illness or fasting when omega oxidation of fats occurs in microsomes with the resultant production of dicarboxylic acids that appear in the urine.

Confirmation of the specific disorder, particularly the long chain fat oxidation defects VLCAD and LCHAD, requires fat oxidation studies in cultured skin fibroblasts. CPT1 deficiency and CTD are not detected by this method. CTD is diagnosed by measuring the fractional excretion of carnitine in urine and CPT1 requires specific enzymology.

All defects are inherited in an autosomal recessive manner and genotyping is available. Prenatal diagnosis is available for all fat oxidation disorders on chorionic villus sampling or amniocentesis apart from HMG CoA synthase deficiency, which is not expressed in fibroblasts. Molecular methods are now preferred due to their rapid turnaround.

The management principles of fat oxidation defects are based on avoidance of fasting to prevent mobilization of the body's fat stores and the buildup of the toxic fatty acyl-coA intermediates. During acute illnesses this comprises the consumption of glucose polymer drinks every 2–3 hours orally, or via a nasogastric tube or gastrostomy if in place, until the illness has resolved and normal feeding resumed. If this is refused or not tolerated due to vomiting or diarrhea, intravenous 10% dextrose with electrolyte additives (sodium and potassium) is given at maintenance rates until the patient has recovered and normal feeding and drinking are established. In most cases this is no more than 12–24 hours but on occasion may be 48 hours or longer.

Dietary restriction of long chain fat is essential in VLCAD and LCHAD with continuous overnight feeds in infants, which may be replaced by uncooked cornstarch at bed time as a slow release form of glucose in children and adults. Medium chain fatty acids gain direct entry to the mitochondrion bypassing the carnitine cycle and so may be of use as a fuel in long chain fat oxidation defects but should be avoided in short and medium chain fat oxidation defects including MADD and the ketone synthesis defects.

Carnitine supplementation has a clear role in CTD reversing the clinical manifestations of the condition. Its use, however, in fat oxidation defects remains controversial, particularly the long chain fat oxidation defects with the concern that carnitine supplementation enhances entry of long chain fatty acids into the mitochondria and therefore exacerbate the buildup of toxic fatty acyl-CoA intermediates. Riboflavin (100 mg per day) has been used in mild MADD and SCAD with reported favorable outcomes (Olsen et al. 2007), being the cofactor for these enzymes.

Triheptanoin is currently under clinical trial as a new treatment for fat oxidation disorders acting as an anaplerotic substrate (Roe et al. 2002). This is a new approach to treating long chain fat oxidation defects aiming to replace depleted catalytic intermediates of the tricarboxylic acid (TCA) cycle by supplementing medium odd chain fatty acids that are precursors of acetyl-CoA and propionyl-CoA thereby restoring energy production and improving cardiac and skeletal muscle function.

Carnitine Cycle Defects

Long chain fatty acids, unlike medium chain fatty acids, are unable to enter directly into the mitochondrion and therefore require a special transport mechanism utilizing carnitine for entry into the mitochondrion (Figure 26–3). Initially carnitine gains entry into the cell using the carnitine transporter. The free fatty acids are then activated in the cytosol to their fatty acyl-CoA esters that conjugate with carnitine and via the carnitine cycle enter the mitochondrion. The carnitine cycle comprises three enzymes—CPT1, which is the rate-limiting step conjugating the fatty acyl-CoA with carnitine allowing entry to the intermitochondrial space, the carnitine acylcarnitine translocase embedded in the inner mitochondrial membrane, and then CPT2 releases carnitine for recycling and the free fatty acyl-CoA. Defects of CTD, translocase, and CPT2 are all associated with cardiac disease.

Carnitine Transporter Defect (CTD)

CTD is unusual within the family of fat oxidation disorders as the primary presentation is cardiac only. Presentation usually occurs in the first months of life with progressive heart failure and muscle weakness. Infants are usually normal at birth and then develop signs of progressive cardiomyopathy between 1 and 7 years with the median age of 3 years (Tein 2003). Occasionally, patients do

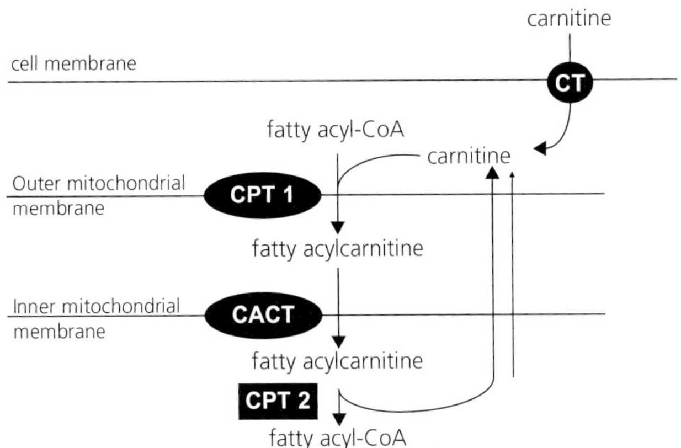

Figure 26–3 The carnitine cycle. CT, carnitine transporter; CPT, carnitine palmitoyl transferase; CACT, carnitine acylcarnitine transferase.

present with hypoglycemic hypoketotic encephalopathy but usually at a younger age. CTD is effectively treated with carnitine supplementation (100–200 mg/kg/day) and the long-term prognosis is good (Cederbaum et al. 2002). Carnitine supplementation is for life and free carnitine levels should be monitored to ensure adequate supplementation aiming to keep concentrations within the normal range. Diagnosis is confirmed by measuring the fractional excretion of carnitine with simultaneous measurement of carnitine in plasma and urine.

The OCTN2 carnitine transporter is encoded by the *SLC22 A5* gene on chromosome 5q. Numerous mutations have been reported (Wang et al. 2001). Sudden death secondary to cardiac arrest has been reported in older patients when carnitine supplementation has been discontinued. Newborn screening has revealed asymptomatic adults who were diagnosed when low free carnitine levels were detected on the infant's routine newborn screen (Schimmenti et al. 2007). Two mothers had minimal symptoms such as fatigue whereas one mother had episodes of syncope with ventricular arrhythmias in pregnancy. Mutation analysis revealed some mutations previously identified in classical patients in those with minimal symptoms (N32S, R282X, R254X, S467C) whereas the completely asymptomatic mothers had mutations not previously reported (P46S, R488C, and T520fsX521).

Carnitine Acylcarnitine Translocase Deficiency (CACT)

CACT deficiency is a rare inborn error presenting in the neonatal period or early infancy with hypoketotic hypoglycemia, encephalopathy, cardiomyopathy, and ventricular arrhythmias with many infants dying in the first months of life (Chalmers et al. 1997). Milder cases with fasting hypoglycemia have been reported. Diagnosis is suggested by the combination of decreased free carnitine with pronounced elevations of long chain acylcarnitines. Successful prospective management of CACT deficiency with medium chain triglyceride (MCT), low fat diet, and carnitine supplementation in a sibling has been reported (Pierre et al. 2007).

Carnitine Palmitoyltransferase-2 Deficiency (CPT2)

CPT2 deficiency may be divided into three clinical presentations: adult, infantile, and neonatal forms. The adult form is the most common and usually presents with rhabdomyolysis in the second and third decades of life. Cardiac arrest has, however, been reported following strenuous exercise (Ratliff et al. 2002).

Cardiac involvement occurs in approximately 50% of the infantile form either as dilated or hypertrophic cardiomyopathy or as arrhythmias and conduction disorders. Histology and electron microscopy revealed lipid accumulation in the heart and other organs (North et al. 1995; Guertl 2000). Age of onset is between 6 months and 2 years, the majority presenting in the first year of life. Patients present with recurrent attacks of acute liver dysfunction with hypoketotic hypoglycemia and coma. The neonatal onset form is associated with congenital brain and renal malformations including cystic dysplasia, polymicrogyria, glial heterotopias, and hemorrhages. The symptom-free interval between birth and the onset of acute metabolic decompensation ranges from a few hours to the first few days of life characterized by hypoglycemic seizures with hepatomegaly, cardiomegaly with associated arrhythmias with marked metabolic acidosis, and hyperammonemia with a rapidly fatal outcome (Bonnefont et al. 2004).

Diagnosis in all three forms is suggested by reduced free carnitine levels in plasma with higher than normal levels of acylcarnitine intermediates, especially palmitoyl-carnitine (C16) and linoleoylcarnitine (C18:1), with confirmation on fibroblast fat oxidation studies, the residual flux through the fat oxidation pathway correlating well with the severity of the disease. Specific enzymology can be measured on frozen skeletal muscle.

The *CPT2* gene contains five exons and is assigned to chromosome 1p32. Most mutations are missense mutations (Sigauke et al. 2003). Genotype–phenotype correlations have been described with patients with the late onset myopathic form having higher residual activity missense mutations, especially the 338C>T (S113L) mutation, which is the most common mutation in the adult form. The severe neonatal presentation is associated with nonsense mutations or deletions whereas the intermediate infantile form is usually associated with one copy of the severe mutation and one milder mutation (Thuillier et al. 2003). CPT2 is managed like other fat oxidation defects with avoidance of prolonged fasting and glucose polymer remains the mainstay of therapy. MCT supplementation is also recommended. Investigation of triheptanoin anaplerotic therapy is under investigation and bezafibrate has been shown to restore both CPT2 activity and long chain fat oxidation in fibroblasts from patients with the adult form (Djouadi et al. 2003). In rats, theophylline has been shown to increase cardiac and renal CPT activity by an unknown mechanism (Alhomida 2001). Sodium valproate is contraindicated as it may trigger rhabdomyolysis.

β Oxidation Defects

The β oxidation cycle has four steps: acyl-CoA dehydrogenase, enoyl-CoA hydratase, L-3-hydroxy acyl-CoA dehydrogenase, and 3-keto-acyl-CoA thiolase. Each turn of the cycle reduces the fatty acid chain length by two carbons that are converted to acetyl-CoA. The very long chain acyl-CoA dehydrogenase and the trifunctional protein bearing all three of the enzyme activities (enoyl-CoA hydratase, L-3-hydroxy acyl-CoA dehydrogenase, and 3-keto-acyl-CoA thiolase) are bound to the inner mitochondrial membrane. The simultaneous production of reduced cofactors donates electrons to the respiratory chain for ATP synthesis.

Very Long Chain Acyl-CoA Dehydrogenase Deficiency (VLCAD)

VLCAD is the rate-limiting step in long chain fat oxidation. Patients present with hypoketotic hypoglycemia or with chronic cardiomyopathy and weakness. In a review of 30 cases, 30% presented within the first 2 days of life and 82% by the end of the first year (Vianey-Saban et al. 1998). Although hypoketotic hypoglycemia was the commonest presenting symptom (43%), 36% presented with hypertrophic cardiomyopathy and a further 18% with arrhythmias or cardiac arrest. Overall 47% developed hypertrophic cardiomyopathy (age range 2.5–10 months). Prognosis is related to the severity of the initial illness with 30% dying during the course of the first episode, but only 13% dying later. Hypertrophic cardiomyopathy is often associated with pericardial effusion and this was responsible for most deaths. Like CPT2, VLCAD may be divided into three phenotypes with a severe lethal neonatal presentation with cardiac involvement either dilated or hypertrophic, a later milder delayed onset with hypoketotic hypoglycemia but no cardiac involvement and a later adolescent/adult form where muscle symptoms and rhabdomyolysis dominate.

Diagnosis is suggested by elevated tetradecenoyl-carnitine (C14:1) and is confirmed on fibroblast fat oxidation studies. Such studies have revealed two profiles with the hypoglycemic phenotype characterized by mainly dodecenoyl-carnitine (C12) while the cardiomyopathic form is characterized by mainly myristoyl-carnitine (C14) and palmitoyl-carnitine (C16). A genotype–phenotype correlation has been defined with milder disease associated with higher residual activity missense mutations and severe disease associated with nonsense mutations and deletions (Andresen et al. 1999). Management comprises avoidance of prolonged fasting with frequent feeds during the day and continuous overnight feeds in the infant with the use of uncooked cornstarch as an alternative from the age of 18 months. This is used in conjunction with dietary long chain fat restriction and the use of MCT. Anaplerotic therapy with triheptanoin has been reported. The use of triheptanoin in a 6-year-old girl led to resolution of her hypertrophic cardiomyopathy with improvement of her fractional shortening from 19% to 30% within a month of starting treatment and reduction in the intraventricular septum thickness and posterior wall of the left ventricle (Roe et al. 2002).

Long Chain Hydroxy Acyl-CoA Dehydrogenase Deficiency (LCHAD) and the Mitochondrial Trifunctional Protein deficiency (TFP)

The mitochondrial TFP consists of four α and four β subunits. The α subunit contains both the long chain enoyl-CoA hydratase and LCHAD activities whereas the β subunit contains the long chain 3-keto-acyl-CoA thiolase (LCAT). Some patients have the isolated LCHAD deficiency whereas others are also deficient in the hydratase and LCAT (TFP deficiency). The clinical phenotype is broad ranging from a mild condition not dissimilar to MCADD with fasting hypoketotic hypoglycemia, to the more typical long chain presentation like VLCAD. Cardiac manifestations include cardiomegaly with poorly contracting left ventricle, hypertrophic cardiomyopathy, dilated poorly contracting left ventricle and cardiac dysrhythmias such as sinus node dysfunction and atrioventricular block (Guertl et al. 2000). In a review of 50 cases, cardiomyopathy was present in 46% of cases (den Boer et al. 2002). Four-fifths of cases presented with acute metabolic decompensation of which 18% had arrhythmias, 21% cardiorespiratory arrest, and 9% sudden death. The overall mortality was high with deaths occurring prior to diagnosis or within 3 months of the diagnosis. The age of onset of clinical symptoms ranged from 1 day to 26 months (mean 5.8 months). Fifteen percent presented within the neonatal period. Patients who did not present with acute decompensation presented with chronic liver disease, growth faltering, feeding difficulties, and/or hypotonia. Following diagnosis and follow-up, no patient subsequently developed cardiomyopathy. Some patients develop pigmentary retinopathy and/or peripheral neuropathy.

Diagnosis is suggested by long chain hydroxyacylcarnitines on tandem mass spectrometry and long chain hydroxydicarboxylic acids on urine organic acid analysis. Diagnosis is confirmed on fat oxidation studies in fibroblasts.

Patients may be screened for the common G1528C mutation in exon 15 of the HADHA gene (Rakheja et al. 2002), which affects the NAD^+ binding site of LCHAD leading to loss of enzyme activity. TFP, which is less common, may be caused by mutations affecting either the HADHA or HADHB genes. Complete loss of activity is associated with mutations leading to truncated proteins or affecting the stability of the interaction between the α and β subunits. There is a well-established association with the HELLP syndrome and AFLP. Although only a small proportion of cases will be associated with a mother carrying an affected fetus with a long chain fat oxidation defect, all infants born to mothers with HELLP or AFLP should be screened with a plasma acylcarnitine sample in the first few days of life to screen for this possible diagnosis. LCHAD and TFP are managed along similar lines to VLCAD.

Electron Transfer Defects

Multiple Acyl-CoA Dehydrogenase Deficiency (MADD)

MADD results in a block of transfer of electrons not only from fat oxidation but also the oxidation of branched chain amino acids, sarcosine, and lysine. Clinically, patients present with hypoketotic hypoglycemia and metabolic acidosis, hypotonia, cardiomyopathy, and coma in the neonatal period. Some neonates have associated congenital anomalies including facial dysmorphism, polycystic kidneys, anomalies of external genitalia, and muscular defects of the anterior abdominal wall. Most patients die within the first few months of life. Treatment with riboflavin, carnitine, and diets low in protein and fat have had limited success when used in milder or later onset disease (Frerman and Goodman 2001). Case reports using ketone body supplementation (D,L-3-hydroxybutyrate) have shown some promise (Van Hove et al. 2003).

Diagnosis is suggested by a diagnostic urinary organic acid profile with the presence of ethylmalonate, glutarate, and isovalerate in conjunction with multiple acylcarnitine abnormalities. The condition is inherited in a recessive manner with the gene located on chromosome 4q32.

Lysosomal Storage Disorders (LSD)

Lysosomes are membrane-bound intracellular organelles containing a large number of hydrolytic enzymes at acid pH whose main function is the degradation of complex macromolecules. The LSDs are each due to a specific enzyme deficiency resulting in abnormal storage of partially degraded macromolecules in the lysosomes. Around 40 distinct lysosomal disorders are known and, apart from Fabry, Danon, and Hunter's diseases, which are X-linked, all are inherited in an autosomal recessive pattern.

The clinical spectrum of the storage disorders is wide, ranging from prenatal hydrops fetalis to mild disease in adulthood. Suggestive signs may include coarsening of facial features, neurological deterioration, and hepatosplenomegaly. Patients with storage disorders often have a characteristic skeletal dysplasia (dysostosis multiplex) with a large skull, spinal deformities, and short, thick tubular bones. The liver and spleen are important sites for abnormal lysosomal storage, hence hepatosplenomegaly is a frequent finding, but the clinical picture is often dominated by neurodevelopmental regression.

The heart is frequently affected in this group of disorders. There is abnormal accumulation of complex macromolecules such as glycosaminoglycans in the myocardium, the valves are affected, cardiac rhythm abnormalities have been reported, and in some cases abnormalities are seen in the coronary arteries. Endocardial fibroelastosis is also a feature of some subtypes of LSD. Cardiac abnormalities progress over time and are rarely the reason for the presentation and diagnosis of these conditions. Notable exceptions to this are infantile Pompe disease (GSD II, acid maltase deficiency) where symptoms of severe cardiomyopathy present within the first few weeks of life (Kishnani et al. 2006) and the cardiac variant of Fabry disease where few other features of Fabry are observed (Perrot et al. 2002).

The diagnosis of this group of disorders relies upon specific enzyme assay in leucocytes or fibroblasts. Other investigations that direct diagnosis are urinary glycosaminoglycans and oligosaccharides [mucopolysaccharidoses (MPS), mucolipidoses (ML), mannosidosis, sialidosis], vacuolated cells in peripheral blood smear (GM1 gangliosidosis, Pompe disease), foamy cells on bone marrow aspirate (GM1 gangliosidosis), and dysostosis multiplex on skeletal survey (MPS, GM1 gangliosidosis, ML). The genes responsible for LSD are now largely known and DNA mutation analysis can support both diagnosis in the index case and prenatal diagnosis. Prenatal diagnosis is possible for all this group of disorders.

The lysosomal disorders are chronic, progressive diseases and until recently were regarded as untreatable. However, several LSDs are now treatable through a range of therapies. Bone marrow transplantation (BMT) has been shown to be effective in some disorders, the donor marrow providing a source of the deficient enzyme (Yeager et al. 2002). In addition, the recognition that the enzymes are targeted to the lysosome by mannose-6 phosphate has allowed the development of successful enzyme replacement therapy (ERT) for several lysosomal storage diseases (MPS I, II, VI, Pompe, Gaucher, and Fabry) (Rohrbach et al. 2007). Enzyme injected into peripheral veins will migrate to the lysosome in affected tissues. ERT, however, will not cross the blood–brain barrier and will not therefore treat the neurological effects of the disease. Other new therapies using small molecules have the advantage of blood–brain barrier penetration. Examples of therapies under development include "substrate deprivation" (Winchester et al. 2000; Butters et al. 2003) and "chaperone" therapies. In substrate deprivation therapy, treatment is aimed, not at counteracting the effects of stored product or supplying the deficient enzyme, but at reducing production of the stored lysosomal compound (the substrate) by blocking an earlier step in the pathway. Certain small molecules can act as "chaperones" for a misfolded enzyme that protects the enzyme from being destroyed in the endoplasmic reticulum. This altered enzyme remains active, which may be sufficient to counteract the disease process particularly in the milder variants (Fan 2007). Thus, with these new treatments, the long-term outcome of these disorders is likely to be radically altered over the next few years.

The newer therapies have an impact on cardiac pathology. In general, ERT improves the cardiomyopathy and cardiac function is measurably improved on treatment. Information to date, however, suggests that ERT has a lesser impact on the associated valvular dysfunction (Braunlin et al. 2006). Whilst it may slow disease progression it does not reverse cardiac valve damage. Initial results on the mouse model suggest that chaperone therapy may be successful in the cardiac variant of Fabry disease and human trials are underway (Grabowski 2008).

To aid further discussion of specific clinical features of the various types of LSD it is helpful to categorize them according to the nature of the primary storage product. Using this approach, LSD may be divided into four major groups: mucopolysaccharidoses, ML, sphingolipidoses, and glycoproteinoses.

Mucopolysaccharidoses

The mucopolysaccharidoses (MPS) are a group of progressive multisystem disorders affecting the bones and joints, brain, liver and spleen, heart, upper airways, and eyes. They can be grouped (type I,

II, III, etc.) according to the underlying enzyme deficiency. Although they share several features, they vary in the degree of facial dysmorphism, neurodegeneration, and degree of physical disabilities.

Clinical effects of MPS include recurrent ENT infections, obstructive sleep apnea, deposits on the cardiac valves and infiltration of the cardiac muscle, inguinal and umbilical herniae, spinal cord compression, and pain and stiffness from the skeletal dysplasia. The deposits within the connective tissue cause thickening of the skin giving rise to the characteristic facial coarsening.

The widespread organ involvement in the MPS disorders demands that management involves the input from a multidisciplinary team consisting of cardiology, anesthesia, orthopedics, ENT, neurosurgery, physiotherapy, audiology, and speech therapy. Their care should ideally be coordinated by the pediatrician/physician.

Anesthesia should be undertaken with care in the MPS disorders, more specifically in types I, II, IV, and VI as these children are difficult to intubate due to MPS deposition around the airway (Walker et al. 1994). Intubation is further compromised by the vulnerability of the cervical spinal cord in these subtypes.

MPS I (Hurler Syndrome, Hurler-Scheie and Scheie)

MPS I arises due to deficiency of the lysosomal enzyme iduronidase. There is a wide spectrum of disease from Hurler syndrome (in many ways the prototype of MPS disorders) through to Scheie disease, which may be diagnosed for the first time in adulthood. Children with Hurler disease present around the age of 9 months with coarse facies, skeletal abnormalities such as the gibbus deformity of the lumbar spine, corneal clouding, and recurrent ENT infections. There are usually inguinal and/or umbilical herniae, middle ear disease with hearing impairment, and with time neurodegeneration occurs. The cardiac component of MPS IH is usually cardiac valvular disease, mitral incompetence being the most common defect (Mohan et al. 2002). There may additionally be aortic valve disease and a cardiomyopathy. Endocardial fibroelastosis has been reported leading to early infantile presentation (Stephan et al. 1989). This is an unusual occurrence but justifies urinary glycosaminoglycans in the cardiomyopathy screen as these children may not yet show any other features suggestive of Hurler disease. The natural history of type IH is of progressive skeletal and cardiopulmonary disease with death by age of 10 years. However, bone marrow transplant is offered to suitably matched children before 18 months of age. The results of BMT are good with improvement in cardiopulmonary function, remodeling of the face, reduction in ENT disease, and normalization of the size of the liver and spleen (Hopwood et al. 1993; Peters et al. 1996). The neurodegeneration is avoided but some degree of learning disability may occur. Early transplantation appears to have a more favorable outcome. Certainly, it should be performed before 18–24 months of age. Despite transplant, orthopedic complications progress as the transplanted cells do not prevent the skeletal complications.

MPS IH/S refers to an intermediate form of iduronidase deficiency in which the presenting symptoms are of pain and stiffness due to joint disease. Corneal clouding is usually present, carpal tunnel syndrome is common but intellect is usually normal or nearly so. Cardiac disease is an important factor in the management of this subtype. As in most of the MPS conditions, mitral valve disease is most frequent followed by involvement of the atrial valve. Since these individuals live to adulthood, valve replacement may become necessary.

The later onset of MPS I is known as Scheie disease and both this and MPS I/S are also referred to as the attenuated forms of MPS I. Scheie syndrome may be diagnosed as an adult due to the finding of corneal clouding or joint problems. Valve disease is similar to the previous forms. A recent report also highlights the abnormalities in systolic and diastolic function in these adults (Soliman et al. 2007).

ERT is available to all individuals with the non-neurological forms of MPS I. It reverses organ enlargement, remodels the facial features, reduces ENT problems, and improves joint stiffness (Wraith 2005). It does not penetrate the brain and therefore cannot be a sole treatment for MPS I (Hurler syndrome). It improves the cardiomyopathy but has minimal effect on valvular disease although may slow its progression (Braunlin et al. 2006). ERT has also been used, however, as an adjunct to BMT in order to improve the cardiopulmonary function in young children awaiting a suitable bone marrow donor. Larger studies are needed to measure the value of this approach (Cox-Brinkman et al. 2006). ERT has been useful, however, in an infant with endocardial fibroelastosis whose cardiac function improved sufficiently to proceed to BMT (Hirth et al. 2007). Many mutations are recognized in the α-iduronidase gene and there is evidence of some degree of genotype–phenotype correlation (Bunge et al. 1998). The mutations W402X and Q70X are the most frequently detected in European populations and both cause a Hurler phenotype.

MPS II (Hunter Syndrome)

MPS II is an X-linked disorder that arises due to deficiency of the lysosomal enzyme iduronate-2-sulfatase. It shares many features with Hurler syndrome but the onset is later typically leading to diagnosis between 2 and 4 years of age. The facial appearance, though coarse, differs slightly from Hurler. There are similar somatic problems of recurrent upper airways and middle ear disease, skeletal dysplasia, hepatosplenomegaly, and herniae. There are, broadly speaking, two groups: neurological where neurodegeneration occurs about the age of 6 years and non-neurological in which intellect is maintained. This categorization, however, is a simplification and the disorder is now regarded as a continuum between severe and attenuated forms (Wraith et al. 2008). The cardiac problems are similar to type I with mitral and aortic valve disease and cardiomyopathy (Mohan et al. 2002). Sudden death due to AV block occurs in MPS II (Hishitani et al. 2000). ERT has been available for MPS II in the past few years. The effects are as in other disorders; the organ enlargement is reversed and cardiopulmonary function improves but valvular disease is not reversed. The brain effects are not expected to respond to ERT and it is unknown to what extent ERT will affect the neurological phenotype in terms of life expectancy (Wraith et al. 2008). Non-neurological forms of Hunter disease may live to adulthood and so valve replacement may become necessary in this type. This operation has been successfully performed in an adult with the attenuated form of Hunter disease (Bhattacharya et al. 2005), and it is likely that such treatments will become more frequent as ERT improves longevity. As an X-linked disorder, mutation detection is important in establishing carrier status within families. Over 150 mutations have been described. The presence of major deletions or rearrangements in the gene correlates with severe disease (Wraith et al. 2008).

MPS III (Sanfilippo Syndrome)

MPS III is a severe neurodegenerative disease. There are four subtypes (A–D) each due to a different defective enzyme. The features are similar throughout the range. In Sanfilippo syndrome, the somatic affects are less pronounced and thus the diagnosis is made somewhat later around the age of 4 years when the developmental delay is investigated (Valstar et al. 2008). Although the heart is affected in MPS III, the cardiac pathology is milder than in other MPS types. However, on occasions, it can lead to severe symptoms (Muenzer et al. 1993).

MPS IVA (Morquio Disease)

MPS IVA individuals have normal intelligence but suffer a severe skeletal dysplasia. The storage product is largely keratan sulfate and the condition is caused by deficiency of the lysosomal enzyme N-acetylgalactosamine-6-sulfate sulfatase. The diagnosis is usually made around 4 years of age although symptoms are recognized 2 years earlier. The severe skeletal dysplasia dominates in this syndrome and individuals are very short, with final height around 1.2 m. Physical problems include cardiopulmonary disease secondary to the fixed chest deformity, cervical myelopathy due to odontoid hypoplasia, and joint problems. The hips and knees are dysplastic and there is ligamentous laxity (Montaño et al. 2007). The heart valves are frequently abnormal with both mitral and aortic valve involvement (Mohan et al. 2002). The disease is progressive and is associated with death usually by the third decade. Cardiac valve replacement is possible although attention to the anesthetic is very important here and consideration to the long-term outcome (Nicolini et al. 2008). There are no specific new therapies yet for Morquio disease although animal model work is underway. Morquio disease is extremely heterogeneous and this is represented in the wide range of mutations detected in the gene (Tomatsu et al. 2005). There are some correlations with phenotype.

MPS VI (Maroteax-Lamy Disease)

MPS VI frequently affects the heart. The deficient enzyme is N-acetylgalactosamine-4-sulfatase Affected individuals have normal or near normal intelligence but a severe skeletal dysplasia with short stature. The somatic features are similar to Hurler with hepatosplenomegaly, corneal clouding, and retinal disease. The cardiac effects include cardiomyopathy and valvular disease. This disorder has been treated in the past by BMT and more recently with ERT (Giugliani et al. 2007). Both therapies stabilize cardiac function and valvular damage. Individuals have undergone cardiac valve replacement. It is an extremely rare disorder in the United Kingdom.

MPS VII (Sly Disease)

MPS VII is the most rare of the MPS disorders. However, since the enzyme responsible (β-glucuronidase) was one of the earliest to be purified, studies on Sly disease has generated much of the information that has led to the development of new therapies for the other MPS disorders. It is associated with hydrops fetalis in utero. Outside the perinatal presentation Sly disease usually causes progressive valve disease (Sewell et al. 1982).

Mucolipidoses

The ML includes ML type II, ML type III and IV. ML II and III are due to the same biochemical defect. ML IV is an extremely rare disorder seen mainly in the Ashkenazi Jewish population. It is not known to cause heart disease.

ML II or "I cell" disease presents earlier than Hurler but shares many physical features. It is a severe disease with neurological degeneration and death occurs in early childhood. Corneal clouding is common; there is also a retinal degeneration. Cardiomyopathy is frequently seen in ML II. It can be a life-threatening feature in infancy. Valvular involvement is also common and may cause clinical symptoms early in life. Valve replacement has been successfully undertaken in infants (Daimon and Yamagishi 2005). This is a severe, usually rapidly progressive disease and careful consideration of all facts of the disease progress is advised before any specific cardiac therapeutic intervention.

ML III is more slowly progressive than ML II. The clinical course unfolds over years with diagnosis made around the age of 8–10 years and survival to adulthood is expected. Affected children have stiffening of the joints from early years with slight facial coarsening and kyphoscoliosis. Intellect is relatively well preserved with most children having normal or slight reduction in IQ. They are prone to carpal tunnel syndrome. Cardiac valvular involvement predominates and cardiac follow-up should be part of the multidisciplinary review of these individuals.

ML II/III arises due to abnormal trafficking of lysosomal enzymes into the cell. Since the enzymes are not taken up into the lysosome the diagnosis can be made by finding an increase in circulating plasma lysosomal enzymes. The underlying enzyme deficiency is UDP-N-acetylglucosamine-1-phosphotransferase and mutations in the gene GNPTA that codes for the α/β subunits of this multimeric enzyme have been identified in known patients. Rather than considering ML II and III as separate entities they are best thought of as a continuum with varying ages of onset of symptoms (Bargal et al. 2006). There is no enzyme therapy for this disorder and treatment is symptomatic including ophthalmology, orthopedic, and cardiology reviews.

Glycoprotein Disorders

Glycoproteins are complex compounds composed of a protein and a carbohydrate. The carbohydrate portion of glycoproteins is made of combinations of the oligosaccharides glucose, galactose, mannose, and fucose. Deficiency of the degradative enzymes results in accumulation in the lysosome of these products. Six different diseases caused by a defect in glycoprotein breakdown are recognized: α-mannosidosis, aspartylglucosaminuria, β-mannosidosis, fucosidosis, galactosialidosis, Schindler disease, and sialidosis. These are all extremely rare disorders and their rarity may mean that cardiac aspects are overlooked in the medical literature. Cardiomegaly has been reported in fucosidosis. This is typically a progressive neurodegenerative disease with seizures, mild coarsening of the facies, mild skeletal dysplasia, and angiokeratoma. BMT may be effective if performed early enough in the course of the disease (Vellodi et al. 1995). In sialic acid storage disease there is a block in efflux of sialic acid from the lysosome. There is a range of severity from infantile sialic acid storage disease (ISSD), which is a severe neurodegenerative disorder with Hurler-like physical features and death in infancy to Salla disease in which mental retardation and ataxia are slowly progressive and there is a near normal life span. In ISSD, there may be a cardiomyopathy and conduction defects. There is no specific treatment for this disorder. In galactosialidosis the underlying problem is defective protective protein/cathepsin A. This causes loss of function of two important lysosomal enzymes β-galactosidase and neuraminidase giving rise to a phenotype that combines typical physical lysosomal features of dysostosis multiplex with neurodegeneration. The heart pathology therefore is similar to that of GM1 gangliosidosis, which is due to β-galactosidase deficiency (see next section).

Sphingolipidoses

Sphingolipids are complex membrane lipids composed of sphingosine and a long chain fatty acid. Since these intricate molecules form an integral part of cerebral membranes, the sphingolipidoses, in which the catabolism is deranged, are often associated with relentless neurodegeneration. The hallmark of the neurodegenerative subgroup of sphingolipids is the cherry-red spot. This group includes disorders such as GM2 gangliosidosis (Tay-Sachs and Sandhoff disease), metachromatic leucodystrophy and Krabbe disease. These are all severe neurodegenerative disorders in which cardiac involvement is rare. The disorder in which the heart is affected is GM1 gangliosidosis.

GM1 gangliosidosis arises due to deficient β-galactosidase. Infantile GM1 gangliosidosis causes symptoms early in life with hypotonia from birth. By the age of 6 months children have developmental delay and are developing a coarse physical appearance with puffy skin, maxillary hyperplasia, hypertrophied gums, and macroglossia. They have dysostosis multiplex. About half of the affected children have cherry-red spot. Rapid neurological deterioration is usual and by the second year of life, individuals have seizures and swallowing difficulties. Death usually occurs by 2 years. Dilated and hypertrophic cardiomyopathy has been noted (Simma et al. 1990; Morrone et al. 2000). It is possible that cardiac anomalies are present more commonly than previously reported in this condition as the overwhelming neurological deterioration dictates the need for palliative care and specific attention to cardiac involvement is rare. Interestingly, the *GLB1* gene produces two alternatively spliced transcripts that code β-galactosidase and the elastin-binding protein. It is thought that this effect on elastin correlates with cardiac pathology (Morrone et al. 2000). Although there is currently no curative treatment, new therapies such as chaperone or gene therapy are under research. The advantage of these modalities is the ability to penetrate the blood–brain barrier. Juvenile and adult forms of GM1 gangliosidosis are recognized in which there are no physical changes but a picture of neurological deterioration is observed.

Gaucher Disease

Gaucher disease is caused by deficiency of glucocerebrosidase. There are three forms: 1, 2, and 3. Type 1 is the most common and is a disorder of the hematopoetic system, which causes hepatosplenomegaly, anemia, and bone deformity. Type 2 is a severe neurodegenerative disease. Hepatosplenomegaly is present within the first 6 months of life and neurological involvement is severe with feeding problems, spasticity, and regression. Involvement of the bulbar centers is characteristic and this, with the eye findings of a squint and the severe spasticity, gives the clinical triad of opisthotonus, trismus, and strabismus. In type 3 the hematological features are present but in addition there are neurological features. The characteristic neurological sign is supranuclear ophthalmoplegia. Cardiac involvement in Gaucher disease is rare but cardiomyopathy can occur. In addition, the D409H mutation in the homozygous form has been associated with calcification of the aortic and mitral valves (George et al. 2001).

Fabry Disease

Fabry disease is a lysosomal disease caused by deficiency of the enzyme α-galactosidase A. The defect leads to the intralysosomal accumulation of glycosphingolipids throughout the body. This X-linked metabolic defect causes a multisystem disorder consisting of chronic progressive painful small-fiber neuropathy, renal dysfunction, heart disease, and stroke. Skin lesions known as angiokeratoma corporis diffusum are characteristic of the disorder. They are dark red angiectases and occur on the lower part of the abdomen, buttocks, and scrotum (the bathing trunk area). The eye typically shows cornea verticillata, an appearance of lines radiating from a point near the center of the cornea with a whorl-like appearance. This can also be seen in asymptomatic females. Depression may be an underreported feature (Cole et al. 2007). Fabry disease typically presents in males in late childhood or adolescence with pain in the extremities (acroparesthesia) provoked by exertion or change in temperature. Female heterozygotes may show clinical expression of the disease with acroparesthesia and angiokeratoma. In addition, it is now recognized that females may have cardiac abnormalities. The main life-limiting complications are progressive renal disease, cerebrovascular disease, and hypertrophic cardiomyopathy.

In a minority of cases, heart disease can be the sole manifestation of the disease (the so-called cardiac variant Fabry). This variant is rare, however, but cardiac involvement is common in all individuals with Fabry including women and children. Myocardial abnormalities are characterized mainly by left ventricular (LV) wall thickening without significant dilatation, the most frequent abnormal structural pattern being concentric LV hypertrophy (LVH). Systolic function is largely preserved in a large majority of affected individuals but impairment of diastolic filling is a relatively common finding. Valvular structural abnormalities are frequently found particularly mitral valve infiltration. Valvular regurgitation seems to be relatively frequent but mostly insignificant. Electrocardiographic changes include atrioventricular conduction abnormalities, signs of LVH, and repolarization abnormalities. Cardiac pacing has been necessary in some cases due to severe AV block (Breunig and Wanner 2008). Although more advanced in males, the heart is also affected in women who may suffer cardiac symptoms. Children do not have symptoms attributable to cardiac effects but the heart is larger than normal and shows progressive enlargement over time (Kampmann et al. 2008).

The incidence of Fabry has been estimated at 1 in 40, 000 to 1 in 117, 000 males. However, it may be more common. Prevalence studies in end-stage renal disease or hypertrophic cardiomyopathy clinics indicate prevalences of 1.2% and 4.9 % (male) respectively (Linhart and Elliott 2007).

The gene for α-galactosidase is located on Xq22.1 and more than 350 mutations have been identified throughout all seven exons of the gene. The mutations are generally "private" and result in complete lack of identifiable enzyme. There are three missense mutations most often seen in those with "cardiac" Fabry disease (R112H, R301Q, and G328R).

Fabry disease is amenable to ERT (Desnick et al. 2003). Treatment with intravenous infusion of recombinant enzyme results in an improvement in cardiac function and a measurable reduction in LVH. Cardiac biopsies have shown a reduction in the amount of the storage product globotriaosylceramide (Hughes et al. 2008). ERT is more beneficial to those with mild to moderate renal disease and has little impact on the kidney where ERT is commenced in those with advanced disease. Other beneficial effects of ERT include reduction in likelihood of cerebrovascular events and improvement in pain scores. The use of chaperone therapy is also under development for Fabry disease. This approach is aimed at the milder variants of the disease due to underlying missense mutations in which sufficient residual enzyme activity remains to avoid the multisystem effects of the disorder. Benefits from galactose infusions have been reported in this group (Frustaci et al. 2001).

Pompe Disease (GSD II, Acid Maltase Deficiency, Acid α-Glucosidase Deficiency)

Pompe disease is a progressive neuromuscular disease resulting from deficiency of the lysosomal enzyme acid maltase. This enzyme normally degrades glycogen to glucose within the lysosome. In Pompe disease glycogen accumulates within the lysosome leading to distension and destruction of cellular function. In common with other LSD there is a spectrum of severity but Pompe is usually divided into two entities. This distinction is of importance as it is the presence of cardiomyopathy that is the key distinguishing feature. Thus infantile Pompe is associated with early onset muscle weakness and hypertrophic cardiomyopathy whilst weakness without heart involvement categorizes an individual as having juvenile or adult onset. Biochemically, the presence of cardiomyopathy is associated with lower enzyme levels and infantile Pompe sufferers have acid maltase levels <1% of normal. The diagnosis is suggested by the clinical features, the finding of vacuolated lymphocytes on blood film and confirmed by enzyme assay on white cells, skin fibroblasts, or muscle (Pompe Disease Diagnostic Working Group et al. 2008).

Infantile Pompe presents early in infancy usually by 6 weeks of age with a combination of feeding problems, failure to thrive, respiratory difficulties, paucity of movements, and motor weakness. Cardiomegaly is virtually invariable even from birth. There are characteristic ECG changes of a shortened PR interval, increased QT dispersion, and large LV voltages. Echocardiographically concentric LVH is present. Untreated, the disease progresses rapidly with poor weight gain, macroglossia, and death occurs within the first year of life (van den Hout et al. 2003). The infantile form is a rare disorder with incidence around 1 in 100, 000 in the Caucasian population.

Over the past few years, ERT has been successfully developed for Pompe disease (van der Beek et al. 2006). The most recent results of treating infants age 6 months or younger has shown promising results. All 18 infants had survived until 18 months and the risk of invasive ventilation was reduced by 92%. The cardiomyopathy improves with reduction of LV mass index. ECG abnormalities may be a useful indicator of the severity of cardiac involvement and trend toward normal is observed in serial ECG on enzyme therapy (Ansong et al. 2006). The results of ERT commencing before 6 months of age showed a more promising outcome than earlier studies in which the median age of starting ERT was older (Kishnani et al. 2007) emphasizing the need for early intervention. This point has led to development in newborn screening for Pompe disease. It is possible to detect Pompe in the newborn but not to distinguish the infantile form from later onset varieties on blood-spot testing. A potential approach could include echocardiography on screen-positive samples and this should detect infantile Pompe. However, the ethics of detecting juvenile forms in the newborn period requires careful consideration before population screening could begin.

Many different mutations are recognized in the gene GAA encoding α-glucosidase and some phenotype/genotype pattern is emerging (Hermans et al. 2004).

Danon Disease

Danon disease is an X-linked disorder in which glycogen accumulates in lysosomes but in this disorder acid maltase activity is normal. It arises due to mutations in the lysosomal-associated membrane protein-2 (LAMP-2). It was first recognized as a disorder in 1981 (Danon et al. 1981), but the underlying deficiency of LAMP-2 was only recently understood in 2000 (Nishino et al. 2000). It seems to be extremely rare with only about 40 cases described worldwide. The features include muscle weakness and dilated cardiomyopathy. Although not invariable, learning disability has been a frequent finding. Typically, cases present after the age of 10 years although infantile presentation has been noted. The function of the LAMP-2 gene is not known and thus the pathophysiology of Danon disease is poorly understood. Diagnosis previously required a combination of the following: skeletal and cardiomyopathy, normal acid maltase activity, evidence of vacuolation and glycogen deposition on muscle biopsy, and absence of the LAMP-2 protein. More usually, the diagnosis is confirmed by the finding of a mutation in the LAMP-2 gene. Males appear to have a more severe course of disease than females. As more reports emerge the clinical spectrum is extending and a milder cardiac phenotype has been described (van der Kooi et al. 2008). There is no specific treatment. Cardiac transplantation has been performed on one affected individual (Echaniz-Laguna et al. 2006).

Congenital Disorders of Glycosylation

Congenital disorders of glycosylation are a rapidly growing group of metabolic disorders. They arise from defects in the addition of oligosaccharide chains to glycoprotein or glycolipid compounds. Correct glycosylation of glycoproteins and lipids is essential for their biological function and the sugar chains act as biosignals for a range of cellular functions such as signaling, protein folding, and targeting of proteins. Hypoglycosylation of glycoproteins lead to impaired bioability, decreased activity, and rapid degradation. Given the importance of glycosylation, it is not surprising that a disruption of glycosylation leads to multisystemic and severe diseases. Initially, defects in the N-glycosylation pathway were recognized and are grouped as congenital disorders of glycosylation (CDG), formerly known as carbohydrate-deficient glycoprotein syndromes. More recently, defects in the less well-defined O-glycosylation pathway are being identified and combined glycosylation disorders in which both, the N- and O-glycosylation processes are affected (Grünewald 2007).

Symptoms and signs suggestive of CDG include hypotonia, esotropia, abnormal fat distribution seen especially as fat pads on the buttocks and inverted nipples, psychomotor retardation, and seizures. Ataxia is a frequent finding and the cerebellum is underdeveloped. Liver dysfunction is common and a protein-losing enteropathy may be observed. Endocrine effects include hyperinsulinism and abnormal thyroid function. These are truly multisystem disorders and many other features have been reported albeit in smaller numbers such as microcephaly and stereotypic behaviors. The most common type is CDG Ia due to phosphomannose mutase 2 deficiency. The enzymes involved are known for all subtypes and diagnosis can be confirmed in most either by enzyme assay or mutation detection. The initial biochemical investigation is isoelectric focusing of transferrin and it is upon the pattern of the bands seen that a disorder is categorized as type I or II.

The importance of cardiac involvement in CDG has been recognized only recently. It is thought to be more common in the multisystemic infantile presentation rather than the neurological attenuated form of the disease. Both dilated and hypertrophic cardiomyopathies have been reported (Gehrmann et al. 2003). It is speculated that the pathophysiology of the cardiac effects are due to hypoglycosylation of dystrophin-associated glycoproteins in the sarcolemmal plasma membrane. Accounts of cardiomyopathy have mainly been in cases of CDG Ia (the most common type) but have also been noted in types Ig, Im, and IIe. In some cases, it has been the cardinal symptom leading to the underlying diagnosis of a glycosylation disorder. Pericardial effusion can accompany or even precede the cardiomyopathy. There is a substantial risk of sudden death reported in CDG where cardiomyopathy exists and routine cardiology monitoring is indicated when a diagnosis of CDG is established. Other vascular effects that are seen include stroke-like symptoms and a coagulation disorder. CDG is associated with both increased thrombosis and increased risk of bleeding. Awareness of the hematological complications become important should any cardiac interventions such as ECMO become necessary.

Cholesterol Biosynthesis Defects

Cholesterol is an essential component of cell membranes and the immediate precursor for steroid hormone and bile acid synthesis. Seven disorders in humans have been identified out of the possible 30 in this complex synthetic pathway: Smith-Lemli-Opitz syndrome being the most common, mevalonate kinase deficiency, desmosterolosis, X-linked dominant chondrodysplasia punctata, Child syndrome (congenital hemi-dysplasia with ichthyosiform naevus and limb defects), lathosterolosis, and hydrops-ectopic calcification-moth-eaten skeletal dysplasia (HEM or Greenberg skeletal dysplasia). Cholesterol is inadequately transported through the placenta and therefore cholesterol synthesis occurs very early in the fetus. Disordered embryogenesis is therefore the hallmark of this group of disorders and structural cardiac lesions have been reported in several of these conditions.

Smith-Lemli-Opitz Syndrome

Smith-Lemli-Opitz (SLO) syndrome results from deficiency of the penultimate enzyme in cholesterol synthesis, 3-β-hydroxysterol Δ7-reductase, which converts 7-dehydrocholesterol to cholesterol. This leads to accumulation of 7-dehydrocholesterol, which is the basis for diagnosis and assessment of the 7-dehydrocholesterol:ch olesterol ratio in chorionic villus sampling facilitates biochemical prenatal diagnosis. The *DHCR7* gene is located on the long arm of chromosome 11.

Patients with classical SLO syndrome have characteristic facies with microcephaly, ptosis, anteverted nares, and micrognathia. Developmental delay is common along with growth faltering exacerbated by poor feeding. Syndactyly of the second and third toes is present in the majority of cases including the most mild. Structural cardiovascular malformations have been reported in nearly 50% of patients (Lin 1997). The commonest defects encountered include atrial septal defects, endocardial cushion defects, anomalous pulmonary venous drainage, and patent ductus arteriosus. Cholesterol has a critical role in the formation of normally active hedgehog proteins and therefore the specific defects seen within this group of disorders is thought to result from cholesterol-induced alteration of sonic hedgehog functions (Digilio et al. 2003). Other associated findings secondary to altered sonic hedgehog function includes heterotaxia, postaxial polydactyly, and holoprosencephaly.

CHILD Syndrome

CHILD syndrome is associated with a striking unilateral distribution of anomalies including an ichthyosiform skin lesion present at birth and throughout life and ipsilateral hypoplastic lesions including brain, skeletal structures, lungs, kidneys, and heart. The right side is more commonly affected than the left. The NSDHL gene responsible is inherited in an X-linked dominant fashion and is lethal in the male (Kim et al. 2005).

Desmosterolosis

Only two clinical cases of desmosterolosis have been reported, both with multiple congenital anomalies (Fitzpatrick et al. 1998; Andersson 2002). The cardiac defects seen were total anomalous pulmonary venous return in one case and patent ductus arteriosus in the other. In the first case the child was born at 34 weeks and survived only 1 hour. Dysmorphic features included macrocephaly, a hypoplastic nasal bridge, thick alveolar ridges, gingival nodules, cleft palate, ambiguous genitalia, short limbs with generalized osteosclerosis, and total anomalous pulmonary venous drainage. The second case was diagnosed at 3 years of age with severe microcephaly, agenesis of the corpus callosum, down-slanting palpebral fissures, micrognathia, submucous cleft palate, talipes, and a persistent patent ductus arteriosus. The underlying biochemical block is at the level of 3-β hydroxysterol-Δ 24-reductase secondary to mutations in the *DHCR24* gene inherited in an autosomal recessive fashion. Levels of desmosterol were increased markedly.

X-linked Dominant Chondrodysplasia Punctata

X-linked dominant chondrodysplasia punctata (CDPX2, also called Conradi-Hunerman syndrome) is a rare X-linked disorder with skeletal, skin, and ocular manifestations with presumed male lethality. Structural heart lesions have been reported in approximately 16% of cases, most commonly patent ductus arteriosus and ventricular septal defects (Fourie 1995).

Glycogen Storage Diseases (GSD)

Glycogen is the main storage form of carbohydrate in animals and accumulates in the liver, kidney, and muscle providing a steady supply of energy during fasting. The glycogen storage diseases are due to defects of glycogen synthesis or breakdown, each caused by a specific enzyme defect, and result in abnormal storage and/or deficient mobilization of glycogen. Some enzyme defects are confined to the liver and are associated with hepatomegaly and hypoglycemia, whereas others affect muscle glycogen metabolism and result in muscle cramps, weakness, and (cardio)myopathy. Only certain subtypes of GSD affect the heart. These are GSD II, III, IV, and IX. GSD II and Danon disease were discussed in the lysosomal section.

Glycogen Storage Disease Type III

GSD type III is caused by deficiency of the debrancher enzyme amylo-1,6- glucosidase resulting in accumulation of partially broken down glycogen molecules (limit dextrin). Patients with liver and muscle involvement (GSD IIIa) have a generalized debrancher deficiency that affects liver, muscle, fibroblasts, cardiac muscle, and erythrocytes, whereas patients with GSD IIIb have debrancher deficiency confined to the liver. Type IIIa is more common, occurring in about 80% of patients with GSD III.

The main clinical features are hypoglycemia, hepatomegaly, short stature, skeletal myopathy, hyperlipidemia, and cardiomyopathy. Patients who have muscle involvement often develop slowly progressive skeletal myopathy and wasting, progressing from minimal signs in childhood to severe muscle weakness by the third or fourth decade of life. LVH is common in patients with muscular involvement, and may lead to significant cardiac dysfunction in the long term. Conduction defects have also been noted (Carvalho et al. 1993).

Diagnosis is suggested by the clinical picture and confirmed on enzyme assay either on leucocytes or liver biopsy. GSD III arises due to changes in the AGL gene and many mutations are recognized. Recent work describes the differing isoforms that distinguish types IIIa and IIIb. Mutations in exon 3 are linked to IIIb. Although there are many more frequent mutations described in IIIa there is some genotype–phenotype correlation emerging (Shen and Chen 2002).

General principles of treatment are aimed at maintaining normoglycemia using overnight continuous nasogastric tube glucose feeds or uncooked cornstarch with frequent daytime feeds. Although satisfactory glucose control is associated with catch-up growth and decreased liver size, it does not prevent the development of cardiomyopathy in adolescence or adulthood. Later hepatic complications can also occur with liver failure or hepatic adenomas. However, malignant transformation is rare. Liver transplantation may be indicated for cirrhosis, end-stage liver failure, and/or hepatocellular carcinoma (Davis and Weinstein 2008). For those with GSD IIIa, the prognosis depends on the severity of neuromuscular and cardiac disease. At present, there appears to be no satisfactory way of preventing progressive myopathy.

GSD IV (Brancher Deficiency)

This is an extremely rare form of glycogen storage disorder due to deficiency of the brancher enzyme in which abnormal glycogen known as amylopectin accumulates. It is a highly heterogeneous disorder with several patterns of presentation recognized including severe liver disease in infancy, arthrogryposis, a fatal neonatal neuromuscular disease, hydrops fetalis, and cardiomyopathy (Moses et al. 2002). Several mutations have been found in the GBE gene. Cardiac transplantation has been successfully performed (Ewert et al. 1999).

GSD IX (Phosphorylase Kinase Deficiency)

Phosphorylase kinase deficiency causes hepatomegaly due to accumulation of glycogen. It is a complex enzyme made up of four subunits and inheritance can be X-linked or autosomal recessive. Typically it presents with hepatomegaly and can run a benign course although hypoglycemia and renal tubular leak are associated. A rare form of isolated cardiac phosphorylase kinase has been described with infantile hypertrophic cardiomyopathy. Diagnosis in that case required cardiac biopsy (Regalado et al. 1999).

GSD 0 (Glycogen Synthase Deficiency)

Although strictly not a disorder of glycogen storage, deficiency of glycogen synthase, essential for the production of glycogen, is included in the classification. There are two isoforms with the liver enzyme expression restricted to liver and a muscle enzyme with ubiquitous expression including muscle and heart. The role of muscle and heart glycogen is to provide energy during bursts of activity and sustained work and therefore it is not surprising that cardiomyopathy has been reported in muscle glycogen synthase deficiency (Kollberg et al. 2007). Clinical effects included reduced exercise capacity, hypertrophic cardiomyopathy, and sudden cardiac arrest. Unlike the liver glycogen synthase deficiency, glucose tolerance is normal. The enzyme is encoded by the *GYS1* gene whereas the liver glycogen synthase deficiency is encoded by *GYS2*. The cardiac manifestations have been successfully managed with β-blockers.

Other Metabolic Disorders

Tyrosinemia Type 1

Tyrosinemia type 1 is the commonest inherited block in the metabolism of tyrosine, secondary to fumaryl acetoacetase deficiency. Infants usually present within the first 6 months of life with acute liver failure or in the second 6 months of life with liver disease, growth faltering, phosphaturic rickets, and hypotonia. Rarely patients present after the first year with chronic liver disease, renal disease, rickets, and cardiomyopathy with or without a porphyria-like syndrome. Cardiomyopathy is a frequent incidental finding occurring in 30% of patients but is usually of little clinical consequence (Arora et al. 2006). The cardiomyopathy is asymptomatic although a murmur may be detectable on auscultation. ECG changes are rare and usually indicate ventricular septal hypertrophy. Localized myocardial thickening is more common and may affect the ventricular septum and the ventricular wall. Concentric hypertrophy is less common.

Tyrosinemia type 1 is effectively managed with nitisinone which blocks the catabolism of tyrosine at an earlier point in the pathway prior to the fumarylacetoacetase block. The patients therefore still have high tyrosine levels that necessitate tyrosine restriction with a low tyrosine diet supplemented with a tyrosine-free amino acid supplement, but the toxic metabolites of fumarylacetoacetase and succinylacetone are not produced thereby healing both the liver and kidneys. The cardiomyopathy also responds to this treatment (André et al. 2005).

Tyrosinemia type 1 is inherited in an autosomal recessive fashion secondary to mutations in the FAH gene localized to chromosome 15q23–25. Many mutations have been reported; however, there is a common mutation IVS12 + 5 G > A found in about 25% of alleles worldwide and is frequent in the French Canadian population. IVS6–1 G > T is the predominant mutation in patients from the Mediterranean area. No clear phenotype–genotype correlations have been found.

Diagnosis is based on the presence of a raised tyrosine in plasma with the presence of raised succinylacetone in urine, which is pathognomonic for tyrosinemia type 1. Confirmation of the diagnosis requires either enzyme assay or mutation analysis.

Prognosis has been very much influenced by the introduction of nitisinone which is well tolerated with few side effects, such as thrombocytopenia and neutropenia and transient eye symptoms (Holme and Lindstedt 2000). Hepatic and neurological decompensations are prevented by nitisinone treatment and deterioration of liver function is rare. Previously hepatocellular carcinoma was a common occurrence on dietary treatment alone; however, this risk appears very much reduced, especially when commenced on nitisinone under the age of 6 months. The long-term cognitive outcome in tyrosinemia type 1 patients remains unclear although significant learning difficulties have been found in many patients (Masurel-Paulet et al. 2008).

Propionic Acidemia

Propionic acidemia is caused by a deficiency in propionyl-coA carboxylase, which is essential for the catabolism of isoleucine and valine. Patients can present with a severe neonatal decompensation characterized by encephalopathy, severe acidosis with ketosis, and lactic acidosis. Some patients present with a milder neurological presentation with recurrent attacks of coma or with Reye-like illnesses with hepatomegaly, liver dysfunction, hyperammonemia, and encephalopathy. More chronic progressive forms may present with gastrointestinal disturbances, nonspecific developmental concerns, or seizures. Acute cardiomyopathy may complicate metabolic decompensation and may be rapidly fatal (Massoud and Leonard 1993). Postmortem studies have revealed LVH with histological evidence of increased myofiber size with enlarged hypochromatic nuclei (Mardach et al. 2005). ECG findings are variable with most frequent abnormalities indicating LVH and strain. In one series of 10 patients, 70% had a prolonged QT interval. Holter monitoring revealed a low instance of ventricular dysrhythmia (20%) with no patient showing sustained ventricular tachycardia (Baumgartner et al. 2007). Potential mechanisms for QT prolongation include carnitine-induced electromyocardial changes; however, free carnitine levels are usually low in these patients. Cardiac changes may be secondary to a direct toxic effect of intermediary metabolites building up, secondary to intercardiac depletion of an essential substrate or inhibition of oxidative phosphorylation in mitochondria by propionyl-coA.

Propionic acidemia is suggested by severe metabolic acidosis in association with hyperammonemia, raised lactate, and marked ketosis. Other biochemical findings include transient neutropenia or pancytopenia. Complications include pancreatitis and therefore a plasma amylase should be measured. Diagnosis is confirmed by the finding of raised propionate in urinary organic acids with methylcitrate and 3-hydroxypropionate. Propionyl-carnitine is elevated on acylcarnitine analysis and free carnitine may be secondarily depleted. Diagnosis is confirmed on enzymology and genotyping. Liver transplantation has a role in the long-term management of propionic acidemia abolishing acute decompensations (Rela et al. 2007). There is evidence for transplantation halting the progression of the cardiomyopathy, but no evidence for resolution (Barshes et al. 2006).

Propionic acidemia is an autosomal recessive disorder resulting from mutations in the PCCA or PCCB genes encoding the α and β subunits of propionyl-coA carboxylase. Many mutations have been identified in different populations. Newborn screening in Japan has identified a mild phenotype associated with the Y435C mutation in the PCCB gene (Yorifuji et al. 2002).

Malonic Aciduria

Malonic aciduria results from a deficiency of malonyl-coA decarboxylase in the catabolic pathways of leucine and isoleucine. The clinical presentation is variable with the major manifestations including developmental delay, hypotonia, hypoglycemia, and cardiomyopathy. The exact physiological role of the enzyme remains unclear but it may play a role in the regulation of cytoplasmic malonyl-coA and therefore influence mitochondrial and peroxisomal fatty acid oxidation (Bennett et al. 2001). Echocardiographic findings include dilated and hypertrophic cardiomyopathy (Matalon et al. 1993; Yano et al. 1997).

Diagnosis relies on elevated malonic and methylmalonic acids on urinary organic acid analysis. Total and free carnitine concentration in plasma is low with associated accumulation of malonyl carnitine. Enzymology is confirmed on cultured fibroblasts or genotyping. Malonic aciduria is inherited in an autosomal recessive fashion. The MLYCD gene is located on chromosome 16q24. The specific management of malonic aciduria remains to be determined, but carnitine supplementation appears to correct the carnitine deficiency and has improved cardiomyopathy in some patients (Ficicioglu et al. 2005). The use of a glucose polymer during intercurrent infections is instituted with the aim of reducing the chance of a full-scale decompensation.

D-2-Hydroxyglutaric Aciduria

D-2-hydroxyglutaric aciduria (D-2-HGA) is rare autosomal recessive disorder with a highly variable phenotype. The biochemical basis for the biochemical phenotype is not completely resolved with mutations in the D-2-HGD gene being found in only 50% of the patients (Struys 2006). The severe phenotype is characterized by neonatal or early onset epileptic encephalopathy, hypotonia, developmental delay, and visual impairment. Cardiomyopathy is found in approximately half of all patients with the severe form (van der Knaap 1999), but is rare in the mild phenotype: variable hypotonia and developmental delay. The severe phenotype is also associated with dysmorphic features including a flat face with broad nasal bridge and ear anomalies.

It is thought that the pathophysiological mechanism in D-2-HGA is likely to be secondary to the accumulation of D-2-HG and it has been suggested that potential treatment strategies should focus on lowering these levels.

Maternal Phenyketonuria

Phenylalanine hydroxylase deficiency (PKU) is not associated with cardiac defects; however, it became clear that raised phenylalanine in PKU mothers during pregnancy had a teratogenic effect, including congenital heart disease (Levy et al. 2001). The effect of phenylalanine is independent of the fetus having PKU itself and indeed this is unlikely unless the result of a consanguineous relationship.

The incidence of congenital heart disease in the general population is 0.8% compared to 7.5% in the maternal PKU population (Rouse et al. 2000); especially coarctation of the aorta and hypoplastic left heart syndrome. Phenylalanine control and the time at which control is gained in pregnancy correlate with the likelihood or not of having congenital heart disease in this group. The basal maternal phenylalanine level of >900 μmol/L may be a threshold for congenital heart disease. One aims for preconception counseling and management to keep levels below 250 μmol/L throughout pregnancy with frequent monitoring (3 times per week) and monthly reviews in clinic. Inadequate protein intake during pregnancy appears to have an additive effect on the incidence of congenital heart defects in the presence of elevated blood phenylalanine (Michals-Matalon et al. 2002) along with reduced vitamin B_{12} intakes (Matalon et al. 2003). In the maternal PKU population in the United Kingdom, the congenital heart disease incidence is much lower at 2.4% reflecting the difference in practices between the United Kingdom and the United States and Europe, with a greater number of women achieving good control preconception and throughout pregnancy (Lee et al. 2005).

References

Alhomida AS. Oral theophylline changes renal carnitine palmitoyltransferase activity in rats. *Arch Med Res*. 2001;32:394–399.

Anderson G, Smith VV, Malone M, Sebire NJ. Blood film examination for vacuolated lymphocytes in the diagnosis of metabolic disorders; retrospective experience of more than 2,500 cases from a single centre. *J Clin Pathol*. 2005;58:1305–1301.

Andersson HC, Kratz L, Kelley R. Desmosterolosis presenting with multiple congenital anomalies and profound developmental delay. *Am J Med Genet*. 2002;113:315–319.

André N, Roquelaure B, Jubin V, Ovaert C. Successful treatment of severe cardiomyopathy with NTBC in a child with tyrosinaemia type I. *J Inherit Metab Dis*. 2005;28:103–106.

Andresen BS, Olpin S, Poorthuis BJ, et al. Clear correlation of genotype with disease phenotype in very-long-chain acyl-CoA dehydrogenase deficiency. *Am J Hum Genet*. 1999;64:479–494.

Ansong AK, Li JS, Nozik-Grayck E, et al. Electrocardiographic response to enzyme replacement therapy for Pompe disease. *Genet Med*. 2006;8:297–301.

Arora N, Stumper O, Wright J, Kelly DA, McKiernan PJ. Cardiomyopathy in tyrosinaemia type I is common but usually benign. *J Inherit Metab Dis*. 2006;29:54–57.

Bargal R, Zeigler M, Abu-Libdeh B, et al. When Mucolipidosis III meets Mucolipidosis II: GNPTA gene mutations in 24 patients. *Mol Genet Metab*. 2006;88:359–363.

Barshes NR, Vanatta JM, Patel AJ, et al. Evaluation and management of patients with propionic acidemia undergoing liver transplantation: a comprehensive review. *Pediatr Transplant*. 2006;10:773–781.

Barth PG, Valianpour F, Bowen VM, et al. X-linked cardioskeletal myopathy and neutropenia (Barth syndrome): an update. *Am J Med Gen*. 2004;126:349–354.

Baumgartner D, Scholl-Bürgi S, Sass JO, et al. Prolonged QTc intervals and decreased left ventricular contractility in patients with propionic acidemia. *J Pediatr*. 2007;150:192–197.

Bennett MJ, Harthcock PA, Boriack RL, Cohen JC. Impaired mitochondrial fatty acid oxidative flux in fibroblasts from a patient with malonyl-CoA decarboxylase deficiency. *Mol Genet Metab*. 2001;73:276–279.

Bhattacharya K, Gibson SC, Pathi VL. Mitral valve replacement for mitral stenosis secondary to Hunter's syndrome. *Ann Thorac Surg*. 2005;80:1911–1912.

Bonnefont JP, Djouadi F, Prip-Buus C, Gobin S, Munnich A, Bastin J. Carnitine palmitoyltransferases 1 and 2: biochemical, molecular and medical aspects. *Mol Aspects Med*. 2004;25:495–520.

Braunlin EA, Berry JM, Whitley CB. Cardiac findings after enzyme replacement therapy for mucopolysaccharidosis type I. *Am J Cardiol*. 2006;98:416–418.

Breunig F, Wanner C. Update on Fabry disease: kidney involvement, renal progression and enzyme replacement therapy. *J Nephrol*. 2008;21:32–37.

Bunge S, Clements PR, Byers S, Kleijer WJ, Brooks DA, Hopwood JJ. Genotype-phenotype correlations in mucopolysaccharidosis type I using enzyme kinetics, immunoquantification and in vitro turnover studies. *Biochim Biophys Acta*. 1998;1407:249–256.

Butters TD, Mellor HR, Narita K, Dwek RA, Platt FM. Small-molecule therapeutics for the treatment of glycolipid lysosomal storage disorders. *Philos Trans R Soc Lond B Biol Sci*. 2003;358:927–945.

Carvalho JS, Matthews EE, Leonard JV, Deanfield J. Cardiomyopathy of glycogen storage disease type III. *Heart Vessels*. 1993;8:155–159.

Cederbaum SD, Koo-McCoy S, Tein I, et al. Carnitine membrane transporter deficiency: a long-term follow up and OCTN2 mutation in the first documented case of primary carnitine deficiency. *Mol Genet Metab* 2002;77:195–201.

Chalmers RA, Stanley CA, English N, Wigglesworth JS. Mitochondrial carnitine-acylcarnitine translocase deficiency presenting as sudden neonatal death. *J Pediatr*. 1997;131:220–225.

Clayton P, Winchester B, Di Tomaso E, Young E, Keir G, Rodeck C. Carbohydrate-deficient glycoprotein syndrome: normal glycosylation in the fetus. *Lancet*. 1993;341:956.

Cole AL, Lee PJ, Hughes DA, Deegan PB, Waldek S, Lachmann RH. Depression in adults with Fabry disease: a common and under-diagnosed problem. *J Inherit Metab Dis*. 2007;30:943–951.

Cox-Brinkman J, Boelens JJ, Wraith JE, et al. Haematopoietic cell transplantation (HCT) in combination with enzyme replacement therapy (ERT) in patients with Hurler syndrome. *Bone Marrow Transplant*. 2006;38:17–21.

Daimon M, Yamagishi M. Surgical treatment of marked mitral valvar deformity combined with I-cell disease 'Mucolipidosis II'. *Cardiol Young*. 2005;15:517–519.

Danon MJ, Oh SJ, DiMauro S, et al. Lysosomal glycogen storage disease with normal acid maltase. *Neurology*. 1981;31:51–57.

Davis MK, Weinstein DA. Liver transplantation in children with glycogen storage disease: controversies and evaluation of the risk/benefit of this procedure. *Pediatr Transplant*. 2008;12:137–145.

den Boer ME, Wanders RJ, Morris AA, IJlst L, Heymans HS, Wijburg FA. Long-chain 3-hydroxyacyl-CoA dehydrogenase deficiency: clinical presentation and follow-up of 50 patients. *Pediatrics*. 2002;109:99–104.

Desnick RJ, Brady R, Barranger J, et al. Fabry disease, an under-recognized multisystemic disorder: expert recommendations for diagnosis, management, and enzyme replacement therapy. *Ann Intern Med*. 2003;138(4):338–346.

Digilio MC, Marino B, Giannotti A, Dallapiccola B, Opitz JM. Specific congenital heart defects in RSH/Smith-Lemli-Opitz syndrome: postulated involvement of the sonic hedgehog pathway in syndromes with postaxial polydactyly or heterotaxia. *Birth Defects Res A*. 2003;67: 149–153.

Djouadi F, Bonnefont JP, Thuillier L, et al. Correction of fatty acid oxidation in carnitine palmitoyl transferase 2-deficient cultured skin fibroblasts by bezafibrate. *Pediatr Res*. 2003;54:446–451.

Echaniz-Laguna A, Mohr M, Epailly E, et al. Novel Lamp-2 gene mutation and successful treatment with heart transplantation in a large family with Danon disease. *Muscle Nerve*. 2006;33:393–397.

Ewert R, Gulijew A, Wensel R, et al. Glycogenosis type IV as a seldom cause of cardiomyopathy--report about a successful heart transplantation. *Z Kardiol*. 1999;88:850–856.

Fan JQ. Pharmacological chaperone therapy for lysosomal storage disorders--leveraging aspects of the folding pathway to maximize activity of misfolded mutant proteins. *FEBS J*. 2007;274:4943.

Ficicioglu C, Chrisant MR, Payan I, Chace DH. Cardiomyopathy and hypotonia in a 5-month-old infant with malonyl-coA decarboxylase deficiency: potential for preclinical diagnosis with expanded newborn screening. *Pediatr Cardiol*. 2005;26:881–883.

FitzPatrick DR, Keeling JW, Evans MJ, et al. Clinical phenotype of desmosterolosis. *Am J Med Genet*. 1998;75:145–152.

Fourie DT. Chondrodysplasia punctata: case report and literature review of patients with heart lesions. *Pediatr Cardiol*. 1995;16:247–250.

Frerman FE, Goodman SI. Defects of electron transfer flavoprotein and electron transfer flavoprotein-ubiquinone oxidoreductase: glutaric aciduria type II. In: Scriver CR, Beaudet AL, Sly WS, et al. (eds.). *The Metabolic and Molecular Bases of Inherited Disease*. McGraw-Hill Medical, New York, USA; 2001.

Frustaci A, Chimenti C, Ricci R, Natale L, Russo MA et al. Improvement in cardiac function in the cardiac variant of Fabry's disease with galactose-infusion therapy. *N Engl J Med*. 2001;345(1):25–32.

Gehrmann J, Sohlbach K, Linnebank M, et al. Cardiomyopathy in congenital disorders of glycosylation. *Cardiol Young*. 2003;13:345–351.

George R, McMahon J, Lytle B, Clark B, Lichtin A. Severe valvular and aortic arch calcification in a patient with Gaucher's disease homozygous for the D409H mutation. *Clin Genet*. 2001;59:360–363.

Gilbert-Barness E, Barness LA. Pathogenesis of cardiac conduction disorders in children genetic and histopathologic aspects. *Am J Med Genet A*. 2006;140:1993–2006.

Giugliani R, Harmatz P, Wraith JE. Management guidelines for mucopolysaccharidosis VI. *Pediatrics*. 2007;120:405–418.

Grabowski GA. Treatment perspectives for the lysosomal storage diseases. *Expert Opin Emerg Drugs*. 2008;13:197–211.

Grünewald S. Congenital disorders of glycosylation: rapidly enlarging group of (neuro)metabolic disorders. *Early Hum Dev.* 2007;83: 825–830.

Guertl B, Noehammer C, Hoefler G. Metabolic cardiomyopathies. *Int J Exp Pathol.* 2000;81:349–372.

Hermans MM, van Leenen D, Kroos MA, et al. Twenty-two novel mutations in the lysosomal alpha-glucosidase gene (GAA) underscore the genotype-phenotype correlation in glycogen storage disease type II. *Hum Mutat.* 2004;23:47–56.

Hirth A, Berg A, Greve G. Successful treatment of severe heart failure in an infant with Hurler syndrome. *J Inherit Metab Dis.* 2007;30:820.

Hishitani T, Wakita S, Isoda T, Katori T, Ishizawa A, Okada R. Sudden death in Hunter syndrome caused by complete atrioventricular block. *J Pediatr.* 2000;136:268–269.

Holme E, Lindstedt S. Nontransplant treatment of tyrosinemia. *Clin Liver Dis.* 2000;4:805–814.

Hopwood JJ, Vellodi A, Scott HS, et al. Long-term clinical progress in bone marrow transplanted mucopolysaccharidosis type I patients with a defined genotype. *J Inherit Metab Dis.* 1993;16:1024–1033.

Hughes DA, Elliott PM, Shah J, et al. Effects of enzyme replacement therapy on the cardiomyopathy of Anderson-Fabry disease: a randomised, double-blind, placebo-controlled clinical trial of agalsidase alfa. *Heart.* 2008;94:153–158.

Ibdah JA, Yang Z, Bennett MJ. Liver disease in pregnancy and fetal fatty acid oxidation defects. *Mol Genet Metab.* 2000;71:182–189.

Johnson RA, Baker SS, Fallon JT, et al. An occidental case of cardiomyopathy and selenium deficiency. *N Engl J Med.* 1981;304:1210–1212.

Kampmann C, Wiethoff CM, Whybra C, Baehner FA, Mengel E, Beck M. Cardiac manifestations of Anderson-Fabry disease in children and adolescents. *Acta Paediatr.* 2008;97:463–469.

Kim CA, Konig A, Bertola DR, et al. CHILD syndrome caused by a deletion of exons 6–8 of the NSDHL gene. *Dermatology.* 2005;211:155–158.

Kishnani PS, Corzo D, Nicolino M, et al. Recombinant human acid [alpha]-glucosidase: major clinical benefits in infantile-onset Pompe disease. *Neurology.* 2007;68:99–109.

Kishnani PS, Hwu WL, Mandel H, et al. A retrospective, multinational, multicenter study on the natural history of infantile-onset Pompe disease. *J Pediatr.* 2006;148:671–676.

Kollberg G, Tulinius M, Gilljam T, et al. Cardiomyopathy and exercise intolerance in muscle glycogen storage disease 0. *N Engl J Med.* 2007;357:1507–1514.

Lee PJ, Ridout D, Walter JH, Cockburn F. Maternal phenylketonuria: report from the United Kingdom Registry 1978–97. *Arch Dis Child.* 2005;90:143–146.

Levy HL, Guldberg P, Güttler F, et al. Congenital heart disease in maternal phenylketonuria: report from the Maternal PKU Collaborative Study. *Pediatr Res.* 2001;49:636–642.

Lieu YK, Hsu BY, Price WA, Corkey BE, Stanley CA. Carnitine effects on coenzyme A profiles in rat liver with hypoglycin inhibition of multiple dehydrogenases. *Am J Physiol.* 1997;272:E359–E366.

Lin AE, Ardinger HH, Ardinger RH Jr, Cunniff C, Kelley RI. Cardiovascular malformations in Smith-Lemli-Opitz syndrome. *Am J Med Genet.* 1997;68:270–278.

Linhart A, Elliott PM. The heart in Anderson-Fabry disease and other lysosomal storage disorders. *Heart.* 2007;93:528–535.

Mardach R, Verity MA, Cederbaum SD. Clinical, pathological, and biochemical studies in a patient with propionic acidemia and fatal cardiomyopathy. *Mol Genet Metab.* 2005;85:286–290.

Massoud AF, Leonard JV. Cardiomyopathy in propionic acidaemia. *Eur J Pediatr.* 1993;152:441–445.

Masurel-Paulet A, Poggi-Bach J, Rolland MO, et al. NTBC treatment in tyrosinaemia type I: long-term outcome in French patients. *J Inherit Metab Dis.* 2008;31:81–87.

Matalon KM, Acosta PB, Azen C. Role of nutrition in pregnancy with phenylketonuria and birth defects. *Pediatrics.* 2003;112:1534–1536.

Matalon R, Michaels K, Kaul R, et al. Malonic aciduria and cardiomyopathy. *J Inherit Metab Dis.* 1993;16:571–573.

Michals-Matalon K, Platt LD, Acosta PP, Azen C, Walla CA. Nutrient intake and congenital heart defects in maternal phenylketonuria. *Am J Obstet Gynecol.* 2002;187:441–444.

Mohan UR, Hay AA, Cleary MA, Wraith JE, Patel RG. Cardiovascular changes in children with mucopolysaccharide disorders. *Acta Paediatr.* 2002;91:799–804.

Montaño AM, Tomatsu S, Gottesman GS, Smith M, Orii T. International Morquio A Registry: clinical manifestation and natural course of Morquio A disease. *J Inherit Metab Dis.* 2007;30:165–174.

Morrone A, Bardelli T, Donati MA, et al. Beta-galactosidase gene mutations affecting the lysosomal enzyme and the elastin-binding protein in GM1-gangliosidosis patients with cardiac involvement. *Hum Mutat.* 2000;15:354–366.

Moses SW, Parvari R. The variable presentations of glycogen storage disease type IV: a review of clinical, enzymatic and molecular studies. *Curr Mol Med.* 2002;2:177–188.

Muenzer J, Beekman RH, Profera LM, Bove EL. Severe mitral insufficiency in mucopolysaccharidosis type III-B (Sanfilippo syndrome). *Pediatr Cardiol.* 1993;14:130–132.

Nicolini F, Corradi D, Bosio S, Gherli T. Aortic valve replacement in a patient with morquio syndrome. *Heart Surg Forum.* 2008;11:E96–E98.

Nishino I, Fu J, Tanji K, et al. Primary LAMP-2 deficiency causes X-linked vacuolar cardiomyopathy and myopathy (Danon disease). *Nature.* 2000;406:906–910.

North KN, Hoppel CL, De Girolami U, Kozakewich HP, Korson MS. Lethal neonatal deficiency of carnitine palmitoyltransferase II associated with dysgenesis of the brain and kidneys. *J Pediatr.* 1995;127: 414–420.

Nugent AW, Daubeney PE, Chondros P, et al. Clinical features and outcomes of childhood hypertrophic cardiomyopathy: results from a national population-based study. *Circulation.* 2005;112:1332–1338.

Olsen RK, Olpin SE, Andresen BS, et al. ETFDH mutations as a major cause of riboflavin-responsive multiple acyl-CoA dehydrogenation deficiency. *Brain.* 2007;130:2045–2054.

Perrot A, Osterziel KJ, Beck M, Dietz R, Kampmann C. Fabry disease: focus on cardiac manifestations and molecular mechanisms. *Herz.* 2002;27:699–702.

Peters C, Balthazor M, Shapiro EG, et al. Outcome of unrelated donor bone marrow transplantation in 40 children with Hurler syndrome. *Blood.* 1996;87:4894–4902.

Pierre G, Macdonald A, Gray G, Hendriksz C, Preece MA, Chakrapani A. Prospective treatment in carnitine-acylcarnitine translocase deficiency. *J Inherit Metab Dis.* 2007;30:815.

Pompe Disease Diagnostic Working Group, Winchester B, Bali D, et al. Methods for a prompt and reliable laboratory diagnosis of Pompe disease: report from an international consensus meeting. *Mol Genet Metab.* 2008;93:275–281.

Rakheja D, Bennett MJ, Rogers BB. Long-chain L-3-hydroxyacyl-coenzyme a dehydrogenase deficiency: a molecular and biochemical review. *Lab Invest.* 2002;82:815–824.

Rashed MS, Ozand PT, Bennett MJ, Barnard JJ, Govindaraju DR, Rinaldo P. Inborn errors of metabolism diagnosed in sudden death cases by acylcarnitine analysis of postmortem bile. *Clin Chem.* 1995;41:1109–1114 .

Ratliff NB, Harris KM, Smith SA, Tankh-Johnson M, Gornick CC, Maron BJ. Cardiac arrest in a young marathon runner. *Lancet.* 2002; 360:542.

Regalado JJ, Rodriguez MM, Ferrer PL. Infantile hypertrophic cardiomyopathy of glycogenosis type IX: isolated cardiac phosphorylase kinase deficiency. *Pediatr Cardiol.* 1999;20:304–307.

Rela M, Battula N, Madanur M, et al. Auxiliary liver transplantation for propionic acidemia: a 10-year follow-up. *Am J Transplant.* 2007; 7:2200–2203.

Roe CR, Sweetman L, Roe DS, David F, Brunengraber H. Treatment of cardiomyopathy and rhabdomyolysis in long-chain fat oxidation disorders using an anaplerotic odd-chain triglyceride. *J Clin Invest.* 2002;110:259–269.

Rohrbach M, Clarke JT. Treatment of lysosomal storage disorders: progress with enzyme replacement therapy. *Drugs.* 2007;67:2697–2716.

Rouse B, Matalon R, Koch R, et al. Maternal phenylketonuria syndrome: congenital heart defects, microcephaly, and developmental outcomes. *J Pediatr.* 2000;136:57–61.

Rowland LP, Hays AP, DiMauro S et al. Diverse clinical disorders associated with morphological abnormalities of mitochondria. In Cerri C, Scarlato G, eds. Mitochondrial Pathology in Muscle Diseases. *Piccin Editore,* Padua, 1983:141–158.

Saudubray JM, Martin D, de Lonlay P, et al. Recognition and management of fatty acid oxidation defects: a series of 107 patients. *J Inherit Metab Dis.* 1999;22:488–502.

Schimmenti LA, Crombez EA, Schwahn BC, et al. Expanded newborn screening identifies maternal primary carnitine deficiency. *Mol Genet Metab.* 2007;90:441–445.

Schulze A, Lindner M, Kohlmüller D, Olgemöller K, Mayatepek E, Hoffmann GF. Expanded newborn screening for inborn errors of metabolism by electrospray ionization-tandem mass spectrometry: results, outcome, and implications. *Pediatrics.* 2003;111:1399–1406.

Sewell AC, Gehler J, Mittermaier G, Meyer E. Mucopolysaccharidosis type VII (beta-glucuronidase deficiency): a report of a new case and a survey of those in the literature. *Clin Genet.* 1982;21:366–373.

Shen JJ, Chen YT. Molecular characterization of glycogen storage disease type III. *Curr Mol Med.* 2002;2:167–175.

Sigauke E, Rakheja D, Kitson K, Bennett MJ. Carnitine palmitoyltransferase II deficiency: a clinical, biochemical, and molecular review. *Lab Invest.* 2003;83:1543–1554.

Simma B, Sperl W, Hammerer I. GM1 gangliosidosis and dilated cardiomyopathy. *Klin Padiatr.* 1990;202:183–185.

Soliman OI, Timmermans RG, Nemes A, et al. Cardiac abnormalities in adults with the attenuated form of mucopolysaccharidosis type I. *J Inherit Metab Dis.* 2007;30:750–757.

Stanley CA. Carnitine disorders. *Adv Pediatr.* 1995;42:209–242.

Stephan MJ, Stevens EL Jr, Wenstrup RJ, et al. Mucopolysaccharidosis I presenting with endocardial fibroelastosis of infancy. *Am J Dis Child.* 1989;143:782–784.

Strauss AW, Johnson MC. The genetic basis of pediatric cardiovascular disease. *Semin Perinatol.* 1996;20:564–576.

Struys EA. D-2-Hydroxyglutaric aciduria: unravelling the biochemical pathway and the genetic defect. *J Inherit Metab Dis.* 2006;29:21–29.

Tein I. Carnitine transport: pathophysiology and metabolism of known molecular defects. *J Inherit Metab Dis.* 2003;26:147–169.

Thuillier L, Rostane H, Droin V, et al. Correlation between genotype, metabolic data, and clinical presentation in carnitine palmitoyltransferase 2 (CPT2) deficiency. *Hum Mutat.* 2003;21:493–501.

Tomatsu S, Montaño AM, Nishioka T, et al. Mutation and polymorphism spectrum of the GALNS gene in mucopolysaccharidosis IVA (Morquio A). *Hum Mutat.* 2005;26:500–512 .

Valstar MJ, Ruijter GJ, van Diggelen OP, Poorthuis BJ, Wijburg FA. Sanfilippo syndrome: a mini-review. *J Inherit Metab Dis.* 2008 (In press).

van den Hout HM, Hop W, van Diggelen OP, et al. The natural course of infantile Pompe's disease: 20 original cases compared with 133 cases from the literature. *Pediatrics.* 2003;112:332–340.

van der Beek NA, Hagemans ML, van der Ploeg AT, Reuser AJ, van Doorn PA. Pompe disease (glycogen storage disease type II): clinical features and enzyme replacement therapy. *Acta Neurol Belg.* 2006;106:82–86.

van der Knaap MS, Jakobs C, Hoffmann GF, et al. D-2-hydroxyglutaric aciduria: further clinical delineation. *J Inherit Metab Dis.* 1999;22: 404–413.

van der Kooi AJ, van Langen IM, Aronica E, et al. Extension of the clinical spectrum of Danon disease. *Neurology.* 2008;70:1358–1359.

van Hove JL, Grünewald S, Jaeken J, et al. D,L-3-hydroxybutyrate treatment of multiple acyl-CoA dehydrogenase deficiency (MADD). *Lancet.* 2003;36:1433–1435.

Vellodi A, Cragg H, Winchester B, et al. Allogeneic bone marrow transplantation for fucosidosis. *Bone Marrow Transplant.* 1995;15(1):153–158.

Vianey-Saban C, Divry P, Brivet M, et al. Mitochondrial very-long-chain acyl-coenzyme A dehydrogenase deficiency: clinical characteristics and diagnostic considerations in 30 patients. *Clin Chim Acta.* 1998; 269:43–62.

Waisbren SE, Albers S, Amato S, et al. Effect of expanded newborn screening for biochemical genetic disorders on child outcomes and parental stress. *JAMA.* 2003;290:2564–2572.

Walker RW, Darowski M, Morris P, Wraith JE. Anaesthesia and mucopolysaccharidoses. A review of airway problems in children. *Anaesthesia.* 1994;49:1078–1084.

Wang Y, Korman SH, Ye J, et al. Phenotype and genotype variation in primary carnitine deficiency. *Genet Med.* 2001;3:387–392.

Winchester B, Vellodi A, Young E. The molecular basis of lysosomal storage diseases and their treatment. *Biochem Soc Trans.* 2000;28:150–154.

Wraith JE. The first 5 years of clinical experience with laronidase enzyme replacement therapy for mucopolysaccharidosis I. *Expert Opin Pharmacother.* 2005;6:489–506.

Wraith JE, Scarpa M, Beck M, et al. Mucopolysaccharidosis type II (Hunter syndrome): a clinical review and recommendations for treatment in the era of enzyme replacement therapy. *Eur J Pediatr.* 2008;167: 267–277.

Yano S, Sweetman L, Thorburn DR, Mofidi S, Williams JC. A new case of malonyl coenzyme A decarboxylase deficiency presenting with cardiomyopathy. *Eur J Pediatr.* 1997;156:382–383.

Yeager AM. Allogeneic hematopoietic cell transplantation for inborn metabolic diseases. *Ann Hematol.* 2002;81(suppl 2):S16–S19.

Yorifuji T, Kawai M, Muroi J, et al. Unexpectedly high prevalence of the mild form of propionic acidemia in Japan: presence of a common mutation and possible clinical implications. *Hum Genet.* 2002;111:161–165 .

27

Heart and Neuromuscular Disease

John P Bourke and Kate Bushby

Introduction

Cardiologists have not usually been involved in the management of patients with most forms of inherited muscle disorders. When they have been consulted about patients with muscular dystrophy, many have been uncertain what to recommend, given the relative lack of a specific evidence base on which to base decisions. This perceived lack of evidence combined with a relative nihilism prompted by the more apparent physical limitations of these patients has been used by cardiologists to justify a lower standard of care in patients with muscular dystrophies than they would provide in other contexts (English and Gibbs 2006). However, as life expectancy has improved in the commoner muscular dystrophies due to an integrated multidisciplinary approach to management and interventions such as correction of scoliosis, corticosteroid therapy, and noninvasive ventilation, the impact of cardiac involvement on prognosis is increasingly appreciated (Eagle et al. 2002; Bushby et al. 2003; Manzur et al. 2004). It is now to be expected that cardiologists play their part in the multidisciplinary management of these complex patients.

The rate of discoveries in genetics and molecular biology have contributed significantly to our understanding of how genetic defects cause some of the phenotypes in primary cardiac and neuromuscular conditions. Seen in this context, there is considerable overlap in underlying mechanisms between some of the commoner inherited muscular dystrophies and primary cardiomyopathies (SOLVD 1991; Pfeffer et al. 1992; Kober et al. 1995; McMurray 1999; Laing 1999, 2007; Lee et al. 2000; Zannad et al. 2001). This chapter will describe the cardiac involvement in some of the more frequent neuromuscular disorders (Table 27–1). Overlaps with cardiac conditions, in which similar genetic defects cause cardiomyopathy or conduction tissue disease/arrhythmias, in the absence of muscle disease, will be highlighted.

Duchenne and Becker Muscular Dystrophy

Duchenne muscular dystrophy (DMD) and Becker (BMD) muscular dystrophy are X-linked recessively inherited neuromuscular disorders caused by a deficiency in the expression of the protein dystrophin on the inner aspect of the cell sarcolemma (Babuty et al., 1999; Darras et al. 1990; Palmieri and Sblendorio 2006, 2007). Both conditions are characterized by progressive weakness of proximal limb-girdle muscles and calf muscle hypertrophy (Ferlini et al. 1999). Individuals with DMD typically lose ambulation and become wheelchair dependent before the age of 13 years and die from cardiorespiratory failure at around the age of 20 years (Emery and Skinner 1976; Eagle et al. 2002; Manzur et al. 2004; Parker et al. 2005). Those affected with the milder BMD form have a more varied course, tending to retain ambulation into their third or fourth decade and surviving into their seventh decade (Emery and Skinner 1976).

Dystrophin is a component of the dystrophin-associated sarcoglycan complex of cell membranes (Figure 27–1). This complex contributes to the maintenance of cell membrane stability and force transduction. When dystrophin is deficient (BMD) or absent (DMD), normal levels of mechanical stress result in abnormal cell membrane permeability, loss of membrane integrity, and progressive cell destruction. Progressive myocyte destruction, whether in skeletal or cardiac muscle results in a loss of muscle mass, fibrosis, and clinical evidence of muscle weakness (Barresi et al., 2000).

About 90% of males with DMD and 50% with BMD develop a severe, progressive form of cardiomyopathy (Nigro et al. 1990; Backman and Nylander 1992; Maeda et al. 1995; Ferlini et al. 1990; Figure 27–2). Cardiac involvement usually begins with localized hypokinesis of the posterobasal segments of the left ventricle. Over time, these segments become akinetic and the other areas become involved, left ventricular dimensions enlarge, and measures of global ventricular function deteriorate. Heart failure symptoms typically only develop when left ventricular ejection fraction has fallen to between 10% and 15%. The severity of cardiac involvement in BMD can be out of proportion to the degree of skeletal muscle weakness, so that cardiomyopathy becomes the key determinant of survival (de Visser et al. 1992). In DMD about 20% of patients have evidence of left ventricular impairment on echocardiography by the age of 10 years (Ferlini et al. 1990; Nigro et al. 1990; Backman and Nylander 1992). Abnormalities in left ventricular function are evident in an even larger proportion of patients at all ages when more sensitive imaging techniques, such as tissue Doppler, magnetic resonance, or metabolic imaging are deployed (Mercier 1982; Perloff et al. 1984; Eidem 1998; Crilley et al. 2000; Giglio et al. 2003; Mavrogeni et al. 2005).

In the past, most patients with DMD have tended not to experience heart failure symptoms because of their inability to exercise and the onset of respiratory failure.

Table 27–1a Epidemiology of Cardiac Involvement in Different Forms of Primary Myopathies and Myotonic Dystrophy

Disease	Cardiac Involvement (in Increasing Order of Severity)	% of Patients in Whom Abnormality Likely	Age Range	Morbidity/Mortality
Duchenne muscular dystrophy	ECG abnormalities HCM Dilated cardiomyopathy (DCM)	Abnormal ECG > 90% Abnormal Echo > 90%	ECG abnormalities detectable from age 6, progressive thereafter	Cardiac death in approx 10%–20%, usually in teens
Becker muscular dystrophy	ECG abnormalities HCM DCM	ECG abnormal - 90%, Echo abnormal - 65%	Variable, may be disproportionate to skeletal involvement	Cardiac death in up to 50%
Manifesting carriers of DMD/BMD	ECG abnormalities HCM DCM	Variable estimates 21%–90%	Variable, may be out of proportion to skeletal muscle involvement	DCM in 7%–11%. Several reports of successful cardiac transplantation
XLEDMD	AV block Atrial paralysis Atrial flutter fibrillation	>95% by age 30 years	10–39 years	Sudden death common in non-paced individuals (mean age at pacing 24 yrs, range 14–35)
Myotonic dystrophy	AV conduction disturbances Atrial flutter and fibrillation Ventricular tachy- arrhythmias	Approximately 65% of the adult myotonic dystrophy population have abnormal ECG	Earliest age at which abnormalities become clinically relevant is unclear. Greatest risk is in middle adulthood	Approximately 5% require pacemaker insertion. Risk of sudden death
Sarcoglycanopathies (LGMD2C-2F)	ECG abnormalities HCM and DCM	18.7%	Not established	Impact on overall prognosis unclear
LGMD2I	ECG abnormalities DCM	1/3 of adult onset cases	Over whole spectrum of LGMD2I/ MDC1C probably relates to severity of overall disease	1/3 of adult cases have cardiomyopathy. Further data needed on natural history
MDC1C	DCM	Invariable and clinically significant	Present from early childhood in severe cases	May be a major contributory factor to early death
Laminopathies (including AD-EDMD, LGMD1B)	AV block Atrial paralysis Atrial fibrillation/ flutter	>95 by age 30 years	15–52 years	Mean age at pacing 32 (range 19–57) years 50% of deaths are sudden despite pacing
Laminopathies (including AD-EDMD, LGMD1B)	DCM	35% of all cases	19–55 years	Death from heart failure common, if not transplanted.
Facioscapulohumeral muscular dystrophy	Conduction defects Atrial arrhythmias	Minor ECG changes in up to 30%	Prevalence of cardiac involvement in severe childhood onset disease unclear	Few reports of clinically relevant cardiac involvement
MDC1A	Reduced ejection fraction			No reports to date of clinically significant cardiomyopathy

As life expectancy has improved because of a more integrated approach to management including glucocorticoid steroid therapy to improve muscle strength and prolong ambulation, orthopedic correction of scoliosis, and noninvasive ventilation for respiratory muscle weakness (Eagle et al. 2002; Manzur et al. 2004; Ylmaz et al. 2004; Balaban et al. 2005; Parker et al. 2005; Wells 2006; Bach et al. 2007; Velasco et al. 2007), DMD patients are surviving to an age when cardiac involvement is more advanced and the heart more often contributes directly to death.

1. Effects of Steroid Therapy on Cardiac Involvement

Glucocorticoid steroids are now routinely prescribed in DMD boys to improve muscle strength and prolong ambulation (Manzur et al. 2004). Theoretically, long-term steroid use could adversely affect heart function by causing left ventricular hypertrophy through anabolic effects and aggravation of salt and water retention in those with severely impaired function. Evidence from human and the mdx mouse (a validated animal model of the skeletal muscle DMD phenotype) are contradictory. In one series of 33 patients with DMD (Silversides et al. 2003), the effect of deflazacort (0.9 mg/kg/day) on left ventricular function was assessed by serial echocardiograms and compared with patients who had never received steroid therapy. Eight had moderate to severe left ventricular dysfunction and two had a history of heart failure. Therapy was started at mean age 8.4 ± 2 years of age. Not only was ambulation retained for longer in all those on steroid therapy but also parameters of left ventricular function were better in those on steroids at the end of the study period. In another nonrandomized study, echocardiograms were compared over time of those who had (n = 14) or had never (n = 23) received steroid therapy. Initial cardiac assessments were at 7.5 ± 0.8 years and follow-up at 12 ± 0.7 years. Ninety-three percent of those treated with steroids were free

Table 27–1b Inherited Muscle Diseases with Cardiac Involvement

Autosomal Dominant	Gene/Locus	Protein
Myotonic dystrophy		
DM1	19q13.2-q13.3	Myotonin protein kinase (DMPK)
DM2/PROMM		*Expanded CTG trinucleotide repeats at 3' end*
	3q13.3-q24	Zinc finger protein-9 (ZNF9)
		Expanded CCTG tetranucleotide repeats at promoter end adjoining intron 1
Limb-girdle muscular dystrophy		
LGMD1A	5q31	Myotilin
LGMD1B	1q21.2	Lamin A/C
LGMD1C	3p25	Caveolin-3
Emery-Dreifuss muscular dystrophy	1q11-q21	Lamin A/C
Facioscapulohumeral dystrophy	4q35	Unknown
Bethlem myopathy	21q22, 2q37	CollagenVI (α1;α2), collagenVIα3
Nemaline myopathy		
Desminopathies		
Primary desminopathy	1p36-p35	Desmin
Myofibrillar myopathy (MFM)	2q35	Desmin-related
Autosomal recessive		
Limb-girdle muscular dystrophy		
LGMD2A	15q15.1-q21.1	Calpain 3
LGMD2B	2p13.3-p13.1	Dysferlin
LGMD2C	13q12	γ-sarcoglycan
LGMD2D	17q12-q21	α-sarcoglycan
LGMD2E	4q12	β-sarcoglycan
LGMD2F	5q33	δ-sarcoglycan
LGMD2G	17q11-q12	Telethonin
LGMD2H	9q31-q34	TRIM32
LGMD2I-FKRP	19q13.3	Fukutin-related protein
LGMD2J	2q31	Titin
Congenital muscular dystrophy		
Fukuyama type (MDC1C)	19q13.3	Fukutin
Merosin-deficient type (MDC1A)	6q22-q23	Laminin α-2 (LAMA2)
Merosin-positive type	4p16.3	Merosin
Desminopathies		
RSMD1	1p35-p36	Desmin
Glyocogenoses		
GSD II	17q25.2	Acid α-1,4 glucosidase (GAA)
GSD III	1p21	Glycogen debrancher enzyme (AGL)
GSD IV	3p12	Glycogen branching enzyme (GBE1)
GSD VII	12q13.3	Muscle phosphofructokinase (PFKM)
X-linked		
Xp21 myopathies		
DMD—surviving longer	Xp21	Dystrophin
BMD—more active		
Intermediate DMD/BMD		
X-linked cardiomyopathy		
Xp21 myopathies		
Emery-Dreifuss muscular dystrophy	Xq28	Emerin
Barth syndrome	Xq28	Tafazin
Danon disease	Xq24	LAMP2

From Dr D Kumar (From NCBI/OMIM 30 May 2008)—personal communication.

of cardiac involvement compared to only 53% of those untreated at 1,500 days follow-up (HR 0.16; 95% CI: 0.04, 0.70) (Markham et al. 2008). Conversely, in the mdx mouse model steroids seem to increase left ventricular stiffness and impair diastolic function. Based on human data, glucocorticoid therapy is undoubtedly beneficial for its skeletal muscle effects and, at least, does not appear to aggravate cardiac dysfunction (Bauer et al. 2009).

2. Rationale for Intervention in DMD and BMD Cardiomyopathy

In patients with left ventricular dysfunction following myocardial infarction or with idiopathic forms of DCM, initiating heart failure therapy at the presymptomatic stage has been shown to delay or prevent the onset of cardiac failure and improve prognosis (Thuillez et al. 1990; SOLVD 1991; Pfeffer et al. 1992; Kober et al.

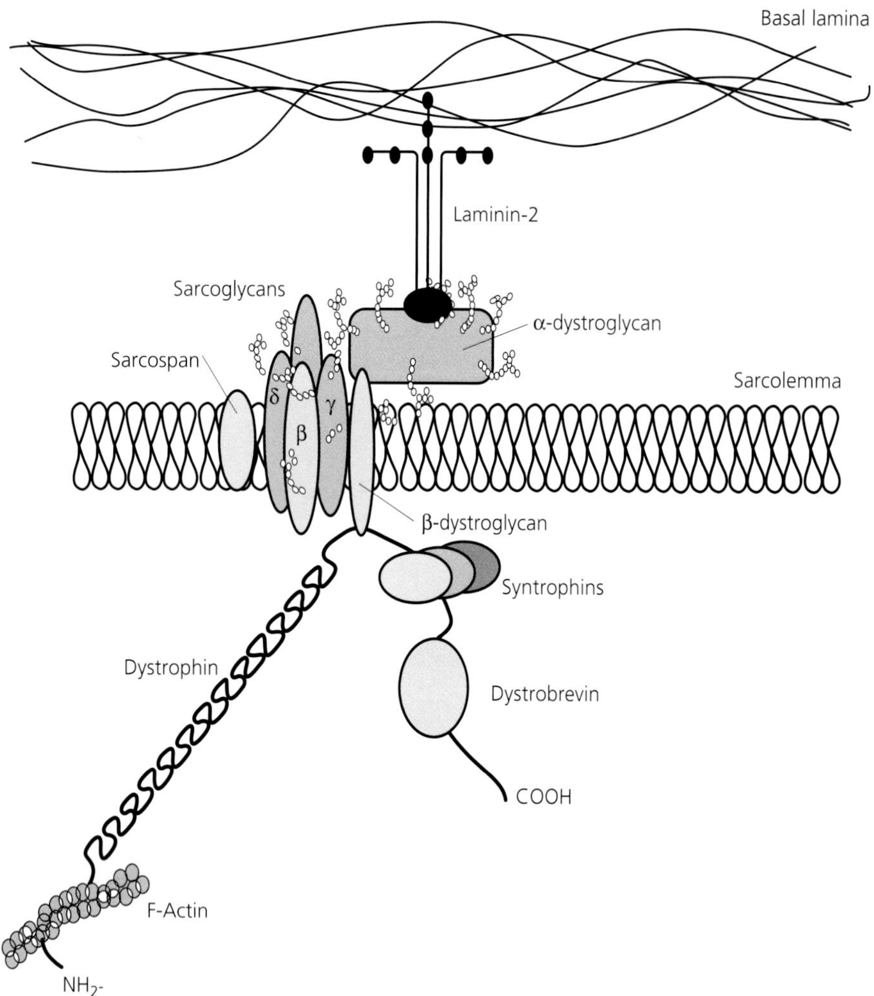

Figure 27–1 Dystrophin–sarcoglycan membrane complex.

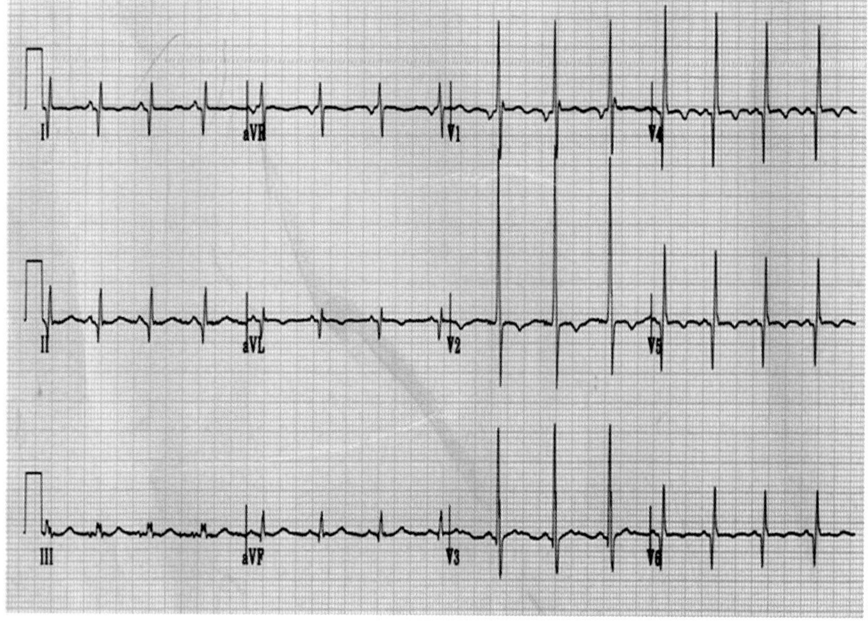

Figure 27–2 ECG in DMD. Abnormal Q waves in lateral (I and aVL), inferior (II, III, aVF), and apical (V5–6) leads. Abnormally tall R waves in right precordial leads (V1–2). Widespread repolarization changes in chest leads.

1994; 1995; MacMahon et al. 1997; Anonymous 1999 ; Hjalmarson et al. 1999; McMurray 1999; Locolley et al. 2001; Zannad et al. 2001, CIBIS II study 1999; Tsutamoto 1999). The use of combination therapy with an angiotensin-converting enzyme (ACE) inhibitor (Thuillez et al. 1990; SOLVD investigators 1991; Pfeffer et al. 1992; Kober et al. 1995), nonselective β-blocker (MacMahon et al. 1997; Hjalmarson et al. 1999; McMurray 1999), and aldosterone antagonist (Locolley et al. 2001; Zannad et al. 2001) is well established by the results of large, multicenter, randomized controlled trials. Extrapolating from this evidence, a consensus multidisciplinary group of experts recommended in 2003 that ACE inhibitors be deployed routinely in cardiac dystrophinopathy (Bushby et al. 2003). This recommendation was based on the assumption that, although ACE-inhibitors and β-blockers would not be expected to correct the underlying cause of cardiomyopathy in DMD/BMD, they should slow the rate of cardiac decompensation.

Since then, evidence of the benefits of ACE-inhibitor and β-blocker therapy in the later stages of dystrophinopathy has been reported by several groups (Ishikawa et al. 1999; Jefferies et al. 2005; Ramaciotti et al. 2006). In a study by Ishikawa et al. (1999) 11 of 85 patients with DMD developed symptomatic left ventricular dysfunction and were treated with ACE inhibitors with or without β-blocker therapy. Symptoms and left ventricular function improved in all patients. Endocrine measures of cardiovascular decompensation such as brain and atrial naturetic peptides and norepinephrine levels also fell with initiation of therapy. In another series, treatment was started at the stage of asymptomatic left ventricular dysfunction in a cohort of 76 boys (69 DMD; 7 BMD), with mean age of 13 years (Murdoch 1997; Jefferies et al. 2005). Thirty-one were started on ACE-inhibitor therapy as soon as abnormalities of left ventricular function were evident on echocardiography (13 ACEi alone) and β-blocker therapy was added after 3 months (ACEi and BB 18) if ventricular function had not improved. Twenty-nine were followed up on single or combined therapy for periods of between 1.6 and 2.7 years. Contrary to the natural history expected, left ventricular function stabilized in 2, improved in 8, and normalized in 19 (Backman and Nylander 1992; Kazuya et al. 1998). Measures of left ventricular dimensions, ejection fraction, wall motion index, and sphericity index were all improved by treatment. In another study (Ramaciotti et al. 2006) of 50 boys and men with DMD, 27 (56%) developed left ventricular dysfunction at age 13 ± 2 years and were started on enalapril therapy. Ten responded to therapy and left ventricular fractional shortening normalized during follow-up ranging 5–58 months. No differences in age, starting left ventricular dimensions, or mutation analyses were identified between those who responded to therapy and those who did not. These discordant findings could be due to inadequate dosages of therapy, the lack of concomitant therapy with β-blockade or, as the authors infer, the fact that response to therapy may not be uniform.

On the basis of current molecular biological understanding of the causes of isolated cardiomyopathies, therapies are more likely to be effective in modifying the progressive course of left ventricular impairment, if started before the process has led to functional abnormalities (Crilley et al. 2000). This could mean that the opportunity to improve prognosis may be reduced if therapy is delayed until cardiomyopathy is already established, even though still at an asymptomatic stage. In the only randomized study of truly prophylactic deployment of cardioactive therapy in DMD to date, the ACE inhibitor perindopril was started before left ventricular dysfunction was evident on radionuclide ventriculography (Duboc et al. 2005). Over a 5-year period of follow-up in a two-phase study of 60 patients, heart function was better preserved in those on perindopril throughout the study compared to those on placebo in phase I and on perindopril in phase II. Although imperfect in design and controversial in its findings the results suggest that by starting ACE-inhibitor therapy even earlier—before the stage of detectable left ventricular dysfunction—the heart may be protected for longer from the effects of dystrophinopathy.

Despite these encouraging reports, it will be many years before the effect, if any, of these agents on survival can be established definitively by ongoing randomized placebo-controlled trials (Duboc et al. 2007). Nevertheless, on the basis of the available evidence, "heart protection" therapy should be initiated—regardless of symptoms—once there is convincing evidence of left ventricular dysfunction. This should comprise ACE-inhibitor therapy and anecdotal evidence supports the superiority of combination therapy with ACEi and β-blockers (Box 27–1).

Box 27–1 DMD/BMD Males

- Patients should have a cardiac investigation (echocardiogram or similar ventricular assessment and ECG) at diagnosis.
- DMD patients should have cardiac investigations before any surgery, every 2 years to age 10 and annually after age 10.
- Respiratory failure is also common in DMD and assessment and treatment of respiratory function should be performed in parallel with the cardiac investigations.
- Patients should be treated with ACE inhibitors/angiotensin-receptor blockers initially in the presence of progressive abnormalities. Subsequently, the addition of β-blockers should be considered.
- There is no evidence that the currently used steroid treatment regimes have a detrimental effect on cardiac involvement or are a contraindication for the concurrent use of ACE inhibitors.
- The multiple other complications of DMD including scoliosis and respiratory failure mean that these patients are rarely fit for cardiac transplantation.

Female Carriers of the Abnormal Xp21 Gene

There is unequivocal evidence that some 10% of female carriers of dystrophin mutations—either DMD or BMD—develop overt cardiomyopathy, even in the absence of skeletal muscle involvement (Mirabella et al. 1993; Politano et al. 1996; Hoogerwaard et al. 1999; Grain et al. 2001). The reasons for this remain to be clarified, but all female carriers should be considered vulnerable to cardiomyopathy, triggered perhaps by environmental influences (Lee et al. 2000). Females with muscle symptoms ("muscle manifesting") are probably at even greater risk of cardiomyopathy. Treatment of left ventricular dysfunction should follow the same regime as for DMD-affected males and, in the severest cases, there are reports of carriers undergoing cardiac transplantation successfully Despite the risk of cardiac involvement, however, prognosis and life expectancy for abnormal Xp21 gene carriers has been shown to be comparable to that of the general population in one recent epidemiological study (Holloway et al. 2008; Box 27–2).

Myotonic Dystrophy

Myotonic dystrophy is the commonest inherited muscle disorder in adults with an estimated incidence of 1/8,000 births and a prevalence of 2–14/100,000 population (Mankodi and Thornton 2002; Pelargonio et al. 2002). The classical form (DM1; Steinert's Disease) has autosomal dominant inheritance and the genetic basic for the condition is an expansion of CTG repeats on the *DMPK* gene on chromosome 19. This expansion mutation is highly unstable and the condition becomes more severe in successive generations of a family as the number of CTG repeats increases progressively. Patients typically present between the second and fourth decades of life with slowly progressive symptoms of myotonia, muscle weakness, cataracts, and cardiac conduction abnormalities. It is, however, a multisystem disorder that can have diverse manifestations as outlined in Table 27–2 (Pelargonio et al. 2002).

A second type of myotonic dystrophy [DM2; proximal myotonic myopathy (PROMM)] with similar inheritance is due to

Box 27–2 Female Carriers of the Abnormal DMD/BMD Gene

- All DMD/BMD carriers should have an echocardiogram and ECG at diagnosis or after the age of 16 years.
- Repeat assessment of ventricular function should be recommended every 5 years in those with normal initial test results and more frequently if abnormal.
- Manifesting carriers (muscle symptoms) are at greater risk of cardiomyopathy.
- Once left ventricular dysfunction is confirmed, treatment with ACE inhibitors/angiotensin-receptor blockers and β-blockers should be initiated, regardless of symptoms.
- Ultimately cardiac transplantation may be appropriate.

Table 27–2 Multisystem Effects of Myotonic Dystrophy Type 1

System	Condition/Effect
Eye	Cataracts
Endocrine	Diabetes mellitus; thyroid abnormalities; hypogonadism
Central Nervous	Cognitive impairment; mental retardation
Gastrointestinal	Constipation; gall stones; constipation/pseudoobstruction
Heart:	
Conduction	AV block
Arrhythmias	Supraventricular and ventricular tachyarrhythmias
LV Function	Systolic and diastolic dysfunction

LV = left ventricular.

expansion of CCTG repeats on chromosome 3 (Day et al. 1998; Mankodi and Thornton 2002). Although this can manifest in a multisystem way, similar to that in DM1, it typically starts with proximal muscle weakness, the heart is less often affected and prognosis appears to be better than in DM1 (Mankodi and Thornton 2002; Meola et al. 2002).

Life expectancy is severely reduced in DM1 (Day et al. 1998). In a 10-year follow-up study of 367 patients with confirmed MD, for example, 75 (20%) died. Mean age of death was only 53.2 years (range 24–81). Deaths were attributed to respiratory causes in 32 (43%), cardiovascular disease in 15 (20%), neoplasia in 8 (11%), and 8 (11%) died suddenly—presumably due to bradycardia/asystole or ventricular tachyarrhythmias (Mathieu et al. 1999). Prognosis was worst in childhood onset type and best in the milder phenotypes, with symptom onset typically over 50 years.

The degree of cardiac involvement in a patient with myotonic dystrophy, its age of onset, and rate of progression are now considered to relate to the number of abnormal CTG repeats (Hayashi et al. 1997; Lazarus et al. 1999; Mathieu et al. 1999; Clarke et al. 2001; Groh et al. 2002). Patients with DM1 are probably not at increased risk of developing coronary heart disease compared to age- and sex-matched controls, as was once considered (Moorman et al. 1985; Hayashi et al. 1997; Clarke et al. 2001; Groh et al. 2002).

Cardiac Involvement in DM Type 1

The commonest cardiac effect in myotonic dystrophy (DM1) is conduction system disease (Figure 27–3). In many patients, conduction defects progress in a predictable way over time (Hawley et al. 1991; Finsterer et al. 2001). Histology of hearts from patients with DM1 consistently shows extensive patchy interstitial fibrosis, fatty infiltration, and focal myocarditis (Phillips et al. 1997). The molecular mechanism whereby CTG repeats result in these changes remains unclear (Mankodi and Thornton 2002). The protein kinase encoded by *DMPK* is known to be involved in regulating components of the cytoskeleton and in calcium homeostasis. However, CTG expansion also alters the function of other related genes and these secondary effects—altered conformation of chromatin (Klesert et al. 2000), reduced expression of *DMPK* (Taneja et al. 1995), toxic effects of mutant *DMPK* (Seznec et al. 2001), effects of mutant RNA-binding proteins (Phillips et al. 1998)—may all contribute to the various aspects of DM1.

The *standard 12-lead ECG* provides a readily available and easily repeatable measure of cardiac conduction. Sinus bradycardia, all degrees of AV and bundle branch block, QRS-axis shift, and nonspecific widening of the QRS are evidence of conduction tissue disease (Figure 27–3). In a prospective study of 46 patients with DM1, sinus bradycardia was present in 33%, first-degree AV block in 33%, and QRS longer than 110 ms in 20% (Moorman et al. 1985; Oloffson et al. 1988; Phillips et al. 1997). Obtaining an ECG at diagnosis and repeating it regularly—preferably annually—thereafter is the standard way of detecting the presence and rate of progression of abnormalities of conduction. The importance of comparing ECG results serially, to decide when to recommend prophylactic implantation of a permanent pacemaker, cannot be overstated. Patients who do not comply with regular testing are at greatest risk of sudden death—estimated to be 2%–30%—mainly from unheralded catastrophic failure of the conduction system (Mathieu et al. 1999). For surveillance to be effective, patients need to appreciate the importance of the cardiac aspects of their condition to their well-being and participate actively in surveillance. Surface ECG recordings, however, typically underestimate the severity of conduction abnormalities in DM. A normal surface ECG, for example, does not exclude important infra-Hisian conduction delay and the severity of conduction abnormalities is always much more advanced, when assessed by invasive electrophysiology testing when compared to that by ECG. The implication of infra-Hisian conduction delay is that, if complete heart block occurs, there may be no escape ventricular rhythm and death may occur suddenly due to ventricular asystole.

Holter ECG recordings provide additional information and are frequently required when the 12-lead ECG is abnormal. For example, when new first-degree AV block is present or no old traces are available, Holter recordings may reveal higher grade abnormalities, justifying permanent pacing, or provide the reassurance needed to continue surveillance safely (Lazarus et al. 2002). Similarly, in the case of sinus bradycardia, it is important to distinguish whether this is pathological or physiological. Apart from contributing to exercise intolerance itself, chronotropic incompetence can facilitate the development of atrial flutter or fibrillation and mask progressive abnormalities in AV conduction on surface ECG.

Signal averaging of the ECG has long been used to assess patients at risk of ventricular tachyarrhythmias following myocardial infarction. The presence of late potentials (i.e., QRS duration >120 ms, mean amplitude of terminal 40 ms of QRS <25 μV, terminal QRS below 40 μV >40 ms) indicates areas of slow ventricular activation and inhomogeneous conduction—the substrate for reentrant ventricular tachycardia (Richards et al. 1991). This technique has also been advocated in patients with DM as a way of identifying slow ventricular activation due to the presence of infra-Hisian conduction delay rather than arrhythmia risk (Pelargonio

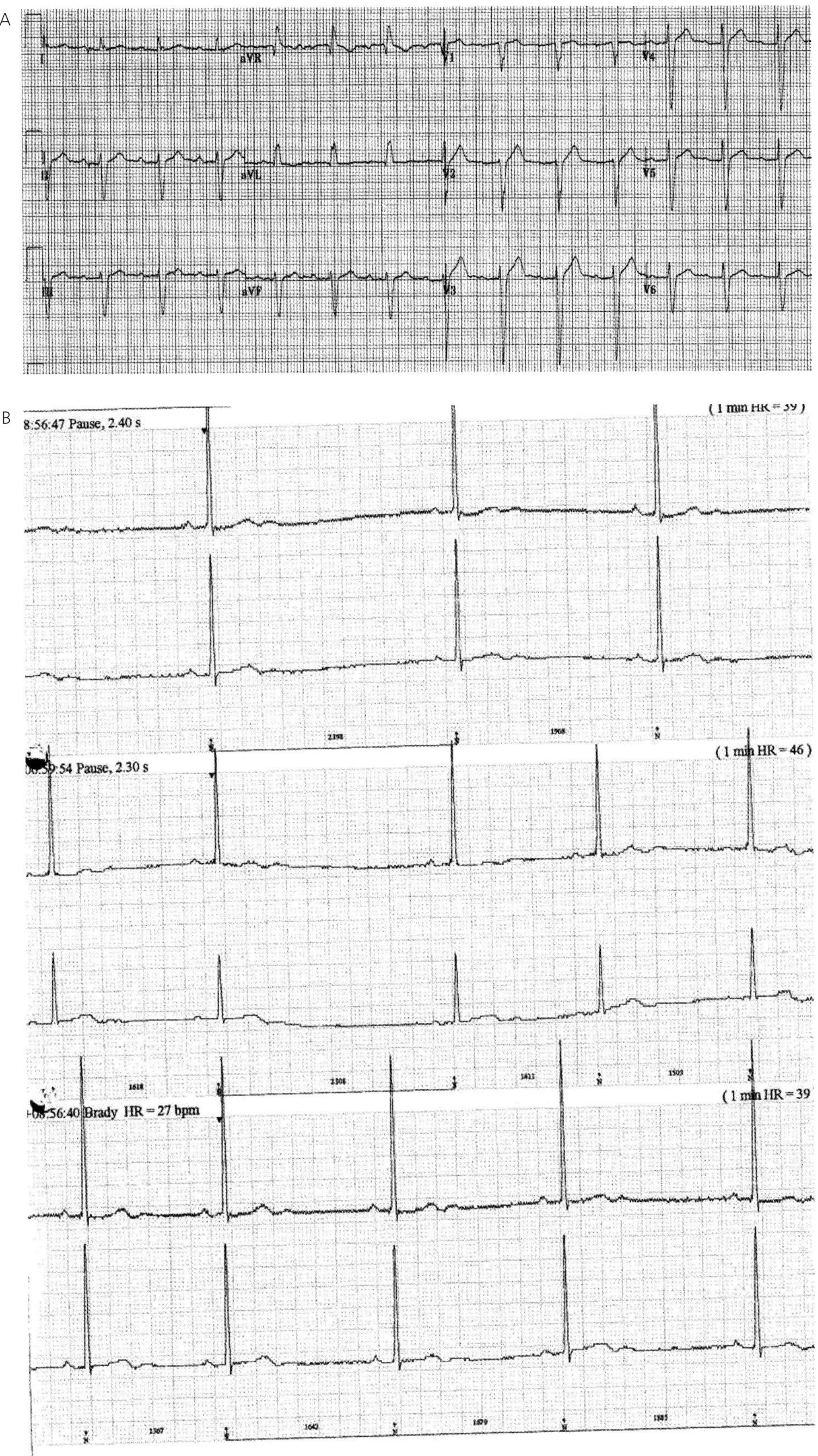

Figure 27–3 ECG examples in myotonic dystrophy. (a) First-degree AV block (PR-interval 260 ms), wide-QRS (> 120 ms) with left axis deviation. (b) Sinus bradycardia (27 bpm) on Holter ECG in DM1 patient.

2002). The presence of late potentials (i.e., QRS duration >100 ms, low amplitude in the last 40 ms of QRS complex >36 μV) correlated with the presence of abnormally prolonged HV interval (>60 ms) with a sensitivity of 80% and specificity of 86% (Babuty et al. 1999). The use of this additional modality of testing, therefore, complements conventional ECG surveillance (Figure 27–4).

Invasive electrophysiology testing is the most accurate way of assessing all aspects of cardiac conduction and propensity to atrial and ventricular tachycardia in patients with DM (Prystowsky et al. 1979; Lazarus et al. 1999). In one study of 83 patients with DM1, AV conduction disturbances were common and typically distal as manifested by a prolonged HV interval (HV 66.2 ± 14 ms) (Lazarus et al. 1999). When the surface ECG showed a prolonged PR interval, the HV interval was always abnormal. However, the HV interval was also abnormally long in 11 of 20 patients, whose PR interval on surface ECG was within normal limits (≤200 ms).

Therefore, invasive electrophysiology testing can be used to assess sinus and AV node conduction and to clarify the need for permanent pacing but in practice it is seldom justified except in a research context. The finding of HV interval of 70 ms or longer is a clear indication for permanent pacing, regardless of symptoms. Atrial and ventricular tachyarrhythmias are often inducible but the degree to which inducible arrhythmias manifest spontaneously during follow-up remains to be determined (Merino 1998; Lazarus et al. 1999). Trials already underway are likely to provide the answer to this important question. At present, therefore, the evidence does not support the use of implantable defibrillators when pacemaker is being implanted for bradycardia or conduction disease indications.

In clinical practice, the nature, duration, and frequency of cardiac surveillance needed in patients with DM1 depend largely on the threshold for recommending permanent pacing. An ECG should be obtained at diagnosis and annually thereafter. More detailed assessment with Holter ECGs may be indicated in adult patients who already have evidence of conduction abnormalities at baseline (i.e., prolonged PR interval, sinus bradycardia, bifascicular block). Similarly, patient-activated or implantable loop recordings should be deployed when needed to document rhythm at time of symptoms suggestive of tachyarrhythmias (e.g., atrial fibrillation, atrial flutter) or in the rare patient reporting, syncope or presyncope (Hadian et al. 2002). When deterioration in conduction is evident on serial ECGs (i.e., new PR prolongation,

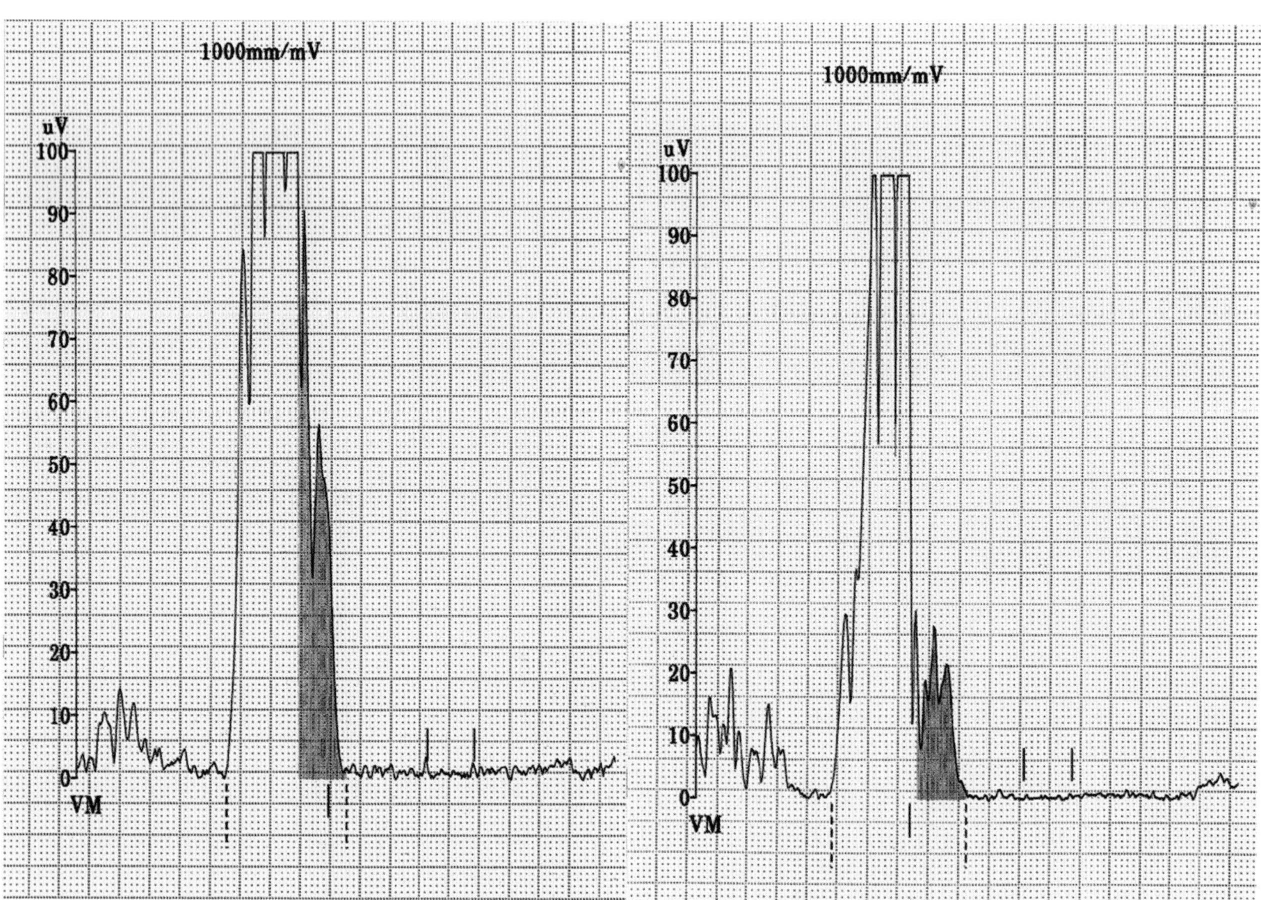

Figure 27–4 Signal-averaged ECG for presence of delayed ventricular activation (late potentials).
Total QRS duration (filtered) = 99 ms
Duration of HFLA signals <40 μv = 15 ms
Mean voltage in terminal 40 ms = 39 μV
Total QRS duration (filtered) = 110 ms
Duration of HFLA signals <40 μV = 46 ms
Mean voltage in terminal 40 ms = 14 μV.

progressive widening of QRS, axis shift in context of lesser prior abnormalities, etc.), the timing of pacemaker implant should be discussed with DM1 patients. Pragmatically, the threshold for pacemaker implant should be low—knowing the natural history of the condition—as an alternative to increasing the frequency of noninvasive testing or submitting the patient to invasive electrophysiology evaluation(s). Except in a research context, invasive evaluation is really only indicated in rare situations where surface ECG is normal and the patient reports syncope, for example.

Current pacemakers can be programmed initially so as to avoid ventricular pacing except when absolutely necessary (i.e., minimum ventricular pacing or similar algorithms). In addition, battery longevity has increased to the point where, with optimal programming, "early prophylactic implant" has fewer disadvantages than might have been the case heretofore. Typically, when patients with DM1 are paced, it is not uncommon for pacing to replace all native AV nodal conduction, which is indicative of the precarious state of conduction in some of these patients (Box 27–3).

1. Left Ventricular Dysfunction in DM1

In most adults with DM1, left ventricular function is normal when assessed by echocardiography. More sensitive assessments can show subclinical abnormalities of systolic and diastolic function in the absence of symptoms (Badano et al. 1993). As AV conduction deteriorates and QRS width increases, a progressive dyssynchrony of contraction can occur within and between cardiac chambers—atrioventricular, interventricular, and intraventricular. However, these rarely result in symptoms to justify specific correction, such as with biventricular pacing, at the time of pacemaker implant for conventional indications.

Congenital Muscular Dystrophy

The congenital muscular dystrophies are a heterogeneous group of autosomal recessively inherited muscle diseases normally present at birth and associated with characteristic changes on muscle biopsy (Kobayashi et al. 1996; Minetti et al. 1996; Voit 1998; Mendell 2001; Baker et al. 2005). Whether cardiac involvement can be expected depends on the specific type (Forsberg et al. 1990; Reardon et al. 1993; Gilhuis et al. 2002). In congenital muscular dystrophy, therefore, defining the genetic basis of the disease determines the most appropriate schedule of cardiac surveillance.

In congenital muscular dystrophy 1C (MDC1C)—due to mutations in fukutin-related protein gene (*FKRP*) cardiac involvement appears common and cardiac surveillance is indicated routinely (Brockington et al. 2001a; Topaloglu et al. 2003). In one report, two of four patients had evidence of cardiomyopathy in their second decade of life (Mercuri et al. 2003). There are also reports of cardiomyopathy in MDC1A but to date this has been nonprogressive (Spyrou et al. 1998; Gilhuis et al. 2002). In other types of CMD, ECG and assessment of ventricular function is recommended at diagnosis and, thereafter, prior to surgery or as clinically indicated.

Emery-Dreifuss Muscular Dystrophy (EDMD)

EDMD is a genetically heterogeneous condition. X-linked EDMD is due to mutations in the STA gene encoding the protein emerin (Emery and Dreifuss 1966; Merlini et al. 1986; Bione et al. 1994; Funakoshi et al. 1999; Wehnert et al. 1999). Autosomal dominant EDMD (EDMD2) is due to mutations in the lamin A/C (LMNA) gene encoding for a nuclear lamina protein (Bharati et al. 1992; Van der Kooi et al. 1997; Bharati et al. 1998; Nelson et al. 1998; Bonne et al. 1999; Buckley et al. 1999; Fatkin et al. 1999; Becane et al. 2000; Bonne et al. 2000; Vohanka et al. 2001). Lamin A/C mutations are also found in a range of other conditions including autosomal recessive EDMD (Di Barletta et al. 2000), LGMD1B, familial DCM (Graham and Owens 1999; Davies 2000), partial lipodystrophy, and peripheral neuropathy (AR CMT2). Variable phenotypes may be seen in the same family. Because of the different implications of laminopathy and emerinopathy both from the point of view of management and genetic counseling, a precise diagnosis should be sought in all patients (Box 27–4).

X-linked EDMD

There is strong evidence for cardiac involvement in X-linked EDMD (XLEDMD) and in this condition and the long-term prognosis is dictated predominantly by cardiac status (Emery and Dreifuss 1966; Merlini et al. 1986; Bione et al. 1994; Funakoshi et al. 1999; Wehnert et al. 1999; Sakata et al. 2005). Postmortem examination of EDMD hearts shows fibrofatty replacement of atrial myocardium in both atria but particularly around the sinus node region. Increased fibrosis around the AV node has also been reported. Loss of atrial muscle results in thinning of chamber walls and biatrial enlargement (Fishbein et al. 1993). This process results in sinus node failure, sometimes

Box 27–3 Myotonic Dystrophy

Cardiac surveillance:

1. Annual ECG from diagnosis for sinus node and AV conduction disease.
2. Holter ECG if initial assessment abnormal or for symptoms.
3. Echocardiogram at diagnosis in congenital myotonic dystrophy.
4. Signal-averaged ECG for *late potentials* increases surveillance sensitivity.
5. Invasive electrophysiology testing rarely indicated.

Treatment:

1. "Low threshold" for permanent pacemaker implantation.
2. Incidence of ventricular tachyarrhythmias does not support use of implantable defibrillator routinely when pacing for brady indications.

Box 27–4 Cardiac Surveillance in X-linked EDMD

- Regular cardiology follow-up advised since ECG abnormalities may be subtle and difficult to interpret.
- 12-lead ECG at diagnosis and annually thereafter.
- Holter monitoring for tachy- or bradyarrhythmia annually.
- Periodic assessment of ventricular function by echocardiography or other modality.
- Permanent pacemaker implantation is justified, even in asymptomatic patients, when ECG begins to show abnormalities of sinus node or AV node disease. Nocturnal AV-Wenkebach may be a normal finding in young people.
- In the presence of sinoatrial or AV nodal conduction abnormalities on surface ECG, invasive electrophysiology testing probably adds little to the decision to or timing of pacemaker implantation. However, such testing may have a role in determining the optimum pacing mode or sites for pacing.
- Full anticoagulation is required with the onset of atrial flutter/fibrillation or following permanent pacing for thromboembolic prophylaxis.

Box 27–5 Limb-Girdle Muscular Dystrophies

- Cardiac surveillance is not indicated routinely in LGMD2A, 2B, 2G, 2H, 2J, 1A, and 1C. Cardiac evaluations at diagnosis and when patients lose independent ambulation seem justified.
- Sarcoglycanopathy patients should be investigated with the same intensity as in patients with DMD/BMD (refer DMD/BMD sections).
- LGMD2I patients are at risk of cardiomyopathy and should be assessed as for DMD/BMD. The severity of cardiomyopathy may be out of proportion to that of skeletal muscle involvement.
- ECG and transthoracic echocardiography are appropriate investigative tools for standard initial clinical assessment and follow-up.
- The incidence of tachy- or bradyarrhythmias appears to be low. Additional arrhythmia surveillance with Holter ECG or similar recordings is justified, if standard ECG or symptoms suggest an arrhythmia.
- Standard therapy—as for DMD/BMD should be equally effective in sarcoglycanopathy-related cardiomyopathy, but given the rarity of the condition, trial evidence of efficacy is lacking.
- Cardiac transplantation may be indicated in selected patients with cardiac failure progressing despite antifailure therapy.
- Smooth muscle dysfunction may facilitate coronary artery spasm and contribute to the development of cardiomyopathy in sarcoglycanopathy. Although data from mouse models suggest a role for calcium antagonists as a specific treatment to improve coronary flow, it will be difficult to establish this in humans.

with complete atrial standstill or the onset of atrial tachycardias, flutter, or fibrillation. Progressive AV nodal conduction defects are also common (Bharati et al. 1992, 1998; Nelson et al. 1998; Becane et al. 2000; Boriani et al. 2003). Sudden death is probably explained by ventricular standstill in most of the cases reported, since in most reports patients had not been paced (Sakata et al. 2005). There are, however, rare reports of DCM (Merchut et al. 1990; Talkop et al. 2002; Muntoni 2003b), congestive heart failure, or sudden death, despite pacemaker implantation (Golzio et al. 2007; Box 27–5).

As with DMD, there may be some *female carriers* of XLEDMD, who manifest cardiac disease (Fishbein et al. 1993). Published cases of manifesting carriers may have been diluted by cases of the dominant form of disease. Carrier status should be established in females at risk and these women offered periodic ECG surveillance to detect sinoatrial or AV nodal conduction disease. There is a need for more systematic study of the natural history of cardiac involvement in XLEDMD carriers.

Laminopathy

Apart from the partial lipodystrophy and CMT phenotypes, there is strong evidence for cardiac involvement in laminopathy and this is progressive with age (Merlini et al. 1986; van der Kooi et al. 1997; Nelson et al. 1998; Fatkin et al. 1999; Funakoshi et al. 1999; Wehnert and Muntoni 1999; Bonne et al. 1999; Buckley et al. 1999; Becane et al. 2000; Vohanka et al. 2001). As with XLEDMD, long-term prognosis is directly related to cardiac status, and investigation of these patients should be performed as outlined for XLEDLD. However, the cardiac management of this group is more complex than XLEDMD. DCM may develop as well as conduction defects (van der Kooi et al. 1997; Buckley et al. 1999; Fatkin et al. 1999; Vohanka et al. 2001). Sudden death is seen in patients even after pacing (Bharati et al. 1992; Nelson et al. 1998; Fatkin et al. 1999; Becane et al. 2000; Bonne et al. 2000; van Berlo et al. 2004; Meune et al. 2006). As a result of accumulating evidence of sudden death despite pacing, the current consensus recommendation is that, when these patients require permanent pacing for bradycardia indications, implantable defibrillators should probably be recommended (Bushby et al. 2003; van Berlo et al. 2004; Meune et al. 2006). However, management of these cases is complex and needs to be individualized. The cost, frequency of device replacement, and expected long-term complications will be greater for implantable defibrillators than for "simpler" pacemakers. These patients should be managed in specialized centers and their data collated to contribute to further evidence in the future (Box 27–6).

Box 27–6 Laminopathies

- Cardiac involvement is typical in this muscular dystrophy.
- Prognosis is determined primarily by cardiac involvement.
- Cardiac involvement consists of progressive conduction abnormalities (sinus and AV node), atrial flutter/fibrillation, and cardiomyopathy.
- Sudden cardiac death can occur even in those paced. When pacing is indicated for bradycardia indications, defibrillator implantation should be recommended.
- Anticoagulation for thromboembolic prophylaxis is required with the onset of atrial flutter/fibrillation and after pacing/ICD implantation.
- Given the rarity of the condition and the complexity of cardiac involvement, regular surveillance is probably best undertaken at a specialist center.

Limb-Girdle Muscular Dystrophies

"Limb-girdle muscular dystrophy" (LGMD) refers to a heterogeneous group of genetic disorders caused by a variety of underlying genetic abnormalities (Bushby 1995, 1999; Bushby et al. 2007). Patients typically present with a face-sparing, predominantly proximal, progressive limb dystrophy in adolescence, which progresses to muscle wasting in adulthood (Gordon and Hoffman 2001; Norwood et al. 2007). Creatine kinase levels are elevated and muscle biopsies show dystrophic changes. LGMD can usually be distinguished clinically from the much commoner dystrophinopathies by older age of onset and slower rate of clinical progression—as well as by the presence of dystrophin on muscle biopsy. LGMDs affect both males and females and the incidence of sarcoglycanopathy in females is approximately the same as of manifesting carriers of the abnormal dystrophin gene. It is crucial, therefore, for appropriate genetic counseling to distinguish between the two conditions (Hoffman et al. 1996). At least five autosomal dominant and ten autosomal recessive gene defects have been identified so far underlying the clinical manifestations of LGMD (Roberts et al. 1994; Wicklund and Hilton-Jones 2003; Bushby et al. 2004). A reclassification of subtypes based on the specific underlying genetic abnormalities has been proposed and is outlined in Table 27–3. Because of the heterogeneity of phenotype, a lack of natural history data, and the rarity of many of these conditions, it is important that patients are seen and assessed regularly (Bushby et al. 2004). In addition to muscle and respiratory assessments, measures of left ventricular function should also be included, typically from ECG and echocardiogram (Bushby et al. 2003).

Table 27–3 Autosomal Recessive Limb-Girdle Muscular Dystrophy and Cardiac Involvement

AR LGMD Forms	Gene Locus	Protein	Medical Implications: Management
LGMD2A	15q15	Calpain-3	Contracture management, rarely require respiratory support
LGMD2B	2p13	Dysferlin	Ankle foot orthoses, rarely require respiratory support
LGMD2C	13q12	γ-Sarcoglycan	Contracture management, scoliosis management, risk of respiratory disease, and cardiomyopathy
LGMD2D	17q21	α-Sarcoglycan	Contracture management, scoliosis management, risk of respiratory disease, and cardiomyopathy
LGMD2E	4q12	β-Sarcoglycan	Contracture management, scoliosis management, risk of respiratory disease, and cardiomyopathy
LGMD2F	5q33	δ-Sarcoglycan	Contracture management, scoliosis management, risk of respiratory disease, and cardiomyopathy
LGMD2G	17q12	Telethonin	Not reported outside Brazil
LGMD2H	9q31–3413.3	TRIM32	Not reported outside Canadian Hutterites
LGMD2I	19q	FKRP	Contracture management, scoliosis management in childhood forms, risk of respiratory failure, and cardiomyopathy
LGMD2J	2q24.2	Titin	Not reported outside Finland
LGMD2K	9q34	POMT1	Rare; may require contracture management, scoliosis management in childhood forms, risk of respiratory failure, and cardiomyopathy
LGMD2L	11p13–12 ?	?	Described in group of Canadian families only
LGMD2M	9q31	Fukutin	Rare; may require contracture management, scoliosis management in childhood forms, risk of respiratory failure, and cardiomyopathy
LGMD2N	14q24	POMT2	Rare; may require contracture management, scoliosis management in childhood forms, risk of respiratory failure, and cardiomyopathy

Source: Table adapted from Guglieri et al. (2008).

In sarcoglycanopathy, since the subunits of the dystrophin-sarcoglycan complex (α-,β-, γ-, δ-) are bound together and functionally interrelated (Figure 27–1) defects in any element can result in dysfunction of the whole complex, although not invariably so. α-, γ-, and δ-sarcoglycans are expressed exclusively in striated and smooth muscle, while β-sarcoglycan is expressed widely, but especially in skeletal and cardiac muscle (Bushby 1995; Muntoni 2003a; Bushby et al. 2003; Guiglieri 2008). The incidence and severity of cardiac involvement in each of the sarcoglycanopathies is probably explained by the specific composition of the subcomplexes in skeletal as compared to those in cardiac muscle (Muntoni 2003a). Animal models of sarcoglycan-deficient cardiomyopathy have been developed in the sarcoglycan null mouse and sarcoglycan-deficient hamster. However, several important differences have emerged between the animal and human phenotypes making extrapolation of results from animal intervention to humans problematic (Kobuke et al. 2008; Bauer et al. 2008).

Cardiomyopathy has now been reported in humans with or suspected of having mutations in α-, β-, γ-, and δ-sarcoglycan genes (Bushby 1995; Bushby et al. 2003; Muntoni 2003a). For example, a particularly severe form of cardiomyopathy has been reported in two young patients with mutations in the β-sarcoglycan gene although milder forms have also been reported in patients with similar defects. LGMD2I due to mutations in the FKRP gene appears to have a frequent association with cardiomyopathy (van der Kooi et al. 1998; Politano et al. 2001; Brockington et al. 2001b; Poppe et al. 2002, 2003; Gaul et al. 2006). In LGMD2I the severity of cardiomyopathy may be out of proportion to that of skeletal muscle involvement. In each of the sarcoglycanopathies, the severity of the phenotype seems to correlate with the amount of protein expressed in each patient. In the most severely affected cases, cardiac transplantation has been required and undertaken successfully (Gaul et al. 2003; Poppe et al. 2004).

In contrast, there is much less evidence for cardiac involvement in calpainopathy (LGMD2A) or dysferlinopathy (LGMD2B) (Pollitt et al. 2001). Similarly, cardiac involvement has not been described to date in the rarer LGMD2H (TRIM 32), LGMD2G (telethoninopathy), or LGMD2J (titin) nor in the dominant form, LGMD1C (caveolin). Although there have been no reports of cardiac involvement in the families described with LGMD1A to date, the possibility of cardiac involvement cannot be excluded because of the relationship of this condition to MFM (refer later). Therefore, the recommendations for cardiac surveillance in this group depend very much on the particular type of LGMD and results of baseline evaluations.

It has been suggested that ischemic myocardial damage may contribute to the cardiomyopathy, particularly in β and δ forms of sarcoglycanopathy, through coronary artery spasm. This could occur as a direct effect of involvement of smooth muscle in arterial walls in the condition. In the mouse model, for example, coronary flow could be improved by reversing coronary spasm by calcium channel blockers (Gnecchi-Ruscone 1999; Durbeej and Campbell 2002). However, in γ -sarcoglycan-deficient mice coronary spasms are known to occur despite the fact that the complex is not disrupted in smooth muscle (McNally et al. 2003). It is more likely therefore that coronary spasm follows the progress of the cardiomyopathy rather than being the primary cause. None the less, calcium channel blockers, as opposed to β-blockers, may have a specific cardioprotective role along with ACE inhibitors or angiotensin-receptor blockers in the management of cardiomyopathy in this condition. There are now reports of successful cardiac transplantation in patients with FKRP (Box 27–7).

Box 27–7 Emery-Dreifuss Muscular Dystrophy

- Cardiac involvement is typical in this muscular dystrophy.
- Prognosis is determined primarily by cardiac involvement.
- Cardiac involvement consists of progressive sinus and AV nodal conduction problems (atrial standstill atrial flutter/fibrillation and AV block).
- Anticoagulation for thromboembolic prophylaxis and permanent ventricular pacing for AV block is usually required.
- There are only rare reports of cardiomyopathy.

Facioscapulohumeral Muscular Dystrophy

Facioscapulohumeral muscular dystrophy (FSHD) is probably not a major cause of cardiac disease (de Visser 1992; Faustmann et al. 1996; Gnecchi-Ruscone et al. 1999; Pollitt et al. 2001). The older literature reporting atrial paralysis in FSHD may have represented cases of misdiagnosed EDMD (Bloomfield and Sinclair-Smith 1965; Caponnetto et al. 1968; Baldwin et al. 1973). There are few large series and few papers with secure genetic data (Kimura et al. 1997; Laforet et al. 1998; Gnecchi-Ruscone et al. 1999). Severe cardiac involvement is exceptional (or not related to the FSHD). There appears to be a low incidence of conduction defect and atrial arrhythmia potentially complicated by embolism (Woelfel et al. 1989; Stevenson et al. 1990). However, data are lacking on the prevalence of cardiac problems in severe childhood disease. In patients with classical FSHD, it is probably advisable to perform an echocardiography or other assessment of ventricular function and 12-lead ECG at diagnosis. Further cardiac follow-up should be dictated by the clinical situation or if abnormalities are detected.

Cardiac Involvement in Rarer Forms of Muscular Dystrophy

1. Myofibrillar Myopathy

The term MFM has been used to link various myopathies with similar light-microscopic biopsy appearances—an accumulation of myofibrillar breakdown products at inappropriate sites within the muscle cells (de Bleecker et al. 1996; Nakano et al. 1997). The proteins expressed include myotilin, desmin, α-BC, dystrophin, and amyolid-related proteins and the particular types predominating can be distinguished by special staining techniques (Edstrom et al. 1990; Goebel 1997; Goldfarb et al. 1998). Appearances on electron microscopy show progressive myofibrillar degeneration from the Z-disk of the myofibril and accumulation of filaments in vacuoles (Engel 1999). The genetic basis for these conditions is as yet incompletely elucidated, but the features are compatible with abnormalities in myofibril- and Z-disk-associated proteins. Z-disk-associated proteins are already implicated in actin myopathy, nemalin myopathies, and some types of LGMD (1A and 2G). Titin mutations cause a form of muscular dystrophy with associated cardiomyopathy.

In one report of 63 patients with MFM, symptoms began over a wide age spectrum (mean age of onset 54 ± 16 years) usually with weakness of both proximal and distal muscles (Selcen et al. 2004). Cardiac involvement was present at diagnosis in 10 (16%) and consisted of symptomatic or asymptomatic degrees of ventricular dysfunction, with or without abnormalities of cardiac conduction or arrhythmias. ECG abnormalities reported included nonspecific repolarization abnormalities and frequent ventricular ectopy, compatible with their underlying cardiomyopathy, paroxysmal atrial fibrillation, or AV conduction delay. In another report a patient with an autosomal dominant form of myofibrillar myopathy developed features of arrhythmogenic right ventricular cardiomyopathy ("dysplasia") (Melberg et al. 1999).

Patients with MFM should undergo periodic assessment of left ventricular function by echocardiography or similar alternatives, and ECG. Management of cardiomyopathy or arrhythmias should be instituted early, even in the absence of symptoms, if identified (see section on DMD/BMD).

2. Central Core Disease

Central core disease (CCD) is a dominantly inherited congenital myopathy related to malignant hyperthermia and caused by mutations in the ryanodine gene (on chromosome 19q13.1) (Shy and Magee 1956; Shuaib et al. 1987; Hayashi 1989; Quinlivan et al. 2003). The variability in clinical presentation and discovery of a recessively inherited form probably means that CCD is genetically heterogeneous (Zhou et al. 2006). Typical clinical features of CCD include hypotonia in infancy, delay in achieving motor milestones due to diffuse muscle weakness, reduced muscle bulk, scoliosis, and congenital dislocation of the hip. The diagnosis is made from muscle biopsy by the appearance of abnormal rounded areas ("cores") throughout the length of type 1 muscle fibers, an excess of fat and connective tissue, and loss of oxidative activity (Hayashi et al. 1989; Monnier et al. 2001). Mutations in *RYR1* are thought to cause failure of calcium release channels in skeletal muscle (Monnier et al. 2001). In the series of 11 patients with ryanodine mutations reported by Qunilivan et al. the degree of disability ranged from clinically normal to never having achieved independent ambulation (Quinlivan et al. 2003). Four (36%) of these patients also had respiratory muscle involvement. Although CCD is considered rare, the fact that some patients have minimal or no clinical features of the condition, that de novo mutations are thought to be common, and that the disease is nonprogressive may mean that some patients may remain undiagnosed in the community (Monnier et al. 2001).

Malignant hyperthermia, an autosomal dominant pharmacological disorder of calcium regulation, is also due to mutations in the ryanodine receptor (MacLennan et al. 1990; McCarthy et al. 1990).

Cardiac involvement in CCD has not been described to date. However, the mutations in *hRyR1* causing central core myopathy and malignant hyperthermia and in *hRyR2* causing primary cardiac conditions are detectable in the same domains (Danieli and Rampazzo 2002). Defects in cardiac ryanodine receptor function (*hRyR2*) and calcium homeostasis are already known to underlie some forms of hypertrophic and right ventricular cardiomyopathies (Tiso et al. 2001; Danieli and Rampazzo 2002), catecholaminergic polymorphic ventricular tachycardia ("Coumel-type" VT) (Coumel et al. 1978; Laitinen et al. 2001; Priori et al. 2001; Sumitomo et al. 2003) and alterations in calcium handling in hearts failing from any etiology (Yano et al. 2006; Yamamoto et al. 2008). This raises the possibility of intriguing common interests between cardiologists and neuromuscular specialists in conditions related to ryanodine receptor disorders. Further discussion of the role of ryanodine receptor dysfunction in primary cardiac disorders is, however, more properly the subject of other chapters of this book (see Chapters 14 and 16).

Conclusions

At the present time, routine cardiac surveillance is justified on the basis that heart involvement is part of many forms of inherited muscle conditions. Substantial progress has been made in recent years in understanding the precise genetic abnormalities underlying muscular dystrophies, and how they translate into specific clinical phenotypes.

In the case of conditions with associated cardiomyopathy, early intervention with ACE inhibitor, angiotensin-receptor blockers, and β-blockers or calcium channel blockers, depending on the particular condition, can slow the rate of progression, delay symptom onset, and prolong life. For conditions with associated conduction defects and arrhythmias, timely deployment of pacemaker or defibrillator therapy can be life saving. Anticoagulation is appropriate in advanced stages of left ventricular dysfunction and in conditions associated with atrial arrhythmias to prevent pulmonary and arterial thromboembolism, respectively. Discoveries in genetics and molecular biology are already providing exciting new possibilities for therapies (Wells 2006), targeted at fundamental aspects of the specific conditions involved. However, the possibilities of exciting treatments in the future should not blind clinicians to the value of deploying therapies already available now to these patients with the aim of preventing or slowing the rate of deterioration of cardiomyopathy and improving prognosis.

References

Assmann PE, Slager CJ, van der Borden SG, Tijssen JG, Oomen JA, Roelandt JR. Comparison of models for quantitative left ventricular wall motion analysis from two-dimensional echocardiograms during acute myocardial infarction. *Am J Cardiol*. 1993;71:1262–1269.

Babuty D, Fauchier L, Tena-Carbi D, et al. Is it possible to detect infrahissian cardiac conduction abnormalities in myotonic dystrophy by non-invasive methods? *Heart*. 1999;82:634–637.

Bach J, Bianchi C, Vidigal-Lopes M, et al. Lung inflation by glossopharyngeal breathing and "air stacking" in Duchenne muscular dystrophy. *Am J Phys Med Rehabil*. 2007;86:295–300.

Backman E, Nylander E. The heart in Duchenne muscular dystrophy: a non-invasive longitudinal study. *Eur Heart J*. 1992;13:1239–1244.

Badano L, Autore C, Fragola PV, et al. Left ventricular myocardial function in myotonic dystrophy. *Am J Cardiol*. 1993;71:987–991.

Baker NL, Morgelin M, Peat R, et al. Dominant collagen VI mutations are a common *cause of Ullrich* congenital muscular dystrophy. *Hum Mol Genet*. 2005;14:279–293.

Balaban B, Matthews D, Clayton G, et al. Corticosteroid treatment and functional improvement in Duchenne muscular dystrophy: long-term effect. *Am J Phys Med & Rehab*. 2005;84:843–850.

Baldwin BJ, Talley RC, Johnson C, Nutter DO. Permanent paralysis of the atrium in a patient with fascioscapulohumeral muscular dystrophy. *Am J Cardiol*. 1973;31:649–653.

Barresi R, Di Blasi C, Negri T, et al. Disruption of heart sarcoglycan complex and severe cardiomyopathy caused by beta-sarcoglycan mutations. *J Med Genet*. 2000;37:102–107.

Bauer R, Macgowan GA, Blain A, Bushby K, Straub V. Steroid treatment causes deterioration of myocardial function in the {delta}-sarcoglycan-deficient mouse model for dilated cardiomyopathy. *Cardiovasc Res*. 2008 (In press).

Bauer R, Straub V, Blain A, Bushby K, MacGowan GA. Contrasting effects of steroids and angiotensin-converting-enzyme inhibitors in a mouse model of dystrophin-deficient cardiomyopathy. *Eur J Heart Fail*. 2009;11:463–471.

Becane HM, Bonne G, Varnous S, et al. High incidence of sudden death with conduction system and myocardial disease due to lamin A and C gene mutation. *PACE*. 2000;23:1661–1666.

Bharati S, Surawicz B, Vidaillet HJ Jr, Lev M. Familial congenital sinus rhythm abnormalities: clinical and pathological correlates. *PACE*. 1992;15:1720–1729.

Bione S, Maestrini E, Rivella S, et al. Identification of a novel X-linked gene responsible for Emery-Dreifuss muscular dystrophy. *Nat Genet*. 1994;8:323–327.

Bloomfield DA, Sinclair-Smith BC. Persistent atrial standstill. *Am J Med*. 1965;39:335–340.

Bonne G, Di Barletta MR, Varnous S, et al. Mutations in the gene encoding lamin A/C cause autosomal dominant Emery-Dreifuss muscular dystrophy. *Nat Genet*. 1999;21:285–288.

Bonne G, Mercuri E, Murchir A, et al. Clinical and molecular genetic spectrum of autosomal dominant Emery-Dreifuss muscular dystrophy due to mutations of the lamin A/C gene. *Ann Neurol*. 2000;48:170–180.

Boriani G, Gallina M, Merlini L, et al. Clinical relevance of atrial fibrillation/flutter, stroke, pacemaker implant and heart failure in Emery-Dreifuss muscular dystrophy: a long-term longitudinal study. *Stroke*. 2003;34:901–908.

Brockington M, Blade DJ, Prandini P, et al. Mutations in the fukutin-related protein gene (FKRP) cause a form of congenital muscular dystrophy with secondary laminin alpha-2 deficiency and abnormal glycosilation of alpha-dystroglycan. *Am J Hum Gen*. 2001a;69:1189–1209.

Brockington M, Yuva Y, Prandini P, et al. Mutations in the fukutin-related protein gene (FKRP) identify limb-girdle muscular dystrophy 21 as a milder allelic variant of congenital muscular dystrophy MDC1C. *Hum Mol Genet*. 2001b;10:2851–2859.

Buckley AE, Dean J, Mahy IR. Cardiac involvement in Emery-Dreifuss muscular dystrophy: a case series. *Heart*. 1999;82:105–108.

Bushby K, Muntoin F, Urtizberea A, et al. Report on the 124th ENMC International Workshop. Treatment of Duchenne muscular dystrophy: defining the gold standards of management in the use of corticosteroids. *Neuromusc Disord*. 2004;14:526–534.

Bushby K, Norwood F, Straub V. The limb-girdle muscular dystrophies—diagnostic strategies. *Biochim Biophys Acta*. 2007;1772:238–242.

Bushby KMD. Diagnostic criteria for the limb-girdle muscular dystrophies: report of the ENMC consortium on limb-girdle dystrophies. *Neuromusc Disord*. 1995;5:71–74.

Bushby KMD. The limb-girdle muscular dystrophies: multiple genes, multiple mechanisms. *Hum Mol Genet*. 1999;341:1759–1762.

Bushby KMD, Muntoni F, Bourke JP. Cardiac involvement in muscular dystrophy and myotonic dystrophy: report on 107th ENMC International Workshop. *Neuromusc Disord*. 2003;13:166–172.

Caponnetto S, Pastorini C, Tirelli G. Persistent atrial standstill in a patient affected by fascioscapulohumeral dystrophy. *Cardiologia*. 1968;53:341–350.

Clarke NRA, Kelion AD, Nixon J, Hilton-Jones D, Forfar JC. Does cytosine-thymine-guanine (CTG) expansion size predict cardiac events and electrocardiographic progression in myotonic dystrophy? *Heart*. 2001;86:411–416.

Coumel P, Fidelle J, Lucet V, et al. Catecholaminergic-induced severe ventricular arrhythmias with Adams-Stokes syndrome in children: report of four cases. *Br Heart J*. 1978;40(suppl):28–37.

Crilley JG, Boehm EA, Rajagopalan B, et al. Magnetic resonance spectroscopy evidence of abnormal cardiac energetics in Xp21 muscular dystrophy. *J Am Coll Cardiol*. 2000;15:1953–1958.

Danieli GA, Rampazzo A. Genetics of arrhythmogenic right ventricular dysplasia. *Curr Opin Cardiol*. 2002;17:218–221.

Darras BT. Molecular genetics of Duchenne and Becker muscular dystrophy. *J Pediatr*. 1990;117:1–15.

Davies MJ. The cardiomyopathies: an overview. *Heart*. 2000;83:469–474.

Day JW, Roelofs R, Leroy B, et al. Clinical and genetic characterisation of a five-generation family with a novel form of myotonic dystrophy (DM2). *Neuromusc Disord*. 1998;9:19–27.

de Bleecker JL, Engel AG, Ert BB. Myofibrillar myopathy with abnormal foci of desmin positivity. II Immunocytochemical analysis reveals accumulation of multiple other proteins. *Neuromusc Disord*. 1996;6:339–349.

de Visser M, de Voogt WC, la Riviere GV. The heart in Becker muscular dystrophy, fascio-scapulo-humeral dystrophy and Bethlem myopathy. *Muscle & Nerve*. 1992;15:591–596.

di Barletta RM, Ricci E, Galluzzi G, et al. Different mutations in the LMNA gene cause autosomal dominant and autosomal recessive Emery-Dreifuss muscular dystrophy. *Am J Genet*. 2000;66:1407–1412.

Duboc D, Meune C, Bertrand P, et al. Perindopril preventive treatment on mortality in Duchenne muscular dystrophy: 10 years' follow-up. *Am Heart J.* 2007;154:596–602.

Duboc D, Meune C, Lerebours G, et al. Effect of perindopril on the onset and progression of left ventricular dysfunction in Duchenne muscular dystrophy. *J Am Coll Cardiol.* 2005;45:855–857.

Durbeej M, Campbell KP. Muscular dystrophies involving the dystrophin-glycoprotein complex: an overview of mouse models. *Curr Opin Genet Dis.* 2002;12:349–381.

Eagle M, Baudouin SV, Chandler C, Giddings DR, Bullock R, Bushby K. Survival in Duchenne muscular dystrophy: improvements in life expectancy since 1967 and the impact of home nocturnal ventilation. *Neuromuscul Disord.* 2002;12:926–929.

Edstrom L, Thornell L-E, Albo J, et al. Myopathy with respiratory failure and typical myofibrillar lesions. *J Neurol Sci.* 1990;96:211–228.

Eidem BW, Tei C, O'Leary PW, Cetta F, Seward JB. Non-geometric quantitative assessment of right and left ventricular function: myocardial performance index in normal children and patient with Ebstein anomaly. *J Am Soc Echo.* 1998;11:849–856.

Emery A, Skinner R. Clinical studies in benign Becker type X-linked muscular dystrophy. *Clin Genet.* 1976;10:189–201.

Emery AED, Dreifuss FE. Unusual type of benign X-linked muscular dystrophy. *J Neurol Neurosurg Psychiatry.* 1966;29:338–342.

Engel AG. Myofibrillar myopathy. *Ann Neurol.* 1999;46:681–683.

English KM, Gibbs JL. Cardiac monitoring and treatment for children and adolescents with neuromuscular disorders. *Dev Med Child Neurol.* 2006;48:231–235.

Fatkin D, MacRae C, Sasaki T, et al. Missense mutations in the rod domain of the lamin A/C gene as causes of dilated cardiomyopathy and conduction-system disease. *N Engl J Med.* 1999;341:1715–1724.

Faustmann PM, Farahati J, Rupilius B, et al. Cardiac involvement in fascio-scapulo-humeral muscular dystrophy: a family study using Thallium-201 single- photon-emission-computer tomography. *J Neurol Sci.* 1996;144:59–63.

Ferlini A, Sewry C, Melis MA, Mateddu A, Muntoni F. X-linked dilated cardiomyopathy and the dystrophin gene. *Neuromuscul Disord.* 1999;9:339–346.

Finsterer J, Gharchbaghi-Schnell E, Stollberger C, et al. Relation of cardiac abnormalities and CTG-repeat size in myotonic dystrophy. *Clin Genet.* 2001;59:350–355.

Fishbein MC, Siegel RJ, Thompson CE, Hopkins LC. Sudden death of a carrier of X-linked muscular dystrophy. *Ann Intern Med.* 1993;119:900–905.

Forsberg H, Olofsson BO, Eriksson A, Andersson S. Cardiac involvement in congenital myotonic dystrophy. *Br Heart J.* 1990;63:119–121.

Funakoshi M, Tsuchiya Y, Arahata K. Emerin and cardiomyopathy in Emery-Dreifuss muscular dystrophy [Review]. *Neuromusc Disord.* 1999;9:108–114.

Gaul C, Deschauer M, Tempelmann C, et al. Cardiac involvement in limb-girdle muscular dystrophy 2I: conventional cardiac diagnostic and cardiovascular magnetic resonance. *J Neurol.* 2006;253:1317–1322.

Giglio V, Pasceri V, Messano L, et al. Ultrasound tissue characterization detects preclinical myocardial structural changes in children affected by Duchenne muscular dystrophy. *J Am Coll Cardiol.* 2003;42:309–316.

Gilhuis HJ, Donkelaar HJ, Tanke RB, et al. Nonmuscular involvement in merosin-negative congenital muscular dystrophy. *Paediatr Neurol.* 2002;26:30–38.

Gnecchi-Ruscone T, Taylor J, Mercuri E, et al. Cardiomyopathy in Duchenne, Becker, and sarcoglycanopathies: a role for coronary dysfunction? *Muscle & Nerve.* 1999;22:1549–1556.

Goldfarb LG, Park KY, Cervenakova L, et al. Missense mutations in desmin associated with familial cardiac and skeletal myopathy. *Nat Genet.* 1998;19:402–403.

Golzio PG, Chiribiri A, Gaita F. Unexpected sudden death avoided by implantable-defibrillator in Emery-Dreifuss patient. *Europace.* 2007;9:1158–1160.

Gordon ES, Hoffman EP. The ABC's of limb-girdle muscular dystrophy: alpha-sarcoglycanopathy, Bethlem myopathy, calpainopathy and more. *Curr Opin Neurol.* 2001;14;567–573.

Graham RM, Owens WA. Pathogenesis of inherited forms of dilated cardiomyopathy. *N Engl J Med.* 1999;341:1759–1762.

Grain L, Cortina-Borja M, Forfar C, et al. Cardiac abnormalities and skeletal muscle weakness in carriers of Duchenne and Becker muscular dystrophies and controls. *Neuromusc Disord.* 2001;11:186–191.

Groh W, Lowe M, Zipes D. Severity of cardiac conduction involvement and arrhythmias in myotonic dystrophy type 1 correlates with age and CTG repeat length. *J Cardiovasc Electrophysiol.* 2002;13:444–448.

Guglieri M, Straub V, Bushby K, Lochmuller H. Limb-girdle muscular dystrophies. *Curr Opin Neurol.* 2008;21:576–584.

Hadian D, Lowe MR, Scott LR, et al. Use of implantable loop recorder in a myotonic dystrophy patient. *J Cardiovasc Electrophysiol.* 2002;13:72–73.

Hawley RJ, Milner MR, Gottdiener JS, et al. Myotonic heart disease: a clinical follow-up. *Neurology.* 1991;41:259–262.

Hayashi K, Miller G, Brownell AK. Central core disease: ultrastructure of the sarcoplasmic reticulum and T-tubules. *Muscle Nerve.* 1989;12:95–102.

Hayashi Y, Ikeda U, Kojo T, et al. Cardiac abnormalities and cytosine-thyamine-guanine repeats in myotonic dystrophy. *Am Heart J.* 1997;134:292–297.

Hjalmarson A, Goldstein S, Fagerberg B, et al. Effect of metoprolol CR/XL in chronic heart failure: metoprolol CR/XL randomized intervention trial in congestive heart failure (MERIT-HF). *Lancet.* 1999;353:2001–2007.

Hoffman EP, Pegoraro E, Scacheir P, et al. Genetic counselling of isolated carriers of Duchenne muscular dystrophy. *Am J Med Genet.* 1996;28:573–580.

Holloway SM, Wilcox DE, Wilcox A, et al. Life expectancy and death from cardiomyopathy amongst carriers of Duchenne and Becker muscular dystrophy in Scotland. *Heart.* 2008;94:633–636.

Hoogerwaard EM, van der WouwPA, Wilde AA, et al. Cardiac involvement in carriers of Duchenne and Becker muscular dystrophy. *Neuromusc Disord.* 1999;9:347–351.

Ishikawa Y, Bach JR, Minami R. Cardio-protection for Duchenne's muscular dystrophy. *Am Heart J.* 1999;137:895–902.

Jefferies JL, Eidem BW, Belmont JW, et al. Genetic predictors of remodeling of dilated cardiomyopathy in muscular dystrophy. *Circulation.* 2005;112:2799–2804.

Kazuya S, Sakata K, Kachi E, Hirata S, Ishihara T, Ishikawa K. Sequential changes in cardiac structure and function in patients with Duchenne type muscular dystrophy: A two-dimensional echocardiographic study. *Am Heart J.* 1998;135:937–944.

Kimura T, Moriwaki T, Sawada J, et al. A family with fascioscapulohumeral muscular dystrophy and hereditary long-QT syndrome (Japanese). *Rinsho Shinkeigaku - Clin Neurol.* 1997;37:690–692.

Klesert TR, Cho DH, Clarke JI, et al. Mice deficient in Six5 develop cataracts. implications for myotonic dystrophy. *Nat Genet.* 2000;25:105–109.

Kobayashi O, Hayashi Y, Arahata K, et al. Congenital muscular dystrophy: clinical and pathological study of 50 patients with the classical (Occidental) merosin-positive form. *Neurology.* 1996;46:815–818.

Kober L, Torp-Pedersen C, Carlsen J, Videbaek R, Egeblad H. An echocardiographic method for selecting high risk patients shortly after acute myocardial infarction, for inclusion in multi-centre studies. *Eur Heart J.* 1994;15:1616–1620.

Kober L, Torp-Petersen C, Carlsen JE, et al. A clinical trial of the angiotensin-converting-enzyme inhibitor, trandolapril in patients with left ventricular dysfunction after myocardial infarction. *N Eng J Med.* 1995;333:1670–1676.

Kobuke K, Piccolo F, Garringer KW, et al. A common disease-associated missense mutation in alpha-sarcoglycan fails to cause muscular dystrophy in mice. *Hum Mol Gen.* 2008;17:1201–1213.

Laforet P, de Toma C, Eymard B, et al. Cardiac involvement in genetically confirmed fascioscapulohumeral muscular dystrophy. *Neurology.* 1998;51:1454–1456.

Laing NG. Inherited disorders of sarcomeric proteins. *Current Opinion in Neurology* 1999;12:513–18.

Laing NG. Congenital myopathies. *Curr Opin Neurol.* 2007;20:583–589.

Laitinen PJ, Brown KM, Piippo K, et al. Mutations of the cardiac ryanodine receptor (RyR2) gene in familial polymorphic ventricular tachycardia. *Circulation.* 2001;103:485–490.

Lazarus A, varin J, Babuty D, Anselme F, Coste J, Duboc D. Long-term follow-up of arrhythmias in patients with myotonic dystrophy treated byb pacing: A multicenter diagnostic pacemaker study. *J Am Coll Cardiol.* 2002;40:1645–1652.

Lazarus A, Varin J, Ounnoughene Z, et al. Relationships among electrophysiological findings and clinical status, heart function and extent of DNA mutation in myotonic dystrophy. *Circulation.* 1999;99:1041–1046.

Lee G-H, Badorff L, Knowlton KU. Dissociation of sarcoglycans and the dystrophin-carboxyl terminus from the sarcolemma in enteroviral cardiomyopathy. *Circ Res.* 2000;87:489–495.

Locolley P, Safar ME, Lucet B, Ledudal K, Labet C, Benetos A. Prevention of aortic and cardiac fibrosis by spironolactone in old normotensive rats. *J Am Coll Cardiol.* 2001;37:662–667.

MacLennan DH, Duff C, Zorzato F, et al. Ryanodine receptor gene is a candidate for predisposition to malignant hyperthermia. *Nature.* 1990;343:559–561.

MacMahon S, Sharpe N, Doughty R, et al. Randomised, placebo-controlled trial of carvedilol in patients with congestive heart failure due to ischaemic heart disease. *Lancet.* 1997;349:375–380.

Maeda M, Nakao S, Miyazato H, et al. Cardiac dystrophin abnormalities in Becker muscular dystrophy assessed by endomyocardial biopsy. *Am Heart J.* 1995;129:702–707.

Mankodi A, Thornton CA. Myotonic syndromes. *Curr Opin Neurol.* 2002;15:545–552.

Manzur AY, Kuntzer T, Pike M, Swan AV. Glucocorticoid corticosteroids for Duchenne muscular dystrophy. *Cochrane Database of Systematic Reviews* 2007, Issue 4. Art. No.: CD003725. DOI: 10.1002/14651858.CD003725.pub3.

Markham LW, Kinnett K, Wong BL, et al. Corticosteroid treatment retards development of ventricular dysfunction in Duchenne muscular dystrophy. *Neuromusc Disord.* 2008;18:365–370.

Mathieu J, Allard P, Potvin L, Prevost C, Begin P. A 10-year study of mortality in a cohort of patients with myotonic dystrophy. *Neurology.* 1999;52:1658–1662.

Mavrogeni S, Tzelepis G, Athanasopoulos G, et al. Cardiac and sternocleidomastoid muscle involvement in Duchenne muscular dystrophy: an MRI study. *Chest.* 2005;127:143–148.

McCarthy TV, Healy JMS, Heffron JJA, et al. Localization of the malignant hyperthermia locus to human chromosome 19q12–13.2. *Nature.* 1990;343:562–564.

McMurray JJ. Major beta-blocker mortality trials in chronic heart failure: a critical review. *Heart.* 1999;82(suppl IV):IV14–IV22.

McNally E, Allikian M, Wheeler MT, et al. Cytoskeletal defects in cardiomyopathy. *J Mol Cell Cardiol.* 2003;35:231–241.

Melberg A, Oldfors A, Blomstrom-Ludqvist C, et al. Autosomal dominant myofibrillar myopahty with arrhythmogenic right ventriuclar cardiomyopathy linked to chromosome 10q. *Ann Neurol.* 1999;46:684–692.

Mendell J. Congenital muscular dystrophy: searching for a definition after 98 years. *Neurology.* 2001;56:993–994.

Meola G, Sansone V, Marinou K, et al. Proximal myotonic myopathy: a syndrome with favourable prognosis? *J Neurol Sci.* 2002;193:89–96.

Merchut MP, Zdonczyk D, Gujrati M. Cardiac transplant in female Emery-Dreifuss muscular dystrophy. *J Neurol.* 1990;237:316–319.

Mercier JC, DiSessa TG, Jarmakani JM, et al. Two-dimensional echocardiographic assessment of left ventricular volumes and ejection fraction in children. *Circulation.* 1982;65:962–969.

Mercuri E, Brockington M, Straub V, et al. Phenotypic spectrum associated with mutations in the fukutin-related protein gene. *Ann Neurol.* 2003;53:537–542.

Merino JL, Carmona JR, Fernandez-Lazano I, et al. Mechanism of sustained ventricular tachycardia in myotonic dystrophy. *Circulation.* 1998;98:541–546.

Merlini L, Granata C, Dominici P, Bonfiglioli S. Emery-Dreifuss muscular dystrophy: report of five cases of a family and review of the literature. *Muscle & Nerve.* 1986;9:481–485.

Meune C, Van Berlo JH, Anselme F, et al. Primary prevention of sudden death in patients with lamin A/C Gene mutations [Letter]. *N Eng J Med.* 2006;354(2):209–210.

Minetti C, Bado M, Morreale G, et al. Disruption of muscle basal lamina in congenital muscular dystrophy with merosin deficiency. *Neurology.* 1996;46:1354–1358.

Mirabella M, Servidei S, Manfredi G, et al. Cardiomyopathy may be the only clinical manifestation in female carriers of Duchenne muscular dystrophy. *Neurology.* 1993;43:2342–2345.

Monnier N, Romero NB, Lerale J, et al. Familial and sporadic forms of central core disease are associated with mutations in the C-terminal domain of the skeletal muscle ryanodine receptor. *Hum Mol Genet.* 2001;10:2581–2592.

Muntoni F. Cardiomyopathy in muscular dystrophies. *Curr Opin Neurol.* 2003a;16:577–583.

Muntoni F. Cardiac complications of childhood myopathies. *J Child Neurol.* 2003b;18:191–202.

Murdoch DR, Byrne J, Morton, et al. BNP is stable in whole blood and can be measured using a simple rapid assay: implications for clinical practice. *Heart.* 1997;78:594–597.

Nakano S, Engel AG, Akiguchi I, Kimura J. Myofibrillar myopathy. III. Abnormal expression of cyclin-dependent kinases and nuclear proteins. *J Neuropathol Exp Neurol.* 1997;56:850–856.

Nelson SD, Sparks EA, Graber HL, et al. Clinical characteristics of sudden death victims in heritable (Chromosome 1p1–1q1) conduction and myocardial disease. *J Am Coll Cardiol.* 1998;32:1717–1723.

Nigro G, Comi LI, Politano L, Bain RJI. The incidence and evolution of cardiomyopathy in Duchenne muscular dystrophy. *Int J Cardiol.* 1990;26:271–277.

Norwood F, de Visser M, Eymard B, et al. EFNS guideline on diagnosis and management of limb-girdle muscular dystrophies. *Eur J Neurol.* 2007;14:1305–1312.

Oloffson B, Forsberg H, Andersson S, et al. Electrocardiographic findings in myotonic dystrophy. *Br Heart J.* 1988;59:47–52.

Palmieri B, Sblendorio V. Duchenne muscular dystrophy: an update, part I. *J Clin Neuromusc Dis.* 2006;8:53–59.

Palmieri B, Sblendorio V. Duchenne muscular dystrophy: an update, part II. *J Clin Neuromusc Dis.* 2007;8:122–151.

Parker AE, Robb SA, Chambers J, et al. Analysis of an adult Duchenne muscular dystrophy population. *QJM.* 2005;98:729–736.

Pelargonio G, Dello Russo A, Sanna T, De Martino G, Bellocci F. Myotonic dystrophy and the heart. *Heart.* 2002;88:665–670.

Perloff JK, Henze E, Schelbert HR. Alterations in regional myocardial metabolism, perfusion and wall motion in Duchenne muscular dystrophy studied by radionuclide imaging. *Circulation.* 1984;69:33–42.

Pfeffer MA, Braunwald E, Moye LA, et al. Effect of captopril on mortality and morbidity in patients with left ventricular dysfunction after myocardial infarction: results of the Survival and Ventricular Enlargement Trial. *N Engl J Med.* 1992;327:669–677.

Phillips AV, Timchenko LT, Cooper TA. Disruption of splicing regulated by a CUG-binding protein in myotonic dystrophy. *Science.* 1998;280:737–741.

Phillips MF, Harper PS. Cardiac disease in myotonic dystrophy. *Cardiovasc Res.* 1997;33:13–22.

Politano L, Nigro V, Nigro V, et al. Development of cardiomyopathy in female carriers of Duchenne and Becker muscular dystrophy. *JAMA.* 1996;275:1335–1338.

Politano L, Nigro V, Passamano L, et al. Evaluation of cardiac and respiratory involvment in sarcoglycanopathies. *Neuromusc Disord.* 2001;11:178–185.

Pollitt C, Anderson LV, Pogue R, Davison K, Pyle A, Bushby KMD. The phenotype of calpainopathy: diagnosis based on multidisciplinary approach. *Neuromusc Disord.* 2001;11:287–296.

Poppe MJ, Cree L, Bourke J, et al. The phenotype of limb-girdle muscular dystrophy type 2I. *Neurology.* 2003;60:1246–1251.

Poppe MJ, Eagle M, Bourke J, et al. Respiratory and cardiac involvement are an important part of limb-girdle muscular dystrophy. *Neuromusc Disord.* 2002;12:732–733.

Priori SG, Napolitano C, Tiso N, et al. Mutations in the cardiac ryanodine receptor gene (hRyR2) underly catecholaminergic polymorphic ventricular tachycardia. *Circulation.* 2001;103:196–200.

Prystowsky EN, Pritchett ELC, Roses AD, Gallagher J. The natural history of conduction system disease in myotonic muscular dystrophy as determined by serial electrophysiology studies. *Circulation.* 1979;60:1360–1364.

Quinlivan RM, Muller CR, Davis M, et al. Central core disease: clinical, pathological and genetic features. *Arch Dis Child.* 2003;88:1051–1055.

Ramaciotti C, Heistein LC, Coursey M, et al. Left Ventricular Function and Response to Enalapril in Patients With Duchenne Muscular Dystrophy During the Second Decade of Life. *Am J Cardiol.* 2006;98:825–827.

Reardon W, Newcombe R, Fenton I, Silbert J, Harper PS. The natural history of congenital myotonic dystrophy: mortality and long term clinical aspects. *Arch Dis Child.* 1993;68:177–181.

Richards DA, Byth K, Ross DL, Uther JB. What is the best predictor of spontaneous ventricular tachycardia and sudden cardiac death after myocardial infarction? *Circulation.* 1991;83:756–763.

Roberts SL, Leturcq F, Allamand V, et al. Missense mutations in the adhalin gene linked to autosomal recessive muscular dystrophy. *Cell.* 1994;78:625–633.

Sakata K, Shimizu M, Hidekazu I, et al. High incidence of sudden cardiac death with conduction disturbances and atrial cardiomyopathy caused by a nonsense mutation in the STA gene. *Circulation.* 2005;111:3352–3358.

Selcen D, Ohno K, Engle AG. Myofibrillar myopathy: clinical, morphological and genetic studies in 63 patients. *Brain.* 2004;127:439–451.

Seznec H Agbulut O, Sergeant N, et al. Mice transgenic for the human myotonic dystrophy region with expanded CTG repeats display muscular and brain abnormalities. *Hum Mol Genet.* 2001;10:2717–2726.

Shuaib A, Paasuke RT, Brownell AKW. Central core disease: clinical features in 13 patients. *Medicine.* 1987;66:389–396.

Shy GM, Magee KR. A new congenital non-progressive myopathy. *Brain.* 1956;79:610–621.

Silversides CK, Webb GD, Harris VA, et al. Effects of deflazacort on left ventricular function in patients with Duchenne muscular dystrophy. *Am J Cardiol.* 2003;91:769–772.

SOLVD. The effect of enalapril on survival in patients with reduced left ventricular ejection fraction and congestive cardiac failure. *N Eng J Med.* 1991;325:293–302.

Spyrou N, Philpot J, Foale R, et al. Evidence of left ventricular dysfunction in children with merosin-deficient congenital muscular dystrophy. *Am Heart J.* 1998;136:474–476.

Stevenson WG, Perloff JK, Weiss JN, Anderson TL. Fascioscapulohumeral muscular dystrophy: evidence for selective genetic electrophysiologic cardiac involvement. *J Am Coll Cardiol.* 1990;15:292–299.

Sumitomo N, Harada K, Nagashima M, et al. Cathecholaminergic polymorphic ventricular tachycardia: electrocardiographic characteristics and optimal therapeutic strategies to prevent sudden death. *Heart.* 2003;89:66–70.

Talkop UA, Tabrik I, Sonajak M, et al. Early onset of cardiomyopathy in two brothers with X-linked Emery-Dreifuss muscular dystrophy. *Neuromusc Disord.* 2002;12:978–981.

Taneja KL, McCurrach M, Schalling M, et al. Foci of trinucleotide repeat transcripts in nuclei of myotonic dystrophy cells and tissues. *J Cell Biol.* 1995;128:995–1002.

The cardiac insufficiency bisoprolol study II (CIBIS II): a randomized trial. *Lancet.* 1999;11:138–142.

Thuillez C, Richer C, Loueslati H, et al. Systemic and regional haemodynamic effects of perindopril in congestive heart failure. *J Cardiovasc Pharmacol.* 1990;15:527–535.

Tiso N, Stephan DA, Nava A, et al. Identification of mutations in the cardiac ryanodine receptor gene in families affected by arrhythmogenic right ventricular cardiomyopathy type 2 (ARVD2). *Hum Mol Genet.* 2001;10:1890–1894.

Topaloglu H, Brokington M, Yuva Y, et al. FKRP mutations cause congenital muscular dystrophy, mental retardation and cerebral cysts. *Neurology.* 2003;60:988–992.

Tsutamoto T, Wada A, Maeda K, et al. Plasma BNP level as a biochemical marker of morbidity and mortality in patients with asymptomatic or minimally symptomatic left ventricular dysfunction. Comparison with plasma angiotensin II and endothelin-1. *Eur Heart J.* 1999;20:1799–1807.

van Berlo JH, Duboc D, Pinto YM. Often seen but rarely recognised: cardiac complications of lamin A/C mutations [Editorial]. *Eur Heart J.* 2004;25:812–814.

van der Kooi AJ, de Voogt WG, Barth PG, et al. The heart in limb-girdle muscular dystrophy. *Heart.* 1998;79:73–77.

van der Kooi AJ, van Meegen M, Ledderhof TM, McNally EM, de Visser M, Bolhuis PA. Genetic localization of a newly recognized autosomal dominant limb-girdle muscular dystrophy with cardiac involvement (LGMD1B) to chromosome 1q11–21. *Am J Hum Genet.* 1997;60:891–895.

Velasco M, Colin A, Zurakowski D, et al. Posterior spinal fusion for scoliosis in Duchenne muscular dystrophy diminishes the rate of respiratory decline [Miscellaneous Article]. *Spine.* 2007;32:459–465.

Vohanka S, Vytopil M, Beanarik J, et al. A mutation in the X-linked Emery-Dreifuss muscular dystrophy gene in a patient affected with conduction cardiomyopathy. *Neuromusc Disord.* 2001;11:411–413.

Voit T. Congenital muscular dystrophies: 1997 update. *Brain & Dev.* 1998;20:65–74.

Wehnert M, Muntoni F. 60th ENMC International Workshop: non X-linked Emery-Dreifuss muscular dystrophy 5–7 June 1998;Naarden, The Netherlands. *Neuromusc Disord.* 1999;9:115–121.

Wells DJ. Therapeutic restoration of dystrophin expression in Duchenne muscular dystrophy. *J Muscle Res Cell Motil.* 2006;27:387–398.

Wicklund MP, Hilton-Jones D. The limb-girdle muscular dystrophies: genetic and phenotypic definition of a disputed entity. *Neurology.* 2003;60:1230–1231.

Woelfel A, Cascio W, Smith SW. Cerebral embolization in two young patients with fascioscapulohumeral muscular dystrophy and atrial dysrhythmias. *Am Heart J.* 1989;118:632–633.

Yamamoto T, Yano M, Xu X, et al. Identification of target domains of the cardiac ryanodine receptor to correct channel disorder in failing hearts. *Circulation.* 2008;117:762–772.

Yano M, Yamamoto T, Ikeda Y, et al. Mechanisms of disease: ryanodine receptor defects in heart failure and fatal arrhythmias. *Nat Clin Pract Cardiovasc Med.* 2006;3:43–52.

Ylmaz O. Karaduman A, Topaloglu H. Prednisolone therapy in Duchenne muscular dystrophy prolongs ambulation and prevents scoliosis. *Eur J Neurol.* 2004;11:541–544.

Zannad F, Alla F, Dousset B, Perez A, Pitt B. Limitation of excessive extracellular matrix turn over may contribute to survival benefit of spironolactone therapy in patients with congestive heart failure: insights from the randomized aldosterone evaluation study (RALES). RALES investigators. *Circulation.* 2001;102:2700–2706.

Zhou H, Yamaguchi N, Xu L, et al. Characterisation of recessive RYR1 mutations in core myopathies. *Hum Mol Genet.* 2006;15:2791–2803.

28

Cardiovascular Complications in Ehlers-Danlos Syndromes

Michael F Pope

Introduction

Ehlers-Danlos syndromes (EDS) are a complex group of inherited disorders of connective tissue (IDCTs), particularly of skin, ligaments, and the vasculature, but also affecting the gastrointestinal tract, and other structural tissues, such as bones, cartilage, teeth, gums, cornea, vitreous humor, pleuroperitoneal linings, and various basement membranes (Pope and Burroughs 1997). Other IDCTs include osteogenesis imperfecta, the Marfan syndrome, Stickler syndrome, Cutis Laxa, and pseudoxanthoma elasticum, all of which are distinguished from EDS by virtue of its typical cutaneous fragility. Nevertheless, all of them and particularly benign hypermobile syndrome (EDS III) overlap with other common population variants, such as arterial aneurysms, osteoporosis, osteoarthritis, astigmatism, and keratoconus (Figure 28–1).

General Properties of Connective Tissue

Connective tissue ground substance is produced by fibroblasts, osteoblasts, chondrocytes, adipocytes, and epithelial cells, mostly arising from differentiated mesenchymal stem cells. The ground substance contains both fibrous proteins and a more amorphous ground substance (Grays Anatomy 1973). The protein component of ground substance includes collagen and elastic tissue proteins such as elastin, fibulin, and fibrillin, whilst the amorphous portion includes glycosaminoglycans and various other glycoproteins such as laminin, entactin, and the tenascins.

Collagens are very diverse, with more than 20 proteins coded by 30 genes. All are triple helical polymers of (Gly XY) repeats forming distinct subsets such as the fibrillar, FACIT, short-chain, basement membrane, and membrane-bound collagens (Kielty and Grant 2002). The fibrillar group, defects of which cause several distinctive EDS subgroups, have perfect central triple helices and similar, cleavable, N- and C-terminal extensions, which are removed in the process of extracellular fibril assembly. Defects of other collagens cause inherited defects of basement membranes, myopathies, growth and skeletal development, or of epithelial adhesion, whilst many more await discovery.

Nearly all of the recognized EDS subtypes disturb connective tissue organization and most of them affect collagen fibril organization, composition, or stability by several distinctive mechanisms (see below). Specifically, they are caused by errors in helical collagen sequence (EDS types I, II, III, IV, VIB), processing (EDS VII), or posttranslational modification (EDS VIA), or protein–protein interaction (some EDS III homozygotes).

History of EDS

Eponymously attributed to Ehlers (1901) and Danlos (1908), who independently described the unusual bruising, excessive cutaneous extensibility, and molluscoid pseudotumors (Figure 28–2), it was actually first described earlier by Tschernogobow (1892). In 1967, Barabas first proposed three separate subtypes, including classical, venous, and arterial subgroups (Barabas 1967a), whilst Beighton (1968) had independently subdivided the classical into severe (gravis) and milder (mitis) variants. He also described an X-linked variety (Beighton 1968a, 1968b, 1993). McKusick (1972) added hydroxylysine-deficient and procollagen-peptidase-deficient variants, as originally described by Pinnell et al.(Pinnell et al. 1972) and later confirmed by Lichtenstein et al. (1973). The addition of the common hypermobile type completes the present-day classification of types I, II, III, IV, VI, and VII, from which Beighton's X-linked variant (type V) has been excluded from the modern Villefranche classification (Beighton et al. 1997; Table 28–1). EDS types VIII and X are also excluded from the general classification as both are too closely overlapping or too rare.

Genetics of EDS

Although the vertical transmission consistent with autosomal dominant inheritance in EDS was noticed very early, a convincing five-generation British/Canadian family was published in 1949 (Johnson and Falls 1949) (see Figure 28–3). Subsequently, autosomal recessive inheritance has been clearly described in EDS types VIA and VIIC, as well as tenascin X-deficient EDS III, all of which are either homozygous or doubly heterozygous. The previously described X-linked recessive inheritance of EDS V is rather

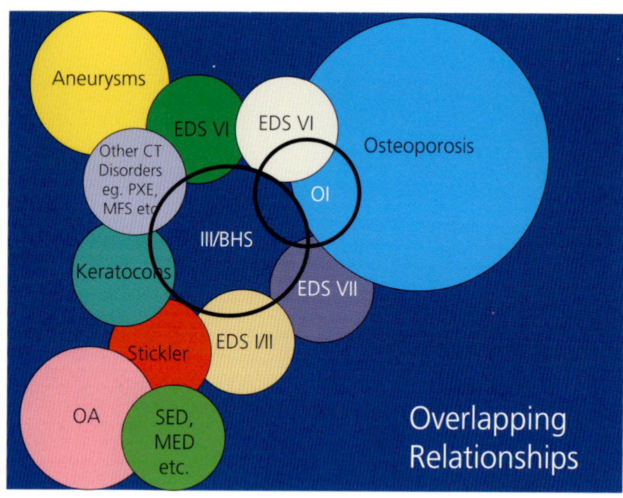

Figure 28–1 Overlapping relationships. Venn diagram showing overlaps between the commonest EDS III/BHS variant, with other common disorders such as osteoporosis, arterial aneurysms, osteoarthritis, and uncommon single gene disorders, such as EDS I/II, IV, VI, VII, Osteogenesis Imperfecta, Stickler Syndrome, Marfan Syndrome, and Pseudoxanthoma Elasticum.

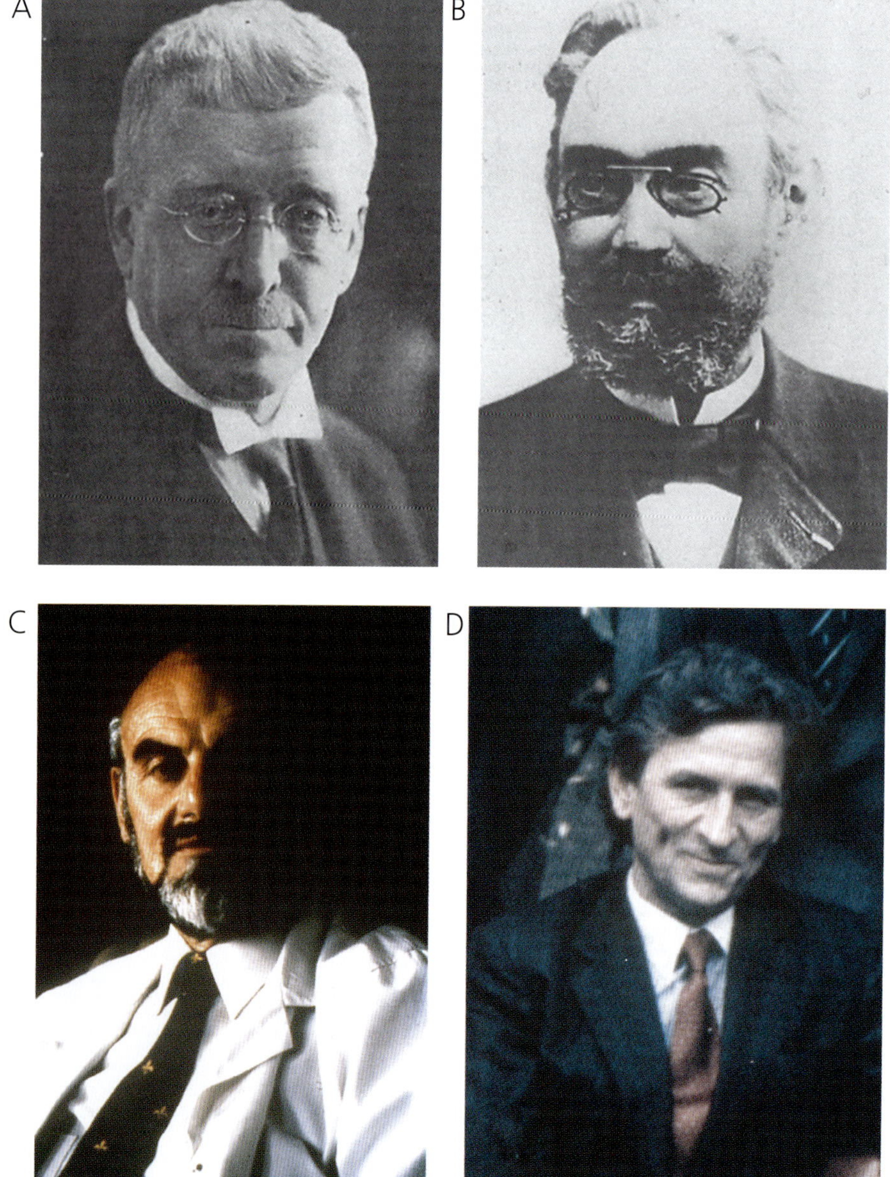

Figure 28–2 (a–d) Clinical pictures. Clinical pictures of Drs. Ehlers and Danlos who separately described the distinct clinical entity now recognized as the Ehlers-Danlos syndrome. Drs Beighton and Barabas who made major contributions to the recognition of clinical diversity of EDS are shown in Figures 28–2 c and d.

Table 28–1 The Classification of EDS

Villefranche	Type	Synonym	McKusick No.	Special Features	Histology Electron Microscopy	Basic Defect
Classical	EDS I	Gravis type	AD 130000	Widespread scarring, bruising, especially forehead, chin, and shin. Molluscoid pseudotumors	Cauliflower fibrils	COL5A1 linked in some families. Mutations include exon skips and a translocation and a cysteine substitution
Classical	EDS II	Mitis type	AD 130010	Similar but less severe	Cauliflower fibrils	
Hypermobility	EDS III	Hypermobile type	AD 130020	No cutaneous scars	Nonspecific	Unknown
Vascular	EDS IV	Vascular type IVA acrogeric IVB acrogeric IVC ecchymotic	AD 130050 AR 22535 AD 130050	Nearly always type III collagen deficient Risk of arterial rupture highest in acrogeric subtypes	Collagen depletion, variation of fiber size	COL3A1 mutations. Numerous point mutations and exon skips, rarely deletions
Other	EDS V	X-linked type	XL 305200	Very rare; not lysyl oxidase deficient. Resembles EDS I, II, and III		
Kyphoscoliotic	EDS VI	Ocular scoliotic VIA decreased lysyl hydroxylase levels VIB normal levels	AR 225400	Muscular hypotonia, often muscular dystrophy suspected (slow motor milestones) Persistent premature scoliosis Arterial rupture in 30%	Nonspecific	Lysyl hydroxylase point mutations or exon skips (homozygosity)
Arthrochalatic	EDS VII A,B,C	Arthrochalasis multiplex congenita	AD 130060	Extremely lax joints with congenital hip dislocation Occasionally mild facial cutis laxa Some types have skin fragility, mandibular hyperplasia	Fibrils vary from angular in A and B, to hieroglyphic C	Types A and B specific exon skips or deletions of COL1A1, 1A2 either pNa1(I) or pNa2(I) retained. Type C procollagen peptidase deficiency
Dermatosparactic			AR 224510	Severe generalized cutis laxa in humans; dermatosparaxis in cattle, sheep, and cats		Both pNa1(I) and pNa2(I) extensions retained
Other	EDS VIII EDS IX EDS X	Periodontitis type Vacant Fibronectin abnormality	AD 130080 AR 225310	Allelic variation with variable expression Fibronectin deficient	Nonspecific	Some are COL3A1 others not Association with FN may be coincidental

Note: Combined Villefranche and traditional-type-specific classification of the EDS.

doubtful, as no other families have subsequently been identified and the segregation pattern of affected males and apparent carrier females may have been autosomal dominant with relatively more severe clinical phenotype in the affected males.

Current Classification of EDS

This is based on both the 1988 and 1997 International Classifications (Beighton et al. 1988, 1997) consisting of types I to VII (1988), in which types I and II were merged, whilst types VIIA and VIIB were separated from type VIIC in the 1997 classification (Villefranche proposals). This information is summarized in Table 28–1 but for clarity the older type I to VII notation has been mainly retained.

Molecular Abnormalities

Most mutations disrupt collagen fibril assembly, either directly by alteration of collagen α-chain translational, or post-translational sequence, or by altering crucial interactive molecules that secondarily interfere with normal collagen fibrillogenesis. There are three broad categories:

1. Altered collagen α-chain sequence, as in EDS types I, II, (COL5A1, 5A2), IV (COL3A1), and occasionally, type III (COL3A1).
2. Abnormal collagen or procollagen processing, EDS VIA (lysyl hydroxylase deficiency, caused by PLOD1 mutations), EDS VIIA and B (persistent pNα1 and pNα2 sequences caused by exon 6 missplicing of COL1A1 or COL1A2), EDS VIIC (deficiency of the ADAMS TS2 gene coding for the

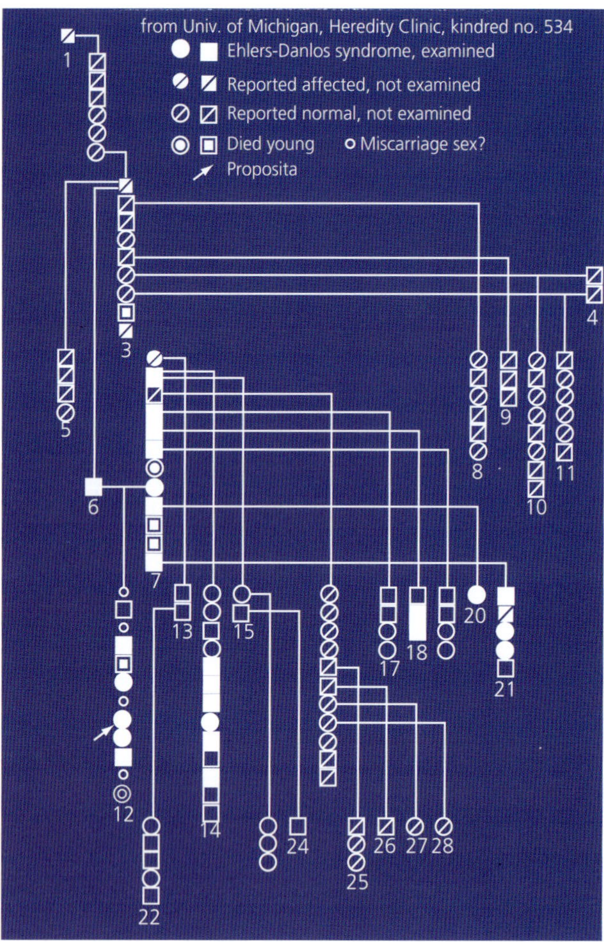

Figure 28–3 Early pedigree of Canadian family of British origin. This clearly shows autosomal dominant inheritance of what was retrospectively an EDS I/II phenotype. Reprinted from Johnson SAF, Falls HF. Ehlers-Danlos syndrome: a clinical and genetic study. *Arch Derm Syphilol.* 1949;60:82–105, with permission.

processing peptidase causes persistence of both pNα1 and pNα2 chains).

3. Other defective interactive noncollagenous molecules causing secondary impairment of collagen fibrillogenesis, as in tenascin-X mutations in homozygous EDS type III.

Brief Clinical Features of the Various Subtypes

1. EDS Types I and II

Typical features include hyperextensible, doughy but fragile skin, with atrophic pigmented scarring over knees, shins, elbows, forehead, and chin. Pretibial ecchymoses and hemosiderosis are also common and the earlier that the cutaneous splitting first occurs, the more severe and persistent the subsequent scarring. Broad hands and feet (mesomorphism) may also feature, as do epicanthic folds, blue sclerae, varicose veins, fibrous nodules of knees, shins, and ankles. Mutations of COL5A1 or COL5A2, include glycine substitutions, exon skips, and larger deletions (Pope and Burroughs 1997), whilst haploinsufficiency of COL5A1 is relatively common (Wenstrup et al. 2000). Electron microscopy shows the characteristic cauliflower fibrils, whilst protein analysis is only occasionally helpful (Figures 28–4c), as when the responsible mutation shortens the secreted protein. More usually, there are subtle variations in protein intensity, as at least 50% of COL5A1 mutants are haploinsufficient.

2. EDS Type III

This is the commonest, and clinically simplest of all the EDS subtypes. Paradoxically, it is also the least well understood at the biochemical and molecular levels and may also be the most molecularly heterogeneous. Unlike all other EDS subtypes, the skin is not fragile, but it is variably hyperextensible. Scarring is rare and minimal, whilst the main and most striking feature is the very obvious joint hypermobility. This typically has a Beighton score in excess of 3/9. Overlaps occur with almost all other EDS subtypes (Figures 28–1 and 28–4e), as well as common forms of osteoporosis, osteoarthritis, and occasional arterial or gastrointestinal fragility. There is an irregularly penetrant and puzzling association with chronic pain syndromes in some families, but more usually, the hypermobility is mechanically beneficial in the fields of athletics, dancing, and gymnastics.

EDS III is the commonest EDS variant and is clearly autosomal dominant. Potential homozygotes occur in very large EDS III pedigrees, whilst the heterozygous parents of homozygous EDS VI are clinically indistinguishable from autosomal dominant EDS III phenotypes. Furthermore, only occasional mutations have been identified in EDS III, for example, a COL3A1 glycine substitution (Narcisi et al. 1994) described in a family with EDS III manifesting with premature osteoarthritis, but with normal arteries. Homozygous tenascin-X mutations caused severe homozygous EDS III (Schalkwijk et al. 2001), and certain homozygous COL5A1 mutations can cause mild EDS II, whilst the heterozygote carriers are clinically normal (Giunta et al. 2002). Paradoxically, Zweers et al 2006 have also described high serum levels of Tenascin-X with lowered amounts of the latter in common forms of abdominal aortic aneurysms.

3. EDS Type IV (Vascular EDS)

Vascular fragility dominates this subtype often causing lethal arterial rupture or dissection. More severe types have pretibial ecchymoses and hemosiderosis, thereby sometimes causing confusion with EDS types I/II and EDS VIII. However, in contrast the skin is generally prematurely thinned and is much less extensible than in EDS type I/II. Skin thinning may be focal and limited to the face, shoulders, and forearms or more generalized and even complete. Usually, widespread thinning is accompanied by specific facial features, including large eyes, variably thin lips, lobeless ears (the Madonna face) (Figure 28–5a). The combination of prematurely thin skin over the dorsum of hands and feet together with the facial appearance is termed acrogeria (Figures 28–5a and b). Sometimes the extensive premature acral dermal atrophy and bruising is accompanied by metacarpal subluxations and can be misdiagnosed as rheumatoid degeneration with steroid atrophy (Figure 28–5b). When accompanied by premature thinning of scalp hair (metageria) it can be confused with progeria (Figure 28–5c). Other more variable clinical signs include acroosteolysis, elastosis perforans serpiginosa, keloid scars, premature hip or other joint dislocations, bilateral premature talipes in children, or spontaneous colonic perforations in adults. Vascular pathology includes aneurysms of small- and medium-sized arteries, such as the renal, splenic, coeliac axis, brachial, subclavian, femoral, popliteal, internal carotid, and carotid cavernous sinus vessels (Figures 28–5d–g). Occasionally, coronary aneurysms have also been described. Aortic aneurysms involving the aortic arch, descending, and abdominal aorta are much more frequent than coronary pathology and fatal aortic dissections are common.

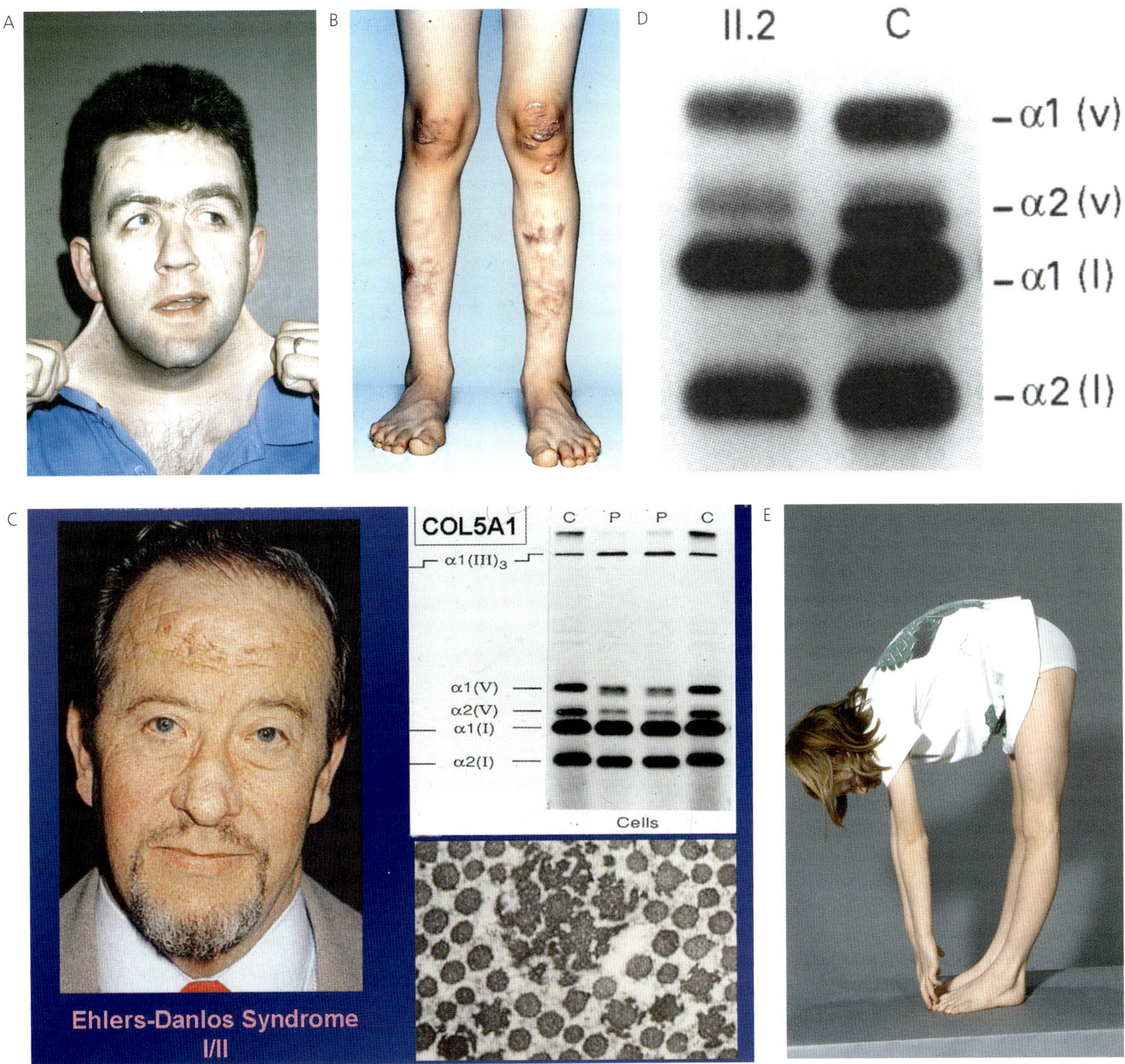

Figure 28–4 (a–e) EDS. Fragile, hyperextensible, doughy skin typical of EDS I/II (a), the pretibial scarring is especially typical (b). Compound montage showing the typical forehead scars of EDS I/II (c); the collagen protein analysis shows a double α1(V) component, the lower of which has a deleted fragment (Nicholls et al. 1994); there is also electron microscopy of skin, showing characteristic fused cauliflower fibrils, caused by misregulated fibril assembly and misaggregation of collagen type I and III fibrils (c). Haploinsufficiency of typeV α2 collagen chains, from a family with EDS II (d). The athletic pose of uncomplicated EDS III/BHS, with striking flexibility with recurving of the knees (e).

Light microscopy characteristically shows marked dermal thinning, collagen depletion, and elastic proliferation (Figure 28–5h) and is sufficiently specific as to be diagnostic (Pope et al. 1996). Similarly, electron microscopy of dermal collagen fibers shows altered collagen fibril diameters, in contrast to the normal evenly distributed size (Figure 28–5i). Protein chemistry shows two patterns of collagen type III depletion (Figure 28–5j and k). In the more severe dominant-negative type only 1/8th of collagen trimers are normal and abnormal trimers remain intracellular. In the haploinsufficient type, collagen type III secretion is close to 50% and abnormal protein is not produced or retained (Figure 28 5k). Generally, protein patterns match the general clinical appearance and overall severity. Collagen type III, *COL3A1* mutations include triple helical glycine substitutions (Figure 28–l), exon skips, and small and large deletions. Occasional nonhelical C propeptide mutations have also been described (Pope et al. 1996; Pepin et al. 2000; Malfait et al. 2007).

4. EDS Type VI

There are two types of EDS type VI of which the molecular pathology of type VIA is well understood. Here, extreme ligamentous laxity combines with severe progressive premature scoliosis, ocular fragility with retinal detachment, and extreme joint laxity with severe valgus rotation, and pes planus of the feet (Figures 28–6a

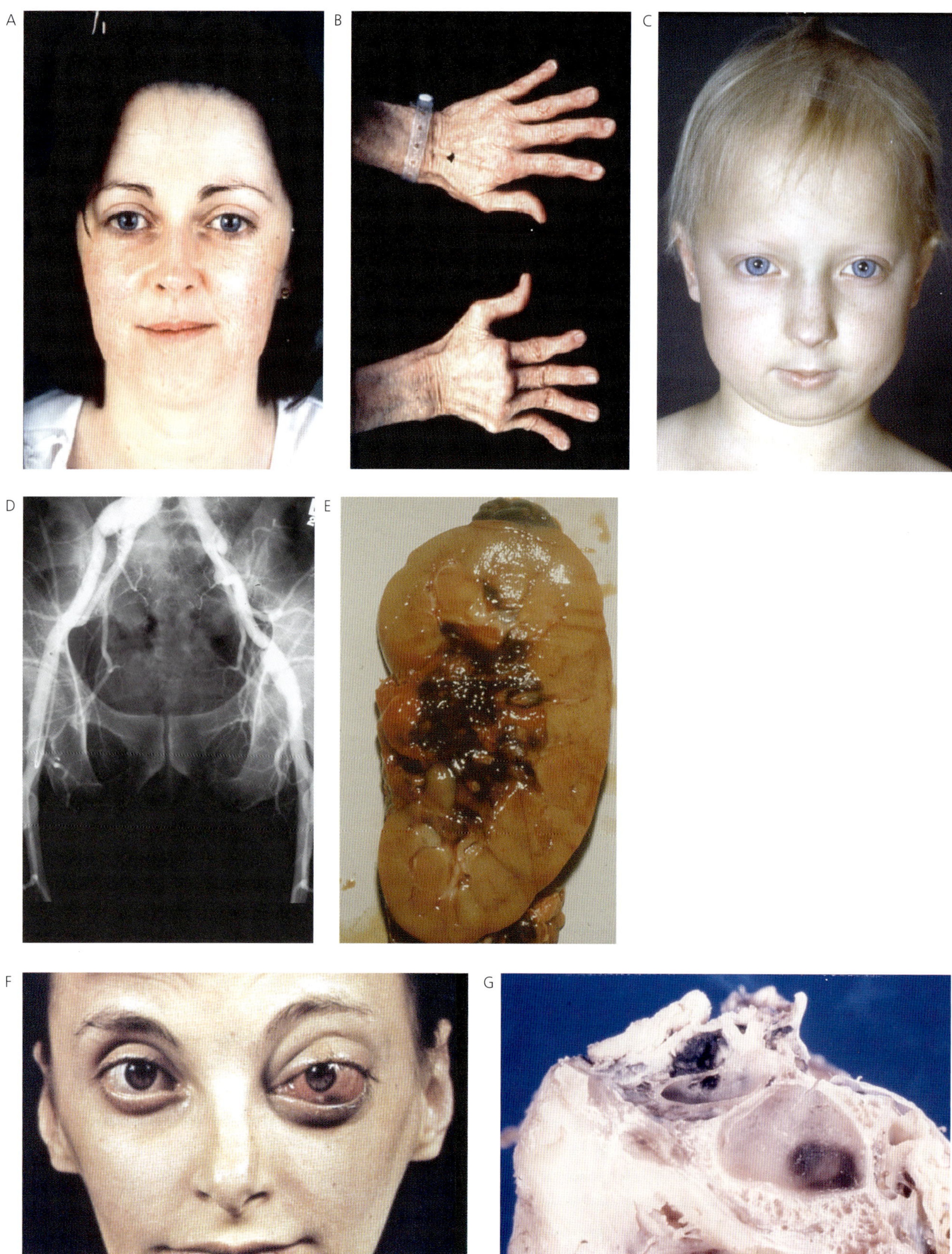

Figure 28–5 (Continued)

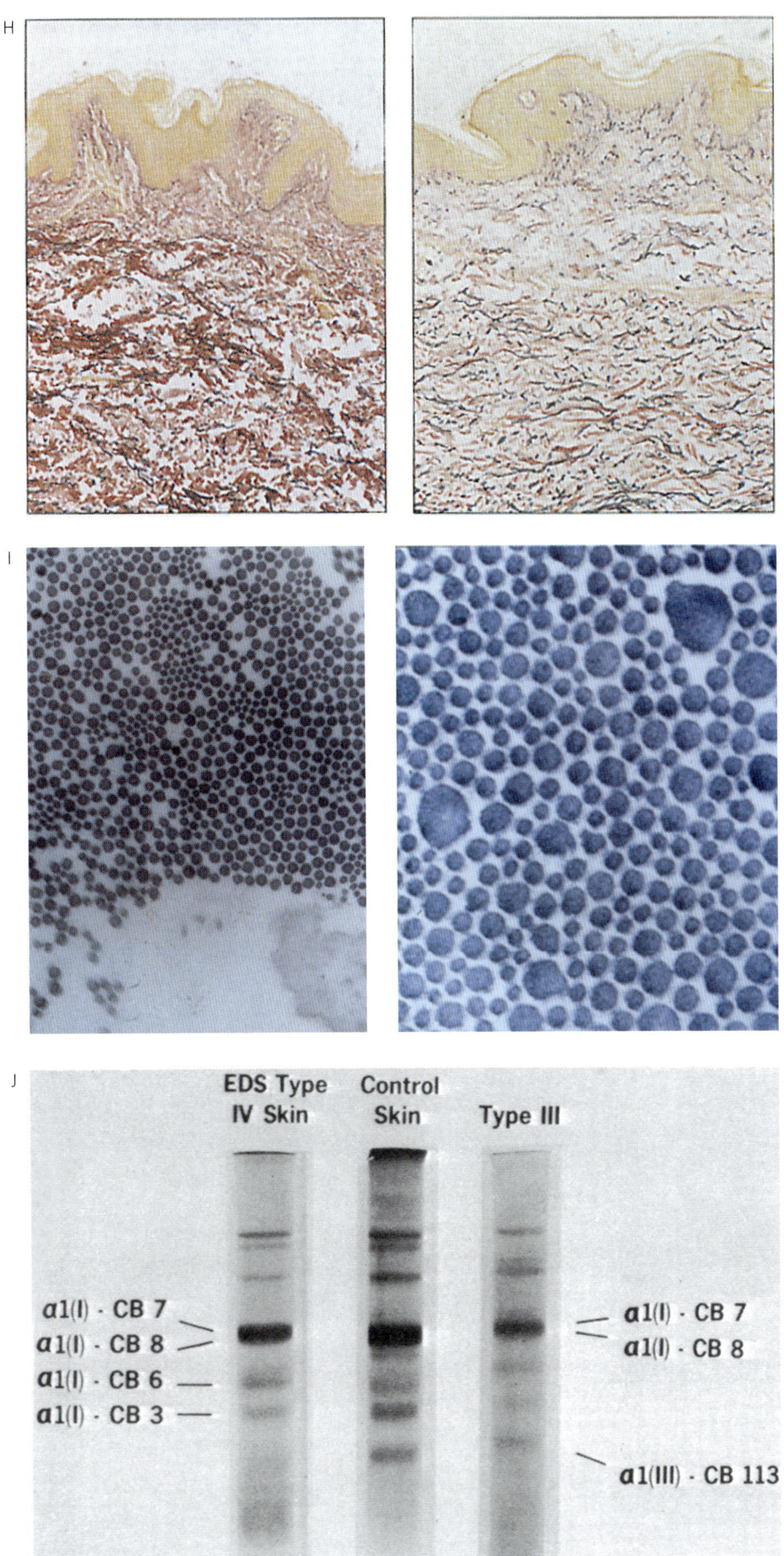

Figure 28–5 (Continued)

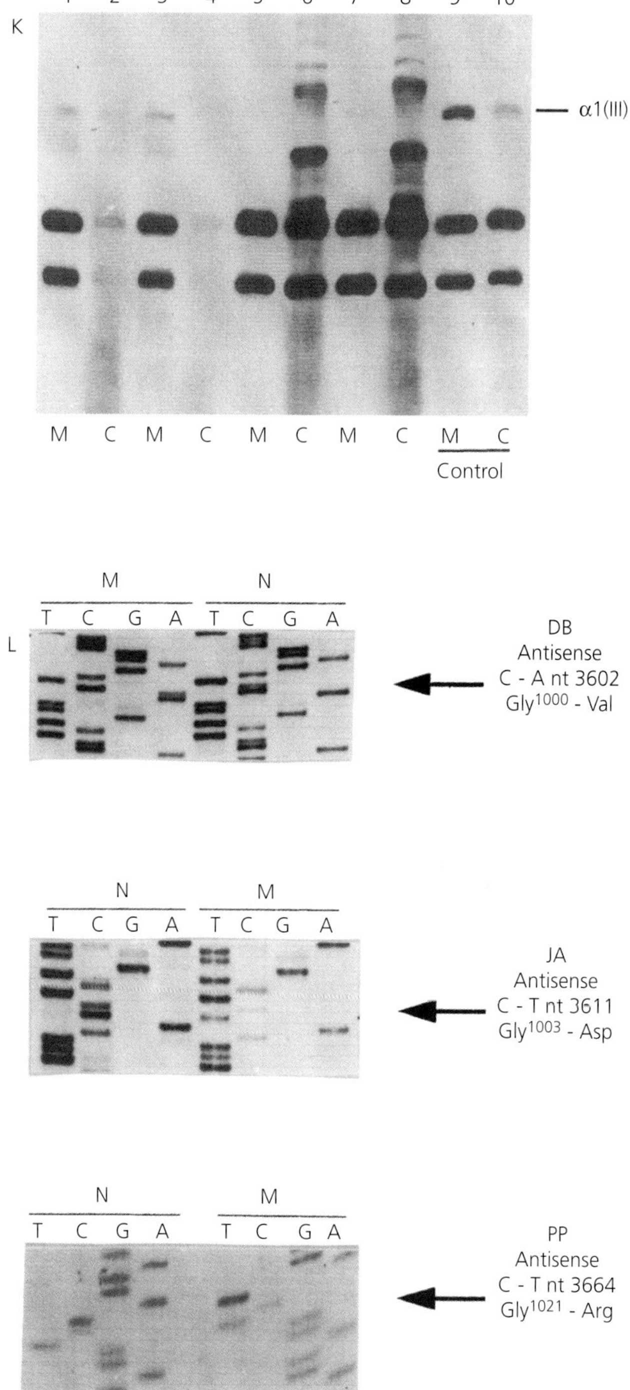

Figure 28–5 (a–l) (a) Madonna face of 25-year-old female acrogeric EDS IV patient. (b) Her prematurely aged hands clearly demonstrate the remarkable dermal thinning, reminiscent of steroid atrophy. The striking multiple MCP subluxations were, understandably, confused with rheumatoid arthritis. (c) Diffuse hair loss characterizes the so-called metageric phenotype, though the general facial pattern is very similar to (a). (d) Arterial pathology includes diffuse aorto-iliac tortuosity and dilatation; (e) a medium-sized ruptured renal artery necessitating total nephrectomy to control bleeding; (f) acute unilateral exophthalmos, following a carotid cavernous-sinus aneurysm (g). (h) Light microscopy of acrogeric skin with collagen depletion and elastic proliferation (L), compared with normal skin (R), whilst electron microscopy (i) shows variably sized collagen fibrils in both arterial (L) and skin samples (R). (j) Direct collagen protein analysis directly from tissue samples or (k) from radiolabeled cultured skin fibroblasts, show collagen type III deficiency. The radiolabeling distinguishes two patterns: a haploinsufficient one where collagen type III secretion is diminished by 50% (tracks 1–4), and a dominant-negative pattern in which only 1/8th of normal collagen is secreted whilst 7/8ths is retained and overmodified intracellularly (tracks 5–8), compared with normal (tracks 9 and 10). Amplified and sequencing of *COL3A1* cDNA fragments of the collagen type III gene *COL3A1*, shows specific glycine substitutions (l). Reproduced with permission: Figures h, i, k, l, from Pope FM, Narcisi P, Nicholls AC et al. *COL3A1* mutations cause variable clinical phenotypes including acrogeria and vascular rupture *Br J Dermatol.* 1996;135(2):163–181. and Figure j from Pope et al. 1975.

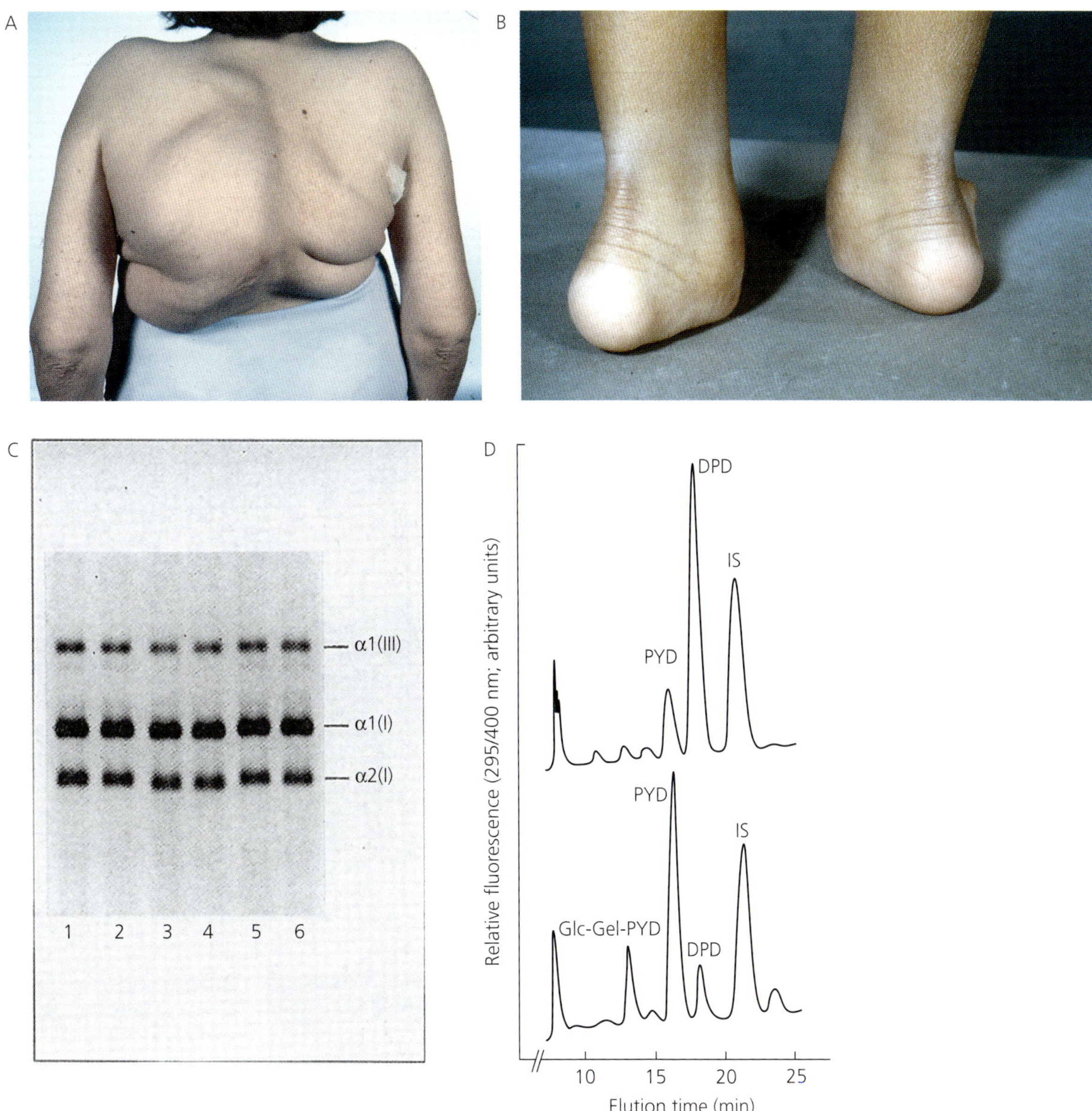

Figure 28–6 (a–d) (a) Typical severe kyphoscoliosis of EDS VIA. (b) The marked valgus rotation of the heels and very severe bilateral pes planus. (c) Subsequent to PLOD1 enzyme deficiency, both collagen types I and III are underhydroxylated and migrate further than normal on polyacrylamide gels. (d) Alternatively, urinary collagen cross-linking patterns are disturbed showing reversal of the normal hydroxylated/unhydroxylated pattern, of lysyl pyridinoline ratios (Courtesy of Professor Simon Robins).

and b). There may also be short stature and moderate to severe premature osteoporosis and clear autosomal recessive inheritance (Krane et al. 1972; Pinnell et al. 1972). Occasionally, overlapping the vascular pathology of EDS IV, there may be premature arterial rupture, dilatation, or arteriovenous fistulae (Debnath et al. 2007). The ligamentous laxity is so early and severe that motor milestones are very seriously delayed and congenital muscular dystrophy often suspected. Muscle biopsy is invariably normal or sometimes nonspecific. The disorder is caused by deficiency of lysyl hydroxylase (procollagen lysyl 2 oxoglutarate 5 deoxygenase), causing deficient or even complete underhydroxylation of specific collagen lysine residues. Consequently, hydroxylysine-hydroxylysine condensation cross-links, especially of type I collagen are absent, with resulting tissue instability.

The underhydroxylated collagen type I can be detected either by collagen type protein analysis, when underhydroxylated collagen type I α chains migrate further than normal chains (Figure 28–6c). Alternatively, lysine-derived cross-link patterns can be tested on fresh urine samples (Figure 28–6d). In both instances homozygous or doubly heterozygous mutations of the *PLOD1* gene coding for the hydroxylase are causative (Hyland et al. 1992). Heterozygote parents are clinically unaffected but often closely resemble EDS III/BHS heterozygotes, with obviously hypermobile joints and increased Beighton scores. In the case of EDS VIB, the physical signs are milder and enzyme levels, collagen hydroxylation, urinary cross-links, and *PLOD1* gene analyses are normal. Occasional homozygous *COLIA1* or *COL1A2* helical mutations, without bone fractures, but with osteoporosis have been identified indicating both causal and clinical overlap with osteogenesis imperfecta (Nicholls et al. 2001). In our experience, EDS VIB is more than 20 times commoner than EDS VIA and is mostly of unknown cause (Pope and Robins 2007).

5. EDS Type VII (Types A, B, and C)

These are a subset of focal type I collagen mutations or modifications, thereby also having clinical and causal overlaps with osteogenesis imperfecta and other osteoporoses. EDS type VII A and VIIB are very rare with less than 20 cases published worldwide (Dalgliesh 2007). Clinically, the cutaneous features overlap with both EDS I/II and mild cutis laxa. Distinctive features include severe premature ligamentous laxity, with congenital hip dislocations (Figures 28–7a and b). Distinguishing features from EDS I/II include small stature, severe deforming ligamentous laxity, osteoporosis with fractures, and occasional dentinogenesis imperfecta. There have been no recorded examples of cardiac or cardiovascular complications.

Very specific protein abnormalities arise from the failure to excise type I procollagen N terminal propeptides. This is either due to deletion of the enzyme cleavage sequence of either α1(I) or α2(I), N terminal propeptides, or is caused by homozygous deficiency of the cleavage enzyme. In EDS VIIA this causes the longer pNα1(I) chains to persist and in EDS VIIB, pNα2 chains remain. They are detectable by their pepsin-resistant pNα2 fragments by PAGE (Figure 28–7c). Because collagen type I heterotrimers contain twice as many α1 as α2 chains, EDS VIIA (75% of trimers abnormal) is more severe than EDS VIIB (50% of trimers abnormal). This is reflected in more disrupted collagen fibril packing in the former compared with the latter (Figure 28–7d and e). At EM level type VIIA collagen fibers are significantly more distorted than type VIIB fibers. They are at their most abnormal, when neither pNα1 nor pNα2 extensions are cleaved (Figure 28–7d). Molecularly, *COL1A1* or *COL1A2* exon 6 deletions are caused by splice junction acceptor, donor, or nearby intronic substitutions, all resulting in the deleted protein cleavage errors.

In the case of EDS VIIC, in which both ligamentous laxity, skin fragility, cutis laxa osteoporosis, and general collagen disorganization is greatest, the cleavage enzyme coded by the *ADAMSTS2* gene is faulty (Colige et al. 2004). Consequently, both pNα1(I) and pNα2 chains persist, all collagen type I triple helices are faulty. Electron microscopy shows flanged rods rather than collagen cylinders, visible as hieroglyphic fibers (Figures 28–7d and e). Lethal animal mutations in sheep, cattle, and cats cause so-called dermatosparaxis.

6. EDS Type VIII

Although excluded from the 1992 Villefranche classification because of its clinical overlap with EDS types I/II and IV, some EDS VIII families are unique. Clinically, however, the pretibial ecchymoses, hemosiderosis, cutaneous scarring, and moderate to severe periodontal involvement may also occur in other EDS subtypes. However, they are distinguishable, either by the other characteristic clinical or biochemical gene sequence or EM features. Furthermore, convincing gene linkage data define a causative locus at chromosome12p13, independent of any other known connective structural or other locus (Rahman et al. 2003).

Cardiovascular Complications of EDS

Cardiac as opposed to cardiovascular complications of EDS are relatively rare. Thus McKusick in the 1972, 4th Edition of *Inherited Defects of Connective Tissue*, describes only occasional cardiac complications, including left bundle branch block, partial right bundle branch block, aortic stenosis and incompetence, floppy mitral valve, combined mitral and tricuspid regurgitation, nodular thickening of the mitral valve, combined mitral incompetence with aortic stenosis, and combinations of ASD, VSD, and tetralogy of Fallot. However, he did not correlate these changes with particular EDS subtypes, with the exception of BHS/EDS III in which he noted that mitral valve prolapse (MVP) was common in EDS III. Similarly, Peter Beighton's EDS monograph (Beighton 1970), recorded only inconsistent associations, including benign systolic murmurs (10%), mitral incompetence (1%), ASD (1%), right-sided aortic arch (1%), aortic stenosis and incompetence (1%), and mitral incompetence (1%). He also quoted that 13/300 previously published EDS families (4.3%) had assorted cardiac problems, without any consistent pattern. His own studies tabulated 29% of EDS patients with possible cardiac abnormalities, which included four with pulmonary systolic murmurs, who may or may not have had significant pulmonary stenosis. He also made a detailed study of the existing literature upon previously published cardiac complications in EDS (Table 28–2).

Contrastingly, the vascular complications of arterial fragility were well described, and clearly separated from other EDS subtypes by both Barabas (1967a and b) and Beighton (1968a) They were quickly incorporated into the EDS classification, by McKusick, as the vascular variant, or EDS type IV. Although, preceded by Sack (1936) and also Mories (1960), both Barabas (1967a and b) and Beighton (1968a) had independently separated the vascular from other ecchymotic subtypes, such as EDS types I, II, and later EDS VIII. Amongst key features enumerated by McKusick were spontaneous intestinal perforation, rectal bleeding, hemoperitoneum, sigmoid colonic rupture, dissecting aneurysm of the aorta with cystic medial necrosis, proximal aortic dilatation with aortic valvular incompetence (rarely), popliteal, subclavian, iliac and carotid aneurysms, and arteriovenous fistulae, especially of intracranial and carotid cavernous-sinus vessels. Barabas (1967) had also very clearly described the arterial fragility, characteristic of this subtype, which he separated from more benign phenotypes.

EDS VIA is only rarely complicated by arterial fragility, or cardiac problems and even then, usually late in life (McKusick 1972). His original case with severe microcornea, glaucoma, and bilateral retinal detachment eventually died from a late aortic rupture. In contrast to arterial EDS, ruptured arteries are very uncommon in EDS VIA, although both carotid and aortic rupture have been described and documented, as well as mitral incompetence complicated by subacute bacterial endocarditis and congestive heart failure. Similarly, aortic root echocardiography shows that up to 40% of haploinsufficient COL5A1 defective EDS I/II probands have significant aortic root dilatation. However, in the author's experience, aortic rupture is extremely rare, only one such example reported in more than 100 affected families. That is not to say that careful monitoring, β-blockade, and good blood pressure control are not prudent. Nevertheless, COL3A1 deficient EDS IV is both the main cause of arterial fragility and the most dangerous of EDS subtypes, susceptible to cardiovascular sequelae. Thus, amongst 180 published examples quoted by PUB MED between 1987 and 2008, 100 (56%) were caused by EDS IV, with two each respectively of EDS II (Alvarez et al. 1992; Fernandez-Garcia et al. 2004), and OI (Okamura et al. 1995) and a single example of tenascin deficiency in EDS III/BHS (Peeters et al. 2004). As regards OI, author has personal experience of a single dominant Sillence type I OI family, in which an affected brother and sister and their two daughters all had similar combinations of aortic dilatation, aortic

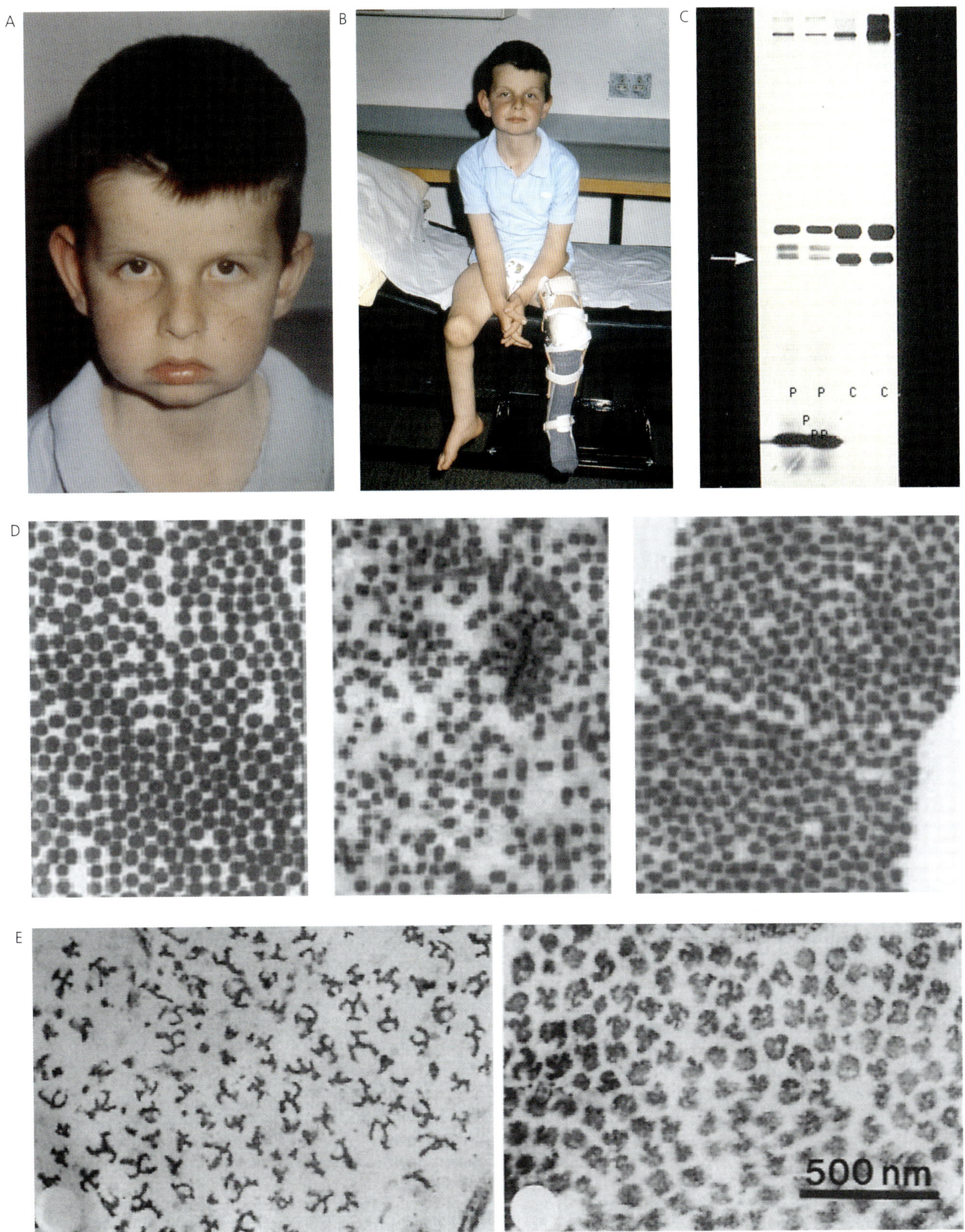

Figure 28–7 (a–e) (a) Face of 7-year-old male with EDS VIIB, showing mild, but obvious cutis laxa.(b) He was also abnormally hypermobile, with early instability of his knees. (c) Radiolabeled collagen analysis showing a pepsin-resistant pNα2(I) fragment, caused by a heterozygous exon 6 deletion of his *COL1A2* gene. (d and e) Disturbed collagen fibril assembly causes distortions of fibril shape seen in cross section as angulated fibrils (EDS VIIB), to swing wing fibrils (EDS VIIA) and hieroglyphical fibrils (EDS VIIC). Patterns of altered shape are dictated entirely by the numbers of pNα extensions remaining uncleaved.

Table 28–2 Comparative Studies of the Echocardiographic Complications of EDS

Reference	EDS Subtype	Numbers	Male/Female	Mitral Valve Prolapse	Aortic Dilatation, SVAR, etc.	Miscellaneous	Conclusion
McDonnell et al. 2006	I/II	16	7/31	1/38		↓LV function, 13/38 ↑PA pressure 3/38 Mild AI 2/38	Mild aortic root dilatation is common
Wenstrup et al. 2002	I/II/III	71	28/43	–	28% 33% EDS I/II 17% EDS III		Unexpectedly high ARD that is stable, rather than rapidly progressive like MFS
Dolan et al. 1997	I/II/III IV	30 3	6/27	6% EDS 7% Control	None	Atypical chest pain: 48% Palpitations: 39% Dyspnea (exertion): 30%	Benign, no aortic root dilatation MVP similar to controls
Tiller et al. 1998	I/II/III	5	114	4/5 (80%)	4/5 (80%)	Mitral incompetence	Although a selected cohort, EDS I/II and III, potentially significant aortic pathology

Note: Summary of the previously published cases with cardiovascular complications of EDS.
Source: Reprinted from Beighton P *The Ehlers Danlos Syndrome*. Chapter VI.
Cardiovascular Complications, William Heinemann Medical Books Limited SBN 433 02150 0; 1970, with permission.

incompetence, and aortic valve replacements, in addition to their frequent fractures.

Illustrative Case Reports

Whilst vascular complications in EDS are very common, these only rarely affect the heart directly. Instead, vascular fragility, especially of the aorta, carotid, and cerebral circulation is common, although any large- or medium-sized artery may be implicated. Occasionally, there may be direct valvular or perfusion abnormalities of the heart itself. The cases described below have been previously published either by the author's group or others, except those unreferenced ones, which are from the author's clinical archives.

1. Vascular Complications in EDS IV

I. Case 1 (Pope et al. 1996) A 27-year-old female had successive spontaneous right or left pneumothoraces, in teenage. Later she developed acute central abdominal pain, which at laparotomy revealed a left renal artery hematoma and peritoneal bleeding. Except for troublesome tendoachilles contractures, following an awkward fall, she made an otherwise trouble-free recovery, until unexpectedly dying from a ruptured aorta, 18 years later. She had a heterozygous glycine to glutamic acid 1021 substitution in exon 49 of *COL3A1* gene.

II. Case 2 (Pope et al. 1996) A 7-year-old proband was noticed by her dentist to have unusual bruising of her shins. Although nonaccidental injury was suspected, clinical examination showed acrogeric EDS IV. She had both an affected mother and brother, although her mother's two pregnancies had been uncomplicated. Her brother died unexpectedly in teenage of a spontaneously ruptured pulmonary vein, dissecting backward to produce mediastinal compression and a hemothorax. The mother died in middle age of a spontaneous aortic dissection. After trouble-free teenage and early adulthood, the proband spontaneously dissected and died from a lower abdominal aortic aneurysm, 3 months after delivery by Caesarian section of her daughter. The family had a heterozygous glycine to glutamic acid 1006 substitution in exon 48 of COL3A1.

2. *COL3A1* gene

III. Case 3 (Pope et al. 1996) A 30-year-old lady died suddenly following investigations for suspected cholecystitis. After conservative observation she was discharged, but shortly afterward collapsed and died. Postmortem examination showed a large perisplenic hematoma, with blood in the peritoneal cavity. Unknown to her surgeons, she had a past history of a ruptured liver, following the birth of her only (but normal) daughter. Childhood clinical pictures and her later clinical appearance were diagnostic of acrogeric EDS IV. She had a heterozygous glycine to arginine 1003 substitution in exon 48 of *COL3A1* gene.

IV. Case 4 (Fox et al. 1988; Pope et al. 1996) A 22-year-old bookseller developed sudden roaring and tinnitus in his left year with intermittent swelling of his left eyelid. Clinical examination showed a pulsatile left sided exophthalmos with a dilated left pupil (Horner's Syndrome). Bilateral carotid angiograms showed a left sided carotid cavernous-sinus fistula, which was successfully closed by intraarterial coil embolization. He subsequently made a full recovery, and also later survived a myocardial infarction caused by a coronary aneurysm, before eventually succumbing to the systemic complications of a spontaneous colonic rupture almost 20 years later. Whilst he showed subtle generalized cutaneous features of EDS IV, his parents and brother were clinically normal. He had a heterozygous glycine to glutamic acid 847 substitution, in exon 43 of his *COL3A1* gene.

V. Case 5 (Pope et al. 1996) A 37-year-old man presented to the vascular surgeons with a ruptured popliteal aneurysm. Angiography showed iliac and femoral dilatation with diffuse aneurysms. His mother had died of acute pancreatitis, but was not examined postmortem. Her wedding photographs showed acrogeric features similar to her son's. Both her granddaughters were also affected. The proband had a heterozygous glycine to glutamic acid 736 substitution in exon 40 of his *COL3A1* gene.

VI. Case 6 A young man had an aortic valve replacement at the age of 21 years for progressive aortic dilatation. Second and then a third aortic valve replacements were required because of recurrent leakage. Whilst Marfan syndrome was excluded clinically, the main clinical features were those of EDS III (BHS), segregating amongst other affected family members as an autosomal dominant trait, and in association with collagen type III deficiency.

VII. Case 7 (Pope et al. 1996; Tsai-Goodman et al. 2002) A 15-year-old female had presented with an unexplained cardiac murmur at the age of 6 years. Subsequently, this progressed and was diagnosed as progressive pulmonary stenosis, which was monitored by Doppler recordings. She had a grade 3 pulmonary systolic murmur and right ventricular hypertrophy. Given the potential hazards of open surgical correction, eventually, she required pulmonary valvuloplasty using a 90% balloon/annulus angioplasty balloon. Although technically uncomplicated, this was rapidly followed by early mild restenosis. Her clinical phenotype and family history was that of EDS IV with keloid scarring. Her mother had died of a ruptured intraabdominal aneurysm, having survived several cerebral aneurysms. Her mother's brother and at least one of his children also had the external EDS IV phenotype, with numerous widespread keloid scars and associated severe Dupuytren's contacture in her uncle's case.

VIII. Case 8 (Jazayeri et al. 2002) A 31-year-old woman developed a left perirenal hematoma with bilateral renal artery dissection. Transthoracic and esophageal cardiac echocardiography showed a pericardial effusion and localized hematoma of the ascending aorta. Situs solitus with dextrocardia was also evident on the chest X-ray and in the echocardiogram. Because of right ventricular compression, drainage of the hematoma was undertaken. Twenty-four hours later, this was complicated by perihepatic and rectus abdominis hematomas. A spontaneous pneumothorax followed and she subsequently died from a pseudomonas pulmonary infection 72 hours later. This paper emphasized the hazards of invasive interventional procedures of hollow organs and the potential hemorrhagic complications of EDS IV. The dextrocardia was a chance association.

IX. Cases 9 and 10 (Kitazono et al. 1989) This report describes two separate examples of premature myocardial infarction in vascular EDS IV. The first was in a 30-year-old female with previously unexplained hip dislocations and spontaneous idiopathic hematemeses. Coronary angiography was complicated by exceptionally fragile femoral and brachial arteries. Cardiac catheterization was consequently abandoned.

The second example was a 32-year-old male who, following a mild but unspecified sternal injury, developed central chest pain with ST elevation. ECG and enzyme levels confirmed an anterior myocardial infarction. Digital subtraction angiography also showed an old abdominal aortic aneurysm. Both patients had biochemical collagen type III deficiency, whilst the authors considered that only the first patient had definitive clinical signs of EDS IV.

X. Case 11 (Pope et al. 1996) This 28-year-old lady developed an acutely swollen right calf, following a prolonged car journey. A deep venous thrombosis was suspected and she was anticoagulated with warfarin and heparin. This greatly worsened her pain and swelling and surgical exploration of the posterior compartment of her lower limb showed a very large hematoma, complicated by Volkmann's ischemic contracture. She had the typical generalized facial features of vascular EDS and although remaining well for 15 years, eventually died of a spontaneous lower aortic rupture. She had a heterozygous deletion of exon 43 of the *COL3A1* gene.

XI. Case 12 (Pope et al. 1996) A 52-year-old woman survived multiple ruptured aneurysms, before eventually succumbing to a lethal descending aortic aneurysm. Her mother and brother had also suffered lethal aortic aneurysms. She was deleted for exon 37 of the *COL3A1* gene.

XII. Case 13 (Pope et al. 1996) A 37-year-old female doctor had numerous arterial complications, including renal, iliac, and cerebral aneurysms, before eventually suffering fatal aortic rupture. Her external features suggested, but were not diagnostic of EDS IV. She deleted exon 7 from one of her *COL3A1* genes, probably accounting for the relatively nonspecific clinical phenotype. Very probably, the deletion of the most N terminal and first of the COL3A1 helical exons, made this mutation relatively mild, both clinically, as regards its external clinical phenotype, but also biochemically, with respect to its disruption of collagen type III misassembly, but was nevertheless still eventually lethal.

3. Cardiovascular Manifestations in Vascular EDS (EDS IV)

Generally, there are three distinctive patterns of cardiovascular pathology in EDS IV (see Table 28–3), which include premature coronary artery disease, MVP, and pulmonary stenoses. Although

Table 28–3 Cardiological Manifestations in of EDS Based on Patients Published by Tiller et al. (1998)

Sex	Age	Skin	Joints	EDS Subtype	Echo	Family History
Female	4 years	Lacerations Widened scars	Beighton 9/9	EDS I	ARD ↑ ▶ 2SD ASD ↑ ▶ 2SD	N/A
Female	4 years	Velvety skin	Beighton 6/9	EDS III	MVP, MI incompetence LV + midsystolic click	N/A
Female	8 years	Velvety skin	Beighton 6/9 Bendy fingers	EDS III	MVP (no MI murmur) ARD ↑ ▶ 2SD Bicuspid aortic valve	N/A
Male	35 years	Doughy Skin Elastic arms Striae Fingers Astigmatic	Beighton 9/9 Bendy	EDS II	MVP myxomatous anterior leaflet ARD ↑ 42 mm ▶ 3SD	N/A
Female	51 years	Soft velvety skin High arched palate	Beighton 8/9 Unstable knees	MFS queried, EDS III,	MVP (asymptomatic) Dilated ascending aorta Aortic root 52 mm ▶ 4SD Aortic aneurysm Unexplained sudden death	3 affected children Unexplained sudden death

Note: Tabulation of previously published cardiovascular complications of EDS IV.

Table 28–4 Cardiological Manifestations in of EDS

EDS Subtype	Reference	Cardiac Abnormality
I	McKusick 1972	Aortic incompetence
II	Leier et al. 1980	
III	Tiller et al. 1998	
IV	Tiller et al. 1998	
Unspecified	Tiller et al. 1998 Wenstrup et al. 1989 Hata et al. 1988 Nicholls et al. 1994 Seny et al. 1988	Aortic incompetence
IV	Beighton 1970 Barabas 1967 Kuivaniemi et al. 1990 Kontusaari 1990	Dilatation and/or sudden rupture. Ascending aorta and occasionally descending aorta. Other medium-sized arteries.
I	Leier et al. 1980	Dilated sinus of valsalva
III	Tucker et al. 1963 Leier et al. 1980	

Note: Summary of various echocardiographical studies of EDS types I, II, III, and IV.

premature coronary aneurysms or dissection are by far the most spectacular published cardiovascular manifestation of EDS IV premature coronary artery disease is actually very rare (see also Table 28–4). Thus less than half a dozen cases of premature coronary artery disease in EDS IV have been published, whilst there have also been a few unpublished examples in our own series. Whilst quite clearly, the arterial fragility of EDS IV is caused by collagen type III deficiency, recent MRI evidence suggests that this causes both increased arterial atheroma, increased mural thickening, increased stiffness, and reduced vessel distensibility (Kerwin et al. 2008). These radiological observations do not tally with the limited postmortem data available, in which EDS IV coronary arteries and aortas are thinner than normal and generally free from atheromatous plaque (Pope et al. 1977; Pope 2008). The earliest recorded association of coronary arterial pathology in EDS IV are the two cases published by Kitazono and colleagues (Kitazono et al. 1989). The first was a 30-year-old female with central chest pain and ECG abnormalities and increased cardiac enzymes, in which attempted cardiac catheterisation via the femoral route caused severe femoral bleeding at the first attempt and brachial arterial rupture following a subsequent attempted recatherisation. The second was a 32-year-old male with an acute myocardial infarction who synthesized low type III collagen in fibroblast culture. Here, a superficial temporal artery biopsy showed scanty collagen fibrils. They rightly warned against coronary angiography because of underlying arterial fragility. Di Mario and colleagues (1988), described a 48-year-old man with transient T-wave inversion, in whom further angiography revealed multiple coronary aneurysms, MVP and regurgitation, fusiform dilatation of the ascending aorta with aortic valve regurgitation, and left anterior hemiblock. A very detailed clinical and biochemical study of a 16-year-old Australian adolescent with a spontaneous dissection of the left anterior descending coronary artery followed by an anterior myocardial infarction was published by Ades et al. (1995). His cardiac history included gradual central chest pain, whilst at rest and Q-waves in leads I, aVL, and V3–4, with a 10-fold elevation of creatine kinase levels. Coronary angiography demonstrated a dissection of the proximal left anterior descending coronary artery. He also demonstrated the typical external phenotype of EDS IV with prominent eyes, thin skin, keloid scar formation, and bilateral talipes equinovarus. He also had an affected brother, with a similar external phenotype, who had ruptured his spleen with a resulting hemoperitoneum and their mother who had similar external facial and cutaneous features had died prematurely, aged 28 years, of a spontaneous bowel perforation followed by a right vertebral aneurysmal rupture. The clinical diagnosis was confirmed biochemically, by convincing collagen type III deficiency. The authors. rightly caution against hasty angiography in EDS IV, quoting a 65% frequency of associated complications, such as hemorrhage, rupture, or dissection. Catanese et al. (1995) published in the same year another example of a spontaneous coronary artery dissection in a 33-year-old male also with a family history of EDS IV. Unlike the Australian teenager, this patient died from coronary arterial rupture. The authors emphasized the difficulties of investigating and treating coronary artery occlusion in EDS IV, as both thrombolysis and coronary angiography are potentially lethal.

Another example of coronary artery dissection is in the patient illustrated earlier as Case 4 (Fox et al. 1988; Pope et al. 1996), whose coronary artery dissection and resultant myocardial infarction almost incidentally followed his spectacular recovery from a carotid cavernous-sinus aneurysm. Sadly, his charmed-life recoveries failed to save him from the lethal septicemic complications of a colonic perforation.

Athanassiou and Turrentine (1996) described a patient with myocardial infarction and coronary artery dissection complicating premature labor at the 30th week of pregnancy. Labor was successfully suppressed with terbutaline, but was followed 72 hours later by a coronary artery dissection and spontaneous myocardial infarction. The authors concluded that betamimetic tocolytics should be avoided in premature labor-complicating EDS IV.

Pulmonary valvular or pulmonary arterial stenoses have also occasionally been reported in EDS IV (Tsai-Goodman et al. 2002; D'Aloia et al. 2008). One of author's patients (Tsai-Goodman et al. 2002) was operated upon at 15 years of age for progressive pulmonary valvular stenosis, first diagnosed at the age of 6 years. She was a member of a three-generational family with a clear history of arterial fragility, keloid scarring, and spontaneous arterial ruptures. Like other family members, she was procollagen type III deficient, showing in addition the typical facial vascular phenotype. There was both X-ray and ECG evidence of right ventricular hypertrophy, whilst echocardiography confirmed severe valvular pulmonary stenosis with pulmonary and tricuspid regurgitation. Pulmonary valvuloplasty successfully improved but did not abolish the stenosis, which remained stable over the next 18 months.

A second intriguing example of multiple pulmonary arterial stenoses was recently published by D'Aloia et al. (2008). In this instance two affected sisters, aged 20 and 21 years, with multiple pulmonary arterial stenoses were described. The paper, which detailed the clinical features of the younger proband, described early right ventricular hypertrophy with severe pulmonary arterial hypertension. Arteriography showed multiple bilateral pulmonary arterial stenoses and poststenotic lesions. In addition, there was elongation, kinking, and coiling of aortic, carotid, and vertebral vessels. Whilst the authors considered the family to show typical EDS features (type unspecified), they also mentioned but did not specify a mutation in the *GLUT10* gene that causes the arterial tortuosity syndrome. Their conclusion was that the sisters had two coincident disorders (i.e., EDS and arterial tortuosity). They also commented that pulmonary arterial stenoses affect other inherited connective tissue disorders, such as Noonan, Williams, Alagilles, and Apert Syndromes, as well as the arterial tortuosity syndrome (see also Chapter 9).

Lastly, MVP, whilst very common in some forms of EDS, is rare in EDS IV and only occasional examples have been published (Watanabe et al. 1988; Seve et al. 2005). This contradicts the earlier views of Jaffe et al. (1981), in which 6 of 8 patients in a family with collagen type III deficiency had detectable MVP by two-dimensional (2D) M-mode echocardiography. There was complete concordance, in this family, between collagen type III depletion and MVP. The patient with EDS IV and associated dextrocardia is both exceptional and coincidental, and there have been no other published examples (Jazayeri et al. 2002).

4. Management of Aortic Dissection in Vascular EDS

Aortic dissection is predominantly a specific problem of EDS IV, compared with other EDS subtypes. In EDS IV, catastrophic and frequently fatal arterial rupture or dissection is common, but very few examples are published of this problem in other EDS subtypes, despite the relatively common occurrence of aortic root dilatation in EDS types I, II, and III (Fox et al. 1988; Bade et al. 2007). Unlike the Marfan syndrome in which the value of aortic root diameter monitoring and prophylaxis with either β-blockade or TGF-β inhibitors in retarding aortic dilatation is well proven, EDS IV produces sudden arterial failure without prior evidence of gradual deterioration. Those few studies of arterial morphology in EDS IV (Kerwin et al. 2008), whilst showing stiffened, poorly distensible arteries show only scanty evidence of aortic root dilatation, in cross-sectional studies. Whether prospective image analysis on a rolling basis would retard or delay vascular rupture of small, medium, or large arterial lesions is currently unknown. It therefore follows that the management of the arterial complications of EDS IV are immediate and not in any way prospective.

5. Small- or Medium-Sized Aneurysms

There are several examples of carotid cavernous sinus aneurysms, causing acute exophthalmos and III cranial nerve paresis with Horner's syndrome (Fox et al. 1988; Pope et al. 1996; Pope 2008); all of them were successfully managed by coil embolization. The same is not true of smaller aneurysms at other sites, which have to be managed by conservative control of bleeding, resection of aneurysms within hematomas, and very careful, preferably nonangiographic arteriography, to localize the source. Vascular surgery is potentially hazardous, as hemostasis can be very difficult to establish, given the friability of the aneurysmal or dissected vessels. For the similar reasons, varicose vein surgery should be avoided whenever possible.

6. Friability of Large Arteries

There are plenty of published examples of large arterial rupture or dissection in EDS IV (Barabas 1967; Beighton 1968; Beighton 1993; McKusick 1972; Pope et al. 1996; Pepin et al. 2000) many of which are rapidly fatal and always life threatening. Unlike the Marfan syndrome, in which the aortic dilatation is slow and progressive and also retarded by β-blockade, the aneurysms of EDS IV are unpredictable and probably unpreventable. Conservative management is a less frequent option than with smaller arterial disease, but there are frequent published examples of conventional grafting as well as successful endovascular repair (Serry et al. 1988; Ascione et al. 2000; Bade et al. 2007; Tonnessen et al. 2007). Sometimes associated bleeding could only be controlled with factor VIIA infusions (Faber et al. 2007). Type A dissections of the proximal aorta in common with those of the Marfan syndrome, bicuspid aortic valve, coarctation of the aorta, and other pathological processes, such as vasculitis, trauma, or arteriography, are surgical emergencies with very high mortality (Nienaber and Eagle 2003).

7. Cardiovascular Complications of EDS Types I, II, and III

EDS types I, II, and III are very much more benign clinical variants than type IV EDS, nevertheless cardiac complications can occur (see Tables 28-4 and 28-5). In contrast to EDS IV, they are late and only slowly progressive. Two very important recent cross-sectional studies have documented the frequency of cardiac complications in classical EDS I/II and BHS/EDS III (Dolan et al. 1997; Wenstrup et al. 2002). Other very important papers addressing this issue include those of McDonnell et al. (2006) and Tiller et al. (1998). These papers were important in systematically documenting the frequency of mitral and aortic disease in certain EDS variants, but had several contradictory findings.

The Dolan paper studied 36 EDS patients who fulfilled the Berlin Nosology diagnostic criteria. Of these 30 were classified as EDS I/II or EDS III/ BHS, whilst three had EDS IV. There was a female to male ratio of 4.5/1, suggesting bias of ascertainment in favor of females. They used a standard 2D ECHO via a parasternal approach and measured aortic profiles at four sites, including the annulus, sinotubular arch, and abdomen. The frequency of MVP was only 6.1% rather than 78%, which had been previously quoted. Similarly 12.1% of patients had abnormal ECHOs, compared with the control frequency of 6.05%. The abnormal ECHOs included 1 ASD, 1 bicuspid prolapse, and 2 true MVP. A further five patients had possible MVP, either by auscultation or M-mode echocardiography. Other observations included MVP with mitral incompetence in EDS/III, tricuspid incompetence in EDS III, MVP in EDS III, and aortic stenosis with poststenotic aortic aneurysmal dilatation. They also recorded atypical chest pain (48%), palpitations (39%), and unexplained dyspnea (30%). There were two MVP patients with atypical chest pain. In contrast, to the later studies of Wenstrup et al. (2002) and McDonnell et al. (2006) and earlier studies by Leier (1980), Dolan et al. found no evidence of aortic root dilatation in any of their 33 subjects. They concluded that cardiac complications in EDS were both rare and mostly benign.

The Wenstrup paper, written 5 years later, and studying aortic root dilatation by 2D echocardiography in a similar EDS spectrum showed very contrasting changes. Thus, 20/71 (28%) had aortic root dilatation by 2D echocardiography, of which 14/42 (33.33%) had classical EDS and 6/29 (20.7%) had EDS III/BHS. The female to male ratio of 1.6/1 in this study was much lower than in that by Dolan et al. In contrast to Dolan et al. they concluded that aortic root dilatation (ARD) is unusually common in EDS types I, II, and III and is much commoner than MVP. It is, however, very substantially less common and much more slowly progressive than in the Marfan syndrome where the frequency of ARD is 80%.

The later 2006 study of McDonnell et al. largely confirmed the original Wenstrup observations. It studied 38 patients with a female to male ratio of 4.4/1, so much resembling the Dolan study (Dolan et al. 1997). In this study there were almost equal numbers of EDS I/II and EDS III patients. Significant sinus of valsalva, aortic root, or proximal aortic dilatation were observed in 13%, which was only half the frequency of the earlier Wenstrup study (Wenstrup et al. 2002), but much higher than Dolan's observations. Other findings were MVP 2.6%, mild mitral with aortic regurgitation (21%), increased pulmonary pressure 7.8%, and poor left ventricular relaxation in 7.8%. There was also impaired left ventricular relaxation in 13%. They concluded that mild aortic root dilatation is common in EDS types I, II, and III. The explanation

Table 28–5 Clinical Examples of EDS with Cardiac Manifestations

Reference	Clinical	Cardiac	Genetics	Chemistry	Comments
Ades et al. 1995	Classical EDS IV Keloids, acrogeria, bilateral talipes Male aged 16 years	LAD coronary artery dissection, myocardial infraction	Autosomal dominant, brother died of ruptured spleen, mother died of vertebral aneurysm	Classical dominant-negative collagen type III deficiency	Angiography hazardous
Athanassiou and Turrentine 1996	EDS IV	Coronary artery dissection 30th week of pregnancy	N/A	N/A	Avoid β mimetic tocolytlcs to delay delivery
D'Aloia et al. 2008	EDS type unspecified	Multiple pulmonary arterial stenoses, pulmonary hypertension RV +	Autosomal dominant, with affected sister	Possible GLUT 10 mutation Collagen type III status unknown	Kinking of carotid, vertebral, and aortic arteries
Pope case 4, this Article and Pope et al. 1996	Classical acrogeric EDS IV M22	Presented with carotid/ cavernous sinus aneurysm Later, myocardial infarction from coronary dissection	Mother mosaic, but clinically normal	Collagen type III deficient, dominant-negative pattern Gly-Glu847 COL3A1	Eventually died of perforated colon, with septicemia
Pope case 6, this Article and Pope et al. 1996	EDS III/BHS, M21	Progressive aortic dilatation, 3 successive aortic valves replaced	Autosomal dominant	Collagen type III deficient	
Pope 2008 Unpublished	EDS III/BHS, F28	Acute coronary artery dissection, myocardial infarction	Sporadic Collagen type III	Declined testing, for insurance reasons	
Jaffe et al. 1981	Classical EDS IV	6/8 affected, all with MVP	Autosomal Dominant	Collagen type III	Exception frequency of MVP
Watanabe et al. 1988	EDS IV	MVP	N/A	N/A	
Seve et al. 2005	EDS IV	Acute papillary Muscle rupture with acute mitral incompetence	N/A	N/A	Very rare cardiac complication
Tsai-Goodman et al. 2002	Classical acrogeric EDS IV F15	Very early pulmonary stenosis, requiring mechanical endovascular correction	Clear autosomal dominant, with keloids, Dupuytren's contractures, and lethal arterial	Collagen type III deficient, dominant-negative pattern fragility	Early onset pulmonary pathology exceptional
Jazayeri et al. 2002	Classical EDS IV F 30	Incidental dextrocardia	N/A	N/A	Draining of pericardial effusion followed by lethal bilateral renal artery dissection
Kitazono T et al. 1989	(i) Possible EDS IV, F 30	Central chest pain, cardiac infarction, bled from ruptured brachial artery, (arteriography) acute myocardial infarction	N/A	N/A	Phenotype ill defined Superficial temporal artery biopsy histologically collagen depleted
	(ii) EDS III/IV, M 32		N/A femoral	Collagen type IIII deficient	

Note: Tabulation of the five cases of cardiac complications published by Tiller et al. (1998).

of the disparity between the two studies is not obvious, but it may be due to bias of ascertainment of the two cohorts.

The Tiller paper (Tiller et al. 1998) described five cases of EDS types I, II, and III in which cardiovascular complications included MVP, ruptured medium-sized aneurysms, varicose veins, capillary fragility, dilatation or rupture of the sinus of valsalva and ruptured aorta. The case histories included a 4-year-old EDS I girl with aortic root dilatation, another 4-year-old female with congestive heart failure secondary to MVP, an 8-year-old EDS III female with MVP, mitral incompetence, and aortic root dilatation, a 35-year-old female with EDS II and MVP, and a 51-year-old female with MVP, aortic dilatation, and an aortic murmur.

These are tabulated below and include patients with EDS I, II, III, and VI with aortic incompetence, dilatation of the ascending aorta or aortic arch (McKusick 1972; Leier et al. 1980; Haita et al. 1988; Wenstrup et al. 1989; Nicholls et al. 1994; Tiller et al. 1998), dilatation or rupture of the ascending aorta in EDS IV (Barabas 1967; Beighton 1970; Serry et al. 1988; Kuivaniemi et al. 1990; Kontusaari et al. 1990), and dilatation of the sinus of valsalva in EDS types I and III (Tucker 1963; Leier et al. 1980). Tiller also thoroughly reviewed the existing literature (Tucker et al. 1963; Leier et al. 1980; Seny et al. 1988; Wenstrup et al. 1989; Nicholls et al. 1994; Tiller et al. 1998) of several previously published cardiac complications and drew attention to the association of aortic dilatation with

Table 28–6 Previously Published Cardiac Complications of EDS (Beighton 1970)

Reference	Male/Female	Cardiac Features	Comments
Freeman 1950	Female 13 years	Atrial septal defect	
Sestak 1962	Female 43 years	Atrial septal defect, RBBB Tricuspid incompetance	
Fantl et al. 1961	Female 11 years	Partial AV canal, cleft mitral and tricuspid leaflets	
Wallach and Burkhart 1950	Female 26 years	Tetralogy of Fallot, RBBB	
Rubinstein and Cohen 1964	Female 2 years	Congenital heart disease unspecified	Mother died of internal carotid aneurysm, EDS IV likely
Bopp et al. 1965	Male 10 years	Bifid pulmonary artery, aortic arch abnormality	
Robitaille et al. 1964	Male 28 years	Abnormal aortic arch	Sudden death, unspecified
McKusick 1966	Male 40 years Female 25 years	Aortic stenosis/mitral incompetence Systolic/diastolic murmurs	Dilated right heart
McFarland and Fuller 1964	Male 17 years	Bicuspid tricuspid valve	Fatal subclavian rupture, ED IV?
Madison et al. 1963	Male 17 years	Mitral/tricuspid incompetence	Died CCF
Tucker et al. 1963	Female 42 years	Aneurysm sinus of Valsalva/AI	Probably EDS I/II or III
Margarot et al. 1933	Male 9 years	Pulmonary hypertension Systolic murmurs	Thoracic deformity (pectus?)

Note: Summary tabulation of the various previously published cardiac complications by EDS subtype, referred to by Tiller et al. (1998).

classical EDS. Furthermore, Tiller clearly distinguished between the extreme fragility of the cardiovascular tree in EDS type IV, compared with the relatively sturdy vessels of EDS types I, II, and III (Table 28–6; see also Tables 28–4 and 28–5). Rupture of both spinal segmental arteries, iliac artery and vein were described as complications of spinal repair in EDS IV by Akpinar et al. 2003.

Later, the Wenstrup haploinsufficient *col5a1* mouse model successfully inactivated one of the two mouse *col5a1* genes, to produce a dosage model (Wenstrup et al. 2006). Correlation of the dosage of collagen V α chains with consequent disruption of type I and III collagen fibrillogenesis could then be studied in both heterozygotes and homozygotes (Roulet et al. 2007). In turn this could be correlated with clinical and pathological effects upon skin, ligaments, and the vasculature. Collagen biochemistry could then be correlated with fibrillogenesis and biophysical changes in the animals and their tissue composition. There were objectively demonstrable reductions of aortic stiffness, tensile strength that correlated with decreased cutaneous extensibility. The authors were also able to rationalize how the 50% reduction in mouse collagen type I protein visibly misregulated type I and III collagen fibril accretion and growth. The aberrant misassembly disrupts normal linear and lateral fibril growth producing abnormal fibrils with dysfunctional fibril nucleation and growth. All of the subsequent cardiac and cutaneous pathology directly arises from this disturbance.

A largely unexpected observation was that certain *COL1A2* mutations with a general clinical phenotype resembling EDS III also produced significant aortic and mitral valve pathology rather than fragile, easily fractured bones, and severe OI, which are very well recognized effects of such genetic errors. Thus in 2004, Schwarze et al. described three unrelated patients with the combination of autosomal recessively inherited EDS, cutaneous and joint hypermobility, and *COL1A2* nonsense-mediated mRNA decay. Patient 1 had recurrent childhood shoulder dislocations, small joint hypermobility, pectus deformities, scarring of the knees, shins, and chin, and inguinal hernias. He also had anterior MVP with mitral regurgitation, left ventricular hypertrophy, and an aortic root diameter at the upper limits of normal. He died after mitral and aortic valve replacements dehisced. Patient 2 had EDS II, with generally soft, doughy skin and bruisability. She survived mitral valve replacement uneventfully. Patient 3 had neonatal bilateral inguinal hernias, generalized joint laxity, and soft extensible skin. He had an atrial septal defect, mitral and aortic regurgitation. His brother with similar clinical features had required early aortic valve replacement. All affected individuals were homozygous or doubly heterozygous null COL1A2 exon skips. In 2006, Malfait et al. described a 6-year-old boy with otherwise unremarkable BHS/EDS, who had MVP, as well as complete collagen α2(I) deficiency. Both the Schwarze and Malfait papers describe a mild connective tissue phenotyope with unexpected cardiac complications. More usually, COL1A2 homozygous deletions cause severe progressive OI (Nicholls et al. 1979; Pihlajaneimi et al. 1984). However COL1A2 deficient mice have defective thoracic aortae (Pfeiffer et al. 2005).

There have been rare examples of similar aortic valvular incompetence and proximal aortic dilatation in occasional autosomal dominant OI families (see case history below). Schwarze et al. (2004) also considered an earlier Japanese patient to have been similarly affected (Sasaki et al. 1987) and have also suggested that our pair of affected sisters with homozygous COL1A2 deficiency are at risk of cardiac mitral and aortic valve disease. So far, the children are healthy and have normal hearts (Nicholls et al. 2001). Vascular fragility is rare in EDS VI, but can present with aortic or carotid territory rupture (McKuisick 1972), whilst cardiac complications are even rare. The patient described by Takano et al. (2005), in which severe mitral incompetence with left ventricular hypertrophy required mitral valve replacement, had deficient biochemical data. Thus, neither hydroxylysine amino acid analysis nor lysyl hydroxylase levels had been measured. This paper contained useful information on the excellent results of mitral valve replacement in Marfan syndrome (Fuzeloler et al. 1998) and the early papers on replacement in other EDS subtypes (Edmondson et al. 1979; Kitagawa et al 1984; Avlonitis and Large 1999).

In contrast, no cardiac complications have so far been documented in EDS types VIB, VIIA, B, C, or VIII. At least some of these subtypes overlap with OI, both clinically and also by the general type of underlying DNA mutations. Thus certain EDS VIB, VIIA and B phenotypes all have demonstrable abnormalities of the *COL1A1* and/or the *COL1A2* gene, with absent α2(I) chains (Pope and Burroughs 1997; Nicholls et al. 2001; Dalgliesh 2007).

8. Bicuspid Aortic Valves

Whilst there are occasional examples of bicuspid valves in EDS (Cecconi et al. 2006) bicuspid aortic valve (BAV) is a distinctive connective syndrome with specific mortality risks. Dilatation of the proximal thoracic aorta is frequently complicated by aortic dilatation, aneurysmal dilatation, or dissection. DellaCorte and colleagues (Dellacorte et al. 2007) studied 280 patients with isolated bicuspid aortic valve, in which the ratio of aortic root to ascending aorta often exceeded one to one. Aortic dilatation of the root or ascending aorta affected 83.7%. A small root occurred in only 5.7%, whilst the 50–60-year age group had the most frequent dilatation with the severest problems in the over 60 year-old males. Aortic stenosis and/or hypertension increase the severity of dilatation. Pathological changes are concentrated in the midascending aorta, in which there is ectasia and elastic degeneration. Aortic root dilatation in younger men most probably has a different pathogenesis. The population frequency of BAV was recently studied by Guntheroth et al. (2008). They kept a registry of affected individuals, with a mean age of 63 years. The population frequency was 3%, of which 72% were hypertensive and the late mortality rate was 10%. Ortiz et al. (2006) noted a high frequency of aortic stenosis, severe valvular dysfunction, and the risks of bacterial endocarditis. The biophysics of BAV has been studied in detail by Schaefer and colleagues (2008). They deduced parameters such as aortic stiffness and distensibility correlated with systolic blood pressure and mean aortic pressures. In general, they observed decreased distensibility, raised aortic pressures, and increased stiffness of the affected valve and proximate aortic wall. Schaefer et al. (2008) studied 191 patients and could distinguish two patterns: type I, in which affected males had normal aortic morphology, but large aortic sinuses, and type II, in which there is ascending aortic dilatation and myxomatous mitral valve disease. In a second study (2007), they identified two echocardiographic phenotypes in both the anteroposterior and right to left dimensions. The former showed larger stiffer sinuses of valsalva and smaller aortic root diameters.

The mechanism of the aortic changes is obscure but using 2D electrophoresis, mass spectometry, and phosphostaining, Matt and colleagues (2007) showed decrease in the endoplasmic reticulum chaperone protein Hsp 27. Three other phosphoproteins were also altered, including RhoGDP, Calponin S, and Myosin regulatory protein 2.

The clinical and molecular overlaps between BAV and EDS are presently unclear, but are certainly worthy of more detailed systematic analysis, using clinical protocols similar to those of the Marfan (Ghent) and EDS (Villefranche) criteria. Similarly genome-wide searches will also be required to examine whether common genetic mechanisms are shared between these various IDCT disorders and BAV.

9. Cardiovascular Complications in Other Inherited Disorders of Connective Tissue

The cardiovascular complications of EDS certainly overlap with other inherited defects of connective tissue, such as the Marfan syndrome, Loeys-Dietz syndrome, arterial tortuosity syndrome, cutis laxa, Williams syndrome, and other inherited defects of elastin, such as supravalvar aortic stenosis, and pseudoxanthoma elasticum, as well as Stickler syndrome and osteogenesis imperfecta, all of which can be differentiated by clinical, histopathological, or molecular DNA analyses. Nevertheless, all of them overlap by virtue of defects in connective tissue components shared among the various EDS subsets.

References

Ades LC, Waltham RD, Chiodo AA, et al. Myocardial infarction resulting from coronary artery dissection in an adolescent with Ehlers Danlos Syndrome type IV due to a collagen type III mutation. *Br Heart J.* 1995;74(2):112–116.

Akpinar S, Gogus A, Talu U, et al. Surgical Management of Spinal deformity in EDS VI. *Eur Spine J.* 2003;12(2):135–140.

Alvarez C, Gonzalez-Gay MA, Fernandez CB, et al. Ehlers Danlos syndrome type II. A family study. *Annals Med Interna.* 1992;9(6):285–286.

Ascione R, Gomes WJ, Bates M, et al. Emergency repair of type A aortic aneurysm in type IV Ehlers Danlos Syndrome. *Cardiovasc Surg.* 2000;8(1):75–78.

Athanassiou AM, Turrentine MA. Myocardial infarction and coronary artery dissection during pregnancy, associated with Ehlers-Danlos Syndrome. *Am J Perinatol.* 1996;13(3):181–183.

Avlonitis VS, Large SR. Ehlers Danlos Syndrome: surgical management of mitral regurgitation and atrial fibrillation. *J Heart Valve Dis.* 1999;8(4):463–465.

Bade MA, Queral LA, Mukherjee D, et al. Endovascular abdominal aortic aneurysm repair in a patient with Ehlers Danlos Syndrome. *J Vasc Surg.* 2007;46(2):360–362.

Barabas AP. Heterogeneity of the Ehlers-Danlos syndrome: description of three clinical types and a hypothesis to explain the basic defect(s). *Br Med J.* 1967a;2(5552):612–615.

Barabas AP. Vascular complications in the Ehlers Danlos Syndrome, with special reference to the "arterial type or Sack's Syndrome. *J Cardiovasc Surg.* 1967b;13(2):160–167.

Beighton P. Lethal complications of the Ehlers-Danlos syndrome. *Br Med J.* 1968a;3(5619):656–659.

Beighton P. X-linked recessive inheritance in the Ehlers Danlos syndrome. *Br Med J.* 1968b;3(5615):09–11.

Beighton P. *The Ehlers Danlos Syndrome.* Chapter VI Cardiovascular Complications. William Heinemann Medical Books Limited; 1970.

Beighton P. *McKusick's Heritable Disorders of Connective Tissue.* 5th ed. St Louis, MO: Mosby; 1993. London.

Beighton P, De Paepe A, Danks D, et al. International nosology of heritable disorders of connective tissue. *Am J Med Genet.* 1988;29(3):581–594.

Beighton P, De Paepe A, Steinmann B, et al. Ehlers-Danlos syndromes: revised nosology, Villefranche, 1997. Ehlers-Danlos National Foundation (USA) and Ehlers Danlos Support Group UK. *Am J Med Genet.* 1998;77(1):31–37.

Bopp P, Hatam K, Bussat P, et al. Cardiovascular aspects of the Ehlers Danlos syndrome. Report of a case with pulmonary artery bifidity and aortic arch anomaly. *Circulation.* 1965;32(4):602–607.

Catanese V, Venot P, Lemesle F, et al. Myocardial infarction, by spontaneous dissection of coronary arteries in a subject with type IV Ehlers Danlos Syndrome. *Presse Med.* 1995;24(29):1345–1347.

Cecconi M, Nistri S, Quarti A, et al. Aortic dilatation in patients with bicuspid aortic valve. *J Cardiovasc Med (Hagerstown).* 2006;7(1):11–20.

Colige A, Nuytinck L, Hausser I, et al. Novel types of mutation responsible for the dermatosparactic type of Ehlers Danlos syndrome (type VIIC) and common polymorphisms in the ADAMSTS2 gene. *J Invest Dermatol.* 2004;123(4):656–663.

D'Aloia A, Vizzardi E, Zanini G, et al. Young woman affected by a rare form of Familial Connective Tissue Disorder associated with multiple arterial pulmonary stenosis and severe pulmonary hypertension. *Circ J.* 2008;72(1):164–167.

Dalgliesh R. A database of human type I and type III collagen mutations: http://www.le.ac/ge/collagen/2007.

Danlos M. Un cas de cutis laxa avec tumeures par contusion chronique des coudes et des genoux (xanthome juvenile pseudo-diabetique. *Bulletin Societie Medicine de Dermatologie et Syphiligraphie.* 1908;19:70–72.

Debnath UK, Sharma H, Roberts D, et al. Coeliac axis thrombosis after surgical correction of spinal deformity in type VI Ehlers Danlos Syndrome. *Spine.* 2007;32(18):E528–E531.

Dellacorte A, Baricone C, Quanto C, et al. Predictions of ascending aortic dilatation with bicuspid aortic valve:a wide spectrum of disease expression. *Eur J Cardiovasc Surg.* 2007;31(3):397–404.

Dermal Connective Tissue: Section In: Warner R, Williams PL, ed. *Grays Anatomy*, 35th ed. Longman; 1973:32–41.

Di Mario C, Zanchetta M, Maiolino P. Coronary aneurysms in a case of Ehlers Danlos Syndrome. *Jpn Heart J.* 1988;29(4):491–496.

Dolan AL, Mishra MB, Chambers JB, et al. Clinical and echocardiographic survey of the Ehlers Danlos Syndrome. *Br J Rheumatol.* 1997;36(4);459–462.

Edmondson P, Nellen M, Ross DN. Aortic valve replacement in a case of Ehlers Danlos Syndrome. *Br Heart J.* 1979;42(1):103–105.

Ehlers E. Cutis Laxa neigung zu hamorrhagien in der haut, lockerung mehrerer artikulationem. *Dermatologische Zeitschrifte.* 1901;14:76.

Faber P, Craig WL, Duncan JL, et al. The successful use of recombinant Factor VIIa in a patient with vascular-type Ehlers Danlos Syndrome. *Acta Anaesthesiol Scand.* 2007;51(9):1277–1279.

Fantl P, Morris KN, Sawers RJ. Repair of a cardiac defect in a patient with Ehlers Danlos Syndrome and deficiency of Hageman factor. *Br Med J.* 1961;1(5234):1202–1204.

Fernandez-Garcia R, Ramos-Zabala A, Perez-Mencia T, et al. Subarachnoid anesthesia for cesarean section in a patient with Ehlers-Danlos Syndrome type II. *Rev Esp Anestesiol Reanim.* 2004;51(5):268–271.

Fox R, Pope FM, Narcisi P, et al. Spontaneous carotid cavernous fistula in the Ehlers Danlos Syndrome. *J Neurol Neurosurg Psychiatry.* 1988;51(7):984–986.

Freeman JT. Ehlers Danlos syndrome. *Am J Dis Child.* 1950;79(6): 1049–1056.

Fuzellier JF, Chauvaud SM, Fornes P, et al. Surgical management of mitral regurgitation associated with Marfan's syndrome. *Ann Thorac Surg.* 1998;66(1):68–72.

Giunta C, Nuytinck L, Raghanuth M, et al. Homozygous gly530Ser substitution in COL5A1 causes mild classical Ehlers-Danlos syndrome. *Am J Med Gen*et. 2002;109(4):284–290.

Guntheroth WG. A critical review of the American College of Cardiology/American Heart Association practice guidelines on bicuspid aortic valve with dilated ascending aorta. *Am J Cardiol.* 2008;102(1):107–110.

Hata R, Kurata S, Shinkai A. Existence of malfunctioning pro alpha2(I) collagen genes, in a patient with proalpha2(I) chain defective variant of Ehlers Danlos Syndrome. *Eur J Biochem.* 1988;174:231–237.

Hyland J, Ala-Kokko L, Royce P, et al. A homozygous stop codon in the lysyl hydroxylase gene in two siblings with Ehlers-Danlos syndrome type VI. *Nat Genet.* 1992;2(3):228–231.

Jaffe AS, Geltman EM, Rodney GE, et al. Mitral valve prolapse: a consistent manifestation of type IV Ehlers Danlos Syndrome. The pathogenetic role of the abnormal production of type III collagen. *Circulation.* 1981;64(1):121–125.

Jazayeri S, Gomez MC, Tatou E, et al. Fatal cardiovascular complications in a patient with Ehlers Danlos syndrome type IV and dextrocardia. *Cardiovasc Surg.* 2002;10(6):640–643.

Johnson SAF, Falls HF. Ehlers-Danlos syndrome: a clinical and genetic study. *Arch Derm Syphilol.* 1949;60(1):82–105.

Kerwin W, Pepin M, Mitsumori L, et al. MRI of great vessel morphology and function in Ehlers Danlos Syndrome type IV. *Int J Cardiovasc Imaging.* 2008;24(5):519–528.

Kielty CM, Grant ME. The collagen family: structure, assembly and organisation of extracellular matrix: Chapter 2. In: Royce PM, Steinmann B, ed. *Connective Tissue and Its Heritable Disorders*, 2nd ed. 2002: 159–221. Wiley-Liss, Newyork.

Kitagawa M, Nagagawa Y, Shibairi M, et al. Mitral valve replacement in a case of Ehlers-Danlos syndrome. *Nippon Kyoba Geka Gakkai Zasshi.* 1984;32(7):1073–**1077.**

Kitazono T, Imaizumi T, Imavama S, et al. Two cases of myocardial infarction in type IV Ehlers Danlos Syndrome. *Chest.* 1989;95(6):1274–1277.

Kontusaari S, Tromp G, Kuivaniemi H, et al. Inheritance of the RNA splicing mutation G+IVS 20, in the type III procollagen gene COL3A1 in a family having aortic aneurysms and easy bruisability: phenotypical overlap between familial arterial aneurysms and Ehlers–Danlos Syndrome type IV. *Am J Hum* Genet. 1990;47(1):112–120.

Krane SM, Pinnell SR, Erbe RW. Lysyl procollagen hydroxylase deficiency in fibroblasts from siblings with hydroxylysine deficient collagen. *Proc Natl Acad Sci USA.* 1972;69(10):2899–2903.

Kuivaniemi H, Kontusaari S, Tromp G, et al. Identical G+1 to A mutations in three different introns of the type III procollagen gene (COL3A1) produce different patterns of RNA splicing in three variants of Ehlers Danlos Syndrome type IV. An explanation for exon skipping some mutations and not others. *J Biol Chem.* 1990;265(20):12067–12074.

Kurata A, Oka H, Ohmomo T, et al. Successful stent placement for cervical artery dissection associated with Ehlers Danlos Syndrome. Case report and review of the literature. *J Neurosurg.* 2003;99(6):1077–1081.

Leier CV, Call TD, Fulkerson PK, et al. The spectrum of cardiac defects in Ehlers-Danlos Syndrome types I and III. *Ann Intern Med.* 1980;92(2 Pt1):171–178.

Lichtenstein JR, Martin GR, Kohn LD, et al. Defect in the conversion of procollagen to collagen in a form of Ehlers-Danlos syndrome. *Science.* 1973;182(109):292–300.

Madison WM (Jr), Bradley EJ, Castillo EJ. Ehlers Danlos Syndrome with cardiac involvement. *Am J Cardiol.* 1963;11:689.

Malfait F, Symoens S, Coucke P, et al. Total absence of the alpha2(I) chain of collagen type I causes a rare form of Ehlers Danlos Syndrome with hypermobility and propensity to cardiac valvular problems. *J Med Gen*et. 2006;43(7):e36.

Malfait F, Symoens S, De Backer J, et al. Three arginine to cysteine substitutions in the pro-alpha1-collagen chain cause Ehlers Danlos syndrome with a propensity to arterial rupture in early adulthood. *Hum Mutat.* 2007;28(4):387–395.

Margarot J, Deveze P, De Carrera C. Hyperlaxite cutanee et articulaire (syndrome de danlos) existant chez trois membres d'une meme famille. *Bulletin Societe Francaise Dematologie et Syphiligraphie.* 1933;40:277.

Matt P, Carrel T, Huso DL, et al. Proteomic alterations in heat shock protein 27 and identification of phosphoproteins in ascending aortic aneurysm associated with bicuspid and tricuspid aortic valve. *J Mol Cell Cardiol.* 2007; 43(6):792–801.

McDonnell NB, Gorman BL, Mandel KW, et al. Echocardiographic findings in classical and hypermobile Ehlers-Danlos syndromes. *Am J Med Gen*et. 2006;140(2):129–136.

McFarland W, Fuller DE. Mortality in Ehlers Danlos Syndrome due to spontaneous rupture of large arteries. *N Eng J Med.* 1964;271:1309–1310.

McKusick VA. Ehlers Danlos Syndrome in Heritable Disorders of Connective Tissue 3rd ed. St Louis, MO: Mosby; 1966:179–229.

McKusick VA. *Ehlers Danlos Syndrome in Heritable Disorders of Connective Tissue* 4th ed. St Louis, MO: Mosby; 1972:292–371.

Mories A. Ehlers Danlos Syndrome with report of a fatal case. *Scott Med J.* 1960;5:269–272.

Narcisi P, Richards AC, Ferguson SD, et al. A family with Ehlers-Danlos syndrome type III/articular hypermobility syndrome has a glycine 637 to serine substitution in type III collagen. *Hum Molec Gen.* 1994;3(9):1617–1620.

Nicholls AC, McCarron S, Narcisi P, et al. Molecular abnormalities of collagen in two patients with Ehlers Danlos Syndrome. *Am J Hum Gen.* 1994;5523b.

Nicholls AC, Pope FM, Schloon HG. Biochemical heterogeneity of osteogenesis imperfecta: new variant. *Lancet.* 1979;(I):(8127):1193.

Nicholls AC, Valler D, Wallis S, et al. Homozygosity for a splice site mutation of the COL1A2 gene yields a non-functional pro(alpha)2(I) chain and an EDS/OI clinical phenotype. *J Med Gen.* 2001;38(2):132–136.

Nienaber CA, Eagle KA. Aortic dissection: new frontiers in diagnosis and management. Part II: therapeutic management and follow-up. *Circulation.* 2003;108(6):772–778.

Okamura T, Yamamato M, Ohta K, et al. A case of ruptured cerebral aneurysm associated with fenestrated vertebral artery in osteogenesis imperfecta. *No Shinkei Geka.* 1995;23(5):451–455.

Ortiz JY, Shin DD, Rajamannan NM. Approach to the patient with bicuspid aortic valve and ascending aorta aneurysm. *Curr Trans Options Cardiovasc Med.* 2006;8(6):461–467.

Peeters AC, Kucharekova M, Timmermans J, et al. A clinical and cardiovascular survey of Ehlers Danlos syndrome patients with complete deficiency of tenascin-X. *Neth J Med.* 2004 ;62(5):160–162.

Pepin M, Schwarze U, Superti-Furga A, et al. Clinical and genetic features of Ehlers-Danlos type IV, the vascular type. *N Eng J Med.* 2000;342(10):673–680.

Pfeiffer BJ, Franklin CL, Hsieh FH, et al. Alpha2(I) collagen deficient *oim* mice have altered biomechanical integrity, collagen content and collagen cross linking of their thoracic aorta. *Matrix Biol.* 2005;24(7):451–458.

Pihlajaneimi T, Dickson LA, Pope FM, et al. Osteogenesis imperfecta; Cloning of a proalpha2(I) collagen gene with a frameshift mutation. *J Biol Chem.* 1984;259(21):12941–12944.

Pinnell SR, Krane SM, Kenzora J, et al. A heritable disorder of collagen, with hydroxylysine deficient collagen disease. *N Eng J Med.* 1972;286(19):1013–1020.

Pope FM. Unpublished data. 2008. Personal communication.

Pope FM, Burroughs NP. Ehlers-Danlos syndrome has varied molecular mechanisms. *J Med Gen.* 1997;34(5):400–410.

Pope FM, Martin GR, Lichtenstein JR, et al. Patients with Ehlers-Danlos syndrome type IV lack type III collagen. *Proc Natl Acad Sci USA.* 1975;72(4):1314–1316.

Pope FM, Martin GA, McKusick VA. Inheritance of Ehlers-Danlos type IV Syndrome. *J Med Gene*t. 1977;14(13):200–204.

Pope FM, Narcisi P, Nicholls AC, et al. COL3A1 mutations cause variable clinical phenotypes including acrogeria and vascular rupture. *Br J Dermatol.* 1996;135(2):163–181.

Pope FM, Robins SR. Unpublished data upon 52 UK EDS VI patients. 2007.

Rahman N, Dunstan T, Teare MD, et al. Ehlers-Danlos syndrome with severe early-onset periodontal disease (EDS-VIII), is a distinct, heterogeneous disorder with one predisposition gene at chromosome 12p13. *Am J Hum Gene*t. 2003;73(1):198–204.

Robitaille GA. Ehlers-Danlos syndrome and recurrent haemoptysis. *Ann Intern Med.* 1964;61:716–721.

Roulet F, Ruggierro F, Karsenty G, et al. A comprehensive study of the spatial and temporal expression of the col5a1 gene in the mouse embryos: a clue for understanding collagen V function in developing connective tissues. *Cell Tissue Res.* 2007;327(2):323–332.

Rubinstein MK, Cohen NH. Ehlers Danlos Syndrome associated with multiple intracranial aneurysms. *Neurology.* 1964;14:125–132.

Sack G. Status Dysvascularis;ein falle von beisonderer. *Zerreisslichkeit der Blutgefasse Deutsch Archiv Klinische Med.* 1936;178:663–666.

Sasaki T, Arai K, Ono M, et al. Ehlers Danlos Syndrome. A variant characterised by deficiency of pro alpha 2 chain of type I procollagen. *Arch Dermatol.* 1987;123(1):76–79.

Schaefer BM, Lewin MB, Stout KK, et al. Usefulness of bicuspid aortic valve phenotype to predict elastic properties of the ascending aorta. *Am J Cardiol.* 2007;99(5):688–690.

Schaefer BM, Lewin MB, Stout KK, et al. The bicuspid aortic valve: an integrated phenotypic classification of leaflet morphology and aortic root shape. *Heart.* 2008;94(12):1634–1638. Epub 2008.

Schalkwijk J, Zweers MC, Steijlen PM, et al. A recessive form of the Ehlers-Danlos syndrome caused by Tenascin-X deficiency. *N Eng J Med.* 2001;345:1167–1175.

Schwarze U, Hata R, McKusick VA, et al. Rare autosomal recessive cardiac valvular form of Ehlers-Danlos Syndrome results from mutations in the COL1A2 gene that activate the nonsense-mediated RNA decay pathway. *Am J Hum Gene*t. 2004;74(5):917–930.

Serry C, Agomuoh OS, Goldin MD. Review of Ehlers-Danlos syndrome: successful repair of rupture and dissection of abdominal aorta. *J Cardiovasc Surg* (Torino). 1988;29(5):530–534.

Sestak Z. Ehlers-Danlos syndrome and cutis laxa: an account of families in the Oxford area. *Ann Hum Genet.* 1962;25:313.

Seve P, Dubreuil O, Farhat F, et al. Acute mitral regurgitation caused by papillary muscle rupture in the immediate postpartum period revealing Ehlers Danlos Syndrome type IV. *J Thorac Cardiovasc Surg.* 2005;129(3):680–681.

Takano H, Miyamoto Y, Sawa Y, et al. Successful mitral valve replacement in a patient with Ehlers-Danlos Syndrome type VI. *Ann Thorac Surg.* 2005;80:320–322.

Tiller GE, Cassidy SB, Wensel C, et al. Aortic root dilatation in Ehlers-Danlos syndrome types I, II and III. A report of five cases. *Clin Genet.* 1998;53(6):460–465.

Tonnessen BH, Sterrnbergh WC 3rd, Mannava K, Money SR. Endovascular repair of an iliac artery aneurysm in a patient with Ehlers Danlos Syndrome type IV. *J Vasc Surg.* 2007;45(1):177–179.

Tsai-Goodman B, Martin RP, Pope FM, et al. Pulmonary valvuloplasty in a case of vascular Ehlers Danlos Syndrome. *Catheter Cardiovasc Interv.* 2002;57(1):92–94.

Tschernogobow A. Cutis Laxa Monatschrifte Praktische. *Dermatologie.* 1892;14:76.

Tucker DH, Miller DE, Jacoby WJ Jr. Ehlers Danlos Syndrome with sinus of valsalva aneurysm and aortic insufficiency simulating rheumatic heart disease. *Am J Med.* 1963;35:715–720.

Wallach EA, Burkhart EF. Ehlers Danlos Syndrome associated with the tetralogy of Fallot. *Arch Derm Syphilol.* 1950;61(5):750–752.

Watanabe S, Ishimitsu T, Inoue K, et al. Type IV Ehlers Danlos Syndrome associated with mitral valve prolapse: a case report. *J Cardiol Suppl.* 1988;18:97–105.

Wenstrup RJ, Florer JB, Davidson JM, et al. Murine model of the Ehlers-Danlos Syndrome COL5A1 haploinsufficiency disrupts collagen fibril assembly at multiple stages. *J Biol Chem.* 2006;281(18):12888–12895.

Wenstrup RJ, Florer JB, Willing MC, et al. COL5A1 haploinsufficiency is a common molecular mechanism underlying the classical form of EDS. *Am J Hum Gen.* 2000;66(6):1766–1776.

Wenstrup RJ, Murad S, Pinsella SR. Ehlers-Danlos Syndrome Type VI, clinical manifestations of collagen lysyl hydroxylase deficiency. *J Pediatr.* 1989;115(3):405–409.

Wenstrup, RJ, Meyer RA, Lyle JS, et al. Prevalence of aortic root dilatation in the Ehlers Danlos Syndrome. *Genet Med.* 2002;4(3):112–117.

Zweers MC, Peeters AC, Graafsma S, et al. Abdominal Aortic Aneurysm is associated with high serum levels of Tenascin-X and decreased aneurysmal tissue tenascin-X. *Circulation.* 2006;113(13);1702–1707.

29

The Heart in the Inherited Diseases of Hemoglobin and the Hemochromatosis Syndromes

Malcolm J Walker and Constantinos O'Mahony

Introduction

Abnormalities of hemoglobin synthesis due to genetic defects are common and often associated with heart disease. In many the prime pathophysiology involves excessive deposition of iron in the myocardial tissues, either as a direct consequence of the hemoglobinopathy, or due to the need for treatment by regular transfusion, which leads to increased red cell destruction and liberation of large amounts of iron, which overwhelms the body's very limited excretory capacity for this ion. In sickle cell disease, heart injury may occur not only from endothelial dysfunction and microvascular occlusion by the adhesion of deformed or hemolyzed erythrocytes but also from iron overload, as there is an increasing trend to treat this disease with exchange transfusion. This means that like in the thalassemias, iatrogenic iron overload may cause an increasing frequency of cardiovascular complications. In many of the conditions the clinical picture is complicated and aggravated by the additional effects of chronic anemia, blood viscocity changes, abnormal clotting, pulmonary hypertension and associated diabetes or other endocrinopathies, liver disease, renal impairment, and the long-term consequences of reduced physical activity.

Iron Overload, a Common Thread

Iron is a necessary constituent for cellular function, but it is rarely found unbound due to its highly reactive nature and ability to generate or catalyze the formation of toxic free radicals. It has an important role as a cofactor associated with many proteins that have redox, catalytic, and regulatory functions. Many are situated within mitochondria, but some appear in the cytosol and within cytosolic organelles. The uptake of iron by cells and its homeostasis is complex, very tightly regulated, and incompletely described. Recently, the understanding of the "iron cycle" has improved through genetic studies of patients with inherited disorders such as Friedreich's ataxia, hemochromatosis, and the hemoglobinopathies, combined with analysis of mutant strains of mice, rats, zebra fish, and even simpler organisms (Andrews 2000; Walker et al. 2001; Figure 29-1).

The tissue distribution of iron overload in the hemoglobinopathies is similar to that observed in hemochromatosis; organs with high mitochondrial activity face a particularly heavy burden of iron. In the refractory anemias, iron overload of the tissues, including the heart, occurs as a consequence of transfusion therapy. This is amply demonstrated in thalassemia, the most common of the inherited hemoglobinopathies, where the requirement for blood transfusion begins in infancy. In thalassemia the iron burden is significantly exacerbated by an inappropriately increased intestinal iron absorption rate despite the high body iron stores. Mutations of the *HFE* gene are the commonest cause of the clinical syndrome of hereditary hemochromatosis, which is characterized by abnormal intestinal absorption of dietary iron (Townsend and Drakesmith 2002). Escape from a negative feedback loop within the enterocyte means that iron absorption remains high despite ever-increasing stores of iron. The consequence is that the normal iron storage systems that sequester and safely store iron become overwhelmed and excess iron is deposited in the tissues, and particularly damaging free iron (nontransferrin bound iron—NTBI) appears in the blood. The organs preferentially affected are the liver, the pancreas, and the heart (Philpott 2002).

Sickle cell disease is frequently complicated by involvement of the heart, producing arrhythmias, pulmonary hypertension, and ventricular failure in some cases. The tendency now is to treat sickle cell disease with regular transfusion regimes, in order to reduce the incidence of painful and tissue-injuring crises and other complications, particularly stroke in childhood. This adds myocardial iron overload to the potential mechanisms of myocardial damage that can lead to cardiac morbidity and mortality in this important hemoglobinopathy.

The Chronic Refractory Anemias—Thalassemia

Thalassemia is a monogenetic disorder affecting globin chain synthesis (Hill 1992) with a heterozygote frequency varying from 3% to 30%. High prevalence is centered on the Mediterranean and spreads in a broad central swathe eastward to Thailand and New Guinea. It is divided into α- or β-thalassemia syndromes, according to the globin chain involved. Human hemoglobin is a

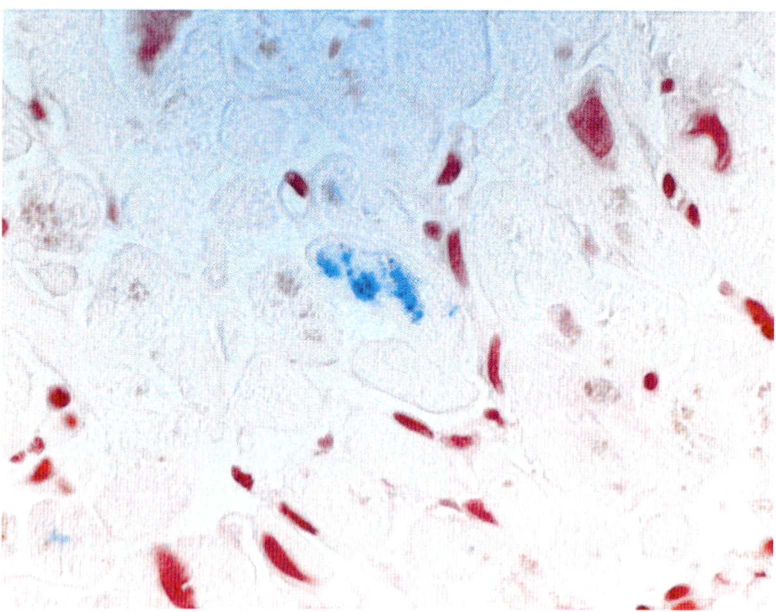

Figure 29–1 A myocardial biopsy stained with Perls' stain, which reveals in blue, scanty iron granules within the myocytes. This was taken from a β thalassemia major patient with a previous history of heart failure 10 years before the biopsy was performed to exclude an active myocarditis.

tetrameric molecule composed of two globin dimers and in the fetus the major hemoglobin is HbF ($\alpha_2\gamma_2$) and in the adult HbA ($\alpha_2\beta_2$). An important consequence of diminished globin production, which is central to the pathogenesis of thalassemia, is the excessive accumulation of the unaffected globin chain. In β-thalassemia the excess α-globin chains are unstable and precipitate within erythrocytes and their precursors, leading to ineffective erythropoiesis and reduced erythrocyte survival. This process is responsible for the anemia that characterizes the thalassemias. Profound anemia leads to increased erythropoietin production, which in turn stimulates bone marrow expansion with the development of characteristic skeletal deformities. The massive erythroid expansion poses excessive metabolic demands on developing children who fail to thrive. The abnormal circulating erythrocytes are trapped in the spleen leading to splenomegaly, which in turn exacerbates the anemia by pooling a higher portion of circulating erythrocytes and by plasma expansion. The expanded plasma volume and the anemia lead to increased cardiovascular demands and affected individuals have a hyperdynamic circulation (Higgs et al. 2001b).

Although α- and β-thalassemia share the same pathogenic basis, they have at least one fundamental difference. In general terms, ineffective erythropoiesis is more severe in β-thalassemia since the excess α chains are more unstable than the excess β and γ chains encountered in α-thalassemia. This leads to significantly less dependence on blood transfusions and hence less aggressive iron loading in α-thalassemia with a few exceptions (Gibbons et al. 2001).

Box 29–1

The thalassemia syndromes

Thalassemias are common monogenic disorders characterized by reduced and imbalanced globin production causing ineffective erythropoiesis and hemolysis.

They are classified into α-thalassemias or β-thalassemia depending on the globin gene affected.

The globin gene defect interacts with other genetic polymorphisms and environmental factors to determine the severity of the hematological phenotype.

The severity and nature of the hematological phenotype determines the cardiological manifestations.

α-Thalassemia—Genetics

The α-like globin genes form a linked cluster on the short arm of chromosome 16. They are arranged, like the β-globin gene cluster in the order of their developmental expression, 5′-ζ-ψζ-ψα-α2-α1-θ-3′. The α-globin gene cluster is embedded in two highly homologous duplication regions that permit misalignment during meiosis and improper recombination leading to a variation in the number of globin genes. ψβ, ψζ, and ψα are pseudogenes, thought to be evolutionary remnants with no functional products. θ is transcribed at low levels but is not a functional globulin. There are two α-globin genes, each with three exons and two introns and share the same coding properties as the for β-globin exons. The α1 and α2 gene products are identical but are expressed at a ratio of 1:3 throughout life. Since α2 expression is more dominant, mutations affecting the α2 gene result in more severe phenotypes. The major α-globin regulatory element is the hypersensitive site −40 kb to the ζ gene (HS-40). In contrast to β-thalassemia, the phenotype of becomes apparent in early life with the formation of tetramers of excess γ chains in the fetus (γ_4 or Hb Bart's) since α chains are expressed in HbF ($\alpha_2\gamma_2$). Post partum, the HbF production switches to HbA ($\alpha_2\beta_2$) and β chains form tetramers leading to (β_4 or HbH) (Higgs et al. 2001a).

Some pathogenic mutations cause α^0-thalassemia haplotypes characterised by the absence of α-globin production whilst other mutations cause α^+-thalassemia haplotypes which retain some residual α-globin production. In contrast to β-thalassemia, where most alleles arise by point mutations, most α-thalassemia alleles are caused by variable deletions of the α-globin gene cluster, which have the potential to abolish one or both of the α-globin genes. α^+-thalassemia haplotypes are caused by deletions of one of the two α-globin genes secondary to reciprocal recombination of misaligned chromosomes during meiosis, which produces one chromosome with a single α-globin gene (−α) and another with three(ααα). α-globin gene deletions causing α^0-thalassemia haplotypes are of variable length and arise by nonhomologous recombination during meiosis. The deletions found in the Mediterranean

($—^{MED}$) and south east Asia ($—^{SEA}$) are the commonest examples. Deletion of HS-40 and surrounding sequences results in severe downregulation of the α-globin genes and leads to α^0-thalassemia despite having normal α-globin genes (Higgs et al. 2001c).

Nondeletional types of α-thalassemia (α^T variants) are rarer but well described. Point mutations affect the α2 globin genes more often than $\alpha 1_1$ and because α2 is more expressed than α1 such mutations confer a more severe phenotype.. Mutations affecting RNA splicing, processing, and translation have also been reported (Higgs et al. 2001c).

The inheritance of α-thalassemia is more complicated than β-thalassemia since there are two α genes per haplotype. The normal complement is therefore αα/αα. In α^0 thalassemia both α-globin chains are not produced, either because of deletions, or nondeletional mutations. In α^+-thalassemia alleles only one of the two α genes is deactivated either because of a deletion (–α) or a deactivating mutation ($\alpha^T\alpha$ or $\alpha\alpha^T$). The different combinations between these alleles give rise to the different α-thalassemia syndromes. In general, inheritance of the normal αα haplotype with any of the α^0- or α^+-thalassemia haplotypes leads to α-thalassemia trait which is a silent carrier state. Inheritance of two α^0 alleles results in hemoglobin Bart's, hydrops fetalis syndrome, which is lethal. Inheritance of α^0 with α^+ alleles causes mostly HbH disease. Coinheritance of two α^+ alleles causes a spectrum of phenotypes that ranges mostly between α-thalassemia trait and HbH disease (Gibbons et al. 2001).

The Population Genetics of α-Thalassemia

The α-thalassemias are frequently encountered in the Mediterranean basin, West Africa, the Middle East, the Indian subcontinent, and throughout Southeast Asia to the Pacific. This distribution is thought to arise as a result of the advantage gained by the heterozygotes who have some protection from malaria. α^0 alleles are mostly found in the Mediterranean and Southeast Asia whilst α^+ alleles are found in West Africa, the Indian subcontinent, and the Pacific islands. The geographical distribution of the α^0 and α^+ alleles thus defines the phenotypes encountered at a particular locality; for example, in Southeast Asia 1 in 200–2,000 births is affected by hemoglobin Bart's hydrops fetalis, which is not as prevalent in areas where the α^0 alleles are not commonly found (Gibbons et al. 2001).

Clinical and Cardiological Manifestations of α-Thalassemia

HbH disease is the only clinically significant entity, as α-thalassemia trait is asymptomatic and hemoglobin Bart's hydrops fetalis syndrome is lethal. The majority of individuals with HbH disease remain well. Some require intermittent blood transfusions, particularly at times of stress, and rarely some individuals develop severe disease later in life, requiring regular blood transfusions. The iron overload affecting transfusion-dependent β-thalassemics is thus not typically encountered in HbH disease (Cohen et al. 2004). However, markedly elevated levels of ferritin are found in over 70% of adult HbH patients and are, associated with increasing age but not clearly to the number of previous blood transfusions. Accumulation of excess iron in HbH disease probably occurs as a consequence of increased intestinal absorption (Chui et al. 2003). Heart failure has been reported in a small proportion of HbH patients and has been attributed to iron overload causing diastolic dysfunction with elevated E/A ratios and short isovolumic relaxation times (IVRT) that correlate with increasing ferritin levels in the absence of blood transfusions (Chen et al. 2000). Whether treatment of HbH patients with elevated ferritin levels and diastolic dysfunction with chelating agents improves diastolic dysfunction is not known(Chan et al. 2006).

Box 29–2

The α-thalassemia syndromes

Primarily a result of gene deletions rather than point mutations in the α-globin gene cluster on chromosome 16, each chromosome carrying two α-globin genes.

In general α-thalassemia is less severe than β-thalassemia as excess β-globin chains are less pathogenic than excess α chains encountered in β-thalassemia.

Deletion of all 4 α-globin genes is lethal (Hb Bart's hydrops fetalis).

HbH disease is characterized by the formation of β-chain tetramers and behaves in a similar fashion to β-thalassemia intermedia.

HbH disease has been linked with diastolic dysfunction and iron overload secondary to excess GI iron absorption.

Deletion of one or two α-globin genes result in a silent carrier state or α-thalassemia trait.

β-Thalassemia Genetics

The β-like globin genes form a cluster on the short arm of chromosome 11. They are arranged in the order of their developmental expression, 5′-ε-Gγ-Aγ-ψβ-δ-β-3′. The β-globin gene itself contains three exons and two introns. The middle exon codes for the hem-binding portion and as well as β-globin regions involved in αβ dimmer formation, whilst the adjacent exons 1 and 3 code for the non-hem-binding regions. Amino acid moieties involved in the binding to 2,3-disphosphoglycerate and the Bohr effect are coded by exon 3. This general gene structure is shared by all other genes in the β-globin region as well as the α-globin genes. There are two γ-globin genes, each producing a γ chain distinguished by the presence of glycine (Gγ) or alanine (Aγ) at position 136 of the γ chain. Untranslated regions (UTR) at the 5' and 3' ends are necessary for gene transcription. The β locus control region (LCR) is found upstream of the cluster and is critical in the expression of all the β-like globin genes. As β-globin expression commences postpartum, the β-thalassemia phenotype develops as γ chain production declines and β-chain deficiency becomes evident with the precipitation of the normally formed α chains in inclusion bodies (Higgs et al. 2001b).

Mutations resulting in the absence of β-globin production cause β^0-thalassemia haplotypes, whilst mutations that retain residual β-globin production cause β^+-thalassemia haplotypes. The vast majority of β-thalassemia alleles arise by substitutions, insertions, or deletions within the β-globin gene or its immediate flanking sequences that affect β-globin gene expression by interrupting either DNA transcription, posttranscriptional RNA processing, or RNA translation.

Mutations that impair transcription are single-base substitutions that affect the β-globin promoter region, which binds to the transcription machinery at the 5' of the β-globin gene. These mutations do not completely silence β-globin expression but reduce the production to 10% to 25% of normal resulting in β^+-thalassemia haplotypes.

Mutations affecting RNA processing involve invariant dinucleotides at the splice junctions between introns and exons, which are crucial to the splicing process responsible for removing the noncoding introns from the primary RNA transcript prior to translation. These mutations allow normal transcription to take place but the abnormally spliced mRNA does not translate to functional β-globin chains leading to $β^0$-thalassemia alleles. Alternatively, mutations leading to abnormal splicing can involve conserved consensus sequences that flank the invariant dinucleotides at the splice junctions rather than the invariant dinucleotides themselves. Such mutations activate cryptic splice sites in introns and exons that are normally present but silent leading to inefficient splicing by competing with the normal splice site by variable degrees depending on the particular mutation. This consequently leads to a phenotype that ranges from mild to severe. Mutations in the 3'UTR AATAAA conserved sequence, which has the important function of signaling for the 3' cleavage of the primary RNA transcript, poly(A) tail attachment, and enhancement of translation lead to unstable elongated mRNA transcripts causing as a general rule mild $β^+$-thalassemia. Other 3'UTR sequence mutations causing abnormal splicing have also been recognized.

Mutations affecting RNA translation constitute more than half of β-thalassemia mutations and almost invariably cause $β^0$-thalassemia. They are mostly nonsense or frameshift mutations, which cause premature termination of translation and thus no functional β-globin is produced. The vast majority of these mutations involve exons 1 and 2,. Interestingly, rare mutations in exon 3 give rise to a dominantly transmitted form of β-thalassemia caused by "viable" β-globin variants that precipitate in erythroid cells producing a more severe phenotype. A few mutations affecting the initiation codon of the β-globin gene have also been indentified and lead to $β^0$-thalassemia alleles.

β-thalassemia alleles secondary to deletions involving part of the β-globin gene or the β-LCR components have also been described but are not common. Deletions involving the ε, Gγ, Aγ, ψβ, δ, and variable portions of the β-globin genes cause εγδβ-thalassemia and heterozygotes develop a β-thalassemia trait phenotype in adult life. The homozygotes state is not viable beyond early gestation. Such deletions of the β-globin gene are rare and private.

Approximately 1% of thalassemia alleles have not been characterized and are likely to involve the upstream β-LCR, β-globin enhancer region, or other non-β-globin regions.

β-Thalassemia Population Genetics

β-thalassemia is found in areas that used to be endemic for malaria. In Cyprus, β-thalassemia trait is found in 17.2% of the population, and a comparably high frequency in Sardinia. In Greece and Italy there seems to be a patchy distribution with low altitude areas having a higher incidence than high altitude regions and the β-thalassemia carrier frequency is 6%–7% but with large regional variation. It is postulated that β-thalassemia heterozygotes have a selective advantage and are protected against severe forms of malaria (Hill et al. 1987). It appears that β-thalassemia alleles have been amplified independently at separate locations and maintained at high frequency by the selection pressure imposed by malaria. The mechanism by which malarial protection is afforded in β-thalassemia is not clear (Weatherall 1997).

In the United Kingdom there are approximately 800 transfusion-dependent patients with homozygote β-thalassemia; historically, the disease affected Greek, Cypriot, and Turkish communities who congregated in north London. Prenatal counseling has led to a reduction in affected births in these groups (Modell et al. 2000a). The disease is now moving northward, fueled by a rapidly increasing incidence of homozygote thalassemic births amongst residents of Pakistani origin (Modell et al. 2001). Globally the situation is potentially much more demanding with an estimated 30,000 to 60,000 homozygous thalassemia births per year (Weatherall and Clegg 2001).

Genotype/Phenotype Relationship

The hallmark of β-thalassemia is the ineffective production of β-globin chains resulting in an imbalance in globin chains. Homozygous or compound heterozygotes may have a severe form of the disease requiring blood transfusions from an early age, whilst others with the same disease have a milder phenotype. Similarly, most heterozygote carriers show minimal phenotypic expression but rarely heterozygotes can exhibit severe disease in a pattern that suggests dominant transmission. The phenotypic heterogeneity of β-thalassemias is therefore large, and is accounted by the large number of mutations affecting the β-globin gene, interacting with other genetic and environmental factors.

More than 200 β-globin mutations have been identified. In general, mutations that result in a complete lack of β-globin chains cause a more severe phenotype than mutations that result in a reduction of β-globin production. The majority of the mild mutations of the β-globin gene result from mutations in the promoter region, poly(A) cleavage sites, cryptic splice sites in exons, and consensus sequences in introns. In heterozygotes such mutations will result in no or mild clinical disease. In homozygotes, however, intermediate severity disease can be encountered, whilst the combination with a severe allele in the compound heterozygote state will result in major or intermediate disease severity (Weatherall 2001).

Since the phenotype of β-thalassemia depends on the severity of the anemia produced by the accumulation of excess α-globin chains during erythopoiesis, any condition that minimizes the excess of α chains will ameliorate the phenotype for a given β-thalassemia genotype. Therefore, coinheritance of α-thalassemia can ameliorate the severity of β-thalassemia. Since both α- and β-thalassemia alleles frequently coexist in many populations, they are not uncommonly coinherited and the interaction between the two conditions can explain some of the phenotypic heterogeneity encountered in β-thalassemia. This experiment of nature also provides an insight into the major underlying pathophysiological mechanism in the thalassemias, which is not reduced hemoglobin production itself but the imbalance between the globin chains produced (Weatherall 2001). On a similar note it has been documented that some patients with homozygous $β^0$-thalassemia have a milder clinical course with persistence of high levels of HbF. The γ chains are able to mop up the excess α chains, thus reducing the imbalance in globin chain production and ineffective erythropoiesis. Hereditary persistence of fetal hemoglobin secondary to mutations in the β-globin gene or the promoter regions of the γ-globin gene is rare, but a polymorphism at position 158 in the Gγ-gene (C→T change)appears to be important in promoting HbF production at times of hemopoietic stress in homozygotes. Since this polymorphism is common, it can modify the phenotype of β-thalassemia. Additional genetic factors on chromosome 6 and the X chromosome have also been identified that promote HbF production (Weatherall 2001).

End-organ damage associated with iron overload in thalassemia is caused not only by blood transfusions but also by enhanced gastrointestinal iron absorption. Genes that modulate iron absorption such as the *HFE* gene, may affect the degree of iron overload and therefore the natural history of thalassemia, although such interactions have not been consistently documented in some studies (Weatherall 2001; Jazayeri et al. 2003). Similarly, polymorphisms in the vitamin D receptor and estrogen receptor may modify the development of osteoporosis in thalassemia patients. Gallstone disease secondary to hemolysis is another clinical feature of thalassemia and a polymorphism in the promoter region of UDP-glucuronosyltransferase has been implicated in higher levels of bilirubin and gallstone disease. The role of environmental factors in modifying the phenotype in thalassemia is even less well understood.

Clinical and Cardiological Manifestations of α-Thalassemia

Thalassemia major is a lethal disease unless treatment with blood transfusions is initiated early. Until effective therapy for its management was developed, β-thalassemia major was considered to be a pediatric condition. Prior to the era of blood transfusions, high output cardiac failure was the leading cause of death in first decade of life. Treatment with blood transfusions prior to the development of chelation treatment leads to a different form of cardiac disease, heart failure due to ventricular dysfunction, secondary to iron overload. Iron overload in thalassemic patients occurs as a consequence of blood transfusions that are central to the treatment of severe disease, which not only corrects the anemia but also suppresses bone marrow expansion. Unfortunately, there is no dedicated iron excretion pathway that can increase the rate of excretion of iron in response to iron loading. Each unit of blood contains 200 mg of iron and regular blood transfusions rapidly lead to iron overload by the age of 11 years in patients with high transfusion requirements. Inappropriately increased intestinal iron absorption also contributes to iron loading. The advent of chelation treatment controlled cardiac complications secondary to iron overload, but unfortunately these complications have not been completely eliminated.

Clinically, the condition is categorized as thalassemia major if the phenotype is severe, or minor if the phenotype is mild. Practically, this division may be made by quantifying transfusion requirements, >8 transfusions per year being accepted as severe, or thalassemia major. Thalassemia intermedia describes individuals with a phenotypic expression of the disease lies between the two ends of the spectrum. There exists a dichotomy in the cardiac manifestations of thalassemia major and intermedia. Heart failure in thalassemia major is caused primarily by left ventricular (LV) dysfunction, whilst in thalassemia intermedia heart failure is produced by right heart dysfunction and pulmonary hypertension (Aessopos et al. 2001). In asymptomatic thalassemia intermedia patients cardiac dimensions, LV mass, LV shortening and ejection fractions, and cardiac output are higher than in thalassemia major patients (Aessopos et al. 2005) and up to 23% have cardiac iron deposits.

In thalassemia intermedia, which makes up a quarter of β-thalassemia patients, approximately half the patients do not receive blood transfusions, and a quarter receive only intermittent transfusions. Pulmonary hypertension is believed to develop as a result of chronic hemolysis leading to vasoconstriction by reducing nitric oxide levels, degeneration of the vascular tree and in situ thrombosis in the pulmonary vasculature. These changes are associated with a high cardiac output, which is a consequence of tissue hypoxia secondary to the anemia and the presence of HbF, which has a high affinity for oxygen (Aessopos et al. 2007).

Although thalassemia intermedia has historically been managed without regular transfusion, affected individuals have increased intestinal iron absorption, driven by the high erythropoeitic drive and probably mediated by a deficiency in hepcidin (Origa et al. 2007). The implication of this is that by the third or fourth decade of life patients with thalassemia intermedia face an iron burden which is not dissimilar to that of transfusion-dependent patients. Deferoxamine treatment not only chelates iron but it also reduces intestinal absorption (Pippard et al. 1977, 1979). Eventhough thalassemia intermedia patients tolerate and manage with chronically low hemoglobin levels, it has become accepted that complications of the disease, including disfiguring erythroid marrow expansion can be avoided by a regular transfusion regime. Thus adoption of transfusion to diminish erythropoeitic drive and conventional chelation to prevent iron accumulation, appear to provide the most likely hope for prevention of disease complications in this group with a "milder" thalassemic phenotype.

The thalassemias are associated with a hypercoagulable state and arterial and venous thrombosis is not uncommon, with a four-fold increase in the risk of thromboembolism in intermedia compared to thalassemia major. Arterial embolization occurs more commonly in thalassemia major whilst venous thrombosis is more frequent in thalassemia intermedia (Taher et al. 2006). Multiple abnormalities contribute to the hypercoagulable state including chronic platelet and endothelial activation, with reduced levels of proteins C and S leading to chronic activation of the coagulation cascade. Subclinical thrombosis in the pulmonary vasculature may thus contribute to the development of pulmonary hypertension and right ventricular dysfunction (Eldor and Rachmilewitz 2002).

Treatment of Thalassemia

Regular blood transfusion, varying from 2 to 4 units every 3 to 5 weeks is generally required to keep hemoglobin levels within the recommended range of 9 to 11 g/dL. Maintaining this level of pretransfusion hemoglobin comes at the price of exposure to a potentially toxic iron load, from 7.5 to 15 g per year in a 65 kg individual (Rebulla and Modell 1991). For the growing child and the family, the advantages of frequent blood transfusions are immediate in terms of well-being and improved growth. It also avoids the development of the skeletal deformities caused by erythroid marrow expansion, which lead to the characteristic facial appearance and distorted body habitus of some affected patients. Adoption of

Box 29–3

The β-thalassemia syndromes

Commonly caused by point mutations leading to impaired transcription and translation of the β-globin genes on chromosome 11.

Mutations cause absent (β^0) or partial (β^+) β-globin synthesis.

β-thalassemia major or Cooley's anemia is caused by the severe deficiency of β chains (β^0/β^0, β^+/β^+, β^+/β^0) and if untreated leads to high output cardiac failure during the second decade of life.

In β-thalassemia, major blood transfusions and increased GI iron absorption rapidly lead to cardiac iron overload with lethal cardiac complications unless chelation treatment is used.

In β-thalassemia intermedia the β-chain deficiency is less severe than the major form of the disease (β^0/β, β^+/β^+) and is not transfusion dependent. The β-thalassemia intermedia disease spectrum includes a wide range of phenotypes that range between the major and minor forms.

β-thalassemia intermedia is complicated primarily by pulmonary hypertension and right ventricular dysfunction and occasionally by excess gastronitestinal iron absorption.

β-thalassemia trait/minor (β^+ or β^0 heterozygotes) causes mild microcytic anemia with no specific cardiac manifestations.

regular blood transfusion, and the adoption of chelation with deferoxamine (desferrioxamine, Desferal; DFO) to induce iron excretion (Sephton Smith 1962), has meant that survival into adulthood can now be expected for the majority of affected individuals. Nevertheless, even in countries, such as the United Kingdom, where treatment with deferoxamine has been freely available, there remains a dramatic rate of mortality and morbidity that begins in adolescence and leads to about 40% of the affected individuals dying before the age of 35 years (Borgna-Pignatti et al. 1998, 2005; Modell et al. 2000b). The majority of these deaths are due to heart failure with a small proportion of sudden, presumed arrhythmic, deaths (Engle et al. 1964; Bannerman et al. 1967; Sanyal et al. 1975; Zurlo et al. 1989).

Detecting Iron Overload in the Heart

Once clinical evidence of cardiac failure is apparent in iron overloaded hearts, the prognosis is poor, with mean survivals in the region of 3 months in historical reports (Engle et al. 1964). Our own experience is that the acute mortality of overt cardiac failure is high, at approximately 50%, but if aggressive chelation is undertaken successfully, subsequent survival is good with normalization of ventricular function to be expected (Figures 29–2 and 29–3). The clinical imperative is therefore to identify iron overloaded hearts early, before severe myocyte failure occurs. In the past this has been difficult. The at-risk population can be identified, however. Amongst the thalassemia population these would be the individuals, aged from teenage to early twenties, often with a history of difficulty with compliance to the DFO infusion regime (Aldouri et al. 1990). Low-risk individuals would tend to have long-term average ferritin levels under 1,500 with the absence of other organ involvement (Telfer et al. 2000). These patients are usually nondiabetic, with normal secondary sexual development, normal growth, and endocrine function. Unfortunately, within any clinical service dealing with thalassemia tragic exceptions occur all too frequently. Patients who ostensibly were expected to be at low risk may rapidly decompensate and die, often precipitated by non-cardiac infections or other illnesses. In the United Kingdom, where the community of thalassemics is relatively small and close knit, such unexpected deaths of young people can have enormous effects on the morale and motivation of the remaining group to continue to comply with a very demanding, often painful and socially debilitating form of treatment that DFO infusions continue to be. The development of an MRI-based noninvasive method to measure tissue iron accumulation has transformed our ability to adequately risk stratify the thalassemic patient population (Anderson et al. 2001). The previous most accurate assessment of total iron burden relied upon quantitative iron measurement in liver biopsies. However, the relationship between liver iron content and heart iron content is not predictable in an individual. So finding a clear liver biopsy does not identify some individuals, who are at great risk due to high heart iron content. Myocardial biopsy has been used to risk stratify patients (Borgna-Pignatti and

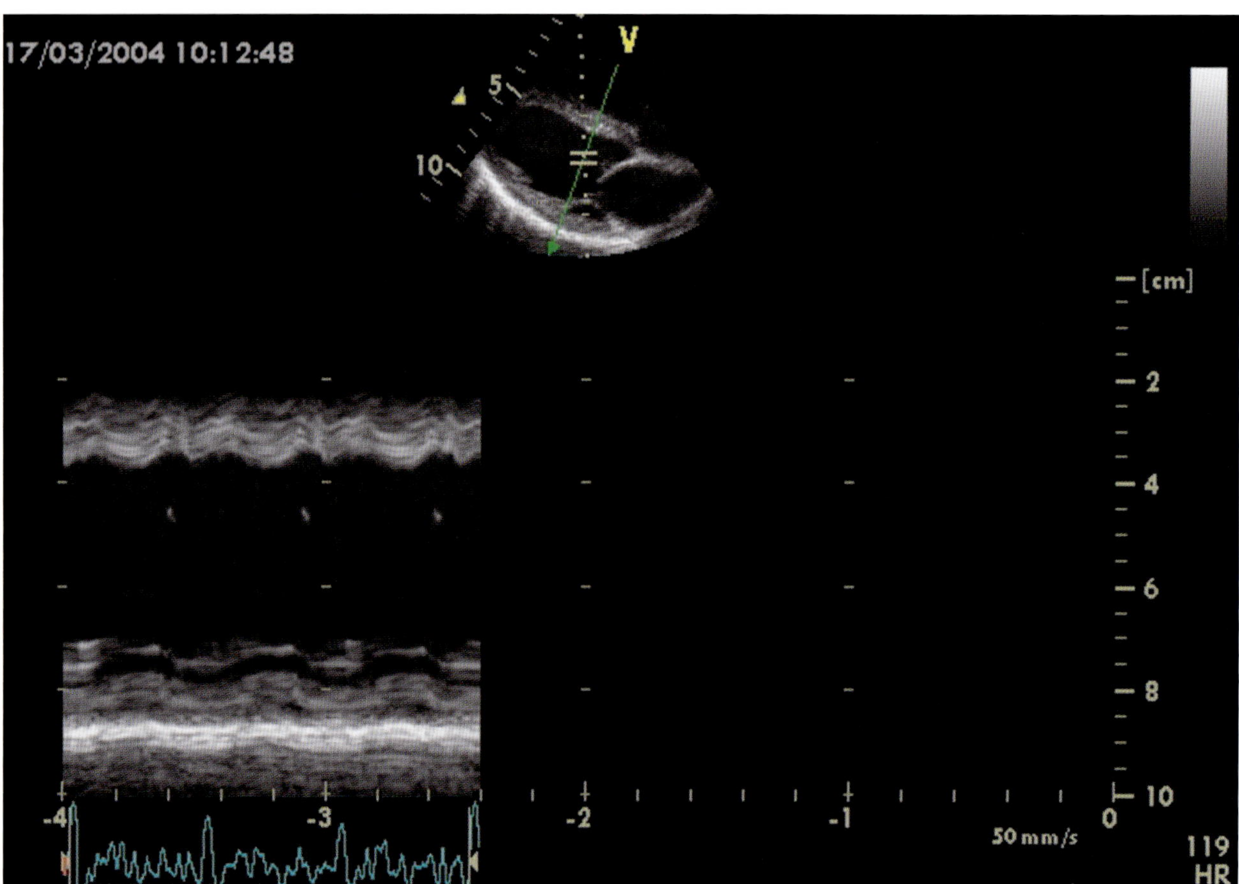

Figure 29–2 The parasternal long axis 2-D and m-mode echo from a 31-year-old woman with β–thalassemia major and an intermittently poor history of chelation with deferoxamine (DFO). She presented to clinic with signs of severe biventricular failure. The echo demonstrates very poor LV function, with LVedd 4.5 cm, LVes 4.0 cm, and FS 12%.

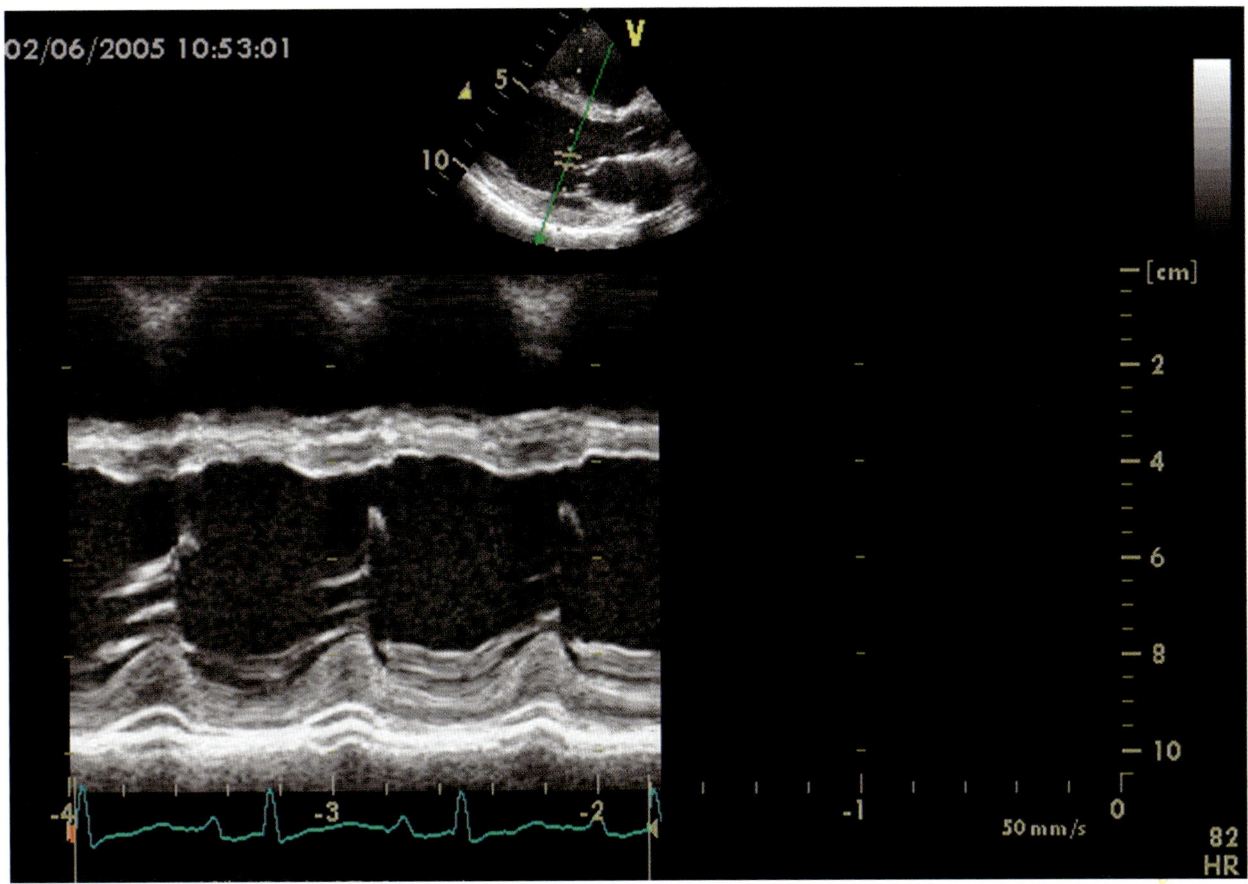

Figure 29–3 The patient mentioned in Figure 29–2 reviewed in clinic 14 months later. She had made a rapid recovery with conventional antifailure treatment and intensified chelation with 24-hour subcutaneous infusions of DFO followed by combination treatment of DFO plus oral deferiprone. The echo reveals virtual normalization of function with LVedd 4.8 cm, LVes 3.5 cm, and FS 28%.

Castriota-Scanderbeg 1991), but its invasive nature and a concern over potential sampling errors precludes its routine use (Fitchett et al. 1980).

The Clinical History in Thalassemia

The nonspecific nature of symptoms attributable to myocardial dysfunction reduces their reliability as discriminators, between high- and low-risk patients. The chronic anemia alone may account for much exercise limitation, although many patients with thalassemia will be able to detect a progressive deterioration across time, which cannot be accounted for by their hemoglobin levels. Chest pain of a nonspecific nature, often sharp, or pleuropericarditic, often worse around the time of lowest hemoglobin, or even immediately after transfusion, is admitted by many patients (29% of patients attending our clinic). Rarely is the pain of any clinical significance. Pericarditis and myocarditis are reported, and may be more prevalent in some areas, such as mainland Greece (Kremastinos et al. 1995), but remain uncommon elsewhere. Peripheral edema, ascites, or hepatic congestion are all late symptoms, usually manifest once advanced biventricular failure has occurred.

Since iron overloaded hearts are susceptible to arrhythmia, it is not surprising that palpitations are a relatively frequent complaint (48% of patients in our clinic), as they are in any general cardiology service. They occasionally are due to life-threatening ventricular tachycardia (VT), but this is usually in grossly iron overloaded hearts with established ventricular impairment. VT may be the first symptom that appears when the heart is seriously iron loaded. Atrial fibrillation (AF) is fairly common (documented episodes in 8% of our clinic population); again it usually occurs in patients who have developed significant iron overload. AF has previously been associated with the risk of impending cardiac failure, but may occur in very mildly affected patients, presumably due to variations in the distribution of iron deposition in the heart. The problem facing the clinician is differentiating between sinister arrhythmias and the more common benign palpitations experienced by a young population, often anxious, who have first-hand experience of the outcomes of some of their less fortunate peers. Having a quantitative estimate of cardiac iron content, by cardiac magnetic resonance (CMR) T2*, will help make this distinction more accurate, especially in those patients with normal ventricular function by conventional assessment.

Investigations

ECG

The ECG is frequently abnormal in thalassemic patients (Figure 29–4). Unfortunately, the abnormalities are nonspecific and have not proven useful in reliably identifying patients with a high iron load. Clearly the ECG may uncover other pathologies, for example, the progressive development of RV overload in a patient with chronic pulmonary emboli from an un-anticoagulated

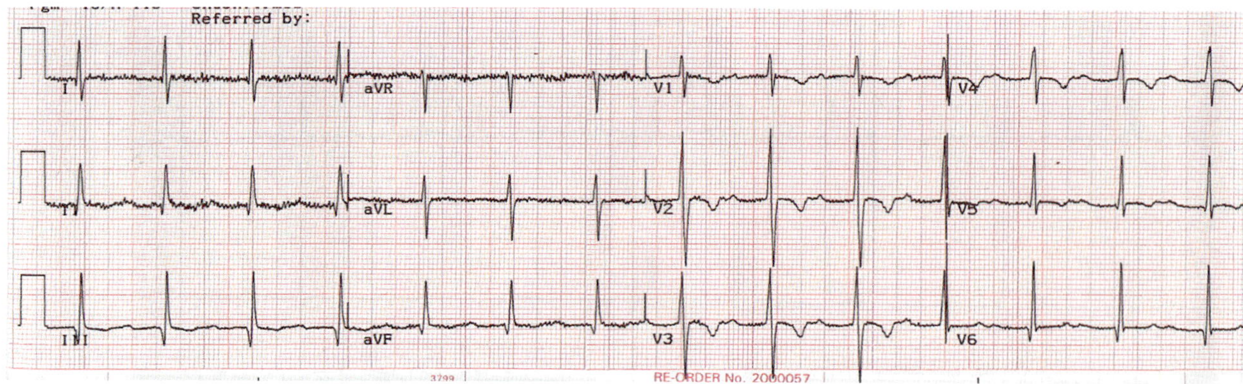

Figure 29–4 The ECG from an asymptomatic β–thalassemia patient of 34 years with no detectable myocardial iron, by MRI (T2* >30 ms), but with a history of heart failure and poor compliance with chelation treatment between teenage and his early twenties. It shows the commonly observed, but nonspecific T-wave changes and a tendency for a high V lead transition point.

in-dwelling central venous line. Exercise testing has also proven to be largely unhelpful, except in isolated cases of exercise-induced arrhythmia, or as a stressor to gauge changes in echocardiography or nuclear ventriculography. Holter or 24-hour ECG monitoring is not valuable as a screening tool in our experience. Its use would follow the pragmatic experience in general cardiology, in that it remains a useful method to investigate symptomatic patients, acting either as a method of providing reassurance about the benign nature of some symptoms or as a guide treatment in those situations where significant arrhythmias are captured.

Echocardiography

Cardiac ultrasound has been used extensively to detect cardiac involvement in thalassemia. Its ease of application and the very widespread availability of the technique and the skills to use it will ensure that it will remain the most useful modality to assess progress in these patients. Its major flaw remains that it cannot be used to reliably exclude potentially serious iron overload, prior to this causing ventricular failure or catastrophic sudden decompensation (usually as a response to an intercurrent illness). This is an indispensable but complementary tool to the MRI-derived iron quantification measurement. The echocardiogrpahic changes in thalassemia may consist of subtle abnormalities of diastolic function (Kremastinos et al. 1993) through to systolic dysfunction, ventricular dilatation, and all the features of a severe dilated cardiomyopathy.

Dilatation of the ventricles, to a mild degree, is a frequent finding in thalassemic patients and, when associated with normal systolic and diastolic function, is likely to be due to the associated moderate anemia rather than to myocardial failure (Intragumtornchai et al. 1994). Increases in ventricular mass index occur (Lattanzi et al. 1996) and changes in the reflectivity of ventricular myocardium have been attributed to iron overload (Lattanzi et al. 1993). The difficulty in correlating the findings on echocardiography with indirect indices of body iron load, such as the number of blood transfusions received and serum ferritin, has led some to suggest that iron loading is not the cause of LV failure (Kremastinos et al. 1984, 1985; Kremastinos 2007). These authors have demonstrated that myocarditis occurred in about 5% of a thalassemic cohort observed over 10 years, and had severe implications for LV function (Kremastinos et al. 1995). However, myocarditis is unlikely to account for many patients who develop severe LV impairment as a consequence of iron overload and its occurrence should not deflect clinicians from aggressively treating patients with heart failure with enhanced iron chelation, since in many cases this will lead to a resolution of ventricular impairment (Anderson et al. 2004).

More sophisticated ultrasound techniques, such as stress echocardiography and Doppler tissue imaging(DTI), may be able to identify problems before they progress to a life-threatening phase. We have shown that DTI can demonstrate regional abnormalities of LV function in a group of asymptomatic thalassemic patients, who had normal LV function by conventional methods of assessment (Vogel et al. 2003). It remains to be demonstrated that there is a relationship between DTI abnormalities and cardiac iron content measured by MRI and that these findings correlate with increased risk. Being able to measure myocardial iron content, using the MRI T2*, it should now be possible to clarify which ecchocardiographic parameters reliably reflect iron content and thus risk (Figures 29–5 and 29–6).

Nuclear Medicine

Radionuclear ventriculography, in particular the MUGA scan, has been used extensively in the past to define cardiac involvement in thalassemia, but suffers from the same criticism as echocardiographic-derived assessments of ventricular function that they identify a problem very late. Stress protocols, with dobutamine or exercise, should be able to detect changes earlier, but these have not often been employed.

Cardiac Magnetic Resonance/Imaging (CMR/MRI)

Magnetic resonance images decay with time along a monoexponential curve, which can be described by its time constant (T2). As the images decay they become darker. Magnetizable, or polar ions in tissues, such as iron, cause this decay to occur faster, thus have smaller T2 values. This susceptibility artifact produced by polar ions has been used to measure, noninvasively, the tissue content of iron including the heart (Johnston et al. 1989; Blankenberg et al. 1994; Mavrogeni et al. 1998; Ooi et al. 1999; Papanikolaou et al. 2000; Mavrogeni et al. 2007). Initially, gradient MRI was used to measure hepatic iron content having the capacity for increased sensitivity to low levels of iron content (Ernst et al. 1997). Modifications of these MRI protocols to measure a T2* parameter has allowed the measurement of intracardiac iron in a large cohort of thalassemia patients (Anderson et al. 2001; Westwood et al. 2003). The T2* measurement is related to T2, but

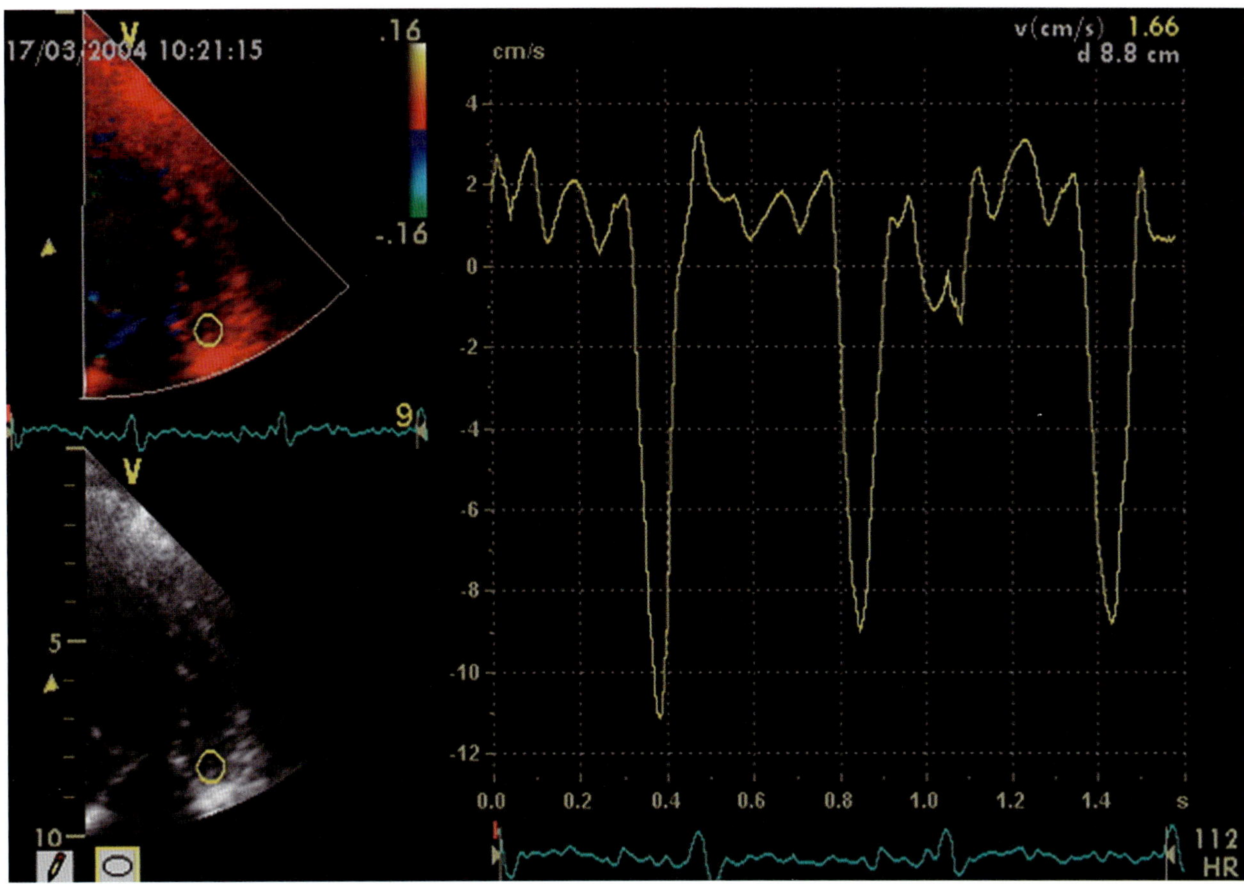

Figure 29–5 The same patient as shown in Figure 29–2, illustrating the technique of Doppler tissue imaging (DTI) used in this instance to measure mitral annular velocity. The panel on the right shows the velocity profile with a virtual absence of a systolic component (upward deflection of waveform) with a slowed and single downward diastolic phase.

was adopted due to its superiority over T2, in that fewer motion artifacts were generated, the heart images were much improved, and the length of time patients had to hold breath was greatly diminished. There is a highly significant correlation between MRI $T2^*$ and biopsy-assayed liver iron content (Anderson et al. 2001). It is a reasonable assumption that cardiac $T2^*$ will have a similar relationship to physical iron content as has been shown for the liver. Increasing iron content, as shown by low $T2^*$ are associated with increasingly impaired ventricular function (Tanner et al. 2006). The $T2^*$ also responds predictably to increased chelation treatment by showing a progressive rise toward normality associated with a slow improvement in ventricular function (Tanner et al. 2007). Impaired LV function was only seen in individuals with high iron content, but, importantly, a group with preserved function and high iron content was identified, who are at high risk of developing cardiac complications; it is this group that should attract the intensified treatment regimes known to improve cardiac outcomes (Aldouri et al. 1990). Unfortunately, the capital cost and lack of availability of MRI scanners in many nations will rule out MRI for many of the potential patients who would benefit from this technology.

Where possible we would advocate the use of MRI in all patients diagnosed with a condition likely to put them at risk of myocardial iron deposition. This imaging technique also lends itself to monitoring progress in individuals after changes in their treatment. Perhaps its greatest importance, however, will be the ability to systematically investigate different treatment strategies and their effectiveness in achieving the logical goal of reducing heart iron content. There is evidence that the oral iron chelator deferiprone may be better at preventing myocardial iron accumulation than DFO, although in the same cohort of patients this oral treatment appeared to be less effective at reducing liver iron content than DFO (Anderson et al. 2002; Tanner et al. 2006, 2007).

Treatment of Myocardial Iron Overload

The mainstay of treatment for iron overload remains the parenteral administration of DFO, using prolonged subcutaneous or intravenous infusions (Borgna-Pignatti and Cohen 1997). The dose should be 20 to 50 mg/kg/day infused over at least 8 to 24 hours on at least 5 to 7 days per week, (Gabutti and Piga 1996). The injections are made subcutaneously with the drug being injected by a mechanical pump, or more conveniently by pressure driven prefilled balloon containers (Lombardo et al. 1996; Canatan et al. 1999). On these doses the majority, but not all patients will achieve a negative iron balance. The treatment is difficult to administer, expensive, and hard to comply with, particularly by adolescents and young adults. Patients at high risk of complications, or those with established evidence of cardiac dysfunction need a more aggressive regime of treatment, which usually means constant 24-hour infusions for 7 days per week (Aldouri et al. 1990; Porter et al. 2005). These can be achieved using subcutaneous infusions, but more often, particularly in the more severely ill patients, constant

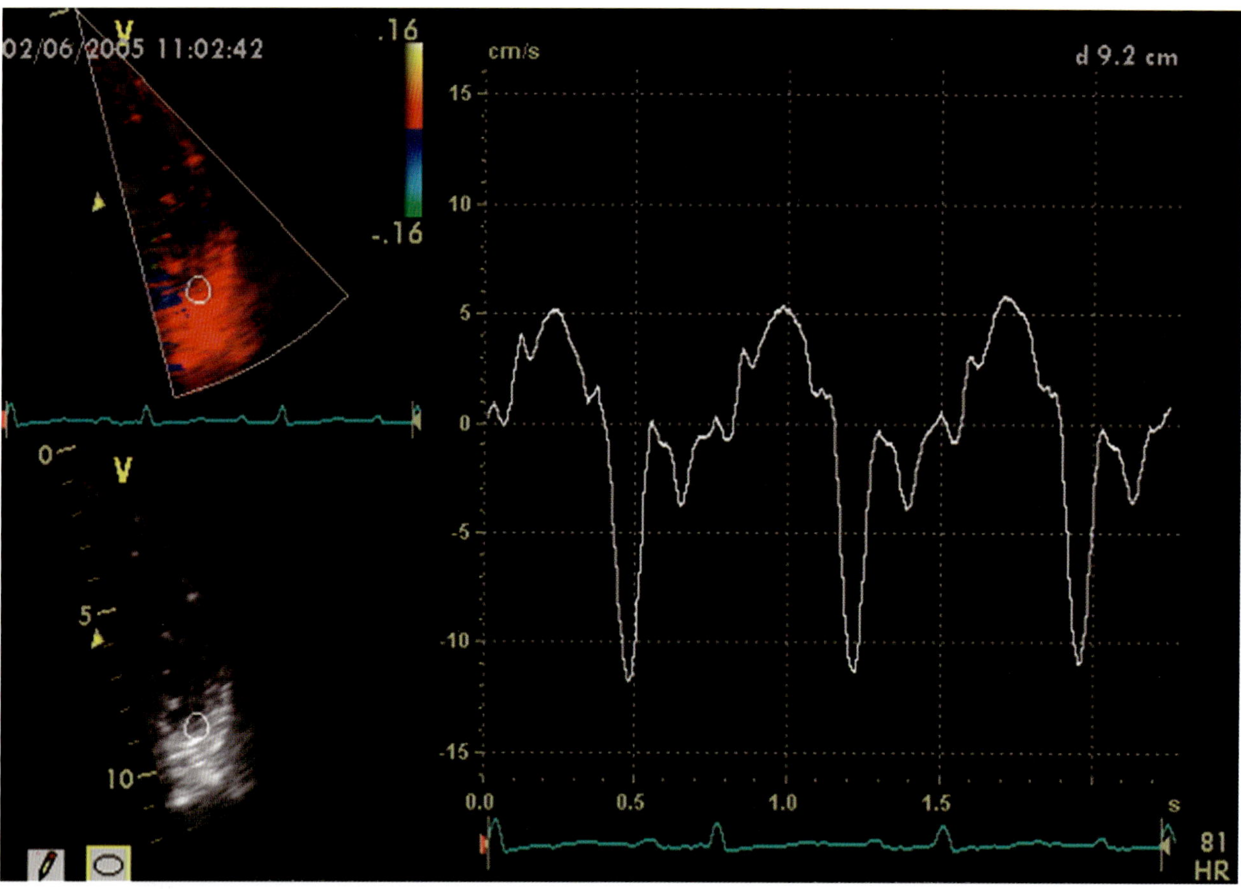

Figure 29–6 The same patient 14 months after intensive treatment now reveals a normal triphasic mitral annular velocity profile. The upward systolic wave is followed by downward E and A waves, all of which approximate normal values for thalassemia patients.

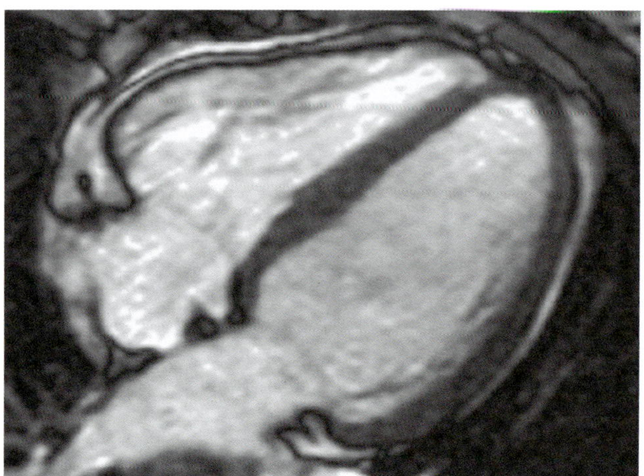

Figure 29–7 CMR long axis views of the heart of patients with severe β–thalassemia major. The figure shows an individual with little or no myocardial iron overload producing a high T2* value (>20 ms). The myocardium appears pale gray and the heart has normal wall thickness; the cine reconstruction revealed normal function with an ejection fraction (EF) of 65%.

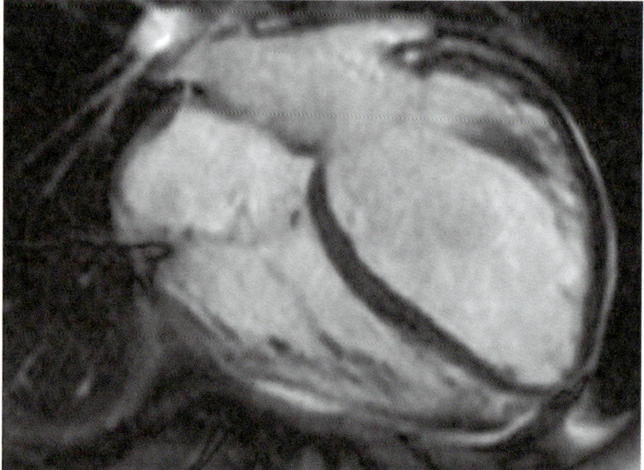

Figure 29–8 A patient with a more dilated ventricle with thin walls (poor EF of 48%) and dark color of the muscle due to iron overload, the T2* value was 8 ms.

intravenous infusions are more effective (Davis and Porter 2000). Chronic indwelling venous catheters or subcutaneous ports (Port-a-Cath) are preferable, since the chronic intravenous treatment may have to be continued for years to achieve effective iron removal from the tissues. Focusing the most intensive regimes on those at greatest risk is an important clinical aim. To this end, aggressive treatment regimes can easily be justified in patients with established myocardial dysfunction or symptoms. With the advent of MRI T2* encouraging such intensification of chelation treatment in patients with high heart iron content, before there is any evidence of ventricular impairment, is necessary.

Deferoxamine is not only difficult to use, but also remains very expensive and a proportion of patients develop allergies. An oral iron chelator, deferiprone (Ferriprox, ApoPharma; L1) has been available for some years (al-Refaie et al. 1995). Initially heralded as a great advance, it subsequently attracted adverse publicity from some quarters (Olivieri and Brittenham 1998). This negative data has been contrasted with positive results in several other studies, both retrospective (Anderson et al. 2002; Borgna-Pignatti et al. 2006) and prospective (Tanner et al. 2007). Deferiprone may have an advantage over DFO in its ability to enter the cell (Shalev et al. 1995) and remove accumulated iron from the cytosol and probably from mitochondria. Combining treatment with DFO and deferiprone may have a particular advantage (Hershko et al. 2004; Piga et al. 2005; Piga 2006; Tanner et al. 2007). The most recent addition to the chelation therapeutic field is another oral agent (desferasirox, Exjade; ICL370), which has been licensed for use by the FDA and the European regulatory authorities, although its clinical role has not yet been clarified (Shashaty et al. 2006; Barton 2007).

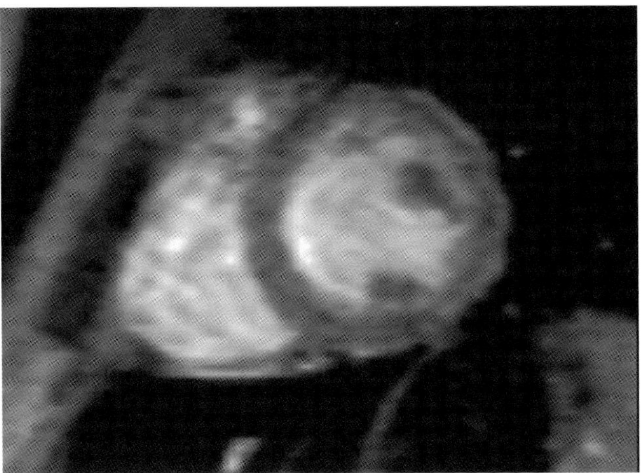

Figure 29–9 The short axis views through the left ventricles of the same patients as shown in Figures 29–7 and 29–8. The difference in myocardial gray coloration between the two patients is more obvious. The liver is glimpsed, underneath the heart in this figure and is very darkly colored. This patient had little or no myocardial iron but a heavily overloaded liver.

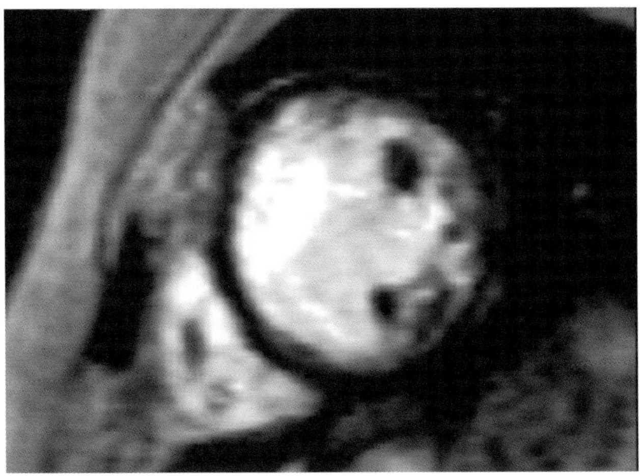

Figure 29–10 The short axis views through the left ventricles of the same patients as shown in figures 29–7 and 29–8. The difference in myocardial gray coloration between the two patients is more obvious. The liver is glimpsed, underneath the heart in Figure 29–9 and is very darkly colored. This patient had little or no myocardial iron but a heavily overloaded liver.

Specific Cardiological Care

The essence of treatment of cardiac disease should be aggressive chelation therapy to rapidly counteract iron toxicity and progressively remove excessive iron deposits (Davis and Porter 2000, 2002). In recent years, there has been a consistent trend to treat patients with thalassemia who have mild ventricular dysfunction with agents known to improve myocardial function in other forms of cardiomyopathy. Treatment of myocardial dysfunction is best undertaken using angiotensin-converting enzyme inhibitors (ACE inhibitors). In controlled trials, these agents have been shown to reduce mortality in nonthalassemic patients with established cardiomyopathy and to reduce the rate of appearance of heart failure in those with asymptomatic LV dysfunction. These results are very promising, and while their extension to heart failure in thalassemia remains conjectural, it is widely applied in clinical practice. The usual precautions for initiating treatment in patients who are well hydrated and starting at low doses are recommended. The dose should be increased to the maximum tolerated, limited by hypotension in patients with thalassemia.

Certain patients are unable to tolerate ACE inhibitors due to the development of chronic cough. Consideration should be made to treat these individuals with the angiotensin II receptor antagonists.

Digoxin may have a role as an inotropic agent in patients with cardiac dilatation accompanied by low blood pressure. Digoxin has a very specific role in the maintenance of reasonable ventricular rates in patients with established atrial fibrillation.

Diuretics are the mainstay in producing symptomatic improvement in those individuals who develop pulmonary congestion or signs of right-sided heart failure. Loop diuretics produce a reduction in circulating volume, which may considerably decrease preload. Therefore, these diuretics should be used with caution in patients with thalassemia. The tendency for thalassemia patients to have restrictive physiology, with impaired diastolic function, means that the reduction in preload due to a loop diuretic can produce a sudden fall in cardiac output. These effects

Table 29–1 Cardiac Investigations in Iron Overload Conditions

Investigation	Indication	Frequency	Justification
ECG	Baseline and all reviews	At least annual	Often nonspecific, but reveals progressive change, e.g., RVH/PHT
ECHO	Baseline	Annual if normal. To investigate change in status at any time.	Symptoms of cardiac failure often late, serial echo may give warning of high risk. Screening for PHT.
CMR	From age 11 years onward	May be needed up to twice yearly for T2* = <10 ms; yearly for T2* 11 to 20 ms; every 2 to 5 years if T2* >>20 ms	Only objective measure of myocardial iron burden. Identifies subgroup at high risk, in need of intensified Rx.

may precipitate prerenal failure. Loop diuretics should therefore be used cautiously and mainly in the late stages of disease.

Recent evidence supports the use of spironolactone as adjunctive treatment in nonthalassemic patients with cardiac failure. This and related agents reduce potassium depletion induced by loop diuretics and counteract the associated hyperaldosteronism. Potassium sparing agents can be used with ACE inhibitors, but require careful monitoring of electrolytes.

When dealing with severe congestive cardiac failure in hospital, it is advantageous to use constant intravenous infusions of loop diuretics. This aids careful titration of the doses of diuretic, on an hour to hour basis, according to the urine output, thus avoiding the dangerous situation of excessive diuresis, volume depletion, fall in cardiac output, and worsening of renal function. Inotropic support may be indicated in severe cases.

Managing these patients can be aided by utilizing biochemical markers of heart failure, BNP or pro-N-terminal BNP. Values are high in decompensated heart failure and fall in response to treatment; there is data to support delaying hospital discharge in patients until the BNP levels have reverted to normality.

In many instances, the use of drugs to treat relatively benign but symptomatic arrhythmias may produce greater morbidity and mortality than in untreated individuals. The decision to treat arrhythmias in patients with thalassemia must be carefully considered, bearing in mind that iron toxicity is the primary cause of this complication. Intensive chelation treatment can reduce arrhythmias (Davis and Porter 2000). In the majority of instances, the arrhythmias are supraventricular, although ventricular tachycardia may occur in seriously ill individuals. The development of arrhythmia may be associated with deteriorating ventricular function and can be improved by addressing the latter problem. For most supraventricular arrhythmias, reassurance of the patient is generally appropriate, whereas patients with ventricular arrhythmias require urgent attention to their associated high myocardial iron load, by the intensification of chelation.

β-blocking agents can also be used to control many arrhythmias and are indicated in patients with stabilized heart failure, as they improve the medium- to long-term prognosis. Dosages should be low at first with careful slow upward titration over days and weeks. In heart failure, Carvidelol and Bisoprolol have a special role and Sotalol may have advantages for the prophylactic treatment of AF.

Amiodarone has a very wide spectrum of effectiveness against supraventricular and ventricular arrhythmias and produces a survival benefit in nonthalassemic individuals with life-threatening ventricular dysrhythmias. It does, however, have an enormous potential for side effects. Among these side effects, disturbances of thyroid function are of particular relevance in patients with thalassemia.

The role of other drugs such as calcium antagonists and class I antiarrhythmic agents has yet to be established. Generally, these agents should be avoided, since they have a tendency to be negatively inotropic. Their use has not been widespread, since arrhythmias tend to be associated with more severe levels of myocardial impairment. Without more formal study, the use of such drugs cannot yet be recommended to patients with thalassemia. In patients who fail to respond to iron chelation therapy and pharmacological intervention, cardioversion may be considered. Increasingly patients with paroxysmal or established AF are being offered the opportunity of electrophysiological investigation and ablation therapy where indicated. The use of these technologies is set to increase in this cohort of patients.

A few patients have undergone cardiac transplantation for severe, irreversible cardiac damage, and this procedure has also been combined with liver transplantation (Olivieri et al. 1994). The outcome of transplant in patients with thalassemia needs to be carefully studied to determine the effectiveness of this approach. The presence of iron-induced damage to other organs may adversely affect the outcome of heart transplant. If surgery is successful, intensive chelation therapy is still required to remove iron from other organs and prevent iron accumulation in the transplanted heart.

Hemochromatosis

Hemochromatosis was first described in the 19th century as a disease characterized by the constellation of diabetes, bronze pigmentation of the skin, and hepatic cirrhosis. The hereditary nature of the disease was subsequently recognized and finally the *HFE* gene responsible for the disease was identified in 1996. In addition to the classic *HFE*-related hemochromatosis, mutations in other non-*HFE* genes involved in iron metabolism can result in iron overload states.

Classic *HFE*-related hemochromatosis exhibits autosomal recessive transmission and is caused by mutations in *HFE* gene on chromosome 6p21.3. The function of the HFE protein is not clearly understood. It structurally bears resemblance to human leukocyte antigen (HLA) type I proteins but is not capable of binding antigenic peptides or iron. Under normal circumstances the HFE protein combines with β_2-microglobulin to form a heterodimer, in a manner similar to other HLA I proteins, , and is then expressed on the cell surface of many cells involved in iron metabolism including duodenal crypt cells and macrophages. Once expressed on the cell surface, HFE interacts with transferin receptor 1 and other proteins to modulate the uptake of transferin-bound iron (Andrews 1999; Pietrangelo 2004a). More than half a century after von Recklinghausen coined the term hemochromatosis in 1889, the inherited nature of the disease was described by Sheldon in 1935 (Edwards and Kushner 1993). Initial studies to identify the genetic cause of hemochromatosis established a link within HLA-A3 region on chromosome 6. It was recognized that particular HLA-A3 genes were coinherited with the then unidentified hemochromatosis gene, and segregated in affected families. Pedigree analysis finally demonstrated that hemochromatosis was inherited as an autosomal recessive condition. The breakthrough came with the identification of the HFE gene in 1996 (Feder et al. 1996).A single point mutation of 845 G→A causes the substitution of cysteine to tyrosine at position 282 (C282Y) of the HFE protein. This mutation disrupts the normal interaction with β_2-microglobulin. This in turn prevents the expression of the HFE-β_2-microglobulin heterodimer to the cell surface and hence the interaction with the transferin receptor 1 involved in iron uptake. Another point mutation of 187C→G results in the substitution of histidine by aspartic acid at position 63 (H63D) of the HFE protein. The H63D mutation, however, unlike C282Y does not affect cell surface expression of HFE. The exact mechanism by which these mutations result in iron overload is not fully understood (Feder et al. 1996; Pietrangelo 2004a). The *HFE* genotype in clinically diagnosed hemochromatosis probands varies depending on the geographical population studied. In Ireland 2.6 % of clinically diagnosed individuals were found to be heterozygotes for C282Y, 89.7% were C282Y homozygotes, 1.3% were H63D heterozygotes, none were H63D homozygotes, 3.9% were compound heterozygotes

C282Y/H63D, and in 2.6% neither mutation was identified. In Great Britain, 0.9% of clinically diagnosed probands were found to be heterozygotes for C282Y; 91% were C282Y homozygotes, none were H63D heterozygotes, 0.9% were H63D homozygotes, 2.6% were compound heterozygotes C282Y/H63D, and in 4.3% of probands neither mutation was identified. In Italy, a different picture is seen with 5.9% of clinically diagnosed individuals found to be heterozygotes for C282Y; 64.5% were C282Y homozygotes, 8.6% were H63D heterozygotes, 1.6% were H63D homozygotes, 5.4% were compound heterozygotes C282Y/H63D, and in 14% neither mutation was found (Hanson et al. 2001). The frequency of C282Y in the general population has also been studied. In Europe as a whole, the average prevalence of C282Y heterozygosity is 9.2% whilst the homozygous state is found in 0.4% of the general population. However, the C282Y mutation is more frequently encountered in northern European populations rather than in south and eastern Europe. In Ireland, the prevalence of the C282Y heterozygote state is a staggering 28.4%, in Iceland the frequency is 6.5% to 10%, and in Denmark the frequency is 11% to 13.7%. South and eastern European populations have a much lower frequency, and in Spain the C282Y heterozygote prevalence is 3.8% to 4.5%, in Greece 2.5% and this allele is not found at all in Turkey. In Asian, African, Middle East, and Australian populations C282Y homozygotes are not reported and the C282Y heterozygotes are rare (Hanson et al. 2001). It is likely that the C282Y mutation arose from a single Celtic or Viking ancestor approximately 2,000 years ago and spread via migration to other European populations (Pietrangelo 2004a). It is postulated that there are selection pressures favoring the *HFE* mutations. Lack of the HFE protein on the cell surface may provide protection from infectious agents that exploit the HFE protein as a receptor to gain entry into the cells. Similar protective mechanisms have been proposed for cystic fibrosis where homozygosity to the most common mutation results in absent cystic fibrosis transmembrane regulator (CFTR) proteins on cell surfaces. *Salmonella typhii* uses CFTR protein to enter the enterocytes, and therefore in heterozygotes with reduced CFTR expression intracellular infection is hampered. Another selective advantage of the HFE mutations is protection against anemia from a variety of pathologies including multiple pregnancies, diet, malaria, and intestinal parasites (Rochette et al. 1999). H63D carrier frequency is 22% in Europe, and ranges from 9% in Greenland to 32.3% in Spain. In North America the H63D allele frequency was 23%. In Africa and Asia, however, the incidence is lower, 5.4% and 2.8% respectively (Hanson et al. 2001).

Two processes contribute to iron overload in haemochromatosis, the enhanced gastrointestinal absorption of dietary iron and the excessive release of iron into the circulation from macrophages. Both processes are thought to be caused by low hepcidin levels demonstrated in all of the haemochromatosis syndromes. Hepcidin is an iron regulatory hormone and inhibits iron release in the circulation from the intestine and macrophages by interacting with the main iron export protein, ferroportin. It is thought that haemojuvelin, transferrin receptor 2, and HFE modulate the hepcidin-ferroportin axis and thus mutations in these genes also cause hereditary haemochromatosis (Pietrangelo et al. 2006b).

Clinical Features of HFE-Related Hemochromatosis

Phenotypic expression is variable, and difficult to define. It is not clear whether biochemical evidence of disease on the basis of high transferin saturations provides an adequate marker of expression of phenotype or whether the development of end-organ involvement provides a more appropriate definition. Irrespective of the measure used for phenotypic expression, there is considerable penetrance. Most homozygotes for C282Y evolve insidiously from the initial stage of high plasma iron, characterized by high transferin saturations, to the next stage of hemochromatosis, characterized by high tissue iron levels illustrated biochemically by elevated ferritin levels, and finally to the expression of clinically evident end-organ damage. Some C282Y homozygotes never exhibit even the earliest biochemical abnormalities of iron metabolism. This variable penetrance depends on a number of other genetic as well as environmental factors, which modify the phenotypic expression of a particular hemochromatosis genotype. Females of child-bearing age have a third of the rate of end-organ involvement as males, presumably due to the influence of menses and/or multiple pregnancies attenuating progressive iron overload. Intestinal infections such as hookworm, which cause chronic anemia, will delay the development of end-organ disease in certain populations. The rate of iron tissue deposition is affected by the expression of other genes that are involved in iron metabolism such as hepcidin (Pietrangelo and Trautwein 2004) and haptoglobulin, whilst end-organ damage is modified by the expression of genes that control fibrosis, tissue repair, and oxidative stress.

More recently it was hypothesized that carriage of the *HFE* gene mutations might increase the susceptibility to ischemic heart disease, but these suggestions have been refuted by several large studies (Gunn et al. 2004; Ellervik et al. 2005; Goland and Malnick 2006).

The presence of other genetic diseases such as hereditary spherocytosis, β-thalassemia minor, idiopathic refractory sideroblastic anemia, or sporadic porphyria cutanea tarda affects the development of iron overload in homozygotes or heterozygotes for hemochromatosis (Edwards and Kushner 1993). Similarly, the presence of *HFE* mutations can modify the course of other diseases. In hepatitis C infection the presence of the C282Y or H63D mutations increases the risk of cirrhosis and hepatic fibrosis (Erhardt et al. 2003; Pietrangelo 2003). The complex interplay of *HFE* mutations with modifier genes, and environmental factors, make the translation of molecular genetic findings to clinical phenotypes challenging.

The incidence of hemochromatosis-related arthropathy, cirrhosis, and deranged liver function tests in clinically unselected homozygote relatives of homozygote probands has been investigated. Of the male relatives screened for hemochromatosis-related disease, 85% were found to have iron overload and 38% had at least one of the above mentioned hemochromatosis-related conditions. Of the female homozygote relatives screened, 68% were found to have evidence of iron overload, and 10% had at least one disease-related condition. Interestingly, male relatives of probands that were diagnosed after the development of end-organ damage were more likely to develop disease when compared to male relatives of probands that were diagnosed via screening, which occurred prior to clinically significant end-organ involvement. Male probands that were diagnosed via screening, as well as male homozygote relatives were also younger than clinically diagnosed probands, with a mean age of 37, 41, and 51 years respectively. This relationship, however, did not hold for the respective female groups. Ferritin levels were higher in the clinically affected probands in both males and females. Transferrin saturation was not significantly different in clinically affected probands, probands detected by screening, and relatives of probands in males, but in females the homozygote relatives were found to have a lower transferring saturation. Fifty two percent of male homozygote relatives aged >40 years developed hemochromatosis-related conditions whilst, 16% of female homozygote relatives >50 years developed such complications. Unfortunately, the incidence of hemochromatosis-related cardiac disease, as well as diabetes was not investigated, as it was difficult to be certain that hemochromatosis was the only underlying cause for these conditions. This study clearly illustrates the effects of sex and age on the incidence of disease, as well as other unidentified genetic and environmental parameters in the phenotypic expression of disease (Bulaj et al. 2000).

Similarly, development of cardiac disease is not inevitable in hemochromatosis. Cardiac disorders have been reported on 52% of death certificates of patients with hemochromatosis (Yang et al. 1998). It is estimated that up to 35% of patients with hemochromatosis experience congestive cardiac failure and 36% develop arrhythmias (Hanson et al. 2001). However, the incidence of lethal cardiomyopathy appears to be variable [3 of 53 patients in one series (Niederau et al. 1985)], although still far in excess of the incidence expected in a normal population (Niederau et al. 1996).

In addition to biventricular dilation and dysfunction similar to that seen in idiopathic dilated cardiomyopathy, haemochromatosis has been associated with isolated right or left ventricular impairment (Dabestani 1984). Diastolic dysfunction, increased left ventricular wall thickness and mass may be early manifestations. Restriction has also been reported but is not common (Cutler et al. 1908). The haemodynamic effects of cirrhosis, another common complication of haemoachromatosis should be considered when evaluating the cardiac status of patients with haemochromatosis. The presence of cirrhosis is associated with a hyperdynamic circulation with a high cardiac output and low systemic vascular resistance. The blood pressure tends to be low and accompanied by tachycardia. Systolic function at rest is typically normal but cardiac reserve in response to exercise is limited. Diastolic dysfunction is also common (Moller et al. 2002). These changes are not related to cardiac iron overload.

Other Forms of Hemochromatosis

HFE mutations account for most, but not all cases of hereditary hemochromatosis. Since the identification on the *HFE* mutations, other non-*HFE*-related genetic defects have subsequently been identified. Currently, the Online Mendelian Inheritance in Man (OMIM) database (http://www.ncbi.nlm.nih.gov/sites/entrez) includes four types of non-HFE-related hemochromatosis caused by mutations in genes involved in iron metabolism. *HFE*-related hemochromatosis is classified as type 1 hemochromatosis. The four main types of non-*HFE* hereditary hemochromatosis are caused by mutations in the hemojuvelin, hepcidin, transferrin receptor 2, and ferroportin genes.

Hemochromatosis type 2A (or juvenile hereditary hemochromatosis) is an autosomal recessive disease caused by mutations in the hemojuvelin (HJV) gene on chromosome 1q21. It was first identified in 2004, in 12 unrelated families of French, Greek, and Canadian origins and six different mutations were described (Papanikolaou et al. 2004). Since then many other mutations have been identified, which are mostly private and restrict themselves to specific families. However, some mutations such as the G320V substitution found in the majority of family members from the seminal study of Greek, French, and Canadian families in 2004 are more widespread, but the significance of this finding is unclear (Wallace and Subramaniam 2007). The function of hemojuvelin is not known. It is expressed in the liver, heart, and skeletal muscle. Hepcidin levels are low in patients with hemojuvelin mutations, and hemojuvelin is thought to be involved in hepcidin regulation and hence iron metabolism (Papanikolaou et al. 2004). Juvenile hemochromatosis produces a more aggressive disease than the classic *HFE*-related form of hemochromatosis. Transferin saturation and ferritin levels tend to be higher, with a mean age of presentation of 23.5 years with both sexes being equally affected. Hypogonadism is the commonest presenting complication, and there is a higher incidence of cardiomyopathy and impaired glucose metabolism when compared to *HFE*-related hemochromatosis, but the incidence of cirrhosis and arthropathy is similar. Survival is significantly affected, and it is not uncommon for patients to succumb to cardiac complications before the fourth decade of life. However, heterozygote relatives do not show evidence of iron overload (De Gobbi et al. 2002).

Hemochromatosis type 2B is another juvenile hereditary hemochromatosis syndrome, but it is rarer than the 2A form. It is also an autosomal recessive disease caused by mutations in the gene encoding hepcidin antimicrobial peptide (HAMP) on chromosome19q13. Two mutations (93delG and 166C→T) were originally described in 2003 when affected individuals from two families were investigated (Roetto et al. 2003). Hepcidin is a protein produced by hepatocytes, which regulates iron absorption in gut and iron release from macrophages, probably through an interaction with ferroportin. When plasma iron levels are high, hepcidin production increases leading to a suppression of iron release from enterocytes and macrophages. The reverse occurs in iron-deficient state. Hepcidin may be acting as an iron regulatory hormone. Type 2B hemochromatosis shares the same aggressive phenotype with type 2A, mirroring the importance of both genes in regulating iron metabolism (Pietrangelo 2004a).

Hemochromatosis type 3 (HFE3) is an autosomal recessive disorder, caused by mutations in the transferrin receptor 2 (*TFR2*) gene on chromosome 7q22. A nonsense mutation causing astop signal at position 250 (Y250X), was first described in a Sicilian family. None of the family members were homozygous for the C282Y mutation, and all affected individuals were found to be homozygous for Y250X, whilst the obligate carriers were Y250X heterozygotes (Camaschella et al. 2000). This was the first non-*HFE*-related hemochromatosis described. Subsequently, further mutations involving the transferrin receptor 2 gene have been identified (Hofmann et al. 2002). The mechanism by which *TFR2* mutations cause hemochromatosis is not known. The TFR2 protein is similar to the TFR1 protein, which is responsible for the uptake of transferrin bound iron to the intracellular compartment. TFR2 is likely to be involved in regulating iron metabolism via hepcidin but is not directly involved in iron transport itself. A few cases of TFR2-related hemochromatosis have been reported and the clinical features appear similar to the ones encountered in the classic *HFE*-related form, with gradual iron overload and primarily hepatic, endocrine, and cardiac involvement, during the fourth and fifth decade of life, although with variable penetrance (Pietrangelo 2004a).

Hemochromatosis type 4 (HFE4), unlike the other types of hereditary hemochromatosis is an autosomal dominant disease caused by mutations of the *SLC40A1* gene (also known as *IREG1*, *MTP1*, and *SLC40A3*) on chromosome 2q32, which encodes for ferroportin. An alternative name for type 4 hemochromatosis is thus ferroportin disease(s). Autosomal dominant transmission of hemochromatosis had been well recognized but the underlying genetic cause was elusive for many years. The breakthrough came when a large Dutch family exhibiting autosomal dominant transmission of hemochromatosis was investigated, and an A→C transversion at position 734 was found in all clinically affected patients.

This transversion results in the substitution of a highly conserved asparagine by histidine at position 144 (N144H) of ferroportin (Njajou et al. 2001; Hofmann et al. 2002). Ferroportin is a transmembrane iron transporter that is found on enterocytes and is involved in the transfer of iron through the gut wall to the blood; it is also found on hepatocytes and the reticuloendothelial system, where ferroportin is involved in iron recycling. Ferroportin downregualtion is controlled by hepcidin (Wallace and Subramaniam 2007). Since the original description, more ferroportin mutations have been identified in patients with autosomal dominant hemochromatosis (Cremonesi et al. 2005). Most *SCL40A1* mutations confine themselves to specific families. However, some mutations such as the V162del are more widespread and affect families in Greece, Italy, the United Kingdom, Sri Lanka, Australia, and Austria, but the significance of this broader geographical distribution is unclear (Wallace and Subramaniam 2007).

The clinical course of ferroportin diseases is variable and different from the classic form of the disease; in the typical form of ferroportin disease, the early stages are characterized by an elevation in ferritin but not transferrin saturation. There is accumulation of iron, primarily in the Kupffer cells of the liver rather than hepatic parenchyma. With disease progression the transferrin saturation rises with eventual deposition of iron in the hepatic parenchyma (Pietrangelo 2004b; Cremonesi et al. 2005). In addition, whilst venesection is well tolerated in *HFE*-related hemochromatosis, some patients with typical ferroportin disease develop anemia. An atypical form of ferroportin disease with a clinical course similar to the classic *HFE*-related hemochromatosis is also encountered. The atypical presentation is thought to be the result of mutations impairing the interaction with hepcidin leading to increased iron absorption and release from the reticuloendothelial system (Wallace et al. 2007).

Management of Hemochromatosis

Despite a long history of clinical recognition, there is surprisingly scant data on optimal management of hemochromatosis patients. Regular venesection (500 mL removed every 1 to 2 weeks, until ferritin normalizes or patient becomes anemic) is the mainstay of therapy (Crosby 1991), but prospective or controlled studies are not available (Whitlock et al. 2006). Survival is good and improvement in most clinical features of the disease follows treatment. In particular, cardiac involvement has been shown to improve (Cutler et al. 1980; Candell-Riera et al. 1983). However, some symptoms such as exhaustion and joint pains may not improve to the same degree. The presence of cirrhosis has historically been shown to carry an adverse prognosis even after removal of accumulated iron (Niederau et al. 1996). With the advent of noninvasive methods to assess tissue iron burden, particularly of the heart, more objective prospective clinical assessment becomes a possibility (Pietrangelo et al. 2006). Extending our observations for thalassemia patients to iron overload in hemochromatosis our experience would support the use of chelation to help clear iron stores quickly and avoid complications of cardiac failure,; this approach has already been reported in a severe case of juvenile hemochromatosis (Fabio et al. 2007).

Box 29–4 Hemochromatosis

Classic *HFE* hemochromatosis is an autosomal recessive disease characterized by mutations of the *HFE* gene on chromosome 6.

HFE gene product modulates iron metabolism by an unknown mechanism.

C282Y is the commonest HFE mutation.

Phenotypic expression is variable and depends on other genetic and environmental factors that affect iron metabolism and end-organ damage.

Approximately, one third of patients develop congestive heart failure and arrhythmias.

Non-*HFE* hemochromatosis is caused by mutations affecting a variety of other genes involved in iron metabolism.

Non-*HFE* hemochromatosis is less common but can be more aggressive.

Sickle Disease

In contrast to the thalassemias where there is a reduction of the rate of production of a particular globin chain, sickle cell disease and other related disorders are caused by mutations resulting in a change in the structure of the globin chains, which leads to loss of normal function. These disorders include the heterozygote state sickle cell trait (HbAS), , the homozygote state sickle cell disease (HbSS), and the compound heterozygote state when the sickle mutation is combined with other structurally abnormal hemoglobins such as HbSC, HbSE, as well as in combination with the thalassemias.

Sickle hemoglobin was first described by Linus Pauling in 1949 based on the abnormal electrophoretic properties of HbS, conferred by the substitution of the negatively charged glutamic acid by the nonpolar valine at position 6 of the β-globin chain. This results from a point mutation of the β-globin gene on chromosome 11. The glutamic to valine amino acid substitution leads to a fundamental change in the physical and chemical properties of sickle hemoglobin ($\alpha_2\beta^s_2$) under conditions of hypoxia. In the deoxygenated state $\alpha_2\beta^s_2$ undergoes a conformational change, which allows hydrophobic regions of $\alpha_2\beta^s_2$, formed by the substitution of glutamate by valine, to bond with each other and form polymers. The process of polymerization is cooperative and results in the formation of rope-like strands composed of 14 $\alpha_2\beta^s_2$ units arranged in seven pairs. When these bundles orient themselves with the long axis of a red blood cell the characteristic sickle shape is produced. It is the ability of deoxygenated sickle hemoglobin to polymerize that initiates a cascade of events responsible for the clinical manifestations of sickle cell disease (Bunn 1997).

Box 29–5 Sickle Cell Syndromes

- Sickle cell anemia—homozygous HbSS.
- Coinheritance with abnormal globin genes.
  - HbC gene—HbSC disease.
  - β-thalassemia genes (β^0 or β^+)—Sickle β-thalassemia (β^0 or β^+)
  - β-globin structural variants—e.g., HbSD disease, HbSO arab.
- Subcatergorization by α-genotype.
  - 65% HbSS have normal α-genotype.
  - 30% HbSS have 1 α-gene deletion.
  - 5% HbSS have 2 α-gene deletions.
- α-gene deletions lead to milder anemia but increased frequency of painful crises.

Apart from the development of deoxygenated HbS, $\alpha_2\beta^s_2$ polymerization is modulated by a number of other factors that have the potential to change the severity of disease. High intracellular HbS concentrations facilitate the polymerization. During sickling the red cell membranes are damaged leading to deregulation of intracellular volume homeostasis. The damaged red cell membranes allow excess cytosolic Ca^{2+} to develop, which in turn enhances intracellular K^+ and water loss via Ca^{2+}-dependent K^+ channels. Enhanced K^+/Cl^- cotransporter activity in red blood cells containing $\alpha_2\beta^s_2$ also contributes to intracellular dehydration. Intracellular dehydration increases HbS intracellular concentration and therefore the tendency for sickling (Bunn 1997). HbF ($\alpha_2\gamma_2$) persisting post partum prevents polymerization of $\alpha_2\beta^s_2$ by interfering with the crosslinking $\alpha_2\beta^s_2$. In vitro experiments have shown that HbS and HbF form an asymmetric $\alpha_2\beta^s\gamma$ tetramer that interrupts the intratetrameric contacts of HbS preventing sickling. Similar effects have been noted with HbA_2 ($\alpha_2\beta^s\delta$) (Nagel et al. 1979).

Once red blood cells undergo sickling they adhere to the vascular endothelium and cause the vasoocclusion responsible for many of the clinical manifestations of sickle cell disease, particularly painful crises and end-organ damage. The severity of the vasoocclusive crises has been associated with the strength of erythrocyte endothelial adhesion. Sickle cells adhere to vascular endothelium 20 times more powerfully than normal red cells. Adhesion to vascular endothelium causes trapping of the sickle cells in the microvasculature, which increases their transit time under hypoxic conditions promoting even more sickling and therefore vascular occlusion (Kaul et al. 1989). Adhesion to the vasculature occurs either directly or via bridging proteins and stimulates the expression of even more vascular adhesion molecules and further vasoconstriction. In addition, there is activation of the coagulation system and platelets during crises exacerbating blood vessel occlusion. Intravascular hemolysis leads to nitric oxide consumption by the hemolyzed sickle cells, encouraging local vasoconstriction. The resultant failure of vasoregulation accounts particularly for some of the clinical features of sickle cell disease, such as pulmonary hypertension, priapism, and leg ulcers and contributes to the most devastating complication, stroke (Switzer et al. 2006; Kato et al. 2007). White blood cells are also involved in the process of vascular obstruction. They are found in increased numbers and in a state of activation in sickle cell disease. They adhere to the vascular endothelium, to each other, to red blood cells, and platelets. Due to their bigger size, leukocytes may be contributing more to vasoocclusion mechanically than the smaller sickle cells (Okpala 2004, 2006).

Hemoglobinopathies such as sickle cell disease are commonly found in malarial endemic areas. The highest frequency for the sickle hemoglobin allele is found in equatorial Africa, where >20% of the population of Cameroon, Zaire, Uganda, and Kenya are carriers. A similar frequency is observed in eastern Saudi Arabia and parts of India. Around the Mediterranean, the Middle East, and Iran it is generally seen in <5% of the population, but variations within populations exist. In the New World, sickle hemoglobin allele is found only in immigrants who originate from the Old World and the mutation has never been reported in native American Indians (Flint et al. 1998).

The geographical distribution and the high incidence of sickle cell disease can be explained by the advantage conferred to heterozygotes in populations residing in endemic regions with falciparum malaria. Falciparum malaria causes high childhood mortality and has been one of the most powerful selective pressures in recent human evolution. The heterozygote carrier state has a 10-fold reduction in the risk of developing life-threatening malaria, which offsets the fatalities caused by the homozygote state. The HbS allele is found in 10% of the native population in malaria endemic regions testifying the strength of the selection pressure imposed by malaria. It appears that different populations living in malaria endemic regions have developed HbS independently, resulting in four different haplotypes. The mechanism by which sickle trait protects against severe malaria is not fully understood. It may involve suppression of malarial growth or enhanced clearance of infected red cells by the spleen. HbE also protects against malaria and has developed independently in Southeast Asia, whilst HbS is mostly found in Africa. Within Africa however, there is more variability and the Dogon people of Mali have a higher incidence of HbC rather than HbS, which also confers an advantage against severe malaria. The persistence and high frequency of HbE, HbC, and HbS are all driven by malaria, but the reason behind the geographical distribution of each allele is unclear. Glucose 6 phosphate dehydrogenase deficiency, ovalocytosis, and Duffy negative blood group are other examples of polymorphisms that have developed as a result of the selection pressure of malaria in different populations (Kwiatkowski 2005).

The underlying hemoglobin genotype remains an important determinant of disease severity, affecting both morbidity and mortality. Patients with HbSS and $HbS\beta^o$ disease have a more severe phenotype than patients with HbSC (β6 Glu→Lys) and $HbS\beta^+$-thalassemia. Those with HbSS and $HbS\beta^0$ suffer a higher incidence of painful crises and acute chest syndromes. HbSS patients have also been shown to have a higher incidence of cerebrovascular accidents as well as bacteremia, which carries a higher mortality rate, when compared to non-HbSS patients (Gill et al. 1995). However, certain complications of such as renal papillary necrosis, proliferative retinopathy, and thromboembolic events are more abundant in HbSC than in HbSS subjects (Ashley-Koch et al. 2000).

The effects of the hemoglobin genotype on mortality are also evident. In a US cohort of pediatric patients the incidence of death in patients with HbSS was 0.62 per 100 person-years compared to 0.2 per 100 person-years for HbSC patients. Approximately 85% of HbSS patients were expected to survive to the age of 20 years of age compared to 95% of HbSC patients. The peak incidence of death in HbSS patients was between the ages of 1and 3 years and related to infections. No deaths were reported in sickle thalassemia patients ($HbS\beta^+$ or $HbS\beta^o$) (Leikin et al. 1989). These mortality figures are based on patients treated in the United States and these findings may not apply in other populations. Overall survival in adulthood is also compromised by sickle cell disease, even in the most advanced societies, with a median age of death of 42 years for males and 48 years for females, with only very few patients reaching their 60s. Patients with HbSC have a median age of death of 60 and 68 years for males and females respectively. The risk of death was higher in more symptomatic patients. Improved survival was seen with higher HbF levels (Platt et al. 1994). The survival of sickle cell patients is increasing with improved medical care, and the "medical environment" is modifying the course of the disease.

When considering $\alpha_2\beta^s_2$ homozygotes only, there is still a large phenotypic variation in disease expression. In a cohort of 280 pediatric HbSS patients in Jamaica who were enrolled at birth after umbilical cord blood screening, 15% had a benign course that was arbitrarily defined as having less than four sickle-related complications by the age of 13 years. Four out of the 43 patients with "benign" sickle cell anemia had no sickle anemia complications at all by the age of 13 years. This benign phenotype associated with the presence of the normal complement of α-globin genes and higher HbF levels (Thomas et al. 1997). Pleiotropic genes have polymorphisms that modify the phenotype either independently or by interacting with other similar genes. These modifier or epistatic genes account for some of the interindividual variability seen in sickle cell anemia. Therefore, HbSS is a monogenic defect but sickle cell anemia is a multigenic disease, which further interacts with environmental factors to result in a spectacular phenotypic variability (Nagel 2001). An increasing number of modifier genes is being recognized. High levels of HbF have been associated with milder phenotypes in HbSS. HbSS is coinherited with one of four major β-globin-like gene clusters that contain regulatory genes affecting HbF expression. Coinheritance of the Senegal or the Arab-Indian haplotype, characterized by a single nucleotide polymorphism at 158 nucleotides 5' to the Gγ-globin gene in patients with HbSS leads to higher HbF and a tendency for milder disease when compared to inheritance of the Bantu haplotype which is associated with lower HbF levels. Other regulatory components of HbF expression probably exist within the β-globin-like cluster as well as other chromosomes but have not yet been clearly defined. Coinheritance of α-thalassemia occurs in 30% of HbSS patients as both gene defects are common in malaria endemic populations. Coinheritance of α-thalassemia has the effect of reducing $\alpha_2\beta^s_2$ concentration and thus reducing vasoocclusive complications of sickle cell anemia such as cerebrovascular accidents. Additional genes regulating secondary pathological phenomena in sickle cell disease such as inflammation, vasoreactivity, and cell adhesion are also likely to play a role in modifying disease expression and a number of single nucleotide polymorphisms have been linked to some phenotypes (Steinberg and Adewoye 2006). Our knowledge of the environmental factors modulating sickle cell disease is much more limited.

Clinical Complications and Management

Sickle cell disease is characterized by a normocytic, normochromic anemia with an increased reticulocyte count and evidence of chronic hemolysis. The tendency for autosplenectomy means that there is frequently an increased platelet count and marrow activity resulting in elevated white cell numbers. Folate deficiency complicates the situation and is prevented by prophylactic supplementation, which also serves to diminish homocystine concentration. Blood transfusion may be indicated in particular circumstances but, increasingly, exchange transfusion aiming to reduce the level of HbS to <30% is offered, particularly in the treatment of painful crisis, prior to planned surgery and to prevent stroke. Alternative approaches to transfusion include the use of erythropoietin or hydroxyurea to increase the proportion of fetal hemoglobin (HbF).

Acute pain syndromes vary in frequency and severity between patients and in the same patient at different times. They generally produce pain in the long bones and in joints, but may involve the scalp, face, chest, or abdomen, and are sometimes preceded by a prodromal phase of milder symptoms, including paresthesiae. The acute chest syndrome is the commonest cause of death in HbSS and may accompany or follow a painful crisis. They are characterized by chest pain, fever, hypoxia, dyspnea, pulmonary infiltrates, and worsening anemia. Although primarily an acute pulmonary condition, pleural and pericardial effusion, hypoxemia, myocardial injury, and pulmonary embolism can result in heart failure or exacerbate preexisting heart failure. Treatment is generally supportive, but exchange transfusion can shorten the duration of the acute illness and thus reduce mortality.

Box 29–6 Sickle Cell Syndromes

An autosomal recessive hemoglobinopathy caused by a point mutation of the β-globin gene on chromosome 11.

Sickle hemoglobin has an abnormal structure and behavior under hypoxic conditions.

Variable phenotypic expression as a result of interactions with other genes and the environment.

Sickle cell disease is associated with pulmonary hypertension.

The life expectancy in the United States is 30 years less for HbSS sufferers than for normal black population.

Pulmonary hypertension has been increasingly recognized as an important complication of sickle cell disease, with between 10% and 30% of adults having evidence of elevated pulmonary pressures, usually detected by echocardiography and indicated by an increased tricuspid valve regurgitant jet velocity (>2.5 m/s) (Gladwin and Kato 2005; Barnett et al. 2008). Despite most of the increases in pulmonary pressure being relatively modest, in the context of sickle cell disease an increased mortality of up to 40% within 40 months has been reported. Acute pulmonary hypertension complicating severe acute chest syndromes has long been recognized and attributed to vascular occlusion, but the more insidious chronic pulmonary hypertension is of more complex origin. It is likely that it follows a generalized endothelial dysfunction precipitated by intravascular hemolysis (Gladwin and Kato 2005). The risk of development of pulmonary hypertension seems to be independent of the number of painful sickle crises, and a number of genetic polymorphisms in genes of the TGFβ pathway have been suggested as candidates for identifying sickle cell patients at risk of developing pulmonary hypertension (Ashley-Koch et al. 2008). Treatment of this complication remains largely hematological, increasing hemoglobin by exchange transfusion and aiming to diminish hemolysis. Pharmacological treatment with sildenafil, the phosphodiesterase-5 inhibitor appears to be a potentially useful approach, but its long-term safety, particularly in a group susceptible to priaprism, has yet to be established (Machado et al. 2005).

Pulmonary hypertension, as a relatively newly recognized and potentially the most serious complication of sickle cell disease and other hemoglobinopathies, will provide an enormous challenge to health services worldwide. Fortunately, the methods required to screen for elevated pulmonary pressure with echocardiography are relatively straightforward, even if the sensitivity of the technique is not ideal. Managing the condition once detected will also be taxing, but more data and prospective trials of the available candidate treatments will soon become available.

Conclusions

Disorders of hemoglobin generate diseases of great complexity, which span medical specialisms. They are of undoubted worldwide importance, there being an estimated 400 million people who are heterozygous for a hemoglobinopathy. For most cardiologists, the cardiomyopathy of thalassemia remains an infrequently observed clinical curiosity, but worldwide, and for its potential impact on young individuals, this is an important cause of morbidity and mortality. It also affords the opportunity to understand myocardial adaptive processes and extend experience from this to other, rarer and less well-studied forms of iron overload cardiomyopathy. This is a unique group of patients with an identifiable cause for cardiac failure, which develops with an incidence of 3%–5% per year even in those well-chelated adults with thalassemia. Many of the mutations causing β-thalassemia have been identified, and some of the reasons behind the very variable phenotypic expression of this monogenetic disorder are being unravelled (Weatherall 2001; Weatherall and Clegg 2001). Managing these patients optimally will still require careful clinical observation, measurement, and well-planned trials of new therapies. A multidisciplinary approach has greatly benefited the survival for β-thalassemia patients. This experience may be applied to the other conditions illustrated in this review. It is to be hoped that by better understanding of the underlying mechanisms and, in particular, an expanding knowledge of the genetic basis of these diseases, the opportunity will arise to treat cardiovascular complications more rationally and, hopefully, more effectively. Only the most common of the diseases have been highlighted in this review, but many of the pathophysiological principles will be common to other examples of hemoglobin disorder, such as the rarer conditions: Diamond Blackfan anemia, acquired aplastic anemia, and Fanconi's anemia. Improved management of iron overload can be translated to long-term survivors from myelodysplastic syndromes and other situations requiring long-term transfusion, many of whom are surviving long enough to be affected by iatrogenic iron overload.

References

Aessopos A, Farmakis D, Deftereos S, et al. Thalassemia heart disease: a comparative evaluation of thalassemia major and thalassemia intermedia. *Chest*. 2005;127(5):1523–1530.

Aessopos A, Farmakis D, Karagiorga M, et al. Cardiac involvement in thalassemia intermedia: a multicenter study. *Blood*. 2001;97(11):3411–3416.

Aessopos A, Kati M, Farmakis D. Heart disease in thalassemia intermedia: a review of the underlying pathophysiology. *Haematologica*. 2007;92(5):658–665.

Aldouri MA, Wonke B, Hoffbrand AV, et al. High incidence of cardiomyopathy in beta-thalassaemia patients receiving regular transfusion and iron chelation: reversal by intensified chelation. *Acta Haematol*. 1990;84(3):113–117.

al-Refaie FN, Hershko C, Hoffbrand AV, et al. Results of long-term deferiprone (L1) therapy: a report by the International Study Group on Oral Iron Chelators. *Br J Haematol*. 1995;91(1):224–229.

Anderson LJ, Holden S, Davis B, et al. Cardiovascular T2-star (T2*) magnetic resonance for the early diagnosis of myocardial iron overload. *Eur Heart J*. 2001;22(23):2171–2179.

Anderson LJ, Westwood MA, Holden S, et al. Myocardial iron clearance during reversal of siderotic cardiomyopathy with intravenous desferrioxamine: a prospective study using T2* cardiovascular magnetic resonance. *Br J Haematol*. 2004;127(3):348–355.

Anderson LJ, Wonke B, Prescott E, Holden S, Walker JM, Pennell DJ. Comparison of effects of oral deferiprone and subcutaneous desferrioxamine on myocardial iron concentrations and ventricular function in beta-thalassaemia. *Lancet*. 2002;360(9332):516–520.

Andrews NC. Disorders of iron metabolism. *N Engl J Med*. 1999;341(26):1986–1995.

Andrews NC. Intestinal iron absorption: current concepts circa 2000. *Dig Liver Dis*. 2000;32(1):56–61.

Ashley-Koch A, Yang Q, Olney RS. Sickle hemoglobin (HbS) allele and sickle cell disease: a HuGE review. *Am J Epidemiol*. 2000;151(9):839–845.

Ashley-Koch AE, Elliott L, Kail ME et al. Identification of genetic polymorphisms associated with risk for pulmonary hypertension in sickle cell disease. *Blood*. 2008;111(12):5721–5726.

Bannerman RM, Keusch G, Kreimer-Birnbaum M, Vance VK, Vaughan S. Thalassemia intermedia, with iron overload, cardiac failure, diabetes mellitus, hypopituitarism and porphyrinuria. *Am J Med*. 1967;42(3):476–486.

Barnett CF, Hsue PY, Machado RF. Pulmonary hypertension: an increasingly recognized complication of hereditary hemolytic anemias and HIV infection. *JAMA*. 2008;299(3):324–331.

Barton JC. Chelation therapy for iron overload. *Curr Gastroenterol Rep*. 2007;9(1):74–82.

Blankenberg F, Eisenberg S, Scheinman MN, Higgins CB. Use of cine gradient echo (GRE) MR in the imaging of cardiac hemochromatosis. *J Comput Assist Tomogr*. 1994;18(1):136–138.

Borgna-Pignatti C, Cappellini MD, De SP, et al. Survival and complications in thalassemia. *Ann N Y Acad Sci*. 2005;1054:40–47.

Borgna-Pignatti C, Cappellini MD, De SP, et al. Cardiac morbidity and mortality in deferoxamine- or deferiprone-treated patients with thalassemia major. *Blood*. 2006;107(9):3733–3737.

Borgna-Pignatti C, Castriota-Scanderbeg A. Methods for evaluating iron stores and efficacy of chelation in transfusional hemosiderosis. *Haematologica*. 1991;76(5):409–413.

Borgna-Pignatti C, Cohen A. Evaluation of a new method of administration of the iron chelating agent deferoxamine. *J Pediatr*. 1997;130(1):86–88.

Borgna-Pignatti C, Rugolotto S, De SP, et al. Survival and disease complications in thalassemia major. *Ann N Y Acad Sci*. 1998;850:227–231.

Bulaj ZJ, Ajioka RS, Phillips JD, et al. Disease-related conditions in relatives of patients with hemochromatosis. *N Engl J Med*. 2000;343(21):1529–1535.

Bunn HF. Pathogenesis and treatment of sickle cell disease. *N Engl J Med*. 1997;337(11):762–769.

Camaschella C, Roetto A, Cali A, et al. The gene TFR2 is mutated in a new type of haemochromatosis mapping to 7q22. *Nat Genet*. 2000;25(1):14–15.

Canatan D, Temimhan N, Dincer N, Ozsancak A, Oguz N, Temimhan M. Continuous desferrioxamine infusion by an infusor in thalassaemia major. *Acta Paediatr*. 1999;88(5):550–552.

Candell-Riera J, Lu L, Seres L, et al. Cardiac hemochromatosis: beneficial effects of iron removal therapy. An echocardiographic study. *Am J Cardiol*. 1983;52(7):824–829.

Chan JC, Chim CS, Ooi CG, et al. Use of the oral chelator deferiprone in the treatment of iron overload in patients with Hb H disease. *Br J Haematol*. 2006;133(2):198–205.

Chen FE, Ooi C, Ha SY, et al. Genetic and clinical features of hemoglobin H disease in Chinese patients. *N Engl J Med*. 2000;343(8):544–550.

Chui DH, Fucharoen S, Chan V. Hemoglobin H disease: not necessarily a benign disorder. *Blood*. 2003;101(3):791–800.

Cohen AR, Galanello R, Pennell DJ, Cunningham MJ, Vichinsky E. Thalassemia. *Hematology Am Soc Hematol Educ Program*. 2004;14–34.

Cremonesi L, Forni GL, Soriani N, et al. Genetic and clinical heterogeneity of ferroportin disease. *Br J Haematol*. 2005;131(5):663–670.

Crosby WH. A history of phlebotomy therapy for hemochromatosis. *Am J Med Sci*. 1991;301(1):28–31.

Cutler DJ, Isner JM, Bracey AW, et al. Hemochromatosis heart disease: an unemphasized cause of potentially reversible restrictive cardiomyopathy. *Am J Med*. 1980;69(6):923–928.

Dabestani A. Primary Hemochromatosis: anatomic and physiologic characteristics of the Cardiac Ventricles and Their Response to Phlebotomy. *Am J Cardiol*. 1984;54:153–159.

Davis BA, Porter JB. Long-term outcome of continuous 24-hour deferoxamine infusion via indwelling intravenous catheters in high-risk beta-thalassemia. *Blood*. 2000;95(4):1229–1236.

Davis BA, Porter JB. Results of long term iron chelation treatment with deferoxamine. *Adv Exp Med Biol*. 2002;509:91–125.

De Gobbi M, Roetto A, Piperno A, et al. Natural history of juvenile haemochromatosis. *Br J Haematol*. 2002;117(4):973–979.

Edwards CQ, Kushner JP. Screening for hemochromatosis. *N Engl J Med*. 1993;328(22):1616–1620.

Eldor A, Rachmilewitz EA. The hypercoagulable state in thalassemia. *Blood*. 2002;99(1):36–43.

Ellervik C, Tybjaerg-Hansen A, Grande P, Appleyard M, Nordestgaard BG. Hereditary hemochromatosis and risk of ischemic heart disease: a prospective study and a case-control study. *Circulation*. 2005;112(2):185–193.

Engle MA, Erlandson M, Smith CH. Late cardiac complications of chronic, severe, refractory anemia with hemochromatosis. *Circulation*. 1964;30:698–705.

Erhardt A, Maschner-Olberg A, Mellenthin C, et al. HFE mutations and chronic hepatitis C: H63D and C282Y heterozygosity are independent risk factors for liver fibrosis and cirrhosis. *J Hepatol.* 2003;38(3):335–342.

Ernst O, Calvo M, Sergent G, Mizrahi D, Carpentier F. Breath-hold MR cholangiopancreatography using a HASTE sequence: comparison of single-slice and multislice acquisition techniques. *AJR Am J Roentgenol.* 1997;169(5):1304–1306.

Fabio G, Minonzio F, Delbini P, Bianchi A, Cappellini MD. Reversal of cardiac complications by deferiprone and deferoxamine combination therapy in a patient affected by a severe type of juvenile hemochromatosis (JH). *Blood.* 2007;109(1):362–364.

Feder JN, Gnirke A, Thomas W, et al. A novel MHC class I-like gene is mutated in patients with hereditary haemochromatosis. *Nat Genet.* 1996;13(4):399–408.

Fitchett DH, Coltart DJ, Littler WA, et al. Cardiac involvement in secondary haemochromatosis: a catheter biopsy study and analysis of myocardium. *Cardiovasc Res.* 1980;14(12):719–724.

Flint J, Harding RM, Boyce AJ, Clegg JB. The population genetics of the haemoglobinopathies. *Baillieres Clin Haematol.* 1998;11(1):1–51.

Gabutti V, Piga A. Results of long-term iron-chelating therapy. *Acta Haematol.* 1996;95(1):26–36.

Gibbons R, Olivieri NF, Wood WG. Part 3 Clinical features of the thalassaemias: the thalassaemias and their interaction with structural haemoglobin variants. In: Weatherall DJ, Clegg JB, (eds.). *The Thalassaemia Syndromes.* 4 ed. Blackwell Science; 2001: 484–526.

Gill FM, Sleeper LA, Weiner SJ, et al. Clinical events in the first decade in a cohort of infants with sickle cell disease. Cooperative Study of Sickle Cell Disease. *Blood.* 1995;86(2):776–783.

Gladwin MT, Kato GJ. Cardiopulmonary complications of sickle cell disease: role of nitric oxide and hemolytic anemia. *Hematology Am Soc Hematol Educ Program.* 2005:51–57.

Goland S, Malnick SD. Letter regarding article by Ellervik et al. "hereditary hemochromatosis and risk of ischemic heart disease: a prospective study and a case-control study". *Circulation.* 2006;113(1):e10.

Gunn IR, Maxwell FK, Gaffney D, McMahon AD, Packard CJ. Haemochromatosis gene mutations and risk of coronary heart disease: a west of Scotland coronary prevention study (WOSCOPS) substudy. *Heart.* 2004;90(3):304–306.

Hanson EH, Imperatore G, Burke W. HFE gene and hereditary hemochromatosis: a HuGE review. Human Genome Epidemiology. *Am J Epidemiol.* 2001;154(3):193–206.

Hershko C, Cappellini MD, Galanello R, Piga A, Tognoni G, Masera G. Purging iron from the heart. *Br J Haematol.* 2004;125(5):545–551.

Higgs DR, Thein SL, Wood WG. Part 2 The biology of the thalassaemias: human haemoglobin. In: Weatherall DJ, Clegg JB, (eds.). *The Thalassaemia Syndromes.* Blackwell Science; 2001a: 65–121.

Higgs DR, Thein SL, Wood WG. Part 2 The biology of the thalassaemias: the pathophysiology of the thalassaemias. In: Weatherall DJ, Clegg JB, (eds.). *The Thalassaemia Syndromes.* 4 ed. Blackwell Science; 2001b: 192–237.

Higgs DR, Thein SL, Wood WG. Part 2 The biology of the thalassaemias: the molecular pathology of the thalassaemias. In: Weatherall DJ, Clegg JB, (eds.). *The Thalassaemia Syndromes.* 4 ed. Blackwell Science; 2001c: 133–191.

Hill AV. Molecular epidemiology of the thalassaemias (including haemoglobin E). *Baillieres Clin Haematol.* 1992;5(1):209–238.

Hill AV, Flint J, Weatherall DJ, Clegg JB. Alpha-thalassaemia and the malaria hypothesis. *Acta Haematol.* 1987;78(2–3):173–179.

Hofmann WK, Tong XJ, Ajioka RS, Kushner JP, Koeffler HP. Mutation analysis of transferrin-receptor 2 in patients with atypical hemochromatosis. *Blood.* 2002;100(3):1099–1100.

Intragumtornchai T, Minaphinant K, Wanichsawat C, et al. Echocardiographic features in patients with beta thalassemia/hemoglobin E: a combining effect of anemia and iron load. *J Med Assoc Thai.* 1994;77(2):57–65.

Jazayeri M, Bakayev V, Adibi P, et al. Frequency of HFE gene mutations in Iranian beta-thalassaemia minor patients. *Eur J Haematol.* 2003;71(6):408–411.

Johnston DL, Rice L, Vick GW III, Hedrick TD, Rokey R. Assessment of tissue iron overload by nuclear magnetic resonance imaging. *Am J Med.* 1989;87(1):40–47.

Kato GJ, Gladwin MT, Steinberg MH. Deconstructing sickle cell disease: reappraisal of the role of hemolysis in the development of clinical subphenotypes. *Blood Rev.* 2007;21(1):37–47.

Kaul DK, Fabry ME, Nagel RL. Microvascular sites and characteristics of sickle cell adhesion to vascular endothelium in shear flow conditions: pathophysiological implications. *Proc Natl Acad Sci USA.* 1989;86(9):3356–3360.

Kremastinos DT. Heart failure in beta-thalassaemia: a local or universal health problem? *Hellenic J Cardiol.* 2007;48(3):189–190.

Kremastinos DT, Rentoukas E, Mavrogeni S, Kyriakides ZS, Politis C, Toutouzas P. Left ventricular filling pattern in beta-thalassaemia major—a Doppler echocardiographic study. *Eur Heart J.* 1993;14(3): 351–357.

Kremastinos DT, Tiniakos G, Theodorakis GN, Katritsis DG, Toutouzas PK. Myocarditis in beta-thalassemia major. A cause of heart failure. *Circulation.* 1995a;91(1):66–71.

Kremastinos DT, Toutouzas PK, Vyssoulis GP, Venetis CA, Avgoustakis DG. Iron overload and left ventricular performance in beta thalassemia. *Acta Cardiol.* 1984;39(1):29–40.

Kremastinos DT, Toutouzas PK, Vyssoulis GP, Venetis CA, Vretou HP, Avgoustakis DG. Global and segmental left ventricular function in beta-thalassemia. *Cardiology.* 1985;72(3):129–139.

Kwiatkowski DP. How malaria has affected the human genome and what human genetics can teach us about malaria. *Am J Hum Genet.* 2005;77(2):171–192.

Lattanzi F, Bellotti P, Picano E, et al. Quantitative ultrasonic analysis of myocardium in patients with thalassemia major and iron overload. *Circulation.* 1993;87(3):748–754.

Lattanzi F, Bellotti P, Picano E, et al. Quantitative Texture Analysis in Two-Dimensional Echocardiography: application to the Diagnosis of Myocardial Hemochromatosis. *Echocardiography.* 1996;13(1):9–20.

Leikin SL, Gallagher D, Kinney TR, Sloane D, Klug P, Rida W. Mortality in children and adolescents with sickle cell disease. Cooperative Study of Sickle Cell Disease. *Pediatrics.* 1989;84(3):500–508.

Lombardo T, Frontini V, Ferro G, Sergi P, Guidice A, Lombardo G. Laboratory evaluation of a new delivery system to improve patient compliance with chelation therapy. *Clin Lab Haematol.* 1996;18(1):13–17.

Machado RF, Anthi A, Steinberg MH et al. N-terminal pro-brain natriuretic peptide levels and risk of death in sickle cell disease. *JAMA.* 2006;296(3):310–318.

Mavrogeni S, Gotsis ED, Berdousi E, et al. Myocardial and hepatic T2* magnetic resonance evaluation in ex-thalassemic patients after bone-marrow transplantation. *Int J Cardiovasc Imaging.* 2007;23(6):739–745.

Mavrogeni SI, Maris T, Gouliamos A, Vlahos L, Kremastinos DT. Myocardial iron deposition in beta-thalassemia studied by magnetic resonance imaging. *Int J Card Imaging.* 1998;14(2):117–122.

Modell B, Harris R, Lane B, et al. Informed choice in genetic screening for thalassaemia during pregnancy: audit from a national confidential inquiry. *BMJ.* 2000a;320(7231):337–341.

Modell B, Khan M, Darlison M. Survival in beta-thalassaemia major in the UK: data from the UK Thalassaemia Register. *Lancet.* 2000b;355(9220):2051–2052.

Modell B, Khan M, Darlison M, et al. A national register for surveillance of inherited disorders: beta thalassaemia in the United Kingdom. *Bull World Health Organ.* 2001;79(11):1006–1013.

Møller S, Henriksen JH. Cirrhotic cardiomyopathy: a pathophysiological review of circulatory disfunction in liver disease. *Heart.* 2002;87:9–15.

Nagel RL. Pleiotropic and epistatic effects in sickle cell anemia. *Curr Opin Hematol.* 2001;8(2):105–110.

Nagel RL, Bookchin RM, Johnson J, et al. Structural bases of the inhibitory effects of hemoglobin F and hemoglobin A2 on the polymerization of hemoglobin S. *Proc Natl Acad Sci USA.* 1979;76(2):670–672.

Niederau C, Fischer R, Purschel A, Stremmel W, Haussinger D, Strohmeyer G. Long-term survival in patients with hereditary hemochromatosis. *Gastroenterology.* 1996;110(4):1107–1119.

Niederau C, Fischer R, Sonnenberg A, Stremmel W, Trampisch HJ, Strohmeyer G. Survival and causes of death in cirrhotic and in noncirrhotic patients with primary hemochromatosis. *N Engl J Med.* 1985;313(20):1256–1262.

Njajou OT, Vaessen N, Joosse M, et al. A mutation in SLC11A3 is associated with autosomal dominant hemochromatosis. *Nat Genet.* 2001;28(3):213–214.

Okpala I. The intriguing contribution of white blood cells to sickle cell disease—a red cell disorder. *Blood Rev.* 2004;18(1):65–73.

Okpala I. Leukocyte adhesion and the pathophysiology of sickle cell disease. *Curr Opin Hematol.* 2006;13(1):40–44.

Olivieri NF, Brittenham GM. Long-term trials of deferiprone in Cooley's anemia. *Ann N Y Acad Sci.* 1998;850:217–222.

Olivieri NF, Liu PP, Sher GD, et al. Brief report: combined liver and heart transplantation for end-stage iron-induced organ failure in an adult with homozygous beta-thalassemia. *N Engl J Med.* 1994;330(16):1125–1127.

Ooi GC, Chen FE, Chan KN, et al. Qualitative and quantitative magnetic resonance imaging in haemoglobin H disease: screening for iron overload. *Clin Radiol.* 1999;54(2):98–102.

Origa R, Galanello R, Ganz T, et al. Liver iron concentrations and urinary hepcidin in beta-thalassemia. *Haematologica.* 2007;92(5):583–588.

Papanikolaou G, Samuels ME, Ludwig EH, et al. Mutations in HFE2 cause iron overload in chromosome 1q-linked juvenile hemochromatosis. *Nat Genet.* 2004;36(1):77–82.

Papanikolaou N, Ghiatas A, Kattamis A, Ladis C, Kritikos N, Kattamis C. Non-invasive myocardial iron assessment in thalassaemic patients. T2 relaxometry and magnetization transfer ratio measurements. *Acta Radiol.* 2000;41(4):348–351.

Philpott CC. Molecular aspects of iron absorption: insights into the role of HFE in hemochromatosis. *Hepatology.* 2002;35(5):993–1001.

Pietrangelo A. Hemochromatosis gene modifies course of hepatitis C viral infection. *Gastroenterology.* 2003;124(5):1509–1523.

Pietrangelo A. Hereditary hemochromatosis—a new look at an old disease. *N Engl J Med.* 2004a;350(23):2383–2397.

Pietrangelo A. The ferroportin disease. *Blood Cells Mol Dis.* 2004b;32(1):131–138.

Pietrangelo A. Hereditary hemochromatosis. *Biochimica et Biophysica Acta.* 2006;1763:700–710.

Pietrangelo A, Corradini E, Ferrara F, et al. Magnetic resonance imaging to identify classic and nonclassic forms of ferroportin disease. *Blood Cells Mol Dis.* 2006;37(3):192–196.

Pietrangelo A, Trautwein C. Mechanisms of disease: the role of hepcidin in iron homeostasis--implications for hemochromatosis and other disorders. *Nat Clin Pract Gastroenterol Hepatol.* 2004;1(1):39–45.

Piga A. Survival improvement in thalassemia: who should take the credit? *Haematologica.* 2006;91(9):1154B.

Piga A, Roggero S, Marletto F, Sacchetti L, Longo F. Combined use of oral chelators and desferrioxamine in thalassemia. *Hematology.* 2005;10(Suppl 1):89–91.

Pippard MJ, Callender ST, Warner GT, Weatherall DJ. Iron absorption in iron-loading anaemias: effect of subcutaneous desferrioxamine infusions. *Lancet.* 1977;2(8041):737–739.

Pippard MJ, Callender ST, Warner GT, Weatherall DJ. Iron absorption and loading in beta-thalassaemia intermedia. *Lancet.* 1979;2(8147):819–821.

Platt OS, Brambilla DJ, Rosse WF, et al. Mortality in sickle cell disease. Life expectancy and risk factors for early death. *N Engl J Med.* 1994;330(23):1639–1644.

Porter JB, Rafique R, Srichairatanakool S, et al. Recent insights into interactions of deferoxamine with cellular and plasma iron pools: implications for clinical use. *Ann N Y Acad Sci.* 2005;1054:155–168.

Rebulla P, Modell B. Transfusion requirements and effects in patients with thalassaemia major. Cooleycare Programme. *Lancet.* 1991;337(8736):277–280.

Rochette J, Pointon JJ, Fisher CA, et al. Multicentric origin of hemochromatosis gene (HFE) mutations. *Am J Hum Genet.* 1999;64(4):1056–1062.

Roetto A, Papanikolaou G, Politou M, et al. Mutant antimicrobial peptide hepcidin is associated with severe juvenile hemochromatosis. *Nat Genet.* 2003;33(1):21–22.

Sanyal SK, Johnson W, Jayalakshmamma B, Green AA. Fatal "iron heart" in an adolescent: biochemical and ultrastructural aspects of the heart. *Pediatrics.* 1975;55(3):336–341.

Sephton Smith R. Iron excretion in thalassaemia major after administration of chelating agents. *BMJ.* 1962;2:1577–1580.

Shalev O, Repka T, Goldfarb A, et al. Deferiprone (L1) chelates pathologic iron deposits from membranes of intact thalassemic and sickle red blood cells both in vitro and in vivo. *Blood.* 1995;86(5):2008–2013.

Shashaty G, Frankewich R, Chakraborti T, et al. Deferasirox for the treatment of chronic iron overload in transfusional hemosiderosis. *Oncology (Williston Park).* 2006;20(14):1799–1806, 1811.

Steinberg MH, Adewoye AH. Modifier genes and sickle cell anemia. *Curr Opin Hematol.* 2006;13(3):131–136.

Switzer JA, Hess DC, Nichols FT, Adams RJ. Pathophysiology and treatment of stroke in sickle-cell disease: present and future. *Lancet Neurol.* 2006;5(6):501–512.

Taher A, Isma'eel H, Mehio G, et al. Prevalence of thromboembolic events among 8,860 patients with thalassaemia major and intermedia in the Mediterranean area and Iran. *Thromb Haemost.* 2006;96(4):488–491.

Tanner MA, Galanello R, Dessi C, et al. A randomized, placebo-controlled, double-blind trial of the effect of combined therapy with deferoxamine and deferiprone on myocardial iron in thalassemia major using cardiovascular magnetic resonance. *Circulation.* 2007;115(14):1876–1884.

Tanner MA, Galanello R, Dessi C, et al. Myocardial iron loading in patients with thalassemia major on deferoxamine chelation. *J Cardiovasc Magn Reson.* 2006;8(3):543–547.

Telfer PT, Prestcott E, Holden S, Walker M, Hoffbrand AV, Wonke B. Hepatic iron concentration combined with long-term monitoring of serum ferritin to predict complications of iron overload in thalassaemia major. *Br J Haematol.* 2000;110(4):971–977.

Thomas PW, Higgs DR, Serjeant GR. Benign clinical course in homozygous sickle cell disease: a search for predictors. *J Clin Epidemiol.* 1997;50(2):121–126.

Townsend A, Drakesmith H. Role of HFE in iron metabolism, hereditary haemochromatosis, anaemia of chronic disease, and secondary iron overload. *Lancet.* 2002;359(9308):786–790.

Vogel M, Anderson LJ, Holden S, Deanfield JE, Pennell DJ, Walker JM. Tissue Doppler echocardiography in patients with thalassaemia detects early myocardial dysfunction related to myocardial iron overload. *Eur Heart J.* 2003;24(1):113–119.

Walker BL, Tiong JW, Jefferies WA. Iron metabolism in mammalian cells. *Int Rev Cytol.* 2001;211:241–278.

Wallace DF, Dixon JL, Ramm GA, Anderson GJ, Powell LW, Subramaniam VN. A novel mutation in ferroportin implicated in iron overload. *J Hepatol.* 2007;46(5):921–926.

Wallace DF, Subramaniam VN. Non-HFE haemochromatosis. *World J Gastroenterol.* 2007;13(35):4690–4698.

Weatherall DJ. Thalassaemia and malaria, revisited. *Ann Trop Med Parasitol.* 1997;91(7):885–890.

Weatherall DJ. Phenotype-genotype relationships in monogenic disease: lessons from the thalassaemias. *Nat Rev Genet.* 2001c;2(4):245–255.

Weatherall DJ, Clegg JB. Inherited haemoglobin disorders: an increasing global health problem. *Bull World Health Organ.* 2001;79(8):704–712.

Westwood M, Anderson LJ, Firmin DN, et al. A single breath-hold multiecho T2* cardiovascular magnetic resonance technique for diagnosis of myocardial iron overload. *J Magn Reson Imaging.* 2003;18(1):33–39.

Whitlock EP, Garlitz BA, Harris EL, Beil TL, Smith PR. Screening for hereditary hemochromatosis: a systematic review for the U.S. Preventive Services Task Force. *Ann Intern Med.* 2006;145(3):209–223.

Yang Q, McDonnell SM, Khoury MJ, Cono J, Parrish RG. Hemochromatosis-associated mortality in the United States from 1979 to 1992: an analysis of Multiple-Cause Mortality Data. *Ann Intern Med.* 1998;129(11):946–953.

Zurlo MG, De SP, Borgna-Pignatti C, et al. Survival and causes of death in thalassaemia major. *Lancet.* 1989;2(8653):27–30.

30

Familial Amyloidoses and the Heart

Claudio Rapezzi, Candida Cristina Quarta, Letizia Riva, Fabrizio Salvi, Paolo Ciliberti, Simone Longhi, Elena Biagini, and Enrica Perugini

Introduction

Amyloid heart disease is the most frequent type of cardiomyopathy with restrictive physiology in Western countries. It is a complex entity with very varied pathophysiology. Even though a definitive diagnosis can readily be made from histological findings in involved tissues, amyloid heart disease is still frequently under diagnosed for at least two reasons. First, electrocardiographic and echocardiographic findings are often misleading, since they can simulate many other diseases, including hypertrophic cardiomyopathy and coronary artery disease. Second, since the clinical manifestations of systemic amyloidosis are manifold, patients may be referred to any one of a variety of specialists (especially hematologists, nephrologists, and neurologists) without necessarily coming to the attention of a cardiologist.

The familial amyloidoses constitute an extremely heterogeneous group of diseases. The form linked to transthyretin (TTR) mutations (conventionally abbreviated as ATTR) is by far the most common variety of familial amyloidosis. This chapter provides an overview of current knowledge regarding the pathogenesis, diagnosis, and treatment of familial amyloid heart disease in general, and of ATTR-related cardiomyopathy in particular. Cardiac involvement in ATTR will necessarily be considered within the context of the broader spectrum of clinical manifestations of the disease. The section dedicated to therapy will address separately questions of general supportive care, liver transplantation (including combined heart-liver transplantation), and the current state of pharmacologic research. Finally, we briefly summarize the clinical aspects of the other (non-TTR-related) forms of familial amyloidosis in which heart disease can occur.

The Amyloidogenic Process

The term amyloidosis refers to a large group of disorders caused by the extracellular deposition of insoluble amyloid fibrils composed of misfolded proteins. These disorders can affect many proteins (to date, at least 21) (Falk et al. 1997; Merlini and Bellotti 2003), but the fibrillary deposits share distinctive structural and tinctorial properties: namely, an amorphous eosinophilic appearance under light microscopy using routine histological stains; an "apple-green" birefringence after Congo-red staining under a polarized light microscope (Figure 30–1); presence of rigid nonbranching fibrils 7.5–10 nm in diameter on electron microscopy; and a predominantly antiparallel β-sheet secondary structure visible under infrared and X-ray diffraction (Falk et al. 1997; Merlini and Bellotti 2003).

The mechanisms by which different monomers with different biomechanical properties bind together to form regular amyloid fibrils is not understood, but three pathogenetic steps in amyloid formation are recognized: (1) a peculiar short amino acid sequence within the precursor protein; (2) an adequate supply of an amyloid precursor protein to allow deposition; and (3) a slow but constant turnover of the resulting amyloid deposits (Merlini and Bellotti 2003; Merlini and Westermark 2004; Hou et al. 2007). The primary structure of fibril precursor proteins is undoubtedly a major determinant of their amyloidogenicity, but it is possible that any protein is intrinsically capable of producing amyloid fibrils in the presence of particular conditions (Merlini and Bellotti 2003; Merlini and Westermark 2004; Hou et al. 2007). There are several ways in which potentially pathogenic misfolded proteins can form. The protein may have an intrinsic propensity to assume a pathologic conformation during aging (e.g., TTR in systemic senile amyloidosis) or at persistently high concentrations in serum (β_2 microglobulin in patients undergoing long-term hemodialysis). Another mechanism involves the replacement of a single amino acid in the protein, such as in hereditary amyloidosis. A third mechanism stems from proteolytic remodeling of the protein precursor, as in the case of β-amyloid precursor protein in Alzheimer's disease. These mechanisms can act independently or in conjunction with (and in addition to) the intrinsic amyloidogenic potential of the pathogenic protein. Other factors may act synergistically in amyloid deposition. For example, the

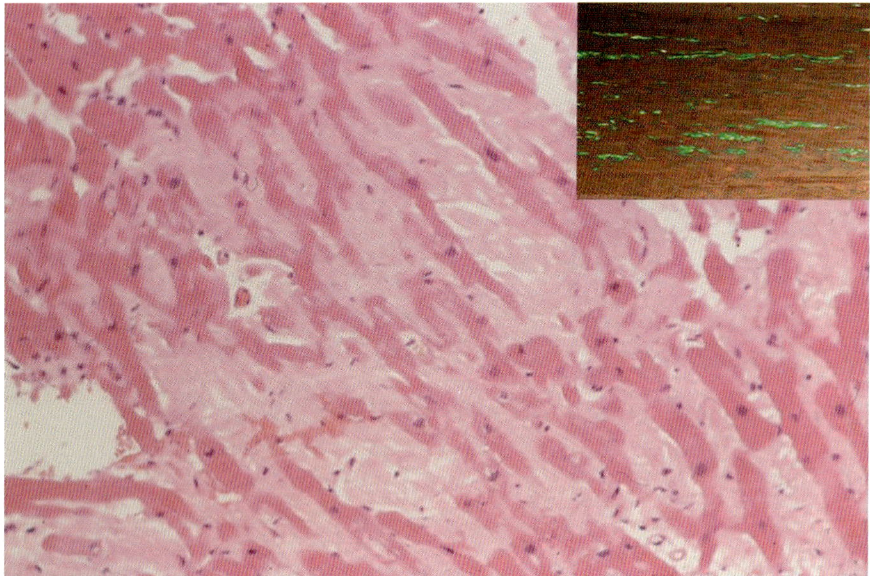

Figure 30–1 Characteristic histological findings in the myocardium of a patient with amyloidotic cardiomyopathy. The amyloid deposits (pale pink with hematoxylin and eosin staining) diffusely infiltrate the myocardial tissue, anatomically and functionally separating the cells from one another. The typical apple-green appearance (inset) can be seen at Congo-red staining under polarized light (photograph kindly provided by Dr Ornella Leone).

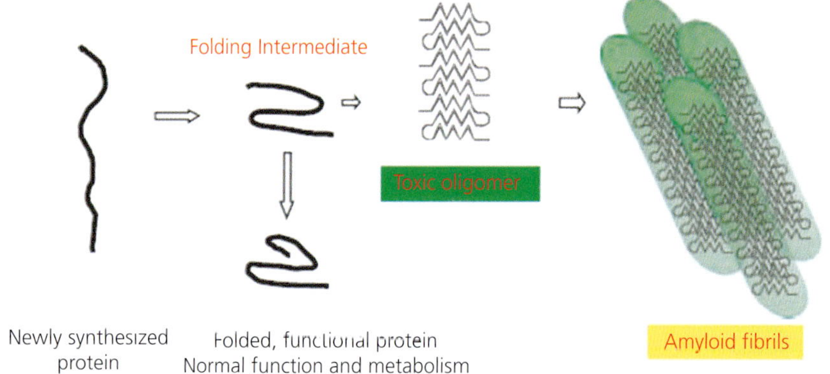

Figure 30–2 Example of how an amyloid filament is thought to be formed. For many amyloid fibril proteins, the aggregation is believed to start from intermediates in the folding process, giving rise to a nucleus from which filament formation proceeds. There is strong evidence that oligomeric aggregates (also called protofibrils), which occur before mature fibrils are formed, exert toxic effects on cells whilst the full-blown fibrils are more inert. Amyloid fibrils usually consist of two or several thin filaments (indicated to the right in the figure) twisted around each other. The width of the definite amyloid fibril is around 10 nm. Reprinted from Hou X, Aguilar MI, Small DH. Transthyretin and familial amyloidotic polyneuropathy. Recent progress in understanding the molecular mechanism of neurodegeneration. *FEBS J*. 2007;274:1637–1650, with permission.

protein precursor must reach a critical local concentration to trigger fibril formation, a process enhanced by local environmental factors and by interactions with extracellular matrices. Some peptides are highly fibrillogenic at high concentrations, while others are normally incorporated in larger protein precursors and become available for fibril formation only after proteolytic cleavage, such as the Aβ-peptide in Alzheimer's disease (Merlini and Westermark 2004).

In the case of TTR protein, evidence suggests that under particular conditions (including pH, ionic strength, and protein concentration), its native structure can be destabilized by amyloidogenic mutations. Such protein mutations induce conformational changes leading to dissociation of the TTR tetramers into partially unfolded nonnative monomers capable of forming high molecular-mass soluble aggregates and self-assembling into amyloid fibrils (Figure 30–2; Hou et al. 2007).

Mechanisms of Amyloid-Induced Tissue Damage

Amyloid can cause organ and tissue damage in several ways. A major factor is the replacement of normal tissue by amyloid, leading to loss of the organ's mechanical function. However, infiltration cannot by itself completely explain the spectrum of clinical, instrumental, and biological manifestations of amyloid diseases. For instance, it has been observed that similar or lesser amounts of cardiac amyloid deposits (as evaluated by echocardiography) have significantly worse functional and prognostic impact in patients with light-chain amyloidosis than in patients with TTR amyloidosis (Dubrey et al. 1997; Hou et al. 2007). Furthermore, the amount of amyloid in an organ does not provide an accurate indicator of the clinical consequences of the disease. For example, patients with AL amyloidosis without hepatic failure may harbor abundant protein deposits in their livers. By contrast, in ATTR small amounts of amyloidotic infiltration of the peripheral nerves may be

Table 30–1 Nomenclature and Classification of Amyloidosis

Amyloidosis	Protein Precursor	Systemic/Localized	Clinical Syndrome/Association
AL	Immunoglobulin light-chain (κ or λ)	S, L	• Primary • Myeloma-associated
AH	Immunoglobulin heavy-chain	S, L	• Primary • Myeloma-associated
AA	(Apo) serum AA	S	• Secondary • Reactive
ATTR	TTR	S L?	• Senile (TTR wild-type) • Familial (TTR mutated) • Tenosynovium
AApoAI	Apolipoprotein-AI	S L	• Familial • Aortic
AApoAII	Apolipoprotein-AII	S	• Familial
AGel	Gelsolin	S	• Familial
ALys	Lysozyme	S	• Familial
AFib	Fibrinogen α-chain	S	• Familial
ACys	Cystatin C	S	• Familial
ABri	ABriPP	S L?	• Familial dementia (British)
Aβ	Aβ-protein precursor (AβPP)	L	• Alzheimer's disease • Aging
APrP	Prion protein	L	• Spongioform encephalopathies
Aβ_2M	β_2–microglobulin	S L?	• Hemodialysis • Joints
ACal	(Pro)calcitonin	L	• C-cell thyroid tumors
AIAPP	Islet amyloid polypeptide	L	• Islets of Langherans • Insulinomas
AANF	Atrial natriuretic factor	L	• Cardiac atria
APro	Prolactin	L	• Aging pituitary • Prolactinomas
AIns	Insulin	L	• Iatrogenic
AMed	Lactadherin	L	• Senile aortic
AKer	Kerato-epithelin	L	• Familial cornea

accompanied by severe neurologic impairment. In vitro, synthetic amyloidotic fibrils can exert lethal toxic effects on various cell types (Yankner et al. 1989; May et al. 1993; Jordan et al. 1998) always via induction of apoptosis (Wang et al. 2001). Although the underlying mechanisms remain unclear, a variety of factors, including oxidative stress (Schubert et al. 1995; Goodman and Mattson 1996), cell membrane destruction (Engström et al. 1995; Janson et al. 1999), and formation of pathological ion channels (Engström et al. 1995; Mirzabekov et al. 1996) have been implicated. It is now thought that cell toxicity largely occurs in the early stages of fibril formation. Experiments with several amyloid fibril proteins manufactured in vitro (Janson et al. 1999) suggest that smaller oligomeric aggregates (so-called protofibrils or intermediate-sized toxic amyloid particles) are probably toxic whereas the mature fibrils from the same peptides may not be (Kayed et al. 2003).

Classification of Amyloidosis

The modern classification of amyloidosis, proposed by the World Health Organisation nomenclature subcommittee (Table 30–1), is based on the precursor protein (Westermark et al. 2002). According to this classification, the amyloid protein is designated "protein A" followed by a suffix (e.g., ATTR), where A stands for amyloid and the suffix specifies the protein (this name is also used to identify the disease). The types of amyloidosis are subdivided into acquired or hereditary. Amyloid distribution may be focal, localized, or systemic. The most common form of systemic amyloidosis is AL (where L stands for light-chain immunoglobulin), which was formerly known as "primary amyloidosis." The incidence of AL in Western countries is approximately 1 new case per 100,000 person-years (Gertz et al. 1999). Hereditary systemic amyloidoses are much less common; they are secondary to deposition of various proteins, including TTR, apolipoprotein A-I and A-II, lysozyme, gelsolin, cystatin C, and fibrinogen A α-chain. Senile systemic amyloidosis stems from deposition of amyloid derived from wild-type TTR (i.e., with a normal amino acid sequence). For reasons that remain unclear, senile systemic amyloidosis is almost exclusively a disorder of old men and mainly affects the heart.

TTR-Related Familial Amyloidosis

TTR-related familial amyloidosis (hereafter referred to as ATTR) is the most frequent form of hereditary systemic amyloidosis. TTR is a tetrameric plasma transport protein for the thyroid hormone and retinol-binding protein/vitamin A, which is synthesized in the liver (and in small amounts in the choroidal plexus and retinal epithelium). TTR is a single polypeptide chain of 127 amino acid residues encoded by a single gene on chromosome 18, which spans approximately 7 kb and has four exons (Merlini and Westermark 2004; Hou et al. 2007).

ATTR is inherited in an autosomal dominant fashion with balanced sex distribution and variable penetrance. Over 80 different amyloidogenic mutations have been identified around the world, many of which have been found in single individuals or families ("private mutations") (Merlini and Westermark 2004; Benson and Kincaid 2007; Hou et al. 2007). Most ATTR carriers are heterozygous for a pathogenic mutation and express both normal and variant TTR. The majority of TTR mutations derive from a single nucleotide substitution (Benson and Kincaid 2007; Hou et al. 2007). An exception is the deletion of an entire 3-base codon (Val122Ile) (Jacobson et al. 1996; Uemichi et al. 1997). Development of the disease is probably the result of changes in primary structure of the protein, modulated by various genetic and possibly also environmental factors (although present in the blood from birth, variant TTR does not start to produce amyloid until adulthood) (Harats et al. 1989).

A few of the TTR mutations are found in extended kindreds in particular locations around the world. The most common of these is the substitution of methionine for valine at position 30 (Val30Met), which leads to "type I familial amyloid polyneuropathy" (FAP) (Andrade 1952). The Val30Met variety of ATTR amyloidosis has major geographical clusters in Portugal, Sweden, and Japan with smaller clusters in more than a dozen other countries (Ando et al. 2005; Figure 30–3). These three countries are geographically distant, and a consanguineous relationship between populations has not been identified. The issue of whether there is a common origin for a mutant allele has not been completely resolved. The hypothesis that the worldwide clusters of FAP (Val30Met) all originate from a mutant allele in the Portuguese kindred was based on historically documented commercial relations. Recently, Ohmori et al. compared haplotypes in several cohorts of patients with FAP and concluded that a common founder could conceivably link Portuguese and Japanese patients and Portuguese and Spanish patients, but could not account for Swedish and other patients (Ohmori et al. 2004).

The prevalence of Val30Met genotype is particularly high (about 1.5%) in northern Sweden, although the penetrance is only about 2% (Ando et al. 2005). In Portugal the disease prevalence rate is estimated at 1 in 1,000 (Ando et al. 2005). In Japan, Val30Met families with early onset neuropathy were initially identified in two limited areas (Arao district and Ogawa village), while a late onset nonendemic type of Val30Met ATTR was reported in a wide distribution throughout the country (Ando et al. 2005). In Sweden, in addition to the endemic foci of Val30Met, Ala45Ser and Tyr69His mutations have been observed (Suhr et al. 2003). The Leu111Me mutation has been reported in Denmark, where it is the cause of so-called familial amyloidotic cardiomyopathy (FAC) (Ranløv et al.1992; Svendsen et al. 1998). TTR Ala60 and it is the most common cause of ATTR in the United Kingdom and Ireland (Reilly et al. 1995). In France, a large population of Portuguese Val30Met families coexists with families of French descent (in these families prevalence of Val30Met is no higher than 40%) (Adams et al. 1992; Planté-Bordeneuve et al. 2003, 2007). High genotypic heterogeneity is also apparent in Italy, where at least 15 different TTR mutations have been identified [about 35% of affected families have Val30Met and Glu89Gln also appears to be relatively frequent (Rapezzi et al. 2006)]. Certain mutations are mainly observed in the United States (Ando et al. 2005; Planté-Bordeneuve et al. 2007): Leu58His (in families originating in Germany), Thr60Ala (in families of Irish descent), and Val122Ile, which is present in 4% of black people (Jacobson et al. 1996, 1997). The high prevalence of Val122Ile within the large Afro-American community probably makes this variety not only the most common familial amyloid cardiomyopathy, but perhaps also the most frequent form of amyloid heart disease (including AL) (Jacobson et al. 1996).

Clinical Profiles and Genotype–Phenotype Correlations

ATTR is characterized by a high degree of phenotypic as well as genotypic heterogeneity. Phenotypic heterogeneity is linked to at least three different factors: (1) the type of TTR mutation; (2) geographic distribution; and (3) the type of aggregation (endemic or nonendemic).

In the "classic" endemic TTR Val30Met type of FAP, prevalent in Portugal and Japan, the disorder is inherited as an autosomal dominant trait with balanced sex distribution. Sensorimotor polyneuropathy is the prominent feature. The neuropathy usually starts at 30–35 years of age with small-fiber dysfunction in the lower limbs very similar to the neuropathy of diabetes mellitus;

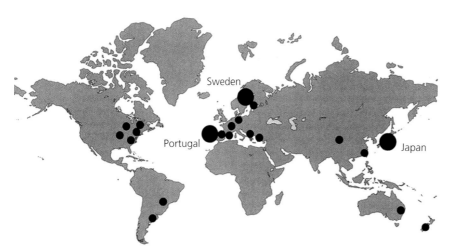

Figure 30–3 Distribution of FAP in the world. Locations of clusters of patients with FAP amyloidogenic mutated transthyretin Val30Met described in previous reports and obtained from personal communications are presented. The size of the circles is related to the number of patients at each location. Reprinted from Ando Y, Nakamura M, Araki S. Transthyretin-related familial amyloidotic polyneuropathy. *Arch Neurol.* 2005;62:1057–1062, with permission.

lack of thermal appreciation despite tactile sensitivity preservation (syringomyelic-like sensory dissociation) is often an early feature (Ando et al. 2005; Benson and Kincaid 2007). Painful paraesthesias and dysesthesias may be prominent. Motor function tends to be well maintained until the sensory neuropathy has reached an advanced phase. Sensory loss in the lower extremities slowly progresses upward from the feet and ankles to the knees and beyond, with similar symptoms eventually developing in the upper extremities. Autonomic neuropathy tends to occur relatively early and leads to severe orthostatic hypotension, disturbed bowel movement with constipation and diarrhoea, erectile dysfunction in men, bladder retention, and urinary incontinence (Ando et al. 2005; Benson and Kincaid 2007). In some men, sexual impotence is the initial clinical symptom. Nerve conduction studies can be a valuable tool for detecting peripheral nerve involvement.

Electrophysiological findings can help distinguish polyneuropathy from localized abnormalities, such as median neuropathy at the wrist (carpal tunnel syndrome). Serial studies can help follow the course of peripheral nerve abnormality (Ando et al. 2005; Benson and Kincaid 2007).

In the subgroup of Japanese and Portuguese patients with the nonendemic, "late onset" Val30Met TTR mutation, autonomic dysfunction is milder, and sensory loss and cardiomyopathy are more common than in early onset cases of FAP (Ando et al. 2005; Benson and Kincaid 2007). The clinical profile of Swedish patients is different in that the average age at onset is the mid-fifties, penetrance at around 50%, and progression of the disease considerably slower than in Japanese and Portuguese patients (Suhr et al. 2003; Ohmori et al. 2004).

The carpal tunnel syndrome is a relatively frequent feature of ATTR irrespective of a particular mutation and occasionally may be the only clinical manifestation. Vocal hoarseness can occur due to recurrent laryngeal nerve palsy, and the "scalloped pupil" deformity, which is essentially pathognomonic for FAP, is due to amyloid deposition in ciliary nerves of the eye (Benson and Kincaid 2007). Vitreous opacities accompany about 20% of TTR mutations, and may be the first manifestation of FAP (Goren et al. 1980; Yazaki et al. 2002). TTR amyloid in the vitreous is probably the result of synthesis by the retinal pigment epithelium. Amyloid fibrils in the vitreous are predominantly (about 90%–95%) composed of variant TTR, which is less prevalent (60%–65%) in fibrils found in nerve and cardiac tissue (Benson and Kincaid 2007).

In a characteristic, oculoleptomeningeal form of FAP, which can be induced by several TTR mutations, cerebral amyloid angiopathy and ocular amyloidosis are common (Goren et al. 1980). Cerebral amyloid angiopathy is characterized by amyloid deposition in the cortex and leptomeninges (Goren et al. 1980; Benson and Kincaid 2007). Typical clinical central nervous system manifestations include stroke, seizures, hydrocephalus, spastic paralysis, spinal cord infarction or, later, cerebral hemorrhage (Goren et al. 1980; Benson and Kincaid 2007). Although amyloid deposits in the meningocerebrovascular system were thought to be the cause of central nervous system symptoms, the precise mechanism of amyloid formation remains to be elucidated. Renal involvement is generally not a feature of TTR-associated cardiac amyloidosis.

Amyloidotic Cardiac Involvement

Amyloid can infiltrate various cardiovascular structures, including the conduction system, the atrial and ventricular myocardium, valvular tissue, the coronary arteries, and the large arteries (Falk et al. 1997; Hattori et al. 2003; Merlini and Bellotti 2003; Ikeda 2004; Falk 2005; Selvanayagam et al. 2007). The conduction system is commonly affected in cardiac amyloidosis, leading to sinoatrial node disease, atrial fibrillation, atrioventricular and bundle branch block, and ventricular tachycardia. Myocardial infiltration progressively increases the thickness of left and right ventricular walls and of the interatrial septum (Figure 30–4). Involvement of cardiac valves leads to formation of nodules or diffuse thickening of the leaflets accompanied by a variable degree (generally mild) of valvular regurgitation. Deposition in the coronary arteries most frequently involves intramural arteries and may lead to myocardial ischemia in spite of angiographically normal epicardial vessels.

Cardiac amyloidosis is generally considered to be a myocardial disease with "hypertrophic phenotype" and restrictive physiology that leads to diastolic heart failure (Klein et al. 1989; Elliott et al. 2008). However, any representative cohort of patients with amyloid heart disease will display a spectrum of diastolic filling abnormalities, with the restrictive pattern seen only in advanced stages of the disease. The left ventricular filling pattern generally evolves from an abnormal relaxation pattern, through a pseudonormal phase, to a restrictive pattern (Klein et al. 1989; Falk 2005). Left ventricular systolic function can be impaired in patients with overt heart failure, although the left ventricular ejection fraction is often only mildly reduced (without left ventricular enlargement). Abnormalities in long-axis function of both ventricles (detectable at tissue Doppler echocardiography) are frequent and appear earlier (Klein et al. 1989; Koyama et al. 2002; Palka et al. 2002; Elliott et al. 2008). Microvascular amyloidotic coronary infiltration can occur even in the absence of ventricular wall thickening, and may lead to systolic/diastolic "ischemic" dysfunction in the context of a dilated nonhypertrophic left ventricle. This presentation of amyloidosis is rare, probably being found in less than 1%–2% of patients with cardiac involvement (Falk 2005; Pasotti et al. 2006).

Prevalence and Clinical Spectrum of Cardiac Involvement in ATTR

In ATTR, the frequency and type of cardiac involvement is related to the specific TTR mutation, geographic area (Portugal, Japan, Sweden, other countries), and endemic/nonendemic aggregation.

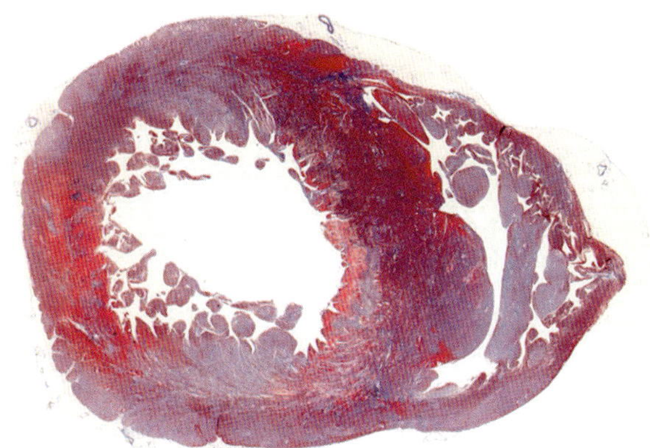

Figure 30–4 Macrosopic cross-section at the mid-ventricular level of a heart explanted from an ATTR patient during combined heart-liver transplantation. The amyloid (pale pink with hematoxylin and eosin staining) has diffusely infiltrated the myocardium, and in many areas has completely replaced the normal myocardial tissue (photograph kindly provided by Dr. Ornella Leone).

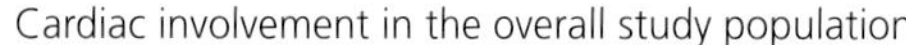

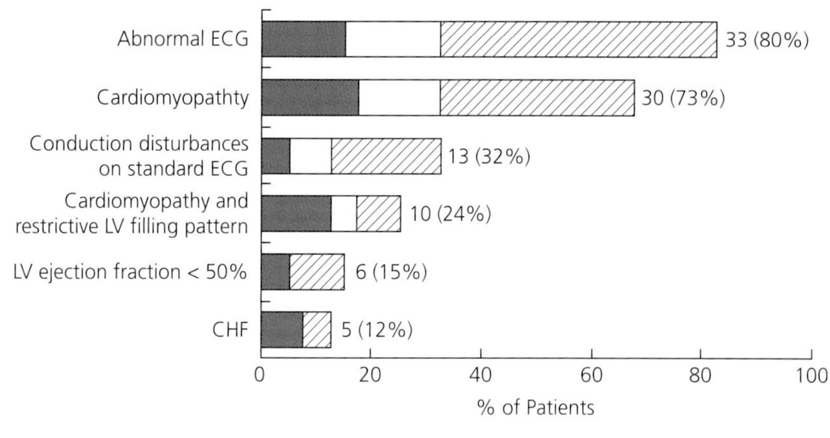

Figure 30–5 Prevalence of different manifestations of cardiac involvement in a series of 41 ATTR patients referred to a specialized Italian tertiary center. Reprinted from Rapezzi C, Perugini E, Salvi F et al. Phenotypic and genotypic heterogeneity in TTR-related cardiac amyloidosis: toward tailoring of therapeutic strategies? *Amyloid.* 2006;13:143–153, with permission.

Table 30–2 List of the Main TTR Mutations Subdivided According to Three Prevalent Clinical Profiles

Prevalent polyneuropathy	Cys10Arg, Asp18Glu, Ala25Ser, Ala25Thr, Val28Met, Val30Ala, Val30Leu, Val30Met, Phe33Ile, Phe33Leu, Phe33Val, Arg34Thr, Lys35Asn, Ala36Pro, Asp38Ala, Phe44Ser, Ala45Asp, Gly47Arg, Gly47Val, Thr49Ala, Thr49Ile, Ser50Arg, Ser52Pro, Glu54Gly, Glu54Lys, Leu55Pro, Leu55Gln, Leu58Arg, Thr59Lys, Glu61Lys, Lys70Asn, Val71Ala, Ile73Val, Ser77Phe, Ile84Thr, Glu89Lys, Ala91Ser, Ser112Ile, Tyr114His, Tyr116Ser, Val122Ala.
Prevalent myocardial involvement	Asp18Asn, Val20Ile, Ser23Asn, Pro24Ser, Phe33Cys, Glu42Asp, Glu42Gly, Ala45Ser, Ala45Thr, Gly47Ala, Thr49Pro, Ser50Ile, Glu51Gly, His56Arg, Leu58His, Thr60Ala, Phe64Leu, Ile68Leu, Tyr69Ile, Ser77Tyr, Ala81Thr, Ile84Asn, Ile84Ser, Glu89Gln, Gln92Lys, Ala97Gly, Arg103Ser, Ile107Val, Leu111Met, Ala120Ser, Val122Ile.
Prevalent leptomeningeal involvement	Leu12Pro, Asp18Gly, Val30Gly, Gly53Glu, Phe64Ser, Ile84Ser, Tyr114Cys.

Severity of cardiac involvement ranges widely from asymptomatic atrioventricular and bundle branch blocks to severe, rapidly progressive heart failure secondary to restrictive cardiomyopathy.

As a general rule, patients with the Val30Met mutation who come from endemic foci tend to have less severe heart involvement in comparison with individuals who carry the same mutation but come from a nonendemic area or have mutations other than Val30Met (Hattori et al. 2003; Ikeda 2004; Ando et al. 2005). In endemic areas of Portugal and Japan, conduction disturbances are the single most frequent form of cardiac involvement, whereas congestive heart failure due to amyloidotic cardiomyopathy is a rare, age-related manifestation. Patients in nonendemic areas of the same countries are more prone to develop severe cardiac amyloidosis (Hattori et al. 2003; Ikeda 2004; Ando et al. 2005). Elsewhere, the likelihood and severity of cardiomyopathy varies with the type of mutation. In an Italian setting, a broad spectrum of cardiac abnormalities was observed (Figure 30–5), with prevalence ranging from 24% for cardiomyopathies with restrictive physiology to 80% for any type of ECG abnormality (Rapezzi et al. 2006). Remarkably, cardiomyopathy of varying degrees of severity was found in the context of all but one of the TTR mutations encountered in this specialist center. Notably, in many non-Val30-Met mutations, amyloidotic cardiomyopathy was the predominant or the exclusive clinical manifestation of ATTR (Table 30–2). In some of these mutations, neurological manifestations can be mild or absent with low penetrance, thereby simulating sporadic forms of non-ATTR amyloidotic cardiomyopathy or even hypertrophic cardiomyopathy caused by sarcomeric protein gene mutations.

Diagnostic Examinations

1. Electrocardiography

The ECG is rarely normal in patients with cardiac amyloidosis (Carroll et al. 1982; Hamer et al. 1992; Rahman et al. 2004; Murtagh et al. 2005). About 10%–15% of patients present with atrial fibrillation. The spectrum of QRS and repolarization alterations includes low ECG voltage (presence of QRS voltage amplitude ≤0.5 mV in all limb leads, or ≤1 mV in all precordial leads), pseudoinfarct patterns (anterior, inferior, or lateral) (Figure 30–6), left anterior hemiblock, right bundle branch block, and ischemic-type or nonspecific T-wave abnormalities (Carroll et al. 1982; Hamer et al. 1992; Rahman et al. 2004; Murtagh et al. 2005). Low QRS voltage is considered the most typical ECG finding in cardiac amyloidosis, especially when coexistent with increased left ventricular wall thickness. In a series of patients with cardiomyopathy of suspected amyloidotic origin, the combination of low QRS voltage and interventricular septal thickness >1.98 cm provided a sensitivity of 72% and a specificity of 91% for a biopsy-proven diagnosis of (mainly AL) cardiac amyloidosis (Rahman et al. 2004). Our experience (unpublished data) of patients affected by amyloidotic

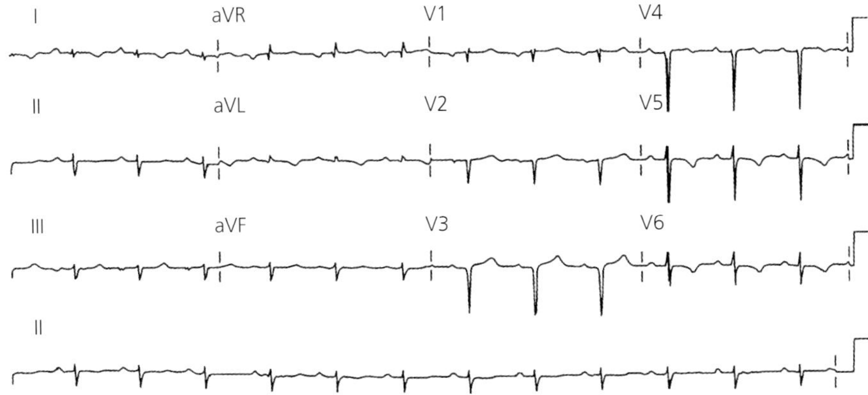

Figure 30–6 Characteristic ECG from an ATTR patient with amyloidotic cardiomyopathy. The most striking features are low QRS voltage in the limb leads, anterior "pseudoinfarction" pattern, and diffuse "ischemic" T-wave abnormalities.

cardiomyopathy suggests that the prevalence of low QRS voltage at presentation may be significantly lower in ATTR than in AL (about 30% vs. 50%). This observation underlines the importance of pursuing any clinical suspicion of ATTR amyloidotic cardiomyopathy, even in the absence of reduced QRS voltage.

2. Echocardiography

Echocardiography is the main noninvasive instrumental examination for detection of cardiac involvement, since it can reveal several features that are suggestive of cardiac amyloidosis (Figure 30–7) (Cueto-Garcia et al. 1984; Klein et al. 1991; Simons and Isner 1992; Trikas et al. 1999; Lachmann et al. 2002; Demir et al. 2005; Gertz et al. 2005). It has to be remembered, however, that such features commonly appear only in the later stages of disease (Falk 2005; Selvanayagam et al. 2007). Thus, echocardiographic images must be interpreted in the context of the clinical picture and other examinations, and they cannot be used in isolation for diagnostic confirmation. The most frequent echocardiographic finding is increased thickness of the interventricular septum and of the left ventricular free wall. This finding is often erroneously referred to as "hypertrophy," whereas in reality it corresponds to amyloidotic myocardial infiltration. Other characteristic echocardiographic findings include

- increased right ventricular wall thickness;
- increased interatrial septal thickness;
- diffuse granular appearance of the myocardium;
- atrioventricular valve thickening;
- pericardial effusion.

Much stress has been laid on the diagnostic relevance of the granular or speckled appearance of the ventricular myocardium at echocardiography. However, recognition of a "granular pattern" remains subjective and current imaging technology may enhance myocardial echogenicity while at the same time attenuating granularity (Selvanayagam et al. 2007). Nevertheless, the current definition of amyloidotic cardiomyopathy (Gertz et al. 2005) is based on echocardiographic criteria: end-diastolic thickness of the interventricular septum >1.2 cm (in the absence of any other cause of ventricular hypertrophy) plus two or more of the following: (1) homogeneous atrioventricular valve thickening, (2) atrial septum thickening, and (3) sparkling/granular appearance of the ventricular septum.

The ventricles are usually not dilated in amyloidotic cardiomyopathy. The left ventricular ejection fraction tends to be normal or only slightly reduced, but the wall thickening velocity is frequently depressed. Similarly, the long-axis function of the left ventricle is often reduced even in the early phases of the disease when radial fractional shortening is still conserved (Demir et al. 2005; Falk 2005). Echo-Doppler evaluation provides particularly relevant information regarding the diastolic phase of ventricular function. The frequency and types of diastolic abnormalities are related to the different phases of the disease. In particular, a true "restrictive filling pattern" is generally encountered only in advanced amyloidotic cardiomyopathy.

3. Magnetic Resonance Imaging

Magnetic resonance imaging (MRI) with delayed gadolinium enhancement is useful for detection of amyloidotic myocardial infiltration (Maceira et al. 2005; Perugini et al. 2006; Thomson 2008; Vogelsberg et al. 2008). Gadolinium tends to accumulate within the interstitium infiltrated by amyloid (Figure 30–8), leading to a late enhancement effect, most often in the subendocardium (Maceira et al. 2005), and less commonly in localized and transmural distributions (Perugini et al. 2006). A unique feature of delayed-enhancement MRI in amyloidotic cardiomyopathy is the dark appearance of the blood pool, due to similar T1 values of the myocardium and blood (produced by high myocardial uptake and fast blood pool washout) (Maceira et al. 2005). Although MRI certainly provides relevant information in the diagnostic work up, its diagnostic accuracy and predictive value have not yet been studied in real-world situations where a variety of primary/secondary myocardial diseases have to be considered in the differential diagnosis.

4. Nuclear Scintigraphy

Scintigraphy is another important noninvasive examination for diagnosis and monitoring of amyloidosis (Hawkins 2002; Falk 2005; Perugini et al. 2005; Selvanayagam et al. 2007). I^{123}-labeled serum amyloid P (SAP) specifically binds with all types of fibril (via a calcium-mediated mechanism). Its consequent accumulation in all amyloid deposits provides valuable information on the presence and topography of amyloid deposits in the body, making it possible to monitor progression and therapeutic response (Hawkins 2002). Unfortunately, SAP scanning is restricted to very few centers and it cannot image the beating heart. Recently, we have provided preliminary evidence that ^{99m}Tc-3,3-diphosphono-1,2-propanodi-carboxylic acid (^{99m}Tc-DPD) scintigraphy is capable of imaging amyloid deposition in the myocardium in the context of TTR-related amyloidosis but not in AL amyloidosis (Perugini et al. 2005). This specific imaging characteristic may facilitate

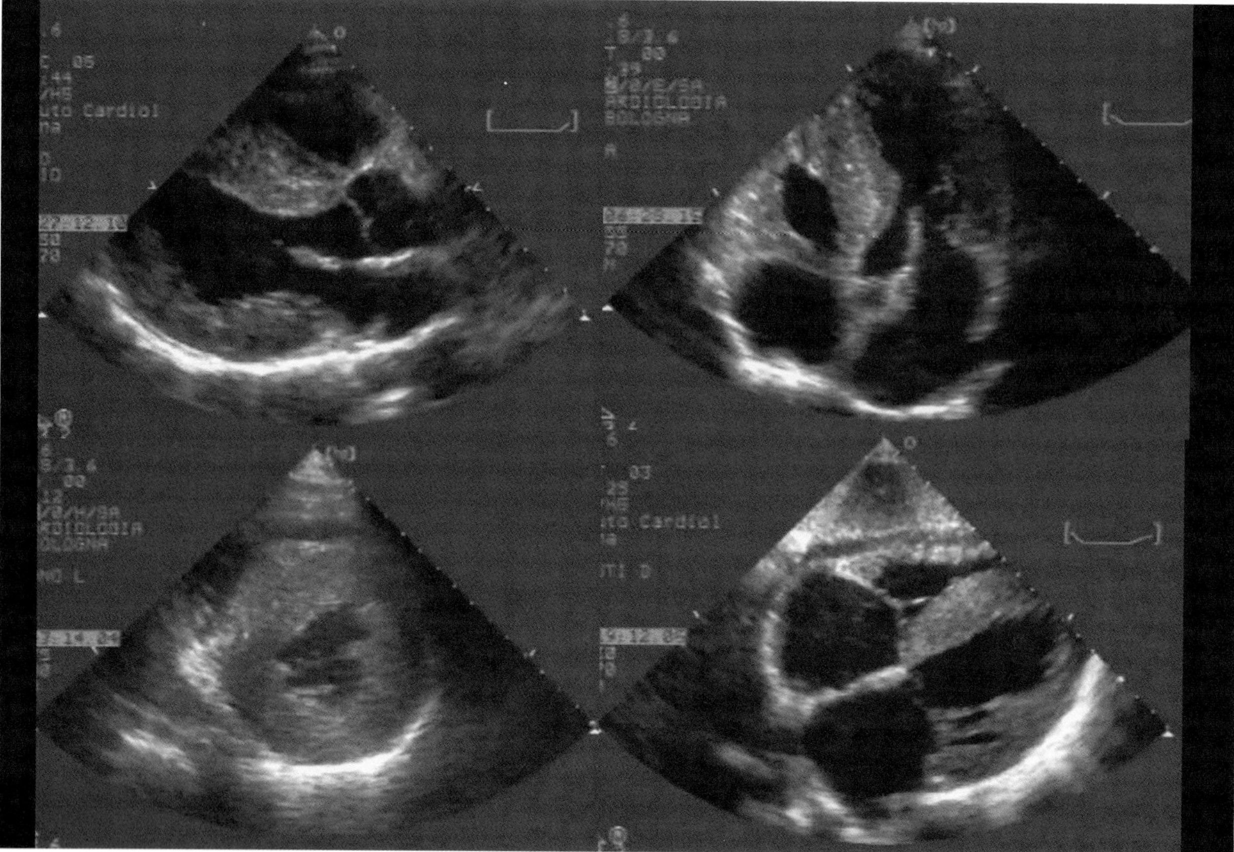

Figure 30–7 Characteristic echocardiograms from four different ATTR patients affected by amyloidotic cardiomyopathy. The most striking shared feature is the increased thickness of the interventricular septum and free left ventricular wall. In the top right panel (four-chamber view), thickening of the mitral valve is also apparent. In the bottom right panel (subcostal view), thickening can also be seen in the free right ventricular wall and interatrial septum.

differential diagnosis between TTR and AL cardiac amyloidosis in routine practice (Figure 30–9)

5. Endomyocardial Biopsy

Endomyocardial biopsy readily provides histological evidence of amyloid heart disease; false negatives are uncommon given the widespread myocardial diffusion of amyloid deposits (Crotty et al. 1995; Gertz et al. 1997; Ardehali et al. 2004). Since the ventricular walls are commonly thickened, biopsy carries a very low risk of cardiac perforation.

Biomarkers

In AL cardiac amyloidosis, troponin T and B-natriuretic peptide (BNP) plasma concentrations both tend to be elevated, even in the context of only limited ventricular dysfunction and mild or absent symptoms of congestive heart failure (Dispenzieri et al. 2003, 2006; Palladini et al. 2003, 2006; Suhr et al. 2008). Both troponin and BNP values can be useful to stratify the prognosis of AL patients and monitor their response to therapy (Dispenzieri et al. 2003, 2006; Palladini et al. 2003, 2006). Fewer biomarker data are available for ATTR (Suhr et al. 2008). In one of the few studies dedicated to ATTR-related cardiomyopathy, the frequency and entity of raised BNP and troponin values were less than those reported for AL. This observation is in line with the hypothesis that TTR amyloid exerts a less toxic effect on myocytes than AL amyloid (Schubert et al. 1995; Suhr et al. 2008).

ATTR Amyloidosis versus AL and Systemic Senile Amyloidosis

Hitherto, we have mainly considered amyloidotic cardiac involvement in the broad context of a systemic amyloidosis that infiltrates the heart. Although ATTR, AL, and systemic senile cardiac amyloidosis share many features, there are some important differences (Table 30–3) (Dubrey et al. 1997; Ng et al. 2005). Compared to AL cardiac amyloidosis (the most common form), ATTR seems to be characterized by slightly greater ventricular wall thickness, less pronounced systolic and diastolic cardiac dysfunction with lower ventricular filling pressures, and lower prevalence of low QRS voltage. Furthermore, ATTR cardiac amyloidosis patients less often develop heart failure symptoms or die from cardiovascular complications.

Diagnosis of ATTR Cardiac Amyloidosis

1. Clinical Suspicion

From the cardiologist's standpoint, two main clinical scenarios can be distinguished in ATTR: (1) a clinical picture characterized by neurological impairment or a preexisting diagnosis of FAP; (2) heart muscle disease in the absence of a neurological diagnosis. If there is a strong suspicion or an existing diagnosis of FAP, the cardiologist's role is to look for signs of cardiac involvement. In such situations, ECG and echocardiography generally provide all the necessary diagnostic information. To recognize very early signs of

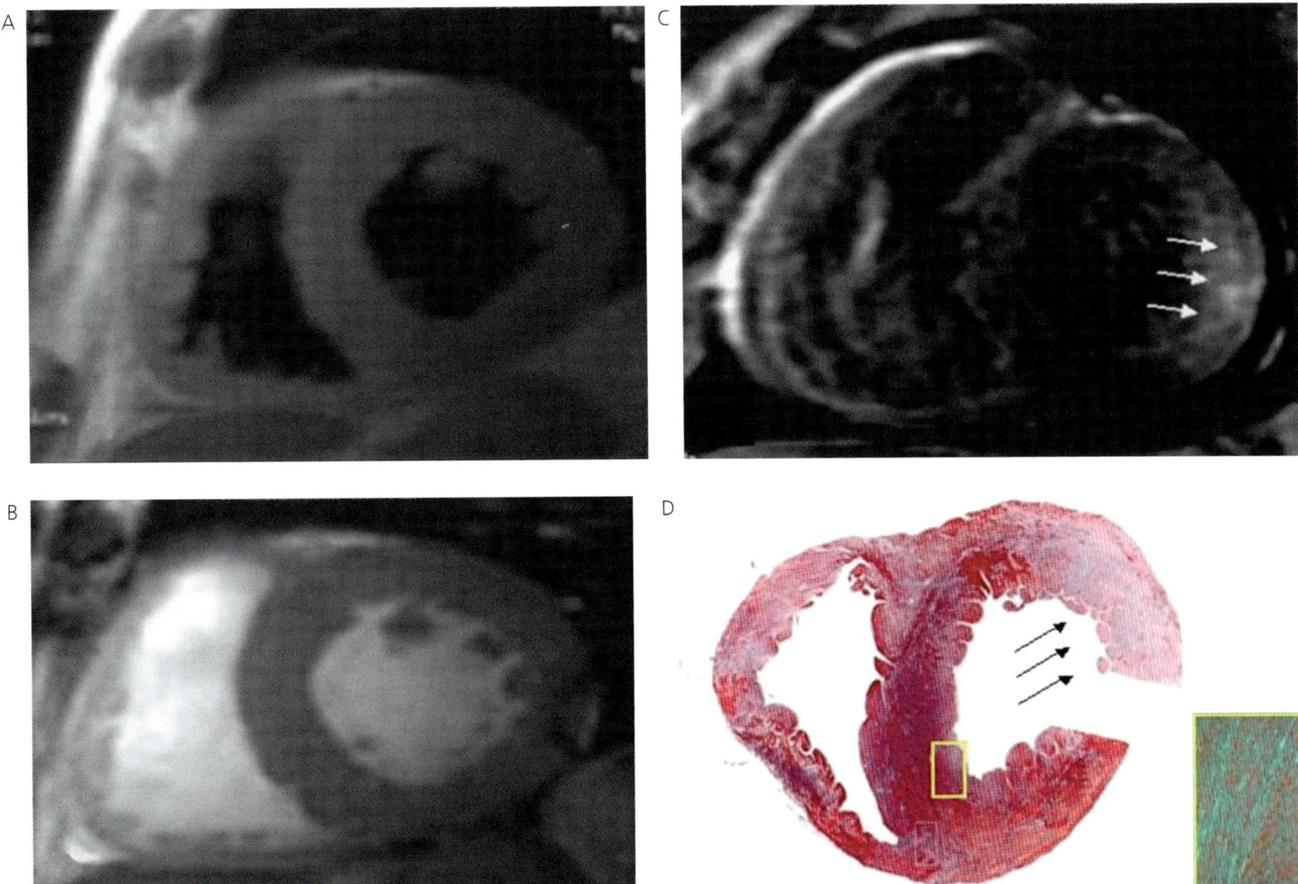

Figure 30–8 In a 43-year-old man with familial TTR-related cardiac amyloidosis, conventional cardiac magnetic resonance (CMR) with (A) black blood fast spin echo and (B) bright blood fast gradient echo sequences shows increased left and right ventricular thicknesses. (C) Gadolinium inversion recovery fast gradient echo also shows a large transmural zone of strong, patchy hyperenhancement (arrows). (D) After combined heart and liver transplantation, myocardial histological analysis showed diffuse amyloid deposition with characteristic green birefringence on Congo-red staining (inset) and an area of massive infiltration (arrows) corresponding to the strong, patchy enhancement seen on Gd-CMR. With permission from Perugini E, Rapezzi C, Piva T, et al. Noninvasive evaluation of the myocardial substrate of cardiac amyloidosis by gadolinium cardiac magnetic resonance. *Heart.* 2006;92:343–349.

Table 30–3 Comparison of the Characteristics of the Three Main Forms of Systemic Cardiac Amyloidosis: Summary of the Literature (and the Authors' Experience)

	AL	Systemic Senile Amyloidosis	ATTR
Ventricular walls	Mild thickening	Greatly thickened	Moderate thickening
AV valve involvement	Sometimes	Sometimes	Frequent
Diastolic dysfunction	Often moderate	Often mild	Sometimes
Systolic dysfunction	Sometimes	Frequent	Occasionally
Low QRS voltage	Frequent	Occasionally	Sometimes
Left bundle branch block	Sometimes	Occasionally	Sometimes
^{99m}Tc-DPD myocardial uptake	Absent/weak	Strong	Strong
Severe heart failure	Very frequent	Frequent	Occasionally
Prognosis	Poor	Fair	Fair

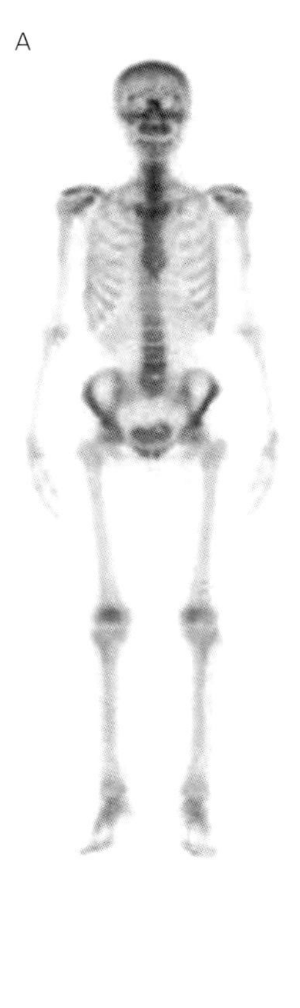

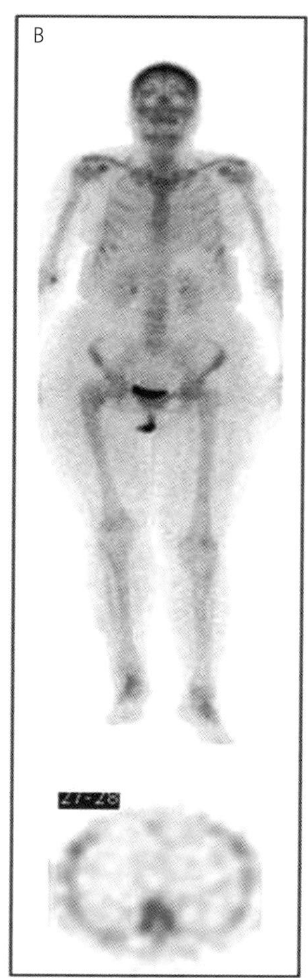

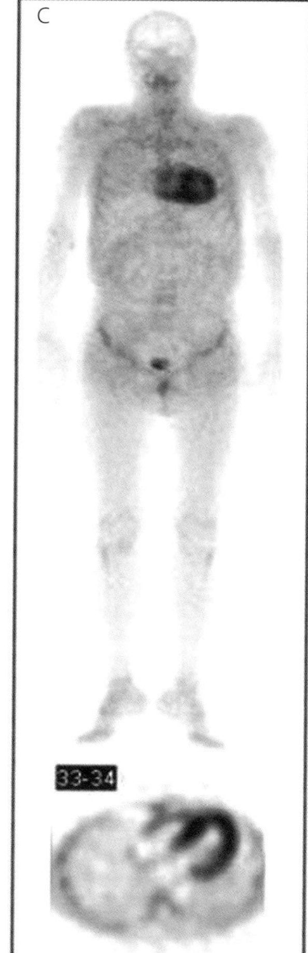

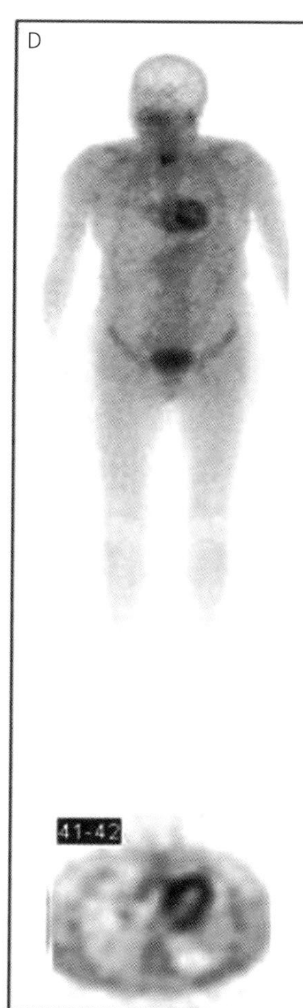

Figure 30–9 Representative examples illustrating the spectrum of ^{99m}Tc-DPD uptake among patients with TTR-related or AL cardiac amyloidosis and unaffected controls (top row: whole-body scans, anterior view; bottom row: cross-sectional views of cardiac SPECT in the same patients). (A) Unaffected control subject without visually detectable uptake. (B) Patient with AL amyloidosis and echocardiographic documentation of cardiac involvement without any visually detectable sign of myocardial ^{99m}Tc-DPD uptake; mild uptake of the tracer is visible only at soft tissue level. (C and D) Two patients with TTR-related amyloidosis and echocardiographic documentation of cardiac involvement, both showing strong myocardial ^{99m} Tc-DPD uptake (with absent bone uptake); in one of the patients (D), splanchnic uptake is also visible. Perugini E, Guidalotti PL, Salvi F, et al. Noninvasive etiologic diagnosis of cardiac amyloidosis using 99mTc-3,3-diphosphono-1,2-propanodicarboxylic acid scintigraphy. *J Am Coll Cardiol.* 2005;46:1076–1084.

myocardial involvement, careful observation of the longitudinal left ventricular function with tissue Doppler echocardiography is particularly revealing.

The situation in which there is no neurological suspicion of FAP is much more challenging for cardiologists. Patients may be present with heart failure symptoms, arrhythmias, syncope, orthostatic hypertension, or ECG/echocardiographic abnormalities in the absence of symptoms. Differentiation from cardiomyopathies of other etiology can be difficult and not infrequently results in misdiagnosis of cardiac amyloidosis as familial hypertrophic cardiomyopathy. However, the particular echocardiographic signs described above should raise suspicion of amyloidotic etiology once "hypertrophic cardiomyopathy" has been recognized. Perhaps the single most useful sign is the presence of low or normal QRS voltage despite increased left ventricular wall thickness (Figure 30–10). Unfortunately, this highly specific sign is not very sensitive and is more frequent in AL than in TTR-related amyloidosis.

Apart from evident neurological manifestations, other clinical pointers for a diagnosis of hereditary ATTR amyloidosis include

- familial neurological disease (even in the absence of a precise diagnosis of FAP);
- a personal history of carpal tunnel syndrome;
- sensorimotor peripheral neuropathy;
- unexplained intense muscular pain in the leg and burning sensations;
- autonomic nervous system dysfunction (e.g., dyshydrosis, erectile dysfunction, diarrhoea alternating with constipation);
- vitreous opacity.

Since some of these signs can be very mild, and not necessarily self-reported by the patient, an active search is mandatory.

2. Tissue Diagnosis

Table 30–4 summarizes the main features that can facilitate a differential etiological diagnosis between the three main forms of systemic amyloidosis. Since AL amyloidosis is the most common form of the disease, a search for clonal plasma-cell dyscrasia is generally the first step. A detailed description of the sequence of

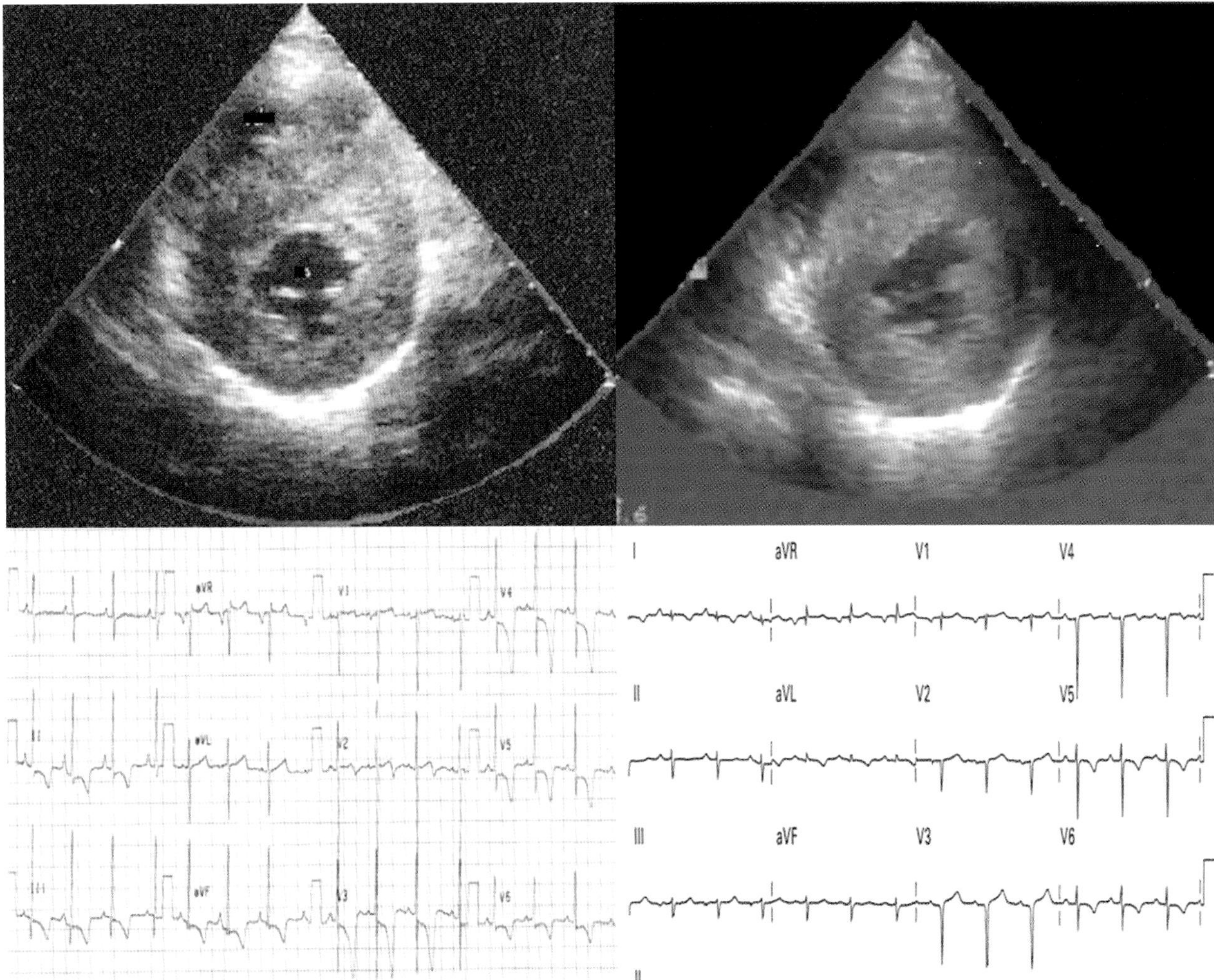

Figure 30–10 Echocardiograms and ECG from a patient with sarcomeric hypertrophic cardiomyopathy (left) and amyloidotic cardiomyopathy (right). Despite similar degrees of left ventricular "hypertrophy" at echocardiography, the ECG are profoundly different (left ventricular hypertrophy and strain in the patient with sarcomeric hypertrophic cardiomyopathy vs. low QRS voltage in the patient with amyloidotic cardiomyopathy).

diagnostic tests used for plasma-cell dyscrasia can be found elsewhere (Merlini and Bellotti 2003; Falk 2005; Gertz et al. 2005). Histological evidence of amyloid deposits is essential for a final diagnosis of amyloidosis. In cases of AL amyloidosis, abdominal fat aspiration is generally regarded as preferable to other forms of biopsy. Immunohistochemical staining of biopsies from involved tissues or abdominal fat using specific antibodies can reliably distinguish between AL and ATTR. However, abdominal fat analysis is less sensitive for TTR-related forms of systemic amyloidosis (Falk 2005; Selvanayagam et al. 2007). In theory, an endomyocardial biopsy is necessary to reach a definitive histological diagnosis. However, in a patient with a genetically proven diagnosis of ATTR, echocardiographic identification of unexplained ventricular hypertrophy provides clinical evidence of the specific disease.

Therapy

The Pharmacological Approach to the Amyloidogenic Process

Ideally, treatment of systemic amyloidosis would halt amyloid deposition and promote resorption of the abnormal protein in order to recover the impaired organ function. Unfortunately, no such pharmacological option is yet available in clinical practice. However, there is increasing interest in the use of small molecules that impede fibril formation (Miroy et al. 1996; Merlini and Bellotti 2003; Merlini and Westermark 2004). As amyloid fibril formation partially depends on the concentration of the amyloidogenic precursor, it may be sufficient to reduce the concentration of the precursor below a critical threshold in order to arrest deposition (and possibly promote resorption of the deposits). Since several types of amyloidosis stem from impaired folding of the protein precursor, there has been a search for ligands that could restabilize the precursor, thereby preventing its aggregation and fibril formation. Following the initial observation that the natural ligand thyroxin can inhibit fibril formation in vitro by stabilizing the TTR tetramer (Miroy et al. 1996), several structurally distinct families of similar ligands have been identified (Baures et al. 1998; Peterson et al. 1998), including some commonly used nonsteroidal antiinflammatory drugs. The current challenge is to develop ligands that are highly selective for TTR in plasma (without binding to albumin). Availability of such compounds could pave the way to a pharmacological treatment of TTR-related disease, as well as other types of amyloidosis where the protein precursor is amenable to stabilization.

Table 30–4 Main Features that can Facilitate a Differential Etiological Diagnosis between the Tree Main Forms of Systemic Amyloidosis

Suggestive clinical/instrumental signs	AL present	ATTR present	Systemic Senile Amyloidosis present
Histological finding of amyloid in biopsy from affected organ or abdominal fat	positive	positive	positive (myocardium)
Plasma-cell dyscrasia	present	absent	absent
Transthyretin mutation	absent	present	absent
Immunoistochemistry	positive for κ or λ light chains	positive for TTR	positive for TTR
Characteristic neurological signs	Sometimes	Yes	Sometimes
Echocardiographic findings suggestive of amyloidotic cardiomyopathy	Sometimes	Sometimes	Yes

Another potential pharmacological approach involves disruption of the process of self-aggregation of proteins/peptides, which drives the formation of amyloid fibrils. Molecules that have shown to be capable of inhibiting fibrillogenesis in vitro could theoretically also be applied to other forms of amyloidosis. However, several problems still need to be addressed, including low specificity and toxicity (Wolfe 2002).

Several compounds can directly target amyloid deposits to induce their resorption or disassembly. Iodinated anthracycline (4'-iodo-4'-deoxydoxorubicin) preferentially binds with amyloid fibrils of various biochemical types. This molecule reduces the formation of AA-amyloid deposits in mice (Merlini et al. 1995) and promotes amyloid fibril disaggregation in vitro (Merlini et al. 1995; Sebastiao et al. 2000; Cardoso et al. 2003). However, early clinical trials indicate that when used alone this drug induces transient responses in only a small proportion of patients (Gianni et al. 1995; Gertz et al. 2002) and its real utility remains uncertain. In animal models, less toxic compounds such as tetracyclines have been shown to inhibit fibril formation and disassemble preformed fibrils (Forloni et al. 2001; Cardoso et al. 2003).

Prevention and Treatment of Cardiovascular (and Other) Complications

In the absence of specific treatments for any of the etiologically distinct forms of cardiac amyloidosis, the main therapeutic aims are to relieve symptoms, treat congestive heart failure, and prevent arrhythmic and thromboembolic complications (Falk 2005; Selvanayagam et al. 2007). Diuretics are essential for treatment of venous congestion. However, their use must be judicious, as preload reduction in patients with overt restrictive physiology may reduce ventricular filling pressures, leading to decreased cardiac output and hypotension. Large resistant pleural effusions (particularly frequent in AL) may indicate the presence of pleural amyloidotic involvement (Berk et al. 2003), occasionally necessitating recurrent pleural taps or even pleurodesis. Digoxin must be used with caution, due to its high arrhythmogenicity in the amyloidotic substrate (Falk et al. 1997). Indeed, the high propensity of this drug to bind with amyloid fibrils (Rubinow et al. 1981) can easily lead to clinical manifestations of digoxin toxicity, even in the presence of apparently "therapeutic" serum levels (Falk 2005). Maintenance of sinus rhythm is important, since development of atrial fibrillation worsens diastolic dysfunction, and a rapid ventricular response may further compromise the pumping function.

The decision whether or not to start antithrombotic therapy is complex, particularly in AL where risk of hemorrhage is high. In ATTR, hemorrhagic events appear to be less common. Anticoagulation with warfarin is mandatory for patients with paroxysmal or permanent atrial fibrillation and flutter. It has also been suggested that transesophageal echocardiography is useful to identify patients that have atrial dysfunction despite sinus rhythm (by revealing spontaneous echo contrast or atrial appendage Doppler velocities below 40 cm/s). In such cases, warfarin may be indicated in view of the risk of thrombus formation in the atrial appendage (Klein et al. 1989).

No controlled study is available regarding the effects of β-blocker used in amyloidosis, whether for rate control of atrial fibrillation or for treatment of heart failure, but rate reduction with β-blockers can cause a critical decrease in cardiac output without providing benefits in terms of reverse ventricular remodeling. Calcium channel blockers are contraindicated, since these drugs often exert relevant negative inotropic effects (Gertz et al. 1985; Pollak and Falk 1993).

In heart failure generally, ACE inhibitor or angiotensin-receptor blockers are standard therapy. However, for patients with cardiac amyloidosis these drugs must be administered with extreme caution due to the elevated risk of inducing or exacerbating hypotension.

Although sudden death is frequent in amyloidosis (Falk et al. 1984; Wright et al. 2006), very little is known about the underlying cause of most events. Sudden death has reportedly been caused by advanced atrioventricular block, ventricular tachycardia/fibrillation, and electromechanical dissociation. Implantable cardiac defibrillators have been used only in a small number of cases in the absence of any documented effect on survival. Although some centers use amiodarone to try to prevent arrhythmias and sudden death in patients with amyloidotic cardiomyopathy, studies of efficacy are lacking. If cardioversion is performed to treat atrial fibrillation, use of a temporary prophylactic pacemaker is advisable due to the risk that the abnormal sinus node may fail. When amyloidosis patients present with bradyarrhythmias, clinicians may feel justified to proceed to prophylactic pacemaker implantation earlier than they normally would with other patients. In the presence of restrictive physiology, dual-chamber devices should be preferred (Falk et al. 1984).

Neurogenic orthostatic hypotension is difficult to prevent and treat. General prophylactic nonpharmacologic measures and midodrine, a peripheral, selective, direct α1-adrenoreceptor agonist (the only medication approved by the U.S. Food and Drug Administration for the treatment of orthostatic hypotension) are the only palliative treatments that can be offered to patients (Freeman 2008). Phosphodiesterase inhibitors can be used to treat erectile dysfunction (Obayashi et al. 2000).

Orthotopic Liver Transplantation

Since the liver is mainly responsible for TTR production, orthotopic liver transplantation (OLT) can provide a "surgical gene therapy" for ATTR amyloidosis. OLT promotes a rapid and stable decrease of circulating mutated TTR in the serum and stabilizes symptoms.

According to the FAP World Transplant Registry, more than 700 OLT procedures have been performed in a total of 12 different countries. (Herlenius et al. 2001) Prophylactic preoperative pacemaker implantation is widely performed in patients with evidence of cardiac autonomic involvement. Long-term survival after OLT (77% at 5 years) appears to compare favorably with that of patients undergoing OLT due to liver disease. However, the continued production of variant TTR in the choroid plexus, which occurs with some TTR mutations, and patients' differing rates of amyloid turnover may both contribute to adverse outcomes after OLT. The outcomes of ATTR patients affected by the Val30Met mutation, who account for the vast majority (over four-fifths) of all the OLT procedures, were significantly better than those of patients with other mutations (overall survival, 80% vs. 59% at 5 years) (Suhr et al. 2000; Dubrey et al. 2001; Herlenius et al. 2001; Olofsson et al. 2002). More favorable 5-year survival figures were also recorded for patients with shorter (<7-year) prior histories of neurological symptoms (80% vs. 60%) and for those with better nutritional status (83% vs. 60%) (Herlenius et al. 2001). Furthermore, improvements in sensorimotor neuropathy (reported by 44% of OLT recipients) or neuromuscular status (reported by 41%) tended to be more common in patients with mild symptoms of recent onset (Herlenius et al. 2001). Gastrointestinal symptoms also improved in about half the recipients; about two-fifths of the ATTR patients who had poor nutritional status at the time of OLT subsequently became better nourished. Experience of OLT in oculoleptomeningeal amyloidosis is limited to a handful of patients carrying the Pro52, Cys114, and His69 TTR mutations; survival has been poor with only about half the patients living after 3 years of onset of symptoms.

Taken together, the FAP World Transplant Registry data support the concept that the first clinical improvements after OLT regard autonomic neuropathy (gastrointestinal symptoms) and are followed by benefits in terms of nutritional status, reduced orthostatic hypotension, improvements in cardiac sympathetic function, resolution of anhydrosis, and possibly also some restoration of bladder and erectile function in certain patients (Herlenius et al. 2001). Issues regarding the course of cardiac disease after OLT are more complex (see below).

Since TTR-related familial amyloidosis is an unrelenting progressive disease, OLT must be considered as soon as possible for all patients with clinically evident, molecularly confirmed disease (no indication exists for healthy carriers). Moreover, as OLT seems primarily to halt disease progression without fully reversing the clinical manifestations, this strategy cannot be reasonably proposed for patients in advanced stages of the disease (Ando et al. 2005; Falk 2005).

Domino Liver Transplantation

Since liver function is preserved in ATTR amyloidosis and the amyloid deposition is a slow process, domino transplantation can be considered. Most data regarding domino liver transplantation come from the FAP World Transplant Registry. Between 1995 and 2002, a total of 210 domino transplantations were performed with livers that had been explanted from ATTR patients, which were mainly reused for patients with hepatocellular carcinoma (Herlenius et al. 2001). The procedural results and posttransplant outcome of the domino procedures did not appear to differ from those of other heart transplantations for the underlying diseases, and none of the recipients documented in the currently available FAP Transplant Registry reports appears to have developed amyloid-related clinical manifestations (Herlenius et al. 2001). However, it has subsequently been reported that a single patient who received a liver from a domino donor with Val30Met ATTR did develop (at 8 years from OLT) progressive peripheral neuropathy, with TTR amyloid deposits being found in nerve and rectal biopsies (Stangou et al. 2005).

Combined Heart-Liver Transplantation

Cardiac involvement can affect the success of OLT and the patient's postoperative outcome in at least two different ways. Patients with amyloidotic cardiomyopathy have an increased perioperative morbidity and mortality. Indeed, any cardiological complication that leads to low cardiac output or increased filling pressure in the perioperative phase can fatally damage the transplanted liver, thereby threatening the life of the recipient and wasting a precious life-saving organ. Cardiovascular complications account for about two-fifths of deaths after OLT (almost half of which occurs within the first 3 months) (Stangou et al. 2005). The second major problem is progression of cardiomyopathy even after successful OLT. This phenomenon has been echocardiographically documented, especially (though not exclusively) in patients with mutations other than Val30Met. After OLT, some patients with the Leu30 variant of ATTR have shown an increased proportion of amyloid derived from wild-type TTR in their myocardial tissue (Ikeda 2004). Furthermore, slow but progressive amyloidotic cardiomyopathy has been observed after OLT even in patients whose cardiac involvement was only mild up to the time of transplantation. It is currently thought that although wild-type TTR is only weakly amyloidogenic, its potential for myocardial deposition can increase dramatically in the presence of a preexisting template of amyloid in the heart. These considerations provide the rationale for combined heart-liver transplantation in selected patients (Ruygrok et al. 2001; Arpesella et al. 2003). The number of such interventions is currently limited (with no more than 30 reports available in the literature). Combined heart-liver transplantation is a technically challenging procedure, which is necessarily the province of a few highly specialized centers. The degree of neurological impairment and the patient's nutritional status are thought to be the two major factors influencing long-term outcome (Herlenius et al. 2001). Encouragingly, the cardiac grafts do not appear to be affected by amyloid during follow-up.

The main indication for combined heart-liver transplantation is presence of severe heart failure due to amyloidotic cardiomyopathy in a patient without advanced neurological involvement. Combined heart-liver transplantation has also been proposed as a therapeutic option for patients affected by mutations other than Val30Met who are candidates for OLT and who have an echocardiographic diagnosis of cardiomyopathy (even in the absence of major cardiovascular symptoms) (Rapezzi et al. 2006).

Other Hereditary Amyloidoses

Other mutated genes that can induce systemic disease with variable patterns of organ involvement and clinical severity include apolipoprotein A-I (AApoAI), apolipoprotein A-II (AApoAII), lysozyme (ALys), gelsolin (AGel), fibrinogen Aa (AFib), and Cystatin C (ACys). Clinically relevant cardiac involvement mainly occurs in patients with apolipoprotein A-I mutation.

Apolipoprotein A-I Amyloidosis (AApoAI)

Apolipoprotein A-I is the main constituent of high-density lipoprotein particles (the *ApoAI* gene is located on chromosome 11). About half of apolipoprotein A-I is synthesized in the liver and the other half in the small intestine (Nichols et al. 1990; Benson and Kincaid 2007). Twelve different *ApoAI* gene mutations (mostly single nucleotide substitutions) have been associated with deposition of apolipoprotein A-I amyloid (Benson 2003; Merlini and Westermark 2004). All forms of apolipoprotein A-I amyloidosis are inherited as autosomal dominant traits, but clinical onset varies from the third decade of life to advanced age and the penetrance is not known (although it is probably greater than 50%). Unlike ATTR, the kidney is the most frequently affected organ, and death is usually caused by renal failure. Other sites of involvement include liver, spleen, and occasionally the heart. In rare cases, cardiac involvement can lead to massive hypertrophy with very diminutive ventricular cavities (Hamidi et al. 1999). In contrast to most cases of AL, in apolipoprotein A-I amyloidosis proteinuria is usually very limited.

Apolipoprotein A-II Amyloidosis (AApoAII)

Like apolipoprotein A-I, apolipoprotein A-II is predominantly synthesized by the liver and the intestines. Apolipoprotein A-II amyloidosis is the most recently discovered hereditary systemic form of the disease. It is an autosomal dominant amyloidosis caused by point mutations in the *ApoAII* gene. Clinically, it is characterized by early adult onset of progressive renal failure. Dialysis and renal transplantation are currently the only two therapeutic options, both of which are palliative (Magy et al. 2003). After transplantation, recurrence of amyloid deposition in the graft is rare and progression of any other organ involvement tends to be very slow (Magy et al. 2003).

Lysozyme Amyloidosis (ALys)

Lysozyme is a ubiquitous bacteriolytic enzyme present in both external secretions and in leukocytes, macrophages, gastrointestinal cells, and hepatocytes; its physiologic role is not clear. Lysozyme amyloidosis is an autosomal dominant "nonneuropathic" form of hereditary amyloidosis, associated with four different lysozyme gene mutations (Trp64Arg, Ile56Thr, Asp67His, Phe57Ile) (Granel et al. 2006). Gastrointestinal involvement has been seen in nearly all reported cases of lysozyme amyloidosis, varying from mild abdominal discomfort to severe malabsorption syndrome (Granel et al. 2006). Megaloblastic anemia due to acid folic deficiency secondary to amyloid deposition in the small intestine (Yood et al. 1983) and bleeding of the gastrointestinal tract have also been described.

Renal manifestations are frequent in lysozyme amyloidosis (Simon and Moutsopoulos 1979; Yood et al. 1983). Other clinical manifestations that have been described include "sicca syndrome" (Valleix et al. 2002), bone marrow infiltration (Granel et al. 2002), and heart involvement (Gillmore et al. 1999; Booth et al. 2000).

Gelsolin (AGel)

Gelsolin amyloidosis is rather common in Finland (Sack et al. 1981; Sunada et al. 1993; Benson and Kincaid 2007) but very rare elsewhere. This type of amyloidosis stems from a mutation (Asp187Asn) in plasma gelsolin, an actin-modulating protein that takes part in the clearance of actin filaments (Levy et al. 1990; Maury et al. 2006). The main clinical manifestations are corneal lattice dystrophy, cranial neuropathy, and cutis laxa. Peripheral and autonomic neuropathy, and cardiac or renal involvement can also occur (Chastan et al. 2006). Lattice corneal dystrophy is pathognomonic, greatly facilitating diagnosis of the condition (Meretoja 1973).

Fibrinogen Amyloidosis (AFib)

Fibrinogen amyloidosis (AFib) is an autosomal dominant disease with low penetrance, caused by point mutations in the fibrinogen A α-chain gene (about six amyloidogenic mutations in the fibrinogen A α-chain have been identified, the most common being Glu526Val) (Tennent et al. 2007). Kidneys are the main sites of amyloid deposition. Cardiac involvement has yet to be reported.

Cystatin C Amyloidosis (ACys)

This disease, documented in a seven-generation pedigree in northwest Iceland (hereditary cerebral hemorrhage with amyloidosis, Icelandic type, HCHWA-I) is a rare, fatal, autosomal dominant condition, directly linked to a Leu68Gln mutation in the cystatin C protein sequence, a cysteine protease inhibitor (Olafsson and Grubb 2000). Mutant cystatin C forms amyloid in brain arteries and arterioles, and to a lesser degree in tissues outside the central nervous system such as the skin, lymph nodes, testis, spleen, submandibular salivary glands, and adrenal cortex.

Key Points

1. Systemic amyloidoses are complex entities, which are widely underdiagnosed.
2. ATTR (i.e., transthyretin-related familial amyloidosis) is the most frequent form of hereditary systemic amyloidosis. It is characterized by a high degree of genotypic (over 80 different amyloidogenic mutations) and phenotypic heterogeneity. The clinical spectrum of ATTR ranges from almost exclusive neurologic involvement (within a clearly familial context) to apparently sporadic cases with a strictly cardiological presentation.
3. Phenotypic heterogeneity is linked to at least three different factors: the type of TTR mutation, the geographic distribution, and the type of aggregation (endemic or non-endemic).
4. Cardiac amyloidosis is generally considered to be a myocardial disease with "hypertrophic phenotype" and restrictive physiology. However, any representative cohort of patients with amyloid heart disease will display a spectrum of diastolic filling abnormalities, with the restrictive pattern manifesting only in advanced stages of the disease.
5. The single most useful sign to arouse diagnostic suspicion of cardiac amyloidosis is the presence of low or normal QRS voltage at ECG despite increased left ventricular wall thickness at echocardiography.

6. Histologic evidence of amyloid deposits is essential for a final diagnosis of amyloidosis. However, in a patient with a genetically proven diagnosis of ATTR, echocardiographic identification of unexplained ventricular hypertrophy provides clinical evidence of the specific disease.
7. Since the liver is mainly responsible for TTR production, orthotopic liver transplantation can provide a "surgical gene therapy" for ATTR and must be considered as soon as possible for all patients with clinically evident, molecularly confirmed disease
8. Combined heart-liver transplantation can be offered to patients with severe heart failure due to amyloidotic cardiomyopathy, or to patients affected by mutations other than Val30Met who are candidates for OLT and who have an echocardiographic diagnosis of cardiomyopathy (even in the absence of major cardiovascular symptoms).

References

Adams D, Reilly M, Harding AE, Said G. Demonstration of genetic mutation in most of the amyloid neuropathies with sporadic occurrence. *Rev Neurol (Paris).* 1992;148:736–741.

Ando Y, Nakamura M, Araki S. Transthyretin-related familial amyloidotic polyneuropathy. *Arch Neurol.* 2005;**62**:1057–1062.

Andrade C. A peculiar form of peripheral neuropathy. Familial atypical generalized amyloidosis with special involvement of the peripheral nerves. *Brain.* 1952;75:408–427.

Ardehali H, Qasim A, Cappola T, et al. Endomyocardial biopsy plays a role in diagnosing patients with unexplained cardiomyopathy. *Am Heart J.* 2004;147:919–923.

Arpesella G, Chiappini B, Marinelli G, et al. Combined heart and liver transplantation for familial amyloidotic polyneuropathy. *J Thoracic Cardiovascular Surg.* 2003;125:1165–1166.

Baures PW, Peterson SA, Kelly JW. Discovering transthyretin amyloid fibril inhibitors by limited screening. *Bioorg Med Chem.* 1998;6:1389–1401.

Benson MD. The hereditary amyloidoses. *Best Pract Res Clin Rheumatol.* 2003;17:909–927.

Benson MD, Kincaid JC. The molecular biology and clinical features of amyloid neuropathy. *Muscle Nerve.* 2007;36:411–423.

Berk JL, Keane J, Seldin DC, et al. Persistent pleural effusions in primary systemic amyloidosis: etiology and prognosis. *Chest.* 2003;124:969–977.

Booth DR, Pepys MB, Hawkins PN. A novel variant of human lysozyme (T70N) is common in the normal population. *Hum Mutat.* 2000;16:180.

Cardoso I, Merlini G, Saraiva MJ. 4¢-iodo-4¢-deoxydoxorubicin and tetracyclines disrupt transthyretin amyloid fibrils in vitro producing noncytotoxic species: screening for TTR fibril disrupters. *FASEB J.* 2003;17:803–809.

Carroll JD, Gaasch WH, McAdam KP. Amyloid cardiomyopathy: characterization by a distinctive voltage/mass relation. *Am J Cardiol.* 1982; 49:9–13.

Chastan N, Baert-Desurmont S, Saugier-Veber P, et al. Cardiac conduction alterations in a French family with amyloidosis of the Finnish type with the p.Asp187Tyr mutation in the GSN gene. *Muscle Nerve.* 2006;**33**:113–119.

Crotty TB, Li C-Y, Edwards WD, et al. Amyloidosis and endomyocardial biopsy: correlation of extent and pattern of deposition with amyloid immunophenotype in 100 cases. *Cardiovasc Pathol.* 1995;4:39–42.

Cueto-Garcia L, Tajik AJ, Kyle RA, et al. Serial echocardiographic observations in patients with primary systemic amyloidosis: an introduction to the concept of early (asymptomatic) amyloid infiltration of the heart. *Mayo Clin Proc.* 1984;59:589–597.

Demir M, Paydas S, Cayli M, et al. Tissue Doppler is a more reliable method in early detection of cardiac dysfunction in patients with AA amyloidosis. *Ren Fail.* 2005;27:415–420.

Dispenzieri A, Kyle RA, Gertz MA, et al. Survival in patients with primary systemic amyloidosis and raised serum cardiac troponins. *Lancet.* 2003;361:1787–1789.

Dispenzieri A, Lacy MQ, Katzmann JA, et al. Absolute values of immunoglobulin free light chains are prognostic in patients with primary systemic amyloidosis undergoing peripheral blood stem cell transplantation. *Blood.* 2006;107:3378–3383.

Dubrey SW, Burke MM, Khaghani A, et al. Long-term results of heart transplantation in patients with amyloid heart disease. *Heart.* 2001;85:202–207.

Dubrey SW, Cha K, Skinner M, et al. Familial and primary (AL) cardiac amyloidosis: echocardiographically similar diseases with distinctly different clinical outcomes. *Heart.* 1997;78:74–82.

Elliott P, Andersson B, Arbustini E, et al. Classification of the cardiomyopathies: a position statement from the European Society Of Cardiology Working Group on Myocardial and Pericardial Diseases. *Eur Heart J.* 2008;29:270–276.

Engström I, Ronquist G, Pettersson L, Waldenström A. Alzheimer amyloid beta-peptides exhibit ionophore-like properties in human erythrocytes. *Eur J Clin Invest.* 1995;25:471–476.

Falk RH. Diagnosis and management of the cardiac amyloidoses. *Circulation.* 2005;**112**:2047–2060.

Falk RH, Comenzo RL, Skinner M. The systemic amyloidoses. *N Engl J Med.* 1997;337:898–909.

Falk RH, Rubinow A, Cohen AS. Cardiac arrhythmias in systemic amyloidosis: correlation with echocardiographic abnormalities. *J Am Coll Cardiol.* 1984;3:107–113.

Forloni G, Colombo L, Girola L, Tagliavini F, Salmona M. Anti-amyloidogenic activity of tetracyclines: studies in vitro. *FEBS Lett.* 2001;487:404–407.

Freeman R. Neurogenic orthostatic hypotension. *N Engl J Med.* 2008;358:615–624.

Gertz MA, Comenzo R, Falk RH, et al. Definition of organ involvement and treatment response in immunoglobulin light chain amyloidosis (AL): a consensus opinion from the 10th international symposium on amyloid and amyloidosis. *Am J Hematol.* 2005;79:319–328.

Gertz MA, Falk RH, Skinner M, Cohen AS, Kyle RA. Worsening of congestive heart failure in amyloid heart disease treated by calcium channel–blocking agents. *Am J Cardiol.* 1985;55:1645.

Gertz MA, Grogan M, Kyle RA, Tajik AJ. Endomyocardial biopsy proven light chain amyloidosis (AL) without echocardiographic features of infiltrative cardiomyopathy. *Am J Cardiol.* 1997;80:93–95.

Gertz MA, Lacy MQ, Dispenzieri A. Amyloidosis. *Hematol Oncol Clin North Am.* 1999;13:1211–1233.

Gertz MA, Lacy MQ, Dispenzieri A, et al. A multicenter phase II trial of 4¢-iodo-4¢-deoxydoxorubicin (IDOX) in primary amyloidosis (AL). *Amyloid.* 2002;9:24–30.

Gianni L, Bellotti V, Gianni AM, Merlini G. New drug therapy of amyloidoses: resorption of AL-type deposits with 4¢-iodo-4¢-deoxydoxorubicin. *Blood.* 1995;86:855–861.

Gillmore JD, Booth DR, Madhoo S, Pepys MB, Hawkins PN. Hereditary renal amyloidosis associated with variant lysozyme in a large English family. *Nephrol Dial Transplant.* 1999;14:2639–2644.

Goodman Y, Mattson MP. K+ channel openers protect hippocampal neurons against oxidative injury and amyloid b-peptide toxicity. *Brain Res.* 1996;706:328–332.

Goren H, Steinberg MC, Farboody GH. Familial oculoleptomeningeal amyloidosis. *Brain.* 1980;103:473–495.

Granel B, Serratrice J, Valleix S, et al. A family with gastrointestinal amyloidosis associated with variant lysozyme. *Gastroenterology.* 2002;123:1346–1349.

Granel B, Valleix S, Serratrice J, et al. Lysozyme amyloidosis: report of 4 cases and a review of the literature. *Medicine (Baltimore).* 2006; 85:66–73.

Hamer JP, Janssen S, van Rijswijk MH, et al. Amyloid cardiomyopathy in systemic non-hereditary amyloidosis. Clinical, echocardiographic and electrocardiographic findings in 30 patients with AA and 24 patients with AL amyloidosis. *Eur Heart J.* 1992;13:623–627.

Hamidi L, Liepnieks JJ, Hamidi K, et al. Hereditary amyloid cardiomyopathy caused by a variant apolipoprotein A1. *Am J Pathol.* 1999;154: 221–227.

Harats N, Worth RM, Benson MD. Hereditary amyloidosis: evidence against early amyloid deposition. *Arthritis Rheum.* 1989;32:1474–1476.

Hattori T, Takei Y, Koyama J, Nakazato M, Ikeda S. Clinical and pathological studies of cardiac amyloidosis in transthyretin type familial amyloid polyneuropathy. *Amyloid.* 2003;**10**:229–239.

Hawkins PN. Serum amyloid P component scintigraphy for diagnosis and monitoring amyloidosis. *Curr Opin Nephrol Hypertens.* 2002; 11:649–655.

Herlenius G, Larsson M, Ericzon BG. FAP World Transplant Register and domino/sequential register update. *Transplant Proc.* 2001;331–367.

Hou X, Aguilar MI, Small DH. Transthyretin and familial amyloidotic polyneuropathy. Recent progress in understanding the molecular mechanism of neurodegeneration. *FEBS J.* 2007;**274**:1637–650.

Ikeda S. Cardiac amyloidosis: heterogenous pathogenic backgrounds. *Intern Med.* 2004;**43**:1107–1114.

Jacobson DR, Pastore R, Pool S, et al. Revised transthyretin Ile 122 allele frequency in African-Americans. *Hum Genet.* 1996;98:236–238.

Jacobson DR, Pastore RD, Yaghoubian R, et al. Variant-sequence transthyretin (isoleucine 122) in late-onset cardiac amyloidosis in black Americans. *N Engl J Med.* 1997;336:466–473.

Janson J, Ashley RH, Harrison D, McIntyre S, Butler PC. The mechanism of islet amyloid polypeptide toxicity is membrane disruption by intermediate-sized toxic amyloid particles. *Diabetes.* 1999;48:491–498.

Jordan J, Galindo MF, Miller RJ, Reardon CA, Getz GS, LaDu MJ. Isoform-specific effect of apolipoprotein E on cell survival and beta-amyloid-induced toxicity in rat hippocampal pyramidal neuronal cultures. *J Neurosci.* 1998;18:195–204.

Kayed R, Head E, Thompson JL, et al. Common structure of soluble amyloid oligomers implies common mechanism of pathogenesis. *Science.* 2003;300:486–489.

Klein AL, Hatle LK, Burstow DJ, et al. Doppler characterization of left ventricular diastolic function in cardiac amyloidosis. *J Am Coll Cardiol.* 1989;13:1017–1026.

Klein AL, Hatle LK, Taliercio CP, et al. Prognostic significance of Doppler measures of diastolic function in cardiac amyloidosis. A Doppler echocardiography study. *Circulation.* 1991;83:808–816.

Koyama J, Ray-Sequin PA, Davidoff R, et al. Usefulness of pulsed tissue Doppler imaging for evaluating systolic and diastolic left ventricular function in patients with AL (primary) amyloidosis. *Am J Cardiol.* 2002;89:1067–1071.

Lachmann HJ, Booth DR, Booth SE, et al. Misdiagnosis of hereditary amyloidosis as AL (primary) amyloidosis. *N Engl J Med.* 2002;346: 1786–1791.

Levy E, Haltia M, Fernandez-Madrid I, et al. Mutation in Gel gene in Finnish hereditary amyloidosis. *J Exp Med.* 1990;172:1865–1867.

Maceira AM, Joshi J, Prasad SK, et al. Cardiovascular magnetic resonance in cardiac amyloidosis. *Circulation.* 2005;111:186–193.

Magy N, Liepnieks J, Kluvebeckerman B. Renal transplantation for apolipoprotein AII amyloidosis. *Amyloid.* 2003;10:224–228.

Maury CPJ, Kere J, Tolvanen R, de la Chapelle A. Finnish hereditary amyloidosis is caused by a single nucleotide substitution in the Gel gene. *FEBS Lett.* 1990;276:75–77.

May PC, Boggs LN, Fuson KS. Neurotoxicity of human amylin in rat primary hippocampal cultures: similarity to Alzheimer's disease amyloid-b neurotoxicity. *J Neurochem.* 1993;61:2330–2333.

Meretoja J. Genetic aspects of familial amyloidosis with corneal lattice dystrophy and cranial neuropathy. *Clin Genet.* 1973;4:173–185.

Merlini G, Ascari E, Amboldi N, et al. Interaction of the anthracycline 4¢-iodo-4¢- deoxydoxorubicin with amyloid fibrils—inhibition of amyloidogenesis. *Proc Natl Aca Sci USA.* 1995;92:2959–2963.

Merlini G, Bellotti V. Molecular mechanisms of amyloidosis. *N Engl J Med.* 2003;349:583–596.

Merlini G, Westermark P. The systemic amyloidoses: clearer understanding of the molecular mechanisms offers hope for more effective therapies. *J Intern Med.* 2004;**255**:159–178.

Miroy GJ, Lai Z, Lashuel HA, Peterson SA, Strang C, Kelly JW. Inhibiting transthyretin amyloid fibril formation via protein stabilization. *Proc Natl Acad Sci USA.* 1996;93:15051–15056.

Mirzabekov TA, Lin M, Kagan BL. Pore formation by the cytotoxic islet amyloid peptide amylin. *J Biol Chem.* 1996;271:1988–1992.

Murtagh B, Hammill SC, Gertz MA, et al. Electrocardiographic findings in primary systemic amyloidosis and biopsy-proven cardiac involvement. *Am J Cardiol.* 2005;95:535–537.

Ng B, Connors LH, Davidoff R, et al. Senile systemic amyloidosis presenting with heart failure: a comparison with light chain-associated amyloidosis. *Arch Intern Med.* 2005;165:1425–1429.

Nichols WC, Gregg RE, Brewer HB, Benson MD. A mutation in apolipoprotein A-I in the Iowa type of familial amyloidotic polyneuropathy. *Genomics.* 1990;8:318–323.

Obayashi K, Ando Y, Terazaki H, et al. Effect of sildenafil citrate (Viagra) on erectile dysfunction in a patient with familial amyloidotic polyneuropathy ATTR Val30Met. *Auton Nerv Syst.* 2000;12:89–92.

Ohmori H, Ando Y, Makita Y, et al. Common origin of the Val30Met mutation responsible for the amyloidogenic transthyretin type of familial amyloidotic polyneuropathy. *J Med Genet.* 2004;41:51–55.

Olafsson I, Grubb A. Hereditary cystatin C amyloid angiopathy. *Amyloid.* 2000;7:70–79.

Olofsson BO, Backman C, Karp K, et al. Progression of cardiomyopathy after liver transplantation in patients with familial amyloidotic polyneuropathy, Portuguese type. *Transplantation.* 2002;73:745–751.

Palka P, Lange A, Donnelly E, et al. Doppler echocardiographic features of cardiac amyloidosis. *J Am Soc Echocardiogr.* 2002;15:1353–1360.

Palladini G, Campana C, Klersy C, et al. Serum N-terminal pro-brain natriuretic peptide is a sensitive marker of myocardial dysfunction in AL amyloidosis. *Circulation.* 2003;107:2440–2445.

Palladini G, Lavatelli F, Russo P, et al. Circulating amyloidogenic free light chains and serum N-terminal natriuretic peptide type B decrease simultaneously in association with improvement of survival in AL. *Blood.* 2006;107:3854–3858.

Pasotti M, Agozzino M, Concardi M, Merlini G, Rapezzi C, Arbustini E. Obstructive intramural coronary amyloidosis: a distinct phenotype of cardiac amyloidosis that can cause acute heart failure. *Eur Heart J.* 2006;**27**:1810.

Perugini E, Guidalotti PL, Salvi F, et al. Noninvasive etiologic diagnosis of cardiac amyloidosis using 99mTc-3,3-diphosphono-1,2-propanodicarboxylic acid scintigraphy. *J Am Coll Cardiol.* 2005;**46**:1076–1084.

Perugini E, Rapezzi C, Piva T, et al. Non-invasive evaluation of the myocardial substrate of cardiac amyloidosis by gadolinium cardiac magnetic resonance. *Heart.* 2006;92:343–349.

Peterson SA, Klabunde T, Lashuel HA, Purkey H, Sacchettini JC, Kelly JW. Inhibiting transthyretin conformational changes that lead to amyloid fibril formation. *Proc Natl Acad Sci USA.* 1998;95:12956–12960.

Planté-Bordeneuve V, Carayol J, Ferreira A, et al. Genetic study of transthyretin amyloid neuropathies: carrier risks among French and Portuguese families. *J Med Genet.* 2003;40:e120.

Planté-Bordeneuve V, Ferreira A, Lalu T, et al. Diagnostic pitfalls in sporadic transthyretin familial amyloid polyneuropathy (TTR-FAP). *Neurology.* 2007;**69**:693–698.

Pollak A, Falk RH. Left ventricular systolic dysfunction precipitated by verapamil in cardiac amyloidosis. *Chest.* 1993;104:618–620.

Rahman JE, Helou EF, Gelzer-Bell R, et al. Noninvasive diagnosis of biopsy-proven cardiac amyloidosis. *J Am Coll Cardiol.* 2004;43:410–415.

Ranløv I, Alves IL, Ranløv PJ, Husby G, Costa PP, Saraiva MJ. A Danish kindred with familial amyloid cardiomyopathy revisited: identification of a mutant transthyretin-methionine111 variant in serum from patients and carriers. *Am J Med.* 1992;93:3–8.

Rapezzi C, Perugini E, Salvi F, et al. Phenotypic and genotypic heterogeneity in transthyretin-related cardiac amyloidosis: towards tailoring of therapeutic strategies? *Amyloid.* 2006;**13**:143–153.

Reilly MM, Staunton H, Harding AE. Familial amyloid polyneuropathy (transthyretin Ala-60) in north west Ireland: a clinical, genetic, and epidemiological study. *J Neurol Neurosurg Psychiatry.* 1995;59:45–49.

Rubinow A, Skinner M, Cohen AS. Digoxin sensitivity in amyloid cardiomyopathy. *Circulation.* 1981;63:1285–1288.

Ruygrok PN, Gane EJ, McCall JL, et al. Combined heart and liver transplantation for familial amyloidosis. *Intern Med J.* 2001;31:66–67.

Sack GH, Dumars KW, Gummerson KS, Law A, McKusick VA. Three forms of dominant amyloid neuropathy. *Johns Hopkins Med J.* 1981;149:239–247.

Schubert D, Behl C, Lesley R, et al. Amyloid peptides are toxic via a common oxidative mechanism. *Proc Natl Acad Sci USA*. 1995;92:1989–1993.

Sebastiao MP, Merlini G, Saraiva MJ, Damas AM. The molecular interaction of 4¢-iodo-4¢-deoxydoxorubicin with Leu-55Pro transthyretin "amyloid-like" oligomer leading to disaggregation. *Biochem J*. 2000; 351:273–279.

Selvanayagam JB, Hawkins PN, Paul B, Myerson SG, Neubauer S. Evaluation and management of the cardiac amyloidosis. *J Am Coll Cardiol*. 2007; 50:2101–2110.

Simon BG, Moutsopoulos HM. Primary amyloidosis resembling sicca syndrome. *Arthritis Rheum*. 1979;22:932–934.

Simons M, Isner JM. Assessment of relative sensitivities of non-invasive tests for cardiac amyloidosis in documented cardiac amyloidosis. *Am J Cardiol*. 1992;69:425–427.

Stangou AJ, Heaton ND, Hawkins PN. Transmission of sistemi transthyretin amyloidosis by means of domino liver transplantation. *N Engl J Med*. 2005;352:235–236.

Suhr OB, Anan I, Backman C, et al. Do troponin and B-natriuretic peptide detect cardiomyopathy in transthyretin amyloidosis? *J Intern Med*. 2008;263:294–301.

Suhr OB, Herlenius G, Friman S, et al. Liver transplantation for hereditary transthyretin amyloidosis. *Liver Transpl*. 2000;6:263–276.

Suhr OB, Svendsen IH, Andersson R, Danielsson A, Holmgren G, Ranløv PJ. Hereditary transthyretin amyloidosis from a Scandinavian perspective. *J Intern Med*. 2003;**254**:225–235.

Sunada Y, Shimizu T, Nakase H, et al. Inherited amyloid polyneuropathy type IV (Gel variant) in a Japanese family. *Ann Neurol*. 1993;33: 57–62.

Svendsen IH, Steensgaard-Hansen F, Nordvåg BY. A clinical, echocardiographic and genetic characterization of a Danish kindred with familial amyloid transthyretin methionine 111 linked cardiomyopathy. *Eur Heart J*. 1998;19:782–789.

Tennent GA, Brennan SO, Stangou AJ, O'Grady J, Hawkins PN, Pepys MB. Human plasma fibrinogen is synthesized in the liver. *Blood*. 2007;109:1971–1974.

Thomson LE. Cardiovascular magnetic resonance in clinically suspected cardiac amyloidosis: diagnostic value of a typical pattern of late gadolinium enhancement. *J Am Coll Cardiol*. 2008;**51**:1031–1032.

Trikas A, Rallidis L, Hawkins P, et al. Comparison of usefulness between exercise capacity and echocardiographic indexes of left ventricular function in cardiac amyloidosis. *Am J Cardiol*. 1999;84:1049–1054.

Uemichi T, Liepnieks JJ, Waits RP, Benson MD. A trinucleotide deletion in the transthyretin gene (V122) in a kindred with familial amyloidotic polyneuropathy. *Neurology*. 1997;48:1667–1670.

Valleix S, Drunat S, Philit JB, et al. Hereditary renal amyloidosis caused by a new variant lysozyme W64R in a French family. *Kidney Int*. 2002;61:907–912.

Vogelsberg H, Mahrholdt H, Deluigi CC, et al. Cardiovascular magnetic resonance in clinically suspected cardiac amyloidosis: noninvasive imaging compared to endomyocardial biopsy. *J Am Coll Cardiol*. 2008;51:1022–1030.

Wang C-N, Chi C-W, Lin Y-L, Chen C-F, Shiao Y-J. The neuroprotective effects of phytoestrogens on amyloid b protein-induced toxicity are mediated by abrogating the activation of caspase cascade in rat cortical neurons. *J Biol Chem*. 2001;276:5287–5295.

Westermark P, Benson MD, Buxbaum JM, et al. Amyloid protein fibril nomenclature–2002. *Amyloid*. 2002;9:197–200.

Wolfe MS. Therapeutic strategies for Alzheimer's disease. *Nat Rev Drug Discov*. 2002;1:859–866.

Wright BL, Grace AA, Goodman HJ. Implantation of a cardioverter-defibrillator in a patient with cardiac amyloidosis. *Nat Clin Pract Cardiovasc Med*. 2006;3:110–114.

Yankner BA, Dawes LR, Fisher S, Villa-Komaroff L, Oster-Granite ML, Neve RL. Neurotoxicity of a fragment of the amyloid precursor associated with Alzheimer's disease. *Science*. 1989;245:417–420.

Yazaki M, Connors LH, Eagle RC Jr, Leff SR, Skinner M, Benson MD. Transthyretin amyloidosis associated with a novel variant (Trp41Leu) presenting with vitreous opacities. *Amyloid*. 2002;9:263–267.

Yood RA, Skinner M, Rubinow A, Talarico L, Cohen AS. Bleeding manifestations in 100 patients with amyloidosis. *JAMA*. 1983;249:1322–1324.

31

Cardiac Involvement in Mitochondrial Disease

Patrick F Chinnery and Grainne Gorman

Introduction

Mitochondria are ubiquitous double-membrane intracellular organelles that are involved in many different cellular processes, including calcium signaling and the initiation of one process of apoptosis (programmed cell death) through the release of cytochrome *c*. Mitochondria enzymes are also involved in intermediary metabolism (fatty acid β-oxidation and the tricarboxylic acid cycle). However, the term "mitochondrial encephalomyopathy" or "mitochondrial disorder" usually means a disease that is primarily due to an abnormality of the final common pathway of energy metabolism—the mitochondrial respiratory chain, which is linked to the production of adenosine triphosphate (ATP) by oxidative phosphorylation (OXPHOS). The respiratory chain is essential for aerobic metabolism, and respiratory chain defects characteristically affect tissues and organs that are heavily dependent on oxidative metabolism (such as the central nervous system, the eye, skeletal muscle, and endocrine organs).

Normal cardiac function is critically dependent on adequate levels of ATP, which is required for myofibril contraction and the maintenance of ionic gradients needed for electrical conduction. This chapter will focus on the cardiac complications of primary disorders of OXPHOS with an established, or presumed primary genetic basis. Secondary impairment of mitochondrial function has been implicated in the pathophysiology of a number of different cardiac diseases—both inherited (e.g., Friedreich's ataxia) and sporadic (e.g., myocardial ischemia)—and age-related mitochondrial damage may contribute to unexplained cardiac failure with aging (presbycardia). These so-called secondary mitochondrial cardiomyopathies do not fall within the scope of this chapter.

Mitochondrial Biogenesis: Biochemistry and Genetics

The metabolism of carbohydrates, amino acids, and fatty acids generates the reduced cofactors NADH, NADPH, and $FADH_2$, which transfer electrons to the mitochondrial respiratory chain. The respiratory chain is a group of approximately 100 proteins arranged into five complexes on the inner mitochondrial membrane (Figure 31–1). Electrons enter the respiratory chain through complexes I and II, and are passed through complexes III and IV, pumping protons out of the mitochondrial matrix into the intermembrane space. This creates an electrochemical gradient that is coupled by complex V (ATP synthase) to generate ATP from ADP and Pi (adenosine diphosphate and inorganic phosphate). Each respiratory chain complex contains many polypeptide subunits, some of which are coded by genes within the nucleus and some of which are encoded by the mitochondrial genome. Thirteen essential polypeptides synthesized within mitochondria from small circles of DNA present within the mitochondrial matrix (mtDNA). However, the majority of proteins are synthesized from nuclear genes, some of which have yet to be characterized.

The mitochondrial genome (Figure 31–2) has 16,569 base pairs (bp) and encodes seven complex I subunits (NADH-ubiquinone oxidoreductase), one of the complex III subunits (ubiquinol-cytochrome *c* oxidoreductase), three of the complex IV (cytochrome *c* oxidase, or COX) subunits, and the ATPase 6 and ATPase 8 subunits of complex V (Anderson et al. 1981; Andrews et al. 1999). Interspaced between the protein-encoding genes are two ribosomal RNA genes (12S and 16S rRNA), and 22 transfer RNA genes that provide the necessary RNA components for the mitochondrial translation machinery. The remaining polypeptides, including all of the complex II subunits (succinate dehydrogenase, SDH), are synthesized from nuclear gene transcripts within the cytosol. These are subsequently imported into the mitochondria through the specialized import machinery: the inner and outer membrane translocation complexes. Currently, there are estimated to be approximately 1,000 mitochondrial proteins; many of these are involved in mitochondrial biogenesis, the maintenance, transcription and translation of mtDNA, and assembly of the respiratory chain. Mitochondrial diseases can therefore be due to mutations in either mtDNA or the nuclear genome.

Mitochondrial Genetics

There are major differences between nuclear DNA and mtDNA that are central to our understanding of the pathogenesis, which also have direct clinical implications.

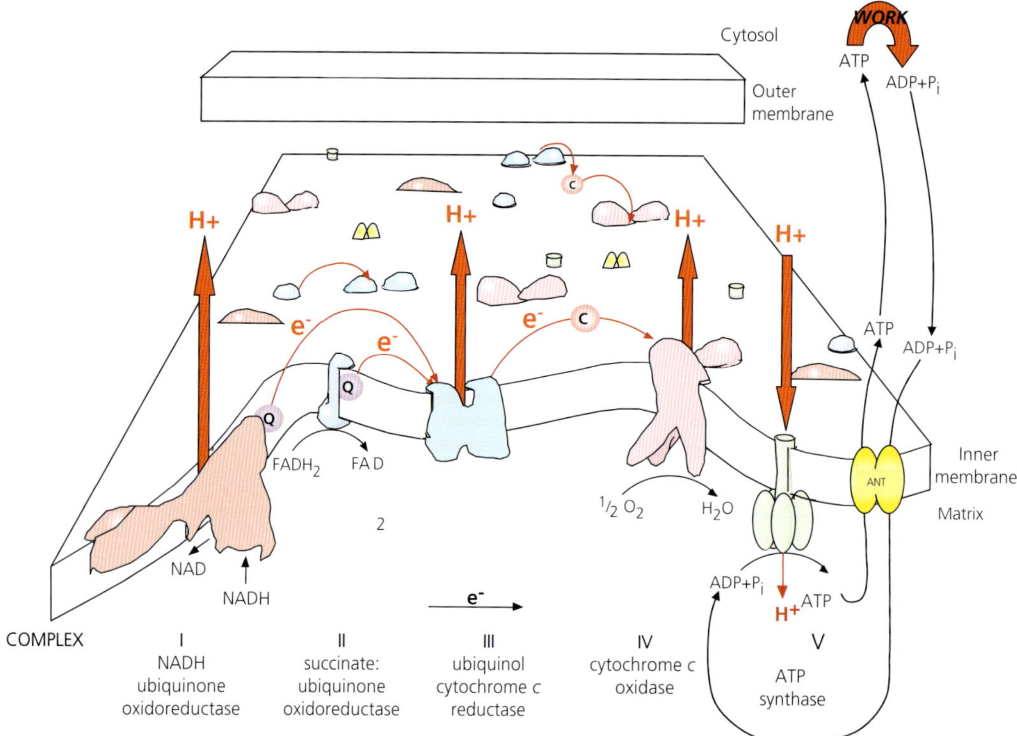

Figure 31–1 The mitochondrial respiratory chain. Schematic diagram of the respiratory chain. Reduced cofactors (NADH and $FADH_2$) are produced from the intermediary metabolism of carbohydrates, proteins, and fats. These cofactors donate electrons (e^-) to complex I (NADH-ubiquinone oxidoreductase) and complex II (succinate-ubiquinone oxidoreductase). These electrons flow between the complexes down an electrochemical gradient (black arrow), shuttled by ubiquinone (Q) and cytochrome *c* (C), involving complex III (ubiquinol-cytochrome *c* oxidase reductase) and complex IV (cytochrome *c* oxidase, or COX). Complex IV donates an electron to oxygen, which results in the formation of water. Protons (H^+) are pumped from the mitochondrial matrix into the intermembrane space (red arrows). This proton gradient generates the mitochondrial membrane potential, which is harnessed by complex V to synthesize ATP from ADP and Pi. ANT = adenine nucleotide translocator that exchanges ADP for ATP across the mitochondrial membrane (Our thanks to Dr. Z. Chrzanowska-Lightowlers for providing the figure).

Multicopy Genome, Heteroplasmy, and the Threshold Effect

Each human cell contains many copies of mtDNA, with the precise amount varying from organ to organ, and between different cell types within the same organ. Being heavily energy dependent, each cardiomyocyte contains approximately 10,000 copies of mtDNA. In healthy subjects, these are usually all identical at birth (identical = homoplasmy). By contrast, patients with mtDNA disease often harbor a mixture of mutated and wild-type (normal) mtDNA—this is called mtDNA heteroplasmy. Individual cells are able to tolerate large amounts of mutated mtDNA (Schon et al. 1997). They only express an OXPHOS defect when the proportion of mutated mtDNA exceeds a critical threshold level. This is associated with the loss of wild-type mtDNA, which may ultimately be responsible for the biochemical defect. The precise threshold, whether it is the proportion of mutated mtDNA or the absolute amount of wild-type mtDNA, varies from tissue to tissue (Taylor and Turnbull 2005). Different organs, and even adjacent cells within the same organ, often contain different amounts of mutated mtDNA. These factors explain why some organs are preferentially affected in patients with mtDNA disease. In general, postmitotic (nondividing) tissues such as neurons, skeletal and cardiac myocytes, and endocrine organs harbor much higher levels of mutated mtDNA, which results in organ dysfunction and disease. Rapidly dividing tissues such as bone marrow are only rarely clinically affected (DiMauro and Schon 2003).

Pathogenic mtDNA Mutations

The first pathogenic mutations of mtDNA were identified in 1989 (Holt et al. 1988; Wallace et al. 1988). Since then a large number of different pathogenic mutations have been identified (Table 31–1; Servidei 2004). Mutations fall into one of two groups: point mutations and rearrangements. Pathogenic point mutations affect the protein-encoding genes impairing the function of the corresponding respiratory chain complex, or they involve individual RNA genes and cause a generalized defect of protein synthesis within the mitochondrion. Two forms of rearrangement have been described. Deletions can be small and fall within a protein-encoding gene or RNA gene, exerting a similar effect to a point mutation. Large deletions remove one or more genes, and often involve an RNA gene, leading to a defect of intra-mitochondrial protein synthesis. Duplications often coexist with deletions. They are not thought to be directly pathogenic, but they are thought to form deletions in affected tissues.

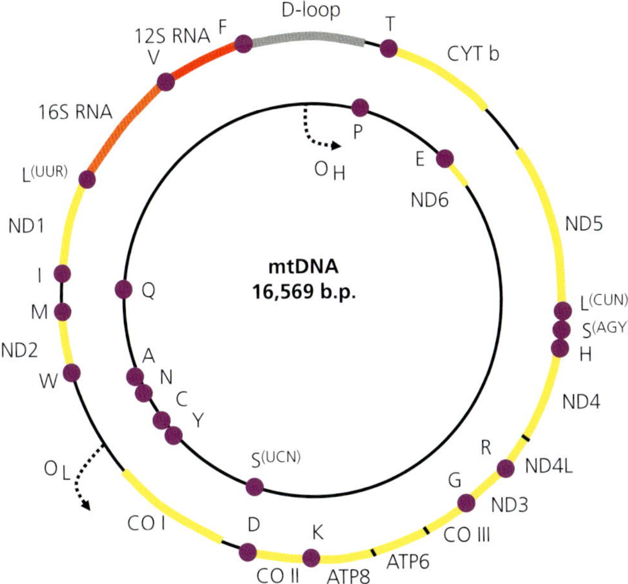

Figure 31–2 The human mitochondrial genome. The human mitochondrial genome (mtDNA) is a small 16,569 kb molecule of double-stranded DNA. mtDNA encodes for 13 essential components of the respiratory chain. ND1–ND6 and ND4L encode seven subunits of complex I (NADH-ubiquinone oxidoreductase). Cyt b is the only mtDNA encoded complex III subunit (ubiquinol-cytochrome *c* oxidase reductase). COX I to III encode for three of the complex IV (cytochrome *c* oxidase, or COX) subunits, and the ATP 6 and ATP 8 genes encode for two subunits of complex V (ATP synthase). Two ribosomal RNA genes (12S and 16S rRNA), and 22 transfer RNA genes are interspaced between the protein-encoding genes. These provide the necessary RNA components for intra-mitochondrial protein synthesis. D-loop = the 1.1 kb noncoding region, which is involved in the regulation of transcription and replication of the molecule, and is the only region not directly involved in the synthesis of respiratory chain polypeptides. O_H and O_L are the origins of heavy and light strand mtDNA replication.

Maternal Inheritance and the Transmission of Heteroplasmy

Mature human oocytes contain approximately 200,000 copies of mtDNA, and sperms contain approximately 200 copies of mtDNA. After fertilization, sperm mitochondria are tagged with ubiquitin and actively destroyed. This is why mtDNA is only transmitted down from mother to offspring. Males with mtDNA disease cannot transmit the genetic defect. mtDNA deletions are rarely transmitted from clinically affected females to their offspring (recurrence risk ~1 in 24) (Chinnery et al. 2004). By contrast, a female harboring a heteroplasmic mtDNA point mutation, or mtDNA duplications, may transmit a variable amount of mutated mtDNA to her children. Unlike nuclear gene mutations (which are homozygous or heterozygous), the transmitted "mtDNA mutation load" can vary from 1% to 100%. Early during development of the female germline, the number of mtDNA molecules within each oocyte is reduced before being subsequently amplified to reach a final number of greater than 100,000 in each mature oocyte (Cree et al. 2007). This is called the mitochondrial "genetic bottleneck," and it leads to different percentage levels of mutation within primary oocytes. This is responsible for the different levels of mutant mtDNA seen in the offspring of a single female, and consequent variation in the severity of the clinical phenotype within a single sibship (Chinnery et al. 2000).

Somatic Mutation of mtDNA

mtDNA is generally considered to have a high mutation rate. This is because it is tethered to the mitochondrial membrane close to the respiratory chain, which is a potent source of free radicals, it is not protected by histone proteins, and mitochondria are relatively deficient in DNA repair mechanisms. mtDNA acquires somatic mutation throughout life. Unlike nuclear DNA, mtDNA is continuously replicated, even in nondividing tissue such as myocardium. This can lead to the propagation of somatic mutations within single cells by a process called clonal expansion (Brierley 1998). If the proportion of mutated mtDNA exceeds the critical threshold level for that mutation and tissue, this leads to an OXPHOS defect. Focal OXPHOS defects (usually demonstrated histochemically by COX staining) are well recognized in skeletal and cardiac muscle. Cardiac muscle appears to be particularly vulnerable to somatic mutation, with the accumulation of many different types of deleted molecule "sublimons" (nonreplicated deletions) (Kajander et al. 2000). The frequency of mutations and the frequency of COX-deficient cardiomyocytes are low when averaged across the whole tissue. There is therefore great debate as to whether these age-related COX-deficient cells have phenotypic consequences or not. By contrast, in patients with high levels of a single mtDNA mutation causing a mitochondrial disorder, the same mechanism of clonal expansion leads to the accumulation of mutated mtDNA in many individual cells (Muller-Hocker et al. 1992). This contributes to disease progression in mtDNA disease.

Nuclear Mitochondrial Genes

A large number of nuclear genes are involved in the synthesis of respiratory chain subunits and essential cofactors required to assemble the respiratory chain. Nuclear-encoded proteins are required for the replication of mtDNA (polymerase gamma, or polγ, synthesized by the *POLG* gene, and its p55 accessory subunit from *POLG2*), along with the mtDNA helicase Twinkle (from *PEO1*). Regulation of the correct balance of nucleotide DNA building blocks within mitochondria is essential for mtDNA maintenance. This is achieved by a group of cytosolic enzymes (thymidine kinase 2, gene *TK2*; dexyguanosine kinase, gene *DGUOK*; and thymidine phosphorylase, gene *TP*) and the mitochondrial membrane translocase, ANT1 (encoded by *SLC25A4*). Mutations in *POLG, POLG2, SLC25A4*, and *PEO1* cause secondary deletions of mtDNA that accumulate in nondividing tissues (Kaukonen et al. 2000; Spelbrink et al. 2001; Van Goethem et al. 2001; Longley et al. 2006). These disorders are usually autosomal dominant, although recessive *POLG* mutations are well described. Mutations in *POLG, TK2, TP, DGUOK, SUCLA2, RRM2B*, and the membrane protein gene *MPV17* cause loss of mtDNA (mtDNA depletion) in affected tissues (Mandel et al. 2001; Saada et al. 2001; Elpeleg et al. 2005; Bourdon et al. 2007), and the diseases are collectively referred to as disorders of mtDNA maintenance.

The transcription and translation of mtDNA is also dependent on a number of nuclear genes (*PUS1, EFG1, EFTu*, and *MRPS16* to name a few that have been associated with disease) (Bykhovskaya et al. 2004; Coenen et al. 2004; Miller et al. 2004; Smeitink et al. 2006; Saada et al. 2007; Valente et al. 2007). Other critical nuclear genes relevant for mitochondrial cardiomyopathies include *TAZ*, which codes for the membrane protein Tafazzin, and is disrupted

Table 31–1 Primary Mitochondrial DNA Defects Causing Human Disease

Rearrangements (Large-Scale Partial Deletions and Duplications)	Inheritance Pattern
Chronic progressive external ophthalmoplegia (CPEO)	S or M
Kearns-Sayre syndrome	S or M
Diabetes and deafness	S
Pearson marrow-pancreas syndrome	S or M
Sporadic tubulopathy	S
Point mutations	
Protein-encoding genes	
LHON (11778G>A, 14484T>C, 3460G>A)	M
NARP/Leigh syndrome (8993T>G/C)	M
tRNA genes	
MELAS (3243A>G, 3271T>C, 3251A>G)	M
MERRF (8344A>G, 8356T>C)	M
CPEO (3243A>G, 4274T>C)	M
Myopathy (14709T>C, 12320A>G)	M
Cardiomyopathy (3243A>G, 4269A>G, 4300A>G)	M
Diabetes and deafness (3243A>G, 12258C>A)	M
Encephalomyopathy (1606G>A, 10010T>C)	M
rRNA genes	
Nonsyndromic sensorineural deafness (7445A>G)	M
Aminoglycoside induced nonsyndromic deafness (1555A>G)	M
Point mutations	
Protein-encoding genes	
LHON (11778G>A, 14484T>C, 3460G>A)	M
NARP/Leigh syndrome (8993T>G/C)	M
tRNA genes	
MELAS (3243A>G, 3271T>C, 3251A>G)	M

M, maternal; S, sporadic; mtDNA nucleotide positions refer to the L-chain, and are taken from the Cambridge reference sequence. LHON, Leber hereditary optic neuropathy; NARP, neurogenetic weakness with ataxia and retinitis pigmentosa; CPEO, chronic progressive external ophthalmoplegia; KSS, Kearns-Sayre syndrome; MELAS. mitochondrial encephalomyopathy with lactic acidosis and stroke-like episodes; MERRF, myoclonic epilepsy with ragged-red fibers.

in Barth syndrome (Bione et al. 1996), and the various components of the coenzyme Q10 biosynthetic pathway (Quinzii et al. 2006). This discussion is far from comprehensive and places emphasis on genes associated with disease. There is a whole array of known genes that are attractive candidates for human diseases. A current catalog of genes involved in OXPHOS diseases is shown in Tables 31–1 and 31–2 compiled in February 2008.

Overview of OXPHOS Diseases

Mitochondrial disorders are highly variable both clinically and at the genetic level. The same genetic defect may present in a variety of different ways—this may involve a multisystem disorder

Table 31–2 Nuclear Genes Causing Mitochondrial Disease

Nuclear genetic disorders of the mitochondrial respiratory chain, mutations in structural subunits:
Leigh syndrome (complex I deficiency—mutations in *NDUFS1, NDUFS4, NDUFS7, NDUFS8, NDUFV1.* Complex II deficiency, *SDHA*)
Cardiomyopathy and encephalopathy (complex I deficiency, mutations in *NDUFS2*)
Optic atrophy and ataxia (complex II deficiency—mutations in *SDHA*)
Hypokalemia and lactic acidosis (complex III, mutations in *UQCRB*)
Nuclear genetic disorders of the mitochondrial respiratory chain, mutations in assembly factors:
Leigh syndrome (mutations in *SURF* I and the mRNA binding protein *LRPPRC*)
Hepatopathy and ketoacidosis (mutations in *SCO1*) Cardiomyopathy and encephalopathy (mutations in *SCO2*)
Leucodystrophy and renal tubulopathy (mutations in *COX10*)
Hypertrophic cardiomyopathy (mutations in *COX15*)
Encephalopathy, liver failure, renal tubulopathy (with complex III deficiency, mutations in *BCS1L*)
Encephalopathy (with complex V deficiency, mutations in *ATP12*)
Nuclear genetic disorders of intra-mitochondrial protein synthesis:
Leigh syndrome, liver failure, and lactic acidosis (mutations in *EFG1*)
Lactic acidosis, developmental failure, and dysmorphism (mutations in *MRPS16*)
Myopathy and sideroblastic anemia (mutations in *PUS1*)
Leukodystrophy and polymicrogyria (mutations in *EFTu*)
Edema, hypotonia, cardiomyopathy, and tubulopathy (mutations in *MRPS22*)
Hypotonia, renal tubulopathy, lactic acidosis (mutations in *RRM2B*)
Nuclear genetic disorders of mitochondrial DNA maintenance (causing multiple mtDNA deletions or mtDNA depletion):
Autosomal progressive external ophthalmoplegia (mutations in *POLG, POLG2, PEO1,* and *SLC25A4*)
Mitochondrial neurogastrointestinal encephalomyopathy (thymidine phosphorylase deficiency—mutations in *ECGF1*)
Alpers-Huttenlocher syndrome (mutations in *POLG* and *MPV*)
Infantile myopathy/spinal muscular atrophy (mutations in *TK2*)
Encephalomyopathy and liver failure (mutations in *DGUOK*)
Hypotonia, movement disorder, and/or Leigh syndrome with methylmalonic aciduria (mutations in *SUCLA2*)
Optic atrophy, ophthalmoplegia, ataxia, peripheral neuropathy (mutations in *OPA1*)
Others:
Coenzyme Q10 deficiency (mutations in *COQ2*)
Barth syndrome (mutations in *TAZ*)
Cardiomyopathy and lactic acidosis (mitochondrial phosphate carrier deficiency, mutations in *SLC25A3*)

that includes cardiac features. Alternatively, the same mutation can present with isolated organ involvement, including isolated cardiomyopathy. On the other hand, a strikingly similar clinical syndrome can be caused by different genetic defects—either affecting nuclear genes or mtDNA. As a general rule, most adults who present with mitochondrial disease are found to have a defect of mtDNA (although this generalization may not hold true when the full spectrum of *POLG* disease has been defined). By contrast,

Table 31–3 Clinical Syndromes Associated with Mitochondrial Disease

Syndrome	Primary Features	Additional Features
Alpers-Huttenlocher syndrome	Encephalopathy with seizures Liver failure	Developmental delay and hypotonia
Chronic progressive external ophthalmoplegia	External ophthalmoplegia and bilateral ptosis	Mild proximal myopathy
Kearns-Sayre syndrome	Progressive external ophthalmoplegia onset before age 20 years with pigmentary retinopathy Plus one of the following: cerebrospinal fluid protein >1 g/l, cerebellar ataxia, or heart block	Bilateral deafness Myopathy Dysphagia Diabetes mellitus Hypoparathyroidism dementia
Pearson's syndrome	Sideroblastic anemia of childhood pancytopenia Exocrine pancreatic failure	Renal tubular defects
Mitochondrial encephalomyopathy with lactic acidosis and stroke-like episodes (MELAS)	Stroke-like episodes before age 40 years Seizures and/or dementia Ragged-red fibers and/or lactic acidosis Pigmentary retinopathy Cerebellar ataxia	Diabetes mellitus Cardiomyopathy Bilateral deafness
Mitochondrial neurogastrointestinal encephalomyopathy (MNGIE)	Gastrointestinal pseudoobstruction Myopathy Leukoencephalopathy Peripheral neuropathy	
Myoclonic epilepsy with ragged-red fibers (MERRF)	Myoclonus Seizures Cerebellar ataxia Myopathy	Dementia Optic atrophy Bilateral deafness Peripheral neuropathy Spasticity Multiple lipomas
Leber's hereditary optic neuropathy	Subacute bilateral visual failure males:females approximately 4:1 Median age of onset 24 years	Dystonia Cardiac preexcitation syndromes
Leigh syndrome	Subacute relapsing encephalopathy with cerebellar and brainstem signs	Basal ganglia lucencies
Infantile myopathy and lactic acidosis	Hypotonia	Cardiomyopathy +/- Toni–Fanconi–Debre syndrome

children often present with different clinical features and are more likely to have a nuclear genetic defect (mtDNA defects account for approximately 15% of childhood OXPHOS disease) (Skladal et al. 2000). It is often possible to identify well-defined clinical syndromes (Table 31–3), but many patients present with a collection of clinical features that are highly suggestive of respiratory chain disease but do not fit into a discrete clinical category. Isolated cardiomyopathy is well recognized, either in a sporadic case, a family with multisystem disease, or with a family history of cardiac involvement.

Defined Clinical Syndromes

A summary of some of the defined clinical syndromes is shown in Table 31–3. Although some of these syndromes seem complex and difficult to remember for routine clinical practice, some core clinical features, such as chronic progressive external ophthalmoplegia (CPEO), are very easy to recognize even from a brief neurological examination. Features such as this may not be associated with any specific symptoms, but may be the first clue to an underlying mitochondrial disorder.

CPEO is a slowly progressive disorder of eye movement often accompanied by bilateral ptosis (PEO) and usually is due to a single deletion of mtDNA. A similar phenotype is also seen in patients with some point mutations, and multiple deletions of mtDNA due to an underlying nuclear gene defect. Patients with CPEO often develop a mild proximal myopathy as the disease progresses.

CPEO can be accompanied by bilateral sensorineural deafness, cerebellar ataxia, pigmentary retinopathy, diabetes mellitus, and cardiac conduction defects leading to complete heart block (Figure 31–3). Typically, this begins in teenage years and is associated with a raised cerebrospinal fluid protein, and is called the Kearns-Sayre syndrome (KSS). Hypoparathyroidism and hypothyroidism are well-recognized features of KSS. The vast majority (>95%) of cases of CPEO and KSS are sporadic. These two syndromes are the extremes of a spectrum of disease and many individuals lie somewhere between the pure extraocular muscle and severe central neurological phenotypes. The presence of deafness or early onset indicates a poor prognosis (Aure et al. 2007). KSS is also usually due to a single deletion of mtDNA.

Although most patients with PEO and KSS are sporadic cases, PEO can also be inherited as either an autosomal dominant (adPEO) or recessive (arPEO) trait. A high incidence of psychiatric disease, a Parkinsonian syndrome (similar, but distinct from idiopathic Parkinson disease, but responding to L-dopa), and primary gonadal failure have also been documented in some

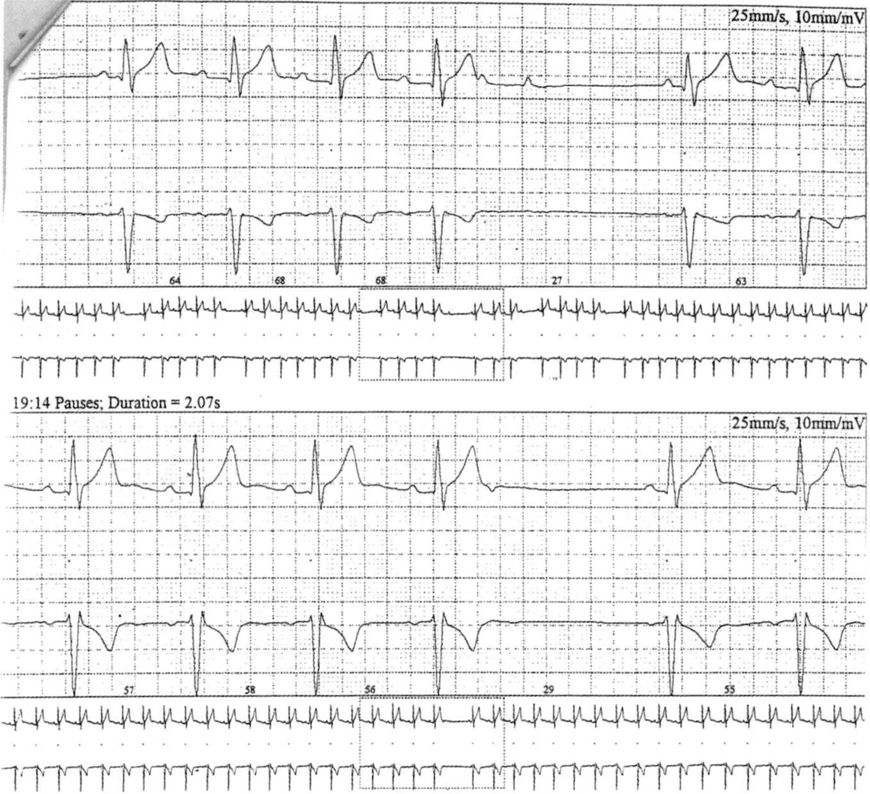

Figure 31–3 Twenty-four-hour electrocardiograph recording of a patient with the Kearns-Sayre syndrome and showing Mobitz type II heart block.

families (Luoma et al. 2004). Cardiomyopathy is well documented in this group (~10% in one series of patients with *POLG* mutations) (Horvath et al. 2006). Some cases have a profound peripheral neuropathy and ataxia (referred to as SANDO, sensory ataxic neuropathy with dysarthria and ophthalmoparesis), and some family members present with adult onset ataxia without ophthalmoplegia (also called mitochondrial recessive ataxia syndrome, MIRAS), which is common in Scandinavia (Hakonen et al. 2005). Mutations in the gene encoding the mitochondrial polymerase (polγ, encoded by the nuclear gene *POLG*) are a major cause of adPEO and arPEO. adPEO can also be caused by mutations in *PEO1* (which codes for the mtDNA helicase, Twinkle), *SLC25A4* (which codes for the adenine nucleotide translocase, ANT1), and *POLG2* (which codes for the accessory subunit of polγ) (Chinnery et al. 2007).

Pearson's syndrome of exocrine pancreatic failure, sideroblastic anemia, and marrow aplasia is usually due to a mtDNA deletion. Pearson's syndrome usually presents in infancy and a number of individuals who survived into later childhood subsequently developed KSS.

Pathogenic point mutations of mtDNA are more common than rearrangements. This is partly because mtDNA deletions cause sporadic disease, whereas many mtDNA point mutations are transmitted down the maternal line. The m.3243A>G mutation in the leucine (UUR) tRNA (*MTTL1*) gene was first described in a patient with MELAS (Goto et al. 1990). Different families harboring the same genetic defect may have different phenotypes. For example, some families harboring m.3243A>G have predominantly diabetes and deafness, some families have CPEO, and some present with hypertrophic cardiomyopathy (Zeviani et al. 1991; Reardon et al. 1992). Maternally inherited cardiomyopathy may be the only feature in some families transmitting m.3243A>G (Zeviani et al. 1991; Reardon et al. 1992). It is currently not known why this is the case but it is likely that additional nuclear genetic factors play an important role in modifying the expression of the primary mtDNA defect. This single mutation is important since it has been estimated that between 0.5% and 1.5% of cases of diabetes mellitus in the general population are associated with the m.3243A>G mutation (Newkirk et al. 1997).

Myoclonic epilepsy, ataxia, optic atrophy, and ragged-red fibers in skeletal muscle (MERRF) may also be due to a point mutation of mtDNA, the most common being m.8344A>G in the mtDNA $tRNA^{Lys}$ gene (*MTTLK*) (Shoffner et al. 1990).

MtDNA mutations are a major cause of visual loss in young adult males. About half of all males who harbor one of three point mutations of mtDNA (m.11778G>A, m.14484T>C, m.3460G>A) develop bilateral sequential visual loss in the second or third decade (Leber hereditary optic neuropathy, LHON, also called Leber optic neuropathy) (Wallace et al. 1988; Howell et al. 1991; Huoponen et al. 1991; Johns et al. 1992). The majority of individuals with these mutations are homoplasmic with only mutated mtDNA. It is not clear why the disease only affects approximately half of the males and 10% of females who inherit the primary mtDNA defect. Environmental factors, such as alcohol and tobacco, may explain the variable penetrance of this disorder; however, additional, as yet unknown, nuclear genetic factors may also be important in modulating the phenotype.

Leigh syndrome (subacute necrotizing encephalomyopathy) is a relapsing encephalopathy with prominent cerebellar and brainstem features that usually presents in childhood and is associated with characteristic low signal in the basal ganglia on MR imaging. Leigh syndrome can be due to a X-linked pyruvate dehydrogenase deficiency or a defect of the mitochondrial respiratory chain. Complex I deficiency or complex IV (COX) deficiency are common causes of Leigh syndrome (Morris et al. 1995). In these patients it may be possible to identify recessive mutations in nuclear complex I genes, or genes involved in the assembly of the respiratory chain complexes (e.g., *SURF 1*). Point mutations at position 8993 in the ATPase 6 gene of mtDNA (m.8993T>C or m.8993T>G) can cause Leigh syndrome, or neurogenic weakness with ataxia and retinitis pigmentosa (NARP), and spinocerebellar ataxia with an axonal sensorimotor neuropathy (Holt et al. 1990; Uziel et al. 1997).

Alpers-Huttenlocher syndrome is a severe autosomal recessive hepatoencephalopathy with intractable seizures and visual failure, which presents in early childhood and is associated with depletion (loss) of mtDNA in affected tissues. Mutations in the *POLG* are a major cause of Alpers-Huttenlocher syndrome (Naviaux et al. 2004). Mutations in *MPV* and *PEO1* also cause an Alper-like disorder (Spinazzola et al. 2006). Other causes of mtDNA depletion include mutations in *TK2* (encoding thymine kinase), which presents with a progressive childhood myopathy or spinal muscular atrophy (Saada et al. 2001), *DGUOK* (encoding dexyguanosine kinase), which presents in childhood with a myopathy and liver failure (Mandel et al. 2001), and *SUCLA2* (coding for ADP-forming succinyl-CoA synthase), which presents in early childhood with an encephalomyopathy (Elpeleg et al. 2005).

COX deficiency may also present in childhood with an infantile myopathy and a severe lactic acidosis, which may also be associated with a cardiomyopathy and the Toni–Fanconi–Debre syndrome. Despite maximal supportive intervention, this is usually a fatal disorder and a severe depletion of mtDNA occurs in a proportion of these cases. It is important to recognize that isolated myopathy and lactic acidosis may be self-limiting, often with a significant improvement by 1 year of age and complete resolution by the age of 3 years.

Coenzyme Q10 deficiency can present in childhood with recurrent myoglobinuria, myopathy, and seizures (Quinzii et al. 2006). In some families it presents with an infantile encephalomyopathy with renal tubular defects. Finally, it may also present with ataxia and variable involvement of other regions of the central nervous system, peripheral nerve, and muscle. Mutations in genes coding for enzymes involved in the biosynthesis of coenzyme Q10 have been found in some families (Mandel et al. 2001). Secondary Q10 deficiency is seen in a number of disorders including defects in the electron-transferring flavoprotein dehydrogenase (*ETFHD*) gene, which can cause cardiomyopathy. (Gempel et al. 2007).

Nonspecific Clinical Presentations

Many patients do not present with a characteristic phenotype, which presents the physician with a major challenge. Children may present in the neonatal period with a metabolic encephalopathy and systemic lactic acidosis, often associated with hepatic and cardiac failure. This may be associated with depletion in the total amount of mtDNA within affected tissues (see above). This syndrome may be fatal, and in some the liver failure is precipitated by exposure to sodium valproate, but it may also be a self-limiting disorder. Childhood presentations may be even less specific, with neonatal hypotonia, feeding and respiratory difficulties, and failure to thrive. A respiratory chain defect should be considered in any patient who has a disease with multiple organ involvement, particularly if there are central neurological features (such as seizures and dementia), a myopathy, cardiomyopathy, and endocrine abnormalities such as diabetes mellitus. Bilateral sensorineural deafness and ocular features (retinopathy, optic atrophy, ptosis, and ophthalmoparesis) are common. Renal tubular defects, gastrointestinal hypomotility, cervical lipomatosis, and psychiatric features are also well described in patients with respiratory chain disease.

Cardiac Involvement in Mitochondrial Diseases

Arrhythmias

Arrhythmias are common in patients with mitochondrial disease, either as an isolated cardiac feature, or associated with cardiomyopathy. In one pediatric cohort, 11% had arrhythmias, most commonly ventricular tachycardia (Scaglia et al. 2004).

Cardiac conduction defects are a defining feature of the KSS (Figure 31–3; Table 31–3). In some patients second-degree heart block remains stable over decades, but sudden death is recognized (Tveskov et al. 1990) and cardiac pacing is usually indicated in patients with second-degree or third-degree atrioventricular block (Anan et al. 1995). Conduction defects may also occur as part of cardiomyopathy in patients with m.3243A>G (Figure 31–4, and see below). Accessory pathways and the Wolff-Parkinson-White Syndrome (WPW) have been documented in patients with LHON (Nikoskelainen et al. 1994), but it is not clear whether this is a direct etiological link or simply a chance finding (Bower et al. 1992). More recently, a high frequency of WPW has been described in patients with m.3243A>G, being found in 13% of 30 patients (Sproule et al. 2007). Asymptomatic individuals do not require active intervention but those with symptomatic tachycardia will require pharmacological management or radio frequency catheter ablation.

Hypertrophic Cardiomyopathy (HCM)

Although previously under-recognized, HCM is a common feature of mitochondrial disease and is actually the most frequent cardiac complication. Point mutations of mtDNA can cause sporadic and maternally inherited HCM, which may be the presenting or only feature in patients with the common m.3243A>G *MTTL1* mutation first described in MELAS (Table 31–3, Figure 31–5). In one study (Vydt et al. 2007), eight m.3243A>G mutation carriers with neurological features had evidence of left ventricular (LV) dysfunction, but none of the participants revealed evidence of arrythmias on electrocardiography or Holter monitoring. Two patients had evidence of LV hypertrophy, five had LV systolic dysfunction, and five had LV diastolic abnormalities. In this study, none of the five asymptomatic carriers had cardiac abnormalities. The natural history of m.3243A>G cardiomyopathy is currently being evaluated. ^{31}P-magnetic resonance spectroscopy (MRS) studies have shown that the myocardial bioenergetic defect precedes the hypertrophic phase (Lodi et al. 2004) and eventually leads to a dilated cardiomyopathy and heart failure, which can be fatal. Anecdotal reports support the use of angiotensin-converting enzyme inhibitors at an early stage. Other point mutations, and mtDNA deletions (Tveskov et al. 1990) can also cause HCM, usually as part of a multisystem disorder. For example, HCM is common in patients carrying the m.8344A>G *MTTK* "MERRF" mutation, and the *MTTI* gene encoding tRNA^{ille} appears to be a mutation hotspot for HCM. HCM can be the sole feature of homoplasmic mtDNA tRNA gene

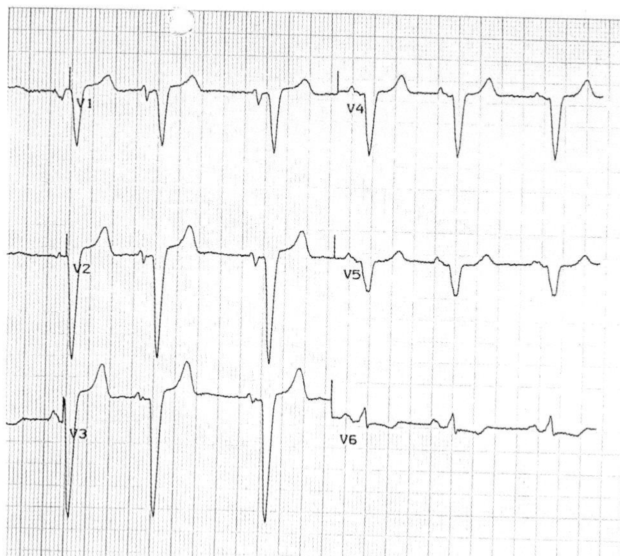

Figure 31–4 Twelve-lead electrocardiograph from a patient with m.3243A>G showing left bundle branch block.

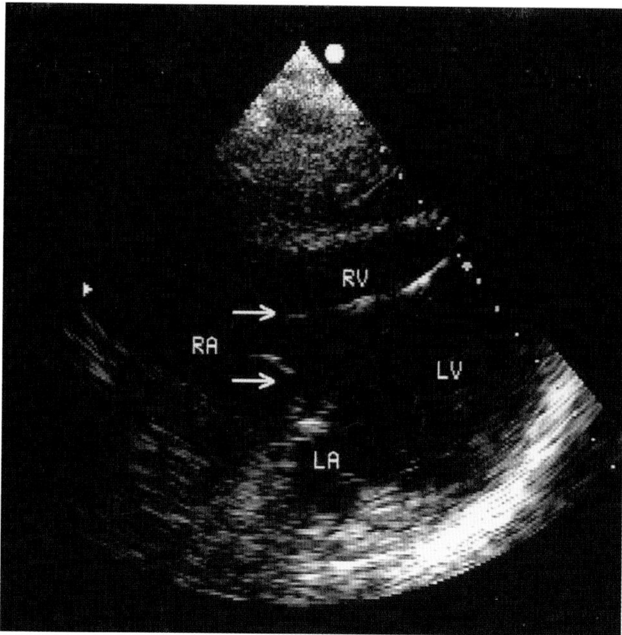

Figure 31–5 Echocardiogram of a patient with m.3243A>G showing septal hypertrophy and LV hypertrophy.

mutations, which characteristically cause tissue-specific phenotypes (Carelli et al. 2003; Taylor et al. 2003).

HCM has also been described in patients with nuclear gene defects causing a secondary defect of mtDNA, especially mutations in *POLG* presenting in childhood as part of Alpers-Huttenlocher syndrome or as late features of autosomal PEO. HCM has also been described in patients with a mutation in *SLC25A4* (which codes for the adenine nucleotide translocase, ANT1) without ophthalmoplegia (Palmieri et al. 2005). This latter finding is mirrored by the cardiomyopathy seen in transgenic ANT1 knockout mice (Graham et al. 1997).

HCM has also been described in Leigh syndrome (LS) (Table 31–3), which can be due to nuclear or mtDNA defects (Pastores et al. 1994; Marin-Garcia et al. 1997; Petruzzella et al. 2001). Infantile HCM dominates the clinical picture in patients with mutations in *SCO2* (Papadopoulou et al. 1999) and COX15 (Antonicka et al. 2003), which also share features of LS; mutations in *ATP12* also cause LS and cardiomyopathy (Houstek et al. 2004). More recently, a mutation in the *SLC25A3* gene resulting in mitochondrial phosphate carrier deficiency was reported in two siblings presenting with lactic acidosis, HCM, and muscular hypotonia who died within the first year of life. An ATP synthase deficiency in muscle mitochondria was identified correlating with the tissue-specific expression of exon 3A (Mayr et al. 2007).

Histiocytoid Cardiomyopathy

Rare forms of cardiomyopathy have been documented in isolated cases of mitochondrial disease, including a histiocytoid cardiomyopathy in patients with mutations in the *MTCYB* gene encoding cytochrome *b* and presenting in early childhood with respiratory chain complex III deficiency and a propensity for dysrhythmias (Andreu et al. 2000).

Left Ventricular Noncompaction (LVNC) and Barth Syndrome

Left ventricular noncompaction is a heterogeneous disease that usually presents with cardiomegaly and congestive cardiac failure in childhood. Some X-linked recessive cases have mutations in *TAZ*, which also causes Barth syndrome (Bione et al. 1996; Ichida et al. 2001), suggesting that the two disorders are allelic. Barth syndrome affects young males and presents with congestive cardiac failure, neutropenia, and skeletal myopathy (Barth et al. 2004), usually associated with abnormal levels of 3-methylglutaconate, 3-methylglutarate, and 2-ethylhydracrylate in the urine (Kelley et al. 1991).

Sengers Syndrome

Sengers syndrome is a rare autosomal recessive mitochondrial disease characterized by congenital cataracts, HCM, and skeletal myopathy with a defect of cytochrome *c* oxidase in muscle (Sengers et al. 1975). The etiology of Sengers syndrome is not known, but presumed secondary abnormalities of ANT have been described at the gene expression and protein levels (Jordens et al. 2002). A patient with HCM due to Sengers syndrome has received a successful cardiac transplant (Robbins et al. 1995).

Congenital Heart Defects (CHD)

Congenital structural defects of the heart have been documented in patients with mitochondrial disease (Farag et al. 2002). Conversely, biochemical abnormalities of mitochondrial function have been described in patients with complex CHDs (Mital et al. 2004; Shinde et al. 2007). These are likely to be secondary to the primary pathology, and their significance has yet to be established.

Do All Mitochondrial Diseases Affect the Heart?

The incidence of cardiomyopathy in mitochondrial disease is not known; however, it is now recognized that characteristic abnormalities are linked to specific mutations. Anan et al. (1995) studied 17 patients with known mitochondrial defects and assessed cardiac involvement using electrocardiography, a chest X-ray, His-bundle electrograms, and echocardiography (Anan et al. 1995).

All three patients with KSS had conduction defects; two of the five MELAS patients had LV hypertrophy; two of the three MERRF patients had cardiomegaly with variable septal wall hypertrophy, with one subsequently developing DCM 2 years later and two of the six ocular myopathy patients with large deletions had ECG abnormalities.

More recently, Debray et al. reviewed the medical notes of 73 children with mitochondrial disease: 29% displayed visceral or cardiac involvement but interestingly this was not an independent prognostic factor with the strongest predictor of mortality being age of onset of symptoms (Debray et al. 2007).

These natural history studies, although limited, are extremely important in aiding our understanding of the incidence and prevalence of cardiomyopathy in mitochondrial disease. To date, particularly in early onset of mitochondrial-related disease, neurological sequelae appear to overshadow other organ symptoms including cardiac. This may relate to the rapid fatality of the primary condition that cardiac manifestations do not have time to develop, or as suggested in the literature that age of onset of symptoms and severity of mitochondrial mutation may determine incidence and degree of cardiac abnormalities.

Best clinical practice would appear to have a high index of suspicion in all cases of mitochondrial disease for the presence of cardiac pathology and to instigate a surveillance policy.

Investigation of Suspected Mitochondrial Disease

The diagnostic approach to suspected mitochondrial disease has a strong clinical foundation. Although ultimately the "holy grail" is a molecular diagnosis, this often takes considerable time, and may never be possible. The first important step is to consider the possibility of a mitochondrial disorder. This is followed by the systematic gathering of clinical data to support the diagnosis, usually involving a detailed family history and standard clinical investigations looking for a pattern of organ involvement consistent with mitochondrial disease. In some cases (such as LHON), it is possible to identify a specific clinical syndrome with a clear maternal family history, leading to a molecular genetic diagnostic test on a blood sample. However, in many instances, this is not appropriate because the clinical features overlap with those of many other disorders. Even if the patient has a mitochondrial disorder, numerous different genetic defects may be responsible, some of which will not be detectable by the analysis of blood samples.

Investigations fall into two main groups: clinical investigations used to characterize the pattern and nature of the different organs involved, and specific investigations to identify the biochemical or genetic abnormality.

General Clinical Investigations

General clinical investigations are used to detect asymptomatic organ involvement in a pattern that is consistent with a mitochondrial disorder, paying particular emphasis on the complications amenable to medical management. Endocrine assessment (oral glucose tolerance test, thyroid function tests, alkaline phosphatase, fasting calcium, and parathyroid hormone levels) and cardiac assessment are mandatory (discussed later). Additional metabolic investigations include urine organic and amino acids, which may point to an underlying tubulopathy (especially in children) but may be abnormal even in patients with normal renal function. High levels of lactate in blood and cerebrospinal fluid can be helpful, but rarely makes a major difference to the diagnostic process in adults because of the many potential causes of lactic acidosis, including fever, sepsis, dehydration, seizures, and stroke. An elevated serum creatine kinase raises the possibility of an associated mitochondrial myopathy, but it is often normal even in patients with a clear-cut metabolic defect in muscle. Peripheral neurophysiological investigations (electromyogram and nerve conduction studies) may identify a myopathy or neuropathy (which is usually axonal and mixed sensorimotor). Electroencephalography may reveal diffuse slow-wave activity consistent with subacute encephalopathy, or it may reveal a predisposition to seizures. Brain imaging can be normal, but may show atrophy, abnormal basal ganglia (including calcification), or a leukoencephalopathy.

Cardiac Investigations

All suspected cases of mitochondrial disease should have a 12-lead electrocardiogram (ECG), and with the exception of LHON, all should have a standard transthoracic echocardiogram to assess chamber and septal dimensions including LV wall thickness. Valve lesions are well documented in patients with mitochondrial disease, particularly when the mitochondrial disorder presents in childhood.

Transesophageal echocardiogram is indicated when there is a suspected septal defect, as has been documented in some cases, but not as a routine. Rhythm monitoring for 24 hours and 48 hours is indicated in patients with paroxysmal symptoms, particularly if there are conduction abnormalities on the 12-lead ECG. There is limited experience of cardiac MRI in patients with mitochondrial cardiomyopathy, although this is likely to change over the next 5 years (Figure 31–6). Given the progressive, and intractable clinical course in many patients with mitochondrial cardiomyopathy, we place great emphasis on the early detection of structural change, leading to generic treatments aimed at preventing remodeling, and cardiac MRI has an important role in this regard. We have studied patients with the common m.3243A>G *MTTL1* mutation and detected structurally abnormal hearts in patients with no symptoms of cardiac disease. The advantage of this technique is that it is possible to study structure and bioenergetic function of the heart simultaneously, using ^{31}P-magnetic resonance spectroscopy (^{31}P-MRS) (Lodi et al. 2004). A defect of myocardial ATP synthesis has been demonstrated in structurally normal hearts in m.3243A>G *MTTL1* mutation carriers, raising the possibility of early treatment before the evolution of structural change or the development of symptoms (see subsequent text). The role of MRS in the routine investigation of suspected mitochondrial cardiomyopathy has yet to be established.

It should be remembered that patients with mitochondrial disease are also vulnerable to developing common cardiac disorders, such as ischemic and hypertensive heart disease. The presence of neurological and muscular disease presents a challenge when investigating these common cardiac diseases, because neurological disability may influence exercise capacity and thus the outcome of exercise testing.

Specific Investigations

These investigations are aimed at demonstrating a biochemical defect of the respiratory chain. In adults, the first approach usually involves a skeletal muscle biopsy. This may not be possible in children, where a less invasive test may be performed (a skin biopsy for fibroblast culture), or a biopsy is taken from an affected tissue (e.g., liver or myocardium). Interpreting myocardial biopsies is difficult because there is limited age-matched control tissue available.

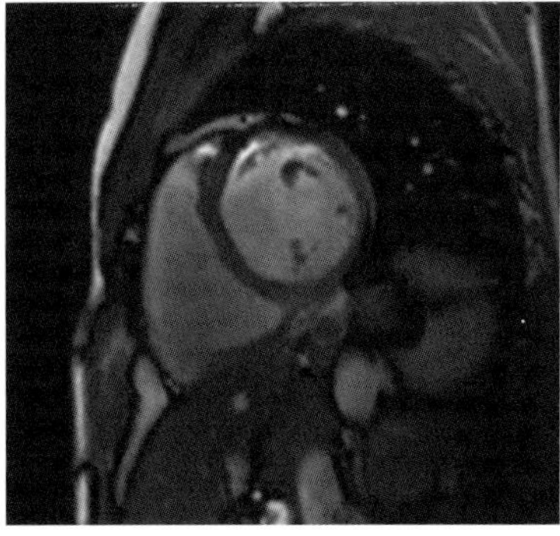
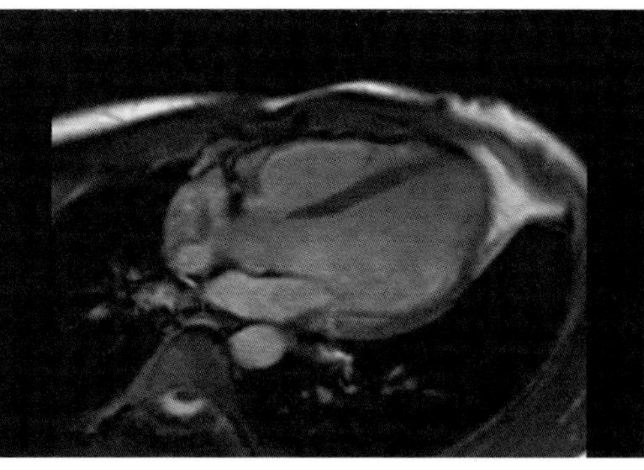

Figure 31–6 Cardiac MRI in a patient with the m.3243A>G mutation. Left panel, sagittal view. Right panel, axial view. Our thanks to Dr Mike Trenell for providing the figure.

Histochemistry and Biochemistry

Histochemistry is carried out on frozen sections of muscle, giving insight into the morphology and function of mitochondria. The accumulation of mitochondria beneath the muscle cell membrane (subsarcolemmal collections, leading to so-called ragged-red fibers), or cytochrome *c* oxidase (COX) deficiency are common in adults. It should, however, be noted that not all patients with suspected mitochondrial disease have abnormal muscle histochemistry, particularly if the phenotype is organ specific and does not involve a myopathy. A mosaic of COX-positive and COX-negative muscle fibers suggests an underlying primary mtDNA defect or a secondary defect of mtDNA as seen in patients with *POLG* mutations. Patients who have COX deficiency due to a nuclear genetic defect often have a global deficiency of COX affecting all muscle fibers, although a mosaic defect can be seen in some patients with nuclear mutation causing a defect of mtDNA maintenance. Electron microscopy may identify paracrystalline inclusions in the intermembrane space, but these may be seen in other nonmitochondrial disorders such as myotonic and other muscular dystrophies. Respiratory chain complex assays can be carried out on various tissues. Skeletal muscle is preferable, but cultured fibroblasts are useful in the investigation of childhood mitochondrial disease. Measurement of the individual respiratory chain complexes determines whether an individual has multiple complex defects that would suggest an underlying mtDNA defect, involving either a tRNA gene or a large deletion. Isolated complex defects may be due to mutations in either mitochondrial or nuclear genes. Coenzyme Q10 can be measured directly in affected tissues.

Molecular Genetics

For some patients, the phenotype is so characteristic that a molecular genetic blood test can be performed early in the investigation of suspected mitochondrial disease. For other patients, the pattern of the histochemical and biochemical defect is an essential guide to subsequent molecular genetic testing. A mosaic histochemical defect points toward a primary mtDNA defect (although there are exceptions; see above). Multiple respiratory chain defects usually indicate a disorder of intra-mitochondrial protein synthesis, which can be of mtDNA or nuclear DNA in origin. Specific isolated complex involvement points to specific mtDNA genes, a nuclear structural subunit gene, or a nuclear-encoded respiratory chain assembly factor. It is important to remember that some mtDNA defects (particularly mtDNA deletions) are not detectable in a DNA sample extracted from blood, and the analysis of DNA extracted from muscle is essential to establish the diagnosis.

In suspected mtDNA disease, the first stage is to look for mtDNA rearrangements or mtDNA depletion by Southern blot analysis, long-range polymerase chain reaction (PCR) or real-time PCR. This is followed by PCR and restriction fragment length polymorphism analysis for common point mutations, and then complete sequencing of mtDNA (which is now part of routine clinical investigation). Interpretation of the sequence data can be extremely difficult because mtDNA is highly polymorphic and any two normal individuals may differ by up to 60 bp. In the strictest sense, a mutation can only be considered to be pathogenic if it has arisen independently several times in the population, it is not seen in controls, and it is associated with a potential disease mechanism. These stringent criteria depend on a good knowledge of polymorphic sites in the background population. If a novel base change is heteroplasmic, this suggests that it is of relatively recent onset. Family, tissue segregation, and single cell studies may show that higher levels of the mutation are associated with mitochondrial dysfunction and disease, which strongly suggests that the mutation is causing the disease. Specific nuclear genes (e.g., *POLG*) are usually sequenced after initial mtDNA analysis identifies a secondary defect of mtDNA (multiple deletions or depletion). Although there may be a corresponding histochemical or biochemical defect, this may not be detectable in readily available tissues.

For suspected nuclear gene defects, blood DNA is adequate. Some of the common nuclear genes (e.g., *POLG*) are screened as part of standard molecular diagnostic procedures—but most (Table 31–2) are only studied in research laboratories at present. A genetic diagnosis is not possible in many patients with suspected nuclear gene defects either because comprehensive screening is not possible, or because the underlying gene defects have not yet been identified.

The Clinical Management of Mitochondrial Disease

There is currently no definitive treatment for patients with mitochondrial disease (Chinnery et al. 2006), except for patients with deficiency of coenzyme Q10 (Quinzii et al. 2006). Management is aimed at minimizing disability, preventing complications, and genetic counseling.

Supportive Care and Surveillance

The multisystem and chronic nature of mitochondrial disease means that many patients require integrated follow-up over many decades, involving the primary physician (often a neurologist, but sometimes a diabetologist or cardiologist, depending on the major phenotype), other specialist physicians (ophthalmology), specialist nurses, physiotherapists, and speech therapists. Management is essentially supportive, as for other phenotypically related disorders.

Genetic Counseling

A precise molecular diagnosis facilitates genetic counseling for patients and their families. Most children with respiratory chain disease are compound heterozygotes with recessive nuclear gene mutations. Some adults have a recessive disorder, or autosomal dominant PEO. In many cases, it is not possible to identify the underlying gene and the counseling is more speculative, and based on the family structure and likely inheritance pattern. For primary mtDNA defects, males cannot transmit pathogenic mtDNA defects. Patients who carry mtDNA deletions rarely have a family history suggestive of mtDNA disease, but there is a small risk that affected women will transmit the mtDNA defect to their offspring. By contrast, women harboring pathogenic mtDNA point mutations may transmit the genetic defect to their offspring. The mitochondrial genetic "bottleneck" leads to a variation in the proportion of mutated mtDNA that is transmitted to any offspring. It is therefore possible for a female to have mildly affected as well as severely affected children. The risk of having affected offspring varies from mutation to mutation, and there does appear to be a relationship between the level of mutated mtDNA in the mother and the risk of affected offspring.

Pharmacological Treatments for Mitochondrial Disease

Standard doses of vitamin C and K, thiamine, riboflavin, and ubiquinone (coenzyme Q10) are reported to be of some benefit in isolated cases and open studies, particularly in patients with isolated Q10 deficiency. Dichloracetate can be used to reduce lactic acid levels but a recent clinical trial showed that the side effects of this treatment are unacceptable (a partially irreversible toxic neuropathy). Moderate exercise is important for patients with mtDNA disease to prevent or reverse deconditioning, which are common in these disorders (Taivassalo et al. 1997).

Management of Mitochondrial Cardiomyopathy

The mainstay of management is surveillance allowing secondary prevention and aggressive treatment of complications. Stringent glycemic control in diabetes associated with m.3243A>G is imperative, as well as instigation of cardioprotective agents such as ACE inhibitors, β-blockers, and statins are indicated in mitochondrial diseases particularly in the setting of large mtDNA mutations. Other complications may require more specialized management such as cardiac pacing in KSS (see above), the treatment of heart failure in cardiomyopathy, and in certain cases cardiac transplantation.

Transplantation

Transplantation as a form of treatment is controversial in the field of mitochondrial disorders. Multiorgan pathology is usually regarded as a contraindication for heart transplantation in metabolic disorders because the prolongation of life achieved by restoring cardiac function could lead to long-term neurological disability. However, it is not unreasonable to consider heart transplantation in mitochondrial cardiomyopathy in cases were the clinical expression of respiratory enzyme deficiency is limited to the myocardium. Neuromuscular weakness can present difficulties during and after anesthesia, but successful orthotopic cardiac transplantations have been reported in such cases. Schmauss et al. reported a case of successful transplantation in a 14-year-old who presented with cardiac failure associated with malignant ventricular arrythmias (Schmauss et al. 2007). More recently, Robbins et al. described successful cardiac transplantation for hypertrophic obstructive cardiomyopathy (HOCM) in Sengers syndrome (Robbins et al. 1995).

Future Treatment Approaches

But perhaps the most challenging and most controversial therapy will lie in gene therapy for the treatment of mitochondrial diseases. To date various attempts have been made to design a delivery system capable of delivering drugs, proteins, peptides, and genes to the site of mitochondria with varying results. Germline therapy raises ethical issues as a possible tool to prevent maternal inheritance of mutant mtDNA. Prevention via genetic counseling and antenatal diagnosis are becoming increasingly used. An experimental method currently in use in France is the use of embryonic screening prior implantation using in vitro fertilization methods (Steffann et al. 2007).

References

Anan R, Nakagawa M, Miyata M, et al. Cardiac involvement in mitochondrial diseases. A study on 17 patients with documented mitochondrial DNA defects. *Circulation.* 1995;91(4):955–961.

Anderson S, Bankier AT, Barrell BG, et al. Sequence and organization of the human mitochondrial genome. *Nature.* 1981;290(5806):457–465.

Andreu AL, Checcarelli N, Iwata S, Shanske S, DiMauro S. A missense mutation in the mitochondrial cytochrome b gene in a revisited case with histiocytoid cardiomyopathy. *Pediatr Res.* 2000;48(3):311–314.

Andrews RM, Kubacka I, Chinnery PF, Lightowlers RN, Turnbull DM, Howell N. Reanalysis and revision of the Cambridge reference sequence for human mitochondrial DNA [letter]. *Nat Genet.* 1999;23(2):147.

Antonicka H, Mattman A, Carlson CG, et al. Mutations in COX15 produce a defect in the mitochondrial heme biosynthetic pathway, causing early-onset fatal hypertrophic cardiomyopathy. *Am J Hum Genet.* 2003;72(1):101–114.

Aure K, Ogier de Baulny H, Laforet P, Jardel C, Eymard B, Lombes A. Chronic progressive ophthalmoplegia with large-scale mtDNA rearrangement: can we predict progression? *Brain.* 2007;130(Pt 6):1516–1524.

Barth PG, Valianpour F, Bowen VM, et al. X-linked cardioskeletal myopathy and neutropenia (Barth syndrome): an update. *Am J Med Genet A.* 2004;126(4):349–354.

Bione S, D'Adamo P, Maestrini E, Gedeon AK, Bolhuis PA, Toniolo D. A novel X-linked gene, G4.5. is responsible for Barth syndrome. *Nat Genet.* 1996;12(4):385–389.

Bourdon A, Minai L, Serre V, et al. Mutation of RRM2B, encoding p53-controlled ribonucleotide reductase (p53R2), causes severe mitochondrial DNA depletion. *Nat Genet.* 2007;39(6):776–780.

Bower SP, Hawley I, Mackey DA. Cardiac arrhythmia and Leber's hereditary optic neuropathy [letter]. *Lancet.* 1992;339(8806):1427–1428.

Brierley EJ, Johnson MA, Lightowlers RN, James OF, Turnbull DM. Role of mitochondrial DNA mutations in human aging: implications for the central nervous system and muscle. *Ann Neurol.* 1998;43(2): 217–223.

Bykhovskaya Y, Casas K, Mengesha E, Inbal A, Fischel-Ghodsian N. Missense mutation in pseudouridine synthase 1 (PUS1) causes mitochondrial myopathy and sideroblastic anemia (MLASA). *Am J Hum Genet.* 2004;74(6):1303–1308.

Carelli V, Giordano C, d'Amati G. Pathogenic expression of homoplasmic mtDNA mutations needs a complex nuclear-mitochondrial interaction. *Trends Genet.* 2003;19(5):257–262.

Chinnery P, Majamaa K, Turnbull D, Thorburn D. Treatment for mitochondrial disorders. *Cochrane Database Syst Rev.* 2006(1):CD004426.

Chinnery PF, DiMauro S, Shanske S, et al. Risk of developing a mitochondrial DNA deletion disorder. *Lancet.* 2004;364(9434):592–596.

Chinnery PF, Thorburn DR, Samuels DC, et al. The inheritance of mitochondrial DNA heteroplasmy: random drift, selection or both? *Trends Genet.* 2000;16(11):500–505.

Chinnery PF, Zeviani M. 155th ENMC workshop: Polymerase gamma and disorders of mitochondrial DNA synthesis, 21–23 September 2007, Naarden, The Netherlands. *Neuromuscul Disord.* 2007.

Coenen MJ, Antonicka H, Ugalde C, et al. Mutant mitochondrial elongation factor G1 and combined oxidative phosphorylation deficiency. *N Engl J Med.* 2004;351(20):2080–2086.

Cree LM, Samuels DC, Chuva de Sousa Lopes S, et al. A reduction in the number of mitochondrial DNA molecules during embryogenesis explains the rapid segregation of genotypes *Nat Genet.* 2007;40:249–254.

Debray FG, Lambert M, Chevalier I, et al. Long-term outcome and clinical spectrum of 73 pediatric patients with mitochondrial diseases. *Pediatrics.* 2007;119(4):722–733.

DiMauro S, Schon EA. Mitochondrial respiratory-chain diseases. *N Engl J Med.* 2003;348(26):2656–2668.

Elpeleg O, Miller C, Hershkovitz E, et al. Deficiency of the ADP-forming succinyl-CoA synthase activity is associated with encephalomyopathy and mitochondrial DNA depletion. *Am J Hum Genet.* 2005;76(6):1081–1086.

Farag E, Argalious M, Narouze S, DeBoer GE, Tome J. The anesthetic management of ventricular septal defect (VSD) repair in a child with mitochondrial cytopathy. *Can J Anaesth.* 2002;49(9):958–962.

Gempel K, Topaloglu H, Talim B, et al. The myopathic form of coenzyme Q10 deficiency is caused by mutations in the electron-transferring-flavoprotein dehydrogenase (ETFDH) gene. *Brain.* 2007;130(Pt 8):2037–2044.

Goto Y, Nonaka I, Horai S. A mutation in the tRNA(Leu)(UUR) gene associated with the MELAS subgroup of mitochondrial encephalomyopathies. *Nature.* 1990;348(6302):651–653.

Graham BH, Waymire KG, Cottrell B, Trounce IA, MacGregor GR, Wallace DC. A mouse model for mitochondrial myopathy and cardiomyopathy resulting from a deficiency in the heart/muscle isoform of the adenine nucleotide translocator. *Nat Genet.* 1997;16:226–234.

Hakonen AH, Heiskanen S, Juvonen V, et al. Mitochondrial DNA polymerase W748S mutation: a common cause of autosomal recessive ataxia with ancient European origin. *Am J Hum Genet.* 2005;77(3):430–441.

Holt I, Harding AE, Morgan-Hughes JA. Deletion of muscle mitochondrial DNA in patients with mitochondrial myopathies. *Nature.* 1988;331:717–719.

Holt IJ, Harding AE, Petty RK, Morgan-Hughes JA. A new mitochondrial disease associated with mitochondrial DNA heteroplasmy. *Am J Hum Genet.* 1990;46(3):428–433.

Horvath R, Hudson G, Ferrari G, et al. Phenotypic spectrum associated with mutations of the mitochondrial polymerase gamma gene. *Brain.* 2006;129(Pt 7):1674–1684.

Houstek J, Mracek T, Vojtiskova A, Zeman J. Mitochondrial diseases and ATPase defects of nuclear origin. *Biochim Biophys Acta.* 2004;1658(1–2):115–121.

Howell N, Bindoff LA, McCullough DA, et al. Leber hereditary optic neuropathy: identification of the same mitochondrial ND1 mutation in six pedigrees. *Am J Hum Genet.* 1991;49(5):939–950.

Huoponen K, Vilkki J, Aula P, Nikoskelainen EK, Savontaus ML. A new mtDNA mutation associated with Leber hereditary optic neuroretinopathy. *Am J Hum Genet.* 1991;48(6):1147–1153.

Ichida F, Tsubata S, Bowles KR, et al. Novel gene mutations in patients with left ventricular noncompaction or Barth syndrome. *Circulation.* 2001;103(9):1256–1263.

Johns DR, Neufeld MJ, Park RD. An ND-6 mitochondrial DNA mutation associated with Leber hereditary optic neuropathy. *Biochem Biophys Res Commun.* 1992;187(3):1551–1557.

Jordens EZ, Palmieri L, Huizing M, et al. Adenine nucleotide translocator 1 deficiency associated with Sengers syndrome. *Ann Neurol.* 2002;52(1):95–99.

Kajander OA, Rovio AT, Majamaa K, et al. Human mtDNA sublimons resemble rearranged mitochondrial genoms found in pathological states. *Hum Mol Genet.* 2000;9(19):2821–2835.

Kaukonen J, Juselius JK, Tiranti V, et al. Role of adenine nucleotide translocator 1 in mtDNA maintenance. *Science.* 2000;289:782–785.

Kelley RI, Cheatham JP, Clark BJ, et al. X-linked dilated cardiomyopathy with neutropenia, growth retardation, and 3-methylglutaconic aciduria. *J Pediatr.* 1991;119(5):738–747.

Lodi R, Rajagopalan B, Blamire AM, Crilley JG, Styles P, Chinnery PF. Abnormal cardiac energetics in patients carrying the A3243G mtDNA mutation measured in vivo using phosphorus MR spectroscopy. *Biochim Biophys Acta.* 2004;1657(2–3):146–150.

Longley MJ, Clark S, Yu Wai Man C, et al. Mutant POLG2 disrupts DNA polymerase gamma subunits and causes progressive external ophthalmoplegia. *Am J Hum Genet.* 2006;78(6):1026–1034.

Luoma P, Melberg A, Rinne JO, et al. Parkinsonism, premature menopause, and mitochondrial DNA polymerase gamma mutations: clinical and molecular genetic study. *Lancet.* 2004;364(9437):875–882.

Mandel H, Szargel R, Labay V, et al. The deoyguanosine kinase gene is mutated in individuals with depleted hepatocerebral mitochondrial DNA. *Nat Genet.* 2001;29:337–341.

Marin-Garcia J, Ananthakrishnan R, Goldenthal MJ, Filiano JJ, Perez-Atayde A. Cardiac mitochondrial dysfunction and DNA depletion in children with hypertrophic cardiomyopathy. *J Inher Metab Dis.* 1997;20(5):674–680.

Mayr JA, Merkel O, Kohlwein SD, et al. Mitochondrial phosphate-carrier deficiency: a novel disorder of oxidative phosphorylation. *Am J Hum Genet.* 2007;80(3):478–484.

Miller C, Saada A, Shaul N, et al. Defective mitochondrial translation caused by a ribosomal protein (MRPS16) mutation. *Ann Neurol.* 2004;56(5):734–738.

Mital S, Loke KE, Chen JM, et al. Mitochondrial respiratory abnormalities in patients with end-stage congenital heart disease. *J Heart Lung Transplant.* 2004;23(1):72–79.

Morris AA, Jackson MJ, Bindoff LA, Turnbull DM. The investigation of mitochondrial respiratory chain disease. *J R Soc Med.* 1995; 88(4):217P–22P.

Muller-Hocker J, Seibel P, Schneiderbanger K, et al. In situ hybridization of mitochondrial DNA in the heart of a patient with Kearns-Sayre syndrome and dilatative cardiomyopathy. *Hum Pathol.* 1992; 23(12):1431–1437.

Naviaux RK, Nguyen KV. POLG mutations associated with Alpers' syndrome and mitochondrial DNA depletion. *Ann Neurol.* 2004;55(5): 706–712.

Newkirk JE, Taylor RW, Howell N, et al. Maternally inherited diabetes and deafness: prevalence in a hospital diabetic population. *Diabet Med.* 1997;14(6):457–460.

Nikoskelainen EK, Savontaus ML, Huoponen K, Antila K, Hartiala J. Pre-excitation syndrome in Leber's hereditary optic neuropathy. *Lancet.* 1994;344(8926):857–858.

Palmieri L, Alberio S, Pisano I, et al. Complete loss-of-function of the heart/muscle-specific adenine nucleotide translocator is associated with mitochondrial myopathy and cardiomyopathy. *Hum Mol Genet.* 2005;14(20):3079–3088.

Papadopoulou LC, Sue CM, Davidson M. Fatal infantile cardioencephalomyopathy with cytochrome c oxidase (COX) deficiency due to mutations in SCO2, a human COX assembly gene. *Nat Genet.* 1999;23: 333–337.

Pastores GM, Santorelli FM, Shanske S, et al. Leigh syndrome and hypertrophic cardiomyopathy in an infant with a mitochondrial DNA point mutation (T8993G). *Am J Med Genet.* 1994;50(3):265–271.

Petruzzella V, Vergari R, Puzziferri I, et al. A nonsense mutation in the NDUFS4 gene encoding the 18 kDa (AQDQ) subunit of complex I abolishes assembly and activity of the complex in a patient with Leigh-like syndrome. *Hum Mol Genet.* 2001;10(5):529–535.

Quinzii C, Naini A, Salviati L, et al. A Mutation in para-hydroxybenzoate-polyprenyl transferase (COQ2) causes primary coenzyme Q10 deficiency. *Am J Hum Genet.* 2006;78(2):345–349.

Reardon W, Ross RJ, Sweeney MG, et al. Diabetes mellitus associated with a pathogenic point mutation in mitochondrial DNA. *Lancet.* 1992;340(8832):1376–1379.

Robbins RC, Bernstein D, Berry GJ, VanMeurs KP, Frankel LR, Reitz BA. Cardiac transplantation for hypertrophic cardiomyopathy associated with Sengers syndrome. *Ann Thorac Surg.* 1995;60(5):1425–1427.

Saada A, Shaag A, Arnon S, et al. Antenatal mitochondrial disease caused by mitochondrial ribosomal protein (MRPS22) mutation. *J Med Genet.* 2007;44(12):784–786 .

Saada A, Shaag A, Mandel H, Nevo Y, Eriksson S, Elpeleg O. Mutant mitochondrial thymidine kinase in mitochondrial DNA depletion myopathy. *Nat Genet.* 2001;29:342–344.

Scaglia F, Towbin JA, Craigen WJ, et al. Clinical spectrum, morbidity, and mortality in 113 pediatric patients with mitochondrial disease. *Pediatrics.* 2004;114(4):925–931.

Schmauss D, Sodian R, Klopstock T, et al. Cardiac transplantation in a 14-yr-old patient with mitochondrial encephalomyopathy. *Pediatr Transplant.* 2007;11(5):560–562.

Schon EA, Bonilla E, DiMauro S. Mitochondrial DNA mutations and pathogenesis. *J Bioenerget Biomemb.* 1997;29:131–149.

Sengers RC, Trijbels JM, Willems JL, Daniels O, Stadhouders AM. Congenital cataract and mitochondrial myopathy of skeletal and heart muscle associated with lactic acidosis after exercise. *J Pediatr.* 1975; 86(6):873–880.

Servidei S. Mitochondrial encephalomyopathies: gene mutation. *Neuromuscul Disord.* 2004;14:107–116.

Shinde SB, Save VC, Patil ND, Mishra KP, Tendolkar AG. Impairment of mitochondrial respiratory chain enzyme activities in tetralogy of Fallot. *CCA; Int J Clin Chem.* 2007;377(1–2):138–143.

Shoffner JM, Lott MT, Lezza AM, Seibel P, Ballinger SW, Wallace DC. Myoclonic epilepsy and ragged-red fiber disease (MERRF) is associated with a mitochondrial DNA tRNA(Lys) mutation. *Cell.* 1990;61(6):931–937.

Skladal D, Bernier FP, Halliday JL, Thorburn DR. Birth prevalence of mitochondrial respiratory chain defects in children. *J Inher Metab Dis.* 2000;23(Suppl 1):138.

Smeitink JA, Elpeleg O, Antonicka H, et al. Distinct clinical phenotypes associated with a mutation in the mitochondrial translation elongation factor EFTs. *Am J Hum Genet.* 2006;79(5):869–877.

Spelbrink JN, Li FY, Tiranti V, et al. Human mitochondrial DNA deletions associated with mutations in the gene encoding Twinkle, a phage T7 gene 4-like protein localised in mitochondria. *Nat Genet.* 2001;28:223–231.

Spinazzola A, Viscomi C, Fernandez-Vizarra E, et al. MPV17 encodes an inner mitochondrial membrane protein and is mutated in infantile hepatic mitochondrial DNA depletion. *Nat Genet.* 2006;38(5):570–575.

Sproule DM, Kaufmann P, Engelstad K, Starc TJ, Hordof AJ, De Vivo DC. Wolff-Parkinson-White syndrome in patients with MELAS. *Arch Neurol.* 2007;64(11):1625–1627.

Steffann J, Gigarel N, Corcos J, et al. Stability of the m.8993T->G mtDNA mutation load during human embryofetal development has implications for the feasibility of prenatal diagnosis in NARP syndrome. *J Med Genet.* 2007;44(10):664–669.

Taivassalo T, De Stefano N, Matthews PM, et al. Aerobic training benefits patients with mitochondrial myopathies more than other chronic myopathies. *Neurology.* 1997;48:A214.

Taylor RW, Giordano C, Davidson MM, et al. A homoplasmic mitochondrial transfer ribonucleic acid mutation as a cause of maternally inherited hypertrophic cardiomyopathy. *J Am Coll Cardiol.* 2003;41(10):1786–1796.

Taylor RW, Turnbull DM. Mitochondrial DNA mutations in human disease. *Nat Rev Genet.* 2005;6(5):389–402.

Tveskov C, Angelo-Nielsen K. Kearns-Sayre syndrome and dilated cardiomyopathy. *Neurology.* 1990;40(3 Pt 1):553–554.

Uziel G, Moroni I, Lamantea E, et al. Mitochondrial disease associated with the T8993G mutation of the mitochondrial ATPase 6 gene: a clinical, biochemical, and molecular study in six families. *J Neurol Neurosurg Psychiatry.* 1997;63(1):16–22.

Valente L, Tiranti V, Marsano RM, et al. Infantile encephalopathy and defective mitochondrial DNA translation in patients with mutations of mitochondrial elongation factors EFG1 and EFTu. *Am J Hum Genet.* 2007;80(1):44–58.

Van Goethem G, Dermaut B, Lofgren A, Martin J-J, Van Broeckhoven C. Mutation of *POLG* is associated with progressive external ophthalmoplegia characterized by mtDNA deletions. *Nat Genet.* 2001;28:211–212.

Vydt TC, de Coo RF, Soliman OI, et al. Cardiac involvement in adults with m.3243A>G MELAS gene mutation. *Am J Cardiol.* 2007;99(2):264–269.

Wallace DC, Singh G, Lott MT, et al. Mitochondrial DNA mutation associated with Leber's hereditary optic neuropathy. *Science.* 1988;242(4884):1427–1430.

Zeviani M, Gellera C, Antozzi C, et al. Maternally inherited myopathy and cardiomyopathy: association with mutation in mitochondrial DNA tRNA $^{Leu(UUR)}$. *Lancet.* 1991;338:143–147.

32

Inherited Cardiac Tumors

Mark D Davies

Introduction

Cardiac tumors are benign or malignant neoplasms of the structures of the heart (pericardium, epicardium, myocardium, endocardium, proximal great vessels, and coronary arteries). Primary tumors of the heart are uncommon with an incidence of approximately 0.1%–0.3% in series of unselected postmortem examinations (Lam et al. 1993; Reynen 1996; Roberts 1997). Frequency and type of primary cardiac tumors vary between children and adults. In children, 90% of primary cardiac tumors are benign with rhabdomyoma being the most common type, followed by teratoma, fibroma, and hemangioma. In adults, approximately 75% of primary cardiac tumors are benign with myxomas accounting for about half of these. In adults and children, the primary malignant tumors of the heart are mainly sarcomas (95%) with a much small proportion being lymphomas and other histological types. A pathological classification of cardiac tumors is given in Table 32–1.

The exact incidence of metastatic disease involving the heart is unknown but is considered to be far more common than primary tumors of the heart. In series of 18,751 unselected autopsies, metastatic disease was found in the heart in 622/18,751 (3.3%), which compares with at least one cancer being found in 7,289 (39%) cases (Bussani et al. 2007). The tumor type with the highest rate of heart metastasis was pleural mesothelioma (48.4%) followed by melanoma (27.8%) and lung adenocarcinoma (21%) with the pericardium being the most common site of cardiac metastasis.

Cardiac tumors present with a variety of signs and symptoms, including those related to mechanical obstruction, arrhythmia, embolism (pulmonary or systemic), and systemic symptoms such as fever or fatigue, thought to be due to tumor production of cytokines and other inflammatory mediators (Butany et al. 2005). The presenting symptom is often related more to the site, size, and mobility of the lesion rather than its pathological nature. Echocardiography is generally the imaging modality of first choice, providing both anatomical and functional information but useful additional information can be provided by cardiac magnetic resonance imaging (MRI) or computed tomography (CT) scans. Surgical resection is generally the treatment of choice except for chemosensitive tumors such as lymphomas.

This chapter will focus on primary cardiac tumors for which a predisposition is inherited in a clear Mendelian manner as a component of a broader tumor predisposition syndrome. These include rhabdomyomas as a component of tuberous sclerosis complex (TSC), myxomas in association with Carney complex, and fibromas in association with nevoid basal cell carcinoma syndrome (NBCCS). Causative genes for these conditions have been identified and this allows molecular genetic testing to be performed, either as a confirmatory diagnostic test, or as a predictive test for asymptomatic adult family members, although this generally requires the pathogenic mutation within a family to be identified, or in prenatal or preimplantation genetic diagnosis, again usually if the familial pathogenic mutation has been identified.

Cardiac Rhabdomyoma

Cardiac rhabdomyomas are the most common primary cardiac tumors during fetal life and childhood, accounting for 60% of such lesions (Beghetti et al. 1997; Uzun et al. 2007). They are benign lesions that predominantly affect the ventricular myocardium but can also occur in the atrial wall and are often multiple. Macroscopically, rhabdomyomas appear uniform, solid, and round with a higher sheen than the surrounding myocardium. Microscopically they consist of abnormal glycogen-filled myocytes. Following routine histological processing loss of the glycogen results in a highly characteristic appearance termed "spider cell," with a radial arrangement of cytoplasm extending from the nucleus (Fenoglio et al. 1976; Grebenc et al. 2000).

They can occur during fetal life, typically appearing between 22 and 28 weeks gestational age and thus can be detected on fetal anomaly scans. Postnatal echocardiography typically shows bright intramural masses with luminal extensions (Figure 32–1). Cardiac rhabdomyomas can cause cardiac arrhythmias, most commonly supraventricular tachycardias. They may extend into a cardiac chamber blocking the outflow tracts or interfere with valve function, leading to cardiac failure or diffusely infiltrate the myocardium, resulting in a dilated cardiomyopathy. Cardiac rhabdomyomas tend to regress with age and complete resolution of greater than 80% of tumors may occur during early childhood

Table 32–1 Classification of Cardiac Tumors

Benign
Myxoma
Rhabdomyoma
Fibroma
Hemangioma
Atrioventricular nodal
Granular cell
Lipoma
Paraganglioma
Mycocytic hamartoma
Histiocytoid cardiomyopathy
Inflammatory pseudotumor
Fibrous histiocytoma
Epitheloid hemangioenothelioma
Bronchogenic cyst
Teratoma
Malignant—Primary
Angiosarcoma
Undifferentiated pleomorphic sarcoma
Osteosarcoma
Leiomyosarcoma
Fibrosarcoma
Myxosarcoma
Rhabdomyosarcoma
Synovial sarcoma
Liposarcoma
Lymphoma
Pericardial mesothelioma

Source: Modified from Roberts WC. Primary and secondary neoplasms of the heart. *Am J Cardiol*. 1997;80(5):671–682.

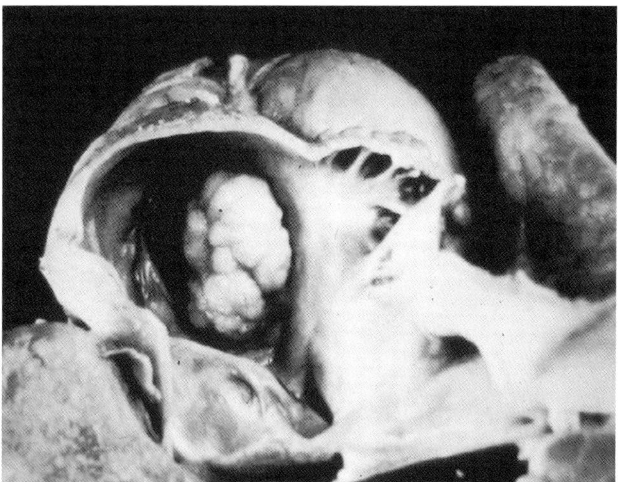

Figure 32–1 Cardiac rhabdomyomas. Cardiac rhabdomyoma as a solitary large irregular mass in the left ventricle detected at postmortem examination. Courtesy of Prof. Julian Sampson, Institute of Medical Genetics, Cardiff University, Cardiff, U.K.

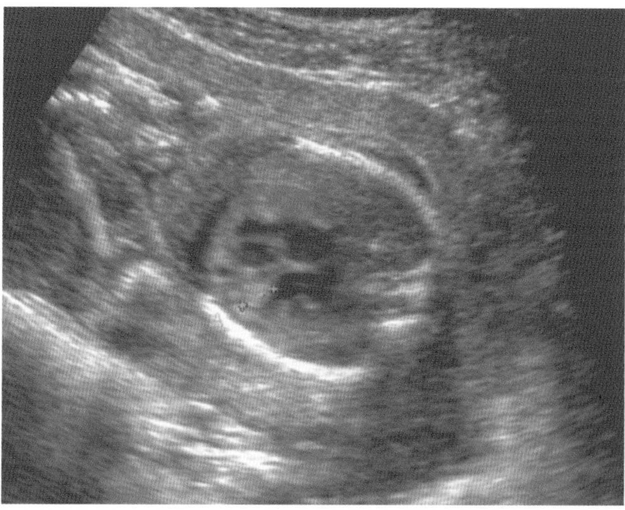

Figure 32–2 Abnormal fetal ultrasound at 19 weeks, 4 days gestation showing a single cardiac rhabdomyoma visible as a single 6.3 mm mass in the left ventricle of the fetal heart (tumor mass lies between the two cross marks). The mother affected with tuberous sclerosis and had a previously affected child. Courtesy of Dr. Susan Morris, Consultant Radiologist, University Hospital of Wales, Cardiff, U.K.

but they can regrow or appear during puberty (Bosi et al. 1996; Jóźwiak et al. 2006).

Surgical intervention may be necessary, particularly when critical valvular obstruction occurs or when medical management fails to control arrhythmias. However, due to their high rate of spontaneous regression these tumors can usually be managed conservatively.

Cardiac rhabdomyomas may be the first manifestation of TSC (OMIM 191100), an autosomal dominant condition that affects approximately 1 in 6,000 individuals (Crino et al. 2006). TSC is characterized by the development of benign tumors in a number of organs, including the brain skin, eye, kidney, and heart. Cardiac rhabdomyomas are observed in about 60% of TS patients less than 2 years old (Jóźwiak et al. 2006). In a case series of 94 patients, the frequency of TSC in patients diagnosed with a single cardiac rhabdomyoma in the fetal or neonatal period was 35%, and in patients diagnosed with multiple tumors the frequency was 95% (Tworetzky et al. 2003). Because of their frequent association with TSC the identification of cardiac rhabdomyoma necessitates a thorough search for other signs of TSC, both in the affected individual and in first-degree relatives. Prenatal genetic testing is possible following the detection of a cardiac rhabdomyoma in a fetus. Amniocentesis allows collection of fetal DNA. If no familial mutation is already known then a genetic testing laboratory may be able to perform a rapid mutation screen that might yield a diagnostic result if a mutation is found, which is known or can be predicted to be pathogenic. Amniocentesis carries a risk of miscarriage and this risk might only be justified if termination of pregnancy would be considered if a pathogenic mutation was found.

The diagnosis of TSC is usually based on clinical and radiological features, using the criteria shown in Table 32–2 (Roach and Sparagana 2004). These are divided into major and minor criteria. As many of the lesions associated with TSC can occur as sporadic lesions the presence of one major feature suggests TSC but is not enough to establish the diagnosis. The minor features are even less

Table 32–2 Diagnostic Criteria for TSC

Definite TSC: Two major features or one major feature plus two minor features

Probable TSC: One major feature plus one minor feature

Possible TSC: One major feature or two or more minor features

Major Features

- Facial angiofibromas or forehead plaque
- Nontraumatic ungual or periungual fibromas
- Hypomelanotic macules (three or more)
- Shagreen patch (connective tissue nevus)
- Multiple retinal nodular hamartomas
- Cortical tuber [1]
- Subependymal nodule
- Subependymal giant cell astrocytoma
- Cardiac rhabdomyoma, single or multiple
- Lymphangiomyomatosis [2]
- Renal angiomyolipoma [2]

Minor Features

- Multiple randomly distributed pits in dental enamel
- Hamartomatous rectal polyps
- Bone cysts
- Cerebral white matter radial migration lines [1]
- Gingival fibromas
- Nonrenal hamartoma
- Retinal achromic patch
- "Confetti" skin lesions
- Multiple renal cysts

Notes: (1) If the cerebral cortical dysplasia and cerebral white matter migration tracts occur together are counted they should be counted as one rather than two features of TSC. (2) When both lymphangiomyomatosis and renal angiomyolipomas are present, other features of TSC must be present before a definite diagnosis is made.
Source: Roach and Sparagana (2004).

specific and no single feature is diagnostic. Because of the variability in expression and the age dependence of some features making the diagnosis of TSC can be difficult.

The characteristic TSC central nervous system lesions are cortical tubers, subependymal nodules (SENs), subependymal giant cell astrocytomas (SEGAs), and white matter abnormalities. These structural abnormalities are likely to contribute the neurological manifestations of TSC, which include seizures, cognitive impairment, and behavioral abnormalities. The cutaneous lesions of TSC include hypomelanotic macules, facial angiofibromas, ungual fibromas, and shagreen patches. One or more of these skin lesions is present in over 90% of individuals with TSC, although none is pathognomonic (Roach et al. 1998). Renal features of TSC include angiomyolipomas (AMLs), simple cysts, polycystic kidney disease, and renal cell carcinoma. The commonest ophthalmologic manifestations of TSC are retinal hamartomas that seldom affect vision. Lymphangioleiomyomatosis (LAM) is a rare disorder of the lungs and lymphatics, which can occur sporadically or in association with TSC. It is characterized by proliferation of abnormal smooth muscle-like cells in the lungs leading to progressive cystic change, recurrent pneumothorax, and progressive respiratory failure.

In individuals suspected to have TSC the following initial assessments should be considered to establish the diagnosis and to identify complication amenable to treatment (Roach and Sparagana 2004):

- Medical history and three-generational family history.
- Clinical examination, including fundoscopy and skin examination under UV light.
- Cranial imaging, for example, MRI.
- Renal ultrasound.
- Electrocardiography in infants.
- Electroencephalography, if seizures are present.
- Neurodevelopmental and behavioral evaluation.
- Chest CT and spirometry for adult females, in the presence of respiratory symptoms.

After initial evaluation the following surveillance has been suggested in TSC patients:

- Renal ultrasonography every 2–3 years, replaced with renal MRI if multiple or large angiomyolipomas are present.
- Cranial MRI every 1–3 years for children and adolescents.
- Electroencephalography, if seizures are problematic.
- Neurological, developmental, and behavioral evaluations.
- Echocardiography, if cardiac symptoms indicate.
- Chest CT, if chest symptoms indicate.

However, the value of performing "routine" cranial and renal imaging in the absence of symptoms or pathology is debatable. An alternative approach is a focused clinical evaluation at regular intervals (e.g., annually) with a focus on neurological, renal, skin, pulmonary, cardiac, developmental, and psychological problems, with investigations directed accordingly, for example, urgent cranial imaging if signs/symptoms suggest raised intracranial pressure.

Molecular Genetics of TSC

TSC is caused by inactivating mutations in either *TSC1* at 9q34 or *TSC 2* at 16p13.3. *TSC1* encodes the protein, hamartin, and *TSC2* the protein, tuberin, which interact to form a functional complex. *TSC2* acts as a GTPase activating protein (GAP) for Rheb (RAS homolog expressed in brain) (Huang and Manning 2008). Like other members of the RAS family, Rheb cycles between an active GTP-bound state and an inactive GTP-bound state. *TSC2* promotes the conversion of Rheb-GTP to Rheb-GDP. Rheb is a key upstream activator of mTORC1, a central component of an intracellular signaling pathway, which integrates growth factor stimulation and cellular environmental cues, such as oxygen and nutrient levels, into the control of fundamental cellular processes such as growth and proliferation (Yang and Guan 2007). Loss of functional hamartin/tuberin complex results in Rheb being maintained in an active form, constitutive activation of mTORC1 and tumor formation.

Consistent with Knudson's two-hit tumor suppressor model, mutation of both alleles of either *TSC1* or *TSC2* appears to be necessary for the formation of most TSC-related tumors although haploinsufficiency probably plays a role in other features of this condition such as the neuronal migration defects (Jozwiak et al. 2008). Loss of heterozygosity (LOH) for *TSC1* or *TSC2* has been consistently observed in the majority of TSC-associated lesions such as subependymal giant cell astrocytomas, angiomyolipomas, and LAM tissue but only in approximately a quarter of TSC cardiac rhabdomyomas (Carbonara et al. 1996; Henske et al. 1996; Sepp et al. 1996; Niida et al. 2001) suggesting other mechanisms may play a role such as phosphorylation and inactivation of *TSC2* by Erk (Jóźwiak et al. 2007; Ma et al. 2007).

Genetic Counseling

TSC is an autosomal dominant condition. Two-thirds of cases arise as new mutations. The condition is fully penetrant but exhibits great variability in clinical features both among and within families. Therefore, the results from molecular genetic testing cannot be used to predict the phenotype. However, sporadic *TSC2* mutations appear to be associated with a more severe phenotype than *TSC1* mutations (Dabora et al. 2001). If one parent is affected the risk for each future child of inheriting TSC is 50%. The parents and siblings of an apparently sporadic case can undergo molecular genetic testing if the disease-causing mutation has been identified. If this is not possible they can be evaluated by

- three-generational family tree;
- skin examination, including the use of a Wood's lamp;
- ophthalmological assessment;
- possible cranial MRI or renal ultrasound.

Even in parents who are clinically unaffected or in whom the pathogenic mutation is not detectable in DNA extracted from leucocytes, there is an approximate 2% risk of recurrence due to the possibility of germline mosaicism.

Cardiac Fibroma

Cardiac fibroma (CF) is the second most common primary cardiac tumor in the general pediatric population, one-third of whom are under 1 year of age at the time of presentation (Burke et al. 1994). However, approximately 15% of CFs occur in adolescents and adults; CFs usually occur as solitary tumors in the interventricular septum or left ventricular free wall and macroscopically appear to be solitary, firm, well-circumscribed lesions. Microscopically, the tumors are composed of spindled cells with variable amounts of collagenized stroma, occasional foci of calcification, and interdigitation of the tumor cells with the normal myocardium (Burke and Virmani 1993). On echocardiography the lesions appear as well-demarcated masses (Grebenc et al. 2000). As with other benign cardiac tumors the fibromas may be assymptomatic or cause symptoms related to mechanical obstruction and arrhythmia.

CFs are thought to be part of the tumor spectrum associated with nevoid basal cell carcinoma syndrome [NBCCS or Gorlin syndrome, OMIM 109400] (Evans et al. 1993; Kimonis et al. 1997, 2004; Gorlin 2004)]. The main features of NBCCS are multiple jaw keratocysts (in approximately 90% of affected individuals, with a peak occurrence in the teenage years), multiple and/or early onset basal cell carcinomas (BCCs), palmer/plantar pits, and a wide range of skeleton abnormalities including rib and vertebral abnormalities and polydactyly. Many affected individuals have a recognizable facial appearance with macrocephaly, bossing of the forehead, a broad nasal root, and mild hypertelorism. Approximately 5% of patients with NBCCS develop medulloblastoma during childhood, typically by 3 years of age. In a study of 105 patients with NBCCS (Evans et al. 1993) cardiac fibromas occurred in 2%, compared to an incidence of less than 0.02% in a cohort of 27,640 children evaluated for cardiac disease by echocardiography (Beghetti et al. 1997). Ovarian fibromas occurred in approximately 25% of affected women. In the same study, eye abnormalities occurred in 26% of patients leading the authors to suggest that eye anomalies (e.g., cataracts, coloboma, microphthalmia) should be included in diagnostic criteria for NBCCS.

Suggested diagnostic criteria for NBCCS are given in Table 32–3 (Kimonis et al. 2004). Examination of the skin, measurement of head circumference, and radiological investigations are useful in establishing the diagnosis of NBCCS in either the putative proband, for example, a child with a cardiac fibroma, or potentially affected relatives. Radiological investigations that could be considered are radiographs of the skull, jaw, chest and ribs, spine, hand and feet, and an ultrasound of pelvis in females. Often imaging allows the diagnosis to be made in children and young adults before the onset of jaw cysts and BCCs. Other investigations that could be performed to either make the diagnosis, to determine the extent of the disease, or to establish baselines to allow future comparisons are

- dental evaluation;
- ophthalmic evaluation;
- echocardiogram in the first year of life.

A number of surveillance strategies have been suggested for patients with or at risk of NBCCS (Evans et al. 1993; Kimonis et al. 1997). In childhood it has been recommended to monitor head circumference and perform regular (e.g., 6 monthly) neurological examinations and developmental assessments in the first few years of life because of the risk of medulloblastoma. Annual brain MRI may be justified up until the age of 7 years. An echocardiogram should be performed soon after birth and repeated if symptoms suggestive of a cardiac fibroma develop. Jaw X-rays have been recommended every 12–18 months in individuals older then 8 years. From puberty, the skin should be examined at least annually by a dermatologist.

Table 32–3 Diagnostic Criteria for NBCCS

NBCCS is diagnosed in individuals with two major diagnostic criteria and one minor diagnostic criterion or one major and two minor diagnostic criteria
Major criteria:
More than two BCCs or one under the age of 20 years
Odontogenic keratocysts of the jaw
Three or more palmar or plantar pits
Lamellar calcification of the falx cerebri
Rib abnormalities
Ovarian fibroma
Medulloblastoma
Flame-shaped lucencies of all phalanges
Brachymetacarpaly in all four limbs
First-degree relative with NBCCS
Minor criteria:
Spina bifida occulta or other vertebral anomalies
Brachymetacarpaly in at least one limb, bossing, "coarse face," moderate or severe hypertelorism
Hypertelorism or telecanthus
Frontal bossing

Source: Kimonis et al. (2004).

Molecular Genetics of NBCCS

The only gene known to be associated with NBCCS is *PTCH1*, a human homolog of the Drosophila segment polarity gene patched (Hahn et al. 1996; Johnson et al. 1996). This encodes for a transmembrane receptor, which is part of the Hedgehog (Hh) signaling pathway (King et al. 2008). The hedgehog signaling pathway plays a role during the development and maintenance of tissues, regulating processes such as cell polarity, differentiation, proliferation, and the maintenance of stem cells. Binding of the Hh ligand to *PTCH1* leads to derepression of smoothened (Smo), a transmembrane protein of the G-protein-coupled receptor family 1 and activation of a signaling cascade that leads, via the Gli family of zinc finger transcription factors, to altered Hh target gene expression.

In NBCCS haploinsufficiency for *PTCH1* is thought to underlie the congenital abnormalities (Ohba et al. 2008) whilst tumor development is thought to reflect loss of residual *PTCH1* function by an acquired second hit (Cowan et al. 1997). Upregulation of Hh signaling has also been found in many sporadic cancers including BCCS (Gailani et al. 1996) and tumors of the brain (Berman et al. 2002), prostate (Karhadkar et al. 2004), ovary (Chen et al. 2007), digestive tract (Berman et al. 2003), and lung (Watkins et al. 2003). Missense mutations in PTCH have been reported in patients with holoprosencephaly, a structural abnormality of the brain. It has been suggested that these mutations result in enhanced repression of the Hh signaling pathway, the converse situation to that found in NBCCS (Ming et al. 2002).

Genetic Counseling

NBCCS is inherited in an autosomal dominant manner, with approximately 20%–30% of probands having a de novo mutation. The condition appears to be completely penetrant. There have been no published phenotype–genotype correlations to date. Identification of a disease causing mutation in the proband allows molecular genetic testing of other family members. If no such mutation has been identified family members can be evaluated by skin examination and X-rays of the skull, jaw, and spine.

Cardiac Myxomas and Carney Complex

Cardiac myxomas are the commonest primary heart tumor in adults, accounting for nearly half of all primary cardiac tumors in this age group but are rarer in children. Cardiac myxomas are benign lesions, thought to arise from multipotential subendocardial mesenychymal cells, that can differentiate within myxomas along a variety of lineages (Ferrans and Roberts 1973; Burke and Virmani 1993). Macroscopically, they are polypoid, often pedunculated masses with a smooth or gently lobulated surface. Microscopically, they are characterized by of a bland myxoid proteoglycan stroma within which stellate cells are scattered, either singly or in small clusters. There may be evidence of multiple cell lineages including foci of extramedullary hemopoesis bone and areas with glandular epithelial-like structures.

Embolism occurs in up to 40% of patients with myxomas (Reynen 1995). Symptoms can arise from mechanical obstruction and systemic complaints such as fever, weight loss, myalgia, and arthralgia occur, thought to be due to secretion of cytokines such as interleukin-6 (Amano et al. 2003). The commonest laboratory findings are anemia, leucocytosis, and raised erythrocyte sedimentation rate (ESR). Nonspecific electrocardiogram abnormalities occur in 20%–40% of patients and include atrial fibrillation or flutter and left and right bundle branch block. On echocardiography cardiac myxomas typically appear as a mobile mass, attached to the endocardial surface by a stalk. Treatment is by surgical resection.

At least 7% cardiac myxomas occur in the context of Carney complex (CNC;OMIM 160980) (Reynen 1995). This is a rare (around 500 known cases) inherited tumor predisposition syndrome, characterized by skin pigmentary abnormalities, cardiac and extra cardiac myxomas, nonmyxomatous extracardiac tumors (pituitary adenomas, psammomatous melanotic schwannomas, Sertoli cell tumors, and breast fibroadenomas), and endocrinopathy. CNC was originally described in 1985 (Carney et al. 1985) and subsequently it has been recognized that patients previously described as having either NAME (nevi, atrial myxomas, myxoid neurofibroma, and ephelides) or LAMB (lentigines, atrial myxoma, mucocutaneous myxoma, and blue nevi) would be more appropriately described by CNC.

Histologically, CNC-related and sporadic cardiac myxomas appear identical but there are differences in clinical behavior. Sporadic myxomas are most frequent between the third and sixth decade of life, occur predominantly in women, and are generally single lesions of left atrial aspect of the interatrial septum, which do not recur after surgical excision. CNC-related cardiac myxomas show no age or gender preference apart from being rare before puberty, and whilst still most likely to occur on the left atrial aspect of the atrial septum, more than a third of tumors occur at other locations within the heart, can be single or multiple, and can recur despite adequate surgical resection, at sites close to or distant from the initial tumor location.

Current diagnostic criteria are based on clinical features supported by histological, biochemical, or radiological findings and are given in Table 32–4 (Stratakis et al. 2001). CNC is considered to be completely penetrant but its manifestations are very variable and have age-related penetrance. There are a number of skin manifestations, the most common of which are lentigines that appear as small brown to black macules and ephelides (freckles), located around the lips, eyelids, conjunctiva ears, and genital area giving rise to an spotty skin pigmentation. Additional pigmented lesions that occur include blue nevi, combined nevi, café-au-lait spots, and depigmented lesions. Cutaneous myxomas in CNC can occur anywhere but most commonly affect the eyelid, external ear canal, breast, and nipples. Myxomas can also be found in the oropharynx and female genitalia.

The commonest endocrine problem in CNC is ACTH-independent Cushing's syndrome due to primary pigmented nodular adrenal disease (PPNAD). This occurs in approximately 25% of CNC patients. PPNAD is so-called because of the macroscopic appearance of the affected adrenals with small (<1 cm) cortisol-secreting pigmented micronodules being found in the adrenal cortex. The hypercortisolism of PPNAD is often insidious in onset evidence with most individuals presenting in the second or third decade, although rarely it can manifest in the first 2–3 years.

Clinically apparent acromegaly due to a pituitary growth hormone-secreting adenoma occurs in about 10% of adults with CNC. Large-cell calcifying Sertoli cell tumors (LCCSCT) are present in most postpubertal males with CNC. The tumors are often multicentric and bilateral, may be hormone secreting, and can affect fertility. The thyroid gland is commonly affected in CNC patients with up to 75% having nonmultiple nonfunctioning thyroid nodules or cysts, of whom around 10% may go on to develop thyroid cancer.

Psammomatous melanotic schwannoma (PMS) is a tumor that occurs very rarely outside the context of CNC. PMS can

Table 32–4 Diagnostic Criteria for CNC

The diagnosis of CNC is made if two or more of the disease manifestations listed below are present or if one disease manifestation is present and one of the supplemental criteria is met.
Spotty skin pigmentation with a typical distribution (lips, conjunctiva and inner or outer canthi of the ear, vaginal and penile mucosa
Blue nevus, epithelioid blue nevus
Cutaneous and mucosal myxoma
Cardiac myxoma.
Breast myxomatosis (including in fat-suppressed MRI of the breast suggestive of this diagnosis, in the absence of a biopsy)
Primary pigmented nodular adrenocortical disease (PPNAD) **or** evidence of adenocortical overactivity demonstrated by a paradoxical positive response of urinary glucocorticosteroids to dexamethasone administration during Liddle's test
Acromegaly due to a growth hormone (GH)-producing pituitary adenoma
Large-cell calcifying Sertoli cell tumor (LCCSCT) or the associated characteristic microcalcification on testicular ultrasonography
Psammomatous melanotic schwannoma (PMS)
Breast ductal adenoma (multiple)
Osteochondromyxoma of bone
Thyroid adenoma or carcinoma **or** multiple, hypoechoic nodules on thyroid ultrasonography
Supplemental criteria
Affected first-degree relative
Inactivating mutation of the *PRKAR1A* gene

Source: Stratakis et al. (2001).

occur anywhere in the central or peripheral nervous system but is most frequently found in the paraspinal parasympathetic chain or the gastrointestinal tract. It is a pigmented tumor due to melanin accumulation, is often multicentric, and rarely can metastasize. Other tumors that have been suggested to occur at an increased frequency in CNC include breast adenomas and osteochondromyxomas.

The clinical diagnosis of CNC can be challenging. The diagnosis may be suggested in a patient with cardiac myxoma if there is a family history of cardiac myxoma, a past medical history of cardiac, extracardiac myxomas, or other unusual tumors (PMS or LCCSCT), endocrinopathy, or spotty pigmentation of the skin.

The following investigations may be useful in making the initial diagnosis of CNC or in establishing the extent of organ involvement:

- Imaging or biochemical screening for endocrine tumors
- Thyroid ultrasound
- Testicular ultrasound in males
- Pelvic ultrasound in females.

Expert opinion recommends that patients with CNC or a genetic predisposition to CNC should have regular screening for manifestations of the disease.

In prepubertal children cardiac echocardiography is recommended in the first 6 months of life and annually thereafter. Growth rate and pubertal status should be monitored, particularly in those with evidence of LCCSCT.

For postpubertal children and adults the following is recommended: annual echocardiogram, annual measurement of urinary free cortisol concentration, and plasma IGF-1. Annual testicular ultrasound is recommended for those with evidence of LCCTS (including testicular microcalicification). Other imaging biochemical investigations may be required according to the developing clinical picture.

Molecular Genetics of CNC

Linkage analysis of CNC families suggested potential loci at 2p16 and 17q24. No causative gene has yet been identified at 2p16 but positional cloning studies of 17q24 locus identified pathogenic mutations in the *PRKAR1A* gene encoding the RIα regulatory subunit of cAMP-dependent protein kinase (also known as PKA) (Kirschner et al. 2000a).

PKA is a key mediator of cAMP signaling and is involved in the regulation of multiple cellular processes including transcription, metabolism, cell cycle progression, and apoptosis. PKA is a tetrameric holoenzyme composed of two regulatory (R) subunits and two catalytic (C) subunits (Taylor et al. 2008). The R subunits bound within the PKA complex inhibit the C subunits. Binding of CAMP to the R units causes them to dissociate freeing the active C units. The C units are serine-threonine kinases, which phosphorylate a wide range of substrate proteins (Sands and Palmer 2008).

Discrete genes encode four different R subunits (*PRKAR1A*, *PRKAR1B*, *PRKAR2A*, and *PRKAR2B*, which encode R1α, R1β, RIIα, and RIIβ proteins, respectively) and three C subunits (*PRKCA*, *PRKCB*, and *PRKCC*, which encode Cα, Cβ, and Cγ proteins respectively). The relative level of expression of the R subunits varies depending on cell type and developmental stage.

In a series of 51 unrelated CNC patients 65% had *PRKAR1A* mutations (Veugelers et al. 2004b). Most of the mutations identified in CNC patients have been nonsense, frame-shift, or spice site, which would be expected to produce mRNA transcripts that would be subject to nonsense-mediated decay (Kirschner et al. 2000b).

The mechanism of *PRKAR1A*-mediated tumorigenesis in CNC is unclear but potentially involves constitutively increased PKA activity due to failure of inhibition of the C subunits or increased cAMP-induced PKA activity, mediated by compensatory increases in levels of other types of R subunits (Robinson-White et al. 2006).

Some but not all types of tumors isolated from patients with CNC exhibit LOH at the *PRKAR1A* locus (Casey et al. 2000; Kirschner et al. 2000a; Bossis et al. 2004; Stratakis et al. 2004; Tsilou et al. 2004) and some data suggest that haploinsufficiency may be sufficient for the development, at least some, of the lesions seen in Carney complex, including cardiac myxomas (Amieux et al. 1997; Griffin et al. 2004; Kirschner et al. 2005).

Mutations in *PRKAR1A* have also been associated with sporadic PPNAD (Groussin et al. 2002), thyroid carcinomas (Sandrini et al. 2002), adrenocortical tumors (Bertherat et al. 2003), and ondontogenic myxomas (Perdigao et al. 2005).

It is likely that CNC is a genetically heterogeneous disease and other disease-causing genes remain to be identified. A family has been described by Veugelers et al. in which typical CNC features cosegregated with trismus-pseudocamptodactyly, a distal arthrogryposis (DA) characterized by an inability to open the mouth fully (trismus) and pseudocamptodactyly in which wrist dorsiflexion produces flexion contracture of the interphalangeal joints (Veugelers et al. 2004a). Affected individuals in this family had no detectable *PRKAR1A* mutations and there was no evidence of linkage to chromosome 17q24.1 or 2p but rather to 17p12–13.1.

A candidate gene strategy identified a missense mutation in *MYH8*, which encodes the perinatal isoform myosin heavy chain (Veugelers et al. 2004a). This mutation had been found in other patients with trismus-pseudocamptodactyly who did not exhibit other features of CNC and their segregation in the pedigree of Veugelers et al. may be coincidental (Toydemir et al. 2006).

Genetic Counseling

CNC is autosomally dominantly inherited, with approximately 30% of patients having a de novo mutation. No genotype–phenotype correlations have been observed for most identified *PRKAR1A* mutations. However, one of the commonest mutations, a small intron 6 deletion that is thought to interfere with splicing is associated with PPNAD but not other features of CNC in most affected individuals (Groussin et al. 2006). If a disease-causing mutation has been identified in a proband, then predictive molecular genetic testing can be offered to potentially at-risk relatives. If a disease-causing mutation hasn't been identified then these relatives can be assessed by taking a medical and family history, performing a physical examination with focus on the skin and on signs of endocrine disease. Imaging and/or biochemical screening can also be considered.

Conclusion

The majority of primary cardiac tumors are sporadic but a number of them occur in patients as part of a broader tumor predisposition syndrome. Identification of such patients allows appropriate management of associated complications and the ascertainment of other affected relatives. An understanding of the genetic pathology of these conditions has enabled molecular testing to be used in either a diagnostic, predictive, or prenatal setting. This understanding has also afforded new therapeutic opportunities in the use of drugs to target aberrant intracellular signaling pathways. For example, sirolimus, a mTORC1 inhibitor, has recently been evaluated in clinical trials as a treatment for renal tumors in patients with TSC and has been shown to reduce the size of these lesions, albeit with low grade side effects (Bissler et al. 2008; Davies et al. 2008). Further refinement of such molecularly targeted approaches may have a significant impact on the morbidity and mortality of tumor predisposition syndromes.

References

Amano J, Kono T, Wada Y, et al. Cardiac myxoma: its origin and tumor characteristics. *Ann Thorac Cardiovasc Surg.* 2003;9(4):215–221.

Amieux PS, Cummings DE, Motamed K, et al. Compensatory regulation of RIalpha protein levels in protein kinase A mutant mice. *J Biol Chem.* 1997;272(7):3993–3998.

Beghetti M, Gow RM, Haney I, Mawson J, Williams WG, Freedom RM. Pediatric primary benign cardiac tumors: a 15-year review. *Am Heart J.* 1997;134(6):1107–1114.

Berman DM, Karhadkar SS, Hallahan AR, et al. Medulloblastoma growth inhibition by hedgehog pathway blockade. *Science.* 2002;297(5586):1559–1561.

Berman DM, Karhadkar SS, Maitra A, et al. Widespread requirement for Hedgehog ligand stimulation in growth of digestive tract tumours. *Nature.* 2003;425(6960):846–851.

Bertherat J, Groussin L, Sandrini F, et al. Molecular and functional analysis of PRKAR1A and its locus (17q22–24) in sporadic adrenocortical tumors: 17q losses, somatic mutations, and protein kinase A expression and activity. *Cancer Res.* 2003;63(17):5308–5319.

Bissler JJ, McCormack FX, Young LR, et al. Sirolimus for angiomyolipoma in tuberous sclerosis complex or lymphangioleiomyomatosis. *N Engl J Med.* 2008;358(2):140–151.

Bosi G, Lintermans JP, Pellegrino PA, Svaluto-Moreolo G, Vliers A. The natural history of cardiac rhabdomyoma with and without tuberous sclerosis. *Acta Paediatr.* 1996;85(8):928–931.

Bossis I, Voutetakis A, Matyakhina L, et al. A pleiomorphic GH pituitary adenoma from a Carney complex patient displays universal allelic loss at the protein kinase A regulatory subunit 1A (PRKARIA) locus. *J Med Genet.* 2004;41(8):596–600.

Burke AP, Rosado-de-Christenson M, Templeton PA, Virmani R. Cardiac fibroma: clinicopathologic correlates and surgical treatment. *J Thorac Cardiovasc Surg.* 1994;108(5):862–870.

Burke AP, Virmani R. Cardiac myxoma. A clinicopathologic study. *Am J Clin Pathol.* 1993;100(6):671–680.

Bussani R, De-Giorgio F, Abbate A, Silvestri F. Cardiac metastases. *J Clin Pathol.* 2007;60(1):27–34.

Butany J, Nair V, Nassemudin A, Nair GM, Catton C, Yau T. et al. Cardiac tumours: diagnosis and management. *Lancet Oncol.* 2005;6(4):219–228.

Carbonara C, Longa L, Grosso E, et al. Apparent preferential loss of heterozygosity at TSC2 over TSC1 chromosomal region in tuberous sclerosis hamartomas. *Genes Chromosomes Cancer.* 1996;15(1):18–25.

Carney JA, Gordon H, Carpenter PC, Shenoy BV, Go VL. The complex of myxomas, spotty pigmentation, and endocrine overactivity. *Medicine (Baltimore).* 1985;64(4):270–283.

Casey M, Vaughan CJ, He J, et al. Mutations in the protein kinase A R1alpha regulatory subunit cause familial cardiac myxomas and Carney complex. *J Clin Invest.* 2000;106(5):R31–R38.

Chen X, Horiuchi A, Kikuchi N, et al. Hedgehog signal pathway is activated in ovarian carcinomas, correlating with cell proliferation: it's inhibition leads to growth suppression and apoptosis. *Cancer Sci.* 2007;98(1):68–76.

Cowan R, Hoban P, Kelsey A, Birch JM, Gattamaneni R, Evans DG. The gene for the naevoid basal cell carcinoma syndrome acts as a tumour-suppressor gene in medulloblastoma. *Br J Cancer.* 1997;76(2):141–145.

Crino PB, Nathanson KL, Henske EP. The tuberous sclerosis complex. *N Engl J Med.* 2006;355(13):1345–1356.

Dabora SL, Jozwiak S, Franz DN, et al. Mutational analysis in a cohort of 224 tuberous sclerosis patients indicates increased severity of TSC2, compared with TSC1, disease in multiple organs. *Am J Hum Genet.* 2001;68(1):64–80.

Davies DM, Johnson SR, Tattersfield AE, et al. Sirolimus therapy in tuberous sclerosis or sporadic lymphangioleiomyomatosis. *N Engl J Med.* 2008;358(2):200–203.

Evans DG, Ladusans EJ, Rimmer S, Burnell LD, Thakker N, Farndon PA. Complications of the naevoid basal cell carcinoma syndrome: results of a population based study. *J Med Genet.* 1993;30(6):460–464.

Fenoglio JJ Jr, McAllister HA Jr, Ferrans VJ. Cardiac rhabdomyoma: a clinicopathologic and electron microscopic study. *Am J Cardiol.* 1976;38(2):241–251.

Ferrans VJ, Roberts WC. Structural features of cardiac myxomas. Histology, histochemistry, and electron microscopy. *Hum Pathol.* 1973;4(1):111–146.

Gailani MR, Stahle-Backdahl M, Leffell DJ, et al. The role of the human homologue of Drosophila patched in sporadic basal cell carcinomas. *Nat Genet.* 1996;14(1):78–81.

Gorlin RJ. Nevoid basal cell carcinoma (Gorlin) syndrome. *Genet Med.* 2004;6(6):530–539.

Grebenc ML, Rosado de Christenson ML, Burke AP, Green CE, Galvin JR. Primary cardiac and pericardial neoplasms: radiologic-pathologic correlation. *Radiographics.* 2000;20(4):1073–1103; quiz 1110–1111, 1112.

Griffin KJ, Kirschner LS, Matyakhina L, et al. A transgenic mouse bearing an antisense construct of regulatory subunit type 1A of protein kinase A develops endocrine and other tumours: comparison with Carney complex and other PRKAR1A induced lesions. *J Med Genet.* 2004;41(12):923–931.

Groussin L, Horvath A, Jullian E, et al. A PRKAR1A mutation associated with primary pigmented nodular adrenocortical disease in 12 kindreds. *J Clin Endocrinol Metab.* 2006;91(5):1943–1949.

Groussin L, Kirschner LS, Vincent-Dejean C, et al. Molecular analysis of the cyclic AMP-dependent protein kinase A (PKA) regulatory subunit

1A (PRKAR1A) gene in patients with Carney complex and primary pigmented nodular adrenocortical disease (PPNAD) reveals novel mutations and clues for pathophysiology: augmented PKA signaling is associated with adrenal tumorigenesis in PPNAD. *Am J Hum Genet.* 2002;71(6):1433–1442.

Hahn H, Wicking C, Zaphiropoulous PG, et al. Mutations of the human homolog of Drosophila patched in the nevoid basal cell carcinoma syndrome. *Cell.* 1996;85(6):841–851.

Henske EP, Scheithauer BW, Short MP, et al. Allelic loss is frequent in tuberous sclerosis kidney lesions but rare in brain lesions. *Am J Hum Genet.* 1996;59(2):400–406.

Huang J, Manning BD. The TSC1-TSC2 complex: a molecular switchboard controlling cell growth. *Biochem J.* 2008;412(2):179–190.

Johnson RL, Rothman AL, Xie J, et al. Human homolog of patched, a candidate gene for the basal cell nevus syndrome. *Science.* 1996;272(5268):1668–1671.

Jozwiak J, Jozwiak S, Wlodarski P. Possible mechanisms of disease development in tuberous sclerosis. *Lancet Oncol.* 2008;9(1):73–79.

Jozwiak J, Sahin M, Jozwiak S, et al. Cardiac rhabdomyoma in tuberous sclerosis: hyperactive Erk signaling. *Int J Cardiol.* 2007;132(1):145–147.

Jóźwiak S, Kotulska K, Kasprzyk-Obara J, et al. Clinical and genotype studies of cardiac tumors in 154 patients with tuberous sclerosis complex. *Pediatrics.* 2006;118(4):e1146–e1151.

Karhadkar SS, Bova GS, Abdallah N, et al. Hedgehog signalling in prostate regeneration, neoplasia and metastasis. *Nature.* 2004;431(7009): 707–712.

Kimonis VE, Goldstein AM, Pastakia B, et al. Clinical manifestations in 105 persons with nevoid basal cell carcinoma syndrome. *Am J Med Genet.* 1997;69(3):299–308.

Kimonis VE, Mehta SG, Digiovanna JJ, Bale SJ, Pastakia B. Radiological features in 82 patients with nevoid basal cell carcinoma (NBCC or Gorlin) syndrome. *Genet Med.* 2004;6(6):495–502.

King P, Guasti L, Laufer E. Hedgehog signalling in endocrine development and disease. *J Endocrinol.* 2008;198(3):439–450.

Kirschner LS, Carney JA, Pack SD, et al. Mutations of the gene encoding the protein kinase A type I-alpha regulatory subunit in patients with the Carney complex. *Nat Genet.* 2000a;26(1):89–92.

Kirschner LS, Kusewitt DF, Matyakhina L, et al. A mouse model for the Carney complex tumor syndrome develops neoplasia in cyclic AMP-responsive tissues. *Cancer Res.* 2005;65(11):4506–4514.

Kirschner LS, Sandrini F, Monbo J, Lin JP, Carney JA, Stratakis CA. Genetic heterogeneity and spectrum of mutations of the PRKAR1A gene in patients with the carney complex. *Hum Mol Genet.* 2000b;9(20):3037–3046.

Lam KY, Dickens P, Chan AC. Tumors of the heart. A 20-year experience with a review of 12,485 consecutive autopsies. *Arch Pathol Lab Med.* 1993;117(10):1027–1031.

Ma L, Teruya-Feldstein J, Bonner P, et al. Identification of S664 TSC2 phosphorylation as a marker for extracellular signal-regulated kinase mediated mTOR activation in tuberous sclerosis and human cancer. *Cancer Res.* 2007;67(15):7106–7112.

Ming JE, Kaupas ME, Roessler E, et al. Mutations in PATCHED-1, the receptor for SONIC HEDGEHOG, are associated with holoprosencephaly. *Hum Genet.* 2002;110(4):297–301.

Niida Y, Stemmer-Rachamimov AO, Logrip M, et al. Survey of somatic mutations in tuberous sclerosis complex (TSC) hamartomas suggests different genetic mechanisms for pathogenesis of TSC lesions. *Am J Hum Genet.* 2001;69(3):493–503.

Ohba S, Kawaguchi H, Kugimiya F, et al. Patched1 haploinsufficiency increases adult bone mass and modulates Gli3 repressor activity. *Dev Cell.* 2008;14(5):689–699.

Perdigao PF, Stergiopoulos SG, De Marco L, et al. Molecular and immunohistochemical investigation of protein kinase a regulatory subunit type 1A (PRKAR1A) in odontogenic myxomas. *Genes Chromosomes Cancer.* 2005;44(2):204–211.

Reynen K. Cardiac myxomas. *N Engl J Med.* 1995;333(24):1610–1617.

Reynen K. Frequency of primary tumors of the heart. *Am J Cardiol.* 1996;77(1):107.

Roach ES, Gomez MR, Northrup H. Tuberous sclerosis complex consensus conference: revised clinical diagnostic criteria. *J Child Neurol.* 1998;13(12):624–628.

Roach ES, Sparagana SP. Diagnosis of tuberous sclerosis complex. *J Child Neurol.* 2004;19(9):643–649.

Roberts WC. Primary and secondary neoplasms of the heart. *Am J Cardiol.* 1997;80(5):671–682.

Robinson-White A, Meoli E, Stergiopoulos S, et al. PRKAR1A mutations and protein kinase A interactions with other signaling pathways in the adrenal cortex. *J Clin Endocrinol Metab.* 2006;91(6):2380–2388.

Sandrini F, Matyakhina L, Sarlis NJ, et al. Regulatory subunit type I-alpha of protein kinase A (PRKAR1A): a tumor-suppressor gene for sporadic thyroid cancer. *Genes Chromosomes Cancer.* 2002;35(2):182–192.

Sands WA, Palmer TM. Regulating gene transcription in response to cyclic AMP elevation. *Cell Signal.* 2008;20(3):460–466.

Sepp T, Yates JR, Green AJ. Loss of heterozygosity in tuberous sclerosis hamartomas. *J Med Genet.* 1996;33(11):962–964.

Stratakis CA, Kirschner LS, Carney JA. Clinical and molecular features of the Carney complex: diagnostic criteria and recommendations for patient evaluation. *J Clin Endocrinol Metab.* 2001;86(9):4041–4046.

Stratakis CA, Matyakhina L, Courkoutsakis N, et al. Pathology and molecular genetics of the pituitary gland in patients with the complex of spotty skin pigmentation, myxomas, endocrine overactivity and schwannomas (Carney complex). *Front Horm Res.* 2004;32:253–264.

Taylor SS, Kim C, Cheng CY, Brown SH, Wu J, Kannan N. Signaling through cAMP and cAMP-dependent protein kinase: diverse strategies for drug design. *Biochim Biophys Acta.* 2008;1784(1):16–26.

Toydemir RM, Chen H, Proud VK, et al. Trismus-pseudocamptodactyly syndrome is caused by recurrent mutation of MYH8. *Am J Med Genet A.* 2006;140(22):2387–2393.

Tsilou ET, Chan CC, Sandrini F, et al. Eyelid myxoma in Carney complex without PRKAR1A allelic loss. *Am J Med Genet A.* 2004;130(4):395–397.

Tworetzky W, McElhinney DB, Margossian R, et al. Association between cardiac tumors and tuberous sclerosis in the fetus and neonate. *Am J Cardiol.* 2003;92(4):487–489.

Uzun, O, DG. Wilson, Vujanic GM, Parsons JM, De Giovanni JV. Cardiac tumours in children. *Orphanet J Rare Dis.* 2007;2:11.

Veugelers M, Bressan M, McDermott DA, et al. Mutation of perinatal myosin heavy chain associated with a Carney complex variant. *N Engl J Med.* 2004a;351(5):460–469.

Veugelers M, Wilkes D, Burton K, et al. Comparative PRKAR1A genotype-phenotype analyses in humans with Carney complex and prkar1a haploinsufficient mice. *Proc Natl Acad Sci USA.* 2004b;101(39):14222–14227.

Watkins DN, Berman DM, Burkholder SG, Wang B, Beachy PA, Baylin SB. Hedgehog signalling within airway epithelial progenitors and in small-cell lung cancer. *Nature.* 2003;422(6929):313–317.

Yang Q, Guan KL. Expanding mTOR signaling. *Cell Res.* 2007; 17(8):666–681.

Part III

Management of Cardiovascular Genetic Diseases

33

The Sudden Arrhythmic Death Syndrome

Pier D Lambiase

Introduction

The diagnosis of the syndromes responsible for the sudden arrhythmic death syndrome (SADS) is a significant challenge as the phenotype of the condition may not be typical and the combined expertise of both electrophysiologists and cardiologists is often required to interpret the screening investigations. In this chapter, the clinical approach to an individual who presents with a family history of SADS or with a primary ventricular fibrillation (VF) arrest under the age of 35 years will be examined. Since the other chapters in this book (Chapters 15–19) have reviewed the genetics and clinical manifestations of these disorders, the role of pharmacological and genetic testing as it applies to screening of SADS families will form the focus of this chapter. This aspect of SADS is increasingly important as both the diagnostic power and clinical utility of pharmacological and genetic testing have improved over the past decade. It is also evident that specific mutations in ion channel genes and myocardial proteins substantially influence prognosis and inform clinical management. Therefore, the identification of disease-causing mutations has a number of advantages over clinical screening alone in determining the pathophysiologic basis of the sudden cardiac death (SCD) as well as directing family screening and therapy. This chapter will discuss the role of clinical and genetic screening in the context of routinely available cardiac investigatory facilities.

Definitions

SADS is defined according to the following criteria: (1) sudden unexplained death at age 1–35 years; (2) no cardiac history; (3) seen alive in the 12 hours before death; (4) normal coroner's autopsy and cardiac pathologist's confirmation of normal heart; and (5) a negative toxicological screen. In postmortem series, the proportion of sudden deaths in the context of a structurally normal heart ranges from 3% to 30% of all deaths depending upon the population studied and the expertise of the pathologist. In published series of SADS cases, family screening using a combination of clinical and genetic assessments identifies an electrical (ion channel related) cause of death in up to 35% (Tan et al. 2005; Tester and Ackerman 2006; Behr et al. 2008).

Clinical Evaluation of SADS Families

The Structure of a SADS Clinic

Figure 33–1 illustrates the sequence of screening processes required in the evaluation of the first-degree relatives of a SADS index case. SADS clinics should be staffed by multidisciplinary teams, capable of providing bereavement and genetic counseling as well as the technical expertise to perform and interpret specific screening investigations. There is no single model for such a team, but the range of staff should include,

1. Bereavement and genetics counselors.
2. Cardiac physiologists to perform resting and exercise ECGs and pharmacologic challenge tests.
3. Echocardiographers trained in contrast echocardiography and tissue Doppler imaging.
4. Arrhythmia nurses.
5. Cardiologists with a specific interest in ion channel disease and arrhythmias—this may encompass individuals with interventional electrophysiological experience and physicians with expertise in the diagnosis and management of inherited cardiac disease.
6. Clinical geneticists.

A considerable amount of preliminary information must be gathered before physically seeing the affected family. Specifically, a detailed postmortem report should be obtained together with clinical information about the index case in life (e.g., an ECG). Whenever possible, tissue sections or preferably the whole heart should be reviewed by an expert cardiac pathologist to look for myocyte disarray suggestive of hypertrophic cardiomyopathy (HCM), fibrosis, and fatty infiltration suggesting arrhythmogenic right ventricular cardiomyopathy (ARVC). Cardiac tissue can also be a valuable source of DNA for subsequent candidate mutation screening, although lymphocytes from the spleen are a more suitable source of DNA.

It is extremely important that the affected family is counseled on the likely implications of clinical and genetic screening tests as a diagnosis may have important consequences for their employment, insurance, psychological health, children, and other close relatives. Outcomes of the initial investigations vary from

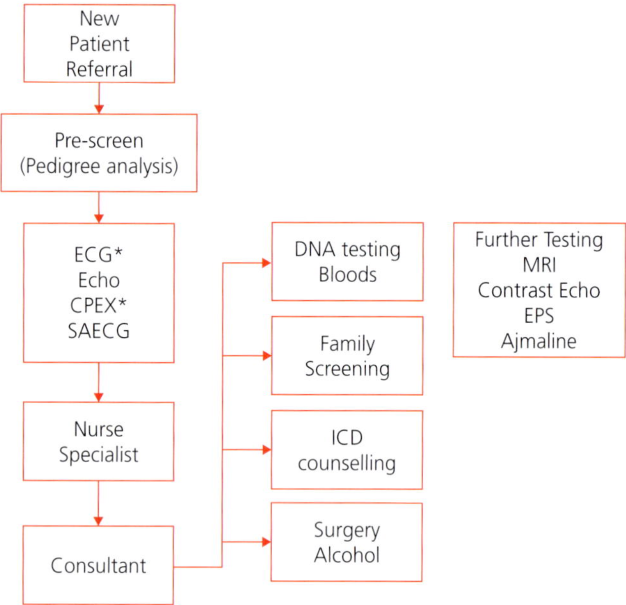

Figure 33–1 Sequence of processes involved in the family screening of a SADS victim. Initial information gathering is followed by preliminary investigations of the family members and subsequent more detailed investigation and treatment based upon the initial findings. "Alcohol" refers to alcohol septal ablation in HCM patients.

Box 33–1 Clinical Details

History
The SADS victim
Mode of death: syncope, sleep, exercise related
Prior medical history
Previous accidents, for example, RTA or syncopal episodes
Prescribed or nonprescribed medications, for example, LQT prolonging drugs
Recreational drug use, for example, cocaine, amphetamines (CPVT, LQT)
Family History
Epilepsy, Cot death
Details of relatives who died under 40 years of age
Available death certification
FHx heart failure or pacemaker implantation, for example, lamin A/C mutations

Box 33–2 Common Causes of SADS

Ion channelopathies
Long QT syndrome
Brugada syndrome
Catecholaminergic polymorphic VT (CPVT)
Lev-Lenegre disease
Short QT syndrome
Cardiomyopathies (may be missed at postmortem)
ARVC
Hypertrophic cardiomyopathy (Troponin T mutations)
Lamin A/C mutations

inconclusive nondiagnostic findings requiring regular follow-up with a 24-hour tape or exercise test on an annual basis to medical therapy with β-blockers for long QT syndrome (LQTS) or an implantable cardioverter-defibrillator (ICD). Counseling should be individualized as each family has its own anxieties and concerns particularly when affected siblings have young children. Therefore, close collaboration with a pediatric cardiologist who has an interest in the field is invaluable.

There is no agreed model for the panel of investigations that should be used in the relatives of sudden death victims. Nevertheless, in most circumstances the following tests are appropriate:

a. Resting 12-lead ECG
b. Exercise ECG
c. Signal averaged ECG
d. Transthoracic echocardiogram
e. Ajmaline or flecainide challenge.

The Consultation

Family screening for SADS begins with a detailed evaluation of the index case. The mode of death may provide useful clues to the etiology. For example, death in the context of swimming is recognized in the LQT 1 subtype (LQT1) and catecholaminergic polymorphic ventricular tachycardia (CPVT). Indeed a recent postmortem series of victims of drowning identified ryanodine receptor 2 (*RYR2*) mutations responsible for CPVT (Choi et al. 2004; Tester et al. 2005) in 20%, suggesting that CPVT may be more common as a cause of sudden death in this context than expected. Exercise is more likely to precipitate ventricular arrhythmia in LQT1 and CPVT. Sudden death during exercise is also recognized in ARVC but the diagnosis can be missed at postmortem, particularly when the right ventricle is not routinely and systematically examined. It is prudent to screen first-degree relatives for ARVC using echocardiography and MRI if there are clinical features to suggest the diagnosis, for example, T-wave inversion in the right precordial leads or late potentials on signal-averaged ECG (Sen-Chowdhry and McKenna 2006). Importantly, such changes may only develop on serial review of first-degree or other close relatives over time as the degree of disease expression advances.

A prior history of syncope in the context of a sudden loud noise, alarm, or fright is characteristic of LQT2. Death during sleep raises the possibility of Brugada syndrome or LQT3. Both conditions are associated with an increased probability of ventricular arrhythmia in the context of increased vagal tone or bradycardia. Detailed questioning of first-degree relatives can be of great value both in terms of ascertaining the details of prior presyncopal or syncopal events and in identifying other family members who are symptomatic with palpitations, presyncope, or syncope. Such individuals may be gene carriers but essentially have subclinical manifestations of the disease.

Investigations

1. Ion Channelopathies

I. Long QT Syndrome LQTS has a prevalence of 1 in 5,000–6,000 (see Chapters 16 & 17). It is caused by mutations in six cardiac ion channel genes. LQT1 is caused by mutations in *KvLQT1* (also *KCNQ1*) the gene encoding the α-subunit of the IKs current (slowly activating potassium current). LQT2 is caused by mutations in *HERG*, the gene encoding the α-subunit of Ikr (rapidly activating potassium current). LQT3 is caused by mutations in *SCN5A*, the cardiac sodium channel gene. LQT4 is caused by mutations in ankyrin-B-a membrane adaptor protein, which interacts with the sodium pump, Na/Ca exchanger, and IP3 receptors. LQT5 is caused by mutations in *KCNE1*, the *minK* gene that encodes the β-subunit for IKs. LQT6 encodes MiRP1, a β-subunit modulating *HERG*. Despite major advances in the genotyping of

LQT—even in the best molecular laboratories—40%–50% of typical LQT patients remain without a molecular diagnosis. The most common LQT genotypes are LQT1, 2, and 3.

i. Clinical Features

The three principal subtypes of LQTS have distinct ECG features that are related to a specific genotype. For example, a bifid T-wave is more common in LQT2. Broad tented T-waves are more common in LQT1 (Figure 33–2). In LQT3 a late onset peaked or biphasic T-wave is a recognized feature. Such typical T-wave patterns are present in 88% of LQT1 and LQT2 patients and 65% of LQT3 (Zhang et al. 2000). Therefore, specific ECG phenotypes are at best only a rough guide to the genotype and by no means a substitute. The triggers for cardiac arrest or syncope seem to track with specific LQT subtypes (Schwartz et al. 2001). In LQT1, exercise accounts for 68% of events and only 15% of events in LQT2. However, predominantly emotional stimuli account for 51% of events in LQT2 versus 28% in LQT1. Sleep and rest without arousal acted as a trigger in 55% of LQT3 cases.

ii. Exercise Testing and Pharmacological Challenge Tests

The principal clinical criteria for LQT are illustrated in Table 33–1. However, clinical diagnosis of LQT can be challenging as conventional clinical criteria only identify 38% of gene-positive cases.

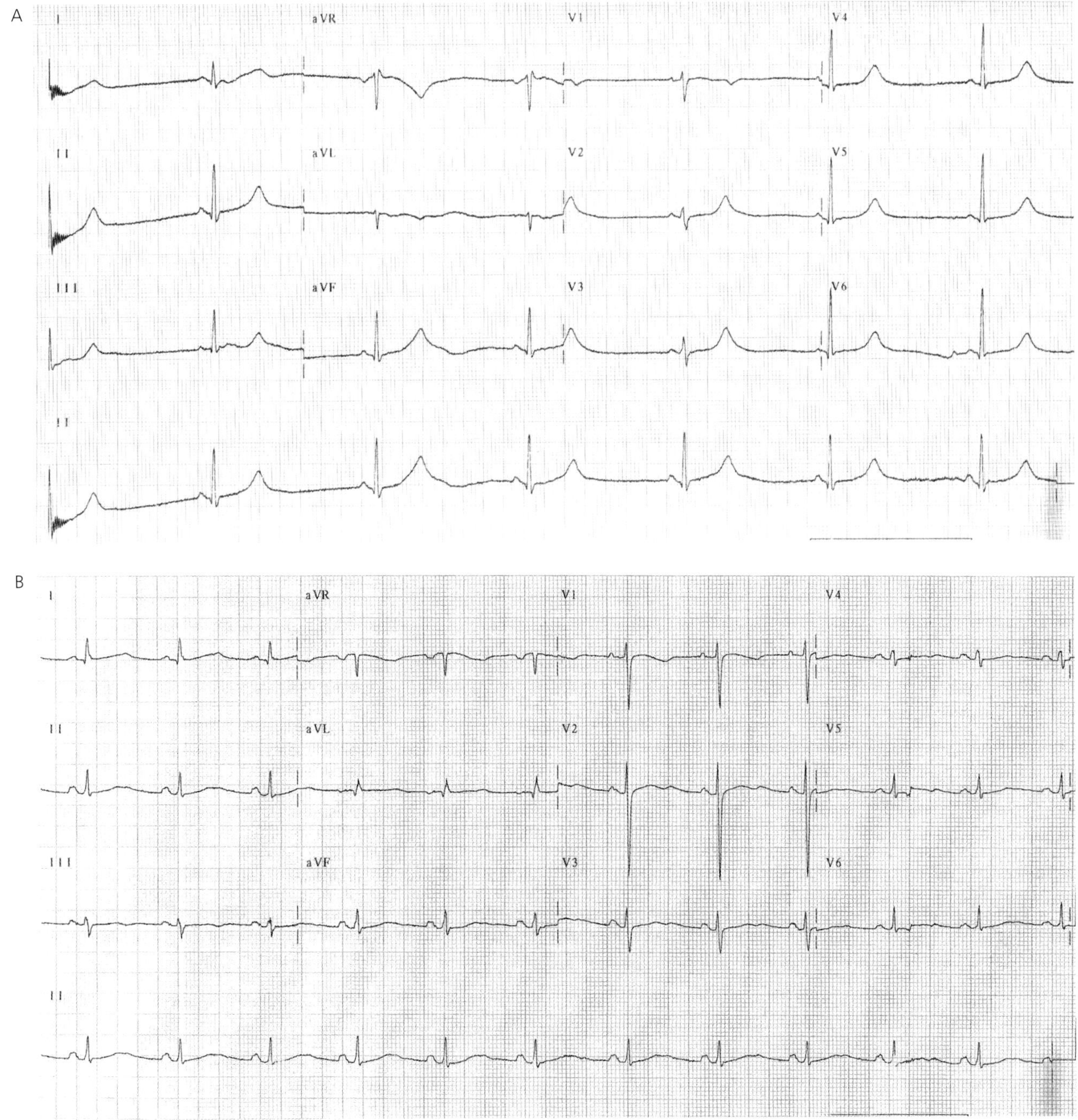

Figure 33–2 (Continued)

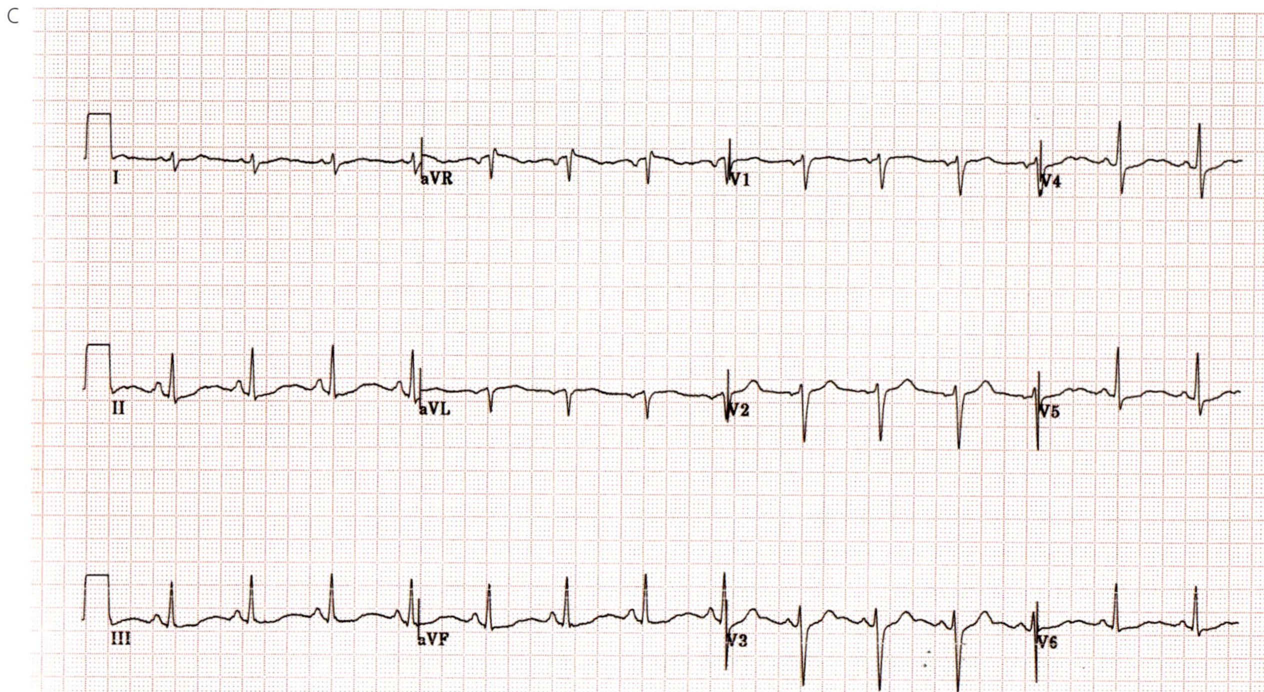

Figure 33–2 (a) Example of an ECG of a patient with LQT1, harboring a *KCNQ1* mutation; QTc = 469 ms; T-waves are broad based with a symmetrical appearance. (b) Example of a patient's ECG with a *KCNH2* mutation (LQT2). The T-waves have a bifid appearance particularly in leads II and V2, QTc = 508 msec (c) Exercise-induced QT prolongation. This ECG recorded immediately upon recovery from exercise illustrates QT prolongation most evident in leads V5 and V6 with the development of a bifid appearance to the T-wave, which was not present at baseline.

Table 33–1 Diagnostic Criteria for LQTS

	Points
Electrocardiographic findings	
QTc[f]	
>480 ms	3
460–470 ms	2
450 (male) ms	1
Torsade de Pointes	2
T-wave alternans	1
Notched T-wave in 3 leads	1
Low heart rate for age[5]	0.5
Clinical history	
Syncope'	
With stress	2
Without stress	1
Congenital deafness	0.5
Family history'	
Family members with definite LQTS[11]	1
Unexplained sudden cardiac death	0.5
Before age 30 years among immediate family members	

Note: Scoring: <1 point = low probability; 2–3 points = intermediate probability; >4 points = high probability.
Source: Adopted from Schwartz PJ, Moss AJ, Vincent GM, and Crampton RS. Diagnostic criteria for the LQTS. An update. *Circulation*. 1993;88:782–784.

On exercise testing the QTc in LQT1 fails to shorten to the same degree during exercise versus controls: this may be more obvious in the recovery phase of exercise in LQT1 but not LQT2 (Figure 33–2). Similarly, at night, LQT3 patients demonstrate marked prolongation of QTc with statistically significant differences between controls and LQT1. Therefore, careful review of the full disclosure of the 24-hour tape may demonstrate significant diurnal changes in QTc and associated changes in T-wave morphology that may not appear at rest.

Further testing to identify LQT subtypes involves the assessment of the response to catecholamines. Intravenous epinephrine prolongs the QTc in LQT1 and this has recently been used to differentiate LQT1 from other subtypes of LQTS (Ackerman et al. 2002). In a recent study of epinephrine challenge in genotyped patients with LQT1, epinephrine had a positive predictive value of 76% and negative predictive value of 96% in the identification of LQT1 versus a non-LQT1 genotype (Vyas et al. 2006). This pharmacological challenge test might be helpful in identifying individuals carrying as yet unidentified LQT1 mutations where the QTc may be normal at rest. The role of this strategy in family screening is yet to be fully evaluated.

II. Brugada Syndrome The resting ECG in Brugada syndrome is pathognemonic of the condition, provided that other secondary causes have been excluded. However, in the majority of families that are screened, first-degree relatives often have normal resting ECGs or very subtle resting changes. Therefore, the key investigation required to identify Brugada syndrome in the family is a pharmacological challenge test employing a Na channel blocker (see Chapter 19).

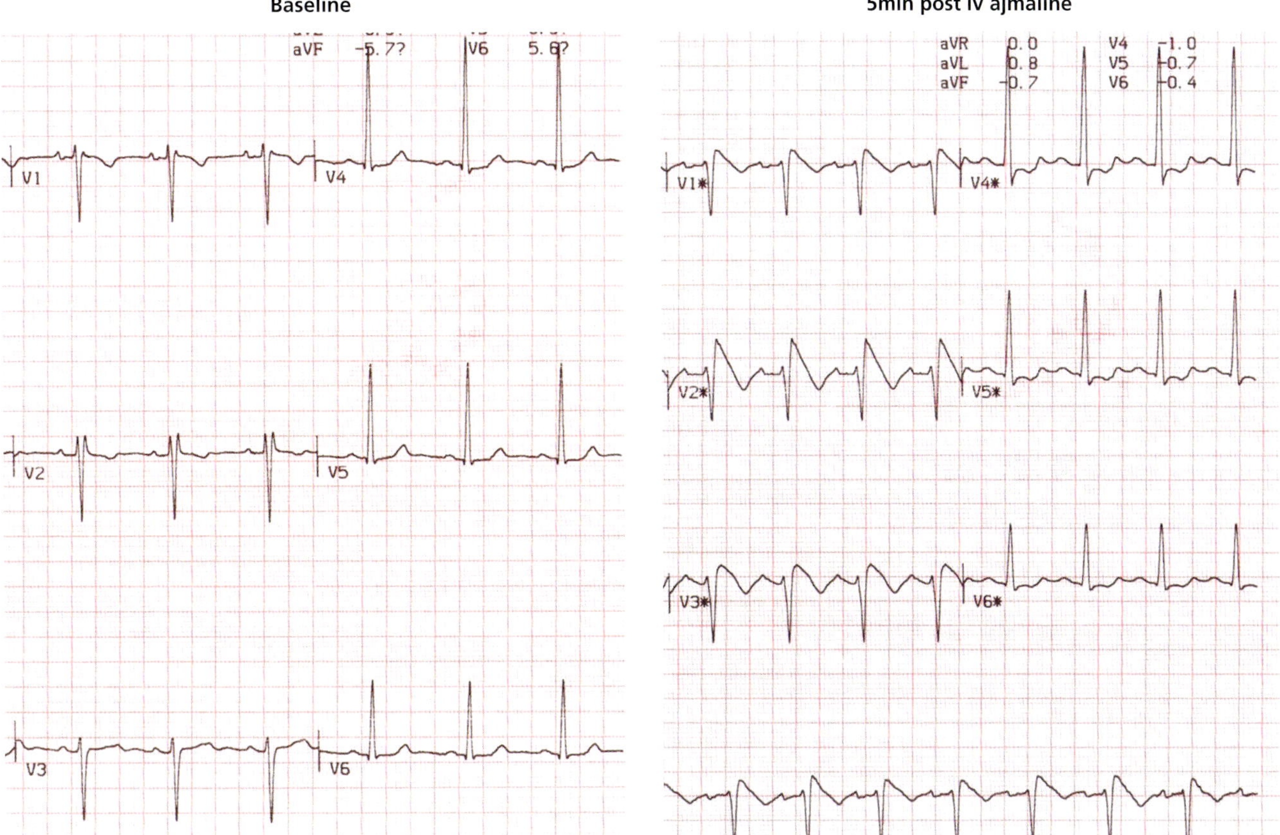

Figure 33–3 Transition from resting changes of Rsr in V1 and minor J point elevation to a type 1 coved ST elevation response to ajmaline indicative of a Brugada phenotype.

iii. Pharmacologic Testing in Brugada Syndrome

Pharmacologic testing must be performed under continuous ECG monitoring and the drug administered with full resuscitation facilities available. In the majority of cases, the facilities in an exercise ECG testing environment are suitable. Figure 33–3 shows a typical type 1 response to an ajmaline challenge test. Particular caution should be exercised in patients with a preexisting atrial or ventricular conduction (or both) disturbances (e.g., suspected cases of Lev or Lenègre disease) or in the presence of wide QRS, wide P-waves, or prolonged PR intervals (i.e., infranodal conduction disease) to avoid the risk of precipitating complete AV block. Electromechanical dissociation has been encountered in isolated cases. Isoprenaline and sodium lactate may be effective antidotes in this setting. Patients at high risk for drug-induced AV block, such as older adults with syncope, should be administered sodium channel blockers in an electrophysiological study (EPS) environment after the insertion of a temporary pacing electrode. For other individuals, especially younger patients, sodium blocker challenge can be safely performed as a bedside test, provided the drug is discontinued as soon as diagnostic ST-segment elevation, QRS widening, or ventricular ectopy is observed. The common agents and doses employed are shown in Table 33–2. The sensitivity, specificity, and positive and negative predictive values of the drug challenge were 80%, 94.4%, 93.3%, and 82.9%, respectively in a group of 147 individuals from four families who had been genetically screened for *SCN5A* mutations (Hong et al. 2004). Penetrance of the disease phenotype increased from 32.7% to 78.6% with the use of sodium channel blockers. In the absence of ST-segment elevation under baseline conditions, a prolonged PR interval, but not incomplete right bundle branch block or early repolarization patterns, indicates a high probability of an *SCN5A* mutation carrier. In another study, J wave elevation >0.16 mV in the right precordial lead -2V(2) was the strongest predictor of a Brugada type response to Na channel blockade challenge when Brugada syndrome was suspected on a baseline ECG (Hermida et al. 2005). Current guidelines regard a positive test as the conversion to type 1 changes on the ECG. Any intermediate change to a type 3 or type 2 ECG is not diagnostic of Brugada syndrome.

Table 33–2 Pharmacological Challenge Tests in Brugada Syndrome

Drug Dosage and Administration
Ajmaline 1 mg/kg over 5 min, IV
Flecainide 2 mg/kg over 10 min, IV (400 mg, PO)
Procainamide 10 mg/kg over 10 min, IV
Pilsicainide 1 mg/kg over 10 min, IV

iv. The Role of EP Studies in Risk Stratification of Brugada

Brugada et al. (2002) have suggested that among asymptomatic patients, the inducibility of VT/VF during EPS predicts the risk of lethal arrythmia. Studies by Priori et al. (2002b), Kanda et al. (2002), and Eckardt et al. (2002, 2007), however, failed to find an association between inducibility and recurrence of VT/VF among both asymptomatic and symptomatic patients with Brugada syndrome. These discrepancies may result from differences in patient characteristics and the use of nonstandardized or noncomparable stimulation protocols. The adverse prognosis and higher predictive value of inducibility by Brugada et al. may, at least in part, be due to more demanding criteria for diagnosing patients with Brugada syndrome and the fact that these cases may be drawn from families with a more malignant family history. It is noteworthy that programmed electrical stimulation-induced VF is observed in 6%–9% of apparently healthy individuals and may represent a false-positive and nonspecific response, particularly when aggressive stimulation protocols are used A protocol involving up to three extrastimuli applied to the right ventricular apex at cycle lengths >200 ms is recommended. If not inducible from the right ventricular apex, then stimulation may be applied to the right ventricular outflow tract (RVOT). The predictive value of EPS is based largely on right ventricular apex stimulation; the value of RVOT pacing for risk stratification is not known. Although inducibility in experimental models is most readily achieved with epicardial stimulation (Fish and Antzelevitch 2003; Yan et al. 2003) clinical data involving this approach are limited (Carlsson et al. 2001). Additional studies are needed to better devise the optimal risk stratification strategy for asymptomatic patients.

III. Catecholaminergic Polymorphic Ventricular Tachycardia CPVT is associated with a completely normal resting ECG but should be suspected following either exercise or catecholamine stress testing that demonstrates ventricular ectopy with bidirectional morphology at heart rates over 120 beats/min (Laitinen et al. 2004; Figure 33–4). This disorder can be very difficult to diagnose clinically as family members may only develop occasional ectopy on exercise testing. One group has recently evaluated the utility of epinephrine challenge in the identification of CPVT in both primary VF survivors and their first-degree relatives (Krahn et al. 2005). This study suggested that adrenaline may be more effective than exercise testing in unmasking diagnostic polymorphic ventricular ectopy and tachycardia, because exercise testing was suggestive in only half of the patients who responded to adrenaline, many with only occasional exercise-induced, isolated ectopy, which was not considered diagnostic. They suggested that this might relate to a combination of sympathetic stimulation and vagal withdrawal during exercise that is less arrhythmogenic than a pure catecholamine trigger during adrenaline infusion in the presence of presumed normal vagal tone.

IV. Short QT Syndrome This syndrome constitutes a new clinical entity that is associated with a high incidence of SCD, syncope, and/or atrial fibrillation even in young patients and newborns. It is characterized by rate-corrected QT intervals <320 ms. Missense mutations in *KCNH2* (*HERG*) linked to a gain of function of the rapidly activating delayed-rectifier current I (Kr) have been identified in the first two reported families with familial SCD (Brugada et al. 2004). Recently, two further gain-of-function mutations in the *KCNQ1* gene (Bellocq, et al. 2004) encoding the α-subunit of the KvLQT1 [I(Ks)] channel and in the *KCNJ2* gene encoding the strong inwardly rectifying channel protein Kir2.1 confirmed a genetically heterogeneous disease (Priori et al. 2005). To date, this condition remains very rare in routine population screening—a recent study of over 100,000 ECGs failed to identify a single case; however, vigilance is required in the context of SADS.

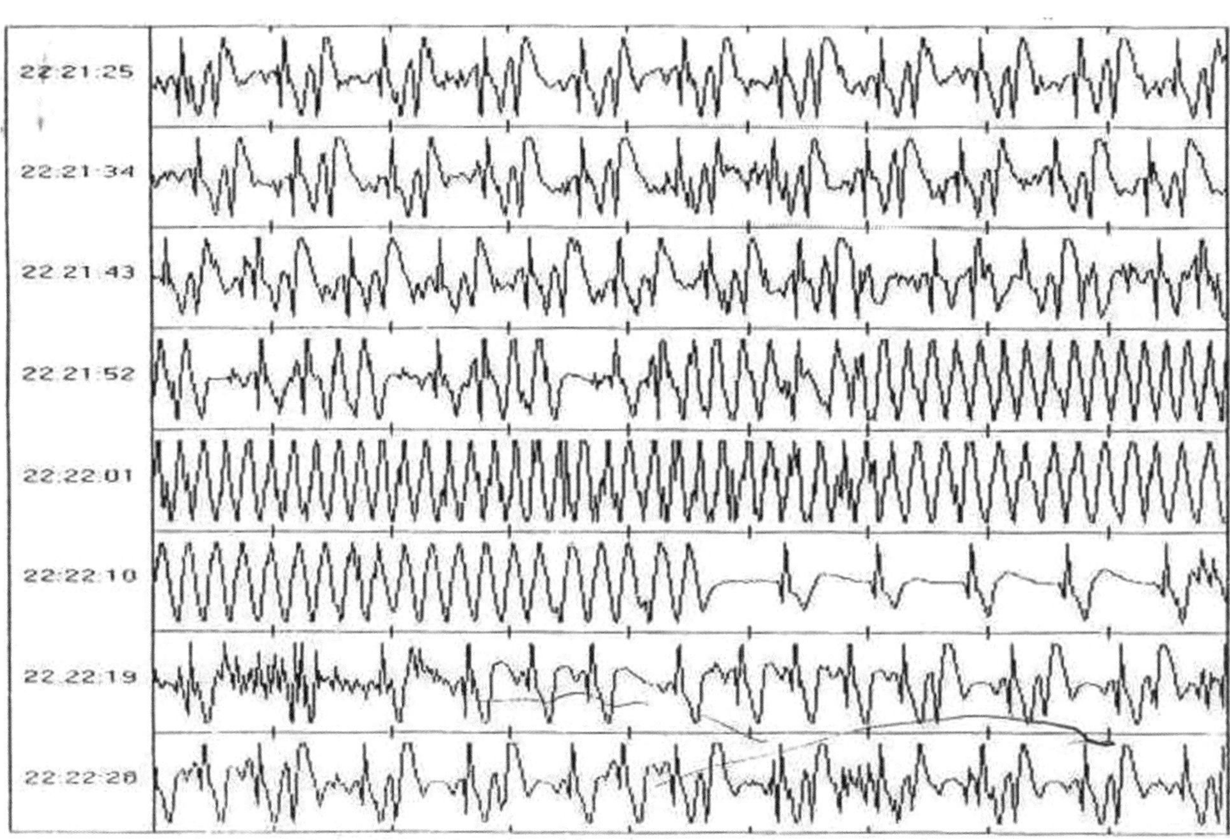

Figure 33–4 A reveal download illustrating ventricular bigemminy developing into VT on exercise.

V. Conduction Disorders In addition to ventricular arrhythmia, inherited conduction disorders—specifically Lev-Lenegre disease and laminopathies—may present with SADS. The former is associated with premature conduction system fibrosis and heart block linked to mutations in *SCN5A* (Napolitano et al. 2003). Detailed family histories often reveal a high incidence of pacemaker implantation. In the case of lamin A/C cardiomyopathy, a disorder of the nuclear envelope, atrioventricular block occurs in the context of a dilated cardiomyopathy (see also Chapter 13). In a recent meta-analysis, cardiac dysrhythmias were reported in 92% of patients after the age of 30 years; heart failure was reported in 64% after the age of 50 years. Sudden death was the most frequently reported mode of death (46%) in both the cardiac and the neuromuscular phenotype. Carriers of lamin A/C gene mutations often received a pacemaker (28%). However, this intervention did not alter the rate of sudden death (Van Berlo et al. 2005). Therefore ICD implnatation is now recommended in lamin A/C mutation carriers due to the risk of lethal ventricular arrhythmia as well as heart block. Family histories usually demonstrate a combination of heart failure, pacemaker implantation, and sudden death.

Genetic Testing of SADS Families

Genetic screening is most valuable in diseases in which mutations can be identified in the majority of cases (e.g., LQTS) but is of limited utility in disorders in which disease-causing mutations are infrequently detected (e.g., Brugada syndrome) (Priori and Napolitano 2006). In the latter case, a clinical diagnostic strategy is more valuable. Genetic testing is usually considered in the following clinical situations:

1. SCD in a proband <35 years old in whom no cause of death was identified at autopsy and the heart was found to be structurally normal. Therefore, a molecular autopsy may inform diagnosis of the cause of SCD and aid screening of first-degree relatives in whom there is limited clinical data to support a diagnosis.
2. First-degree relatives in whom the gene mutation determines prognosis and management of the affected family members. The evidence for this is most robust for LQTS and may inform management in CPVT and Brugada syndrome.
3. Situations where the clinical phenotype is difficult to define or there are large numbers of first-degree relatives who need/request screening. In this case, a single genetic test may prove to be most cost-effective so that further clinical evaluation, risk stratification, and prevention strategies can be focused on gene carriers.
4. Prenatal diagnosis or family planning for families in whom a parent carries a recognized mutation.

The Molecular Autopsy and Role of Molecular Testing in Asymptomatic Family Members

In the United States, 4,000 deaths in the 1–22-year age group occur annually and no diagnosis is made in 50% (Ackerman et al. 2001a; Tester et al. 2005; Tester and Ackerman 2006). Small postmortem series have identified LQT gene mutations as causes of SCD in young probands (Chugh et al. 2004; Di et al. 2004). Recently, Tester completed the largest molecular autopsy series of SADS to date (Tester et al. 2004). Comprehensive mutational analysis of all 60 translated exons in the LQTS-associated genes—*KCNQ1, KCNH2, SCN5A, KCNE1,* and *KCNE2*—and targeted analysis of the CPVT1-associated, *RyR2*-encoded cardiac ryanodine receptor was conducted in a series of 49 SAD probands. Over one-third of SADS cases harbored a presumably pathogenic cardiac ion channel mutation, with mutations in *RyR2* alone accounting for nearly 15% of the cases. In this series, sudden death was the sentinel event in all but four mutation-positive SAD cases. Postmortem genetic testing for cardiac ion channel mutations was recently completed for a large population-based cohort of sudden infant death syndrome (SIDS) cases, revealing mutations in 7% (Ackerman et al. 2001; Tester and Ackerman 2005). A recent review by Ackerman made the point that many deaths in young individuals that occur due to trauma or drowning could be misdiagnosed as noncardiac and a significant proportion of these cases could be secondary to ion channelopathy (Ackerman et al. 2001a). In the LQTS up to 30% of individuals who die suddenly had no preceding symptoms.

In 2003, Behr *et al.* performed a detailed evaluation of 109 first-degree relatives for 32 cases of SAD and showed that 22% of these families had evidence of inherited cardiac disease, with the majority having clinical features suggestive of LQTS. Similarly, in 2005, Tan *et al.* found that 28% of families had an identifiable cardiac channelopathy including CPVT and LQTS following a clinical assessment of first-degree relatives of young SAD victims. Behr's study was expanded in 2008- Thirty families (53%) were diagnosed with inheritable heart disease: 13 definite long QT syndrome (LQTS), three possible/probable LQTS, five Brugada syndrome, five arrhythmogenic right ventricular cardiomyopathy (ARVC), and four other cardiomyopathies. Together, these reports suggest that identifiable and potentially treatable cardiac channelopathies account for approximately one-third of autopsy-negative SAD in young people.

Incomplete penetrance and variable expression are common in arrhythmia syndromes such as LQTS and CPVT and consequently lead to "concealed" forms of these disorders (Priori et al. 1999; Tester et al. 2004). According to Priori *et al.* LQTS has a penetrance of only 25% among families and conventional clinical diagnostic criteria only had 38% sensitivity in correctly identifying carriers of the familial genetic defect. Furthermore, 17% of *RyR2* gene carriers from CPVT families displayed no phenotypic features, and a further 75% of genetically affected parents transmitted the disorder but were asymptomatic (Priori et al. 1999, 2002a; Tester et al. 2004). Therefore, clinical assessment of surviving family members of SADS victims may not be enough to detect LQTS or CPVT in unsuspecting individuals. A molecular diagnosis in the SADS victim involving postmortem cardiac ion channel genetic testing would provide the much needed tool for the pathologist and coroner to explain sudden deaths in young people and subsequently prevent further events in surviving family members. Current data suggest that a diagnosis relevant to family members' prognosis and future management could be made in up to 30% of SAD families independent of expensive and time-consuming undirected family screening.

Gene Testing in Prognostic Evaluation and Clinical Management for Specific Conditions

1. LQT

Probably the most detailed prognostic information available in this field derives from the registry and genetic characterization of LQTS. Schwartz and Priori have produced extensive case series of genotyped patients with LQT1, 2, and 3 (Zareba et al. 1998; Schwartz 2000; Moss et al. 2002; Priori et al. 2003, 2004).

These data have demonstrated significant prognostic differences between the LQT variants and specific activities.

Mortality in LQT1 patients is significantly lower than LQT2 and LQT3 (Priori et al. 2003; Zareba et al. 2003b). Priori et al. demonstrated that the incidence of a first cardiac event before the age of 40 years and before the initiation of therapy was lower among patients with a mutation at the LQT1 locus (30%) than among those with a mutation at the LQT2 locus (46%) or those with a mutation at the LQT3 locus (42%) (Priori et al. 2003). Multivariate analysis showed that the genetic locus and the QTc interval, but not gender were independent predictors of risk in LQT1 and LQT2. The QTc was an independent predictor of risk among patients with a mutation at the LQT1 and the LQT2 loci but not among those with a mutation at the LQT3 locus, whereas gender was an independent predictor of events only among those with a mutation at the LQT3 locus. Therefore, the QTc in isolation cannot be used as an independent predictor of risk. The relative risk of events in LQT2 patients versus LQT1 was 1.6. The highest risk patients are males with LQT 3. LQT3 carries a 1.8-fold relative risk of cardiac events versus LQT1. The inherited genotype is therefore an important determinant of the clinical course of LQTS. The percentage of lethal cardiac events is significantly higher in individuals with mutations involving the *SCN5A* (LQT3) gene than those carrying *KCNQ1* or *HERG* genes. Furthermore, the mutations affecting the pore versus nonpore regions of the ion channel have a greater risk of causing arrhythmia-related events. With nonpore mutations the risk of an event is more dependent on the QTc (Moss et al. 2002). Priori and Schwartz have developed a risk stratification score based upon sex, QTc, and genotype, which facilitates differentiation of high-, intermediate-, and low-risk patients (Priori et al. 2003).

In the Jervell and Lang-Nielson (JLN) syndrome there is evidence that the genotype impacts upon prognosis (Schwartz et al. 2006). Subgroups at relatively lower risk for cardiac arrest and sudden death are identifiable and include females, patients with a QTc <550 ms, those without events in the first year of life, and those with mutations on *KCNE1* as opposed to *KCNQ1*.

The most clear-cut case for genetic testing is that for Timothy syndrome (LQT8), which is caused by a mutation in *CACNA1c* gene. It can be diagnosed by a cheap and accurate genetic test (100%) (Splawski et al. 2004). The condition has an adverse outcome and genetic testing informs prognosis, prenatal diagnosis, family screening, and reproductive counseling.

The clearly demonstrated clinical efficacy of β-blockade in LQTS in observational studies has prevented prospective, randomized placebo controlled trials. The largest retrospective analysis was conducted in 233 LQTS patients, all of whom had been symptomatic with syncope or cardiac arrest. Antiadrenergic therapy (β-blocker or L cervical sympathectomy) reduced mortality to 9% versus 60% in the untreated group over a 15-year follow-up (Schwartz 1985). More recent data illustrates the spectrum of LQTS severity in patients in whom β-blockers were prescribed. The 5-year incidence of cardiac arrest or SCD was below 1% for asymptomatic cases at treatment initiation, 3% in those with a history of syncope, and 13% in cardiac arrest survivors Twenty-five percent of patients that died had stopped β-blockers for a significant time period and many victims were less than 1 year of age. Therefore, in LQTS β-blockade can be very effective; however, it cannot afford total protection following cardiac arrest when the risk of further cardiac arrests remains unacceptably high. Therefore, ICD therapy has been employed in this higher-risk population with clear-cut efficacy (Moss et al. 2000; Zareba et al. 2003a).

Patients with LQT1 and abnormal *IKs* channel function generally demonstrate a good response to β-blocker therapy with either complete resolution of events or a significant reduction in the frequency of syncope (Moss et al. 2000). To date it is not possible to conclude whether β-blockade reduces the frequency of cardiac arrest in LQT1 as the duration of follow-up has not been specified in the published series. In LQT2 β-blockers are particularly effective in preventing events caused by acoustic stimuli. The role of drug therapy in LQT3 is unresolved. Events occur at rest or during sleep and are thought to be bradycardia dependent. Na channel blockers may exert a positive influence on repolarization in these patients where Na channel inactivation may be important, for example, *SCN5A* ΔKPQ deletion (Abriel et al. 2001). Currently a randomized controlled trial of flecainide therapy for this mutation is in progress. Conversely, in the *SCN5A* 1795insD mutation associated with LQT3 and Brugada syndrome, flecainide caused a fourfold delay in recovery from use—dependent flecainide block—thus explaining the proarrhythmic effect of this drug in Brugada syndrome (Viswanathan et al. 2001). The effects of specific mutations upon ion channel kinetics and clinical phenotype are obviously complex, but genotyping may provide a rationale for gene-specific therapies and avoid both frequent cardiac events and the burden of ICD therapy in these populations in the future.

2. Brugada Syndrome

The role of genetic testing in Brugada syndrome is less clear cut as the diagnosis and management is currently based upon clinical criteria. Most mutations that have been identified to be responsible for the condition are in the *SCN5A* gene encoding the α subunit of the human cardiac voltage-gated sodium channel. This is found in up to 30% of affected individuals (Antzelevitch 1998, 1999, 2001; Baroudi et al. 2000, 2001, 2004; Baroudi and Chahine 2000; Kyndt et al. 2001; Clancy and Rudy 2002; Smits et al. 2002; Schulze-Bahr et al. 2003; Chen et al. 2004; Niimura et al. 2004; Shin et al. 2004; Valdivia et al. 2004; Antzelevitch et al. 2005; Arbustini et al. 2005; Hong et al. 2005; Itoh et al. 2005; Makiyama et al. 2005; Todd et al. 2005; Verkerk et al. 2005; Yokoi et al. 2005; Meregalli et al. 2006). Other mutations in SCN5A are responsible for LQTS, Lev-Lenegre disease and sick sinus syndrome (Benson et al 2003), illustrating how abnormalities in different regions of the same gene can result in a variety of phenotypes. Since mutation screening does not currently influence management, its only role is the identification of potentially affected relatives in whom it is known that the proband is a carrier of the *SCN5A* mutation responsible for Brugada syndrome and pharmacological provocation testing is logistically difficult to arrange for geographic reasons or there is a large number of first-degree relatives that may need to be screened.

3. CPVT

Asymptomatic CPVT gene carriers can be at risk of lethal arrhythmia (Priori et al. 2002a; Eldar et al. 2003; Sumitomo et al. 2003; Lahat et al. 2004; Francis et al. 2005; Creighton et al. 2006; Gussak 2006). Approximately 50% of CPVT is due to autosomal dominant *RyR2* mutations and is regarded as type 1 CPVT (CPVT1) (Priori et al. 2001, 2002a; Tester et al. 2004, 2005). A rare subtype of CPVT arises in an autosomal recessive fashion with mutations in calsequestrin encoded by *CASQ2* and is known as type 2 CPVT (CPVT2) (Lahat et al. 2001; Eldar et al. 2003). The lethality of CPVT is illustrated by the presence of a positive family history of young (<40 years) SCD for more than a third of CPVT individuals and in as many as 60% of families hosting *RyR2* mutations (Eldar et al. 2003; Lahat et al. 2003).

Genetic diagnosis may help to inform management in identifying gene carriers at an early age thus ensuring individuals avoid exercise-related triggers and commence prophylactic β-blockade with dose titration guided by treadmill testing. In up to 40% of cases, particularly males, β-blockade is ineffective in the suppression of VT and therefore an ICD may be the indicated management (Priori et al. 2002a; Sumitomo et al. 2003) (Francis et al. 2005). In a mean follow-up of 2 years, half of patients implanted with an ICD on β-blocker therapy had appropriate therapies. Therefore, in high-risk individuals, for example, those who have suffered a VT/VF arrest, unexplained syncope with frequent VEs on Holter, or first-degree relatives of SADS, genetic screening may be informative. There is evidence to support the use of prophylactic β-blockade in these individuals, although the protective effect is currently debated and there is a trend to employ ICDs at an earlier stage in management (Francis et al. 2005). A genetic diagnosis will allow careful follow-up and preventative measures to be undertaken as well as reproductive counseling (see also Chapter 17).

4. Cardiomyopathies

VI. Hypertrophic Cardiomyopathy HCM differs significantly from ion channelopathies since there is far greater genetic heterogeneity in this condition (see also Chapter 13). Approximately 80% of the genotyped HCM patients (60% of all cases) carry mutations in *MYH7* and *MYBPC3* genes. The data regarding prognostic impact of these mutations is, however, limited. Late onset disease is recognized in *MYBPC3* mutations and therefore some patients (but not all) require risk stratification strategies to be concentrated in middle age (Niimura et al. 1998). In the *MYH7* gene R403Q, R719W, and R453C mutations may be higher risk in terms of prognosis whereas normal life expectancy may be anticipated in other allelic variants (Watkins et al. 1992; Anan et al. 1994). Currently, genetic screening in HCM allows presymptomatic diagnosis, identification of silent carriers, and patients in whom prenatal counseling may be appropriate.

VII. Dilated Cardiomyopathy (DCM) Only a small proportion of idiopathic DCM patients have identifiable mutations. However, DCM associated with lamin A/C gene mutations can have important implications for patient prognosis (Bonne et al. 1999; Arbustini et al. 2002). Arbustini reported that 30% of patients with DCM and cardiac conduction defects have mutations in this nuclear membrane protein gene (Arbustini et al. 2002). This mutation causes progressive conduction disease and ventricular arrhythmias and therefore gene-positive individuals should be counseled to receive an ICD in order to avoid the consequences of lethal arrhythmia.

VIII. Arrhythmogenic Right Ventricular Cardiomyopathy (ARVC/ARVD) Approximately 30% of ARVC cases are caused by mutations affecting genes encoding desmosomal proteins (Coonar et al. 1998; Ahmad 2003; Syrris et al. 2006; Tsatsopoulou et al. 2006; van Tintelen et al. 2006). Currently, there are inadequate data correlating genotype with prognosis, but genetic testing helps guide diagnosis in clinically borderline cases (see also Chapter 14). Serial follow-up of gene-positive patients should be undertaken with annual Holter monitoring and echocardiography. Gene carriers should be counseled to report syncope, presyncope, and palpitations, which may be markers of disease progression and herald the onset of prognostically important changes in the ventricle(s).

5. Compound Heterozygotes

It is becoming increasingly evident that heterozygotes harboring ion channel mutations can be protected by polymorphisms of the same gene on the corresponding nonmutant allele. For example, the degree of QT prolongation caused by the ion channel mutation may be attenuated by the effect of the polymorphism of the same nonallelic gene in a given individual. This was recently shown by Crotti et al. who demonstrated that the wild-type polymorphism in *KCNH2* reduced the degree of QT prolongation and arrhythmogenic potential of the *KCNH2* mutation. If this same mutation was coupled with a different (K897T) polymorphism it resulted in a more malignant phenotype in the carrier (Crotti et al. 2005). Similarly, the variation in QT interval between family members inheriting the same ion channel mutations may also be determined by additional mutations in other LQT genes generating a more malignant phenotype (Westenskow et al. 2004). In Brugada syndrome, a specific nonallelic polymorphism may rescue sodium channel function impaired by a *SCN5A* mutation (Poelzing et al. 2006).

Cost-Efficacy of Genetic Screening

There are limited data describing the cost efficacy of genetic screening for ion channelopathies to prevent SCD. Given the fact that lethal events by definition occur under the age of 35 years and these individuals are otherwise fit and well, the identification of at-risk individuals and prevention of lethal arrhythmia in high-risk populations is not difficult to justify. In a recent cost efficacy analysis of the role of ICDs in LQT and HCM, there was clear evidence of a cost benefit in favor of ICD therapy for high-risk individuals (Goldenberg et al. 2005). This study concluded that in appropriately selected patients with inherited cardiac disorders, early intervention with ICD therapy is cost-effective to cost saving due to added years of gained productivity when the lifespan of an individual at risk is considered. The key factors determining the cost efficacy of screening for SADS will relate to the exact costs of the genetic testing and the cost-effectiveness of targeting treatment for gene carriers.

Conclusions and Recommendations

The creation of a SADS clinic to diagnose and manage SADS families is a demanding process requiring considerable expertise from geneticists, genetic counselors, specialist nurses, electrophysiologists, and cardiologists with expertise in cardiomyopathy and cardiac imaging. With the evolution of genetic testing, access to genetic testing facilities is extremely useful for some conditions to make a diagnosis and guide management. One of the key issues in genetic screening is the fact that the identification of an ion channel mutation in a family does not necessarily mean that this mutation is disease causing in a given family member as nonallelic polymorphisms of that gene may be protective. Therefore, careful evaluation of all the clinical data is required to formulate a management plan in any given family. In the future it may be possible to evaluate the entire "electrical gene profile" to assess overall risk but this will require a number of years of meticulous cellular and whole organ-based cardiac research to evaluate the impact of the most common ion channel mutations, polymorphisms, and their interactions. Gene testing may be of benefit in the future for other causes of SAD as our knowledge improves. Table 33–3 summarizes the current evidence adapted from Priori (Priori and

Table 33–3 Summary of Clinical Indications for Genetic Testing in SADS

	Genotyped (%)	Genes	Clinical Score				
			I	II	III	IV	V
Genetic testing should be done							
Timothy syndrome (LQT8)	100	*CACNA1c*		+	+		+
LQTS (Romano Ward)	>50	*KCNq1, KCNH2, SCN5A, KCNE1, KCNE2*	+	+	+	+	+
JLN	>50	*KCNQ1, KCNE1*		+	+		+
Anderson syndrome	50	*KCNJ2*	+	+	+		
DCM-CB	30–50	*LMNA/C*	+	+	+	+	+
HCM		*MYH7, MYL3, MYL2, ACTC, TNNT2, TPM1, TNNI3, MYBPC3, TTNC*	+	+		+	
CPVT	>50	*RyR2, CASQ2*	+	+	+	+	
Genetic testing could be considered							
ARVC	30–50	*PKP2, DSP, JUP*		+	+	+	
Brugada syndrome	<30	*SCN5A*	+	+			
Research only							
Short QT syndrome	0	*KCNQ1, KCNH2, KCNJ2*	+			+	
Progressive cardiac conduction defect	0	*SCN5A*	+			+	
Left ventricular noncompaction	0	*Cypher/ZASP*		+			

Notes: JLN, Jervell-Lange-Nielsen; DCM-CB, dilated cardiomyopathy and conduction block
Clinical Score
I Presymptomatic diagnosis is clinically relevant
II Identification of silent carriers is clinically relevant
III Results influence risk stratification
IV Results influence therapy/lifestyle
V Reproductive counseling is clinically justified.

Napolitano 2006) (c.2007) justifying genetic testing as a means of risk stratification alone in this group of disorders.

References

Abriel H, Cabo C, Wehrens XH, et al. Novel arrhythmogenic mechanism revealed by a long-QT syndrome mutation in the cardiac Na(+) channel. *Circ Res.* 2001;88(7):740–745.

Ackerman MJ, Khositseth A, Tester DJ, Hejlik JB, Shen WK, Porter CB. Epinephrine-induced QT interval prolongation: a gene-specific paradoxical response in congenital long QT syndrome. *Mayo Clin Proc.* 2002;77(5):413–421.

Ackerman MJ, Siu BL, Sturner WQ, et al. Postmortem molecular analysis of SCN5A defects in sudden infant death syndrome. *JAMA.* 2001; 286(18):2264–2269.

Ackerman MJ, Tester DJ, Driscoll DJ. Molecular autopsy of sudden unexplained death in the young. *Am J Forensic Med Pathol.* 2001a;22(2):105–111.

Ahmad F. The molecular genetics of arrhythmogenic right ventricular dysplasia-cardiomyopathy. *Clin Invest Med.* 2003;26(4):167–178.

Anan R, Greve G, Thierfelder L, et al. Prognostic implications of novel beta cardiac myosin heavy chain gene mutations that cause familial hypertrophic cardiomyopathy. *J Clin Invest.* 1994;93(1):280–285.

Antzelevitch C. The Brugada syndrome. *J Cardiovasc Electrophysiol.* 1998;9(5):513–516.

Antzelevitch C. Ion channels and ventricular arrhythmias: cellular and ionic mechanisms underlying the Brugada syndrome. *Curr Opin Cardiol.* 1999;14(3):274–279.

Antzelevitch C. Molecular biology and cellular mechanisms of Brugada and long QT syndromes in infants and young children. *J Electrocardiol.* 2001;34(Suppl):177–181.

Antzelevitch C, Brugada P, Brugada J, Brugada R. Brugada syndrome: from cell to bedside. *Curr Probl Cardiol.* 2005;30(1):9–54.

Arbustini E, Pilotto A, Repetto A, et al. Autosomal dominant dilated cardiomyopathy with atrioventricular block: a lamin A/C defect-related disease. *J Am Coll Cardiol.* 2002;39(6):981–990.

Arbustini E, Scaffino MF, Diegoli M, et al. Gene symbol: SCN5A. Disease: Brugada syndrome. *Hum Genet.* 2005;118(3–4):536.

Baroudi G, Carbonneau E, Pouliot V, Chahine M. SCN5A mutation (T1620M) causing Brugada syndrome exhibits different phenotypes when expressed in Xenopus oocytes and mammalian cells. *FEBS Lett.* 2000;467(1):12–16.

Baroudi G, Chahine M. Biophysical phenotypes of SCN5A mutations causing long QT and Brugada syndromes. *FEBS Lett.* 2000;487(2):224–228.

Baroudi G, Napolitano C, Priori SG, Del Bufalo A, Chahine M. Loss of function associated with novel mutations of the SCN5A gene in patients with Brugada syndrome. *Can J Cardiol.* 2004;20(4):425–430.

Baroudi G, Pouliot V, Denjoy I, Guicheney P, Shrier A, Chahine M. Novel mechanism for Brugada syndrome: defective surface localization of an SCN5A mutant (R1432G). *Circ Res.* 2001;88(12):E78–E83.

Behr E, Wood DA, Wright M, et al. Cardiological assessment of first-degree relatives in sudden arrhythmic death syndrome. *Lancet.* 2003;362(9394):1457–1459.

Behr ER, Dalageorgou C, Christiansen M, Syrris P, Hughes S, Tome Esteban MT, et al. Sudden arrhythmic death syndrome: familial evaluation identifies inheritable heart disease in the majority of families. *Eur Heart J.* 2008;29(13):1670–1680.

Bellocq C, van Ginneken AC, Bezzina CR, et al. Mutation in the KCNQ1 gene leading to the short QT-interval syndrome. *Circulation.* 2004;109(20):2394–2397.

Benson DW, Wang DW, Dyment M, et al. Congenital sick sinus syndrome caused by recessive mutations in the cardiac sodium channel gene (SCN5A). *J Clin Invest.* 2003;112(7):1019–1028.

Bonne G, Di Barletta MR, Varnous S, et al. Mutations in the gene encoding lamin A/C cause autosomal dominant Emery-Dreifuss muscular dystrophy. *Nat Genet.* 1999;21(3):285–288.

Brugada J, Brugada R, Antzelevitch C, Towbin J, Nademanee K, Brugada P. Long-term follow-up of individuals with the electrocardiographic pattern of right bundle-branch block and ST-segment elevation in precordial leads V1 to V3. *Circulation.* 2002;105(1):73–78.

Brugada R, Hong K, Dumaine R, et al. Sudden death associated with short-QT syndrome linked to mutations in HERG. *Circulation.* 2004;109(1):30–35.

Carlsson J, Erdogan A, Schulte B, Neuzner J, Pitschner HF. Possible role of epicardial left ventricular programmed stimulation in Brugada syndrome. *Pacing Clin Electrophysiol.* 2001;24(2):247–249.

Chen JZ, Xie XD, Wang XX, Tao M, Shang YP, Guo XG. Single nucleotide polymorphisms of the SCN5A gene in Han Chinese and their relation with Brugada syndrome. *Chin Med J (Engl.).* 2004;117(5):652–656.

Choi G, Kopplin LJ, Tester DJ, Will ML, Haglund CM, Ackerman MJ. Spectrum and frequency of cardiac channel defects in swimming-triggered arrhythmia syndromes. *Circulation.* 2004;110(15):2119–2124.

Chugh SS, Senashova O, Watts A, et al. Postmortem molecular screening in unexplained sudden death. *J Am Coll Cardiol.* 2004;43(9):1625–1629.

Clancy CE, Rudy Y. Na(+) channel mutation that causes both Brugada and long-QT syndrome phenotypes: a simulation study of mechanism. *Circulation.* 2002;105(10):1208–1213.

Coonar AS, Protonotarios N, Tsatsopoulou A, et al. Gene for arrhythmogenic right ventricular cardiomyopathy with diffuse nonepidermolytic palmoplantar keratoderma and woolly hair (Naxos disease) maps to 17q21. *Circulation.* 1998;97(20):2049–2058.

Creighton W, Virmani R, Kutys R, Burke A. Identification of novel missense mutations of cardiac ryanodine receptor gene in exercise-induced sudden death at autopsy. *J Mol Diagn.* 2006;8(1):62–67.

Crotti L, Lundquist AL, Insolia R, et al. KCNH2-K897T is a genetic modifier of latent congenital long-QT syndrome. *Circulation.* 2005;112(9):1251–1258.

Di Paolo M, Luchini D, Bloise R, Priori SG. Postmortem molecular analysis in victims of sudden unexplained death. *Am J Forensic Med Pathol.* 2004;25(2):182–184.

Eckardt L, Kirchhof P, Schulze-Bahr E, et al. Electrophysiologic investigation in Brugada syndrome; yield of programmed ventricular stimulation at two ventricular sites with up to three premature beats. *Eur Heart J.* 2002;23(17):1394–1401.

Eldar M, Pras E, Lahat H. A missense mutation in the CASQ2 gene is associated with autosomal-recessive catecholamine-induced polymorphic ventricular tachycardia. *Trends Cardiovasc Med.* 2003;13(4):148–151.

Fish JM, Antzelevitch C. Cellular and ionic basis for the sex-related difference in the manifestation of the Brugada syndrome and progressive conduction disease phenotypes. *J Electrocardiol.* 2003;36(Suppl):173–179.

Francis J, Sankar V, Nair VK, Priori SG. Catecholaminergic polymorphic ventricular tachycardia. *Heart Rhythm.* 2005;2(5):550–554.

Goldenberg I, Moss AJ, Maron BJ, Dick AW, Zareba W. Cost-effectiveness of implanted defibrillators in young people with inherited cardiac arrhythmias. *Ann Noninvasive Electrocardiol.* 2005;10(4 Suppl):67–83.

Gussak I. Molecular pathogenesis of catecholaminergic polymorphic ventricular tachycardia: Sex matters! *Heart Rhythm.* 2006;3(7):806–807.

Hermida JS, Denjoy I, Jarry G, Jandaud S, Bertrand C, Delonca J. Electrocardiographic predictors of Brugada type response during Na channel blockade challenge. *Europace.* 2005;7(5):447–453.

Hong K, Brugada J, Oliva A, et al. Value of Electrocardiographic parameters and ajmaline test in the diagnosis of Brugada syndrome caused by SCN5A mutations. *Circulation.* 2004;110(19):3023–3027.

Hong K, Guerchicoff A, Pollevick GD, et al. Cryptic 5' splice site activation in SCN5A associated with Brugada syndrome. *J Mol Cell Cardiol.* 2005;38(4):555–560.

Itoh H, Shimizu M, Takata S, Mabuchi H, Imoto K. A novel missense mutation in the SCN5A gene associated with Brugada syndrome bidirectionally affecting blocking actions of antiarrhythmic drugs. *J Cardiovasc Electrophysiol.* 2005;16(5):486–493.

Kanda M, Shimizu W, Matsuo K, et al. Electrophysiologic characteristics and implications of induced ventricular fibrillation in symptomatic patients with Brugada syndrome. *J Am Coll Cardiol.* 2002;39(11):1799–1805.

Krahn AD, Gollob M, Yee R, et al. Diagnosis of unexplained cardiac arrest: role of adrenaline and procainamide infusion. *Circulation.* 2005;112(15):2228–2234.

Kyndt F, Probst V, Potet F, et al. Novel SCN5A mutation leading either to isolated cardiac conduction defect or Brugada syndrome in a large French family. *Circulation.* 2001;104(25):3081–3086.

Lahat H, Eldar M, Levy-Nissenbaum E, et al. Autosomal recessive catecholamine- or exercise-induced polymorphic ventricular tachycardia: clinical features and assignment of the disease gene to chromosome 1p13–21. *Circulation.* 2001;103(23):2822–2827.

Lahat H, Pras E, Eldar M. RYR2 and CASQ2 mutations in patients suffering from catecholaminergic polymorphic ventricular tachycardia. *Circulation.* 2003;107(3):e29.

Lahat H, Pras E, Eldar M. A missense mutation in CASQ2 is associated with autosomal recessive catecholamine-induced polymorphic ventricular tachycardia in Bedouin families from Israel. *Ann Med.* 2004;36(Suppl 1):87–91.

Laitinen PJ, Swan H, Piippo K, Viitasalo M, Toivonen L, Kontula K. Genes, exercise and sudden death: molecular basis of familial catecholaminergic polymorphic ventricular tachycardia. *Ann Med.* 2004;36(Suppl 1):81–86.

Makiyama T, Akao M, Tsuji K, et al. High risk for bradyarrhythmic complications in patients with Brugada syndrome caused by SCN5A gene mutations. *J Am Coll Cardiol.* 2005;46(11):2100–2106.

Meregalli PG, Ruijter JM, Hofman N, Bezzina CR, Wilde AA, Tan HL. Diagnostic value of flecainide testing in unmasking SCN5A-related Brugada syndrome. *J Cardiovasc Electrophysiol.* 2006; 17(8):857–864

Moss AJ, Zareba W, Hall WJ, et al. Effectiveness and limitations of beta-blocker therapy in congenital long-QT syndrome. *Circulation.* 2000;101(6):616–623.

Moss AJ, Zareba W, Kaufman ES, et al. Increased risk of arrhythmic events in long-QT syndrome with mutations in the pore region of the human ether-a-go-go-related gene potassium channel. *Circulation.* 2002;105(7):794–799.

Napolitano C, Rivolta I, Priori SG. Cardiac sodium channel diseases. *Clin Chem Lab Med.* 2003;41(4):439–444.

Niimura H, Bachinski LL, Sangwatanaroj S, et al. Mutations in the gene for cardiac myosin-binding protein C and late-onset familial hypertrophic cardiomyopathy. *N Engl J Med.* 1998;338(18):1248–1257.

Niimura H, Matsunaga A, Kumagai K, et al. Genetic analysis of Brugada syndrome in Western Japan: two novel mutations. *Circ J.* 2004;68(8):740–746.

Paul M, Gerss J, Schulze-Bahr E, Wichter T, Vahlhaus C, Wilde AA, et al. Role of programmed ventricular stimulation in patients with Brugada syndrome: a meta-analysis of worldwide published data. *Eur Heart J.* 2007;28(17):2126–2133.

Poelzing S, Forleo C, Samodell M, et al. SCN5A polymorphism restores trafficking of a Brugada syndrome mutation on a separate gene. *Circulation.* 2006;114(5):368–376.

Priori SG, Barhanin J, Hauer RN, et al. Genetic and molecular basis of cardiac arrhythmias: impact on clinical management parts I and II. *Circulation.* 1999;99(4):518–528.

Priori SG, Napolitano C. Role of genetic analyses in cardiology: part I: mendelian diseases: cardiac channelopathies. *Circulation.* 2006;113(8):1130–1135.

Priori SG, Napolitano C, Gasparini M, et al. Natural history of Brugada syndrome: insights for risk stratification and management. *Circulation.* 2002b;105(11):1342–1347.

Priori SG, Napolitano C, Memmi M, et al. Clinical and molecular characterization of patients with catecholaminergic polymorphic ventricular tachycardia. *Circulation.* 2002a;106(1):69–74.

Priori SG, Napolitano C, Schwartz PJ, et al. Association of long QT syndrome loci and cardiac events among patients treated with beta-blockers. *JAMA.* 2004;292(11):1341–1344.

Priori SG, Napolitano C, Tiso N, et al. Mutations in the cardiac ryanodine receptor gene (hRyR2) underlie catecholaminergic polymorphic ventricular tachycardia. *Circulation.* 2001;103(2):196–200.

Priori SG, Pandit SV, Rivolta I, et al. A novel form of short QT syndrome (SQT3) is caused by a mutation in the KCNJ2 gene. *Circ Res.* 2005;96(7):800–807.

Priori SG, Schwartz PJ, Napolitano C, et al. Risk stratification in the long-QT syndrome. *N Engl J Med.* 2003;348(19):1866–1874.

Schott JJ, Alshinawi C, Kyndt F, et al. Cardiac conduction defects associate with mutations in SCN5A. *Nat Genet.* 1999;23(1):20–21.

Schulze-Bahr E, Eckardt L, Breithardt G, et al. Sodium channel gene (SCN5A) mutations in 44 index patients with Brugada syndrome: different incidences in familial and sporadic disease. *Hum Mutat.* 2003;21(6):651–652.

Schwartz PJ. Idiopathic long QT syndrome: progress and questions. *Am Heart J.* 1985;109(2):399–411.

Schwartz PJ. Clinical applicability of molecular biology: the case of the long QT syndrome. *Curr Control Trials Cardiovasc med.* 2000;1(2):88–91.

Schwartz PJ, Moss AJ, Vincent GM, Crampton RS. Diagnostic criteria for the LQTS. An update. *Circulation.* 1993;88:782–784.

Schwartz PJ, Priori SG, Spazzolini C, et al. Genotype-phenotype correlation in the long-QT syndrome: gene-specific triggers for life-threatening arrhythmias. *Circulation.* 2001;103(1):89–95.

Schwartz PJ, Spazzolini C, Crotti L, et al. The Jervell and Lange-Nielsen syndrome: natural history, molecular basis, and clinical outcome. *Circulation.* 2006;113(6):783–790.

Sen-Chowdhry S, McKenna WJ. Sudden cardiac death in the young: a strategy for prevention by targeted evaluation. *Cardiology.* 2006;105(4):196–206.

Shin DJ, Jang Y, Park HY, et al. Genetic analysis of the cardiac sodium channel gene SCN5A in Koreans with Brugada syndrome. *J Hum Genet.* 2004;49(10):573–578.

Smits JP, Eckardt L, Probst V, et al. Genotype-phenotype relationship in Brugada syndrome: electrocardiographic features differentiate SCN5A-related patients from non-SCN5A-related patients. *J Am Coll Cardiol.* 2002;40(2):350–356.

Splawski I, Timothy KW, Sharpe LM, et al. Ca(V)1.2 calcium channel dysfunction causes a multisystem disorder including arrhythmia and autism. *Cell.* 2004;119(1):19–31.

Sumitomo N, Harada K, Nagashima M, et al. Catecholaminergic polymorphic ventricular tachycardia: electrocardiographic characteristics and optimal therapeutic strategies to prevent sudden death. *Heart.* 2003;89(1):66–70

Syrris P, Ward D, Asimaki A, et al. Clinical expression of plakophilin-2 mutations in familial arrhythmogenic right ventricular cardiomyopathy. *Circulation.* 2006;113(3):356–364.

Tan HL, Hofman N, van Langen IM, van der Wal AC, Wilde AA. Sudden unexplained death: heritability and diagnostic yield of cardiological and genetic examination in surviving relatives. *Circulation.* 2005;112(2):207–213.

Tester DJ, Ackerman MJ. Sudden infant death syndrome: how significant are the cardiac channelopathies? *Cardiovasc Res.* 2005;67(3):388–396.

Tester DJ, Ackerman MJ. The role of molecular autopsy in unexplained sudden cardiac death. *Curr Opin Cardiol.* 2006;21(3):166–172.

Tester DJ, Kopplin LJ, Creighton W, Burke AP, Ackerman MJ. Pathogenesis of unexplained drowning: new insights from a molecular autopsy. *Mayo Clin Proc.* 2005;80(5):596–600.

Tester DJ, Kopplin LJ, Will ML, Ackerman MJ. Spectrum and prevalence of cardiac ryanodine receptor (RyR2) mutations in a cohort of unrelated patients referred explicitly for long QT syndrome genetic testing. *Heart Rhythm.* 2005;2(10):1099–1105.

Tester DJ, Spoon DB, Valdivia HH, Makielski JC, Ackerman MJ. Targeted mutational analysis of the RyR2-encoded cardiac ryanodine receptor in sudden unexplained death: a molecular autopsy of 49 medical examiner/coroner's cases. *Mayo Clin Proc.* 2004a;79(11):1380–1384.

Todd SJ, Campbell MJ, Roden DM, Kannankeril PJ. Novel Brugada SCN5A mutation causing sudden death in children. *Heart Rhythm.* 2005;2(5):540–543.

Tsatsopoulou AA, Protonotarios NI, McKenna WJ. Arrhythmogenic right ventricular dysplasia, a cell-adhesion cardiomyopathy: insights into disease pathogenesis from preliminary genotype-phenotype assessment. *Heart.* 2006;92(12):1720–1723.

Valdivia CR, Tester DJ, Rok BA, et al. A trafficking defective, Brugada syndrome-causing SCN5A mutation rescued by drugs. *Cardiovasc Res.* 2004;62(1):53–62.

Van Berlo JH, de Voogt WG, van der Kooi AJ, et al. Meta-analysis of clinical characteristics of 299 carriers of LMNA gene mutations: do lamin A/C mutations portend a high risk of sudden death? *J Mol Med.* 2005;83(1):79–83.

van Tintelen JP, Entius MM, Bhuiyan ZA, et al. Plakophilin-2 mutations are the major determinant of familial arrhythmogenic right ventricular dysplasia/cardiomyopathy. *Circulation.* 2006;113(13):1650–1658.

Verkerk AO, Wilders R, Schulze-Bahr E, et al. Role of sequence variations in the human ether-a-go-go-related gene (HERG, KCNH2) in the Brugada syndrome. *Cardiovasc Res.* 2005;68(3):441–453.

Viswanathan PC, Bezzina CR, George AL Jr, et al. Gating-dependent mechanisms for flecainide action in SCN5A-linked arrhythmia syndromes. *Circulation.* 2001;104(10):1200–1205.

Vyas H, Hejlik J, Ackerman MJ. Epinephrine QT stress testing in the evaluation of congenital long-QT syndrome: diagnostic accuracy of the paradoxical QT response. *Circulation.* 2006;113(11):1385–1392.

Watkins H, Rosenzweig A, Hwang DS, et al. Characteristics and prognostic implications of myosin missense mutations in familial hypertrophic cardiomyopathy. *N Engl J Med.* 1992;326(17):1108–1114.

Westenskow P, Splawski I, Timothy KW, Keating MT, Sanguinetti MC. Compound mutations: a common cause of severe long-QT syndrome. *Circulation.* 2004;109(15):1834–1841.

Yan GX, Lankipalli RS, Burke JF, Musco S, Kowey PR. Ventricular repolarization components on the electrocardiogram: cellular basis and clinical significance. *J Am Coll Cardiol.* 2003;42(3):401–409.

Yokoi H, Makita N, Sasaki K, et al. Double SCN5A mutation underlying asymptomatic Brugada syndrome. *Heart Rhythm.* 2005;2(3):285–292.

Zareba W, Moss AJ, Daubert JP, Hall WJ, Robinson JL, Andrews M. Implantable cardioverter defibrillator in high-risk long QT syndrome patients. *J Cardiovasc Electrophysiol.* 2003a;14(4):337–341.

Zareba W, Moss AJ, Locati EH, et al. Modulating effects of age and gender on the clinical course of long QT syndrome by genotype. *J Am Coll Cardiol.* 2003b;42(1):103–109.

Zareba W, Moss AJ, Schwartz PJ, et al. Influence of genotype on the clinical course of the long-QT syndrome. International Long-QT Syndrome Registry Research Group. *N Engl J Med.* 1998;339(14):960–965.

Zhang L, Timothy KW, Vincent GM, et al. Spectrum of ST-T-wave patterns and repolarization parameters in congenital long-QT syndrome: ECG findings identify genotypes. *Circulation.* 2000;102(23):2849–2855.

34

Cardiovascular Pharmacogenomics

Martin C Michel and Dieter Rosskopf

Introduction

What Discriminates Pharmacogenetics from the Genetics of Diseases?

The term *pharmaceogenetics* was coined in the 1950s to describe how some mutant alleles and variations in DNA sequence affect drug disposition or drug action (Motulsky 1957). Identification of a number of Mendelian phenotypes that influence specific drug responses led to some changes in clinical practice. For example, avoidance of primaquine-related drugs in G6PD deficient persons, and restrictive prescribing in patients with acute intermittent porphyria. Greater understanding of the pharmacodynamics of certain drugs helped to minimize the risks of unpleasant side effects, for example, the risk of peripheral neuropathy related to isoniazid antitubercular therapy in slow acetylator individuals. A major shift happened in the early 1990s with rapid advances in genome sciences and new technologies. The term *pharmacogenomics* was then introduced. In contrast to pharmacogenetics, pharmacogenomics refers to the study of the whole genome (genomics, genome-wide analysis), transcriptome, and proteome in order to elucidate disease genes, design drugs, and identify drug targets in specific patient populations. This field received a major boost with the sequencing of the human genome and a number of eukaryotic and prokaryotic genomes. The rapid and powerful developments in bioinformatics, comparative genomics, and several other *omics* have helped enhanced drug discovery and development. Although many authors still use pharmacogenetics and pharmacogenomics interchangeably, pharmacogenomics is the preferred term.

Most chapters in this book cover genetic aspects of cardiovascular diseases. Some chapters relate to monogenic disorders representing for the most part rare syndromes with distinct phenotypes. Here, causal mutations facilitate predictive (deterministic) genetic testing (at least for the family) and provide clues to disease pathophysiology. Other chapters of this book focus on common cardiovascular diseases with complex genetics. In these cases, numerous common genetic polymorphisms [e.g., single nucleotide polymorphisms (SNPs) or insertion/deletion (I/D) variants] have been identified, the alleles of which are differentially distributed between cases and controls. In some instances, analyses of the variant alleles allow for probabilistic estimations of disease risks although these remain controversial.

In this new era of personalized medicine, pharmacogenetics and pharmacogenomics[1] attempt to provide genetic explanations for the observed variances in beneficial and adverse drug effects between individuals. For example, responder rates for contemporary cardiovascular drugs vary between 10% and 90% depending on the definition of therapeutic success (Table 34–1; Figure 34–1). Likewise, susceptibilities to (serious) adverse drug reactions from common drugs vary considerably between individuals. Major drug toxicity accounts for about 2 million hospitalizations per year for serious adverse drug reactions (SADR) and to 100,000 deaths (the fourth leading cause of death in the United States) (Lazarou et al. 1998; Giacomini et al. 2007). Drug responses and toxicities are affected by a multitude of factors including age, sex, body composition, hepatic and renal function, smoking and drinking habits, physical exercise, drug interactions, and adherence to therapy. Nevertheless, genetic mechanisms also contribute significantly to interindividual variances in drug responses. Historically, prime concepts in the field of pharmacogenetics were established on two cardiovascular drugs, the antihypertensive sympatholytic debrisoquine and the antiarrhythmic sparteine (both no longer on the market) for profound genetically determined toxicities (Mahgoub et al. 1977; Eichelbaum et al. 1979; Gonzalez et al. 1988; see also Figure 34–2).

Available evidence suggests that complex genetic diseases display genetic heterogeneity, that is, different genes (or risk variants of different genes) in conjunction with lifestyle factors can lead to the same disease (e.g., hypertension, coronary artery disease; Figure 34–2, upper panel). If a certain drug interacts with a gene variant or pathophysiological pathways directly linked to it, disease gene variants may also govern drug responses. One of the rare examples identified so far is

[1] The term *Pharmacogenetics* was used initially to describe how variations in DNA sequence translate in altered drug disposition or drug action. In contrast, the coverage of *Pharmacogenomics* includes the whole genome (genomics, genome-wide analysis), transcriptome and proteome to elucidate disease genes, design drugs and identify drug targets to specific patient populations. Meanwhile, many authors use *Pharmacogenetics* and *Pharmacogenomics* interchangeably or prefer the term *Pharmacogenomics* for common usage."

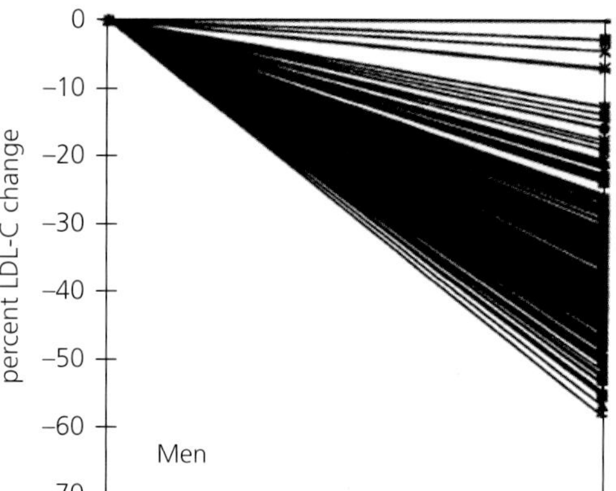

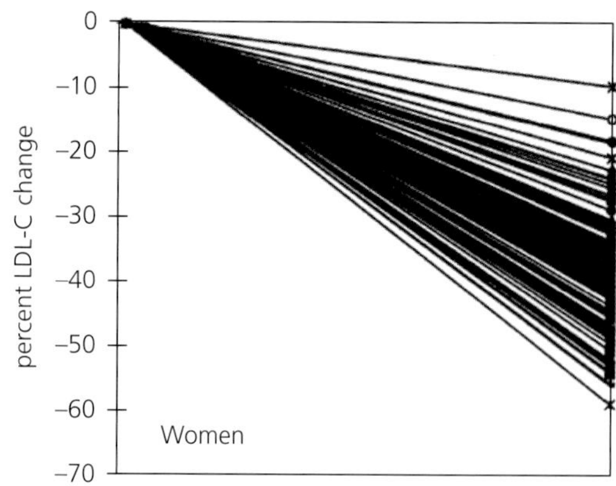

Figure 34–1 Example for varying responder rates. Individual response to a therapy with 10 mg atorvastatin in 195 men and 133 females with hypercholesterolemia. Depicted is the relative decrease in LDL-cholesterol after a therapy with atorvastatin for 1 year. The figure underscores the high variability in the lipid-lowering therapies. From Pedro-Botet et al. 2001 with permission (Atherosclerosis/Elsevier).

Table 34–1 Nonresponder Rates to Drugs Commonly Used in Cardiovascular Patients

Class of Drugs	No or Insufficient Response (%)
ACE inhibitors (heart failure)	10–30
Amiodaron (ventricular tachycardia)	20–30
β-Blockers (heart failure)	15–25
HMG-CoA reductase inhibitors (hypercholesterolemia)	30–70
Antihypertensives (monotherapy); essential hypertension	40–60
β_2-Adrenoceptor agonists; asthma	40–70
Transdermal nicotin; 1 year abstinence	80–90

Note: The classification of "response or nonresponse depends, as a categorical variable, on the definition of relevant effect thresholds explaining the considerable variation shown.
Source: Adapted from Lindpaintner (2002); Eichelbaum et al. (2006); Haefeli (2007).

Liddle's syndrome, a form of monogenic hypertension caused by an inappropriately increased insertion of epithelial sodium channels into the luminal membrane of the cortical collecting duct, ultimately favoring sodium reabsorption and hypertension. Specific blockade of these channels with amiloride or triamterene effectively lowers the increased blood pressure, an effect not observable with these drugs in common forms of hypertension (Rosskopf et al. 2007).

While many genes can contribute to the pathophysiology of a clinical condition, the number of genes potentially involved in mediating effects of a medication tends to be smaller. Typically, they include the gene encoding the molecular target of a drug, for example, the receptor it acts on, and genes involved in its pharmacokinetics, in most cases its metabolism. In some cases, polymorphisms in genes related to the intracellular signal transduction of the drug target may also contribute, but until now this has received little attention (Figure 34–3).

In this chapter we consider pharmacogenetically relevant genes that affect drug action (i.e., *pharmacodynamics*) and the fate of the drug in the organism (i.e., *pharmacokinetics*; Figure 34–3). While these concepts predominantly relate to *therapeutic drug responses,* the situation becomes more complex when the genetics of *adverse drug reactions* are considered. For example, genetically determined alterations in the pharmacodynamics or pharmacokinetics can lead to a toxic increase of the beneficial drug effect (e.g., severe bradycardia upon administration of standard doses of β-agonists). Such reactions are in principle predictable. Drugs also interact with many different additional proteins beside their main drug target and thus cause severe adverse drug reactions that are unrelated to the drugs' main effects. Variants in such unidentified additional "drug targets" can cause an increased susceptibility to these reactions, frequently precipitated by increases in the drug's plasma concentration due to drug interactions, altered lifestyle habits or variants in pharmacokinetically relevant genes. Some of these adverse reactions occur rather frequently (e.g., cough in patients receiving ACE inhibitors). Finally, drugs can cause rare unexplained (idiosyncratic) severe adverse drug reactions such as severe skin reactions, liver failure, and bone marrow disorders. It is plausible that (immuno)genetic mechanisms may contribute to these severe incidents. Efforts are under way to establish a multinational consortium to collect such cases and finally generate the power for refined genetic analyses (Giacomini et al. 2007). Discussion of such rare incidences exceeds the scope of this chapter. Figure 34–4 summarizes the concepts introduced so far.

Pharmacodynamics versus Pharmacokinetics

Within the discipline of pharmacology, two main branches can be distinguished, pharmacodynamics and pharmacokinetics. Pharmacodynamics primarily deals with the question of what a given drug will do to an organism. This relates to the receptors, enzymes, or other molecular targets on which a drug acts as well as other molecules that are involved in the effects of such targets. In this regard, pharmacogenetics studies clearly show how gene polymorphisms in drug targets or their downstream pathways affect drug responses. Genetic polymorphisms in drug targets may be more important for agonists/activators of these targets than for antagonists/inhibitors. There are two key reasons for this: first, if a polymorphism affects the expressed number or activity of a receptor, this will almost always alter the response to an agonist acting on it. On the other hand, the same polymorphism will only affect antagonist responses in the absence of agonist if

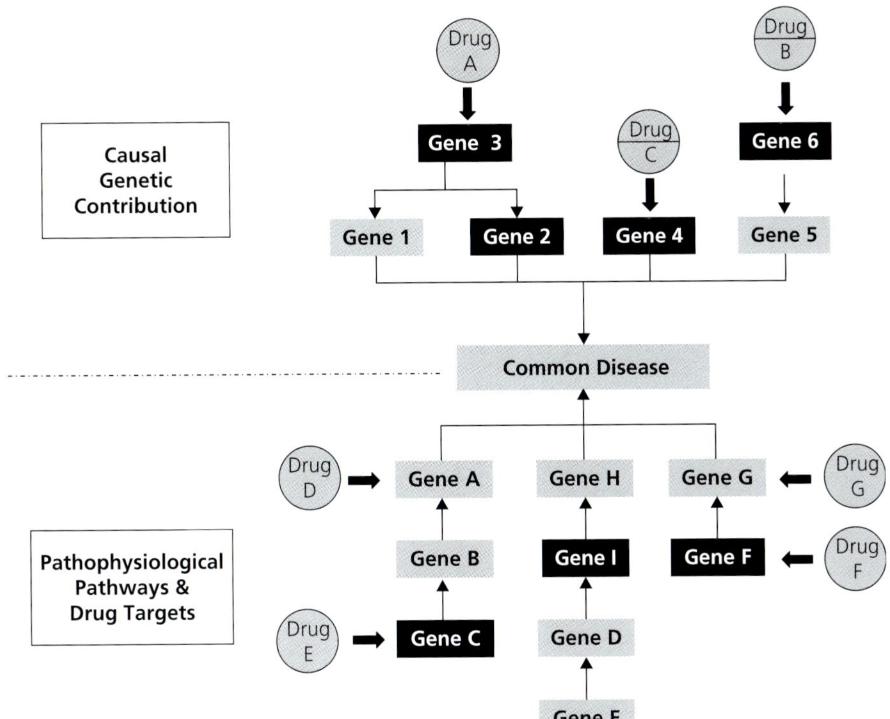

Figure 34–2 Genetic variants and drug actions. Conceptual scheme of how genetic variants affect the therapeutic response to a given drug in common diseases. Many complex diseases exhibit genetic heterogeneity. Drugs may vary in their therapeutic effect depending on their respective actions on the predominant causal mechanisms (upper panel). More frequently, drugs modify pathophysiological pathways involved in the course of the disease. Genetic variants in such target genes affect the therapeutic response to a given drug.

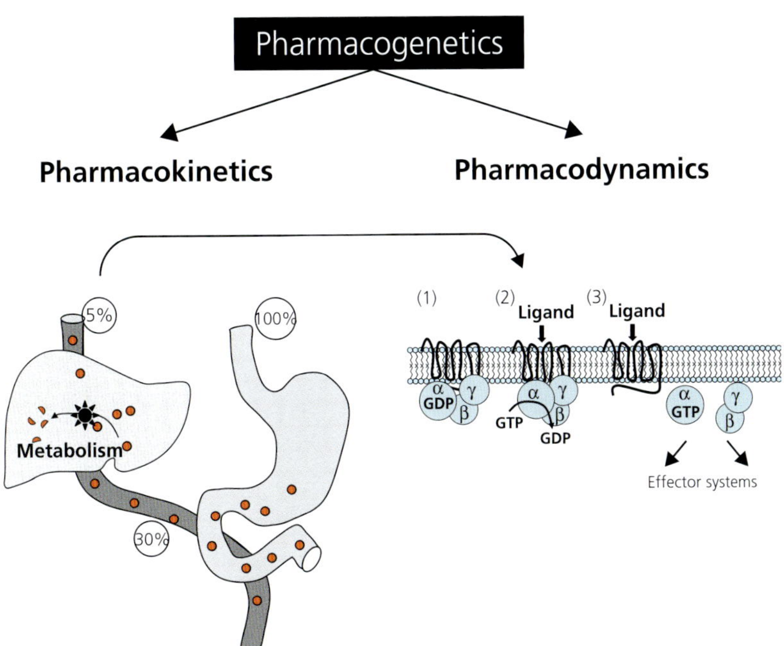

Figure 34–3 Basic distinction of pharmacogenetically relevant systems. *Pharmacokinetics* (left panel) describes how the organism governs the fate of a drug. After *liberation* of the compound from its galenic preparation in the stomach or in the intestine, the drug is *absorbed* in the intestine, frequently by specific drug transporters. While uptake transporters mediate the entry into the enterocyte, efflux pumps mediate the passage from the enterocyte into the portal blood or in a protective mode–back into the enteric lumen. Enterocyte also exhibit considerable *metabolic* activity leading to inactivation or in some instances to the activation of a drug. The central organ for drug metabolism is the liver. Numbers indicate how *metabolic processes* in the gut wall and in the liver affect the fraction of the active compound of a hypothetic drug with low bioavailability (e.g., a statin). Genetic variants in such drug metabolizing enzymes and in drug transporters can distinctly affect the plasma concentration of a given drug. For reasons of simplicity, other pharmacokinetic processes (renal and biliary *elimination*, passages through functional barriers, e.g., the blood–brain barrier, have been omitted). *Pharmacodynamics* (right panel) deals with the actions of a drug on its target structure (here an example for a G-protein-coupled receptor and its downstream effector systems) on molecular, cellular, and systemic levels. Genetic variants in drug targets and their subsequent pathways affect drug responses.

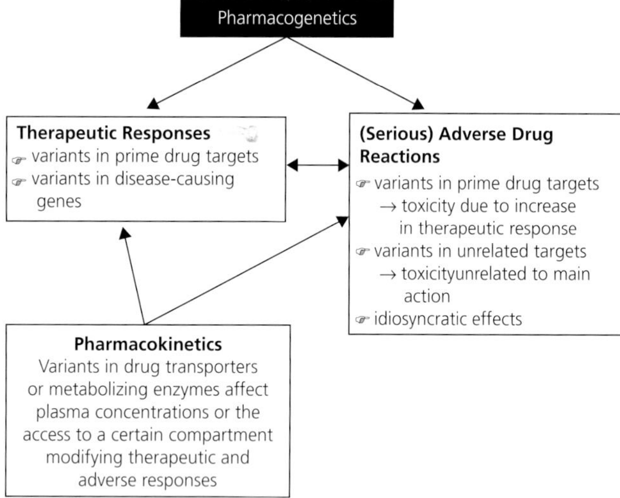

Figure 34–4 Genetic mechanisms affecting drug responses and adverse effects. Genetic variants can affect both therapeutic responses and adverse effects of a specific drug. An increased sensitivity of a key drug target can lead to an improved drug response, which may also manifest as an already toxic effect (e.g., severe bradycardia after administration of β-blockers). Individual susceptibilities for adverse effects unrelated to the main action of the drug may arise from variants in secondary "targets. Alterations in pharmacokinetic mechanisms (drug metabolism or drug transport) may further modify these effects by increasing the plasma concentration to toxic levels.

the antagonist is an inverse agonist[2] and the receptor exhibits relevant constitutive activity. Second, agonists are typically dosed to occupy only a small fraction of receptors, and hence changes in their responsiveness will easily manifest clinically. On the other hand, antagonists and inhibitors are often dosed to largely or even fully occupy a given receptor or enzyme; under these conditions even a major change in receptor activity may not figure prominently as the target is still inhibited. While these key principles of molecular pharmacodynamics apply to many situations some modifications may occur, particularly in clinical settings under chronic dosage regimes. Here, an identical receptor variant may cause an *increased acute* response upon single dose application but may also lead to *enhanced* receptor desensitization processes and, ultimately, to *reduced* responses upon chronic administration, which limits our ability to predict chronic in vivo effects from short-term in vitro investigations. Polymorphisms affecting the β_1- or β_2-adrenoceptor are good examples to illustrate this (see the respective sections).

Pharmacokinetics refers to the effect of an organism on a drug. This includes the processes of absorption, metabolism, distribution, and elimination of a drug. Many of the enzymes and transporters involved in such processes exhibit genetic variability. Thus, variants of the respective genes affect how much of a drug or its metabolites and how long they are available at a given target which, ultimately, contributes to quantitative drug responses. While classical teaching highlighted physicochemical properties of drugs to pass barriers (e.g., from intestine into portal blood), recent developments underscore the significance of highly controlled transport processes that govern the entry of drugs from one compartment (e.g., blood) into another (e.g., the liver cell or the brain). Genetic variants in these systems may have profound effects on individual drug disposition.

Phylogenetically, many metabolizing enzymes and transport proteins evolved to tackle xenobiotics (including drugs) from the environment in order to protect the internal milieu from potentially toxic compounds. Interestingly, many of them have a dual role for endogenous metabolism. Considering the ample chemical diversity of potential foreign substances it is plausible that drug metabolizing enzymes and drug transporters can interact with diverse classes of chemical compounds. This is in contrast to the usually high chemical selectivity of pharmacodynamic drug targets. An advantage of this lower specificity in pharmacokinetic mechanisms for pharmacogenetic research is the possibility to translate evidence about genetic variants in a certain transporter or enzyme obtained with compound A to another compound B, given that it is also a substrate for the respective protein. This further explains why *pharmacokinetic variants* frequently exhibit a pleiotropic pharmacogenetic phenotype, that is, they affect the pharmacokinetics of members of different classes of drugs (e.g., variants in the metabolizing enzyme CYP2D6 affect β-adrenoceptor antagonists, analgesics, antidepressants, neuroleptics, antiarrhythmics). On the other hand, individual members of the same class of drugs (e.g., β-adrenoceptor antagonists, diuretics) may undergo quite different drug metabolism. Hence, genetic variants in pharmacokinetic systems may affect only certain members of a drug class[3]. In contrast, in the pharmacodynamic branch of pharmacogenetics all members of a certain drug class are generally affected similarly from variants in drug targets irrespective of their chemical structure. However, there are exceptions to this rule based upon novel concepts of ligand-directed signaling (also known as biased agonism or protean agonism), which predicts that individual compounds acting on the same receptor will have somewhat different binding pockets within the receptor and, hence, be differentially affected by genetic polymorphisms (Mailman 2007; Michel and Alewijnse 2007). This concept has not been thoroughly tested yet within the framework of pharmacogenetics, but initial examples indicate that it may be relevant in some cases (Rochais et al. 2007).

The limited specificity of metabolizing enzymes and drug transporters explains why these systems can handle a wide variety of xenobiotics as already described. On the other hand, it also illustrates why many drugs are handled by multiple enzymes or transporters and the reason why an altered activity of one of them remains frequently clinically silent as it can be compensated for by the activity of other enzymes. Hence, some pharmacokinetically relevant genetic variants lead to an observable phenotype only for compounds that are predominantly (frequently more

[2] Many receptors are not "silent in the absence of an agonist but display some activity in their basal state. Pure antagonists do not affect the activity of a receptor but prevent an agonist from binding to the receptor (or from activating it). "Inverse antagonists can further diminish the basal activity of a receptor by stabilizing its resting inactive state. Receptor variants can differ in their basal activity and can react differentially to inverse agonists.

[3] The fact that different members of a drug class undergo various metabolic pathways and, thus, have differential susceptibilities for common variants in drug metabolizing enzymes (e.g. CYP2D6) has led to "defensive pharmacogenetics during drug development. Lead compounds and their derivatives are preferred—provided similar pharmacodynamic actions—that do not undergo highly polymorphic metabolism. This procedure reduces the risk for genetically determined toxicities and facilitates dosage recommendation (in the case of CYP2D6 variants, necessary dosages for the same plasma concentration may vary more than a hundredfold, which makes sensible dosage recommendations difficult being applicable only to the majority of a population).

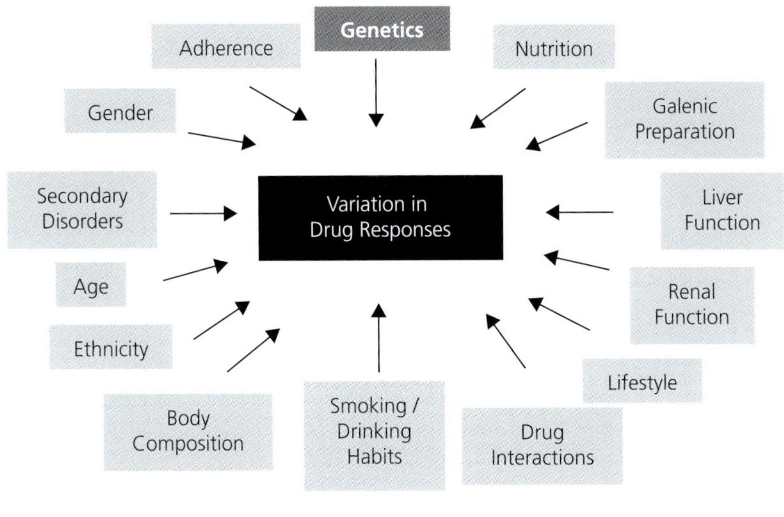

Figure 34–5 Pharmacologic variability, nature, and nurture. The prediction of pharmacologic responses and the explanation of the observed interindividual variability is key concern of pharmacogenetics. This simple scheme illustrates that genetic mechanisms—despite their importance—are a single facet in a complex scenario only. Of note, in *real life* a complex pattern of interactions between these factors (and many more) exists.

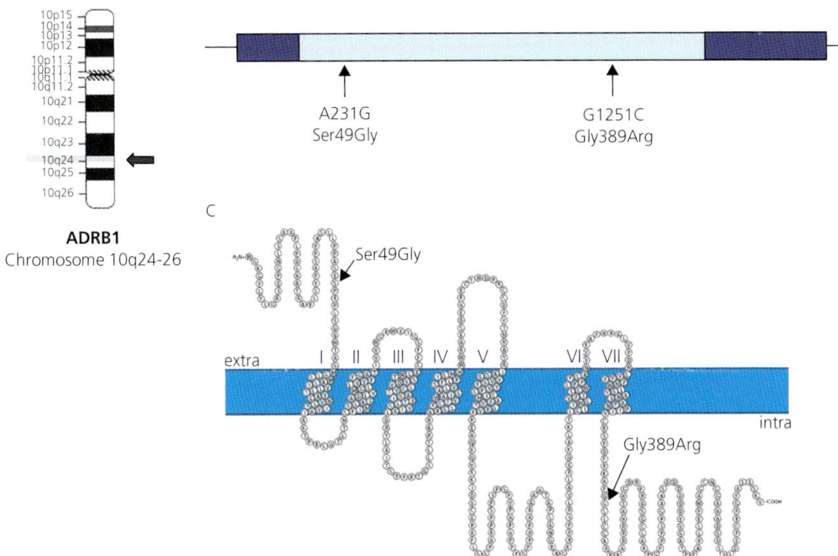

Figure 34–6 Genetics and secondary structure of the β_1-adrenoceptor (ADRB1). This gene is located on chromosome 10 (A) and comprises a single exon (B). Two important common variants exist, Ser49Gly and Gly389Arg. The β_1-adrenoceptor is a typical G protein-coupled receptor comprising seven transmembrane domains (C). The position of the Ser49Gly variant faces the extracellular space while the localization of the Gly389Arg variant is confined to the C terminus, which is implicated in the interaction with G proteins for further signaling.

than 90%) metabolized by a single pathway with no compensatory mechanisms.

On the basis of these introductory remarks we divide the following chapter into two main sections on *pharmacodynamics* and *pharmacokinetics*. The aim is to focus on key concepts of pharmacogenetics and to present instructive examples of prototypical relevance to everyday clinical practice. Despite this focus on genetic and thus *nonmodifiable* mechanisms, one should keep in mind that a major part of such variability arises from simple *modifiable* causes including patient compliance, underlying diagnosis, drug-drug interactions, dosage, and secondary disorders (Figure 34–5).

Genetic Factors Related to Pharmacodynamics

β-Adrenoceptor Agents

The human genome contains three β-adrenoceptor subtypes designated β_1, β_2, and β_3, each encoded by a distinct gene (Bylund et al. 1994). β-Adrenoceptor ligands are used in cardiovascular medicine to treat a range of conditions. Antagonists, mainly targeting β_1-adrenoceptors, are used for the treatment of coronary heart disease, heart failure, arterial hypertension, and arrhythmias and for the prevention of myocardial infarction. Agonists mainly targeting β_1-adrenoceptors are used for acute inotropic support. Selective β_2-adrenoceptors are used in the treatment of obstructive airway disease, where they can have cardiovascular side effects related to vasodilatation. Drugs acting specifically on β_3-adrenoceptors have not yet been introduced into cardiovascular medicine or medicine in general. Polymorphisms have been identified in each of the three β-adrenoceptor genes (Leineweber et al. 2004).

1. β_1-Adrenoceptor Ligands

Several polymorphisms have been described in the human β_1-adrenoceptor gene, of which Ser49Gly and Gly389Arg have been studied most intensively (Leineweber et al. 2004; Figure 34–6). These two SNPs are in linkage disequilibrium, and a haplotype with a homozygous Gly in both positions exists very rarely if at all. The two SNPs are found in about 25% and 27%, respectively, of Caucasian populations (Leineweber et al. 2004), but a somewhat different prevalence has been reported for other ethnicities (Moore et al. 1999; Xie et al. 2001; Belfer et al. 2005; Nonen et al. 2005). Other SNPs within the coding region of the β_1-adrenoceptor gene, such as Ala59Ser, Arg399Cys, His402Arg, Thr404Ala, or Pro418Ala, have allele frequencies of only about 1%, and little information is available about their functional role, particularly with regard to drug action (Leineweber et al. 2004). The functional relevance of the polymorphisms in position 49 and 389 has been studied using transfected cells, isolated tissues from genotyped subjects, clinical pharmacology studies in such subjects, and in patients.

One in vitro study based upon site-directed mutagenesis using physiological expression levels reported that the Ser49 and Gly49 variants respond very similarly to agonists, but that the Gly49 variant is more susceptible to agonist-induced down-regulation (Rathz et al. 2002). Another study using higher and probably supraphysiological expression levels found the Gly49 variant to be constitutively active (Levin et al. 2002); while this was also associated with a greater susceptibility to agonist-induced down-regulation, it also revealed stronger inhibitory responses to the inverse agonist metoprolol. An enhanced susceptibility toward agonist-induced down-regulation may not only manifest during extended treatment with exogenous agonists but may also, due to the presence of endogenous agonist particularly during states of chronically enhanced sympathoadrenal activity, lead to lower expression density in vivo. In contrast, studies comparing the Gly389 and Arg389 variants in vitro upon heterologous expression found that the Gly389 variant exhibited a less effective coupling to the G_s protein and adenylyl cyclase stimulation (Mason et al. 1999). More recent studies reported that the β-adrenoceptor antagonists bisoprolol and metoprolol exhibited similar inverse agonism at both variants, whereas carvedilol showed significantly greater inverse agonism at the Arg389 variant (Rochais et al. 2007). Within the same study, carvedilol also had greater inhibitory effects on spontaneously beating cardiomyocytes transfected with the Arg389 as compared to the Gly389 variant.

These experiments with transfected cells have been extended to ex vivo work with isolated human tissues from genotyped subjects. Using right atria from patients undergoing coronary bypass grafting, one group of investigators demonstrated that the Gly389 variant of the β_1-adrenoceptor was associated with smaller cAMP and inotropic responses (Sandilands et al. 2003), but other investigators did not confirm such differences (Molenaar et al. 2002; Sarsero et al. 2003). Similarly, both genotypes were reported to be associated with similar lipolytic responses to β-adrenergic stimulation in human adipocytes (Ryden et al. 2001).

The next level of evidence is based upon studies in which in vivo responses have been explored in (mostly healthy) genotyped subjects where β-adrenoceptor agonists and antagonists were administered under experimental conditions with measurement of well-defined hemodynamic or hormonal outcome parameters. Some studies have also used endogenously released noradrenaline, as induced by bicycle exercise, to explore the role of β_1-adrenoceptor polymorphisms. Four different studies reported that the Gly389Arg SNP does not affect heart rate, or inotropic or plasma renin activity responses to bicycle exercise (Büscher et al. 2001; Xie et al. 2001; Liu et al. 2003; Sofowora et al. 2003). Similarly, two studies published in abstract form reported that this SNP does affect heart rate or renin response to infusion of the agonist dobutamine, although one of them reported a polymorphism effect on cardiac contractility (Leineweber et al. 2004). On the other hand, it was found in two studies from the same group of investigators that the Gly389Arg SNP was associated with greater reductions of resting heart rate upon administration of atenolol (Sofowora et al. 2003) or metoprolol (Liu et al. 2003).

While lacking direct clinical relevance, the above in vivo studies with healthy volunteers provide mechanistic insight and are an important bridge to the second group of in vivo studies, that is, those measuring clinical outcomes in treated patients. Thus, in confirmation of the healthy volunteer studies, it was reported that the Arg389 genotype was associated with threefold greater metoprolol-induced blood pressure lowering in hypertensive patients (Johnson et al. 2003). Extending these observations to a different phenotype/disease, it was found that Arg389 was also associated with greater improvements of ventricular function upon treatment with the antagonist carvedilol, and similar observations were also made in transgenic mice (Mialat Perez et al. 2003). Similarly, the Arg389Gly polymorphism was also linked to a need for more heart failure medications in metoprolol-treated patients (Terra et al. 2005) or the demand for inotropic catecholamine support following coronary artery bypass grafting (Leineweber et al. 2007).

In conclusion, these data demonstrate that the Gly389 variant of the β_1-adrenoceptor is hypofunctional. Its presence is consistently associated with differences in responses to β-adrenoceptor antagonists, whereas associations with altered agonist responses have been less consistent. While this may be less relevant for the treatment of hypertension, which is driven by the clinical response to be observed within reasonably short time intervals, it may become important for the long-term treatment of congestive heart failure, if the clinical findings in that population can be confirmed by independent investigators.

2. β_2-Adrenoceptor Ligands

Also within the β_2-adrenoceptor gene multiple polymorphisms have been described, among which Arg16Gly, Gln27Glu, and Thr164Ile have been best investigated (Leineweber et al. 2004; Figure 34–7). Among these the Ile164 genotype is rare and has never been reported to occur in a homozygous manner. In contrast Gly16 and Glu27 are each present in about 40% of Caucasian populations but a somewhat different prevalence may exist in other ethnic groups (Hawkins et al. 2006; Lima et al. 2006; Wu et al. 2006). More than a dozen additional SNPs have been reported from the β_2-adrenoceptor gene, but many of them are rare and the available knowledge on their functional relevance is limited for all of them (Leineweber et al. 2004). In contrast, the Arg16Gly, Gln27Glu, and Thr164Ile SNPs have been studied extensively using transfected cells, isolated cells, and tissues from genotyped subjects, clinical pharmacology experiments, and studies with clinical endpoints.

In vitro studies based upon site-directed mutagenesis indicate that Ile164 variant is hypofunctional, that is, exhibits lower agonist affinity in radioligand binding studies and reduced maximal adenylyl cyclase stimulation (Green et al. 1993). On the other hand, the Arg16Gly or Gln27Glu SNPs apparently did not affect agonist affinity or basal or isoprenaline-stimulated adenylyl cyclase activity (Green et al. 1994). However, the Gly16 variant was shown to be more susceptible to agonist-induced down-regulation, whereas the Glu27 variant confers relative resistance to agonist-induced down-regulation (Green et al. 1994). If the two SNPs occur in combination, the Gly16 effects dominate the phenotype, that is, a Gly16/Glu27 double mutant also exhibits enhanced agonist-induced down-regulation; in contrast, the Arg16/Glu27 double mutant was completely resistant to down-regulation (Green et al. 1994).

Ex vivo studies from genotyped subjects have been performed with circulating mononuclear cells (mostly lymphocytes), airway

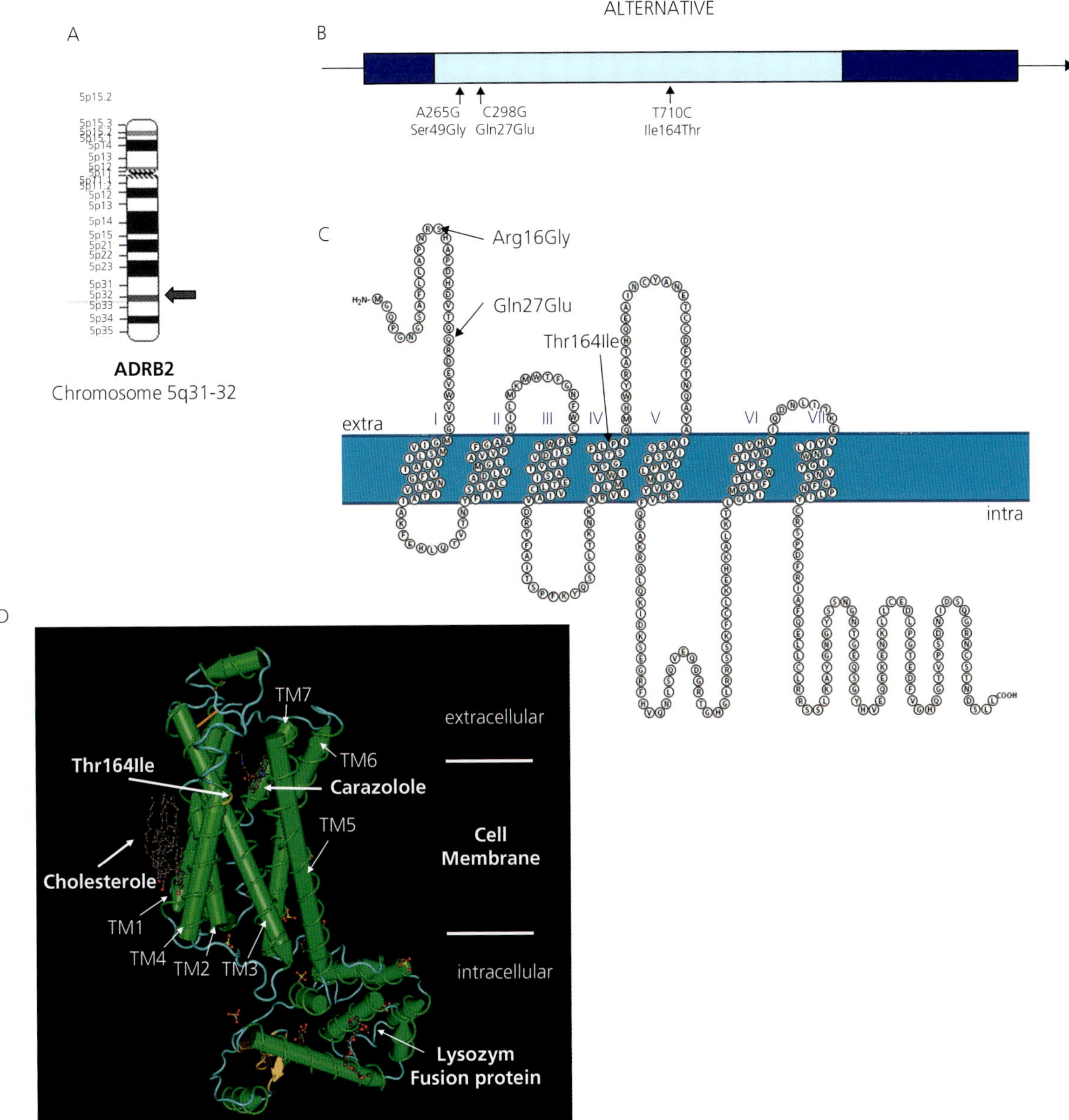

Figure 34–7 Genetics and secondary structure of the β_2-adrenoceptor (ADRB2). This gene is located on chromosome 5 (A) and comprises a single exon (B). Three well-characterized common variants exist, Arg16Gly, Gln27Glu, and Thr164Ile. The β_1-adrenoceptor is a typical G protein-coupled receptor comprising seven transmembrane domains (C). The positions of the Arg16Gly and the Gln27Glu variants face the extracellular space. The position of the Thr164Ile has been predicted to localize to the fourth transmembrane domain. These transmembrane domains are not only important for the insertion of the protein into the cell membrane but are also essential for the correct formation of the binding pocket of the ligand. (D) The predicted localization of the variant Thr164Ile has been confirmed by the recent crystallization and structural analysis of transmembrane domains of the β2-adrenergic receptor, the first available structural analysis of a eukaryotic G protein-coupled receptor. The variants Arg16Gly and Gln27Glu are located on a disordered stretch of amino acids facing the extracellular space that was not amenable to crystallization. For technical reasons a fusion protein of the β_2-adrenoceptor with lysozyme was analyzed. Carazolole is an inverse agonist at the β_2-adrenoceptor. This structure displays the vicinity of the Thr164Ile variant to the binding pocket of the receptor. Figure (D) has been generated with the program Cn3D 4.1 (http://www.ncbi.nlm.nih.gov/Structure/CN3D/cn3d.shtml) using the structure coordinates published by Cherezov et al. (2007) and Rasmussen et al. (2007).

smooth muscle cells, lung mast cells, and adipocytes. Neither the Arg16Gly nor the Gln27Glu SNP appears to affect β_2-adrenoceptor expression (Lipworth et al. 1999). Correspondingly, all available studies indicate that these two SNPs do not affect basal or maximally stimulated adenylyl cyclase activity (Large et al. 1997; Lipworth et al. 1999; Moore et al. 2000; Bruck et al. 2003a). On the other hand, and in line with the findings from transfected cells, the Gly16 genotype exhibited greater agonist-induced desensitization in human airway smooth muscle cells (Moore et al. 2000), although that was not confirmed in a study on human lung mast cells (Chong et al. 2000). A greater agonist-induced desensitization was reported for the Glu27 variant in human airway smooth muscle cells (Moore et al. 2000), whereas less desensitization was found for the same genotype in human lung mast cells (Chong et al. 2000). These data suggest the possibility that the effects of SNPs in the amino terminus of the β_2-adrenoceptor may depend on the cell type in which it is expressed. In contrast, the Thr164Ile SNP (Figure 34–7), even if present only in heterozygotes, was consistently associated with lower potency and/or maximal responses to various β-adrenoceptor agonists in lymphocytes (Büscher et al. 2002), human lung mast cells (Kay et al. 2003), or adipocytes (Hoffstedt et al. 2001).

As few indications exist in cardiovascular medicine for the use of β_2-adrenoceptor agonists, the available in vivo studies largely relate to the experimental use of agonists under well-defined conditions. They have looked at both cardiac (heart rate and contractility) and vascular responsiveness (arterial and venous vasodilatation). Except for one study using salbutamol, which also had elevated baseline values (Gratze et al. 1999), most investigators report a lack of effect of the Arg16Gly or the Gln27Glu SNP on cardiac responsiveness to agonists such as terbutaline (Hoit et al. 2000; Bruck et al. 2003a). With regard to vascular responsiveness, multiple studies demonstrate that the Gln27Glu SNP is associated with higher responsiveness (Cockroft et al. 2000; Dishy et al. 2001), whereas reports on the Arg16Gly SNP are equivocal with lower responsiveness (Gratze et al. 1999; Hoit et al. 2000), no difference (Dishy et al. 2001), or higher responsiveness being reported (Cockroft et al. 2000; Garovic et al. 2003). This apparent contradiction with the in vitro data could be explained by the finding that β_2-adrenoceptors are always exposed to some down-regulation stimuli by endogenous agonist, and the relative resistance toward agonist-induced down-regulation may result in greater responses. In agreement with the in vitro data, the Ile164 variant of the β_2-adrenoceptor was associated with reduced heart rate and contractile in vivo responses to terbutaline in healthy volunteers (Bruck et al. 2003c).

Other studies have assessed whether any of the above genotypes are also associated with alterations in in vivo desensitization upon extended agonist treatment, but the results have remained equivocal. In contrast to some in vitro and ex vivo studies (see above), the Arg16 rather than the Gly16 variant of the β_2-adrenoceptor was reported to be associated with enhanced short-term agonist-induced desensitization in studies using the dorsal hand vein technique (Dishy et al. 2001). In other studies, volunteers were treated orally with terbutaline for up to 2 weeks with subsequent assessment of chronotropic and inotropic response to intravenous terbutaline (Bruck et al. 2003b). In these experiments neither the Arg16Gly nor the Gln27Glu polymorphism affected the extent of agonist-induced desensitization, but the Glu27 homozygotes exhibited a slower desensitization than the other groups. The same group of investigators also reported similar findings for the in vivo down-regulation of lymphocyte β_2-adrenoceptors (Bruck et al. 2003a). On the other hand, the Ile164 variant was not associated with an altered agonist-induced desensitization (Bruck et al. 2003c).

Taken together, the rare Ile164 variant of the β_2-adrenoceptor was consistently reported to be hypofunctional, even in heterozygotes. In contrast, polymorphisms in positions 16 and 27 of the receptor have little direct influence on receptor function; however, they may be associated with alterations in the speed of agonist-induced receptor desensitization but the currently available data are not unequivocal. Overall, β_2-adrenoceptor polymorphisms may not have direct implications for treatment of cardiovascular disease but, if anything, may be associated with quantitative differences in adverse event occurrence. However, they highlight the problem that findings in transfected cells, ex vivo preparations and in vivo responses are not always congruent, and that the impact of genetic factors needs to be assessed at each of those levels.

Angiotensin System and Diuretics

1. Angiotensin-Converting Enzyme Inhibitors

Inhibitors of the angiotensin-converting enzyme (ACE) are used in the treatment of arterial hypertension, congestive heart failure, and for the prevention of diabetic nephropathy. The ACE gene is polymorphic, and an I/D polymorphism of 287 base pairs in intron 16 is the best investigated polymorphism in this gene (Rosskopf et al. 2007; Figure 34–8). The D allele of this polymorphism is associated with a greater enzyme activity (Marre et al. 1994). However, this I/D polymorphism may not directly cause increased enzyme activity but, rather, is in linkage disequilibrium with other polymorphisms directly affecting enzyme activity. In this regard the A2350G SNP shows a tighter correlation with ACE activity than the I/D polymorphism (Narita et al. 2003). However, only little information is available on the role of this SNP in drug responses and most studies have focused on the above I/D polymorphism.

Associations between ACE genotype and clinical response to ACE inhibitors have been tested for a range of diseases. While most studies have focused on blood pressure lowering, many others have looked at prevention of nephropathy (particularly in the context of diabetes) or other uses for this drug class. Associations between I/D genotype and blood pressure responses have been tested for a range of ACE inhibitors including benazepril, captopril, enalapril,

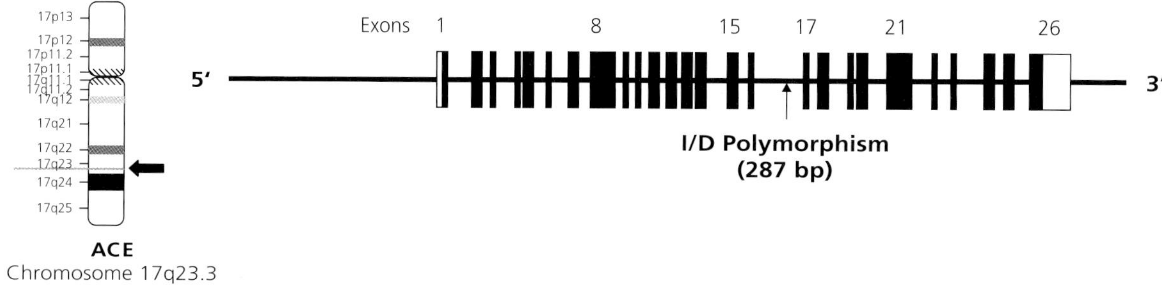

Figure 34–8 Gene structure of the human ACE gene. The ACE gene localized to chromosome 17 harbors 26 exons. Most frequently an insertion/deletion polymorphism in intron 16 has been analyzed. Available evidence suggests that additional polymorphisms confined to the region from exon 17 to exon 26 and potentially in the promoter region, which are in linkage disequilibrium to the insertion/deletion polymorphisms, constitute "causal variants.

fosinopril, quinapril, imidapril, and lisinopril. With regard to the clinical response of blood pressure lowering, a systematic review has reported that out of 11 studies, the D allele was associated with greater ACE inhibitor-induced blood pressure lowering in three studies, whereas it was associated with smaller blood pressure lowering in four other studies; four studies found no difference between genotypes (Koopmans et al. 2003). Using a somewhat different search strategy, other investigators yielded similar conclusions (Mellen and Herrington 2005). However, many of the underlying original studies had been based upon post hoc genotyping and only few had been specifically designed to test genetic effects. Another systematic review has looked at randomized, placebo-controlled trials of ACE inhibitors across a range of cardiovascular and renal indications (Scharplatz et al. 2005). While a trend for greater responses in Caucasian DD carriers as compared to II carriers was observed, pooling of the results from the various studies was considered inappropriate due to heterogeneity in ethnicity, clinical domains, and outcomes. Hence, this analysis also failed to detect a consistent effect for the I/D polymorphism of the ACE gene. Unfortunately, this inconclusive picture based upon published studies remains even when more recent trials are considered (Harrap et al. 2003; Arnett et al. 2005; Bleumink et al. 2005; Schelleman et al. 2005). It also extends to other indications of ACE inhibitors such as coronary artery disease and surrogate markers thereof (Tsikouris and Peeters 2007). Despite these inconsistent results it has been proposed that genotyping for the I/D polymorphism may be cost-effective in the prevention of end-stage renal disease (Costa-Scharplatz et al. 2007).

A polymorphism in the ACE gene could theoretically affect not only responses to ACE inhibitors but, based upon pathophysiological considerations, also to angiotensin receptor type 1 (AT1R) antagonists or diuretics. While the number of available studies in this regard is smaller than that on ACE inhibitors, they also have yielded rather inconsistent results (Kurland et al. 2001, 2002, 2004; Koopmans et al. 2003; Coto et al. 2005).

2. Angiotensin AT_1 Receptor Agents

Similar to the ACE inhibitors, AT1R antagonists are used in the treatment of arterial hypertension and congestive heart failure or in the prevention of diabetic nephropathy. Although more than 600 polymorphisms have been described in the *AT1R* gene (Oro et al. 2007), almost all studies of this gene have investigated the A1166C SNP (Figure 34–9). This SNP is located in the 3' untranslated region of the gene, and its possible functional relevance has long remained elusive. Recent data indicate that this SNP interrupts the repression of receptor expression by microRNA-155 (Martin et al. 2007) and thereby could contribute to the in vivo expression level of the receptor. Among the many other polymorphisms, which have been described within the *AT1R* gene, functional implications have been demonstrated only for one SNP within the coding region of the *AT1R* gene (Hansen et al. 2004), but this polymorphism is very rare. Therefore, the subsequent discussion will be based upon the A1166C SNP.

Similar to the studies on ACE gene polymorphisms, those for AT1R polymorphisms have yielded conflicting results. Compared to the C-allele carriers of the A1166C SNP, homozygous AA carriers showed several blunted losartan responses in one study (Miller et al. 1999). A similarly reduced response was observed in AA carriers for irbesartan-induced regression of heart hypertrophy (Kurland et al. 2002). On the other hand, the opposite, that is, a significantly greater blood pressure lowering response to losartan was reported for AA carriers in another study (Coto et al. 2005). Finally, the blood pressure lowering or reduction of cardiac hypertrophy in response to irbesartan was not related to the A1166C or four other SNPs in the *AT1R* gene (Kurland et al. 2001, 2004; Liljedahl et al. 2004).

Similar to studies in which the effect of ACE gene polymorphisms had been tested for responses to AT1R antagonists, some studies have also assessed the role of AT1R polymorphisms on ACE inhibitor responses. An effect of the A1166C SNP on ACE inhibitor responses was found in some studies (Benetos et al. 1996). On the other hand, no such associations were confirmed in other studies (Hingorani et al. 1995). In three different studies the A1166C SNP was not found to affect the response to diuretics (Mellen and Herrington 2005).

In conclusion, a possible relationship between polymorphisms of the *AT1R* gene and clinical responses to drugs, which work via such receptors or which may involve such receptors indirectly, have not yielded consistent support for the relevance of polymorphisms. Again, it should be noted that almost of all of these studies represent posthoc genotyping and in most cases involved only relatively small patient numbers.

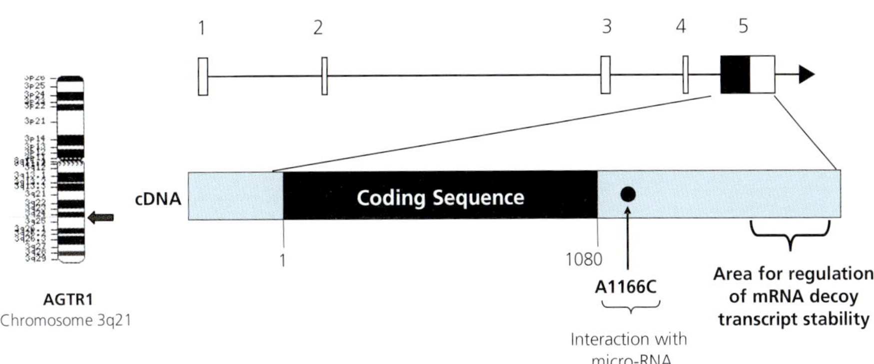

Figure 34–9 Gene structure of the human angiotensin 2 receptor type I gene (*AGTR1*). The gene for this G protein-coupled receptor is confined to chromosome 3. The gene comprises five exons. The last exon codes for part of the 5'-UTR, the coding sequence, and the entire 3'-UTR. Several splice variants pertaining to the 5'-UTR have been reported. A frequent variant consists of exons 1, 2, 3, and 5, another one of exons 1, 2, and 5, and yet another one of exons 1, 3, and 5. A common polymorphism within 3'-UTR of the cDNA (A1166C) has been implicated with mRNA stability and receptor expression. Novel results indicate that a microRNA binds to this region.

3. Diuretics

Thiazide and loop diuretics are a mainstay in the therapy of hypertension and heart failure. Responder rates for common diuretics in the monotherapy of hypertension are in the range of 50%–60% (Materson et al. 1993). Several groups have tried to identify genetic variants that predict the antihypertensive effects of diuretics. Candidate genes involved components of the RAAS system and a common polymorphism in the α-adducin gene.

Available evidence suggests that variants in genes that control renal sodium handling play a major role in the pathogenesis of hypertension, at least for most all forms of monogenic hypertension identified so far (Rosskopf et al. 2007). For common hypertension, polymorphisms in the α-adducin gene have been implicated in its pathogenesis, and alterations in renal sodium homoeostasis have been proposed (Manunta and Bianchi 2006). Adducin is a heterodimeric cytoskeletal protein and comprises an α-subunit and either a β- or a γ-subunit. These subunits are encoded by three different genes (*ADD1*, *ADD2*, and *ADD3*). Adducins are ubiquitously expressed and as end-capping proteins they play an important role in the organization of spectrin-actin lattice through sustained spectrin-actin binding, and controlling the rate of actin polymerization. There is evidence for a contribution to the regulation of the Na^+/K^+ ATPase activity by regulating the endocytosis of this pump and, thus, potentially modulating renal sodium absorption, although these issues await further proof (Efendiev et al. 2004; Manunta and Bianchi 2006; Rosskopf et al. 2007). Common polymorphism in the *ADD1* gene exists (Gly460Trp; Ser586Cys) and the 460Trp allele has been associated with the risk for hypertension, especially hypertension of the low renin phenotype (Cusi et al. 1997). As for many association studies, a considerable controversy subsequently arose with a 50:50 divide supporting and contradicting reports (Bianchi et al. 2005; Rosskopf et al. 2007). Assuming a role in renal sodium reabsorption several groups investigated whether the 460Trp allele alters diuretic responses. Three studies in treatment-naïve hypertensives provided evidence for a greater decline in blood pressure upon administration of hydrochlorothiazide (Cusi et al. 1997; Glorioso et al. 1999; Sciarrone et al. 2003). However, with this selection criterion the number of participants in these studies was small (58, 143, and 86, respectively, for the above reports). In contrast, more extensive population-based studies with 585 to 3,025 individuals reported no effect of the Gly460Trp polymorphism on blood pressure lowering by thiazides (Psaty et al. 2002; Turner et al. 2003; Schelleman et al. 2006). While the extensive study by Psaty et al. with 1,038 managed-care patients with hypertension did not provide evidence for an effect of the 460Trp allele on blood pressure, the therapeutic regime, and the blood pressure achieved by diuretics, there was a significant effect of the 460Trp allele on the therapeutic outcome of a thiazide therapy. In subjects harboring the 460Trp allele, treatment with thiazides dropped the relative risk for myocardial infarction or stroke by 50%, an effect not seen for other antihypertensives or for carriers of the wild-type allele. This effect was *independent* of the blood pressure level attained under therapy. Since the frequency of the 460Trp allele in this study population amounted to 30%, such an effect could be of major significance for the general population. In fact, pharmacoeconomic models suggested that allocation of diuretics depending on the 460Trp status might be cost-effective (Meckley and Veenstra 2006). An independent replication of these results is urgently awaited. Nevertheless, a straightforward interpretation of these results indicates that the α-adducin system affects blood pressure-independent mechanisms in stroke pathogenesis that remain to be elucidated.

Several studies have analyzed whether variants in the ACE gene or the angiotensinogen gene (M235T polymorphism) modify the blood pressure response to thiazides with inconclusive results (Mellen and Herrington 2005). Turner and coworkers (2003) analyzed the effects of six common polymorphisms in 291 African Americans and 294 white Americans with hypertension on thiazide-mediated blood pressure lowering. Among these polymorphisms, the ADD1 Gly460Trp, the ADRB1 Arg389Gly, and the ADRB2 Arg16Gly variants have been reviewed here. Interestingly, only a polymorphism (Glu298Asp) in the endothelial nitric oxide synthase gene was significantly associated with blood pressure response upon statistical adjustment for several confounding factors. The net effect of this polymorphism on the observed variation in blood pressure lowering amounted to 1% and was statistically significant. In contrast, the covariates' gender, ethnicity, age, and waist-to-hip ratio affected the observed variation in systolic and diastolic blood pressure by 26% and 11%, respectively.

For the loop diuretic torasemide, evidence accumulates that common variants in transport proteins may affect its pharmacodynamics and pharmacokinetics. Torasemide is metabolized in the liver by the cytochrome oxidase CYP2C9 (see Chapter 34.3.1.2). CYP2C9*3, a common loss-of-function variant, was associated with reduced torasemide clearance and, in accord, with a slightly increased diuretic effect (Vormfelde et al. 2004). Diuretics are actively transported to and from the renal tubular lumen. Candidate transporters belong to the family of organic anion transporters and in vitro evidence suggests that torasemide is substrate for the isoforms OAT1, OAT3, and OAT4, all of which harbor functionally relevant polymorphisms. Interestingly, variants of the luminally expressed OAT4 affect renal torasemide clearance in controlled clinical trials (Vormfelde et al. 2006). For hepatic metabolism by CYP2C9, torasemide must enter the hepatocyte. There is evidence that the organic anion transport protein OATP1B1 mediates this uptake. There are two frequent loss-of-function variants in OATP1B1 and, with an increasing number of these alleles, torasemide clearance decreased and renal sodium excretion increased. This pattern is in accord with a decreased hepatic torasemide metabolism and, thus, inactivation in carriers of these alleles leading to an increased renal exposure to the drug (Vormfelde et al. 2008). Besides analyzing torasemide pharmacokinetics, the same group also screened common polymorphisms in the renal sodium transporter—studies mostly lacking for thiazides so far. They observed that known genetic variations in the $Na^+/K^+/2Cl^-$ transporter (NKCC2), that is, the specific target for loop diuretics, did not affect the diuretic effect of torasemide. However, a frequent polymorphism in the NaCl cotransporter (NCC; Gly264Ala) and the most frequent haplotype in the β-subunit of the epithelial sodium channel were associated with stronger diuresis, while a certain haplotype of the γ-subunit of the epithelial sodium channel displayed decreased diuresis (Vormfeld et al. 2007).

In conclusion, we begin to understand how the pharmacokinetics and pharmacodynamics of loop diuretics are affected by common genetic variants. However, this relates to scientific understanding of those drugs and does not affect clinical practice. More interesting in this regard is the adducin Gly460Trp polymorphisms. If the results on major genotype-dependent beneficial effects in the prevention of stroke and myocardial infarction in carriers of the 460Trp allele could be reproduced, this could favor routine allocation of thiazides to hypertensive patients with this genotype.

Drugs Affecting Ion Channels

In mammalian heart, the opposing actions of Na^+ and Ca^{2+} ion influx, and K^+ ion efflux through cardiac ion channels determine the action potentials in myocytes, thus controlling the heartbeat. In the last decade many forms of familial arrhythmias have been unravelled by genetic linkage analyses in affected families, and the responsible genes have been identified as cardiac ion channels or as proteins in the regulation thereof. Inherited long QT syndromes have been associated with mutations in α-subunits (*KvLQT1/KCNQ1*; *HERG/KCNH2*) and β-subunits (*MinK/KCNE1*; *MiRP1/KCNE2*) of voltage-gated K^+ channels. Another type of long QT syndrome is caused by mutations in an inward rectifying K^+ channel (*Kir2.1/KCNJ2*), while other forms are caused by mutations in the Na^+ channel SNC5A. Other mutations in this Na^+ channel or in interacting proteins cause Brugada syndrome. These topics are intensively discussed in another chapter of this book. The genetic variants here are typically rare mutations that "run" in families and are of rather limited interest for pharmacogenetics in a broader sense. Interestingly in this context, however, is the observation that individuals with common variants in the ACE, the *AGT*, or the *AGT1R* genes exhibit a higher susceptibility for atrial fibrillation (Tsai et al. 2004). A first pharmacogenetic study recently reported failure to drug response for lone atrial fibrillation of 5%, 41%, and 47% for carriers of the II, ID, and DD genotypes (Darbar et al. 2007). If reproduced, this could be a basis for an optimized allocation of therapies.

Of major importance for practical pharmacology, both for clinical medicine and for pharmaceutical research, is the unpredictable occurrence of drug-induced severe—sometimes fatal—arrhythmias including long QT syndromes or torsades de pointes. Several drugs including the prokinetic cisapride, the antihistamines terfenadine and astemizole, the antibiotic grepafloxacin or the calcium channel blocker mibefradil were removed from the market because of such incidents (Giacomini et al. 2007). In fact, the risk of acquired long QT syndrome is the most common cause of withdrawal or restriction of drugs that have already been marketed. The pathogenesis of such arrhythmias appears to be complex. Evidence suggests that age and gender affect the expression levels of cardiac ion channels, which may explain the significantly increased risk in women (increase two- to threefold) for such drug-induced arrhythmias. In many such cases, drug interactions were identified to have contributed to the event. Owing to some structural peculiarities the HERG channel can bind several types of drugs including antibiotics (sulfamethoxazole, clarithromycin, erythromycin), antidepressants (amitriptyline, imipramine), antihistamines (terfenadine, astemizole), antipsychotics (chlorpromazine, haloperidol), antianginal agents (bepridil), and even Class Ia and Class III antiarrhythmic drugs (Roden 2004; Roden and Viswanathan 2005; Roepke and Abbott 2006). Normally, these interactions are weak and do not contribute to clinically overt arrhythmias. In situations, where the metabolism of such nonspecifically binding drugs is inhibited by the administration of another drug or by nutrients, for example, grapefruit juice, plasma concentrations increase and may lead to significant channel blockade, which results in arrhythmias. This typically occurs for HERG-blocking drugs, which are substrates for CYP3A4 (terfenadine, erythromycin, cisapride, astemizole), the cytochrome oxidase involved in the metabolism of a majority of common drugs (Honig et al. 1992; Ray et al. 2004). The most instructive example is the antihistamine terfenadine that can effectively block HERG channels. Normally, terfenadine is almost completely (>98%) metabolized to fexofenadine presystemically by CYP3A4 in the intestine and in the liver. Fexofenadine is a potent blocker of H1-histamine receptors but lacks HERG-blocking activity. Upon coadministration of potent CYP3A4 inhibitors, for example, erythromycin (which exhibits also some HERG-blocking activity) or azole antimycotics, terfenadine is no longer metabolized and plasma concentrations increase more than 100-fold, finally inducing potentially fatal torsades de pointes in susceptible individuals. This risk is not acceptable for an antihistamine and terfenadine was withdrawn from the market (Woosley et al. 1993).

While plausible for some cases, this scenario does not explain why some individuals suffer arrhythmias while others do not despite the intake of identical drugs and similar plasma concentrations. Emerging evidence suggests that such events are superimpositions of subclinical genetic variations with external factors including drug interactions, age, gender, electrolyte imbalances (hypokalemia), and secondary disorders. Interestingly, a common HERG variant (K897T) affects the QTc interval in women but not in men, exhibiting a gene–gender interaction (Pietila et al. 2002; Bezzina et al. 2003). Other identified HERG variants include the rare HERG R1047L mutation predisposing to torsades de pointes with dofetilide (Sun et al. 2004), the M124T mutation predisposing to long QT syndromes with probucol (Hayashi et al. 2004) or a A561P mutation associated with long QT syndromes induced by clobutinol (Bellocq et al. 2004). Common variants and rare mutations of other ion channels including *MiRP1*, *KCNQ1*, and *SCN5A* have also been implicated in the pathogenesis of severe drug-induced arrhythmias (Roepke and Abbott 2006; Kannankeril and Roden 2007). Of note, a polymorphism (S1102Y) in the sodium channel *SCN5A* gene is associated with an eightfold (95% CI 3.2–23.9) increase in the relative risk for severe arrhythmia especially in the context of drug-induced arrhythmias. The 1102Y variant of this gene occurs in 13% of African Americans and is a good example of genetic risk factors occurring in certain ethnicities only (Splawski et al. 2002).

While the molecular mechanisms detailed so far relate to fortuitous blocking of genetically altered ion channels by common drugs, new findings suggest that drugs can also interfere with the dynamic channel trafficking to the cell membrane in mutated and nonmutated channels (Liu et al. 2005; Kannakeril and Roden 2007). The genetic mechanisms detailed so far affect the pharmacodynamics of specific channel proteins, although the ensuing clinical arrhythmias are frequently triggered by pharmacokinetic influences, predominantly by inhibition of CYP3A4. Table 34–2 summarizes CYP3A4 substrates and inhibitors that have been directly implicated in the pathogenesis of drug-induced arrhythmias. Another CYP enzyme, CYP2D6 is involved in the metabolism of several antiarrhythmics (flecainide, propafenone, metoprolol, propranolol) and antipsychotics (thioridazine, risperidol). CYP2D6 is inhibited by fluoxetine or quinidine. Roughly 7%–10% of whites and African Americans express CYP2D6 variants with no enzymatic activity, as they are poor metabolizers (PM). There is evidence for increased proarrhythmic effects of flecainide, propafenone, and for an increased risk for torsades de pointes in users of thioridazine or risperidol who are PM (Roden and Viswanathan 2005; Kannankeril and Roden 2007).

1. Anticoagulants

Vitamin K antagonists or coumarins, the prototypic oral anticoagulants, are widely used for the primary and secondary prevention of thromboembolism in disorders such as atrial fibrillation, prosthetic heart valve replacement, and venous thrombosis. While in the United States warfarin is the predominant vitamin K antagonist, in some European countries phenprocoumon is preferred.

Table 34–2 CYP3A4 Metabolism and Drug-Induced Arrhythmias

Substance	CYP3A4 Substrate	CYP3A4 Inhibitor	Arrhythmias
Amiodarone	+	+	*
Astemizole	+		++
Azole antimycotics (ketoconazole, itraconazole)	+	+	
Calcium channel blockers	+	(+)	*
Cisapride	+		++
Cyclosporine	+	+	
Grapefruit juice		+	
HIV protease inhibitors	+	+	
HMG Reductase Inhibitors (lovastatin, atorvastatin, simvastatin, fluvastatin,)	+		
Lidocain	+		*
Macrolide antibiotics (erythromycin, clarithromycin)	+	+	+
Mibefradil	+	+	*
Quinidine	+	+	*
Ritonavir	+	+	
Terfenadine	+		++

Note: Selected drugs interact with CYP3A4. The classification between substrate and inhibitor varies between different authors owing to the fact that some inhibitors are metabolized so slowly compared other substrates that this metabolizing appears negligible. * indicates substances that have direct pharmacodynamic effects on cardiac ion channels causing proarrhythmic effects. In this scenario the contribution of CYP3A4 inhibition remains open. Others are known to potentiate the arrhythmogenic effects of coadministered drugs without convincing evidence for own arrhythmogenic potential (e.g., terfenadine vs. azole antimycotics).

Acenocoumarol is another compound in this class (Figure 34–10). In the United States alone more than 20 million prescriptions for warfarin are written each year and 2 million individuals are on warfarin therapy (Rieder et al. 2005; Oldenburg et al. 2007a, 2007b). The management of coumarin therapy, however, is complicated by a narrow therapeutic window and a considerable interindividual variation in therapeutic coumarin doses. Typical warfarin doses range from 2 mg to 10 mg/day, while extremes of the observed dosage range may vary 30-fold. Together, this poses demanding problems. First, a safe and effective stabilizing dose has to be defined during the early weeks of coumarin therapy. Second, maintenance doses have to be regularly controlled by INR measurements and adjusted accordingly. For stroke prevention in atrial fibrillation there is a very narrow window of anticoagulation where the beneficial effects offset the inherent risks, particularly for cerebral hemorrhages. Treatment according to current guidelines aims to prevent 20 ischemic strokes for 1 cerebral hemorrhage. Nevertheless, 1%–2% of all patients on coumarin therapy experience major bleeding events that are fatal in 0.1%–0.7% of all patients. The risk for major bleedings is especially high during the first weeks of dose finding and 10%–17% of all patients suffer from hemorrhages in this period (Kuijer et al. 1999). In another survey, the INR was supratherapeutic more than one-third of the time during the first month of usual care, which underscores the need for better induction management (Beyth et al. 2000).

The considerable interindividual variation in maintenance dose is indicative for genetic mechanisms, although age, body composition, diet, secondary disorders, and coadministered drugs can explain part of this dose variation. Interestingly, major differences in coumarin demand between ethnicities have been observed that are further indicative for genetic mechanism: while more than 95% of Asians require low doses of warfarin, more than 85% of sub-Saharan Africans are treated with high doses and in European cohorts—in the mean—intermediate doses are applied (Oldenburg et al. 2007a).

Coumarins are administered as racemic mixtures of R- and S-enantiomers, the pharmacodynamics and pharmacokinetics of which vary. In general, the anticoagulant effect of the S-enantiomere exceeds that of the R-enantiomere by three- to five-fold (Chan et al. 1994; Takahashi and Echizen 2001). Conversely, the clearance of the S-enantiomeres is more rapid with circulating half-lives of 1.8 versus 6.6 hours for S- and R-acenocoumarol and 24–33 versus 35–58 hours for S- and R-warfarin, respectively. For the enantiomeres of phenprocoumon differences in circulating half-lives are similar with 110–170 hours and 110–156 hours for S- and R-phenprocoumon (Hignite et al. 1980; Ufer 2005; Voora et al. 2005a). S-acenocoumarol in racemic mixtures is so rapidly metabolized that the main anticoagulant effect stems from its R-congener (Thijssen et al. 2000, 2001; Figure 34–10). Coumarins, as highly lipophilic compounds, undergo hepatic metabolism mediated by CYP enzymes. In contrast to acenocoumarol and warfarin, which are metabolized almost entirely, a significant proportion of unchanged phenprocoumon is excreted into bile and urine (Ufer 2005). While CYP2C9 is the key metabolizing enzyme for S-warfarin and S-acenocoumarol (Rettie et al. 1992; Thijssen 2001), S-phenprocoumon is metabolized by both CYP2C9 and CYP3A4 (Ufer 2005). Metabolism of the respective R-enantiomeres involves the CYP enzymes CYP1A1, CYP1A2, and CYP3A4 (Zhang et al. 1995; Kaminsky and Zhang 1997). Common loss-of-function variants of CYP2C9 exist that have a major impact on coumarin disposition, particularly for acenocoumarol and phenprocoumon. CYP2C9 is discussed in detail in the pharmacokinetic section.

It has long been known that coumarins interact with the metabolism of vitamin K and, in turn, inhibit the vitamin K-dependent γ-carboxylation of the coagulation factors II, VII, IX, and X as well as of the anticoagulants C, S, and Z. Here, vitamin

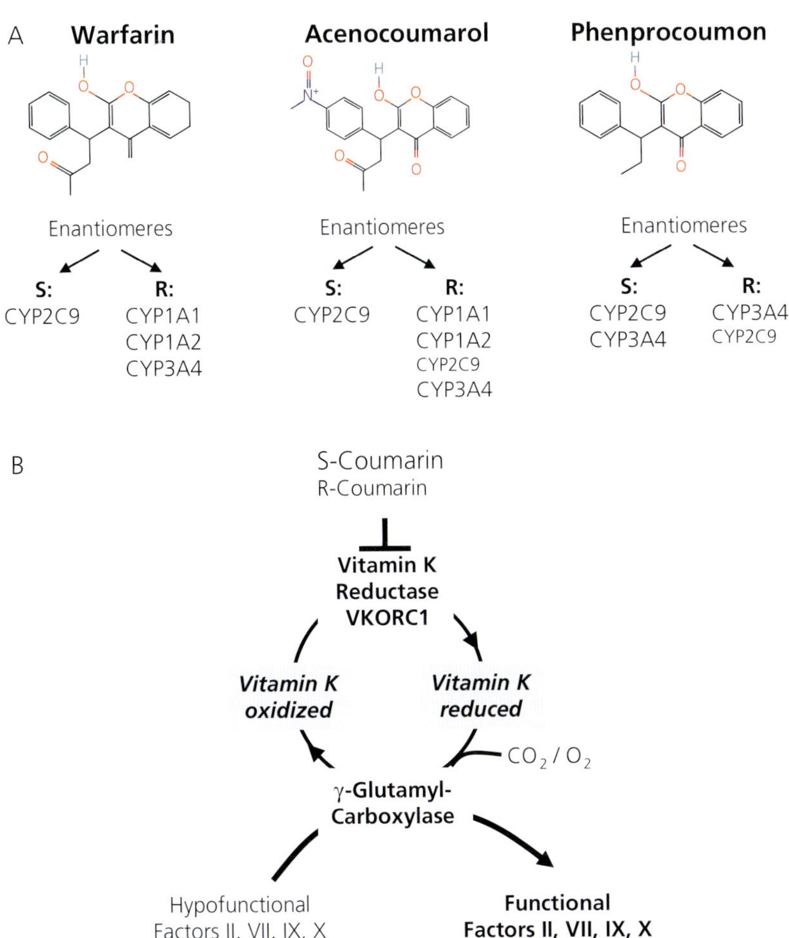

Figure 34–10 Coumarins and oral anticoagulation. Panel A depicts the three different coumarins used for oral anticoagulation and their enantio-selective metabolism. Panel B illustrates the vitamin K cycle, which is necessary for the modification of clotting factors and anticoagulants into functionally active proteins.

K epoxide is generated during γ-carboxylation and is recycled to the active form, vitamin K hydroquinone, by the vitamin K oxidoreductase complex (VKORC) (Figure 34–9). Vitamin K hydroquinone is an essential cofactor for the γ-glutamyl carboxylase (GGCX) mediated carboxylation reaction. Biochemically, this VKORC system was characterized in the 1970s, the proteins involved, however, remaining elusive. Based on two families with vitamin K-responsive bleeding disorders (familial multiple coagulation factor deficiency) from Lebanon and Germany, the *VKORC1* gene encoding for the drug target of coumarins, was identified by positional cloning and mapped to chromosome 16p12. The final identification of the gene was further supported by the parallel identification of an orthologous locus in coumarin-resistant rat strains (Fregin et al. 2002; Rost et al. 2004). Using an elegant siRNA transfection approach, VKORC1 was independently identified by a second group (Li et al. 2004). VKORC1 belongs to a novel class of proteins. It is widely expressed in different tissues including the liver. VKORC1 is confined to the endoplasmic reticulum and secondary structure prediction suggests that VKORC1 is an integral membrane protein (Figure 34–11). With the identification of the drug target gene for coumarins, several groups started intensive searches for variants explaining the considerable variation in coumarin sensitivity. Several groups identified SNPs and haplotypes in the *VKORC1* gene that were associated with varying dose requirements (D'Andrea et al. 2005; Geisen et al. 2005; Rieder et al. 2005; Figure 34–10). Available evidence suggests that six SNPs that are in almost complete linkage disequilibrium define two (three) major haplotypes. These SNPs are located in intronic and promoter regions of the *VKORC1* gene (Geisen et al. 2005; Rieder et al. 2005). While the VKORC1*1 haplotype, the putative ancestral variant, is associated with higher coumarin requirements, the VKORC1*2 haplotype confers enhanced coumarin sensitivity. Interestingly, the distribution of these haplotypes in sub-Saharan Africans (85% VKORC1*1), Asians (95% VKORC1*2), and Europeans (40% VKORC1*2) directly mirrors the observed mean coumarin requirements in these ethnicities. An SNP in the promoter region (G-1639A; rs9923231) is considered the causal SNP since it alters the consensus sequence (E-box) for a transcription factor-binding site in the promoter region. While one group confirmed that the promoter activity was associated with this SNP (Yuan et al. 2005), another group observed identical activities with other reporter gene constructs harboring this SNP (Bodin et al. 2005). Nevertheless, direct quantification of VKORC1 transcript expression in liver tissue by real-time RT-PCR showed a direct association of VKORC1 haplotypes with VKORC1 transcript levels (Rieder et al. 2005). Meanwhile numerous reports have been published that confirmed the association of this genotype with coumarin dose requirements and bleeding risks in different ethnicities (Lee et al. 2006; Kimura et al. 2007; Limdi et al. 2007; Momary et al. 2007; Schelleman et al. 2007). CYP2C9 variants further modulate this effect in all studies conducted so far. While most papers focused on warfarin therapy, a recent paper demonstrates that VKORC1 and CYP2C9 variants also affect phenprocoumon dosing (Schalekamp et al. 2007).

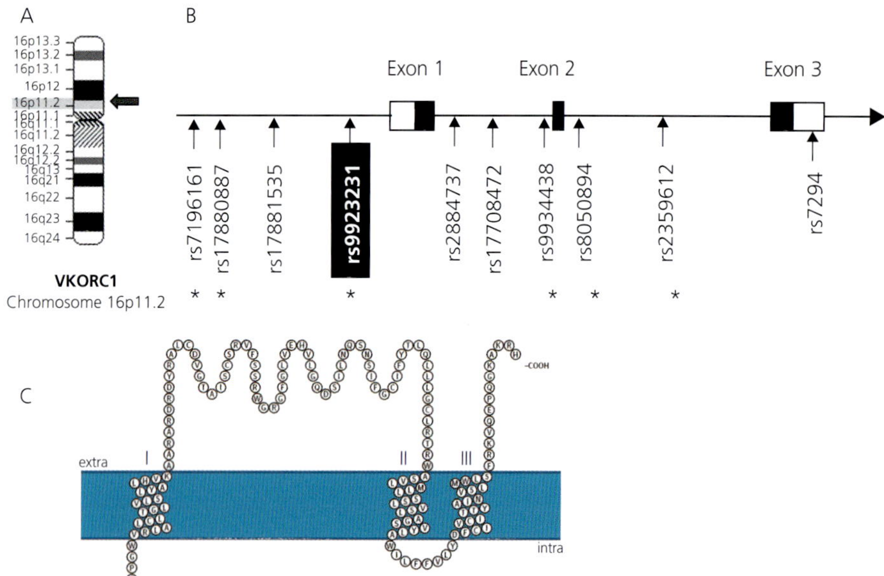

Figure 34–11 *VKORC1* gene and secondary structure prediction. (A) The gene for VKORC1 is localized on chromosome 16. (B) The figure depicts the gene structure and the localization of important polymorphisms. The putative causal polymorphism is indicated in a black box. Asterisks mark those SNPs that are in close linkage disequilibrium (>95%).

In conclusion, genotyping of the VKORC1 variants is a robust method for prediction of coumarin requirements, which can accelerate dose finding and reduce bleeding events. Estimates for acenocoumarol therapy suggest that VKORC1 variants can explain more than 30% of the observed variation in INR reduction and that the combined analysis of VKORC1 and CYP2C9 variants explains 50% of this variation, while the rest is attributed to nutritional and lifestyle factors (Bodin et al. 2005). Other groups reported similar values for warfarin therapy (Gage 2006). There is good evidence that the pharmacogenetic analyses of both variants will be introduced into routine clinical practice. Dosing algorithms have been established that consider these polymorphisms, and can be accessed on a free web site: www.WarfarinDosing.org. Pharmacogenetic analysis may be especially useful together with phenotypic measures in heavily medicated individuals (Michaud et al. 2008). Further, algorithms have been developed for optimized postsurgery warfarin initiation (Millican et al. 2007). Several studies have been initiated that prospectively analyze the (cost-)effectiveness of VKORC1/CYP2C9 genotyping before initiating coumarin therapy. Assuming a two- to threefold increase in major bleeding risks for carriers of the VKORC1*2 haplotype under phenprocoumon therapy as shown in one study (Reitsma et al. 2005), there is a high probability that pharmacogenetic testing is cost-effective (Schalekamp et al. 2006).

Polymorphisms in other genes pertaining to the action of vitamin K-dependent coagulation factors including γ-glutamyl transferase, factor II, and factor VII have not been implicated in the variance of coumarin doses, or exhibit only minor effects (Gage 2006; Oldenburg et al. 2007a).

Genetic Factors Related to Pharmacokinetics

General Considerations

The absorption, distribution, metabolism, and elimination of a drug typically involve many different steps (Figure 34–3). Even within a level, for example, metabolism, frequently multiple enzymes can be involved. For example, a given drug may be concomitantly metabolized by both cytochrome P450 (CYP) 2D6 and 3A4. If the activity of one of the two enzymes is altered by genetic factors, the amount of substrate available for the other can change and hence the net metabolism of a drug may exhibit only small changes. On the other hand, it is possible within the same example that 2D6- and 3A4-generated metabolites exhibit distinct pharmacological profiles, for example, that one is pharmacologically inactive whereas the other is not (Michel and Hegde 2006). In that case, a genetically determined change in the activity of one enzyme may not only alter the amount of drug available at its target but also qualitatively affect drug action. The following chapter will focus on the CYP enzymes CYP2D6 and CYP2C9, which have already been addressed and on variants of two paradigmatic drug transporters, MDR1 (ABCB1, p-glycoprotein, PGP) and OATP1B1. In general, the clinical effects of polymorphisms in genes affecting pharmacokinetics do not primarily depend on the molecular target of a given drug but rather on its chemical structure. On the other hand, drugs acting on the same molecular target may share chemical features and this may lead to an involvement of similar metabolic pathways. For example, many β-adrenoceptor antagonists are CYP2D6 substrates, whereas many Ca entry blockers are CYP 3A4 substrates (Siest et al. 2007).

1. CYP2D6 Variants

Cytochrome P450 enzymes or CYP enzymes are members of a huge superfamily of heme proteins, which is phylogenetically old, since CYP enzymes are also found in bacteria. P450 relates to the fact that the heme group—if complexed to CO—has an absorption peak for light at this wavelength. Typically, CYP enzymes catalyze monooxygenase reactions, that is, they introduce one oxygen atom into an organic substrate. CYP enzymes are normally membrane-bound and confined to the endoplasmic reticulum (microsomes) or mitochondrial membranes. CYP enzymes contribute to the metabolism of both endogenous substrates and of xenobiotics. The Human Genome Project has identified 57 CYP genes and 5 pseudogenes in the human genome. CYP enzymes are named according to their family (e.g., CYP2, CYP3), the letter indicates the subfamily (CYP3A), and the number the individual gene (CYP3A4). Important CYP enzymes for drug metabolism are the CYPs CYP1A1, CYP1A2, CYP2B6, CYP2D6, CYP2C9, CYP2C19, CYP2E1, CYP3A4, and CYP3A5. CYP3A4/5 are involved in metabolism of more than 50% of common drugs and are a "center" for many drug interactions with numerous substrates, inhibitors, and inducers. Pharmacogenetically more relevant are CYP2D6, CYP2C9, and CYP2C19 because common loss-of-function variants affect the metabolism of several drugs. Other CYPs contribute to steroid biosynthesis (CYP11 family) or prostaglandin biosynthesis (CYP5).

CYP2D6 is involved in the metabolism of up to 20% of all clinically used drugs, and can involve O-demethylation, N-demethylation, aromatic, benzylic and aliphatic hydroxylation, N-dealkylation, and sulfoxidation. Its activity, classically determined as debrisoquine/sparteine oxidation, varies widely among individuals. Up to 10% of Caucasian but less than 1% of Asian subjects are PM, that is, basically lack CYP2D6 activity because they have two null alleles. Certain drugs are almost exclusively metabolized by CYP2D6 including debrisoquine or sparteine. Figure 34–11B simulates classical observations for sparteine and instructively shows that in PM enormous increases in plasma concentration occur that lead to serious toxicity. These drugs are almost exclusively metabolized by CYP2D6, which generates a robust phenotype that can be followed in families. In these cases, the CYP2D6 PM state follows a Mendelian inheritance.

On the other hand, some subjects exhibit gene duplication and phenotypically are characterized as ultrarapid metabolizers (UM). The *CYP2D6* gene is highly polymorphic with more than 80 alleles and allelic variants being described. An actual collection of CYP variants and their respective nomenclatures is maintained on www.cypalleles.ki.se. Figure 34–12D displays the CYP2D6 activity distribution in the normal European population. The mathematical analysis of such distributions has led to the definition of extensive metabolizers (EM) and intermediate metabolizers (IM) in addition to UM and PM (Zanger et al. 2004). In a simplified schema one can interpret EM as individuals that harbor at least one "normal CYP2D6 allele. PM have two null alleles. The UM state is generated either by gene duplications or by mutations (e.g., in the promoter area) that augment transcript expression. IM frequently carry one null allele and a second variant allele with reduced enzymatic activity (Meisel et al. 2003; Zanger et al. 2004). While no single polymorphism in the *CYP2D6* gene can reliably predict enzymatic activity, polymorphism patterns are now able to predict the PM phenotype with more than 99% certainty. The most frequent CYP2D6 variants in Caucasians comprise the null allele CYP2D6*4 (allele frequency ~25%; responsible for 70%–90% of PM), which results from a mutation in a splice site acceptor site at the border from intron 3 to exon 4 (Figure 34–11B). This results in transcripts with an insertion of one base and, in turn, to a shift in the reading frame and a premature stop codon. Other inactive CYP2D6 variants are CYP2D6*3 (2549A>del → frame shift) occurring with a frequency of 2%, CYP2D6*5 (gene deletion; frequency 2%), and the rare variants CYP2D6*6 (1707T>del → frame shift; frequency 1%) and CYP2D6*7 (A2935C; His324Pro; frequency 0.1%). CYP2D6 variants with decreased activity (occurring as one copy in IM) comprise CYP2D6*9 (2613–2615delAGA; K281del; frequency 2%). On a molecular level this variant is characterized by reduced heme content. CYP2D6*10 is caused by an amino acid exchange from proline to serine on position 34, that is, in a proline-rich domain that is involved in membrane attachment (Figure 34–12C). It occurs in a frequency of 1.5% in Caucasians. Beside the wild-type CYP2D6*1, CYP2D6*2 is the second most frequent variant in Caucasians occurring in frequencies up to 30%. The CYP2D6*2 variant is characterized by several polymorphisms [-1584G>C, 2850C>T (Arg296Cys), 4180G>C (Ser486Thr)] and the overall enzymatic activity of CYP2D6*2 is reduced. Detailed analyses of such CYP2D6*2 alleles revealed that the activity was diminished to the greatest extent in individuals who harbored a 2988G>A polymorphism in intron 6 in addition to the above signature (Zanger et al. 2004). The molecular mechanism leading to reduced activity may pertain to alternate splicing. This subvariant of CYP2D6*2 has now been termed CYP2D6*41. It occurs in a frequency of 8% in the normal population and roughly 50% of IM have the genotype CYP2D6*0/CYP2D6*41. In addition to PM, genotyping for CYP2D6*41, CYP2D6*9, and CYP2D6*10 allows for the detection of more than 90% of IM (Zanger et al. 2004).

Among cardiovascular drugs, many antiarrhythmics, β-adrenoceptor antagonists and other antihypertensives are substrates for CYP2D6 (Table 34–3). For example, PM and EM exhibit 10- to 15-fold different drug exposures with the same administered dose of nebevilol (Lefebvre et al. 2006), and more than 100-fold differences in plasma concentrations of metoprolol were found among genotypes (Ismail and Teh 2006). Actually, metoprolol is now considered a prototypical substrate of CYP2D6, which can be used as a tool for phenotyping (Frank et al. 2007). The overall role of *CYP2D6* gene polymorphisms in the pharmacokinetics of β-adrenoceptor antagonists has recently been comprehensively reviewed (Shin and Johnson 2007).

An important question is how major genetically determined differences in drug exposure translate into clinical changes of efficacy or tolerability. In this regard the existing studies are not fully conclusive. Some studies have reported that PM were markedly overrepresented among patients experiencing adverse effects while undergoing metoprolol treatment (Wuttke et al. 2002). PM, EM, and UM differed somewhat in metoprolol-induced reductions of resting heart rate (Kirchheiner et al. 2004). Similarly, the modulation of the circadian rhythm of heart rate variability by metoprolol was reported to depend on CYP2D6 genotype (Nozawa et al. 2005). On the other hand, the blood pressure-lowering effect of nebivolol (Lefebvre et al. 2006) or metoprolol (Kirchheiner et al. 2004; Zineh et al. 2004) was not different between PM and EM. Moreover, in several other studies CYP2D6 genotype was not associated with alterations of other efficacy parameters (Terra et al. 2005) or tolerability of metoprolol (Zineh et al. 2004; Fux et al. 2005). In conclusion, genotype of CYP2D6 predicts enzyme activity and this is consistently associated with altered drug exposure to metoprolol. However, whether this translates into alterations of efficacy and/or tolerability of the drug remains under discussion. The effects of CYP2D6 variants in the context of drug-induced arrhythmias have already been discussed elsewhere in this chapter.

2. CYP2C9 Variants

CYP2C9 is another drug metabolizing CYP enzyme for which major pharmacogenetic effects have been described in carriers of common loss-of-function variants. CYP2C9 is involved in the metabolism of 10%–20% of currently marketed drugs and include oral anticoagulants, as already discussed, oral antidiabetics, angiotensin AGTR1 antagonists, and nonsteroidal anti-inflammatory drugs among others (Kirchheiner and Brockmöller 2005). Table 34–4 summarizes these common CYP2C9 substrates. More than 50 CYP2C9 variants have been described so far (see www.cypalleles.ki.se) but only two of them are of major importance, CYP2C9*2 and CYP2C9*3. These variants harbor amino acid exchanges that

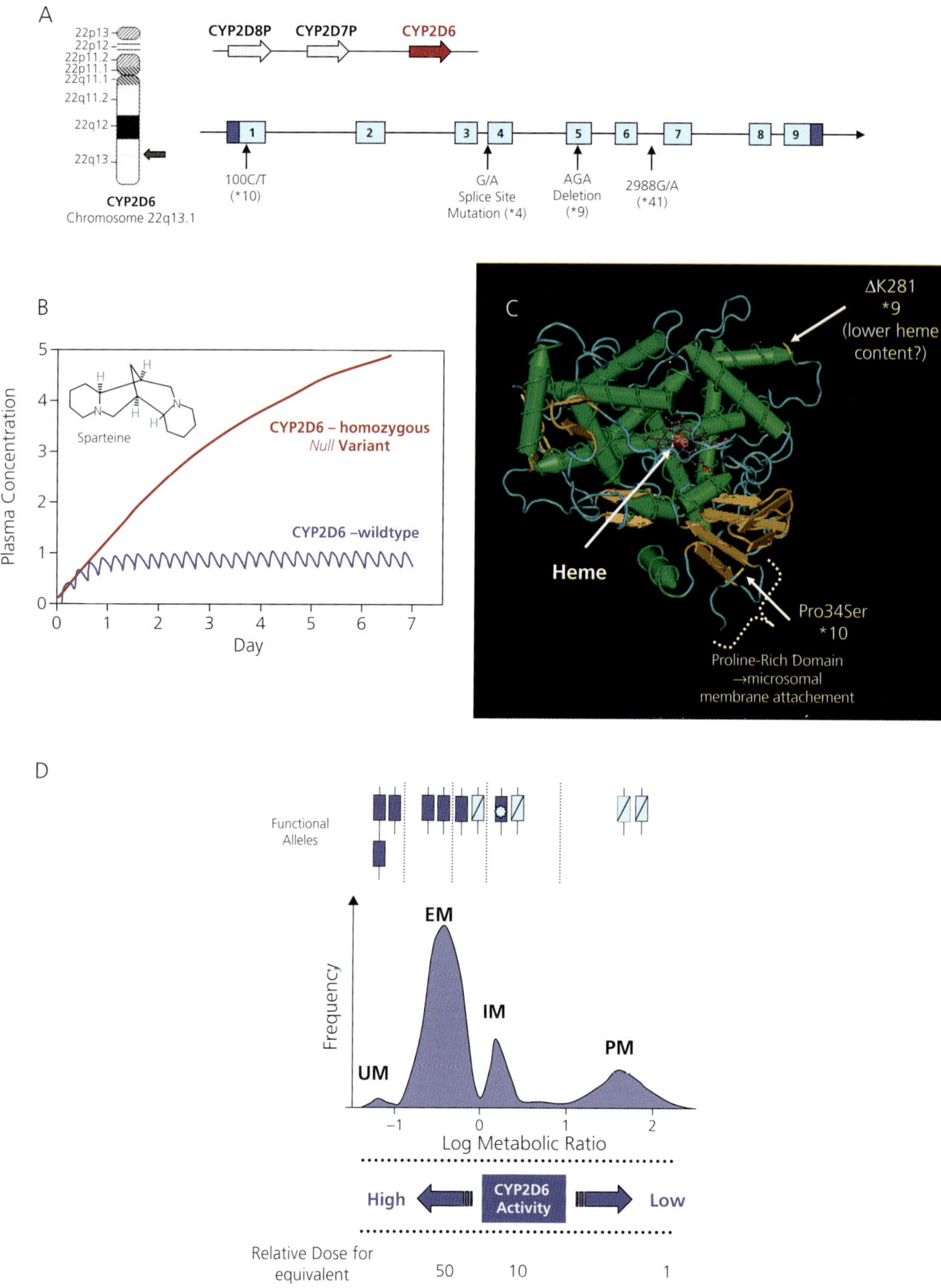

Figure 34–12 Genetics, structure, and function of CYP2D variants. (A) The *CYP2D6* gene is located on chromosome 22q in direct vicinity to two *CYP2D6* pseudogenes. The gene itself consists of 9 exons and 8 introns. Depicted are key polymorphisms of frequent CYP2D6 variants. (B) This panel simulates the plasma concentration for sparteine administration in carriers of the wild-type alleles and in poor metabolizers based on the seminal paper by Eichelbaum et al. 1979. (C) Three-dimensional structure of CYP2D6 showing the essential heme moiety and the localization of two frequent variants associated with the poor metabolizer state. The graph was generated with the program Cn3D4.1 using the structural data generated by Rowland et al. 2006.

cause a dramatically reduced activity of the enzyme (Figure 34–13). Interestingly, both variants have never been detected on one chromosome. CYP2C9*2 occurs with an allele frequency of 11% in the white population, while the allele frequency of CYP2C9*3 amounts to 7%. In Asian subjects the CYP2C9*2 variant is almost absent, while in African populations it occurs with a frequency of approximately 4%. CYP2C9*3 is observed in African and Asian populations in frequencies of 2% and 3%, respectively. The amino acid substitution from Arg to Cys on position 144 in CYP2C9*2 is accompanied by a 50% reduction in enzymatic activity while

Table 34–3 Substrates and Inhibitors of CYP2D6

Substance	CYP2D6 Substrate	CYP2D6 Inhibitor
Ajmaline	+	
Alprenolol	+	
Bupranolol	+	
Carvediolol	+	
Debrisoquine	+	
Dexfenfluramine	+	
Encainide	+	
Flecainide	+	
Flunarizine	+	
Fluoxetine		+
Indoramine	+	
Metoprolol	+	
Mexiletine	+	
Nebivolol	+	
Oxprenolol	+	
Paroxetine		+
Perhexiline	+	
Prajmaline	+	
Procainamide	+	
Propafenone	+	
Propranolol	+	
Quinidine		+
Sparteine	+	
Timolol	+	

Note: Selected cardiovascular drugs that are substrates of CYP2D6. The occurrence of a clinical phenotype in poor metabolizers depends on the exclusivity for a given drug to be metabolized, which is high for debrisoquine or sparteine. Several CYP2D6 inhibitors are also mentioned, which are no substrates for this enzyme. Normal to toxic concentrations of these inhibitors can cause a total inhibition of CYP2D6 that resembles a phenocopy of a poor metabolizer.
Source: Information adapted from Zanger UM, Raimundo S, Eichelbaum M. Cytochrome P450 2D6: overview and update on pharmacology, genetics, biochemistry. *Naunyn-Schmiedeberg's Arch Pharmacol.* 2004;369:23–37.

Table 34–4 CYP2C9 Substrates

Substance
Oral anticoagulants
Acenocoumarol
Phenprocoumon
Warfarin
Oral Antidiabetics
Glimepiride
Glyburide
Tolbutamide
Nateglinide
Angiotensin receptor (AGTR1) antagonists
Losartan
Candesartan
Nonsteroidal anti-inflammatory drugs (NSAID)
Celecoxib
Diclofenac
Ibuprofen
Flurbiprofen
Statins
Fluvastatin
Diuretics
Torasemide

Notes: Cardiovascular drugs that are substrates for CYP2C9. Given their prevalent use in all fields of medicine oral antidiabetics and NSAIDs were included.
Source: Information adapted from Kirchheiner J, Brockmöller J. Clinical consequences of CYP2C9 polymorphisms. *Clin Pharmacol Ther.* 2005;77:1–16.

the substrate affinity remains unaltered. Although the amino acid exchange in CYP2C9*3 from Ile to Leu on position 355 is a conservative one, catalytic activity is significantly reduced for most substrates. Figure 34–13 depicts the localization of these variants in the three-dimensional model of CYP2C9.

Variants of CYP2C9 have a significant effect on the metabolism of common coumarins as already detailed. For both variants, enzymatic degradation of S-warfarin and S-acenocoumarol is dramatically reduced while the metabolism of phenprocoumon is only moderately affected. Hence, in homozygous or compound heterozygotes plasma concentrations of the S-enantiomeres quickly rise to supratherapeutic levels and the risk for bleeding distinctly rises (Chan et al. 1994; Steward et al. 1997; Takahashi et al. 1998a, 1998b; Takahashi and Echizen 2001; Higashi et al. 2002). In one study, patients were divided into two groups according to their warfarin maintenance dose. Those in the low-dose group had a higher risk for supratherapeutic INR episodes, a fourfold increased risk for bleeding and sixfold increased probability to carry one of the loss-of-function variants of CYP2C9 (Aithal et al. 1999). Carriers of CYP2C9*3 variant require 21% to 49% less warfarin, and carriers of the CYP2C9*2 variant 14% to 20% less warfarin per allele (Gage 2006). The effects of these variants are most pronounced during initiation of warfarin therapy (twofold increase in bleeding risk) while their significance for the maintenance therapy, once the right dose has been found, is less clear (Aithal et al. 1999; Taube et al. 2000; Visser et al. 2004a, 2004b; Voora et al. 2005b). An effect of the CYP2C9 variants on phenprocoumon dosing is observable but less pronounced given the fact that considerable amounts of phenprocoumon are excreted unmetabolized (Schalekamp et al. 2004). In conclusion, genotyping of CYP2C9 variants in concert with VKORC1 variants improve dose finding in coumarin therapy, particularly during treatment initiation.

CYP2C9 is also involved in the metabolism of losartan and candesartan. Losartan is metabolized to an active and long-acting metabolite by CYP2C9. A less stable blood pressure reduction in carriers of the *3/*3 genotype has been suggested in one small study (Yasar et al. 2002). For irbesartan, which is inactivated by CYP2C9, there is evidence for an enhanced blood pressure reduction in *1/*2 and *1/*3 genotypes compared to *1/*1 carriers in another small study on 45 individuals (Hallberg et al. 2002). Similarly, the blood pressure reduction upon administration of candesartan was increased for carriers of the *1/*3 genotype (Uchida et al. 2003).

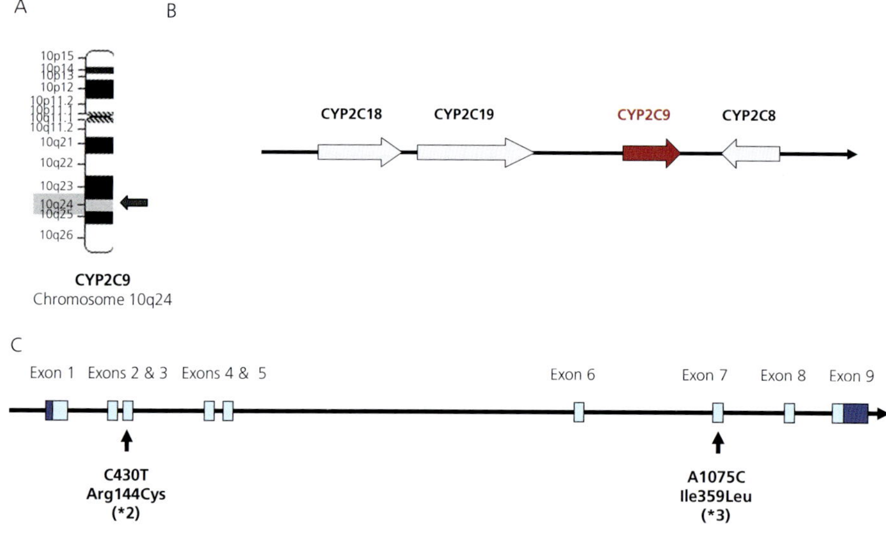

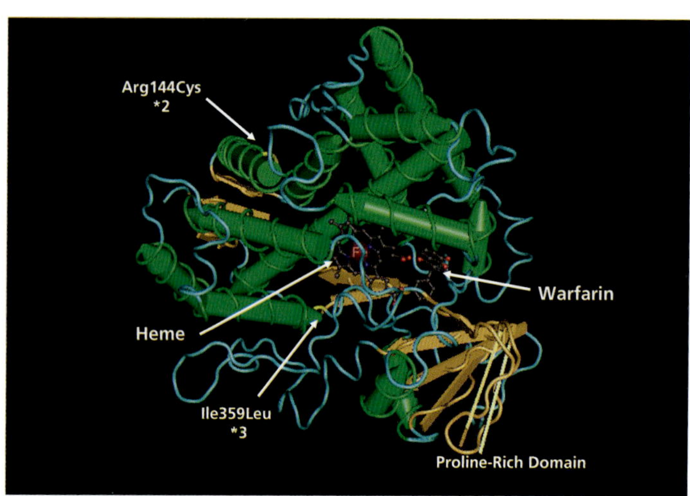

Figure 34–13 Genetics and structure of CYP2C9 variants. (A) The *CYP2C9* gene is located on chromosome 10 in a cluster of other CYP2C enzymes (B). (C) The gene itself consists of 9 exons. The variants *2 and *3 are confined to exons 3 and 7. (D) Three-dimensional structure of *CYP2C9* showing the essential heme moiety and a bound warfarin molecule. The position of the amino acid exchanges in the variants *2 and *3 is indicated. The graph was generated with the program Cn3D4.1 using the structural data generated by Williams et al. 2003.

Genetic Variants in Drug Transporters

While passage of drugs through cell membranes was formerly explained primarily by physicochemical mechanisms as a passive process, the relevance of controlled and regulated vectorial drug transport through cellular barriers mediated by special transport proteins is now a focus of pharmacokinetic research. Basically, one can distinguish efflux transporters from uptake transporters. Usually, this definition relates to the respective cell. From a systemic point of view, both transporter types may contribute to uptake or excretion depending on their respective localization in polarized epithelia. Export transporters belong to the superfamily of ATP-driven export pumps and they are classified as ABC transporters for "ATP-binding cassette," a certain protein motif. The functional identification of the first ABC transporter dates back to the year 1976 when it was observed that colchicin-resistant Chinese hamster ovary cells were also resistant to many structurally unrelated drugs ("multidrug resistance") (Juliano and Ling 1976). This discovery sparked a new field with many hopes to understand and overcome tumor cell resistance. In 1986 the first ABC transporter, that is, the multidrug resistance protein 1 (synonyms MDR1, P-glycoprotein, official name ABCB1) was cloned (Roninson et al. 1986). Today, 49 genes for ABC transporters have been identified that contain either one ("half transporter") or two ATP-binding cassettes (Borst and Elferink 2002; Gerloff 2004). ATP is hydrolyzed and the resulting energy is used for substrate transport against a concentration gradient. Based on their sequence homology, ABC transporters are subdivided into seven subfamilies. Research into the physiology, pharmacology, and pharmacogenetics of such ABC transporter is ongoing at a fast pace and exceeds the scope of this review. ABC transporters involved in drug transport include MDR (ABCB1), MRP1 ("multidrug related protein"; ABCC1), MRP2 (ABCC2), MRP3 (ABCC3), MRP4 (ABCC4), MRP5 (ABCC5), and BCRP ("breast cancer resistance protein"; ABCG2) to name the most important. While the identification and characterization of polymorphisms in such transporter proteins is the subject of current dynamic research, we will focus on well-characterized variants of MDR1. An excellent review on drug transporters and their implications for pharmacotherapy has been provided by Ho and Kim (2005).

While ABC transporter aid in defending the organism from xenobiotics by pumping them back into the intestine, uptake transporter play major roles in vectorial transepithelial transport of important substrates. These carriers belong to the other superfamily of transporters, the solute carriers, which comprises at least

43 families with more than 300 identified genes in the human genome. Many of them serve as transporters for essential substrates including glucose, amino acids, copper, zinc, and nucleosides. SLC transporters exhibit different transport modes, that is, facilitated transport, secondary active transport, or antiport. Several subfamilies of solute carriers are involved in drug transport including members of the OCT ("organic cation transporters) family (OCT1 = SCL22A1; OCT2 = SCL22A2; OCT3 = SLC22A3), the OCTN ("novel organic cation transporters) family (OCTN1 = SLC22A4; OCTN2 = SLC22A5), the OAT ("organic anion transporters) family (OAT1 = SLC22A6; OAT2 = SLC22A7; OAT3 = SLC22A8; OAT4 = SLC22A9), and OATP ("organic anion transport protein) family OATP1B1 = SLCO1B1 = OATP-C; OATP2B1 = SLCO2B1 = OATP-B). This list is far from complete. Here, we will focus on well-characterized variants in SLCO1B1 and their potential role for statin disposition.

1. Polymorphisms in ABCC1 (MDR1; p-Glycoprotein)

MDR1, the first cloned member of the superfamily of ABC transporter is involved in the transport of many xenobiotics. It accepts neutral or cationic compounds with a bulky structure. Interestingly, there is considerable overlap with CYP3A4 substrates, and it has been suggested that MDR1 and CYP3A4 may act in concert in the protection from and detoxification of xenobiotics. MDR1 is expressed on the luminal (apical) side of enterocytes thereby limiting drug entry into the body after oral administration, that is, MDR1 pumps xenobiotics that have entered the enterocyte directly back into the lumen. Once a xenobiotic has reached the blood circulation, MDR1 promotes drug elimination into bile and urine as a result of its expression in the canalicular membrane of hepatocytes and in the luminal membrane of proximal tubule cells in the kidneys, respectively. Once a xenobiotic has reached the systemic circulation, MDR1 limits its uptake into sensitive tissues such as the brain, testis, lymphocytes, and fetal circulation. Details have recently been reviewed by Fromm (2004). For cardiovascular pharmacology, MDR1 activity in the intestine explains why digoxin concentrations increase if quinidine is coadministered. Quinidine is a potent inhibitor of MDR1, which prevents this transporter from pumping digoxin back to the intestinal lumen (Rodriguez et al. 1999).

With respect to its central role in drug absorption, several groups have searched for MDR1 variants that could affect the pharmacokinetics of its substrates. A common synonymous SNP in exon 26 (C3435T) has been identified. The C3435T polymorphism is in linkage disequilibrium with a triallelic G2677T/A polymorphism, which results in amino acid exchanges (Ala893Ser or Ala893Thr; Cascorbi et al. 2001; Kim et al. 2001; Figure 34–14). However, in vitro *data* on the functional consequences of the polymorphism on position 2677 remain controversial, either reporting increased transport activities for the 893Ser variant

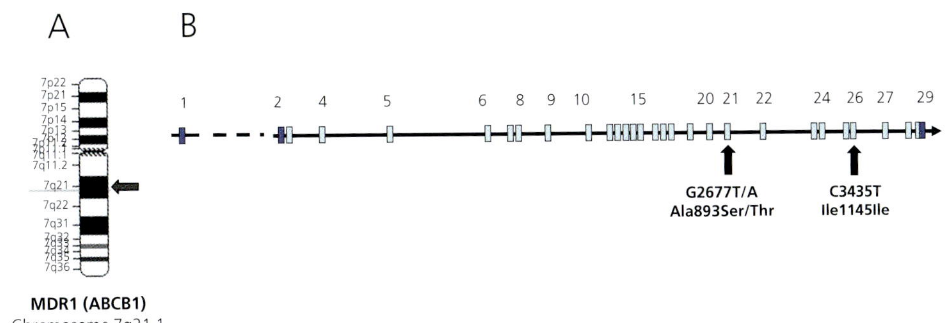

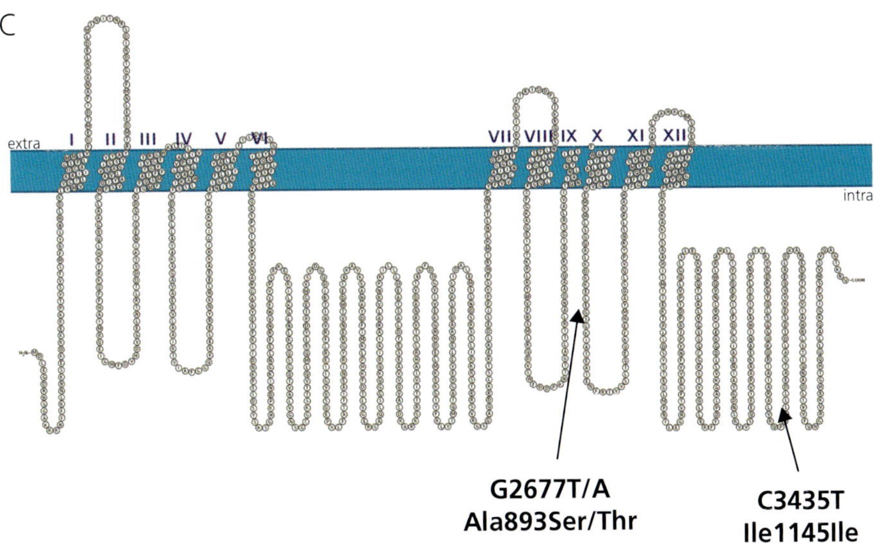

Figure 34–14 Gene structure and predicted secondary structure of MDR1/ABCB1. (A) The *ABCB1* gene is located on chromosome 7. (B) The gene itself consists of 29 exons. The G2677T/A polymorphism is located in exon 21, the C3435T polymorphism in exon 26. (C) Proposed secondary structure of MDR1 with the localization of both polymorphisms.

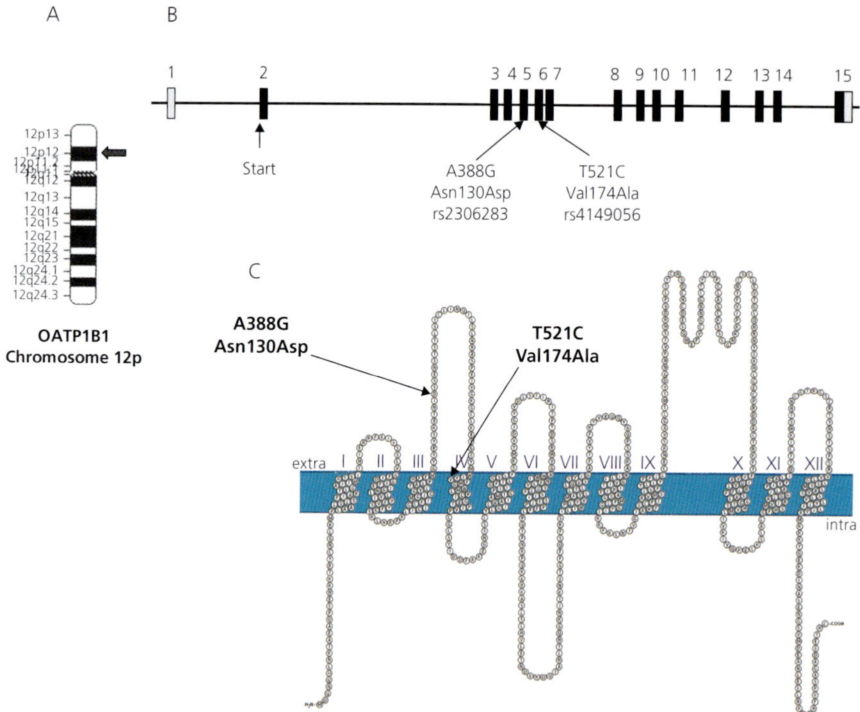

Figure 34–15 Gene structure and predicted secondary structure of OATP1B1. (A) The *OATP1B1* gene is located on chromosome 12. (B) The gene itself consists of 15 exons. The Asn130Asp polymorphism is located in exon 5, Val174Ala polymorphism in exon 6. (C) Proposed secondary structure of OATP1B1 with the localization of both polymorphisms.

(Kim et al. 2001), or activities not different from the wild type (Kimchi-Sarfaty et al. 2002; Morita et al. 2003). The common C3435T variant has been associated with variable expression of MDR1 in the duodenum. In patients homozygous for the T allele, duodenal expression of P-glycoprotein was less than half of that measured in patients with the CC genotype (Hoffmeyer et al. 2000). Interestingly, homozygous carriers of the T allele also had the highest digoxin plasma levels at steady state oral administration (Hoffmeyer et al. 2000; Johne et al. 2002), but not after single dose application (Gerloff et al. 2002). Another group, who analyzed their duodenal samples not only by quantitative RT-PCR but also by immunostaining, observed no association between MDR1 variants and MDR1 transcript or protein expression (Siegmund et al. 2002).

In liver, considerable variation in MDR1 protein expression was observed that was not related to C3435T polymorphism (Owen et al. 2005). For lymphocytes, again basal mRNA levels did not differ between genotypes but transcripts harboring the 3435T allele exhibited an enhanced down-regulation (Markova et al. 2006). MDR1 is also expressed in the heart, confined to the endothelial lumen of capillaries (Meissner et al. 2002). Here, MDR1 mRNA expression as assessed by quantitative RT-PCR was not associated with the C3435T but with the G2677T/A polymorphism (Meissner et al. 2004). For kidney tissue, a reverse association between the 3435T allele and *higher* MDR1 transcripts was recently published (Haenisch et al. 2007).

The MDR C3435T polymorphism has not only been associated with altered drug disposition but it also has been invoked with susceptibility for several disorders, including ulcerative colitis, β-amyloid disposition in Alzheimer's disease, renal carcinoma, and Parkinson's disease, although with considerable controversy (Fromm 2004). Still, the molecular mechanism for the silent C3435T polymorphism to generate a certain phenotype remains elusive. A novel concept suggested that the mRNA stability of MDR1 transcript with the 3435T allele is reduced (Wang et al. 2005, 2006). This issue has been readdressed recently with exciting new results that could have considerable impact on the whole field of genetics (Kimchi-Sarfaty et al. 2007). They expressed the MDR1 variants with the C1236T, the G2677T, and the C3435T polymorphisms either alone or in different haplotypes in various cell types. While expression levels were quite similar the V_{max} of the transporter for the fluorescent substrates rhodamine 123, bodipy-FL-paclitaxel, bodipy-FL-verapamil, daunorubicin, bodipy FL-vinblastine, and calcein-AM were almost identical. However, the MDR1 inhibitors verapamil and cyclosporine A were less effective against all other substrates in cells expressing MDR1 variants with the 3435T allele. In the absence of this allele there was no difference in the potency of the other variants to inhibit the transport of the fluorescent substrates compared to wild-type MDR1. These effects were more pronounced when MDR1 was expressed to higher levels, that is, when more MDR1 plasmid DNA was used resulting in more mRNA. However, there was no genotype-dependent difference in the mRNA levels. The MDR1 protein levels of the different variants were also almost identical. Finally, it was hypothesized that the MDR1 variants differ in their respective conformation, an assumption that was verified using conformation-specific monoclonal antibodies. The binding of this antibody to MDR1 proteins expressing either the 3435T or the 3435C allele varied, both in the absence and in the presence of MDR1 inhibitors. The intriguing mechanism for these astonishing results may relate to the relative synonymous codon usage. The codon ATC is the predominant codon for isoleucine in the human genome (47%), while the codon ATT is used in 35% only. If rare codons are used this can affect the protein translation rate due to reduced supply of the respective infrequent tRNA, and—especially for proteins with complex structure—further processing. These results spark new concepts with broad relevance for other silent mutations: when frequent codons are changed to rare codons in a cluster of infrequently used codons, the timing of cotranslational folding may become affected and may result in altered function (Kimchi-Sarfaty et al. 2007). Another attractive aspect of this concept is the notion that the cellular expression levels and the activity of the translational apparatus may determine whether the variant protein is incorrectly folded or not. Such a concept could easily explain inconsistencies between different studies.

While the investigation of MDR1 has been paradigmatic for the whole field of ABC transporters and despite the fact that the functions of MDR1 variants were initially elucidated with the probe drug digoxin, there is at present little practical benefit from genotyping MDR1 variants in the context of cardiovascular drugs, a conclusion similar to that of a recent review on MDR1 genotype-dependent pharmacokinetics (Sakaeda 2005).

2. Polymorphisms in OATP1B1 (*SLCO1B1*)

The family of human OATP comprises 11 members within the superfamily of solute carriers. They mediate the uptake of a broad range of substances into cells. These substrates include bile salts, sex hormones, statins, cardiac glycosides, and many others. The member OATP1B1 (synonym OATP-C; gene name: *SLCO1B1*) is almost exclusively expressed in the basolateral membrane of hepatocytes. OATP1B1 contributes significantly to the uptake of different drugs from the blood into liver cells where further metabolism occurs. Thus, OATP1B1 plays an essential role in presystemic inactivation. Inactivation of OATP1B1 results in an increased bioavailability of its substrate. The family of OATPB transporters has been reviewed in detail recently (Ho and Kim 2005; König et al. 2006).

Two common polymorphisms in OATP1B1 that lead to amino acid exchanges have been identified and intensively characterized. One of them leads to an exchange of Asn at position 130 for Asp (A388G = Asn130Asp = rs2306283) in the second extracellular loop of the transporter (Figure 34–14). This is most likely associated with altered substrate specificity and most frequently to reduced transport activity.[4] The second variant (T521C = Val174Ala = rs4149056) causes an amino acid exchange in the fourth transmembrane domain, which leads to a sorting defect and a distinctly reduced incorporation of this variant into the membrane, leading to a loss-of-function phenotype (Tirona et al. 2001; Figure 34–15). Both variants are moderately linked and the frequent haplotypes are classified as OATP1B1*1a (130Asn/174Val; wild type), OATP1B1*1b (130Asp/174Val), OATP1B1*5 (130Asn/174Ala), and OATP1B1*15 (130Asp/174Ala). The allele frequencies for the 130Asp and the 174Ala variants in Europeans are approximately 40% and 15%, respectively.

Statins are among the most prescribed drugs today. They are used for the primary and secondary prevention of cardiovascular diseases and aim at lowering LDL-cholesterol. A remarkable interindividual variance in LDL-cholesterol lowering has been observed (see Figure 34–1). Hypercholesterolemia is a complex disorder with lifestyle and nutritional as well as genetic contributors to its pathogenesis. Several reviews have addressed the pharmacogenetics of statins, mostly from a pharmacodynamic point of view (Schmitz et al. 2007; Siest et al. 2007). In one way, statins are special drugs since they exert their therapeutic effect in the hepatocytes (similar to coumarins). While many other drugs are metabolized in the liver and frequently are inactivated, for statins the hepatocyte is the site where they meet their prime drug target, that is, HMG-CoA reductase, and where they undergo metabolic inactivation. It is, therefore, essential for an optimal lipid-lowering effect that a high fraction of an orally administered statin enters the liver cell. OATP1B1 mediates the hepatic uptake of almost all statins. Originally cloned as pravastatin transporter, OATP1B1 also transports rosuvastatin, fluvastatin, atorvastatin, lovastatin, pitavastatin, and cerivastatin. Simvastatin as a lactone is a weak substrate but its active form simvastatin acid is efficiently transported (Nishizato et al. 2003; Mwinyi et al. 2004; Niemi et al. 2004; Chung et al. 2005; Gerloff et al. 2006; Ho et al. 2006; Igel et al. 2006; Pasanen et al. 2006, 2007; Choi et al. 2008). If OATP1B1 mediates the uptake of larger fractions of these statins into the liver, it is plausible to hypothesize that loss-of-function variants, particularly the 174Val allele is associated with reduced statin uptake and inhibition of HMG-CoA reductase and, thus, with increased systemic statin concentrations and a diminished cholesterol-lowering effect. Several studies have addressed this hypothesis in single dose or short-term clinical trials on healthy subjects. With the exception of fluvastatin (the statin with the highest lipid solubility), there is general consensus from these trials that carriers of the *5 and *15 variants display greater AUCs and peak concentrations of the administered statin. In heterozygous carriers of the *15 variant, pravastatin concentrations doubled in single dose trials (Niemi et al. 2004). Since these studies were predominantly conducted with young and healthy individuals the long-term effects on LDL-cholesterol levels were not studied. However, surrogate parameters (lathosterol level) indicate that these pharmacokinetic effects actually affect the main drug effect (Niemi et al. 2004; Gerloff et al. 2006). There is some debate whether carriers of the 130Asp variant (*Ib variant) exhibit an increased uptake of statins into the liver or whether the effect is similar to the wild-type. In conclusion, there is ample evidence that the loss-of-function OATP1B1 174Ala variant is associated with decreased statin uptake into hepatocytes, which results in increased statin plasma concentrations and an enhanced bioavailability of the drug. Long-term trials or careful reanalyses of prospective statin trials are required to investigate whether this translates into a less effective LDL-cholesterol lowering and, ultimately, to a less effective prevention. Since an increase in systemic statin concentrations increase the risk for severe adverse reactions (myopathy and rhabdomyolysis), the OATP1B1 174Ala variant may decrease the benefit/risk ratio of statins.

Conclusions and Clinical Recommendations

Until now reports of altered drug responses based upon gene polymorphisms involving either the pharmacodynamics or the pharmacokinetics of cardiovascular drugs have remained highly controversial. On balance, it appears that the effect of genetics on clinical response is at best small relative to that of other factors affecting cardiovascular drug response (Figure 34–4). If so then it is unlikely that pharmacogenetics will drive the choice of drug and/or dosage in major cardiovascular indications for routine therapy in the near future but anticoagulants may be an exception to this rule. Nevertheless, the concept of personalized cardiovascular medicine remains attractive and may gain clinical relevance in the future (Lichter and Kurth 1997; Roses 2000). Mass genotyping, whole-genome analyses with using arrays for a million different SNPs, the foundation of powerful multinational consortia with thousands of characterized patients and controls, and improved statistical and epidemiological methods have resulted in the discovery of novel genes, loci, or polymorphisms

[4] Of note, for some substrates of OATP1B1 an increased transport activity of the 130Asp has been discussed.

implicated in the pathogenesis of obesity, diabetes mellitus type 2, hyperuricemia, atrial fibrillation, and coronary artery disease (Grant et al. 2006; Frayling et al. 2007; Helgadottir et al. 2006, 2007; Gudbjartsson et al. 2007; Li et al. 2007; McPherson et al. 2007; Samani et al. 2007; Steinthorsdottir et al. 2007; Wellcome Trust Case Control Consortium 2007). While former genetic research in complex diseases predominantly focused on candidate genes, these new approaches facilitate the discovery of novel "anonymous" genes. The FTO gene and its variants in obesity research (Frayling et al. 2007), TCF7L2 transcription factor for the pathogenesis of diabetes type 2 (Grant et al. 2006) and loci on chromosome 9 (in the vicinity of the *CDKN2A* and *CDKN2B* genes) and chromosome 4 in coronary heart disease and atrial fibrillation, respectively are promising candidates in this regard. Further research will show whether these novel disease genes are suitable for the pharmacogenetic prediction of therapeutic responses (Pearson et al. 2007).

The literature search for this chapter ended in December 2007.

References

Aithal GP, Day CP, Kesteven PJL, Daly AK. Association of polymorphisms in the cytochrome P450 CYP2C9 with warfarin dose requirement and risk of bleeding complications. *Lancet.* 1999;353:717–719.

Arnett DK, Davis BR, Ford CE, et al. Pharmacogenetic association of the angiotensin-converting enzyme insertion/deletion polymorphism on blood pressure and cardiovascular risk in relation to antihypertensive treatment. The Genetics of Hypertension-Associated Treatment (GenHAT) study. *Circulation.* 2005;111:3374–3386.

Belfer I, Buzas B, Evans C, et al. Haplotype structure of the beta adrenergic receptor genes in US Caucasians and African Americans. *Eur J Human Genet.* 2005;13:341–351.

Bellocq C, van Ginneken AC, Bezzina CR, et al. Mutation in the KCNQ1 gene leading to the short QT-interval syndrome. *Circulation.* 2004;109:2394–2397.

Benetos A, Cambien F, Gautier S, et al. Influence of the angiotensin II type 1 receptor gene polymorphism on the effect of perindopril and nitrendipine on arterial stiffness in hypertensive individuals. *Hypertension.* 1996;28:1081–1084.

Beyth RJ, Quinn L, Landefeld CS. A multicomponent intervention to prevent major bleeding complications in older patients receiving warfarin. a randomized, controlled trial. *Ann Intern Med.* 2000;133:687–695.

Bezzina CR, Verkerk AO, Busjahn A, et al. A common polymorphism in KCNH2 (HERG) hastens cardiac repolarization. *Cardiovasc Res.* 2003;59:27–36.

Bianchi G, Ferrari P, Staessen JA. Adducin polymorphism. Detection and impact on hypertension and related disorders. *Hypertension.* 2005;45:331–340.

Bleumink GS, Schut AFC, Sturkenboom MCJM, et al. Mortality in patients with hypertension on angiotensin-1 converting enzyme (ACE)-inhibitor treatment is influenced by the ACE insertion/deletion polymorphism. *Pharmacogenet Genomics.* 2005;15:75–81.

Bodin L, Verstuyft C, Tregouet DA, et al. Cytochrome P450 2C9 (CYP2C9) and vitamin K epoxide reductase (VKORC1) genotypes as determinants of acenocoumarol sensitivity. *Blood.* 2005;106:135–140.

Borst P, Elferink RO. Mammalian ABC transporters in health and disease. *Annu Rev Biochem.* 2002;71:537–592.

Bruck H, Leineweber K, Beilfuß A, et al. Genotype-dependent time course of lymphocyte β_2-adrenergic receptor down-regulation. *Clin Pharmacol Ther.* 2003a;74:255–263.

Bruck H, Leineweber K, Büscher R, et al. The Gln[27]Glu β_2-adrenoceptor polymorphism slows the onset of desensitization of cardiac functional responses in vivo. *Pharmacogenetics.* 2003b;13:59–66.

Bruck H, Leineweber K, Ulrich A, et al. Thr164Ile polymorphism of the human β_2-adrenoceptor exhibits blunted desensitization of cardiac functional responses in vivo. *Am J Physiol.* 2003c;285:H2034–H2038.

Büscher R, Belger H, Eilmes KJ, et al. In-vivo studies do not support a major functional role for the Gly389Arg β_1-adrenoceptor polymorphism in humans. *Pharmacogenetics.* 2001;11:199–205.

Büscher R, Eilmes KJ, Grasemann H, et al. β2 adrenoceptor gene polymorphisms in cystic fibrosis lung disease. *Pharmacogenetics.* 2002;12:347–353.

Bylund DB, Eikenberg DC, Hieble JP, et al. IV. International Union of Pharmacology nomenclature of adrenoceptors. *Pharmacol Rev.* 1994;46:121–136.

Cascorbi I, Gerloff T, Johne A, et al. Frequency of single nucleotide polymorphisms in the P-glycoprotein drug transporter MDR1 gene in white subjects. *Clin Pharmacol Therap.* 2001;69:169–174.

Chan E, McLachlan A, O'Reilly R, Rowland M. Stereochemical aspects of warfarin drug interactions: use of a combined pharmacokinetic-pharmacodynamic model. *Clin Pharmacol Ther.* 1994;56:286–294.

Cherezov V, Rosenbaum DM, Hanson MA, et al. High-resolution crystal structure of an engineered human beta2-adrenergic G protein-coupled receptor. *Science.* 2007;318:1258–1265.

Choi JH, Lee MG, Cho JY, Lee JE, Kim KH, Park K. Influence of OATP1B1 genotype on the pharmacokinetics of rosuvastatin in Koreans. *Clin Pharmacol Ther.* 2008;83:251–257.

Chong LK, Chowdry J, Ghahramani P, Peachell PT. Influence of genetic polymorphisms in the β_2-adrenoceptor on desensitisation in human lung mast cells. *Pharmacogenetics.* 2000;10:153–162.

Chung JY, Cho JY, Yu KS, et al. Effect of OATP1B1 (SLCO1B1) variant alleles on the pharmacokinetics of pitavastatin in healthy volunteers. *Clin Pharmacol Ther.* 2005;78:342–350.

Cockroft JR, Gazis AG, Cross DJ, et al. β_2-Adrenoceptor polymorphism determines vascular reactivity in humans. *Hypertension.* 2000;36:371–375.

Costa-Scharplatz M, van Asselt ADI, Bachmann LM, Kessels AGH, Severens JL. Cost-effectiveness of pharmacogenetic testing to predict treatment response to angiotensin-converting enzyme inhibitor. *Pharmacogenet Genomics.* 2007;17:359–368.

Coto E, Marin R, Alvarez V, et al. Pharmacogenetics of angiotensin system in non diabetic nephropathy. *Nefrologia.* 2005;25:381–386.

Cusi D, Barlassina C, Azzani T, et al. Polymorphisms of α- adducin and salt sensitivity in patients with essential hypertension. *Lancet.* 1997;349:1353–1357.

D'Andrea G, D'Ambrosio RL, Di Perna P, et al. A polymorphism in the VKORC1 gene is associated with an interindividual variability in the dose-anticoagulant effect of warfarin. *Blood.* 2005;105:645–649.

Darbar D, Motsinger AA, Ritchie MD, Gainer JV, Roden DM. ACE I/D polymorphism modulates symptomatic response to antiarrhythmic drug therapy in patients with line atrial fibrillation. *Heart Rhythm.* 2007;4:743–749.

Dishy V, Sofowora GG, Xie H-G, et al. The effect of common polymorphisms of the β_2-adrenergic receptor on agonist-mediated vascular desensitization. *N Engl J Med.* 2001;345:1030–1035.

Efendiev R, Krmar RT, Leibiger IB, et al. Hypertension-linked mutation in the adducin α-subunit affects AP2-μ2 phosphorylation and impairs Na^+,K^+-ATPase endocytosis. *Circ Res.* 2004;95:1100–1108.

Eichelbaum M, Ingelman-Sundberg M, Evans WE. Pharmacogenomics and individualized drug therapy. *Annu Rev Med.* 2006;57:119–137.

Eichelbaum M, Spannbrucker N, Steincke B, Dengler HJ. Defective N-oxidation of sparteine in man: a new pharmacogenetic defect. *Eur J Clin Pharmacol.* 1979;16:183–187.

Frank D, Jaehde U, Fuhr U. Evaluation of probe drugs and pharmacokinetic metrics for CYP2D6 phenotyping. *Eur J Clin Pharmacol.* 2007;63:321–333.

Frayling TM, Timpson NJ, Weedon MN, et al. A common variant in the FTO gene is associated with body mass index and predisposes to childhood and adult obesity. *Science.* 2007;316:889–894.

Fregin A, Rost S, Wolz W, Krebsova A, Müller CR, Oldenburg J. Homozygosity mapping of a second gene locus for hereditary combined deficiency of vitamin K-dependent clotting factors to the centromeric region of chromosome 16. *Blood.* 2002;100:3229–3232.

Fromm M. Importance of P-glycoprotein at blood–tissue barriers. *Trends Pharmacol Sci.* 2004;25:423–429.

Fux R, Mörike K, Pröhmer AMT, et al. Impact of CYP2D6 genotype on adverse effects during treatment with metoprolol: a prospective clinical study. *Clin Pharmacol Ther.* 2005;78:378–387.

Gage BF. Pharmacogenetics-based coumarin therapy. *Hematology Am Soc Hematol Educ Program.* 2006;25:467–473.

Garovic VD, Joyner MJ, Diets NM, Boerwinkle E, Turner ST. β_2-Adrenergic receptor polymorphism and nitric oxide-dependent forearm blood flow responses to isoproterenol in humans. *J Physiol (London).* 2003;546:583–589.

Geisen C, Watzka M, Sittinger K, et al. VKORC1 haplotypes and their impact on the inter-individual and inter-ethnical variability of oral anticoagulation. *Thromb Haemost.* 2005;94:773–779.

Gerloff T. Impact of genetic polymorphisms in transmembrane carrier-systems on drug and xenobiotic distribution. *Naunyn-Schmiedeberg's Arch Pharmacol.* 2004;369:69–77.

Gerloff T, Schaefer M, Johne A, et al. MDR1 genotypes do not influence the absorption of a single oral dose of 1 mg digoxin in healthy white males. *Br J Clin Pharmacol.* 2002;54:610–616.

Gerloff T, Schaefer M, Mwinyi J, et al. Influence of the SLCO1B1*1b and *5 haplotypes on pravastatin's cholesterol lowering capabilities and basal sterol serum levels. *Naunyn Schmiedebergs Arch Pharmacol.* 2006;373:45–50.

Giacomini KM, Krauss RM, Roden DM, Eichelbaum M, Hayden MR, Nakamura Y. When good drugs go bad. *Nature.* 2007;446:975–977.

Glorioso N, Manunta P, Filigheddu F, et al. The role of α-adducin polymorphism in blood pressure and sodium handling regulation may not be excluded by a negative association study. *Hypertension.* 1999;34:649–654.

Gonzalez FJ, Skoda RC, Kimura S, et al. Characterization of the common genetic defect in humans deficient in debrisoquine metabolism. *Nature.* 1988;331:442–446.

Grant SF, Thorleifsson G, Reynisdottir I, et al. Variant of transcription factor 7-like 2 (TCF7L2) gene confers risk of type 2 diabetes. *Nat Genet.* 2006;38:320–323.

Gratze G, Fortin J, Labugger R, et al. β-2 Adrenergic receptor variants affect resting blood pressure and agonist-induced vasodilation in young adult Caucasians. *Hypertension.* 1999;33:1425–1430.

Green SA, Cole G, Jacinto M, Innis M, Liggett SB. A polymorphism of the human β_2-adrenergic receptor within the fourth transmembrane domain alters ligand binding and functional properties of the receptor. *J Biol Chem.* 1993;268:23116–23121.

Green SA, Turki J, Innis M, Liggett SB. Amino-terminal polymorphisms of the human β_2-adrenergic receptor impart distinct agonist-promoted regulatory properties. *Biochemistry.* 1994;33:9414–9419.

Gudbjartsson DF, Arnar DO, Helgadottir A, et al. Variants conferring risk of atrial fibrillation on chromosome 4q25. *Nature.* 2007;448:353–357.

Haefeli WE. Therapeutic monitoring, problems of compliance (adherence) and noncompliance. In: Lemmer B, Brune K, (eds.). *Pharmacotherapy–-Clinical Pharmacology*, 13th ed., Springer Heidelberg; 2007: 26–33 (in German).

Haenisch S, Zimmermann U, Dazert E, et al. Influence of polymorphisms of ABCB1 and ABCC2 on mRNA and protein expression in normal and cancerous kidney cortex. *Pharmacogenomics J.* 2007;7:56–65.

Hallberg P, Karlsson J, Kurland L, et al. The CYP2C9 genotype predicts the blood pressure response to irbesartan: results from the Swedish Irbesartan Left Ventricular Hypertrophy Investigation vs Atenolol (SILVHIA) trial. *J Hypertension.* 2002;20:2089–2093.

Hansen JL, Haunso S, Brann MR, Sheikh SP, Weiner DM. Loss-of-function polymorphic variants of the human angiotensin II type 1 receptor. *Mol Pharmacol.* 2004;65:770–777.

Harrap SB, Tzourio C, Cambien F, et al. The ACE gene I/D polymorphism is not associated with the blood pressure and cardiovascular benefits of ACE inhibition. *Hypertension.* 2003;42:303.

Hawkins GA, Tantisira K, Meyers DA, et al. Sequence, haplotype, and association analysis of ADRβ2 in a multiethnic asthma case-control study. *Am J Respir Crit Care Med.* 2006;174:1101–1109.

Hayashi K, Shimizu M, Ino H, et al. Probucol aggravates long QT syndrome associated with a novel missense mutation M124T in the N-terminus of HERG. *Clin Sci. (Lond.).* 2004;107:175–182.

Helgadottir A, Manolescu A, Helgason A, et al. A variant of the gene encoding leukotriene A4 hydrolase confers ethnicity-specific risk of myocardial infarction. *Nat Genet.* 2006;38:68–74.

Helgadottir A, Thorleifsson G, Manolescu A, et al. A common variant on chromosome 9p21 affects the risk of myocardial infarction. *Science.* 2007;316:1491–1493.

Higashi MK, Veenstra DL, Kondo LM, et al. Association between CYP2C9 genetic variants and anticoagulation-related outcomes during warfarin therapy. *JAMA.* 2002;287:1690–1698.

Hignite C, Uetrecht J, Tschanz C, Azarnoff D. Kinetics of R and S warfarin enantiomeres. *Clin Pharmacol Ther.* 1980;28:99–105.

Hingorani AD, Jia H, Stevens PA, Hopper R, Dickerson JE, Brown MJ. Renin-angiotensin system gene polymorphisms influence blood pressure and the response to angiotensin converting enzyme inhibition. *J Hypertension.* 1995;13:1602–1609.

Ho RH, Kim RB. Transporters and drug therapy: implications for drug disposition and disease. *Clin Pharmacol Ther.* 2005;78:260–277.

Ho RH, Tirona RG, Leake BF, et al. Drug and bile acid transporters in rosuvastatin hepatic uptake: function, expression, and pharmacogenetics. *Gastroenterology.* 2006;130:1793–1806.

Hoffmeyer S, Burk O, von Richter O, et al. Functional polymorphisms of the human multidrug-resistance gene: multiple sequence variations and correlation of one allele with P-glycoprotein expression and activity in vivo. *Proc Natl Acad Sci USA.* 2000;97:3473–3478.

Hoffstedt J, Iliadou A, Pedersen NL, Schalling M, Arner P. The effect of the beta_2 adrenoceptor gene Thr164Ile polymorphism on human adipose tissue lipolytic function. *Br J Pharmacol.* 2001;133:708–712.

Hoit BD, Suresh DP, Craft L, Walsh RA, Liggett SB. β_2-Adrenergic receptor polymorphisms at amino acid 16 differentially influence agonist-stimulated blood pressure and peripheral blood flow in normal individuals. *Am Heart J.* 2000;139:537–542.

Honig PK, Woosley RL, Zamani K, Conner DP, Cantilena LR Jr. Changes in the pharmacokinetics and electrocardiographic pharmacodynamics of terfenadine with concomitant administration of erythromycin. *Clin Pharmacol Ther.* 1992;52:231–238.

Igel M, Arnold KA, Niemi M, et al. Impact of the SLCO1B1 polymorphism on the pharmacokinetics and lipid-lowering efficacy of multiple-dose pravastatin. *Clin Pharmacol Ther.* 2006;79:419–426.

Ismail R, Teh LK. The relevance of CYP2D6 genetic polymorphism on chronic metoprolol therapy in cardiovascular patients. *J Clin Pharm Ther.* 2006;31:99–109.

Johne A, Köpke K, Gerloff T, et al. Modulation of steady-state kinetics of digoxin by haplotypes of the P-glycoprotein MDR1 gene. *Clin Pharmacol Ther.* 2002;72:584–594.

Johnson JA, Zineh I, Puckett BJ, McGorray SP, Yarandi HN, Pauly DF. β_1-Adrenergic receptor polymorphisms and antihypertensive response to metoprolol. *Clin Pharmacol Ther.* 2003;74:44–52.

Juliano RL, Ling VA. A surface glycoprotein modulating drug permeability in Chinese hamster ovary cells. *Biochim Biophys Acta.* 1976;455:155–162.

Kaminsky LS, Zhang ZY. Human P450 metabolism of warfarin. *Pharmacol Ther.* 1997;73:67–74.

Kannakeril PJ, Roden DM. Drug-induced long QT and torsade de pointes: recent advances. *Curr Opin Cardiol.* 2007;22:39–43.

Kay LJ, Chong LK, Rostami-Hodjegan A, Peachell PT. Influence of the thr164ile polymorphism in the β_2-adrenoceptor on the effects of β-adrenoceptor agonists on human lung mast cells. *Int Immunopharmacol.* 2003;3:91–95.

Kim RB, Leake BF, Choo EF, et al. Identification of functionally variant MDR1 alleles among European Americans and African Americans. *Clin Pharmacol Ther.* 2001;70:189–199.

Kimchi-Sarfaty C, Gribar JJ, Gottesman MM. Functional characterization of coding polymorphisms in the human MDR1 gene using a vaccinia virus expression system. *Mol Pharmacol.* 2002;62:1–6.

Kimchi-Sarfaty C, Oh JM, Kim IW, et al. A "silent polymorphism in the *MDR1* gene changes substrate specificity. *Science.* 2007;315:525–528.

Kimura R, Miyashita K, Kokubo Y, et al. Genotypes of vitamin K epoxide reductase, gamma-glutamyl carboxylase, and cytochrome P450 2C9 as determinants of daily warfarin dose in Japanese patients. *Thromb Res.* 2007;120:181–186.

Kirchheiner J, Brockmöller J. Clinical consequences of CYP2C9 polymorphisms. *Clin Pharmacol Ther.* 2005;77:1–16.

Kirchheiner J, Heesch C, Bauer S, et al. Impact of the ultrarapid metabolizer genotype of cytochrome P450 2D6 on metoprolol pharmacokinetics and pharmacodynamics. *Clin Pharmacol Ther.* 2004;76:302–312.

König J, Seithel A, Gradhand U, Fromm MF. Pharmacogenomics of human OATP transporters. *Naunyn-Schmiedeberg's Arch Pharmacol.* 2006;372:432–443.

Koopmans RP, Insel PA, Michel MC. Pharmacogenetics of hypertension treatment: a structured review. *Pharmacogenetics.* 2003;13:705–713.

Kuijer PM, Hutten BA, Prins MH, Büller HR. Prediction of the risk of bleeding during anticoagulant treatment for venous thromboembolism. *Arch Intern Med.* 1999;159:457–460.

Kurland L, Liljedahl U, Karlsson J, et al. Angiotensinogen gene polymorphisms: relationship to blood pressure response to antihypertensive treatment. *Am J Hypert.* 2004;17:8–13.

Kurland L, Melhus H, Karlsson J, et al. Angiotensin converting enzyme gene polymorphism predicts blood pressure response to angiotensin II receptor type 1 antagonist treatment in hypertensive patients. *J Hypertension.* 2001;19:1783–1787.

Kurland L, Melhus H, Karlsson J, et al. Polymorphisms in the angiotensinogen and angiotensin II type 1 receptor gene are related to change in left ventricular mass during antihypertensive treatment: results from the Swedish Irbesartan Left Ventricular Hypertrophy Investigation versus Atenolol (SILVHIA) trial. *J Hypertension.* 2002;20:657–663.

Large V, Hellström L, Reynisdottir S, et al. Human beta-2 adrenoceptor gene polymorphisms are highly frequent in obesity and associate with altered beta-2 adrenoceptor function. *J Clin Invest.* 1997;100:3005–3013.

Lazarou J, Pomeranz BH, Corey PN. Incidence of adverse drug reactions in hospitalized patients: a meta-analysis of prospective studies. *JAMA.* 1998;279:1200–1205.

Lee SC, Ng SS, Oldenburg J, et al. Interethnic variability of warfarin maintenance requirement is explained by VKORC1 genotype in an Asian population. *Clin Pharmacol Ther.* 2006;79:197–205.

Lefebvre J, Poirier L, Poirier P, Turgeon J, Lacourciere Y. The influence of CYP2D6 phenotype on the clinical response of nebivolol in patients with essential hypertension. *Br J Clin Pharmacol.* 2006;63:575–582.

Leineweber K, Bogedain P, Wolf C, et al. In patients chronically treated with metoprolol, the demand of inotropic catecholamine support after coronary artery bypass grafting is determined by the Arg389Gly-β_1-adrenoceptor polymorphism. *Naunyn-Schmiedeberg's Arch Pharmacol.* 2007;375:303–309.

Leineweber K, Büscher R, Bruck H, Brodde O-E. β-Adrenoceptor polymorphisms. *Naunyn-Schmiedeberg's Arch Pharmacol.* 2004;369:1–22.

Levin MC, Marullo S, Muntaner O, Andersson B, Magnusson Y. The myocardium-protective Gly-49 variant of the β_1-adrenergic receptor exhibits constitutive activity and increased desensitization and downregulation. *J Biol Chem.* 2002;277:30429–30435.

Li S, Sanna S, Maschio A, et al. The GLUT9 gene is associated with serum uric acid levels in Sardinia and Chianti cohorts. *PLoS Genet.* 2007;3:e194 [Epub ahead of print].

Li T, Chang CY, Jin DY, Lin PJ, Khvorova A, Stafford DW. Identification of the gene for vitamin K epoxide reductase. *Nature.* 2004;427:541–544.

Lichter JB, Kurth JH. The impact of pharmacogenetics on the future of healthcare. *Curr Opin Biotechnol.* 1997;8:692–695.

Liljedahl U, Kahan T, Malmqvist K, et al. Single nucleotide polymorphisms predict the change in left ventricular mass in response to antihypertensive treatment. *J Hypertension.* 2004;22:2321–2328.

Lima JJ, Holbrook JT, Wang J, et al. The C523A β_2 adrenergic receptor polymorphism associates with markers of asthma severity in African Americans. *J Asthma.* 2006;43:185–191.

Limdi NA, McGwin G, Goldstein JA, et al. Influence of CYP2C9 and VKORC1 1173C/T genotype on the risk of hemorrhagic complications in African-American and European-American patients on Warfarin. *Clin Pharmacol Ther.* 2008;83(2):312–321.

Lindpaintner K. The impact of pharmacogenetics and pharmacogenomics on drug discovery. *Nat Rev Drug Discov.* 2002;1:463–469.

Lipworth BJ, Hall IP, Tan S, Aziz I, Coutie W. Effects of genetic polymorphisms on ex vivo and in vivo function of β_2-adrenoceptors in asthmatic patients. *Chest.* 1999;115:324–328.

Liu J, Liu Z-Q, Tan Z-R, et al. Gly389Arg polymorphism of β_1-adrenergic receptor is associated with the cardiovascular response to metoprolol. *Clin Pharmacol Ther.* 2003;74:372–379.

Liu K, Yang T, Viswanathan PC, Roden DM. New mechanisms contributing to drug-induced arrhythmia—Rescue of a misprocessed LQT3 mutant. *Circulation.* 2005;112:3239–3246.

Mahgoub A, Idle JR, Dring LG, Lancaster R, Smith RL. Polymorphic hydroxylation of debrisoquine in man. *Lancet.* 1977;2:584–586.

Mailman RB. GPCR functional selectivity has therapeutic impact. *Trends Pharmacol Sci.* 2007;28:390–396.

Manunta P, Bianchi G. Pharmacogenomics and pharmacogenetics of hypertension: update and perspectives--the adducin paradigm. *J Am Soc Nephrol.* 2006;17:S30–S35.

Markova S, Nakamura T, Sakaeda T, et al. Genotype-dependent downregulation of gene expression and function of MDR1 in human peripheral blood mononuclear cells under acute inflammation. *Drug Metab Pharmacokinet.* 2006;21:194–200.

Marre M, Bernadet P, Gallois Y, et al. Relationships between angiotensin I converting enzyme gene polymorphism, plasma levels, and diabetic retinal and renal complications. *Diabetes.* 1994;43:384–388.

Martin MM, Buckenberger JA, Jiang J, et al. The human angiotensin II type 1 receptor +1166 A/C polymorphism attenuates microRNA -155 binding. *J Biol Chem.* 2007;282:24262–24269.

Mason DA, Moore JD, Green SA, Liggett SB. A gain-of-function polymorphism in a G-protein coupling domain of the human β_1-adrenergic receptor. *J Biol Chem.* 1999;274:12670–12674.

Materson BJ, Reda DJ, Cushman WC, et al. Single-drug therapy for hypertension in men. A comparison of six antihypertensive agents with placebo. The Department of Veterans Affairs Cooperative Study Group on Antihypertensive Agents. *N Engl J Med.* 1993;328:914–921.

McPherson R, Pertsemlidis A, Kavaslar N, et al. A common allele on chromosome 9 associated with coronary heart disease. *Science.* 2007;316:1488–1491.

Meckley LM, Veenstra DL. Screening for the alpha-adducin Gly460Trp variant in hypertensive patients: a cost-effectiveness analysis. *Pharmacogenet Genomics.* 2006;6:139–147.

Meisel C, Gerloff T, Kirchheiner J, et al. Implication of pharmacogenetics for individualizing drug treatment and for study design. *J Mol Med.* 2003;81:154–167.

Meissner K, Jedlitschky G, Meyer zu Schwabedissen H, et al. Modulation of multidrug resistance P-glycoprotein 1 (ABCB1) expression in human heart by hereditary polymorphisms. *Pharmacogenetics.* 2004;14:381–385.

Meissner K, Sperker B, Karsten C, et al. Expression and localization of P-glycoprotein in human heart: effects of cardiomyopathy. *J Histochem Cytochem.* 2002;50:1351–1356.

Mellen PB, Herrington DM. Pharmacogenomics of blood pressure response to antihypertensive treatment. *J Hypertension.* 2005;23:1311–1325.

Mialat Perez J, Rathz DA, Petrashevskaya NN, et al. β_1-adrenergic polymorphisms confer differential function and predisposition to heart failure. *Nat Med.* 2003;9:1300–1305.

Michaud V, Vanier MC, Brouillette D, et al. Combination of phenotype assessments and CYP2C9-VKORC1 polymorphisms in the determination of warfarindose requirements in heavily medicated patients. *Clin Pharmacol Ther.* 2008;83:740–748.

Michel MC, Alewijnse AE. Ligand-directed signaling: 50 ways to find a lover. *Mol Pharmacol.* 2007;72:1097–1099.

Michel MC, Hegde SS. Treatment of the overactive bladder syndrome with muscarinic receptor antagonists--a matter of metabolites? *Naunyn-Schmiedeberg's Arch Pharmacol.* 2006;374:79–85.

Miller JA, Thai K, Scholey JW. Angiotensin II type 1 receptor gene polymorphism predicts response to losartan and angiotensin II. *Kidney Int.* 1999;56:2173–2180.

Millican EA, Lenzini PA, Milligan PE, et al. Genetic-based dosing in orthopedic patients beginning warfarin therapy. *Blood.* 2007;110:1511–1515.

Molenaar P, Rabnott G, Yang I, et al. Conservation of the cardiostimulant effects of (-)-norepinephrine across Ser49Gly and Gly389Arg beta$_1$-adrenergic receptor polymorphisms in human right atrium in vitro. *J Am Coll Cardiol.* 2002;40:1275–1282.

Momary KM, Shapiro NL, Viana MA, Nutescu EA, Helgason CM, Cavallari LH. Factors influencing warfarin dose requirements in African-Americans. *Pharmacogenomics.* 2007;8:1535–1544.

Moore JD, Mason DA, Green SA, Hsu J, Liggett SB. Racial differences in the frequencies of cardiac β_1-adrenergic receptor polymorphisms: analysis of c145A>G and c1165G>C. *Hum Mutat.* 1999;14:271.

Moore PE, Laporte JD, Abraham JH, et al. Polymorphism of the β_2-adrenergic receptor gene and desensitization in human airways smooth muscle. *Am J Respir Crit Care Med.* 2000;162:2117–2124.

Morita N, Yasumori T, Nakayama. Human MDR1 polymorphism: G2677T/A and C3435T have no effect on MDR1 transport activities. *Biochem Pharmacol.* 2003;65:1843–1852.

Motulsky AG. Drug reactions enzymes, and biochemical genetics. *J Am Med Assoc.* 1957;165(7):835–837.

Mwinyi J, Johne A, Bauer S, Roots I, Gerloff T. Evidence for inverse effects of OATP-C (SLC21A6) 5 and 1b haplotypes on pravastatin kinetics. *Clin Pharmacol Ther.* 2004;75:415–421.

Narita I, Goto S, Saito N, et al. Renoprotective efficacy of renin-angiotensin inhibitors in IgA nephropathy is influenced by ACE A2350G polymorphism. *J Med Genet.* 2003;40:e130.

Niemi M, Schaeffeler E, Lang T, et al. High plasma pravastatin concentrations are associated with single nucleotide polymorphisms and haplotypes of organic anion transporting polypeptide-C (OATP-C, SLCO1B1). *Pharmacogenetics.* 2004;14:429–440.

Nishizato Y, Ieiri I, Suzuki H, et al. Polymorphisms of OATP-C (SLC21A6) and OAT3 (SLC22A8) genes: consequences for pravastatin pharmacokinetics. *Clin Pharmacol Ther.* 2003;73:554–565.

Nonen S, Okamoto H, Akino M, et al. No positive association between adrenergic receptor variants of α_{2c}Del322–325, β_1Ser49, β_1Arg389 and the risk for heart failure in the Japanese population. *Br J Clin Pharmacol.* 2005;64:414–417.

Nozawa T, Taguchi M, Tahara K, et al. Influence of CYP2D6 genotype on metoprolol plasma concentration and β-adrenergic inhibition during long-term treatment. A comparison with bisoprolol. *J Cardiovasc Pharmacol.* 2005;46:713–720.

Oldenburg J, Bevans CG, Fregin A, Geisen C, Mller-Reible C, Watzka M. Current pharmacogenetic developments in oral anticoagulation therapy: the influence of variant VKORC1 and CYP2C9 alleles. *Thromb Haemost.* 2007a;98:570–578.

Oldenburg J, Watzka M, Rost S, Müller CR. VKORC1: molecular target of coumarins. *J Thromb Haemost.* 2007;5(Suppl 1):1–6.

Oro C, Qian H, Thomas WG. Type 1 angiotensin receptor pharmacology: signaling beyond G proteins. *Pharmacol Ther.* 2007;113:210–226.

Owen A, Goldring C, Morgan P, Chadwick D, Park BK, Pirmohamed M. Relationship between the C3435T and G2677T(A) polymorphisms in the ABCB1 gene and P-glycoprotein expression in human liver. *Br J Clin Pharmacol.* 2005;59:365–370.

Pasanen MK, Fredrikson H, Neuvonen PJ, Niemi M. Different effects of SLCO1B1 polymorphism on the pharmacokinetics of atorvastatin and rosuvastatin. *Clin Pharmacol Ther.* 2007;82:726–733.

Pasanen MK, Neuvonen M, Neuvonen PJ, Niemi M. SLCO1B1 polymorphism markedly affects the pharmacokinetics of simvastatin acid. *Pharmacogenet Genomics.* 2006;16:873–879.

Pearson ER, Donnelly LA, Kimber C, et al. Variation in TCF7L2 influences therapeutic response to sulfonylureas: a GoDARTs study. *Diabetes.* 2007;56:2178–2182.

Pedro-Botet J, Schaefer EJ, Bakker-Arkema RG, et al. Apolipoprotein E genotype affects plasma lipid response to atorvastatin in a gender specific manner. *Atherosclerosis.* 2001;58:183–193.

Pietila E, Fodstad H, Niskasaari E, et al. Association between HERG K897T polymorphism and QT interval in middle-aged Finnish women. *J Am Coll Cardiol.* 2002;40:511–514.

Psaty BM, Smith NL, Heckbert SR, et al. Diuretic therapy, the alpha-adducin gene variant, and the risk of myocardial infarction or stroke in persons with treated hypertension. *JAMA.* 2002;287:1680–1689.

Rasmussen SG, Choi HJ, Rosenbaum DM, et al. Crystal structure of the human beta2 adrenergic G-protein-coupled receptor. *Nature.* 2007;450:383–387.

Rathz DA, Brown KM, Kramer LA, Liggett SB. Amino acid 49 polymorphisms of the human β_1-adrenergic receptor affect agonist-promoted trafficking. *J Cardiovasc Pharmacol.* 2002;39:155–160.

Ray WA, Murray KT, Meredith S, Narasimhulu SS, Hall K, Stein CM. Oral erythromycin and the risk of sudden death from cardiac causes. *N Engl J Med.* 2004;351:1089–1096.

Reitsma PH, van der Heijden JF, Groot AP, Rosendaal FR, Büller HR. A C1173T dimorphism in the VKORC1 gene determines coumarin sensitivity and bleeding risk. *PLoS Med.* 2005;2:e312.

Rettie AE, Korzekwa KR, Kunze KL, et al. Hydroxylation of warfarin by human cDNA-expressed cytochrome P-450: a role for P-4502C9 in the etiology of (S)-warfarin-drug interactions. *Chem Res Toxicol.* 1992;5:54–59.

Rieder MJ, Reiner AP, Gage BF, et al. Effect of VKORC1 haplotypes on transcriptional regulation and warfarin dose. *N Engl J Med.* 2005;352:2285–2293.

Rochais F, Vilardaga J-P, Nikolaev VO, Bünemann M, Lohse MJ, Engelhardt S. Real-time optical recording of β_1-adrenergic receptor activation reveals supersensitivity of the Arg389 variant to carvedilol. *J Clin Invest.* 2007;117:229–235.

Roden DM. Drug-induced prolongation of the QT interval. *N Engl J Med.* 2004;350:1013–1022.

Roden DM, Viswanathan PC. Genetics of acquired long QT syndrome. *J Clin Invest.* 2005;115:2025–2032.

Rodriguez I, Abernethy DR, Woosley RL. P-glycoprotein in clinical cardiology. *Circulation.* 1999;99:472–474.

Roepke TK, Abott GW. Pharmacogenetics and cardiac ion channels. *Vasc Pharmacol.* 2006;44:90–106.

Roninson IB, Chin JE, Choi KG, et al. Isolation of human mdr DNA sequences amplified in multidrug-resistant KB carcinoma cells. *Proc Natl Acad Sci USA.* 1986;83:4538–4442.

Roses AD. Pharmacogenetics and the practice of medicine. *Nature.* 2000;405:857–865.

Rosskopf D, Schürks M, Rimmbach C, Schäfers RF. Genetics of arterial hypertension and hypotension. *Naunyn-Schmiedeberg's Arch Pharmacol.* 2007;374:429–469.

Rost S, Fregin A, Ivaskevicius V, et al. Mutations in VKORC1 cause warfarin resistance and multiple coagulation factor deficiency type 2. *Nature.* 2004;427:537–541.

Rowland P, Blaney FE, Smyth MG, et al. Crystal structure of human cytochrome P450 2D6. *J Biol Chem.* 2006;281:7614–7622.

Ryden M, Hoffstedt J, Eriksson P, Bringman S, Arner P. The Arg 389 Gly β_1-adrenergic receptor gene polymorphism and human fat cell lipolysis. *Int J Obes Relat Metab Disord.* 2001;25:1599–1603.

Sakaeda T. MDR1 genotype-related pharmacokinetics. Fact or fiction? *Drug Metab Pharmacokinet.* 2005;20:391–414.

Samani NJ, Erdmann J, Hall AS, et al. Genomewide association analysis of coronary artery disease. *N Engl J Med.* 2007;357:443–453.

Sandilands AJ, O'Shaughnessy KM, Brown MJ. Greater inotropic and cyclic AMP responses evoked by noradrenaline through Arg389 β_1-adrenoceptors versus Gly389 β_1-adrenoceptors in isolated human atrial myocardium. *Br J Pharmacol.* 2003;138:386–392.

Sarsero D, Russel FD, Lynham JA, et al. (-)-CGP 12177 increases contractile force and hastens relaxation of human myocardial preparations through a propranol-resistant state of the β_1-adrenoceptor. *Naunyn-Schmiedeberg's Arch Pharmacol.* 2003;367:10–21.

Schalekamp T, Boink GJJ, Visser LE, Stricker BHC, de Boer A, Klungel OH. CYP2C9 genotyping in acenocoumarol treatment: is it a cost-effective addition to international normalized ratio monitoring. *Clin Pharmacol Ther.* 2006;79:511–520.

Schalekamp T, Brass BP, Roijers JF, et al. VKORC1 and CYP2C9 genotypes and phenprocoumon anticoagulation status: interaction between both genotypes affects dose requirement. *Clin Pharmacol Ther.* 2007;81:185–193.

Schalekamp T, Oosterhof M, van Meegen E, et al. Effects of cytochrome P450 2C9 polymorphisms on phenprocoumon anticoagulation status. *Clin Pharmacol Ther.* 2004;76:409–417.

Scharplatz M, Puhan MA, Steurer J, Perna A, Bachmann LM. Does the angiotensin-converting enzyme (ACE) gene insertion/deletion polymorphism modify the response to ACE inhibitor therapy?--A systematic review. *Curr Contr Trials Cardiovasc Med.* 2005;6:16.

Schelleman H, Chen Z, Kealey C, et al. Warfarin response and vitamin K epoxide reductase complex 1 in African Americans and Caucasians. *Clin Pharmacol Ther.* 2007;81:742–747.

Schelleman H, Klungel OH, van Duijn CM, et al. Insertion/deletion polymorphism of the ACE gene and adherence to ACE inhibitors. *Br J Clin Pharmacol.* 2005;59:483–485.

Schelleman H, Klungel OH, Witteman JCM, et al. The influence of the alpha-adducin G460W polymorphism and angiotensinogen M235T polymorphism on antihypertensive medication and blood pressure. *Eur J Hum Genet.* 2006;14:860–866.

Schmitz G, Schmitz-Madry A, Ugocsai P. Pharmacogenetics and pharmacogenomics of cholesterol-lowering therapy. *Curr Opin Lipidol.* 2007;18:164–173.

Sciarrone MT, Stella P, Barlassina C, et al. ACE and alpha-adducin polymorphism as markers of individual response to diuretic therapy. *Hypertension.* 2003;41:398–403.

Shin J, Johnson JA. Pharmacogenetics of β-blockers. *Pharmacotherapy.* 2007;27:874–887.

Siegmund W, Ludwig K, Giessmann T, et al. The effects of the human MDR1 genotype on the expression of duodenal P-glycoprotein and disposition of the probe drug talinolol. *Clin Pharmacol Ther.* 2002;72:572–583.

Siest G, Jeannesson E, Visvikis-Siest S. Enzymes and pharmacogenetics of cardiovascular drugs. *Clin Chim Acta.* 2007;381:26–31.

Sofowora GG, Dishy V, Muszkat M, et al. A common β_1-adrenergic receptor polymorphism (Arg389Gly) affects blood pressure response to β-blockade. *Clin Pharmacol Ther.* 2003;73:366–371.

Splawski I, Timothy KW, Tateyama M, et al. Variant of SCN5A sodium channel implicated in risk of cardiac arrhythmia. *Science.* 2002;297:1333–1336.

Steinthorsdottir V, Thorleifsson G, Reynisdottir I, et al. A variant in CDKAL1 influences insulin response and risk of type 2 diabetes. *Nat Genet.* 2007;39:770–775.

Steward DJ, Haining RL, Henne KR, et al. Genetic association between sensitivity to warfarin and expression of CYP2C9*3. *Pharmacogenetics.* 1997;7:361–367.

Sun Z, Milos PM, Thompson JF, et al. Role of a KCNH2 polymorphism(R1047 L) in dofetilide-induced Torsades de Pointes. *J Mol Cell Cardiol.* 2004;37:1031–1039.

Takahashi H, Echizen H. Pharmacogenetics of warfarin elimination and its clinical implications. *Clin Pharmacokinet.* 2001;40:587–603.

Takahashi H, Kashima T, Nomizo Y, et al. Metabolism of warfarin enantiomers in Japanese patients with heart disease having different CYP2C9 and CYP2C19 genotypes. *Clin Pharmacol Ther.* 1998a;63:519–528.

Takahashi H, Kashima T, Nomoto S, et al. Comparisons between in-vitro and in-vivo metabolism of (S)-warfarin: catalytic activities of cDNA-expressed CYP2C9, its Leu359 variant and their mixture versus unbound clearance in patients with the corresponding CYP2C9 genotypes. *Pharmacogenetics.* 1998b;8:365–373.

Taube J, Halsall D, Baglin T. Influence of cytochrome P-450 CYP2C9 polymorphisms on warfarin sensitivity and risk of over-anticoagulation in patients on long-term treatment. *Blood.* 2000;96:1816–1819.

Terra SG, Pauly DF, Lee CR, et al. β-Adrenergic receptor polymorphisms and responses during titration of metoprolol controlled release/extended release in heart failure. *Clin Pharmacol Ther.* 2005;77:127–137.

Thijssen HH, Drittij MJ, Vervoort LM, de Vries-Hanje JC. Altered pharmacokinetics of R- and S-acenocoumarol in a subject heterozygous for CYP2C9*3. *Clin Pharmacol Ther.* 2001;70:292–298.

Thijssen HH, Flinois JP, Beaune PH. Cytochrome P4502C9 is the principal catalyst of racemic acenocoumarol hydroxylation reactions in human liver microsomes. *Drug Metab Dispos.* 2000;28:1284–1290.

Tirona RG, Leake BF, Merino G, Kim RB. Polymorphisms in OATP-C: identification of multiple allelic variants associated with altered transport activity among European- and African-Americans. *J Biol Chem.* 2001;276:35669–35675.

Tsai, CT, Lai LP, Lin JL, et al. Renin–angiotensin system gene polymorphisms and atrial fibrillation. *Circulation.* 2004;109:1640–1646.

Tsikouris JP, Peeters MJ. Pharmacogenomics of renin angiotensin system inhibitors in coronary artery disease. *Cardiovasc Drugs Ther.* 2007;21:121–132.

Turner ST, Chapman AB, Schwartz GL, Boerwinkle E. Effects of endothelial nitric oxide synthase, alpha-adducin, and other candidate gene polymorphisms on blood pressure response to hydrochlorothiazide. *Am J Hypertens.* 2003;16:834–839.

Uchida S, Watanabe H, Nishio S, et al. Altered pharmacokinetics and excessive hypotensive effect of candesartan in a patient with the CYP2C91/3 genotype. *Clin Pharmacol Ther.* 2003;74:505–508.

Ufer M. Comparative pharmacokinetics of vitamin K antagonists: warfarin, phenprocoumon and acenocoumarol. *Clin Pharmacokinet.* 2005;44:1227–1246.

Visser LE, van Schaik RH, van Vliet M, et al. The risk of bleeding complications in patients with cytochrome P450 CYP2C9*2 or CYP2C9*3 alleles on acenocoumarol or phenprocoumon. *Thromb Haemost.* 2004a;92:61–66.

Visser LE, van Vliet M, van Schaik RH, et al. The risk of overanticoagulation in patients with cytochrome P450 CYP2C9*2 or CYP2C9*3 alleles on acenocoumarol or phenprocoumon. *Pharmacogenetics.* 2004b;14:27–33.

Voora D, Eby C, Linder MW, et al. Prospective dosing of warfarin based on cytochrome P-450 2C9 genotype. *Thromb Haemost.* 2005a;93:700–705.

Voora D, McLeod HL, Eby C, Gage BF. The pharmacogenetics of coumarin therapy. *Pharmacogenomics.* 2005b;6:503–513.

Vormfelde SV, Engelhardt S, Zirk A, et al. CYP2C9 polymorphisms and the interindividual variability in pharmacokinetics and pharmacodynamics of the loop diuretic drug torsemide. *Clin Pharmacol Ther.* 2004;76:557–566.

Vormfelde SV, Schirmer M, Hagos Y, et al. Torsemide renal clearance and genetic variation in luminal and basolateral organic anion transporters. *Br J Clin Pharmacol.* 2006;62:323–335.

Vormfelde SV, Sehrt D, Toliat MR, et al. Genetic variation in the renal sodium transporters NKCC2, NCC, and ENaC in relation to the effects of loop diuretic drugs. *Clin Pharmacol Ther.* 2007;82:300–309.

Vormfelde SV, Toliat MR, Schirmer M, Meineke I, Nürnberg P, Brockmöller J. The Polymorphisms Asn130Asp and Val174Ala in OATP1B1 and the CYP2C9 allele (*)3 independently affect torsemide pharmacokinetics and pharmacodynamics. *Clin Pharmacol Ther.* 2008;83:815–817.

Wang D, Johnson AD, Papp AC, Kroetz DL, Sadée W. Multidrug resistance polypeptide 1 (MDR1, ABCB1) variant 3435C>T affects mRNA stability. *Pharmacogenet Genomics.* 2005;15:693–704.

Wang D, Sadée W. Searching for polymorphisms that affect gene expression and mRNA processing: example ABCB1 (MDR1). *AAPS J.* 2006;8:e61.

Wellcome Trust Case Control Consortium. Genome-wide association study of 14,000 cases of seven common diseases and 3,000 shared controls. *Nature.* 2007;447:661–678.

Williams PA, Cosme J, Ward A, Angove HC, Matak Vinković D, Jhoti H. Crystal structure of human cytochrome P450 2C9 with bound warfarin. *Nature.* 2003;424:464–468.

Woosley RL, Chen Y, Freiman JP, Gillis RA. Mechanism of the cardiotoxic actions of terfenadine. *JAMA.* 1993;269:1532–1536.

Wu H, Tang W, Li H, et al. Association of the β_2-adrenergic receptor gene with essential hypertension in the non-Han Chinese Yi minority human population. *J Hypertension.* 2006;24:1041–1047.

Wuttke H, Rau T, Heide R, et al. Increased frequency of cytochrome P450 2D6 poor metabolizers among patients with metoprolol-associated adverse effects. *Clin Pharmacol Ther.* 2002;72:429–437.

Xie HG, Dishy V, Sofowora G, et al. Arg389Gly β_1-adrenoceptor polymorphism varies in frequency among different ethnic groups but does not alter response in vivo. *Pharmacogenetics.* 2001;11:191–197.

Yasar U, Forslund-Bergengren C, Tybring G, et al. Pharmacokinetics of losartan and its metabolite E-3174 in relation to the CYP2C9 genotype. *Clin Pharmacol Ther.* 2002;71:89–98.

Yuan HY, Chen JJ, LeeMT, et al. A novel functional VKORC1 promoter polymorphism is associated with inter-individual and inter-ethnic differences in warfarin sensitivity. *Hum Mol Genet.* 2005;14:1745–1751.

Zanger UM, Raimundo S, Eichelbaum M. Cytochrome P450 2D6: overview and update on pharmacology, genetics, biochemistry. *Naunyn-Schmiedeberg's Arch Pharmacol.* 2004;369:23–37.

Zhang Z, Fasco MJ, Huang Z, Guengerich FP, Kaminsky LS. Human cytochromes P4501A1 and P4501A2: R-warfarin metabolism as a probe. *Drug Metab Dispos.* 1995;23:1339–1346.

Zineh I, Beitelshees AL, Gaedigk A, et al. Pharmacokinetics and CYP2D6 genotypes do not predict metoprolol adverse events or efficacy in hypertension. *Clin Pharmacol Ther.* 2004;76:536–544.

35

Stem Cell Therapy in Cardiovascular Medicine

Shinsuke Yuasa and Keiichi Fukuda

Introduction

Cardiomyocytes cease to divide immediately after birth and are thought to adapt subsequently to the demands placed on the heart by undergoing hypertrophy without proliferation. Although recent studies have revealed that a low number of cardiomyocytes undergoes cell division immediately after myocardial infarction (MI), these cells appear to have an insufficient impact on heart failure (Beltrami et al. 2001; Yuasa et al. 2004). Cardiovascular regenerative medicine is progressing in terms of investigating the mechanisms underlying cardiomyocyte differentiation. Although significant progress has been achieved, there is no efficient method for generating populations rich in functioning cardiomyocytes from patients. Among the many target diseases for regenerative medicine, heart disease is one of the most important therapeutic targets due to the high mortality rates associated with severe heart failure. Heart failure is the outcome of various cardiac diseases, such as ischemic heart disease, valvular heart disease, congenital heart disease, and cardiomyopathies (dilated cardiomyopathy, hypertrophic cardiomyopathy, and restrictive cardiomyopathy). Although heart transplantation is performed for intractable severe heart failure, it is restricted by a shortage of donors. The replacement of diseased heart tissue with healthy cardiomyocytes through cell transplantation requires potent stem cells with strong proliferation capacities and reliable differentiation abilities.

Stem Cells for Cardiomyocyte Regeneration

Although stem cells are referred to as being pluripotent, they are present in many different developmental stages and organs. Many potential sources of stems cells can be utilized in regenerative cardiac medicine, including bone marrow (BM) stem cells, endothelial progenitor cells, skeletal myocytes, adult cardiac stem cells, and embryonic stem (ES) cells. In 1999, we reported that BM mesenchymal stem cells (MSCs) differentiate into cardiomyocytes (Makino et al. 1999). It is now known that various stem cells present in the body have the ability to differentiate into cardiomyocytes (Fukuda and Yuasa 2006). As each stem cell type has inherent advantages and disadvantages, it is important to understand which stem cells are suitable for cardiac regenerative medicine. Table 35–1 lists the characteristics of representative cells (Evans and Kaufman 1981; Jiang et al. 2002, 2007; Beltrami et al. 2003; Oh et al. 2003; Takahashi and Yamanaka 2006).

Bone Marrow Mesenchymal Stem Cells (BM MSCs) as a Source of Cardiomyocytes

MSCs comprise 0.001%–0.01% of the total nucleated cells in the BM, which is far lower than the percentage of hematopoietic stem cells (HSCs) (Rickard et al. 1994; Prockop 1997). In 1966, MSCs were first identified in the BM as bone formation progenitors (Friedenstein et al. 1966). MSCs have the capacity to differentiate into osteoblasts, chondrocytes, adipocytes, and connective tissues (Prockop 1997; Pittenger et al. 1999; Blanc and Pittenger 2005), and they have been reported to differentiate into skeletal muscle cells, cardiomyocytes (Makino et al. 1999), and neurons (Woodbury et al. 2000). The possibility that marrow stromal cells might also differentiate into cardiomyocytes prompted us to screen for BM stromal cells that could differentiate into cardiomyocytes. We found that BM stromal cells began to beat spontaneously upon exposure to 5-azacytidine (5-AZA), which is a cytosine analog with demethylating activity. The cells isolated from the adult BM stromal cells were termed **c**ardio**m**yo**g**enic (CMG) cells, which differentiate into cardiomyocytes. The use of adult tissue as the source of cardiomyocytes makes this system particularly suitable for the development of cardiomyocytes for transplantation. These experiments were reproducible, although the percentages of differentiated cardiomyocytes differed between the clones.

Cardiomyogenic (CMG) Cells

Phase-contrast microscopy revealed that CMG cells had fibroblast-like morphology before 5-AZA treatment (0 week), a phenotype that was retained despite repeated subculturing under nonstimulating conditions. During 1 week of 5-AZA treatment, the cell morphology gradually changed, with approximately 30% of the cells gradually increasing in size to attain a ball-like appearance or lengthening in one direction to adopt a stick-like morphology. Adjoining cells connected after 2 weeks, and formed myotube-like structures after 3 weeks (Figure 35–1). The differentiated CMG myotubes did not dedifferentiate and they maintained the cardiomyocyte phenotype and beat vigorously for at least 8 weeks

Table 35–1 Classification and Characteristics of Myocardial Stem Cells

	References	Characteristics	Frequency of Occurrence/ Difficulty of Isolation	Differentiation Capacity
ES cells	Evans and Kaufman 1981	Capable of mass culture Immunosuppressive agents required for allogeneic transplantation	Isolation relatively easy Human ES cells have already been established	Can differentiate into wide variety of cells, but cells capable of differentiating in the early embryonic period are easy to obtain in vitro
BM MSCs	Fukuda and Yuasa 2006	Culture method relatively easy	One in several million to several tens of millions in BM	Osteoblasts, chondroblasts, adipocytes, cardiomyocytes, etc.
MAPCs	Verfeille et al. 2002	Culture method extremely difficult. Mass culture impossible	One in a billion (extremely rare) Isolation is difficult, but has been done from human cells	Can differentiate into wide variety of cells including neurons, hepatocytes, skeletal muscle cells, etc.
Bone marrow stem cells (c-Kit cells)	Anversa et al. 2001	Isolation difficult Mass culture impossible	Difficult to use as material for heart tissue Unknown whether possible by biopsy	Myocardium, smooth muscle, vascular endothelial cells
Myocardial tissue stem cells (Sca-1 cells)	Schneider et al. 2003	Isolation difficult Mass culture impossible	Impossible—humans do not possess the Sca-1 antigen	Myocardium
Induced pluripotent stem cells	Yamanaka et al. 2006	Custom use	Induced from adult fibroblast cells	Can differentiate into wide variety of cells, but cells capable of differentiating in the early embryonic period are easy to obtain in vitro

after the final 5-AZA treatment. Most of the other nonmyocytes resembled adipocytes.

Transmission electron microscopy revealed that differentiated CMG myotubes had the typical striation and pale-staining pattern of sarcomeres, with nuclei positioned in the center of the cell rather than beneath the sarcolemma. Membrane-bound dense secretory granules of diameter 70–130 nm were the most conspicuous feature of the differentiated CMG cells. These granules, which were considered to be atrial granules, tended to concentrate within the juxtanuclear cytoplasm, with a few also located near the sarcolemma. These findings suggest that CMG cells have ultrastructures consistent with those of cardiomyocytes. An electrophysiologic study was performed on differentiated CMG cells 2–5 weeks after 5-AZA treatment. Two types of morphologic action potentials were distinguished: sinus node-like potentials (Figure 35–2a), and ventricular myocyte-like potentials (Figure 35–2b). The sinus node-like action potential showed a relative shallow resting membrane potential and late diastolic slow depolarization resembling the

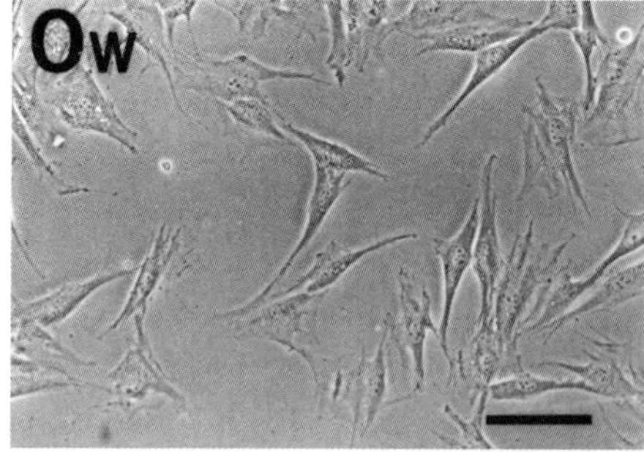

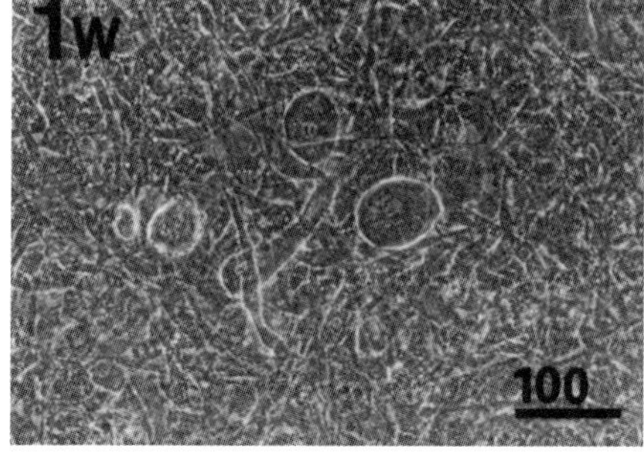

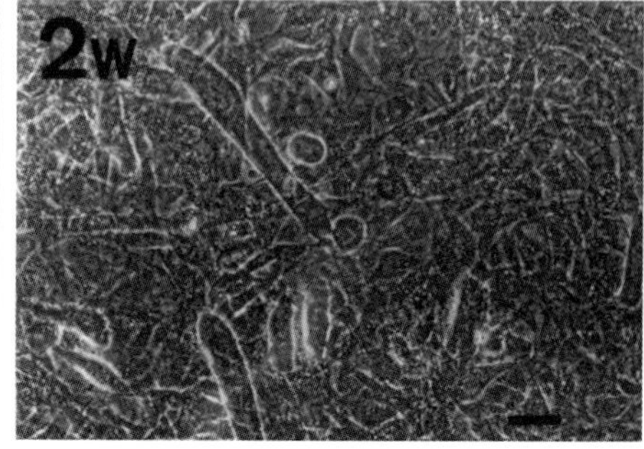

Figure 35–1 Phase-contrast photographs of CMG cells before and after 5-AZA treatment. Upper left, CMG cells show fibroblast-like morphology before 5-AZA treatment (0 week). Upper right, CMG cells at 1 week after the treatment with 5-AZA. Some cells gradually increase in size, becoming ball-like or stick-like in appearance and beginning to beat spontaneously. Lower left, CMG cells at 2 weeks after the treatment with 5-AZA. Ball-like or stick-like cells begin to form connections with adjoining cells and begin to form myotube-like structures. Lower right, CMG cells at 3 weeks after the treatment with 5-AZA. Most of the beating cells have formed connections and myotube-like structures. Bars, 100 μm.

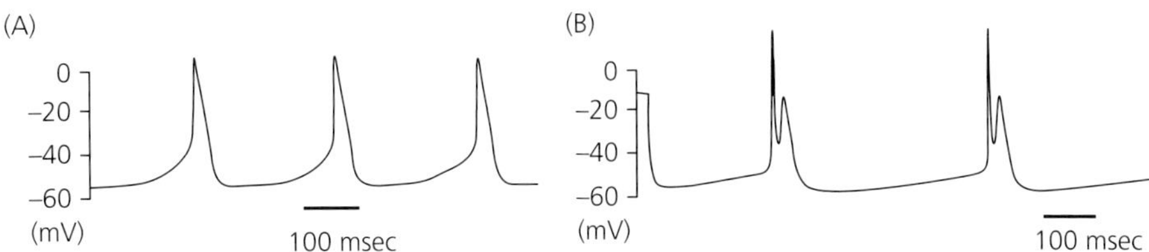

Figure 35–2 a & b Representative tracing of the action potentials of CMG myotubes. Action potentials were recorded with a conventional microelectrode in spontaneously beating cells on Day 28 after 5-AZA treatment. The action potentials are categorized as sinus node-like action potential (a), and ventricular cardiomyocyte-like action potential (b).

potential of a pacemaker. Peak- and dome-like morphologies were observed for the ventricular myocyte-like cells. A cardiomyocyte-like action potential recorded from these spontaneous beating cells had the following properties: relatively long action potential duration or plateau, relatively shallow resting membrane potential, and pacemaker-like late diastolic slow depolarization. Three weeks after 5-AZA treatment, all the action potentials recorded for CMG cells revealed a sinus node-like action potential. It was not until 4 weeks after 5-AZA treatment that ventricular myocyte-like action potentials were initially recorded, and subsequently increased gradually. It is possible that the level of ventricular myocyte-like action potential at 5 weeks was underestimated. Most of the action potentials recorded for differentiated CMG myotubes had a ventricular myocyte-like appearance, although they were difficult to record. Furthermore, the glass microelectrode was frequently damaged because the spontaneous contraction of the differentiated myotubes at 5 weeks was too large.

Differentiated CMG myotubes expressed both the *ANP* and *BNP* genes. Table 35–2 shows a summary of the expression patterns of the cardiac contractile proteins, that is, α- and β-MHC, and α-cardiac and α-skeletal actin genes. Both α-MHC and β-MHC expressions were detected by RT-PCR in differentiated CMG cells, although β-MHC expression was significantly stronger than α-MHC expression. CMG cells expressed both α-cardiac and α-skeletal actin. Northern blot analysis revealed that the α-skeletal actin gene was expressed at markedly higher levels than the α-cardiac actin gene in CMG cells. Interestingly, CMG cells expressed *MLC-2v*, but not *MLC-2a*. Several characteristics of the CMG cell lines support the cardiomyocyte nature of these cells, including the expression of the cardiomyocyte-specific genes *ANP*, *BNP*, *GATA4*, and *Nkx2.5*. In the ventricular muscles of small mammals, there occurs around the time of birth a developmental switch from the expression of β-MHC, which is the predominant fetal form, to the expression of α-MHC. A developmental switch occurs from the expression of α-skeletal actin, which is the predominant fetal and neonatal form, to that of α-cardiac actin, which is the predominant adult form. Differentiated CMG cells express mainly β-MHC and α-skeletal actin. The expression of α-MHC and α-cardiac actin was detected, albeit at low levels. The *MLC-2* genes are expressed specifically in the heart chamber. *MLC-2v* is expressed specifically in ventricular cells, while *MLC-2a* is expressed specifically in atrial cells. Differentiated CMG cells express *MLC-2v*, but not *MLC-2a*. These results suggest that differentiated CMG cells have the fetal ventricular cardiomyocyte phenotype.

Table 35–2 Expression of the Isoforms of the Cardiac Contractile Proteins in CMG Cell

	Atrium		Ventricle			CMG
	Fetal	Adult	Fetal	Neonatal	Adult	
α-actin	Skeletal	Cardiac	Skeletal> cardiac	Skeletal	Cardiac	Skeletal> cardiac
MHC	α>β	α	β>α	α>β	α	β>α
MLC	2a	2a	2v	2v	2v	2v

Notes: MHC, myosin heavy chain; MLC, myosin light chain.

An advantage of deriving cardiomyocytes from BM MSCs is that the patients' own cells can be used, which avoids donor rejection. A drawback is that, while these cells appear to self-replicate throughout life in vivo, the number of passages in vitro is limited. At present, it is not possible to culture large quantities of BM MSCs. Cardiomyocytes that differentiate from BM MSCs initially assume the phenotype of the embryonic ventricular myocardium, but they gradually mature and eventually, they exhibit adult-type gene expression. These cells also express functioning sympathetic and parasympathetic nerve receptors, as do cardiomyocytes in vivo, and they can be successfully transplanted, integrated into the adult heart, and connected to the adult myocardium (Hakuno et al. 2002; Hattan et al. 2005; Tomita et al. 2007).

Other BM Stem Cells

Recent advances in fluorescence-activated cell sorting (FACS) techniques have enabled the isolation of different cell types based on cell surface antigen expression and fluorescent dye efflux characteristics (Osawa et al. 1996; Goodell et al. 1997). FACS analysis has revealed that the HSC population in mice consists of a $CD34^-$ $c\text{-}kit^+$ $Sca\text{-}1^+$ Lin^- tip side population (SP) of cells, whereby c-kit is a stem cell factor receptor, Sca-1 is a stem cell antigen that is expressed in various stem cell populations but only in mice, and Lin is a mixture of antibodies against lineage markers for hematocytes (Matsuzaki et al. 2004). Contrary to some reports, cell surface markers that can be used to isolate MSCs remain to be identified. CD29, CD44, CD105, and murine Sca-1 are widely accepted cell surface markers for MSCs, whereas other potential markers are not universally accepted (Takahashi et al. 1999; Docheva et al. 2007; Phinney and Prockop 2007). In 2001, mitotic cardiomyocytes were observed in a human heart after MI (Beltrami et al. 2001). It is still not clear whether mature cardiomyocytes acquired the ability to proliferate, immature cardiomyocytes (called cardiac stem cells) residing in the adult heart differentiated into proliferating cardiomyocytes, or mature cardiomyocytes acquired the ability to proliferate by fusing with somatic cells that had proliferative ability. In 2001, it was reported that transplanted $c\text{-}kit^+$ Lin^- BM cells could differentiate into cardiomyocytes in peri-infarct tissues after MI (Orlic et al. 2001). In 2002, numerous recipient-derived cardiomyocytes were observed in a donor heart following human heart transplantation, and in 2003, numerous BM-derived cardiomyocytes were shown to be present in the recipient heart after BM transplantation (Quaini et al. 2002; Deb et al. 2003). Subsequently, several studies investigated the differentiation capacities of BM cells, the identities of the BM cell types that are able to differentiate into cardiomyocytes, and other possible mechanisms. Wagers et al. examined a variety of organs after transplanting single GFP-labeled HSC (c-kit^{+}, Lin^{-}, Sca-1^{+}) into irradiated mice, and demonstrated that HSC *trans*-differentiation occurs but it does so rarely (Wagers et al. 2002). Goodell et al. transplanted highly enriched HSCs into lethally irradiated mice, and by following subsequent ischemic reperfusion injury, found that HSCs differentiated into cardiomyocytes in the peri-infarct region at a prevalence of 0.02% (Jackson et al. 2001). In 2004, Balsam et al. investigated whether c-kit^{+} HSCs in the BM are capable of differentiating into cardiomyocytes by injecting BM cells directly into the heart instead of transplanting BM cells after irradiation; thus, they demonstrated that c-kit^{+} HSCs could not differentiate into cardiomyocytes without the effects of irradiation (Balsam et al. 2004). Similar results have been reported by others (Murry et al. 2004). We also examined the differentiation ability of HSCs using a c-kit^{+} Sca-1^{+} CD34^{-} Lin^{-} SP (CD34^{-}KSL-SP) of HSCs (Kawada et al. 2004). Transplantation of whole BM cells, which included both HSCs and MSCs, from GFP-transgenic mice into lethally irradiated mice, followed by the induction of MI, resulted in very few GFP^{+} (BM-derived) cardiomyocytes. Moreover, we confirmed the predominance of MSC-derived GFP^{+} cardiomyocytes in the group transplanted with CMG cells. It should be emphasized that the radiation dose has to be carefully determined in these BM transplantation experiments, since the radiation sensitivity of MSCs is much higher than that of HSCs. We propose that the differentiation of whole BM cells into populations that exclude hematopoietic populations is attributable to MSCs rather than HSCs, and that MSCs are mobilized from the BM.

Clinical Trials using BM Cells

Much clinical research involves the harvesting of mononuclear cells from BM cells or peripheral blood, and then infusing these cells through a catheter into a coronary artery to treat acute MI. Strauer and colleagues were the first to report on the transplantation of BM mononuclear cells after MI, which resulted in slight decreases in the left ventricular end-systolic dimension and infarct region, and increases in the left ventricular ejection fraction (EF) and regional function (Strauer et al. 2002). The TOPCARE-AMI trial allocated 20 patients with reperfused acute MI to receive intracoronary infusion of either BM-derived or circulating blood-derived progenitor cells into the infarct artery, which resulted in a significant increase in the global left ventricular EF and a reduction of the end-systolic left ventricular volume (Assmus et al. 2002). The BOOST trial also involved the transplantation of BM mononuclear cells after acute MI. In most of the studies, transplantation resulted in similar outcomes (Wollert et al. 2004). The REPAIR-AMI trial, which was the first double-blind, placebo-controlled, randomized, multicenter study to evaluate the effect of intracoronary transplantation of BMCs on infarct remodeling, also showed that BMCs improved global left ventricular function in patients with acute MI (Schachinger et al. 2006). However, despite all of these human studies, the mechanistic pathway of BMC differentiation remains unclear. In order for BMC transplantation to become a more powerful tool for regenerative medicine, these mechanisms must be resolved to enable us to improve the effects of BMC transplantation.

Cardiac Stem Cells

Stem cells are present in many adult organs, and they contribute to both the maintenance of physiologic conditions and the repair mechanisms in pathologic states. However, until recently, the existence of stem cells in the heart was unknown. Recent advances in genetic engineering and techniques, such as FACS, are helping to elucidate the populations and properties of stem cells in the heart.

In 2003, it was reported that c-kit^{+} cells in the adult heart were pluripotent and possessed proliferative ability in vitro (Beltrami et al. 2003). These cells are able to differentiate into cardiomyocytes, as well as smooth muscle cells and endothelial cells. Transplantation of these stem cells into a murine MI model confirmed their ability to differentiate into cardiomyocytes in vivo and indicated the existence in the heart of a tissue repair mechanism mediated by stem cells. In 2003, it was reported that Sca-1^{+} cells in the adult mouse heart existed as cardiomyocyte stem cells (Oh et al. 2003). These cells differentiate into cardiomyocytes when exposed to 5-AZA in vitro or when introduced into a murine model of myocardial ischemia. In 2004, Messina et al. isolated from adult human and mouse hearts myocardial stem cells that were capable of proliferating in vitro (Messina et al. 2004). After dissociating the heart with enzymes, they added EGF, bFGF, cardiotrophin-1, and thrombin under low-serum conditions, and revealed a cell population that formed spheroids with proliferation and differentiation abilities.

Recently, we characterized a SP of stem cells in the heart that did not express MHC and that decreased rapidly in number from 4 days after birth (Tomita et al. 2005). FACS analysis revealed the following marker profile for these cells: Ter119^{-}, CD45^{-}, CD13^{-}, CD11b^{-}, CD29^{+}, CD44^{+}, c-kit^{low}, CD34^{low}, CD49e$^{-/low}$, CD49e^{low}, flk-1$^{-\sim low}$ and Sca-1$^{-\sim low}$. Less than 1% of the cardiac SP cells formed floating spheroid colonies upon clonal expansion in serum-free medium that contained FGF-2 and EGF. Immediately after dissociation, the cells from these spheroid colonies expressed markers of neural precursor cells, including nestin, musashi-1, and the p75 NGF receptor. After 14 days in medium that contained 0.5% serum, the cells ceased to express nestin and musashi-1, and some of the cells expressed the neural differentiation markers *MAP2*, peripherin, Neu N, Hu, and P0. Another cell type expressed the cardiac-specific genes *Nkx2.5*, *GATA4*, *MEF2C*, *ANP*, *Cav1.2*, and α-skeletal actin, and a few cells exhibited spontaneous beating (Figure 35–3). These cells displayed a sinus node-like action potential. Other cells expressed GFAP or calponin and α-smooth muscle actin, indicating glial and smooth muscle differentiation. These results suggest that the cardiosphere-forming population of cardiac SP cells has multipotency, with the capacity to differentiate into neurons, glial cells, smooth muscle cells, and cardiomyocytes, and appears to have neural crest-like characteristics.

The neural crest-like characteristics of the cardiosphere-forming population of cardiac SP cells were investigated in vivo by transplanting the cells into the neural crest of a chick embryo. These cells were found to migrate with host-derived neural crest cells and to contribute to cells of the developing peripheral nervous system, such as the dorsal root ganglion and the ventral spinal nerve (Figure 35–4). These cells also entered the lateral migration pathway, which is the usual path taken by ectomesenchymal cells that are neural crest-derived melanocyte precursors. When transplanted directly into the lateral migration pathway, the cardiosphere-forming population of cardiac SP cells entered the outflow tract and conotruncus of the developing heart. Some of these cells expressed the neuronal marker Hu, and a minority expressed the glial marker GFAP. This analysis also revealed a

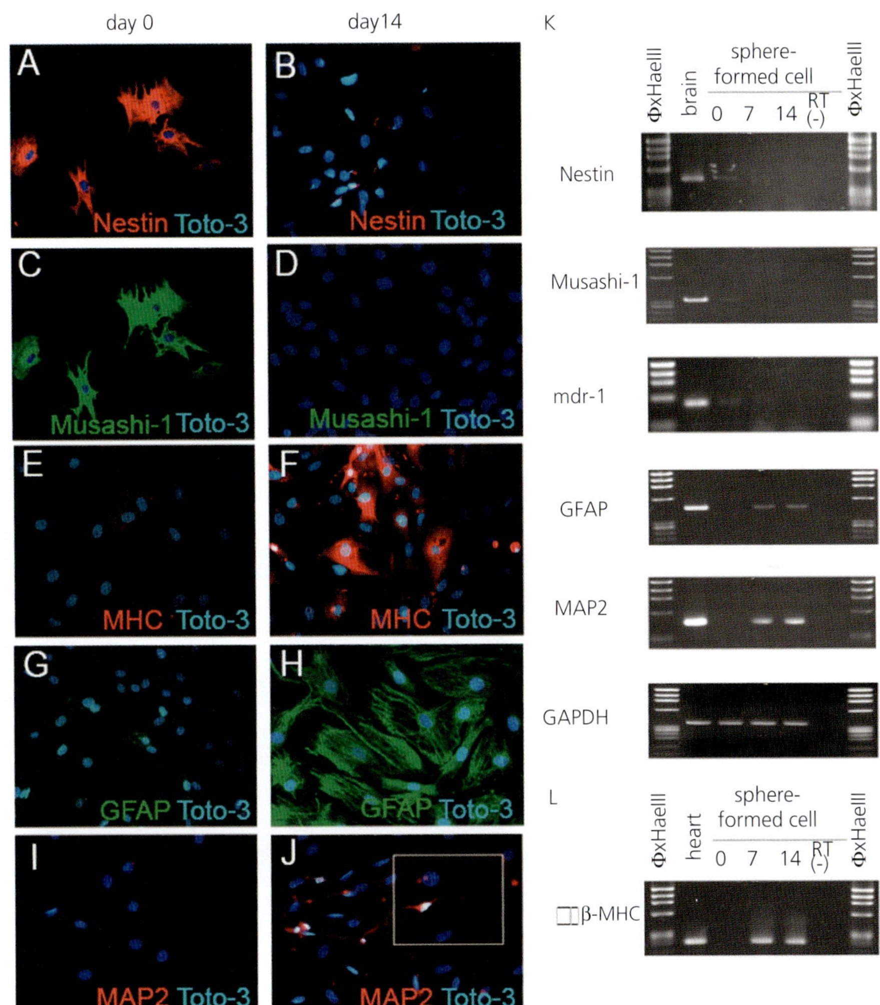

Figure 35–3 Differentiation of cardiosphere-derived cells in vitro. Cardiospheres were obtained from P2 neonates. Dissociated cardiosphere-derived cells were maintained in medium without EGF and FGF-2. At Day 0, almost all of the cells stain positively with the antinestin (a) and antimusashi-1 antibodies (c), but not with the antisarcomeric myosin (MF20), (e, f), anti-GFAP (g), and anti-MAP2 (i) antibodies. At Day 14, the cells show no staining with the antinestin (b) and antimusashi-1 (d) antibodies. In contrast, some cells stain positively with the antisarcomeric myosin (f), anti-GFAP (h), and anti-MAP2 (j) antibodies. The square box in (j) is enlarged in (c). (k) RT-PCR analyses for the *nestin, musashi-1, mdr-1, GFAP,* and *MAP2* genes. Note that the cardiosphere-derived cells at Day 0 express *nestin, musashi-1,* and *mdr-1,* but not *GFAP* or *MAP2.* These stem cell markers are absent at Day 14, and the cells begin to express *GFAP* and *MAP2.* (l) RT-PCR analysis for the *β-myosin heavy chain* (*β-MHC*) gene. Fetal brain or heart was used as a positive control.

subpopulation of cells that contributed to major blood vessels and expressed smooth muscle actin. The contribution of the cardiosphere-forming population of cardiac SP cells to the neural crest-derived tissues in the chick embryo is consistent with the neural crest stem cell characteristics displayed by these cells.

The contribution of neural crest-derived cells to the multipotent cardiac stem cell population has been investigated. For the analysis of the neural crest cell lineage, Yamauchi et al. crossed P0-Cre transgenic mice with CAG-CAT-Z indicator transgenic mice, which carry the *LacZ* gene downstream of a chicken actin promoter and a stuffer fragment flanked by two *loxP* sequences (Yamauchi et al. 1999). In three different transgenic lines, *LacZ* expression was observed in tissues derived from neural crest cells, which included spinal dorsal root ganglia, the sympathetic nervous system, the enteric nervous system, and the ventral craniofacial mesenchyme at developmental stages after E9.0.

Trangenic mice that carried the P0-Cre recombinase and CAG-CAT-EGFP transgenes showed EGFP expression in tissues that were derived from neural crest cells, including the spinal dorsal root ganglia, sympathetic nervous system, enteric nervous system, and ventral craniofacial mesenchyme. EGFP$^+$ cells were concentrated at the outflow tract between the aorta and pulmonary artery and in the aortic valves. These cells were also observed in the intramuscular and subepicardial layers of both ventricles, including the intraventricular septum, free wall, and apex (Figure 35–5), as well as the atrial wall. Triple-immunostaining of the E17.5 heart showed that EGFP$^+$ cells were not stained by the antiactinin antibody but were stained by the anti-GATA4 and antinestin antibodies. In 10-week-old hearts, triple-immunostaining revealed that some EGFP$^+$ cells were actinin$^+$ cardiomyocytes. This result is supported by the finding that cardiospheres obtained from 10-week-old double-transgenic mouse hearts clearly express EGFP. These findings strongly suggest that neural crest-derived cells contribute to various cell types, including cardiomyocytes, in 10-week-old mice and may persist in adult mice.

In 2005, Laugwitz and colleagues reported that *Isl1* (a LIM homeodomain transcription factor), which is a secondary heart field marker, could be used as a cardiomyocyte progenitor marker in the postnatal heart (Laugwitz et al. 2005). These cells are present throughout the heart, in the following order (largest to smallest proportion of total cells): right atrium, left atrium, right ventricle, septum, and left ventricle. *Isl1* expression is down-regulated as soon as the cells adopt a differentiated phenotype, which suggests that this transcription factor delineates a cardiogenic progenitor cell population. In the postnatal heart, *Isl1*-positive cells are capable of self-renewal and readily differentiate into mature cardiomyocytes after clonal selection. ES cells that harbor a reporter gene knock-in in the endogenous *Isl1* locus enabled the isolation of *Isl1*$^+$ cardiac progenitors from murine and human ES cell systems during in vitro cardiogenesis (Moretti et al. 2006). These

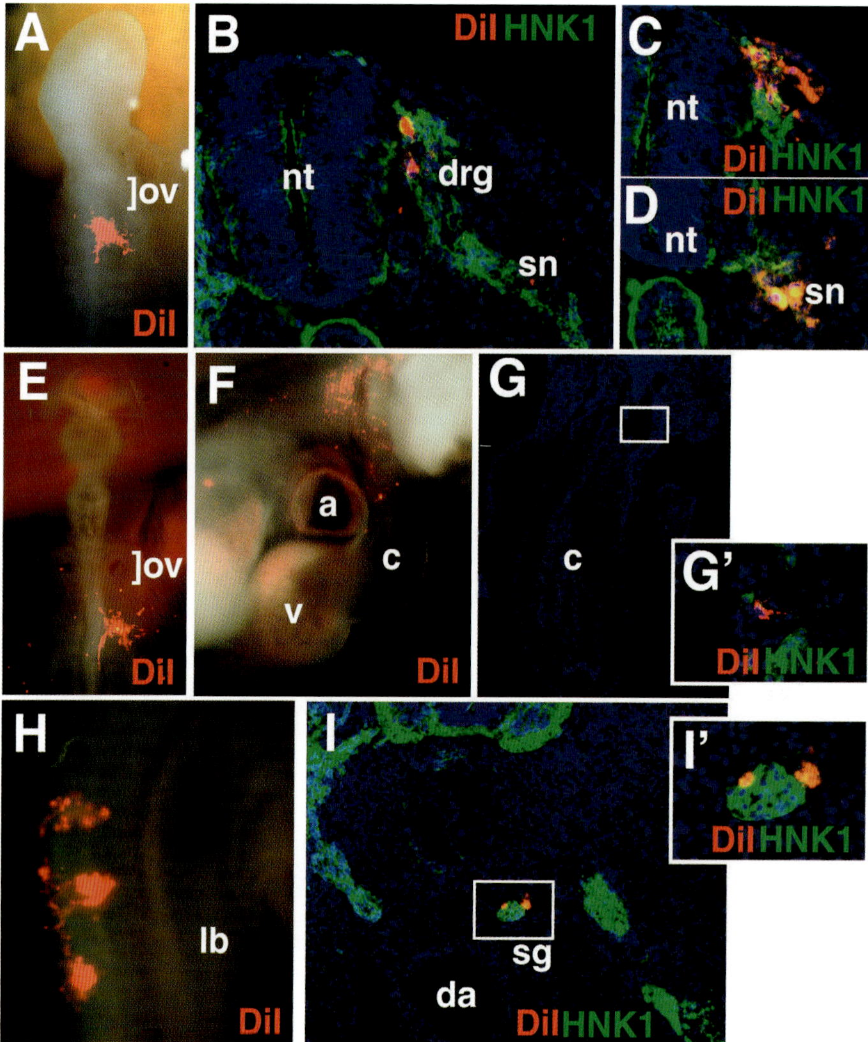

Figure 35–4 Cardiosphere cells act as the neural crest in chicken embryonic environment. Cardiospheres obtained from P2 neonates were labeled with DiI, and were transplanted into the chick neural crest. (a) Dorsal view of a chicken embryo that received cardiosphere cells into the MSA at the second somite level. Cardiosphere-derived cells are well-dispersed 24 hours after transplantation. (b,c) Transverse sections of cardiosphere-transplanted embryos, stained with the anti-HNK1 antibody, which is specific for neural crest-derived cells, and with DAPI, which stains nuclei. DiI-labeled cardiosphere-derived cells contribute to the developing dorsal root ganglia (drg, b), and spinal nerve (sn, d). Many sphere-derived cells also enter the lateral migration pathway (c). (e) Dorsal view of a chicken embryo into which DiI-labeled cardiosphere cells were introduced in the lateral pathway at the second somite level. (f) Side view of an embryo 48 hours after transplantation into the lateral pathway, showing the developing heart. Many cardiosphere-derived cells are entering the outflow tract area. (g) Transverse section of the transplanted embryo, showing the outflow tract and conotruncal region. (g') Higher magnification of the boxed area in (g). A DiI-labeled, sphere-derived cell and a HNK1-positive, host-derived crest cell are visible. (h) Dorsolateral view of an embryo that received three cardiosphere cells into the MSA at the wing limb bud level, 48 hours after transplantation. (i) Transverse section of the transplanted embryo, showing developing sympathetic ganglia (sg). (i') High-magnification view of the boxed area in (i), stained for HNK1 and DAPI. Cardiosphere-derived cells are integrated into the ganglia. Abbreviations: a, atrium; c, conotruncal; da, dorsal aorta; drg, dorsal root ganglia; lb, limb bud; nt, neural tube; ov, otic vesicle; sg, sympathetic ganglia; sn, spinal nerve; v, ventricle.

cells can also contribute to the cardiomyocyte, vascular smooth muscle, and endothelial cell lineages when clonally isolated from differentiating ES cells.

ES Cells as a Source of Cardiomyocytes

The first mouse ES cell line was established by Evans and Kaufman in 1981, and ES cells were initially utilized as a model for the analysis of embryonic development and for generating genetically modified mice (Evans and Kaufman 1981; Manis 2007; Murry and Keller 2008). In the mid-1990s, ES cell research gradually moved toward stem cell-based research and cell transplantation therapy using animal models (Klug et al. 1996; Wobus et al. 1997; Kolossov et al. 1998). In 1998, Thomson and colleagues first reported the establishment of human ES cells, and although ethical issues persist regarding their applications, these cells quickly attracted significant attention as a source of cells for regeneration therapy (Thomson et al. 1998). The development of ES cells for regeneration therapy has two main disadvantages. First, ethical considerations hinder the generation of new human ES cells, as they are derived from preimplantation human embryos (Evans

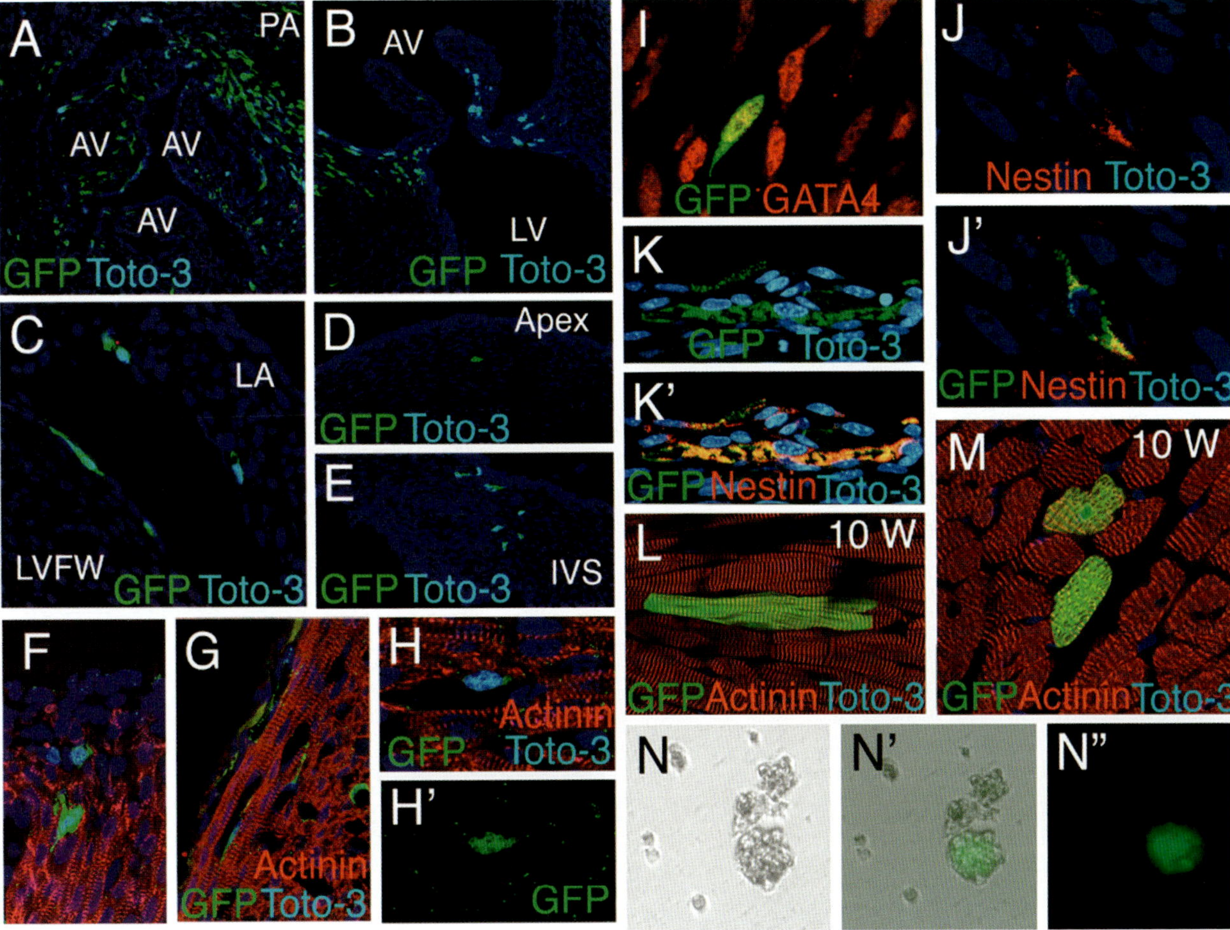

Figure 35–5 Distribution and co-immunostaining of neural crest-derived cells in the heart. (a–e) A P0 Cre/CAG-CAT-EGFP double-transgenic (Tg) mouse heart was immunostained with the anti-TOTO-3 and anti-GFP antibodies. The distribution of EGFP$^+$ cells in the heart is demonstrated. EGFP$^+$ cells are concentrated in the outflow tract and aortic valve (ab), and are also observed in the (c) subepicardial layer and (de) intramuscular layer of the ventricles. EGFP$^+$ cells are observed at the free wall (c), apex (d), interventricular septum (e), and atrium (c). (f–h) Triple-immunostaining for actinin (red), GFP (green), and TOTO-3 (blue) in E17.5 the P0-Cre/CAG-CAT-EGFP double-Tg mouse heart. The EGFP$^+$ cells do not stain with actinin. (h) and (h') show the same field. (i) Double-immunostaining for GATA4 (red) and GFP (green) in the E17.5 double-Tg mouse heart. Some of the EGFP$^+$ cells are stained with the anti-GATA4 antibody. (j,k) Triple-immunostaining for nestin (red), GFP (green), and TOTO-3 (blue) in the E17.5 double-Tg mouse heart. EGFP$^+$ cells are stained with the antinestin antibody. (jj') and (kk') show the same field. (l,m) Triple-immunostaining for actinin (red), GFP (green), and TOTO-3 (blue) in a 10-week-old adult P0-Cre/CAG-CAT-EGFP double-Tg mouse heart. EGFP$^+$ cells express actinin with complete striation, indicative of cardiomyocytes. (n-n") A cardiosphere isolated from a 10-week-old adult P0-Cre/CAG-CAT-EGFP double-Tg mouse heart shows EGFP signals, indicating that it is derived from a neural crest cell.

and Kaufman 1981). Second, ES cell do not show the autologous genotype of the patient. To maintain stem cell characteristics and to avoid ethical issues, many studies have focused on cell fusion and somatic nuclear transplantation, which have resulted in preliminary successes in animal experiments (Wakayama et al. 1997; Wilmut et al. 1997; Cowan et al. 2005; Yang et al. 2007; Tabar et al. 2008). These findings confer the advantage of using somatic cells from patients to produce unique ES cell lines. Subsequent research has focused on investigating the mechanisms underlying the control of ES cell differentiation, to allow the establishment of cell replacement therapy. Many problems related to the clinical applications of this technology remain unsolved.

Differentiation of Cardiomyocytes from ES Cells

The differentiation of mouse ES cells into cardiomyocytes in vitro was first demonstrated in 1985, and it was established that differentiation occurred at a constant rate, as is the case for other cell types (Doetschman et al. 1985). Research into the use of ES cells in cell replacement therapy was initiated in the latter part of the 1990s. In 1996, Field et al. reported that the stable transfection of ES cells with the aminoglycoside phosphotransferase gene under the control of the α-cardiac myosin heavy chain (MHC) promoter facilitated the purification of cardiomyocytes after differentiation in vitro (Klug et al. 1996). This study provided the impetus for the use of ES cells in the clinical setting. The development of methods for differentiating ES cells into cardiomyocytes in more selective and efficient manners using a variety of factors progressed steadily in the late 1990s.

Many methods for the differentiation of ES cells into cardiomyocytes have been reported. The differentiation of ES cells mimics normal embryonic development, thereby providing essential information on developmental processes, including heart development. It is generally accepted that the humoral factors essential for cardiomyogenesis in vivo will also stimulate ES cells to differentiate into cardiomyocytes in vitro. Information from genetically modified mice with cardiac abnormalities has provided information on the factors essential for embryonic heart development. Cardiac anomalies occur in mice that lack the receptor for the vitamin A derivative retinoic acid (RA) or mice that suffer vitamin A deficiency during development, thereby implicating this factor in cardiac differentiation and development (Osmond et al. 1991; Kastner et al. 1994; Dyson et al. 1995). Furthermore, RA induces the differentiation of cardiomyocytes from embryonal carcinoma (EC) cells in vitro, in time- and concentration-dependent manners consistent with normal development (Edwards et al. 1983). Based on these findings, Wobus et al. succeeded in increasing the efficiency of cardiomyocyte induction by exposing ES cells to RA under strictly controlled conditions of concentration and timing (Wobus et al. 1997). This study also showed that the differential induction of ventricular muscle was greater than that of other cardiomyocyte populations (Wobus et al. 1997). Subsequently, the expression of NO synthase in the heart during mouse development and the promotion of cardiomyocyte development by NO were demonstrated, which led to the use of NO donors or inhibitors for the differentiation of ES cell into cardiomyocytes (Kanno et al. 2004). Takahashi et al. screened various compounds and showed that ascorbic acid promotes the induction of cardiomyocyte differentiation (Takahashi et al. 2003). Studies on the differentiation of ES cells into cardiomyocytes using known growth factors and chemical compounds are reviewed elsewhere (Boheler et al. 2002; Sachinidis et al. 2003; Heng et al. 2004).

The differentiation of ES cells into a particular cell lineage is partly dependent upon the regulatory mechanisms underlying normal early development. Although several signaling proteins, including bone morphogenetic proteins (BMPs) (Winnier et al. 1995; Zhang and Bradley 1996; Schlange et al. 2000; Gaussin et al. 2002), Wnts (Marvin et al. 2001; Schneider and Mercola 2001; Foley and Mercola 2005), Notch (Timmerman et al. 2004; Maillard et al. 2005), and FGFs (Mima et al. 1995) are implicated in heart development, little is known about the regulatory signals that mediate the differentiation of ES cells into cardiomyocytes. In murine embryos, cardiac progenitor cells appear at E7.0, and the cardiac crescent is formed by E7.5, which indicates that the growth factors expressed in these regions or in surrounding areas at the relevant developmental stage are important for efficient cardiomyocyte induction.

BMP Signal Inhibition for Cardiomyocyte Differentiation from ES Cells

The BMP family is the largest subfamily of the transforming growth factor-β superfamily. During embryonic development, specific BMPs are expressed before cardioblast formation, as well as during heart organogenesis from the epiblast stage, and they are involved in a broad range of developmental events, including cell proliferation, differentiation, migration, and apoptosis during the progression of development (Hogan 1996; Ray and Wharton 2001; von Bubnoff and Cho 2001; Schneider et al. 2003). At least six BMPs (BMP 2, 4, 5, 6, 7, and 10) are expressed in the heart and have independent and redundant functions (Lyons et al. 1990; Lyons et al. 1995; Andrew and Dudley 1997; Neuhaus et al. 1999). Experiments on genetically modified mice have demonstrated the importance of BMP signaling for heart morphogenesis after the mid-gestation stage. BMPs are expressed in the lateral plate mesoderm, including the anterior lateral plate (cardiogenic mesoderm), and the essential role of these signaling factors is demonstrated by the appearance of heart defects in early stage embryos as a result of *BMP-2* gene targeting (Lyons et al. 1995; Zhang and Bradley 1996). The application of BMP-2-soaked beads in vivo induces the ectopic expression of cardiac transcription factors, and the administration of soluble BMP-2 or BMP-4 to explant cultures induces full cardiac differentiation at chick stages 5 to 7 in the anterior medial mesoderm, which is normally noncardiogenic (Schultheiss et al. 1997). A positive role for BMP has also been shown using pluripotent mouse embryonic carcinoma cells (P19CL6), which could differentiate into cardiac myocyte in vitro (Monzen et al. 1999; Monzen et al. 2001). Noggin, a potent BMP antagonist, when stably transfected into P19CL6 cells inhibited differentiation into cardiac myocytes; BMP downstream signaling molecules rescued cardiac differentiation. However, it has been reported that BMP-2 and BMP-4 suppress cardiomyocyte differentiation in early stage chick embryo explants, which suggests that BMPs inhibit cardiomyocyte development before and around gastrulation (Ladd et al. 1998). Taken together, these findings show that BMPs play critical and dynamic roles in the induction of cardiomyocytes during heart development. In the vertebrate nervous system, Noggin and other BMP inhibitors (Chordin and Follistatin) are involved in neural differentiation and patterning during embryonic development, as well as in adult neurogenesis in a context-dependent fashion (Sasai et al. 1995; Lim et al. 2000).

Although BMP signaling plays crucial roles in mesodermal induction and cardiac development, treatment of ES cells with BMP-2 or BMP-4 did not augment or suppress cardiomyocyte induction in the present study. Previously, we hypothesized that BMP antagonists are involved in cardiomyocyte induction (Yuasa et al. 2005). We performed whole-mount in situ hybridization with probes for various BMP antagonists using mouse embryos at different stages of gastrulation. The BMP antagonist Noggin was transiently but strongly expressed in the heart-forming area (Figure 35–6). Noggin was clearly expressed at the cardiac crescent at E7.5 and in the late crescent stage at E8.0, but it was scarcely detectable in the linear heart tube after E8.5. This expression pattern was also observed in early embryos of the chicken and *Xenopus*, suggesting a conserved mechanism in heart development (Faure et al. 2002; Fletcher et al. 2004). In contrast, notochord expression of Noggin continued after E8.5, as reported previously (Smith and Harland 1992; McMahon et al. 1998). E7.5 and E8.0 whole-mount sections revealed the expression of Noggin in the endodermal and mesodermal layers derived from the primary heart field. This marked difference in the kinetics of Noggin expression between the heart-forming region and notochord suggests that transient expression of Noggin has a role in cardiomyocyte differentiation.

Murine ES cells in suspension culture were stimulated with Noggin under various experimental conditions (Figure 35–7). ES cell cultures were exposed to Noggin before or after embryoid body (EB) formation, so as to model transient and strong expression of Noggin at the early gastrulation stage. The removal of LIF and addition of Noggin before or after EB formation did not increase the incidence of spontaneously beating EB. In contrast, the removal of LIF and addition of Noggin at Day -3 and Day 0 of EB formation slightly but significantly increased the incidence of beating EB, which suggests that the optimal timing for Noggin is both prior to and after EB formation. We also added Noggin on Days -3, 0, +1, +2, and +3, and added LIF prior to EB formation. The addition of Noggin on Day 0 slightly increased the incidence of beating EBs, although this was gradually decreased at the other time points. Based on these results, Noggin was administered on Day -3 and Day 0 of EB formation, resulting in a marked increase (to 95.3%) in the incidence of beating EBs on Day 10, and the

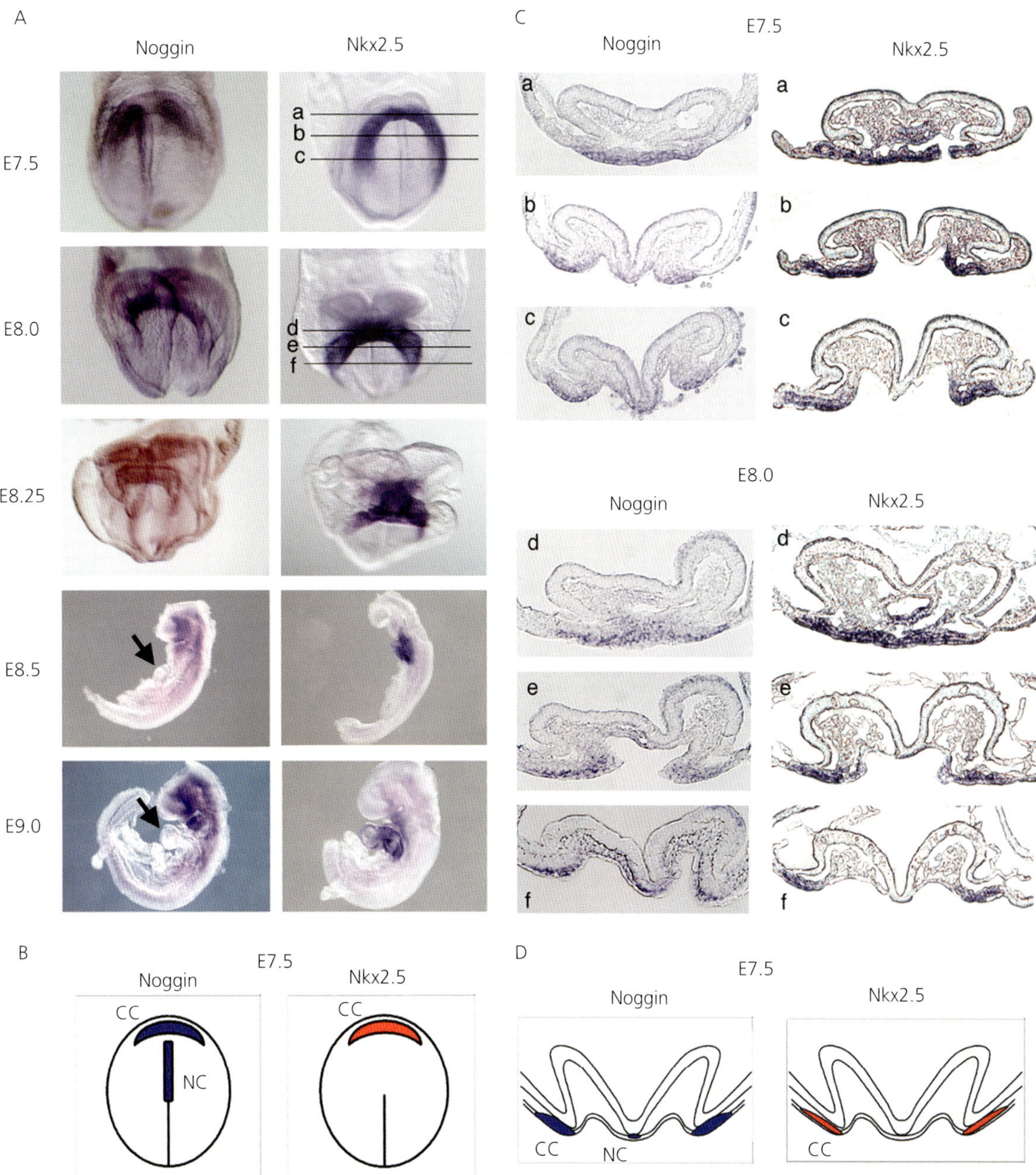

Figure 35–6 Transient expression of Noggin in the heart-forming area. (a) Whole-mount in situ hybridization of Noggin and Nkx2.5 was performed at murine embryo stages E7.5, E8.0, E8.5, and E9.0. Noggin is strongly expressed at the cardiac crescent (E7.5) and linear heart tube (E8.0), but is not detected after E8.5. In contrast, Nkx2.5 is expressed after this stage of development. Arrows indicate the heart. (b) Schematic of Noggin and Nkx2.5 expression at E7.5. CC, cardiac crescent; NC, notochord; LHT, linear heart tube. (c) Sections of samples at E7.5 and E8.0 subjected to whole-mount in situ hybridization. a–f The location of the section shown in Figure 36–1A. (d) Noggin and Nkx2.5 expression at E7.5.

continued growth of the EB to Day 14. Two different ES cell lines gave consistent results, and the optimal concentration of Noggin was found to be 150 ng/mL. These results suggest that the induction of cardiomyocytes by Noggin is restricted to the period from 3 days before to 1 day after EB formation, and that the ES cells must initially be undifferentiated.

To demonstrate specific inhibition of the BMP pathway by Noggin, the ES cells were exposed to various concentrations of BMP-2 on Day 0. Even low doses of BMP-2 strongly inhibited Noggin-dependent cardiomyocyte induction. To confirm that inhibition of BMP signaling early in ES cell differentiation can accelerate cardiomyocyte induction, ES cells were exposed to soluble BMP receptor-1A (BMPR-1A) or to another BMP antagonist, Chordin. Both BMPR-1A and Chordin increased the incidence of beating in individual EBs. However, the administration under the same conditions of various growth factors, including IGF-1, FGF-2, and BMP-2, did not increase cardiomyocyte induction. These results suggest that the inhibition of BMP signaling in

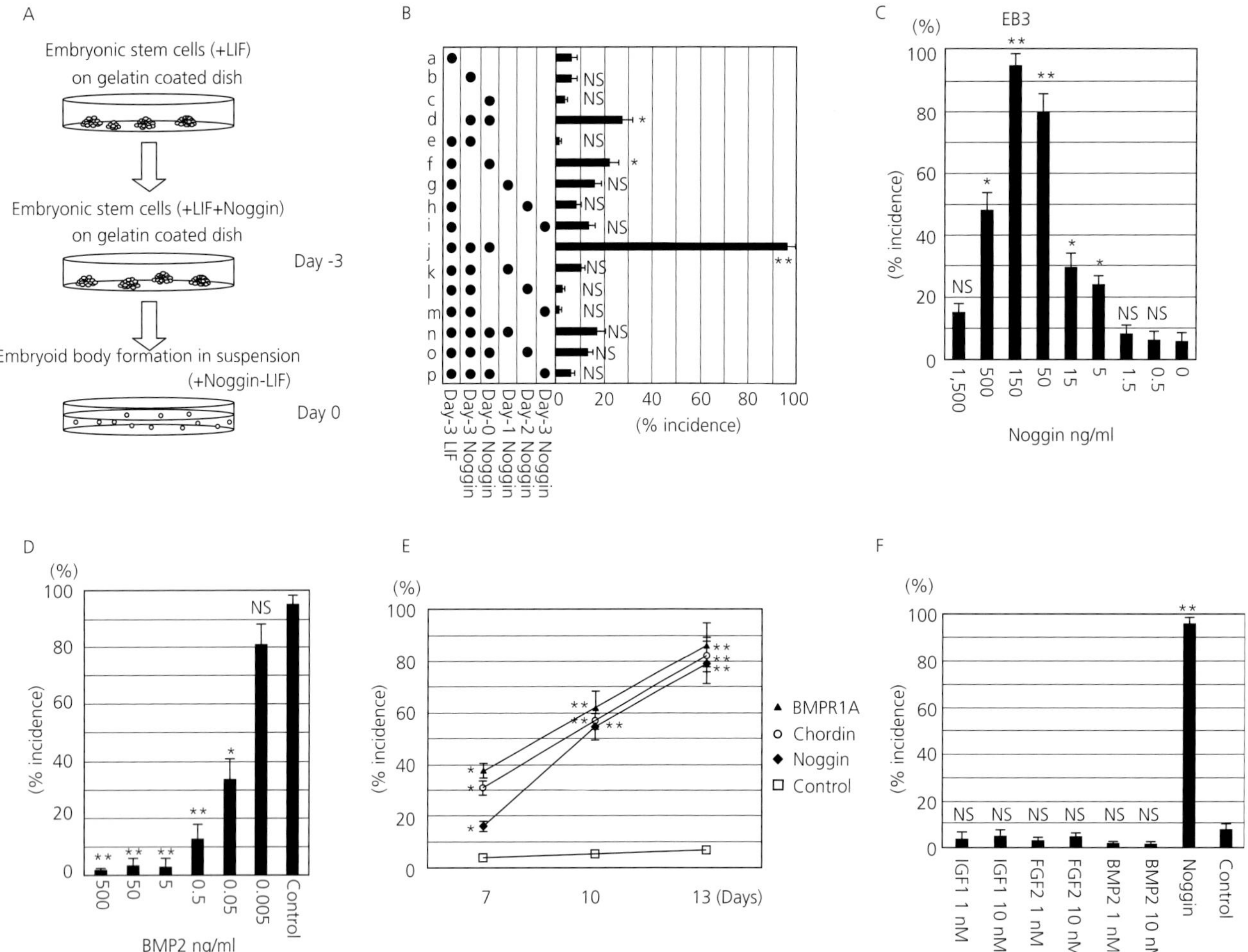

Figure 35–7 Protocol for and efficiency of cardiomyocyte induction from ES cells using Noggin, Chordin, and soluble BMP receptor 1A. (a) Representative protocol used for cardiomyocyte induction from ES cells. (b) Various protocols for Noggin (150 ng/mL) exposure were tested and their efficiencies were compared. (c) Dose-efficiency relationship of Noggin administration using two different ES cell lines, EB3 and R1 (supplemental Figure 1). The two cell lines show the same dose–efficiency relationship. (d) Administration of a low dose of BMP-2 abolishes Noggin induction of cardiomyocytes, which indicates that the BMP-2 concentration is critical for this phenomenon. (e) Effects of the BMP antagonists Chordin and soluble BMPR-1A (BMP neutralizing receptor) on cardiomyocyte induction. Both Chordin and BMPR-1A were administered according to the protocol used for Noggin (150 ng/mL). Both BMP antagonists induced cardiomyocyte induction from ES cells at the same level as Noggin, which indicates that transient suppression of the intrinsic BMP signal is critical for cardiomyocyte induction. (f) Other factors, including IGF-1, FGF-2, and BMP-2, did not affect cardiomyocyte induction when used according to this protocol. *$P < 0.05$; **$P < 0.01$ versus control; NS, not significant.

undifferentiated ES cells or in the early phase of ES cell differentiation is crucial for cardiomyocyte differentiation.

Cardiomyocyte induction by Noggin was quantified by immunostaining for cardiac-specific proteins, followed by confocal LASER microscopy. Most of the cells in the Noggin-treated EBs stained positively for MHC, myosin light chain (MLC), atrial natriuretic peptide (ANP), cardiac troponin I, and sarcomeric actinin (Figure 35–8). In contrast, the levels of these cardiac proteins were markedly lower in the control EBs or in EBs treated with Noggin under different conditions. Synchronous beating of EBs was observed, and isolated cells expressed several cardiac markers and displayed myocyte characteristics. By Day 10, the EBs had attached to the gelatin-coated dishes, stained positively with the anti-MHC antibodies, and contained the cardiomyocytes by 100-fold more than that of the control cells.

The present results suggest that BMP signaling is essential for at least two steps in the cardiomyocyte induction process, that is, mesodermal induction (Winnier et al. 1995) and cardiomyocyte differentiation (Zhang and Bradley 1996). Between these steps, we propose that transient blockage of intrinsic BMP signaling is essential for the determination of CMG differentiation. Recently, it has been shown that short-term BMP treatment and BMP inhibition by Noggin promote cardiac myocyte differentiation from human ES cells, and that long-term BMP treatment results in trophoblast differentiation (Zhang et al. 2008). There are many reports of BMPs and other TGF-β family proteins having strong positive roles in cardiac myocyte differentiation from ES cells, and BMPs clearly play a positive role in cardiomyocyte differentiation (Behfar et al. 2002; Kumar and Sun 2005; Laflamme et al. 2007). The temporal and spatial regulation of BMPs and BMP antagonists reveal crucial involvement in the differentiation of cardiomyocytes during heart development. We conclude that the temporal and spatial expression patterns of Noggin and BMP are important for the in vivo and in vitro differentiation of cardiomyocytes. The

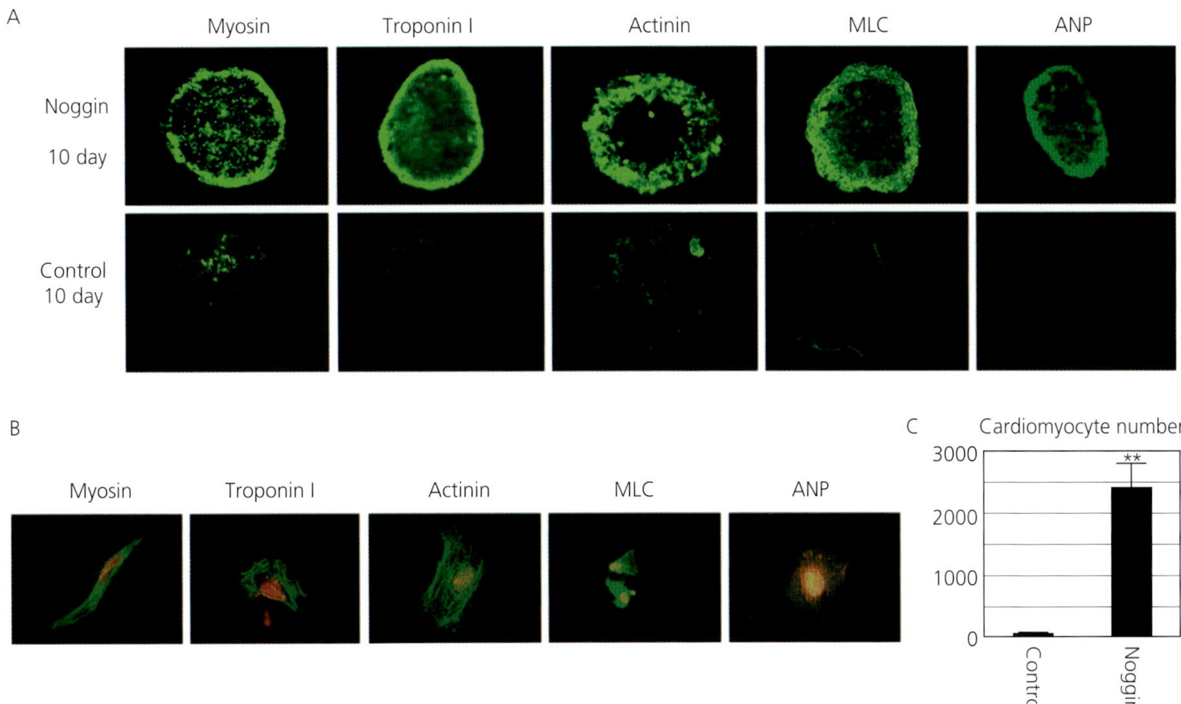

Figure 35–8 Expression of cardiac-specific proteins in Noggin-treated ES cells. (a) Immunostaining with anti-MHC, antitroponin I, anti-ANP, antiactinin, and anti-MLC antibodies is shown. Most of the cells in the whole EBs were stained with cardiomyocyte-specific antibodies. (b) Isolated cells were stained with the same antibodies. Red coloration indicates nuclear staining with PI. In the last immunofluorescence photograph, the ANP, MHC, and nucleolus are stained with rhodamine, FITC, and DAPI, respectively. (c) Dispersed EBs were attached to the gelatin-coated tissue culture plate, stained with the anti-MHC antibody, and the number of cardiomyocytes was evaluated. The number of cardiomyocytes with Noggin-treated cells was 100-fold higher than the number of control cells. $^{**}P < 0.01$ versus control.

protocol used in the present study is predicted to advance the use of ES cell-derived cardiomyocytes in regenerative therapy.

iPS Cell Generation

Takahashi and Yamanaka reported that mouse iPS cells can be generated from adult fibroblasts by genetic transfer of the transcription factors Oct3/4, Sox2, c-Myc, and Klf4 (Takahashi and Yamanaka 2006). Subsequently, Yanamanaka's group and Thomson's group reported that human iPS cells can also be established from human somatic cells by the transfer of a set of four genes,that is, *Oct3/4*, *Sox2*, *c-Myc*, and *Klf4* or *Oct3/4*, *Sox2*, *Nanog*, and *Lin28* (Takahashi et al. 2007; Yu et al. 2007; Park et al. 2008). The morphology, growth characteristics, and pluripotency of iPS cells are similar to those of ES cells. Moreover, the germline competency of iPS cells has been demonstrated using the *cis*-element of Nanog as a selection marker (Okita et al. 2007). Among the introduced transcription factors, there is a risk of tumorigenicity due to reactivation of the oncogene *c-Myc*. iPS cells have been generated from murine and human fibroblasts without *c-Myc*, and these cells do not develop into tumors (Nakagawa et al. 2008). Following the successful establishment of iPS cells, many researchers attempted to clarify the differences in characteristics between iPS cells and ES cells. As genetic and epigenetic abnormalities result in pathogenesis, the genetic and epigenetic statuses of iPS cells have been investigated intensely. The global gene expression patterns are similar but nonidentical between iPS cells and ES cells of the mouse and human (Takahashi and Yamanaka 2006; Takahashi et al. 2007; Lowry et al. 2008; Park et al. 2008). Accumulating evidence reveals that the epigenetic status of iPS cells is highly similar to that of ES cells with regard to the stem cell marker promoter, methylation status, dynamics of X inactivation in female iPS cells, and global patterning of histone methylation (Takahashi and Yamanaka 2006; Maherali et al. 2007; Okita et al. 2007; Takahashi et al. 2007; Hanna et al. 2008; Park et al. 2008). Both murine and human iPS cells differentiate into cardiac myocytes both in vitro and in vivo, as is the case for ES cells (Takahashi and Yamanaka 2006; Maherali et al. 2007; Takahashi et al. 2007; Schenke-Layland et al. 2008).

The many advantages of iPS cells have been reported (Yuasa and Fukuda 2008). Successful reprogramming of differentiated human somatic cells into a pluripotent state would allow the creation of patient- and disease-specific stem cells. For transplantation therapies using stem cells, patient-specific iPS cells would eliminate the possibility of immune rejection. The similarities noted between iPS cells and ES cells have led to methods for the differentiation of ES cells being adapted for the differentiation of iPS cells into cardiomyocytes for clinical applications (Hanna et al. 2007). In drug discovery, human iPS cells should make it easier to generate panels of cell lines that more closely reflect the genetic diversity of a given population. There are many genetic disorders of the heart, such as familial dilated cardiomyopathy, familiar arrhythmia, and congenital heart disease. We are now in the position to be able to examine the development, pathogenesis, and physiologic characteristics of human cardiac myocytes with hereditary disease. This is one of the potent merits of using iPS cells, as it is difficult to obtain high numbers of live diseased cardiomyocytes from patients for drug screening and other analyses.

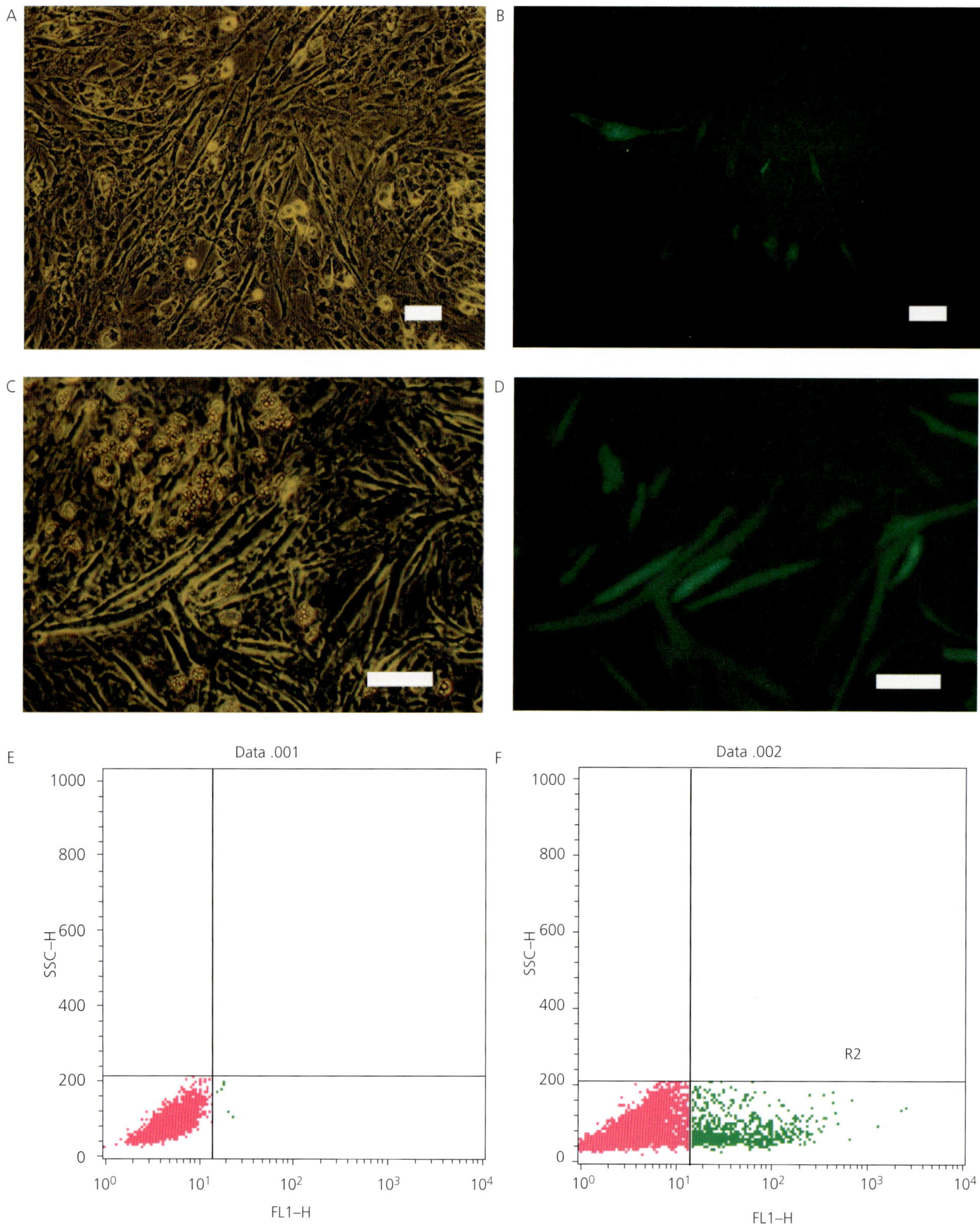

Figure 35–9 Isolation of regenerated cardiomyocytes. BM MSCs were transfected with EGFP under the control of the promoter for a ventricular myocardium-specific protein, myosin light-chain 2v, and induced to differentiate. Some of the cells are GFP-positive 7 days after differentiation (a, b), and the cells start beating at 3 weeks (c, d). When the cells were fractionated with a FACS machine after becoming GFP-positive (e, f), only cardiomyocytes were obtained (g–j). (g, h) Four days, and (i, j) 3 weeks after cell sorting.

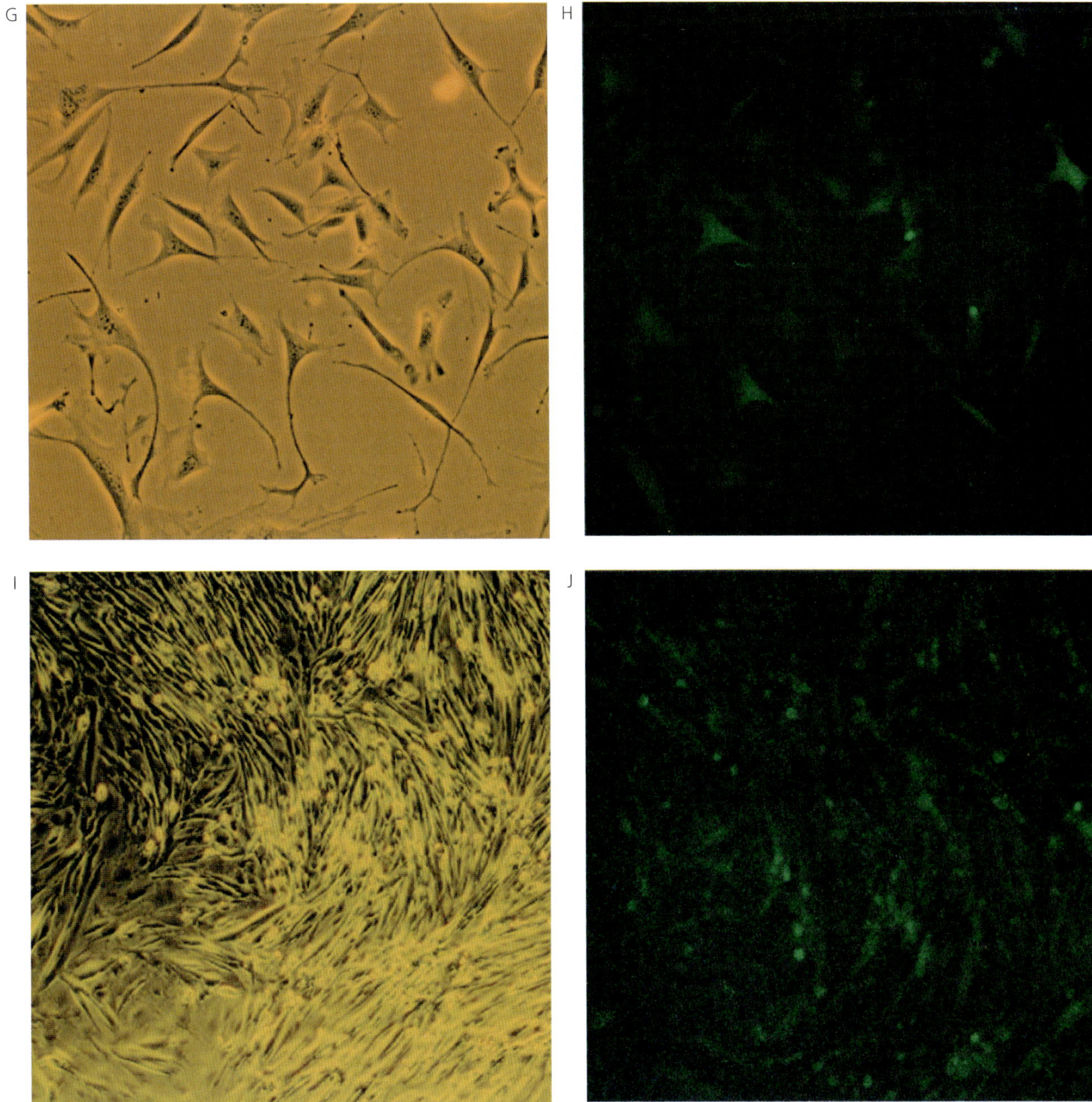

Figure 35–9 (Continued)

Nevertheless, it is important to understand that before iPS cells can be used in a clinical setting, further extensive studies are required to determine whether human iPS cells are safe for clinical use and whether human iPS cell-derived cardiomyocytes are truly identical to normal cardiomyocytes.

Cardiomyocyte Transplantation

The concept of cardiomyocyte transplantation has been advocated since the late 1990s (Li et al. 1996a, 1996b). Fetal or neonatal rat cardiomyocytes were successfully transplanted into the hearts of adult rats, and the transplanted cells were viable within the heart for relatively long periods of time, and formed gap junctions with surrounding recipient cells. Prior to the transplantation of pluripotent ES cell-derived cardiomyocytes into the heart, undifferentiated cells, and cells that have differentiated into other cell types, must be eliminated. Cell sorting methods and the use of drug resistance genes to collect ES cell-derived cardiomyocytes have been reported (Klug et al. 1996; Kolossov et al. 1998; Muller et al. 2000; Moore et al. 2004) and include methods that specifically label cardiomyocytes by introducing into the ES cells GFP (green fluorescent protein) linked to a cardiomyocyte-specific promoter. Previously, we placed GFP under the control of the myosin light-chain gene promoter and introduced this construct into BM MSCs (Hattan et al. 2005). When these cells were induced to differentiate, only the cardiomyocytes produced the GFP signal, so they could be collected with a purity of more than 99% in a FACS cell sorter (Figure 35–9). When these cells were transplanted using a syringe into the hearts of syngeneic mice they moved into the gaps

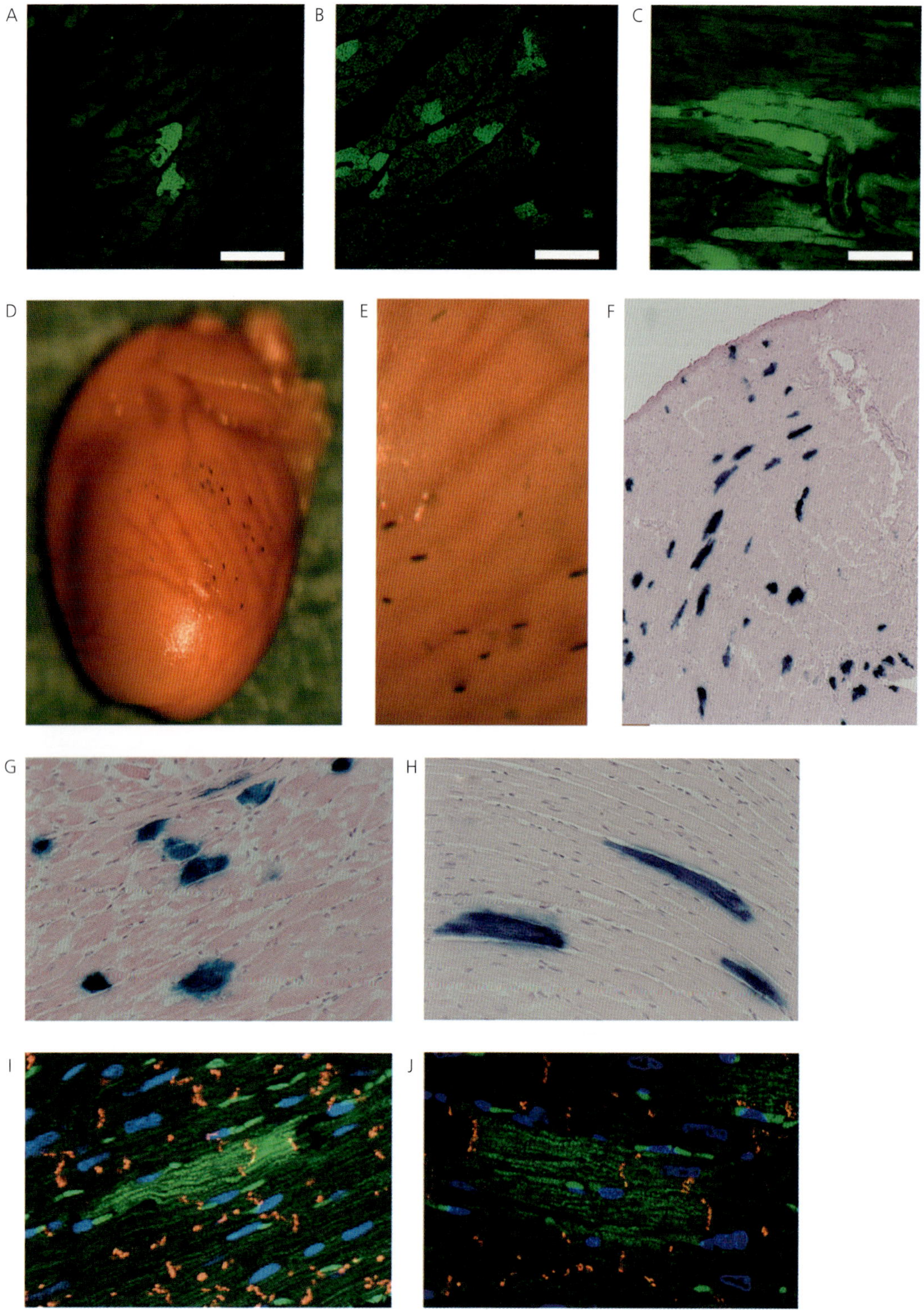

Figure 35–10 Transplantation of regenerated cardiomyocytes. Regenerated cardiomyocytes (Figure 35–2) were transplanted into adult mouse hearts with a syringe. This experiment confirms that transplanted cardiomyocytes reside stably in the heart and survive for a long time. Once injected, the regenerated cardiomyocytes diffuse into the heart-like islands, after which they adhere to the surrounding cardiomyocytes and assume the form of mature cardiomyocytes that look like short strips of paper. (a–c) Cells in which GFP fluorescence was observed; (d–h) cells transfected with the *LacZ* gene and subsequently stained. Coimmunostaining of these cells for connexin 43 reveals that they have formed gap junctions with the surrounding cardiomyocytes (i, j). The green color represents GFP, the blue color represents nuclear staining with TOTO-3, and the red color represents connexin 43.

between recipient cardiomyocytes (Figure 35–10), became connected to surrounding cells via gap junctions, and resided stably in the heart for a long period of time. These results illustrate the potential of regenerated cardiomyocytes as an alternative to fetal or neonatal cardiomyocytes for transplantation.

Although transplanting cells with a syringe is a simple technique, certain disadvantages of this method preclude its clinical application, for example, it is not possible to transplant high numbers of cells, and the transplanted cells have low viability. To improve the clinical applicability of cardiomyocyte transplantation technology, Okano and coworkers produced temperature-sensitive, resin-coated culture dishes. The surfaces of these dishes become hydrophilic when the temperature is lowered, so that cultured cardiomyocytes can be peeled off in sheets (Kikuchi et al. 1998; Shimizu et al. 2002). Using this approach, we developed a novel method for producing cardiomyocyte sheets (Itabashi et al. 2005; Figure 35–11). This new method utilizes polymerized fibrin (fibrin glue), which is normally used in surgical operations. A thin fibrin polymer membrane on the surface of the culture dish is generated by reacting fixed concentrations of fibrinogen and thrombin. When cardiomyocytes are cultured on these dishes, they secrete a variety of endogenous proteases, which break down the fibrin polymer membrane within approximately 3 days, making it possible to obtain cardiomyocytes in sheets. After 7 days of culture, the fibrin is completely degraded. Transplantation of cardiomyocyte sheets is characterized by good cell viability and residence rates (Figure 35–12). Most studies report that less than 10% of cardiomyocytes transplanted using a syringe reside stably in the heart, whereas few cells are lost after transplantation when cardiomyocyte sheets are transplanted subcutaneously. A further advantage of using cardiomyocyte sheets is that they can be layered to vary the thickness of the tissue. These findings support myocardial sheet formation as an important tool for future cell transplantation technology. The efficient clinical application of this technique requires progress in the stimulation of vascularization. Although transplantation is followed by the formation of a microvascular network, large blood vessels are not formed.

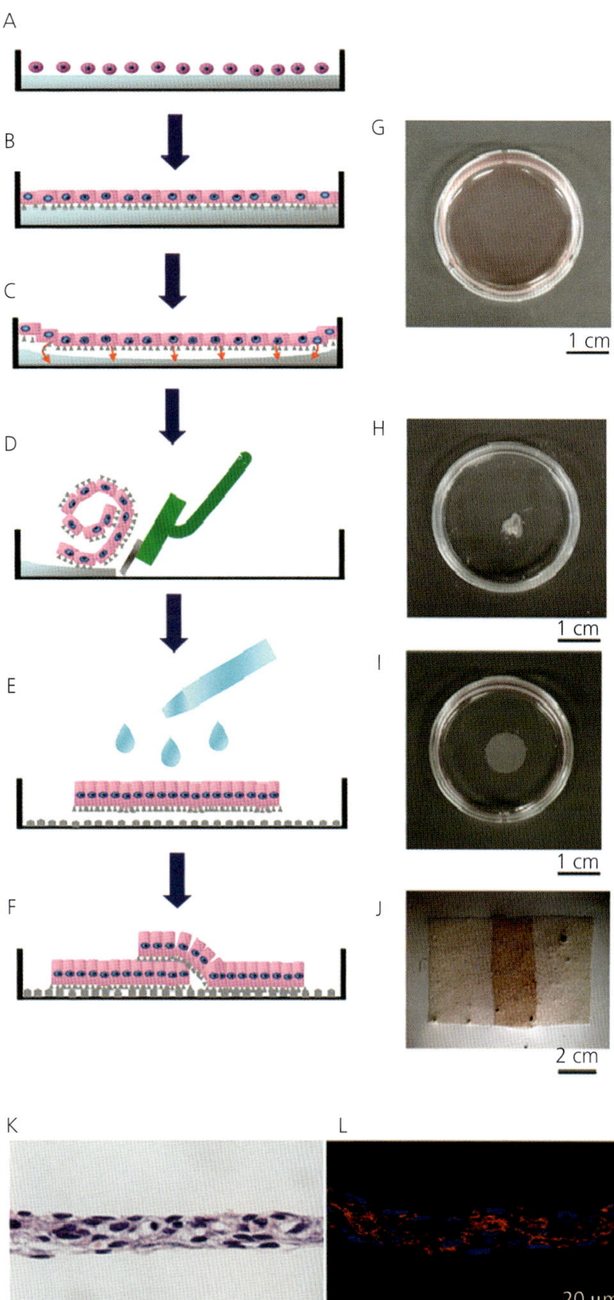

Figure 35–11 Production of myocardial cell sheets. Production of myocardial cell sheets using culture dishes coated with a fibrin polymer membrane. The fibrin polymer is gradually degraded by endogenous proteases secreted by the cardiomyocytes, making it easy to peel the sheet off the surface of the dish. This procedure can be used to produce cardiomyocyte sheets in a convenient manner. (a–f) Illustration of the concept; (g–j) views of the actual process; (k) and (l) show sheets stained with HE and immunofluorescence, respectively. Red, actinin; blue, Toto-3; green, fibrin.

Myocardial Regeneration from Stem Cells in Adults

Research performed to date has demonstrated that BM stem cells differentiate into cardiomyocytes in vitro, although it is not known if they migrate into the heart and differentiate into cardiomyocytes in vivo (Jackson et al. 2001). The pluripotency of HSCs and cell fusion by pluripotent stem cells have been investigated recently (Terada et al. 2002; Ying et al. 2002; Murry et al. 2004). As there is some confusion in the literature regarding the mechanism of in vivo repair used by BM cells, we used an in vivo murine BM transplantation model to investigate the formation of cardiomyocytes by any of the cells in the BM (HSCs or MSCs) (Kawada et al. 2004). In this analysis, GFP-marked HSCs and MSCs were transplanted separately into allogeneic mice that were exposed to a lethal dose of radiation. Individual HSCs were harvested from the GFP-transgenic mice using FACS and the so-called KSL-SP method. These cells were transplanted together with unlabeled radioprotective cells responsible for hematopoiesis. In addition, the MSCs were labeled in such a way that they would express GFP when they differentiated into cardiomyocytes. Transplantation was performed using intra-BM BM transplantation (IBM-BMT). This method was chosen to avoid the possibility of the transplanted MSCs, which are larger than HSCs, becoming trapped in the lungs and other tissues. We induced MI in the mice transplanted with HSCs or MSCs, and analyzed the hearts of these mice 2 months later. In the mice transplanted with HSCs, the frequency of

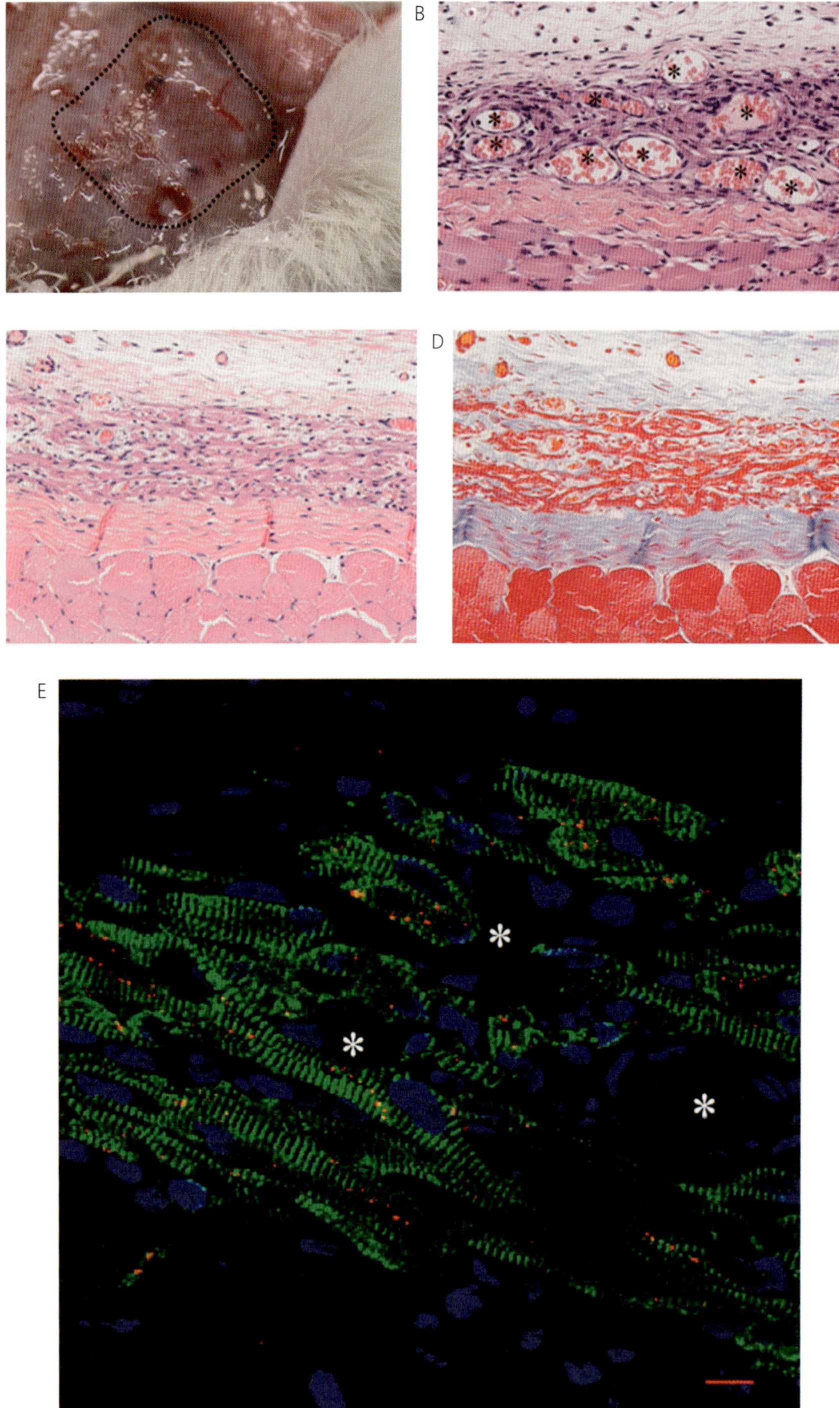

Figure 35–12 Subcutaneous transplantation of cardiomyocyte sheets. (a) External view of a subcutaneously transplanted cardiomyocyte sheet. (b–e) Histologic views; (b, c) HE staining; (d) Azan staining; (e) immunofluorescence staining. Green, actinin; red, connexin 43; blue, nuclei stained with TOTO-3.

GFP-positive was low and the same as that previously reported for cell fusion. In contrast, the mice that were transplanted with MSCs showed actinin-staining GFP-positive cells at the infarct foci. These results suggest that MSCs are mobilized from the BM when an injury occurs that is associated with necrosis of the myocardial tissue, as in MI, and that MSCs are capable of differentiating into cardiomyocytes at infarct foci. We administered the cytokine G-CSF at the time of stem cell mobilization from the BM, since there was a large difference in the number of regenerated cardiomyocytes between the control group and the G-CSF group. G-CSF not only mobilized HSCs in the bloodstream but exhibited the capacity to mobilize MSCs (Figure 35–13).

Although G-CSF is used experimentally and clinically for acute MI, the evaluations remain to be concluded (Kang et al.

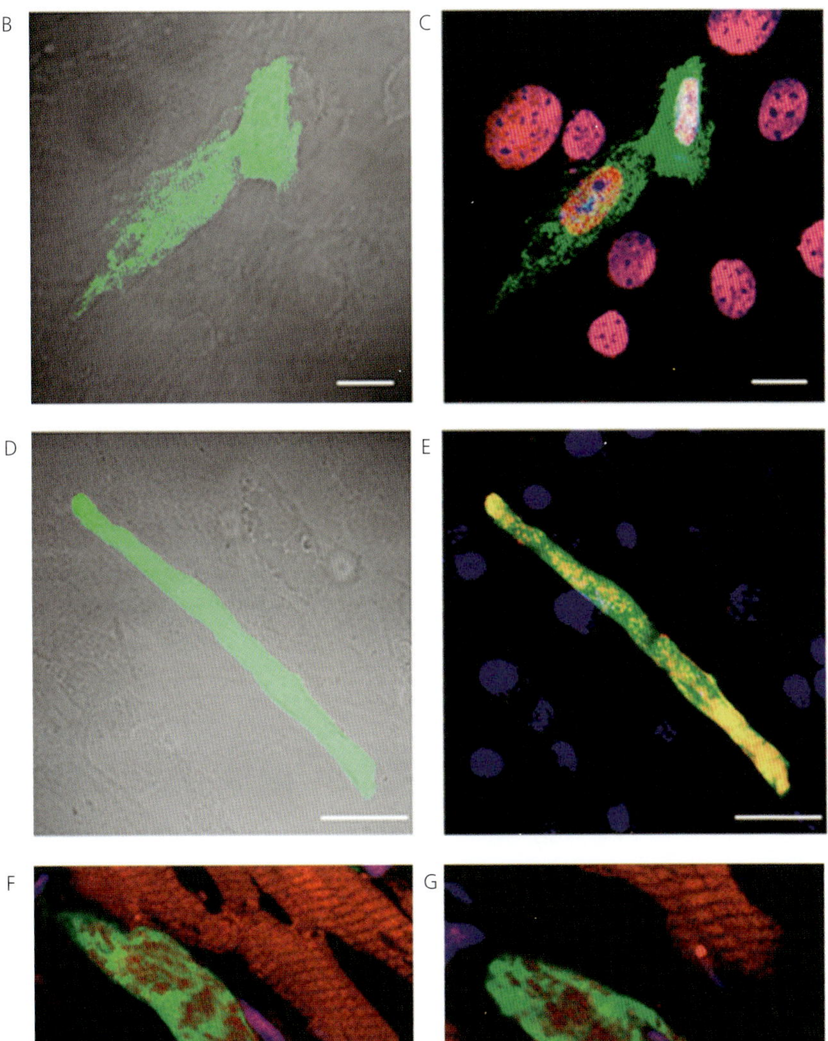

Figure 35–13 BM MSCs are mobilized and differentiate into cardiomyocytes after myocardial infarction in vivo. (a) Experimental protocol. The plasmid described in Figure 35–2 was transfected into BM MSCs, and intra-BM BM transplantation (IBM-BMT) was performed in mice exposed to a lethal dose of radiation. MI was induced in the mice 3 months after the BM had been reconstructed, and the infarct focus was examined. (b–f) Differentiation of cardiomyocyte in vitro. The EGFP-positive cells express *GATA4* (c) and cardiac actinin (e). (g, h) The gene-marked MSCs are mobilized to the infarcted foci and differentiate into cardiomyocytes.

2004; Kovacic and Graham 2004; Harada et al. 2005; Engelmann et al. 2006; Zohlnhofer et al. 2006; Ripa et al. 2007). Furthermore, it is unclear whether MSCs are mobilized in humans to the same extent as in mice, and whether they have the clinical potential for regeneration of heart damage following MI. Further studies are necessary to elucidate the molecular mechanism of G-CSF action before its clinical potential can be fully realized.

Conclusion

Although the concept of stem cell therapy for heart failure is very appealing, it must be based on scientifically sound basic research and should be evaluated objectively. Stem cell research has proceeded at a rapid pace, and it may soon be possible to produce large quantities of cardiomyocytes from ES cells and/or MSCs. Moreover, we can now prepare and use the patients' own iPS cells. Examination of the state of the art for transplantation research is a reminder that this is a period of time when deeper understanding of the issues is needed.

References

Andrew T, Dudley EJR. Overlapping expression domains of bone morphogenetic protein family members potentially account for limited tissue defects in BMP7-deficient embryos. *Dev Dynamics.* 1997;208:349–362.

Assmus B, Schachinger V, Teupe C, et al. Transplantation of progenitor cells and regeneration enhancement in acute myocardial infarction (TOPCARE-AMI). *Circulation.* 2002;106:3009–3017.

Balsam LB, Wagers AJ, Christensen JL, Kofidis T, Weissman IL, Robbins RC. Haematopoietic stem cells adopt mature haematopoietic fates in ischaemic myocardium. *Nature.* 2004;428:668–673.

Behfar A, Zingman LV, Hodgson DM, et al. Stem cell differentiation requires a paracrine pathway in the heart. *FASEB J.* 2002;16:1558–1566.

Beltrami AP, Barlucchi L, Torella D, et al. Adult cardiac stem cells are multipotent and support myocardial regeneration. *Cell.* 2003;114:763–776.

Beltrami AP, Urbanek K, Kajstura J, et al. Evidence that human cardiac myocytes divide after myocardial infarction. *N Engl J Med.* 2001;344:1750–1757.

Blanc KL, Pittenger MF. Mesenchymal stem cells: progress toward promise. *Cytotherapy.* 2005;7:36–45.

Boheler KR, Czyz J, Tweedie D, Yang H-T, Anisimov SV, Wobus AM. Differentiation of pluripotent embryonic stem cells into cardiomyocytes. *Circ Res.* 2002;91:189–201.

Cowan CA, Atienza J, Melton DA, Eggan K. Nuclear reprogramming of somatic cells after fusion with human embryonic stem cells. *Science.* 2005;309:1369–1373.

Deb A, Wang S, Skelding KA, Miller D, Simper D, Caplice NM. Bone marrow-derived cardiomyocytes are present in adult human heart: a study of gender-mismatched bone marrow transplantation patients. *Circulation.* 2003;107:1247–1249.

Docheva D, Popov C, Mutschler W, Schieker M. Human mesenchymal stem cells in contact with their environment: surface characteristics and the integrin system. *J Cell Mol Med.* 2007;11:21–38.

Doetschman TC, Eistetter H, Katz M, Schmidt W, Kemler R. The in vitro development of blastocyst-derived embryonic stem cell lines: formation of visceral yolk sac, blood islands and myocardium. *J Embryol Exp Morphol.* 1985;87:27–45.

Dyson E, Sucov HM, Kubalak SW, et al. Atrial-like phenotype is associated with embryonic ventricular failure in retinoid X receptor α -/- mice. *Proc Natl Acad Sci USA.* 1995;92:7386–7390.

Edwards MK, Harris JF, McBurney MW. Induced muscle differentiation in an embryonal carcinoma cell line. *Mol Cell Biol.* 1983;3:2280–2286.

Engelmann MG, Theiss HD, Hennig-Theiss C, et al. Autologous bone marrow stem cell mobilization induced by granulocyte colony-stimulating factor after subacute ST-segment elevation myocardial infarction undergoing late revascularization: final results from the G-CSF-STEMI (Granulocyte Colony-Stimulating Factor ST-Segment Elevation Myocardial Infarction) trial. *J Am Coll Cardiol.* 2006;48:1712–1721.

Evans MJ, Kaufman MH. Establishment in culture of pluripotential cells from mouse embryos. *Nature.* 1981;292:154–156.

Faure S, de Santa Barbara P, Roberts DJ, Whitman M. Endogenous patterns of BMP signaling during early chick development. *Dev Biol.* 2002;244:44–65.

Fletcher RB, Watson AL, Harland RM. Expression of *Xenopus tropicalis* noggin1 and noggin2 in early development: two noggin genes in a tetrapod. *Gene Expr Patterns.* 2004;5:225–230.

Foley AC, Mercola M. Heart induction by Wnt antagonists depends on the homeodomain transcription factor Hex. *Genes Dev.* 2005;19: 387–396.

Friedenstein AJ, Piatetzky S II, Petrakova KV. Osteogenesis in transplants of bone marrow cells. *J Embryol Exp Morphol.* 1966;16:381–390.

Fukuda K, Yuasa S. Stem cells as a source of regenerative cardiomyocytes. *Circ Res.* 2006;98:1002–1013.

Gaussin V, Van de Putte T, Mishina Y, et al. Endocardial cushion and myocardial defects after cardiac myocyte-specific conditional deletion of the bone morphogenetic protein receptor ALK3. *Proc Natl Acad Sci USA.* 2002;99:2878–2883.

Goodell MA, Rosenzweig M, Kim H, et al. Dye efflux studies suggest that hematopoietic stem cells expressing low or undetectable levels of CD34 antigen exist in multiple species. *Nat Med.* 1997;3:1337–1345.

Hakuno D, Fukuda K, Makino S, et al. Bone marrow-derived regenerated cardiomyocytes (CMG cells) express functional adrenergic and muscarinic receptors. *Circulation.* 2002;105:380–386.

Hanna J, Markoulaki S, Schorderet P, et al. Direct reprogramming of terminally differentiated mature B lymphocytes to pluripotency. *Cell.* 2008;133:250–264.

Hanna J, Wernig M, Markoulaki S, et al. Treatment of sickle cell anemia mouse model with iPS cells generated from autologous skin. *Science.* 2007;318:1920–1923.

Harada M, Qin Y, Takano H, et al. G-CSF prevents cardiac remodeling after myocardial infarction by activating the Jak-Stat pathway in cardiomyocytes. *Nat Med.* 2005;11:305–311.

Hattan N, Kawaguchi H, Ando K, et al. Purified cardiomyocytes from bone marrow mesenchymal stem cells produce stable intracardiac grafts in mice. *Cardiovasc Res.* 2005;65:334–344.

Heng BC, Haider HK, Sim EK-W, Cao T, Ng SC. Strategies for directing the differentiation of stem cells into the cardiomyogenic lineage in vitro. *Cardiovasc Res.* 2004;62:34–42.

Hogan BLM. Bone morphogenetic proteins in development. *Curr Opin Genet Dev.* 1996;6:432–438.

Itabashi Y, Miyoshi S, Kawaguchi H, et al. A new method for manufacturing cardiac cell sheets using fibrin-coated dishes and its electrophysiological studies by optical mapping. *Artif Organs.* 2005;29:95–103.

Jackson KA, Majka SM, Wang H, et al. Regeneration of ischemic cardiac muscle and vascular endothelium by adult stem cells. *J Clin Invest.* 2001;107:1395–1402.

Jiang Y, Jahagirdar BN, Reinhardt RL, et al. Pluripotency of mesenchymal stem cells derived from adult marrow. *Nature.* 2002;418:41–49.

Jiang Y, Jahagirdar BN, Reinhardt RL, et al. Pluripotency of mesenchymal stem cells derived from adult marrow. *Nature.* 2007;447:880–881.

Kang H-J, Kim H-S, Zhang SY, et al. Effects of intracoronary infusion of peripheral blood stem-cells mobilised with granulocyte-colony stimulating factor on left ventricular systolic function and restenosis after coronary stenting in myocardial infarction: the MAGIC cell randomised clinical trial. *Lancet.* 2004;363:751–756.

Kanno S, Kim PKM, Sallam K, Lei J, Billiar TR, Shears LL II. Nitric oxide facilitates cardiomyogenesis in mouse embryonic stem cells. *Proc Natl Acad Sci USA.* 2004;101:12277–12281.

Kastner P, Grondona JM, Mark M, et al. Genetic analysis of RXR [alpha] developmental function: convergence of RXR and RAR signaling pathways in heart and eye morphogenesis. *Cell.* 1994;78:987–1003.

Kawada H, Fujita J, Kinjo K, et al. Nonhematopoietic mesenchymal stem cells can be mobilized and differentiate into cardiomyocytes after myocardial infarction. *Blood.* 2004;104:3581–3587.

Kikuchi A, Okuhara M, Karikusa F, Sakurai Y, Okano T. Two-dimensional manipulation of confluently cultured vascular endothelial cells using temperature-responsive poly(N-isopropylacrylamide)-grafted surfaces. *J Biomat Sci, Polymer Edition.* 1998;9:1331–1348.

Klug MG, Soonpaa MH, Koh GY, Field LJ. Genetically selected cardiomyocytes from differentiating embryonic stem cells form stable intracardiac grafts. *J Clin Invest.* 1996;98:216–224.

Kolossov E, Fleischmann BK, Liu Q, et al. Functional characteristics of ES cell-derived cardiac precursor cells identified by tissue-specific expression of the green fluorescent protein. *J Cell Biol.* 1998;143: 2045–2056.

Kovacic JC, Graham RM. Stem-cell therapy for myocardial diseases. *Lancet.* 2004;363:1735–1736.

Kumar D, Sun B. Transforming growth factor-[beta]2 enhances differentiation of cardiac myocytes from embryonic stem cells. *Biochem Biophys Res Commun.* 2005;332:135–141.

Ladd AN, Yatskievych TA, Antin PB. Regulation of avian cardiac myogenesis by activin/TGFbeta and bone morphogenetic proteins. *Dev Biol.* 1998;204:407–419.

Laflamme MA, Chen KY, Naumova AV, et al. Cardiomyocytes derived from human embryonic stem cells in pro-survival factors enhance function of infarcted rat hearts. *Nat Biotech.* 2007;25:1015–1024.

Laugwitz K-L, Moretti A, Lam J, et al. Postnatal isl1+ cardioblasts enter fully differentiated cardiomyocyte lineages. *Nature.* 2005;433:647–653.

Li RK, Jia ZQ, Weisel RD, et al. Cardiomyocyte transplantation improves heart function. *Ann Thorac Surg.* 1996a;62:654–660.

Li R-K, Mickle DAG, Weisel RD, Zhang J, Mohabeer MK. In vivo survival and function of transplanted rat cardiomyocytes. *Circ Res.* 1996b;78:283–288.

Lim DA, Tramontin AD, Trevejo JM, Herrera DG, Garcia-Verdugo JM, Alvarez-Buylla A. Noggin antagonizes BMP signaling to create a niche for adult neurogenesis. *Neuron.* 2000;28:713–726.

Lowry WE, Richter L, Yachechko R, et al. Generation of human induced pluripotent stem cells from dermal fibroblasts. *Proc Natl Acad Sci USA.* 2008;105:2883–2888.

Lyons KM, Hogan BLM, Robertson EJ. Colocalization of BMP 7 and BMP 2 RNAs suggests that these factors cooperatively mediate tissue interactions during murine development. *Mech Dev.* 1995;50:71–83.

Lyons KM, Pelton RW, Hogan BL. Organogenesis and pattern formation in the mouse: RNA distribution patterns suggest a role for bone morphogenetic protein-2A (BMP-2A). *Development.* 1990;109:833–844.

Maherali N, Sridharan R, Xie W, et al. Directly reprogrammed fibroblasts show global epigenetic remodeling and widespread tissue contribution. *Cell Stem Cell.* 2007;1:55–70.

Maillard I, Fang T, Pear WS. Regulation of lymphoid development, differentiation, and function by the Notch pathway. *Ann Rev Immunol.* 2005;23:945–974.

Makino S, Fukuda K, Miyoshi S, et al. Cardiomyocytes can be generated from marrow stromal cells in vitro. *J Clin Invest.* 1999;103:697–705.

Manis JP. Knock out, knock in, knock down--genetically manipulated mice and the Nobel prize. *N Engl J Med.* 2007;357:2426–2429.

Marvin MJ, Di Rocco G, Gardiner A, Bush SM, Lassar AB. Inhibition of Wnt activity induces heart formation from posterior mesoderm. *Genes Dev.* 2001;15:316–327.

Matsuzaki Y, Kinjo K, Mulligan RC, Okano H. Unexpectedly efficient homing capacity of purified murine hematopoietic stem cells. *Immunity.* 2004;20:87–93.

McMahon JA, Takada S, Zimmerman LB, Fan CM, Harland RM, McMahon AP. Noggin-mediated antagonism of BMP signaling is required for growth and patterning of the neural tube and somite. *Genes Dev.* 1998;12:1438–1452.

Messina E, De Angelis L, Frati G, et al. Isolation and expansion of adult cardiac stem cells from human and murine heart. *Circ Res.* 2004;95:911–921.

Mima T, Ueno H, Fischman DA, Williams LT, Mikawa T. Fibroblast growth factor receptor is required for in vivo cardiac myocyte proliferation at early embryonic stages of heart development. *Proc Natl Acad Sci USA.* 1995;92:467–471.

Monzen K, Hiroi Y, Kudoh S, et al. Smads, TAK1, and their common target ATF-2 play a critical role in cardiomyocyte differentiation. *J Cell Biol.* 2001;153:687–698.

Monzen K, Shiojima I, Hiroi Y, et al. Bone morphogenetic proteins induce cardiomyocyte differentiation through the mitogen-activated protein kinase kinase kinase TAK1 and cardiac transcription factors Csx/Nkx-2.5 and GATA-4. *Mol Cell Biol.* 1999;19:7096–7105.

Moore JC, Spijker R, Martens AC, et al. A P19Cl6 GFP reporter line to quantify cardiomyocyte differentiation of stem cells. *Int J Dev Biol.* 2004;48:47–55.

Moretti A, Caron L, Nakano A, et al. Multipotent embryonic isl1+ progenitor cells lead to cardiac, smooth muscle, and endothelial cell diversification. *Cell.* 2006;127:1151–1165.

Muller M, Fleischmann BK, Selbert S, et al. Selection of ventricular-like cardiomyocytes from ES cells in vitro. *FASEB J.* 2000;14:2540–2548.

Murry CE, Keller G. Differentiation of embryonic stem cells to clinically relevant populations: lessons from embryonic development. *Cell.* 2008;132:661–680.

Murry CE, Soonpaa MH, Reinecke H, et al. Haematopoietic stem cells do not transdifferentiate into cardiac myocytes in myocardial infarcts. *Nature.* 2004;428:664–668.

Nakagawa M, Koyanagi M, Tanabe K, et al. Generation of induced pluripotent stem cells without Myc from mouse and human fibroblasts. *Nat Biotech.* 2008;26:101–106.

Neuhaus H, Rosen V, Thies RS. Heart specific expression of mouse BMP-10 a novel member of the TGF-[beta] superfamily. *Mech Dev.* 1999;80:181–184.

Oh H, Bradfute SB, Gallardo TD, et al. Cardiac progenitor cells from adult myocardium: homing, differentiation, and fusion after infarction. *Proc Natl Acad Sci USA.* 2003;100:12313–12318.

Okita K, Ichisaka T, Yamanaka S. Generation of germline-competent induced pluripotent stem cells. *Nature.* 2007;448:313–317.

Orlic D, Kajstura J, Chimenti S, et al. Bone marrow cells regenerate infarcted myocardium. *Nature.* 2001;410:701–705.

Osawa M, Hanada K-I, Hamada H, Nakauchi H. Long-term lymphohematopoietic reconstitution by a single CD34-low/negative hematopoietic stem cell. *Science.* 1996;273:242–245.

Osmond MK, Butler AJ, Voon FC, Bellairs R. The effects of retinoic acid on heart formation in the early chick embryo. *Development.* 1991;113:1405–1417.

Park I-H, Zhao R, West JA, et al. Reprogramming of human somatic cells to pluripotency with defined factors. *Nature.* 2008;451:141–146.

Phinney DG, Prockop DJ. Concise review: mesenchymal stem/multipotent stromal cells: the state of transdifferentiation and modes of tissue repair current views. *Stem Cells.* 2007;25:2896–2902.

Pittenger MF, Mackay AM, Beck SC, et al. Multilineage potential of adult human mesenchymal stem cells. *Science.* 1999;284:143–147.

Prockop DJ. Marrow stromal cells as stem cells for nonhematopoietic tissues. *Science.* 1997;276:71–74.

Quaini F, Urbanek K, Beltrami AP, et al. Chimerism of the transplanted heart. *N Engl J Med.* 2002;346:5–15.

Ray RP, Wharton KA. Twisted perspective: new insights into extracellular modulation of BMP signaling during development. *Cell.* 2001;104:801–804.

Rickard DJ, Sullivan TA, Shenker BJ, Leboy PS, Kazhdan I. Induction of Rapid osteoblast differentiation in rat bone marrow stromal cell cultures by dexamethasone and BMP-2. *Dev Biol.* 1994;161:218–228.

Ripa RS, Haack-Sorensen M, Wang Y, et al. Bone marrow derived mesenchymal cell mobilization by granulocyte-colony stimulating factor after acute myocardial infarction: results from the Stem Cells in Myocardial Infarction (STEMMI) Trial. *Circulation.* 2007;116: I-24–30.

Sachinidis A, Fleischmann BK, Kolossov E, Wartenberg M, Sauer H, Hescheler J. Cardiac specific differentiation of mouse embryonic stem cells. *Cardiovasc Res.* 2003;58:278–291.

Sasai Y, Lu B, Steinbeisser H, De Robertis EM. Regulation of neural induction by the Chd and Bmp-4 antagonistic patterning signals in Xenopus. *Nature.* 1995;376;333–336.

Schachinger V, Erbs S, Elsasser A, et al. Intracoronary bone marrow-derived progenitor cells in acute myocardial infarction. *N Engl J Med.* 2006;355:1210–1221.

Schenke-Layland K, Rhodes KE, Angelis E, et al. Reprogrammed mouse fibroblasts differentiate into cells of the cardiovascular and hematopoietic lineages. *Stem Cells.* 2008;26(6):1537–1546.

Schlange T, Andree B, Arnold H-H, Brand T. BMP2 is required for early heart development during a distinct time period. *Mech Dev.* 2000;91:259–270.

Schneider MD, Gaussin V, Lyons KM. Tempting fate: BMP signals for cardiac morphogenesis. *Cytokine Growth Factor Rev.* 2003;14:1–4.

Schneider VA, Mercola M. Wnt antagonism initiates cardiogenesis in Xenopus laevis. *Genes Dev.* 2001;15:304–315.

Schultheiss TM, Burch JB, Lassar AB. A role for bone morphogenetic proteins in the induction of cardiac myogenesis. *Genes Dev.* 1997;11:451–462.

Shimizu T, Yamato M, Isoi Y, et al. Fabrication of pulsatile cardiac tissue grafts using a novel 3-dimensional cell sheet manipulation technique and temperature-responsive cell culture surfaces. *Circ Res.* 2002;90, e40–e48.

Smith WC, Harland RM. Expression cloning of noggin, a new dorsalizing factor localized to the Spemann organizer in Xenopus embryos. *Cell.* 1992;70:829–840.

Strauer BE, Brehm M, Zeus T, et al. Repair of infarcted myocardium by autologous intracoronary mononuclear bone marrow cell transplantation in humans. *Circulation.* 2002;106:1913–1918.

Tabar V, Tomishima M, Panagiotakos G, et al. Therapeutic cloning in individual Parkinsonian mice. *Nat Med.* 2008;14:379–381.

Takahashi K, Tanabe K, Ohnuki M, et al. Induction of pluripotent stem cells from adult human fibroblasts by defined factors. *Cell.* 2007;131:861–872.

Takahashi K, Yamanaka S. Induction of pluripotent stem cells from mouse embryonic and adult fibroblast cultures by defined factors. *Cell.* 2006;126:663–676.

Takahashi T, Kalka C, Masuda H, et al. Ischemia- and cytokine-induced mobilization of bone marrow-derived endothelial progenitor cells for neovascularization. *Nat Med.* 1999;5:434–438.

Takahashi T, Lord B, Schulze PC, et al. Ascorbic acid enhances differentiation of embryonic stem cells into cardiac myocytes. *Circulation.* 2003;107:1912–1916.

Terada N, Hamazaki T, Oka M, et al. Bone marrow cells adopt the phenotype of other cells by spontaneous cell fusion. *Nature.* 2002;416:542–545.

Thomson JA, Itskovitz-Eldor J, Shapiro SS, et al. Embryonic stem cell lines derived from human blastocysts. *Science.* 1998;282:1145–1147.

Timmerman LA, Grego-Bessa J, Raya A, et al. Notch promotes epithelial-mesenchymal transition during cardiac development and oncogenic transformation. *Genes Dev.* 2004;18:99–115.

Tomita Y, Makino S, Hakuno D, et al. Application of mesenchymal stem cell-derived cardiomyocytes as bio-pacemakers: current status and problems to be solved. *Med Biol Engin Comput.* 2007;45:209–220.

Tomita Y, Matsumura K, Wakamatsu Y, et al. Cardiac neural crest cells contribute to the dormant multipotent stem cell in the mammalian heart. *J Cell Biol.* 2005;170:1135–1146.

von Bubnoff A, Cho KWY. Intracellular BMP signaling regulation in vertebrates: pathway or network? *Dev Biol.* 2001;239:1–14.

Wagers AJ, Sherwood RI, Christensen JL, Weissman IL. Little evidence for developmental plasticity of adult hematopoietic stem cells. *Science.* 2002;297:2256–2259.

Wakayama T, Hayashi Y, Ogura A. Participation of the female pronucleus derived from the second polar body in full embryonic development of mice. *J Reprod Fertil.* 1997;110:263–266.

Wilmut I, Schnieke AE, McWhir J, Kind AJ, Campbell KHS. Viable offspring derived from fetal and adult mammalian cells. *Nature.* 1997;385:810–813.

Winnier G, Blessing M, Labosky PA, Hogan BL. Bone morphogenetic protein-4 is required for mesoderm formation and patterning in the mouse. *Genes Dev.* 1995;9:2105–2116.

Wobus AM, Kaomei G, Shan J, et al. Retinoic acid accelerates embryonic stem cell-derived cardiac differentiation and enhances development of ventricular cardiomyocytes. *J Mol Cell Cardiol.* 1997;29:1525–1539.

Wollert KC, Meyer GP, Lotz J, et al. Intracoronary autologous bone-marrow cell transfer after myocardial infarction: the BOOST randomised controlled clinical trial. *Lancet.* 2004;364:141–148.

Woodbury D, Schwarz EJ, Prockop DJ, Black IB. Adult rat and human bone marrow stromal cells differentiate into neurons. *J Neurosci Res.* 2000;61L:364–370.

Yamauchi Y, Abe K, Mantani A, et al. A novel transgenic technique that allows specific marking of the neural crest cell lineage in mice. *Dev Biol.* 1999;212:191–203.

Yang X, Smith SL, Tian XC, Lewin HA, Renard J-P, Wakayama T. Nuclear reprogramming of cloned embryos and its implications for therapeutic cloning. *Nat Genet.* 2007;39:295–302.

Ying Q-L, Nichols J, Evans EP, Smith AG. Changing potency by spontaneous fusion. *Nature.* 2002;416:545–548.

Yu J, Vodyanik MA, Smuga-Otto K, et al. Induced pluripotent stem cell lines derived from human somatic cells. *Science.* 2007;318(5858):1917–1920.

Yuasa S, Fukuda K. Recent advances in cardiovascular regenerative medicine: the induced pluripotent stem cell era. *Expert Rev Cardiovasc Ther.* 2008;6:803–810.

Yuasa S, Fukuda K, Tomita Y, et al. Cardiomyocytes undergo cells division following myocardial infarction is a spatially and temporally restricted event in rats. *Mol Cell Biochem.* 2004;259:177–181

Yuasa S, Itabashi Y, Koshimizu U, et al. Transient inhibition of BMP signaling by Noggin induces cardiomyocyte differentiation of mouse embryonic stem cells. *Nat Biotech.* 2005;23:607–611.

Zhang H, Bradley A. Mice deficient for BMP2 are nonviable and have defects in amnion/chorion and cardiac development. *Development.* 1996;122:2977–2986.

Zhang P, Li J, Tan Z, et al. Short-term BMP-4 treatment initiates mesoderm induction in human embryonic stem cells. *Blood.* 2008;111: 1933–1941.

Zohlnhofer D, Ott I, Mehilli J, et al. Stem cell mobilization by granulocyte colony-stimulating factor in patients with acute myocardial infarction: a randomized controlled trial. *J Am Med Assoc.* 2006; 295:1003–1010.

36

Genetic Counseling in Cardiovascular Genetics

Ivan Macciocca

Introduction

The need for genetic counseling in cardiology has grown with the expansion in knowledge of how genetics impacts on a person's cardiovascular risk. The contribution of genetics to cardiovascular disease etiology is growing and becoming more complex—from single gene disorders such as hypertrophic cardiomyopathy and familial hypercholesterolemia to multifactorial conditions such as coronary artery disease (CAD) and congenital heart disease (Cambien and Tiret 2007). Whilst genetic counseling has much to add to the management of multifactorial cardiovascular diseases (Scheuner 2003; Sturm 2004), the focus of this chapter will be genetic counseling for cardiovascular genetic conditions that are typically transmitted in a Mendelian fashion; these include inherited cardiomyopathies and arrhythmias, Marfan syndrome and related conditions as well as inherited lipid disorders (see Box 36-1 for the list of conditions).

Genetic Counseling—What Is It?

It is necessary to define genetic counseling in order to understand what role it can play in helping individuals and their families with cardiovascular genetic conditions. A task force of the National Society of Genetic Counselors in the United States produced the following definition of genetic counseling that is applicable to cardiovascular genetics (Resta et al. 2006):

> Genetic counseling is the process of helping people understand and adapt to the medical, psychological, and familial implications of genetic contributions to disease.

This definition is readily applicable to cardiovascular genetics and demonstrates the diversity of the genetic counselor's role. It includes education, counseling, and working with families to address psychosocial issues they encounter in relation to their disease. Whilst not explicitly stated in this definition, a key aspect of cardiovascular genetic counseling is to assist clients to make informed decisions. Most referrals to genetic counseling are made because the client is considering a decision, either about genetic testing or a related issue. Hodgson and Spriggs propose that as well as providing adequate information to make an assessment of the relative advantages and disadvantages of a decision, it is important for the client to have time to deliberate about their decision (Hodgson and Spriggs 2005). This is where the genetic counselor can engage with the client to assist him or her to understand how their decision fits with their values and the kind of life they want to live now and in the future. Thus genetic counseling always includes provision of information and education about the natural history of the condition in question and basic genetic information including inheritance patterns. Gaps in our knowledge about the cardiovascular genetic condition and limitations of genetic testing are raised so that the clients can make their decision with an awareness of what is known and what is not known.

The psychological, emotional, and practical impact of the condition on the client and his or her family are explored as these factors will influence the client's attitudes, perceptions, and beliefs about the condition. Listening and acknowledging the client's experience allows an assessment of how the client has arrived at his or her view of the condition. This may expose factually incorrect information that has influenced his or her decisions, either positively or negatively.

Genetic counselors will typically work within a multidisciplinary team to achieve these goals in the cardiac setting. Internationally, multidisciplinary cardiogenetic clinics exist, which may include cardiologists, clinical geneticists, genetic counselors, nurses, social workers, and psychologists (Christiaans et al. 2009). In some countries, such clinics do not exist and families are referred to a clinical genetics department for genetic counseling.

Box 36-1 Cardiovascular Genetic Conditions that Are the Focus of this Chapter

- Hypertrophic cardiomyopathy
- Dilated cardiomyopathy
- Arrhythmogenic right ventricular cardiomyopathy
- Restrictive cardiomyopathy
- Long QT syndrome
- Catecholaminergic polymorphic ventricular tachycardia
- Brugada syndrome
- Marfan syndrome
- Familial hypercholesterolemia

The expertise that genetic counselors bring to the cardiac genetics clinic is their understanding of the genetic basis of the conditions, their counseling knowledge and skills, their ability to tune in to family dynamics, their skills in working with the family while respecting the individual, and an awareness that an individual's values, understanding, beliefs, and perceptions about a condition is usually built on their prior experience of the condition.

This chapter is divided into three sections that cover these aspects: genetic testing, processes in genetic counseling, and risk communication. Throughout the rest of the chapter, the individual receiving genetic counseling will be called the consultand, and may or may not be affected with the cardiovascular genetic condition.

Genetic Testing

A key goal of genetic counseling for cardiovascular genetic conditions is to ensure that the consultand understands the clinical utility of genetic tests. There are three main categories of genetic tests for cardiovascular genetic conditions: mutation detection, predictive gene tests, and prenatal gene tests, which are discussed below. Each test type has different limitations and implications.

1. Mutation Detection

Genetic testing for cardiovascular genetic conditions is complicated by the fact that there is more than one causative gene for each condition and that, for the most part, each family has its own unique mutation—the so-called family-specific mutation. Therefore, it is first necessary to test a clinically affected individual from the family to identify the family-specific mutation. This initial step is called mutation detection. If the only affected family member is deceased, tissue may need to be obtained from post-mortem material, or a Guthrie card, if it is available.

It is now well established that a small proportion of families have more than one disease-causing mutation, in either different alleles of the same gene, or different genes. This phenomenon is most widely reported in hypertrophic cardiomyopathy (HCM) and long QT syndrome (LQTS) (Richard et al. 2003; Van Driest et al. 2004; Tester et al. 2005). Therefore, it is recommended that for these conditions, the search for the family-specific mutation in the index case should not cease once a mutation is identified, but should continue to include all of the commonest genes associated with the condition.

Genetic counseling prior to mutation detection should include a discussion about the three possible outcomes of mutation detection:

1. A sequence variation that is believed to be a disease-causing mutation may be identified. The mutation detection success rate will vary depending on the cardiovascular genetic condition (see chapters in other sections of this book for specific mutation detection rates for specific conditions). The vast majority of mutations in cardiovascular genetic conditions are missense (i.e., a single base pair substitution resulting in a change in amino acid) and it can sometimes be difficult to determine whether such changes are pathogenic. The task of determining the pathogenicity of a sequence variation often involves consultation within a multidisciplinary team, with each team member providing different expertise. Molecular geneticists, working together with cardiologists, clinical geneticists, and/or genetic counselors may contribute to the assessment of the pathogenicity of a sequence variation. Sequence variations are generally considered to be disease causing if all, or a subset, of the following set of criteria can be met (Cotton and Scriver 1998):

   I. The sequence variation is absent from a large group of control chromosomes. It is preferable for controls to be ethnically matched to the case.
   II. The sequence variation cosegregates with disease in the family. It may not always be possible to perform cosegregation studies because of small family size or because some affected family members may not wish to have gene testing.
   III. The nature of the amino acid change is significant.
   IV. The sequence variation has been reported in other affected families, with evidence of the mutation cosegregating with disease.
   V. The variant is in an important functional domain of the gene (functional studies may be required to demonstrate this).

   If a disease-causing mutation is identified, this mutation can be used as a "predictive" gene test for relatives who are at risk of the condition, but are asymptomatic. In addition, it can be used as a confirmatory test in other relatives that may be affected by the condition.

2. A second possible outcome of mutation detection is that a sequence variation of unknown significance may be identified. These are variations in the DNA for which there is not enough evidence to clearly categorize the variant as disease causing based on the criteria listed above.

   When a variation of unknown significance is identified, its utility in confirming the diagnosis in a consultand with suspected disease is limited and it cannot be used for predictive gene testing in at-risk relatives. Thus the implication of identifying a sequence variation of unknown significance for first-degree relatives of clinically affected individuals in the family is that predictive gene testing is not available and clinical screening will need to continue.

3. The final possible outcome of mutation detection is that no mutation is identified. There are several explanations for this. It is possible that the disease-causing mutation in the family is present in a gene that was not tested, or in a gene that is yet to be discovered. Alternatively, it is possible that there is a mutation in one of the genes that was tested, but the mutation detection technique employed missed the mutation. For example, gene sequencing is considered the "gold standard" for mutation detection, but even gene sequencing does not detect large deletions or duplications within genes. All laboratory reports should state the testing technique(s) used and the estimated sensitivity and specificity.

   The clinical implications of a gene-negative result, for the individual tested, and the family, are the same as if a sequence variation of unknown significance was identified.

   It is common practice for laboratories to report all variants found in genetic testing, whether they be disease causing, of unknown significance or known polymorphisms. It is incumbent upon both laboratory and clinical services to maintain records of all variants as knowledge of the implications of variants may change with time.

2. Predictive Gene Testing

Predictive gene testing, which is also called asymptomatic gene testing, is possible only if a disease-causing mutation is known in a family. By definition, predictive gene testing is performed in an asymptomatic individual. If the individual were symptomatic, then testing for the family-specific mutation would be considered a confirmatory gene test. As the individual is only being tested for the family-specific mutation, there are only two outcomes of the test; the mutation is present or it is not.

If the family-specific mutation is not present, the risk of developing the condition in question is reduced to population risk and no further cardiac screening is recommended. While it is obvious to health care providers that if the mutation is not present, it cannot be transmitted to offspring, this is not always clear to the consultand who may believe that the gene can "skip generations." Therefore, explicitly stating that the consultand cannot pass on the gene mutation is recommended.

If the mutation is present, the relative is confirmed to be at risk of developing the cardiovascular genetic condition and will need to commence or continue cardiac screening. Serial clinical screening is recommended in gene-positive, phenotype-negative individuals. Prophylactic treatment may be initiated for some conditions and modification of lifestyle risk factors (e.g., participating in competitive sport) may be recommended.

3. Prenatal Testing

A number of reproductive options become available once a consultand is found to have a disease-causing mutation. These include prenatal diagnosis via chorionic villus sampling (CVS) or amniocentesis and preimplantation genetic diagnosis. The number of people utilizing prenatal diagnosis for cardiovascular genetic conditions is likely to be small worldwide; however, the option of prenatal diagnosis should be made known to individuals when they attend for pretest genetic counseling as it may influence decision making about gene testing and family planning.

CVS and amniocentesis are both sampling procedures to obtain tissue from the developing placenta or fetus, which can be used to test for the presence of the family-specific mutation. Both are associated with a risk of miscarriage after the procedure. The risks generally quoted in practice are 0.5% for amniocentesis and 1% for CVS, although emerging literature is beginning to suggest that the risks may be lower (Mujezinovic and Alfirevic 2007). CVS is most commonly performed transabdominally between 11- and 14-weeks gestation, by fine needle aspiration of chorionic cells from which DNA can be extracted and tested. Amniocentesis is also commonly performed transabdominally after 15-weeks gestation by aspiration of amniotic fluid, culture of the cells suspended within the fluid, and extraction of DNA for testing. Culturing of cells can take 1–2 weeks so the result of DNA analysis can take as long as 3 weeks.

As both amniocentesis and CVS are associated with a small risk of miscarriage most couples undergoing such procedures do so with a view to terminating an affected fetus. Given the gravity of such a decision, couples considering prenatal diagnosis should be referred for formal genetic counseling in a prenatal genetic counseling center to assist them through the process.

Preimplantation Genetic Diagnosis

In the past 5–10 years, the use of preimplantation genetic diagnosis (PGD) has become more widespread. In essence, PGD is the process of performing genetic analysis of an embryo for the family-specific mutation that has been identified in one of the parents. Therefore, the couple will need to undergo in vitro fertilization followed by biopsy of one or two cells at the blastocyst stage of any resultant embryos. Testing of the cells will determine which embryos have inherited the family-specific mutation so that an embryo that does not have the mutation is transferred.

The European Society of Human Reproduction and Embryology PGD consortium has not reported any cases of PGD being used for cardiovascular genetic diseases except for Marfan syndrome (Harper et al. 2008). While the rate at which couples are using PGD to select against cardiovascular genetic conditions is currently small, the number of people requesting PGD for cardiovascular conditions is likely to increase as genetic testing for these conditions becomes more widespread.

The users of PGD are most commonly those that have objections to termination of pregnancy or who may have had several terminations for the genetic condition present in the family in the past (Lavery et al. 2002). PGD is often an attractive option to couples when it is first introduced, but there are significant downsides: the invasiveness, cost, and the clinical pregnancy rate per embryo transfer of about 25%–30% (Harper et al. 2008). While the cardiovascular genetic clinic should have as one of its responsibilities to inform consultands about the possibility of using PGD to conceive a pregnancy free of the condition in the family, referral to an IVF center that performs PGD is recommended for detailed counseling.

Processes in Genetic Counseling

The approach to the genetic counseling consultation in cardiovascular genetic conditions is similar to that in other genetic conditions. Two of the commonest reasons for attending are when the consultand has, or is suspected to have, clinically evident disease and presents for diagnostic gene testing and the other is when the consultand is presenting for predictive gene testing. Box 36–2 gives an overview of the content and process of genetic counseling in these settings. Variations to these approaches exist, which will be dependent on the structure and delivery of genetic (or cardiogenetic) services around the world (Charron et al. 2002; van Langen et al. 2004; Ingles et al. 2008; Christiaans et al. 2009).

Box 36–2 Content and Process of Genetic Counseling for Diagnostic/Confirmatory and Predictive Testing for Cardiovascular Genetic Conditions

Diagnostic/confirmatory gene testing

Session 1:

With the consultand +/- partner (or parent if the consultand is a child):

- Ascertain consultand's reason for attending
- Document family history
- Obtain verification of clinical diagnosis
- Ascertain consultand's understanding of the condition and its genetics
- Explain relevant inheritance pattern
- Discuss process of genetic testing including mutation identification success rate and the implications of genetic testing to the individual and his/her relatives (see mutations detection section)
- Raise prenatal diagnosis and preimplantation diagnosis as a potential use of genetic test information if appropriate
- Discuss turnaround time for result and contract for disclosure (aim for face-to-face consultation for disclosure) if consultand decides to proceed with genetic testing
- Assess if any further counseling sessions addressing psychosocial issues are required
- Letter to patient, in lay language, summarizing the consultation

(Continued)

Box 36–2 (Continued)

Session 2—disclosure

With the consultand +/- partner (or parent if a child):

- Explain gene test result and implications for relatives
- Explore impact of the gene test result
- If mutation identified, discuss cascade genetic testing
- If no mutation identified, make/reinforce recommendations for clinical screening of at-risk relatives
- Explore ability of client to communicate implications of the result to his/her relatives. Identify areas of difficulty and offer support and assistance as necessary
- Assess if any further counseling sessions addressing psychosocial issues are required
- Letter to patient, in lay language, summarizing the consultation

Follow-up

Follow-up phone call between 1 and 2 weeks after disclosure to check for understanding and to reinforce cascade screening issues. Check on coping and determine if further follow-up is necessary.

Predictive gene testing

Session 1

With the consultand and partner (or parent if a child):

- Document or review family history
- Explain relevant inheritance pattern
- Explain two possible outcomes of the gene test and discuss the medical implications of each for the consultand and his/her relatives (see the section on Approach to Predictive Testing Counseling)
- Explore potential psychological/emotional and social impacts of the gene testing
- Explore impact on relationship with relatives, potential impact on work, and social activities and insurance
- Assess if any further counseling sessions addressing psychosocial issues are required
- Letter to patient, in lay language, summarizing the consultation

Session 2—disclosure

With the consultand and partner (or parent if a child):

- Explain gene test result and implications for relatives
- If mutation identified, arrange appointment for medical management
- Identify any areas of difficulty and offer support and assistance as appropriate
- Explore impact of the gene test result

Follow-up

Follow-up phone call between 1 and 2 weeks after disclosure to check for understanding and to reinforce cascade screening issues. Check on coping and determine if further follow-up is necessary.

1. Pedigree Drawing and Analysis

The drawing of a pedigree is both a practical and a psychosocial tool. As a practical tool, the pedigree documents the family history in a logical and interpretable manner. It provides an "at a glance" overview of the family; it should be at least three generations and should document who has the cardiovascular genetic condition in question or symptoms that could be related to the condition. Importantly in cardiovascular genetic conditions, there should be a high level of suspicion in relation to any early and unexpected death in the family and where possible, records should be obtained verifying the cause of death, preferably a postmortem report. If a postmortem was not performed, death certificates and medical records may be instructive. Construction and presentation of pedigree should be in accordance with accepted standardized approaches (Bennett et al. 1995, Bennett et al. 2008).

The pedigree may help determine the pattern of inheritance of the condition in question. While the majority of cardiovascular genetic conditions are transmitted in an autosomal dominant fashion, there are rarer autosomal recessive, sex-linked, and mitochondrial forms that may be highlighted by examining the pattern of transmission of disease in the family.

As a psychosocial tool, drawing the pedigree can be used to establish rapport and to gain an understanding of family dynamics, an important factor in facilitating clinical screening of at-risk relatives as well as cascade genetic testing if a disease-causing mutation is known in the family. Drawing the pedigree is an opportunity to explore relationships between relatives thereby assessing how information about clinical screening, or about the availability of a predictive gene test, will be communicated within the family. This may guide the genetic counselor as to which genetic counseling interventions may be required to facilitate dissemination of risk information (see the section on Risk Communication for more details about interventions).

Importantly, the drawing of the pedigree can be used to understand the impact of the condition on the family. For example, how many family members have the condition, how were they diagnosed, what symptoms or events the consultand attributes to the condition or to other causes, and how many sudden deaths there are in the family. This sort of information will shape the consultand's beliefs and understanding of the condition. All this information is important as research from other genetic diseases has shown that severity of the disease manifestations in the family can influence reproductive and genetic testing decisions (Henneman et al. 2001).

2. Family Consultations

Family members tend to want to attend together for genetic counseling. There are advantages to this approach; it can engender a sense of "being in it together," and can facilitate family members providing mutual support. It can be very useful for family members to attend together, particularly when an individual from the family is considering whether to proceed with mutation detection or not. In this context, the genetic counselor can stimulate discussion amongst the family members about their views on genetic testing and how the information from the gene test may or may not be used by different relatives. The aim of this approach is to raise awareness within the family that there may be differing views and to encourage respect for the different views of individuals in the family. The counselor needs to be prepared to deal with such differences and capitalize on these interactions to reinforce the point that there are no correct views, just individual views that should be respected.

3. Approach to Predictive Testing Counseling

There are no specific guidelines about how predictive testing counseling should be performed for cardiovascular genetics conditions. The approach that is taken for predictive testing for cardiovascular genetic conditions is loosely based on guidelines for predictive testing for Huntington disease (HD), an adult onset neurodegenerative condition for which there is no treatment (Charron et al. 2002; Christiaans et al. 2008). The main components of the HD predictive gene testing process are applicable to cardiovascular genetic conditions. Both processes aim to provide the consultand with adequate information to make an informed decision about having the gene test, armed with information about the relative advantages and disadvantages of testing, information about the natural history of the condition in question, and treatment and/or surveillance options if gene positive or gene negative.

An important aspect of predictive testing counseling is giving the consultand time to deliberate about how the genetic information will impact on his or her social circumstances, including family and other relationships, employment and insurance. The consultand also needs time to consider the impact of the test on self, both at a practical and an emotional level. A common strategy in predictive test counseling is to encourage the consultand to imagine what it might be like to be gene positive, and then what it would be like to be gene negative. This strategy aims to prepare the consultand for his or her personal reactions to the gene test result as well as the reaction of others. Most centers would take the approach of meeting with the consultand on at least two occasions, once before testing and once for disclosure, and inviting the consultand to have further sessions for counseling if desired, although variations to this approach do exist (Christiaans 2009a).

When an adult attends for predictive testing it is often suggested that he or she attend with a support person (Tyler et al. 1994). The support person may be a spouse or partner, close friend or family member who is not concurrently undertaking gene testing. As well as providing support to the consultand, this person's views of the test and its implications can be used by the counselor in a circular questioning loop, which involves asking the consultands their views on the impact of the genetic test, and then asking the support person to reflect on these responses. This can be an effective means of exploring how the gene test result may impact on the consultand.

If a family member is attending as a support person, consideration should be given to the ability of the family member to be supportive without his or her own issues about genetic testing interfering in the counseling process. If the support person is a sibling, special thought needs to be given to how the consultand and the sib will each react to the gene test result, particularly if their results are discordant.

While predictive counseling often revolves around the recommended screening and/or treatment for the consultand if they are shown to be gene positive, it is also important to discuss the medical implications of gene-negative results and to reassure the consultand that a gene-negative result means there is no indication for ongoing clinical screening. In one study on familial adenomatous polyposis (FAP), a familial colorectal cancer syndrome, some gene-negative consultands expected to continue with colonoscopic screening (Michie et al. 2002). Similar wishes to continue with cardiac screening have been expressed by the parents of two gene-negative HCM and LQTS adolescent consultands in the clinical practice of the author. Their confidence in the gene result was not complete and they wanted to continue with clinical screening, which they found more reassuring because the results were visible, in the form of the ultrasound images and the tracings of the ECG, forming concrete evidence of their children's wellness.

Experience in clinical practice reveals that the main motivations reported by consultands undergoing predictive testing for cardiovascular genetic conditions is relieving uncertainty about their risk of developing disease and clarifying the risk for children. These anecdotal reports are consistent with those reported in the French and Dutch experience of genetic testing for HCM (Charron et al. 2002; Christiaans et al. 2009a). It is important to point out to the consultands that predictive gene testing may not remove uncertainty if the consultand tests positive. The consultand essentially exchanges uncertainty about his/her gene status with the uncertainties associated with being gene positive. The consultand needs to be aware that disease onset, severity, and progression can not be predicted from the gene test result and that for some inherited cardiovascular conditions there are uncertainties about how a gene-positive asymptomatic individual should be managed medically. If the consultands' motive for predictive testing is to clarify the risk to their children, exploring how they anticipate they will feel about potentially transmitting the condition is instructive in ascertaining how they will cope emotionally with the result. It may also be a catalyst to discuss how they might tell their children about their risk. This type of discussion may raise feelings of guilt, which should be explored openly and normalized (Kessler et al. 1984); even though consultands generally understand that they are not able to control the transmission of their genes, emotionally they may feel responsible.

There is limited research on the impact of predictive gene testing for cardiovascular genetic conditions. The only study of LQTS predictive testing in adults examined the psychological response of those undertaking testing, and their partners, at three time points: before result disclosure and then at 2 weeks and 18 months post disclosure. There were no significant differences in disease-related anxiety and depression scores over the 18-month period. In addition, levels of distress in consultands, which were elevated before disclosure, reduced over the period of the study to normal levels (Hendriks et al. 2008). A cross-sectional Dutch study on quality of life (QOL) of 228 HCM mutation carriers who had predictive testing found that there was no difference in overall QOL and psychological distress compared to Dutch population norms (Christiaans et al. 2009b). These results are largely in keeping with reports on the impact of predictive testing in adult onset neurological diseases and familial cancers (Broadstock et al. 2000; Almqvist et al. 2003). Interestingly, partners of consultands whose predictive gene test was positive had higher levels of disease-related anxiety compared to partners of noncarriers (Hendriks et al. 2008), reinforcing the importance of including partners in the predictive testing counseling, not only to support the consultand but also to have their own concerns addressed.

4. Insurance Considerations in Predictive Testing

Insurance implications of predictive gene test results vary depending on jurisdiction. It is important for consultands to be aware of the local position in relation to insurance and to be cautioned about any potential genetic discrimination that they may face on the basis of a gene test result. For example, in the United Kingdom, a moratorium prohibits the use of predictive gene test results for income protection, life insurance, and critical care policies to specified values. Above these limits only predictive tests that have been approved by the Genetics and Insurance Commission (GAIC) can be used (Department of Health 2008). In the United States, the Genetic Information Nondiscrimination Act (GINA) has recently been passed into law, which will protect Americans against discrimination based on their genetic information when it comes to health insurance and employment.

5. Approach to Genetic Testing in Children and Adolescents

For the purpose of this discussion, I will use the word "children" to describe young people who are developmentally and cognitively unable to participate in the decision-making process about genetic testing. "Adolescents" will be used to refer to those young people who are able to participate in the decision-making process, either independently, or with their parents. They may be able to give consent for testing, or at a minimum, assent for testing.

From a clinical perspective, there is little controversy about genetic testing of children or adolescents who are expressing signs or symptoms of cardiovascular genetic disease, particularly in circumstances where the test is being initiated to confirm a diagnosis, or to ascertain whether the child's condition arose as the result of a de novo mutation, thereby providing information about the risk of disease transmission to other family members. As most of the conditions referred to in this chapter have reduced and/or age-related penetrance, it may not be apparent if a condition was inherited or de novo.

Predictive testing in children should be considered more carefully as consensus about how to treat gene-positive, asymptomatic carriers of cardiovascular genetic diseases has not been reached for all conditions. For the cardiovascular genetic conditions, which are the subject of this chapter, clinical screening of first-degree relatives of an affected person is recommended, in the absence of an identified disease-causing mutation in the family (Maron et al. 2003; Ades 2007; Fatkin 2007; Skinner 2007; Sullivan 2007). Clinical screening for most cardiovascular genetic conditions is usually commenced around the time of puberty although it is often earlier in inherited arrhythmia syndromes. The main argument for performing predictive testing in childhood relates to the fact that clinical screening is recommended in at-risk individuals.

For at-risk adolescents, who will probably already be engaged in a cardiac screening program, gene testing clarifies if they need to continue to be screened if gene positive and enables gene-negative individuals to be spared the time, uncertainty, and anxiety associated with regular screening visits. Performing the predictive test also enables clinical resources to be targeted to those individuals of greatest need.

Adolescents should be included in the counseling process, irrespective of whether a predictive or a confirmatory/diagnostic gene test is being undertaken. In this way, the autonomy of the adolescent is being respected. A qualitative study examining the informational needs of adolescents with genetic conditions found that adolescents do want to participate in their healthcare; in particular, they want to understand how their condition affects them and how to manage it (Szybowska et al. 2007). In practice, some parents have concerns about their child being involved in the genetic counseling process for fear of what they may be told about the risk of sudden death as it applies to the condition in their family. It is useful to preempt this by explaining to the parents the content and process of genetic counseling before their consultation so that their anxieties are addressed. The parent should be encouraged to provide the adolescent with general information about the condition and the ramifications of the gene test in terms of treatment and/or lifestyle modifications, if they have not already done so. The adolescent should know what to expect of the consultation including the length of the consultation, who will they meet, and what investigations they may be asked to have. This preconsultation preparation helps to establish trust with the adolescents and minimize their anxieties about the process.

The adolescent should also be told they will be asked to meet alone with the genetic counselor for at least part of the consultation. This is an important opportunity to elicit any concerns the adolescent feels unable to talk about in the presence of parents. It is not uncommon for adolescents to feel inhibited in the presence of their parents: they do not want to upset their parents by demonstrating that they do have worries about the test or the condition in the family (Meulenkamp et al. 2008). Sometimes their worries are less about the medical impact of the condition and more about how their parents may feel if they test positive. This enables the counselor to talk with the adolescents about the range of responses the counselor has seen and to normalize both the adolescents' fears and the perceived impact their result will have on their parents.

Given that there is some uncertainty about medical management of gene-positive, asymptomatic children and adolescents, it is important to consider the psychological benefits and harms to children, as well as their parents, of genetic testing. A Dutch study investigated the QOL of 35 children and adolescents who had been told they harbor a disease-causing mutation for HCM, familial hypercholesterolemia, and LQTS compared to a reference population of children and adolescents (Smets et al. 2008). The QOL scores of gene-positive children were not different to those of the reference population. Parents tended to relate their children's QOL lower than the children themselves and they also perceived their children to have less positive emotions. The parents also felt that the their gene-positive children experienced less satisfaction with life than the children's own ratings of satisfaction. Despite these differences between parents' and children's perceptions, there was reasonable agreement between parents' and children's overall ratings suggesting that, overall, parents do not grossly overestimate the impact of risk status on their children. The authors speculate that parents' perception of children's QOL may be influenced by their own personal unresolved loss experiences, feelings of guilt, and feelings of helplessness.

Risk Communication

The cardiogenetics consultation is laden with risk information. The types of risks discussed will vary depending on whether the consultand is affected or is an unaffected relative from a family in which there is a cardiovascular genetic disease. The types of risk that may be discussed are:

- the risk of developing clinically symptomatic disease
- the risk that the condition present in a family is inherited or is sporadic. This may not always be evident particularly if there has not been systematic clinical screening of relatives
- the risk that a mutation will be identified in the family
- the risk of inheriting a mutation and the risk of passing on a mutation to (future) offspring
- the risk of sudden death

As many inherited cardiovascular conditions have reduced penetrance and variable expressivity, it is important to highlight the difference between the risk of inheriting a disease-causing mutation and the risk of disease development (or penetrance) which varies according to the cardiovascular genetic condition in the family. Further explicit clarification may be required for some consultands who may equate the risk of disease development to the risk of sudden death, particularly those who have a strong family history of sudden death.

The way in which risk is perceived will vary, even amongst close relatives who share the same family history of the cardiovascular condition. This is because risk perception is not based purely on a numerical figure; it is influenced by the client's experience of the risk, personality traits, coping mechanisms, and beliefs about what can be done to reduce the risk. In the context of predictive testing, the type of relationship (close or distant, for example) consultands have with other affected individuals in the family and their understanding about how the condition has impacted on them will influence how the risk is perceived. In addition, how controllable the risk is, what treatments or management strategies are available to prevent the risk will also impact on how the risk is interpreted. For some cardiovascular genetic conditions there is a treatment or screening strategy available, which may increase the client's sense of control over the situation. For example, for most subtypes of LQTS, treatment with β-blockers plus the use of implantable devices where necessary have been shown to be effective in reducing the risk of sudden death or arrhythmia (Shimizu 2005), in addition to the recommendations for lifestyle medication and avoidance of QT-prolonging drugs.

Given the number of risks that are typically communicated and the variance in the way they are understood, it is useful to ask consultands how they prefer to have risks presented. Risks can be presented as numerical-based representations (e.g., percentages, relative risks, graphical displays) or descriptions of risk categories (e.g., likely, unlikely, high, low). It is recommended that risk information is presented in both quantitative and qualitative manner (McCarthy Veach et al. 2003). Research from the cancer genetics setting has shown that clients find it helpful for a combination of approaches to be used, including visual displays, written information, and numerical risk figures (Lipkus and Hollands 1999). Julian-Reynier et al. recommend providing a context within which the consultand can make sense of the risk (Julian-Reynier et al. 2003). For example, it is often useful to draw on the consultand's family history, where some relatives with the family-specific mutation may have developed severe disease, which can then be contrasted to an elderly relative who must be an obligate carrier who has shown no or little evidence of the disease. This context gives the consultand the range of consequences associated with having the mutation.

1. Communication of Genetic Risk in Families

One of the important roles of genetic counseling in cardiovascular genetics is to facilitate communication of genetic risk in families. As many of the cardiovascular genetic conditions referred to in this chapter have reasonable treatments, can be screened for clinically, and are associated with a risk of sudden death that may be preventable, an active approach to dissemination of risk information in families should be encouraged by the (cardio) genetics clinic. It is typical to rely on family members to communicate information about genetic risk to their relatives. A recent review of the guidelines and position statements of international human genetics societies and bioethics bodies demonstrated that there is consensus that information about genetic risk should be communicated within families (Forrest et al. 2007). This stands to reason as genetic information is a shared commodity within a family.

To aid family communication genetic counselors will identify family members that are at risk of inheriting the condition and make recommendations for clinical screening if the family-specific mutation has not been identified or cascade genetic testing if a mutation is known in the family. Information about how and where relatives can access services by the provision of a letter with such details, and contact details of the health professional, should be provided to facilitate the process.

For many people attending genetic counseling, one of their main motivations in seeking genetic testing is to assist in informing relatives of their risk. In their systematic review on family communication, Gaff et al. concluded that "it appears that communication occurs when a sense of responsibility to provide the family member with potentially important information outweighs concern about harming the individual by imparting "bad" or potentially unwelcome news" (Gaff et al. 2007). In cardiovascular genetic conditions, where there is a risk of sudden death, this tension is particularly apparent and clients frequently comment about their desire, on the one hand, to disseminate information, but also the difficulty of doing so without creating fear and anxiety within the family about sudden death, particularly as it relates to children. Eliciting the consultand's own views on this tension is a beginning point; acknowledgment of his/her concerns about communicating the information may enable the consultand to contemplate talking more broadly in the family about the condition. The counselor should highlight any treatments or surveillance recommendations for the family's condition as this may engender a sense of control within the consultand and his/her family.

In addition to this, exploring family dynamics may tease out some of the issues that may inhibit or enhance communication within the family (Lobb and Gaff, in press). This includes exploring relationships between relatives and inquiring about how current events occurring in the family may influence communication. The counselor may ask the consultand directly about his/her views on the likelihood that certain relatives may present for genetic testing and how they might communicate the information to that relative. This opens a dialog that can encompass strategies about how, when, and what to tell the relative in a way that is consistent with the type of relationship the consultand has with the relatives. Asking if there is a natural matriarch or patriarch in the family who usually takes responsibility for disseminating information in the family may prove fruitful.

One outcome measure used to determine the effectiveness of family communication is uptake of genetic testing. There have only been a few reports of uptake of cascade genetic testing for cardiovascular genetic conditions in the literature. A Dutch study on cascade genetic testing for familial hypercholesterolemia in the 5-year period following the identification of a gene-positive index case reports a participation rate of 90% (Umans-Eckenhausen et al. 2001). In this study, field nurses went to the homes of families, provided information and obtained blood samples for testing, which could explain the high participation rate as well as the reasonably simple and effective treatment that is available for those who test positive. A definition of "participation rate" was not provided, but it is clear from the study that there was enthusiasm for the family screening as 5,442 individuals from 237 families with a LDL receptor gene mutation had gene testing. Another study from The Netherlands (Christians et al. 2008), which reported on uptake of genetic testing for HCM, found 39% of at-risk first-degree relatives, or second-degree relatives when the first-degree relative was deceased, accessed genetic counseling. Of the first- and second-degree relatives that had genetic counseling, 99% proceeded with the predictive gene test. The 39% uptake rate of genetic counseling is similar to that found in other genetic diseases. The mode of disseminating information about the availability of predictive gene testing in this study was by asking the index case to communicate with his or her relatives. This study reports on uptake in mutation-positive families, which only account for approximately 50%–70% of HCM families. Given that a substantial proportion of HCM families are mutation negative, it is equally important to examine uptake of genetic testing in mutation-positive families as well as uptake of clinical screening in mutation-negative families to obtain a true reflection of the communication that occurs in families.

2. Talking About the Risk of Sudden Death

Sudden death is a common feature of the cardiovascular genetic conditions considered in this chapter. In practice, it is the greatest concern of consultands and their families. Genetic counselors need to be able to raise the issue of sudden death while balancing the magnitude of the risk, which is generally small, against the anxiety and fear the discussion may cause. In order for an informed decision about genetic testing to be made, the consultand must be aware of all the ways in which the condition could affect them, including sudden death. It is inevitable that the consultand will be exposed to information about sudden death, whether by other family members or from information on the Internet or other sources. Exploring the issue of sudden death in the context of the clinic provides a safe, contained, environment where immediate responses can be given to questions or concerns about the risk.

Raising the issue of sudden death is confronting for the counselor and the families alike. This is especially so if the consultand is unaware that there is risk of sudden death associated with the condition in the family. Most individuals presenting for counseling will have some awareness of the association with sudden death and the genetic counseling session is an opportunity for their views of the risk to be put into perspective, to correct factual inaccuracies if they exist and to address any fears. Raising the issue of sudden death is also an opportunity to acknowledge that it is frightening, but it also enables the genetic counselor, or other members of the team, to talk about the interventions that may avert sudden death.

One way to raise the issue of sudden death is to ask the consultands to give their understanding of how the condition in their family can affect a person. Typical responses include a description of the more common symptoms of the condition, for example, syncope, breathlessness, and palpitations. The consultand may obliquely refer to sudden death as "blacking out," "your heart stops," "collapsing," or "he just dropped." This is an opening for the counselor to ask the consultand to elaborate. If no reference to sudden death is made by the consultand after questioning, the counselor may probe further by referring to individuals in the family history that may have died suddenly and asking about the consultand's understanding of the cause of death.

If the consultand does not raise the issue of sudden death, one strategy to bring it into the consultation is to begin by describing the other features of the condition, working toward a description of "abnormal heart rhythms" that may cause the "heart to stop suddenly" and then describing what can happen when the this occurs, namely syncope or sudden death. It is important to monitor verbal and nonverbal responses to this and then engage the consultand with further discussion.

Conclusion

The genetic counsellor plays a key role in working with families with cardiovascular genetic conditions, as an information provider, a skilled counselor who explores with the consultands their experience of the disease, their understanding of their risks, and their fears. Genetic testing requires an understanding of the molecular data generated by the test, and the implications for the consultand of a test result. Within the team of health professionals caring for families with cardiovascular genetic conditions, the genetic counselor is well placed to inform consultands of the implications of their condition, work with them on their fears and concerns, and support them through the genetic testing process.

Acknowledgments

The author would like to thank Dr. Susan White, Dr. Smanatha Wake, and Ms. Lisette Curnow for their constructive comments on earlier drafts of this chapter.

References

Ades L. Guidelines for the diagnosis and management of Marfan syndrome. *Heart Lung Circ.* 2007;16:28–30.

Almqvist EW, Brinkman RR, Wiggins S, Hayden MR. Psychological consequences and predictors of adverse events in the first 5 years after predictive testing for Huntington's disease. *Clin Genet.* 2003;64:300–309.

Bennett RL, French KS, Resta RG, Doyle DL. Standardized human pedigree nomenclature: update and assessment of the recommendations of the National Society of Genetic Counselors. *J Genet Couns.* 2008;17:424–433.

Bennett RL, Steinhaus KA, Uhrich SB, et al. Recommendations for standardized human pedigree nomenclature. Pedigree Standardization Task Force of the National Society of Genetic Counselors. *Am J Hum Genet.* 1995;56:745–752.

Broadstock M, Michie S, Marteau T. Psychological consequences of predictive genetic testing: a systematic review. *Eur J Hum Genet.* 2000;8:731–738.

Cambien F, Tiret L. Genetics of cardiovascular diseases: from single mutations to the whole genome. *Circulation.* 2007;116:1714–1724.

Charron P, Heron D, Gargiulo M, et al. Genetic testing and genetic counselling in hypertrophic cardiomyopathy: the French experience. *J Med Genet.* 2002;39:741–746.

Christiaans I, Birnie E, Bonsel GJ, Wilde AA, van Langen IM. Uptake of genetic counselling and predictive DNA testing in hypertrophic cardiomyopathy. *Eur J Hum Genet.* 2008;16(10):1201–1207.

Christiaans I, van Langen IM, Birnie E, Bonsel GJ, Wilde AA, Smets EM. Genetic counseling and cardiac care in predictively tested hypertrophic cardiomyopathy mutation carriers: the patients' perspective. *Am J Med Genet.* 2009a;149A:1444–1451.

Christiaans I, van Langen IM, Birnie E, Bonsel GJ, Wilde AA, Smets EM. Quality of life and psychological distress in hypertrophic cardiomyopathy mutation carriers: a cross-sectional cohort study. *Am J Med Genet.* 2009b;149A:602–612.

Cotton RG, Scriver CR. Proof of "disease causing" mutation. *Hum Mutat.* 1998;12:1–3.

Department of Health U. Genetics and Insurance Committee: sixth Report from January to December 2007, in, Department of Health of the United Kingdom; 2008.

Fatkin D. Guidelines for the diagnosis and management of familial dilated cardiomyopathy. *Heart Lung Circ.* 2007;16:19–21.

Forrest LE, Delatycki MB, Skene L, Aitken M. Communicating genetic information in families—a review of guidelines and position papers. *Eur J Hum Genet.* 2007;15:612–618.

Gaff CL, Clarke AJ, Atkinson P, et al. Process and outcome in communication of genetic information within families: a systematic review. *Eur J Hum Genet.* 2007;15:999–1011.

Harper JC, de Die-Smulders C, Goossens V, et al. ESHRE PGD consortium data collection VII: cycles from January to December 2004 with pregnancy follow-up to October 2005. *Hum Reprod.* 2008;23:741–755.

Hendriks KS, Hendriks MM, Birnie E, et al. Familial disease with a risk of sudden death: a longitudinal study of the psychological consequences of predictive testing for long QT syndrome. *Heart Rhythm.* 2008;5:719–724.

Henneman L, Bramsen I, Van Os TA, et al. Attitudes towards reproductive issues and carrier testing among adult patients and parents of children with cystic fibrosis (CF). *Prenat Diagn.* 2001;21:1–9.

Hodgson J, Spriggs M. A practical account of autonomy: why genetic counseling is especially well suited to the facilitation of informed autonomous decision making. *J Genet Couns.* 2005;14:89–97.

Ingles J, Lind JM, Phongsavan P, Semsarian C. Psychosocial impact of specialized cardiac genetic clinics for hypertrophic cardiomyopathy. *Genet Med*. 2008;10:117–120.

Julian-Reynier C, Welkenhuysen M, Hagoel L, Decruyenaere M, Hopwood P. Risk communication strategies: state of the art and effectiveness in the context of cancer genetic services. *Eur J Hum Genet*. 2003;11:725–736.

Kessler S, Kessler H, Ward P. Psychological aspects of genetic counseling. III. Management of guilt and shame. *Am J Med Genet*. 1984;17:673–697.

Lavery SA, Aurell R, Turner C, et al. Preimplantation genetic diagnosis: patients' experiences and attitudes. *Hum Reprod*. 2002;17:2464–2467.

Lipkus IM, Hollands JG. The visual communication of risk. *J Natl Cancer Inst Monogr*. 1999;25:149–163.

Lobb EA, Gaff C. Communicating genetic risk. In: Kissane D, Bultz B, Butow P, Finlay I, eds. *The Handbook of Communication in Cancer and Palliative Care*. London: Oxford University Press; (In press).

Maron BJ, McKenna WJ, Danielson GK, et al. American College of Cardiology/European Society of Cardiology clinical expert consensus document on hypertrophic cardiomyopathy. A report of the American College of Cardiology Foundation Task Force on Clinical Expert Consensus Documents and the European Society of Cardiology Committee for Practice Guidelines. *J Am Coll Cardiol*. 2003;42:1687–1713.

McCarthy Veach P, LeRoy BS, Bartels DM. *Facilitating the Genetic Counselling Process. A Practice Manual*. New York: Springer-Verlag; 2003.

Meulenkamp TM, Tibben A, Mollema ED, et al. Predictive genetic testing for cardiovascular diseases: impact on carrier children. *Am J Med Genet*. 2008;146A:3136–3146.

Michie S, Collins V, Halliday J, Marteau TM. Likelihood of attending bowel screening after a negative genetic test result: the possible influence of health professionals. *Genet Test*. 2002;6:307–311.

Mujezinovic F, Alfirevic Z. Procedure-related complications of amniocentesis and chorionic villous sampling: a systematic review. *Obstet Gynecol*. 2007;110:687–694.

Resta R, Biesecker BB, Bennett RL, et al. A new definition of Genetic Counseling: National Society of Genetic Counselors' Task Force report. *J Genet Couns*. 2006;15:77–83.

Richard P, Charron P, Carrier L, et al. Hypertrophic cardiomyopathy: distribution of disease genes, spectrum of mutations, and implications for a molecular diagnosis strategy. *Circulation*. 2003;107:2227–2232.

Scheuner MT. Genetic evaluation for coronary artery disease. *Genet Med*. 2003;5:269–285.

Shimizu W. The long QT syndrome: therapeutic implications of a genetic diagnosis. *Cardiovasc Res*. 2005;67:347–356.

Skinner JR. Guidelines for the diagnosis and management of familial long QT syndrome. *Heart Lung Circ*. 2007;16:22–24.

Smets EM, Stam MM, Meulenkamp TM, et al. Health-related quality of life of children with a positive carrier status for inherited cardiovascular diseases. *Am J Med Genet A*. 2008;146:700–707.

Sturm AC. Cardiovascular genetics: are we there yet? *J Med Genet*. 2004;41:321–323.

Sullivan D. Guidelines for the diagnosis and management of familial hypercholesterolaemia. *Heart Lung Circ*. 2007;16:25–27.

Szybowska M, Hewson S, Antle BJ, Babul-Hirji R. Assessing the informational needs of adolescents with a genetic condition: what do they want to know? *J Genet Couns*. 2007;16:201–210.

Tester DJ, Will ML, Haglund CM, Ackerman MJ. Compendium of cardiac channel mutations in 541 consecutive unrelated patients referred for long QT syndrome genetic testing. *Heart Rhythm*. 2005;2:507–517.

Tyler A, Walker R, Went L, Wexler N. Guidelines for the molecular genetics predictive test in Huntington's disease. *J Med Gen*. 1994;31:555–229.

Umans-Eckenhausen MA, Defesche JC, Sijbrands EJ, Scheerder RL, Kastelein JJ. Review of first 5 years of screening for familial hypercholesterolaemia in the Netherlands. *Lancet*. 2001;357:165–168.

Van Driest SL, Vasile VC, Ommen SR, et al. Myosin binding protein C mutations and compound heterozygosity in hypertrophic cardiomyopathy. *J Am Coll Cardiol*. 2004;44:1903–1910.

van Langen IM, Hofman N, Tan HL, Wilde AA. Family and population strategies for screening and counselling of inherited cardiac arrhythmias. *Ann Med*. 2004;36(Suppl 1):116–124.

37

Social and Ethical Issues in Cardiovascular Genetics

Angus Clarke and Siv Fokstuen

The emerging subspecialty of clinical cardiac genetics is learning to assist families as they face some of the most difficult circumstances encountered in the context of medicine and health care. Experience with genetic testing and counseling for these conditions is limited. What has been learned from dealing with other conditions may be applicable in these families too but the context of inherited cardiac disease will present very particular problems, including sudden cardiac death in young adults. In this chapter, we examine some of the social and ethical difficulties that have arisen in relation to other genetic disorders and in relation to the more usual types of "heart disease," before considering how these findings may be relevant to families affected by inherited cardiac disorders.

Family History

The understanding of "heart disease" in most families with an inherited cardiac disorder starts from the same point as in the rest of the population, with an awareness that heart disease is potentially fatal and that it can "run in families." In the more usual types of heart disease, there is sometimes a recognition that individuals' own behaviors contribute to their health or their pattern of disease. Fieldwork in South Wales during the late 1980s revealed the widespread currency of ideas about the type of person who would be at risk of heart disease—the "coronary candidate"—existing alongside notions of luck, fate, destiny, and chaos (Davison et al. 1991, 1992), which notions were reinforced by the observation of counterexamples of individuals whose state of health or disease contradicted the messages of health promotion campaigns. Such simultaneously held but essentially incompatible perspectives can become impregnable systems of belief, allowing adherents to account satisfactorily for any observed pattern of events without their beliefs about heart disease being challenged by cases of, for example, obese smokers living to a ripe old age, succumbing to neither coronary artery disease (CAD) nor lung cancer. Subsequent work in Scotland emphasized the extent to which gender is itself seen as relevant to the risk of heart disease, with men being understood to be at higher risk (Emslie et al. 2001).

This research also showed that the understandings of many lay (nonhealth professional) individuals of "having a family history of heart disease" can differ very substantially from what is understood by heath professionals. In particular, a family history may not be attributed any significance by the individual unless several close relatives have been affected, and the relevance may be discounted if the individual sees himself or herself as being different from the affected person/s in some crucial respect/s (Hunt et al. 2001). Most cardiac risk factors, such as obesity, hypercholesterolemia, or hypertension, do not lead to symptoms until a fatal event occurs. The asymptomatic individuals may therefore regard themselves, comfortingly, as *not* being at increased risk, when professionals might prefer not to give such reassurance. Similar factors operate even for many with cardiac symptoms, who delay seeking medical attention or deny that the symptoms are cardiac, but of course inadequate access to services is another factor not to be ignored in assessing social inequities in health (Tod et al. 2001).

Enquiries into the family history of heart disease in primary health care can be awkward, with professionals not always feeling sufficiently confident to integrate the family history into the context of other risk factors for heart disease and to discuss them together (Hall et al. 2007). The limited evidence available suggests that the interpretation of cholesterol levels is also problematic, with the concept of a continuum of risk being unfamiliar, having not yet replaced the idea of risk thresholds (Adelsward and Sachs 1996). Professionals in U.K. primary health care are more familiar with collecting and interpreting family history information in relation to breast and bowel cancer, for which they have been referring patients appropriately for specialist genetic assessment for some years (Emery et al. 2001). Their confidence may improve in relation to heart disease as the cardiac family history comes to be recorded more frequently and as referral guidelines are developed and promulgated.

An additional practical problem that may arise within some jurisdictions is that of legal restrictions placed upon the collection and storage of information from individuals about their relatives, or at least the self-fulfilling assumption in practice (on the part of health professionals) that such restrictions exist. Such data protection legislation has usually been motivated by a desire to allow individuals effective control over the information held about them by commercial or other organizations but may be unhelpful if applied too rigidly within the context of health care.

If I believe that my Aunt Mabel is affected by a condition X or Y, and I pass that "information" to my physician, is that information mine (about my beliefs) or does it belong to my aunt (as the person about whom the belief is held)? Does the physician have an obligation to check the accuracy of the information? If the information is kept in my medical records and not linked to Mabel's, does that make a difference? There are clearly some tangled issues here that may require unscrambling (Lucassen et al. 2006); these issues will become rapidly more complex as the possibilities for linking the electronic patient records of family members become greater (Temple and Westwood 2006). Family histories of cancer can be checked quite readily within the United Kingdom (UK), without the need to obtain consent from multiple members of each family, because of the established system of cancer registries. Should similar systems be put in place for other disorders, including cardiac disease?

There is another approach to these issues, which has the virtue of treating family situations equitably, whether or not the condition is one where specific information about the mutation in that family would be required for genetic testing to be most effective or at least efficient. This is to distinguish between the fact of the genetic disease being present in the family and the precise nature of that family's mutation. Simply knowing that person X has disease Y is sufficient to make genetic testing available to all who want it in some contexts, but in other contexts it is necessary (or at least very helpful) to know the precise mutation. Knowing that one person has Huntington's disease (HD) or a chromosome translocation would usually be sufficient for family members to have testing, while knowing that a relative has Duchenne muscular dystrophy, cystic fibrosis, or a breast cancer gene mutation would not necessarily be enough. The major Mendelian cardiac disorders are genetically heterogeneous, at the level of the mutations and often the loci too; it is therefore crucial for that group of diseases to identify the mutation in an affected individual before carrying out predictive testing on an unaffected relative. By treating as fully confidential the diagnosis in the affected individual, family members will only become aware of this if the patient chooses to release that information to them. That is what is confidential. Once that information is known in the family, then the mutational basis of the condition can be treated as information that is not an essentially personal item but rather belongs to the laboratory or the health care system. On this understanding, knowledge of the gene locus and the precise mutation should be available for use by the laboratory to test other family members without specific consent from their affected relative (Clarke 2007).

In addition to these questions of information, there may be practical and/or legal restrictions upon access to DNA or tissue stored from deceased family members. The Human Tissue Act in England and Wales has recently introduced a system for regulating access to stored tissue that might be required for pathological analysis or genetic testing. This has been regarded by some as unduly onerous and an obstacle to good research and clinical practice but it is perhaps too early to see how it will function in practice. The situation in other countries varies widely, even within Europe.

Familial Hypercholesterolemia

The first genetic condition to be recognized as an important cause of heart disease, specifically of CAD, was familial hypercholesterolemia (FH). Biochemical testing has been available for decades to confirm the diagnosis of established disease and to assist in dietary and pharmacological management. The more recent advent of molecular genetic testing, although not straightforward, has been most helpful in identifying those with a family history of FH but who do not yet have overt disease and whose biochemical investigations do not establish the diagnosis unequivocally, as can especially occur in the young (Humphries et al. 1997; Heath et al. 2001). Family-based cascade screening of the relatives of known patients is greatly facilitated when a pathogenic mutation has been identified, usually in the *LDLR* gene (Humphries et al. 2006); this has increased the absolute numbers of those diagnosed with the condition in the Netherlands and had a major, beneficial impact on the proportion of known affected persons under appropriate medical management (Umans-Eckenhausen et al. 2001).

Before the advent of safe and effective cholesterol-lowering drugs, one consequence of finding a raised serum cholesterol (not specifically FH) was that some individuals responded paradoxically with unhelpful behaviors—feeling either fatalistically doomed or completely invulnerable (discussion in Clarke 1995, 1997a). The introduction of the newer statin drugs has changed this, so that patients with hypercholesterolemia associated with FH do now regard this as treatable and recognize the need to alter behavior (Senior et al. 2002), although those with FH in whom a causative mutation has been found appear more likely to trust medication than dietary intervention alone (Marteau et al. 2004). This may be an instance of a more general phenomenon, with those at increased risk of disease through an established genetic factor placing more trust in rationally designed pharmacological interventions than in "merely" behavioral or lifestyle changes (Senior and Marteau 2007). There may be lessons here for the conditions under which it may be appropriate to introduce population screening tests for susceptibility to a range of diseases, especially the strength of the evidence that the interpretation of a test result is not only valid but also of clinical utility (Clarke 1997a). The therapeutic effectiveness of statins for treating FH, however, is not in doubt (Scientific Steering Committee on behalf of the Simon Broome Register Group 1999; Smilde et al. 2001), and they are effective in reducing the risk of stroke as well as myocardial infarction (Sever et al. 2008).

Family Cascade Testing

Where there are clear practical benefits from early diagnosis, as with FH, the question arises as to how health services can best be structured with the goal of maximizing the numbers of at-risk people who are identified before they have developed disease complications. They can then decide whether they wish to be investigated or not and take appropriate precautions or not. The strategic choice lies between a population screening approach and a family-based system of offering testing to the first- and second-degree relatives of identified patients, "cascading" out or "snowballing" through the family. The fact that mutation-based genetic testing is much more sensitive and specific than a cholesterol-based population screening test indicates that the family-based approach may be superior, at least for the present. (Once virtually all FH-associated mutations are known in a population, then DNA microarray-based testing may become feasible as a population approach to screening.) For now, however, the family-based approach is more cost-effective (Marks et al. 2002) as well as clinically rational; a population-based screening program for FH using an assay for serum cholesterol would not meet the U.K.'s public health criteria for a screening program (National Screening Committee 2009).

Cascade testing gives families an opportunity to escape from the pattern of disease that has affected previous generations. Because a national scheme for such family-based cascade testing of FH was established in the Netherlands in 1994, we now have the benefit of clinical and research experience with participating families over more than a decade. This has shown that there are some individuals who respond to the offer of cascade testing as inappropriate "meddling" but most individuals welcome it; these responses tend to reflect the pattern of family relationships rather than disrupting them (Horstman and Smand 2008). It is important to note that both parents and children are anxious about the test results of the children, who will often worry about a positive result; they may be anxious about both the potential health implications and the medicalization it will lead to. Cascade testing has also been examined in Norway with encouraging results (Leren 2004). Nevertheless, the question remains as to the practical details of exactly how such testing is offered (Newson and Humphries 2005); even small differences in the operational procedures of a genetic screening program may have a major impact on how it is perceived and the ethical issues it raises (Parsons et al. 2000).

One approach would be for health professionals to contact an index case's relatives directly. While this may in principle be acceptable in some contexts (Wilcke et al. 2000), it will usually be impossible for health services to do so without at least some identifying information from each index case; it then becomes a question of (1) about which relatives the index case gives contact information to the cascade program staff and (2) whether or not the index case contacts his/her relatives in advance of the cascade program doing so. Such a program has operated in the Netherlands for years without causing undue concern (Maarle et al. 2001), although the provision of written information at the time of first contacting the at-risk relatives has been an important part of the program and may have helped to minimize difficulties (Nieuwenhoff et al. 2006); a similar approach has been recommended for general use in the UK after an evaluation project (London IDEAS Genetics Knowledge Park 2007). The clear potential for major health benefits in general outweighs the sense of intrusion that could otherwise result from such unsolicited contact (Suthers et al. 2006). This will not necessarily be the case where the benefits from genetic testing are not so clear and would therefore not be transferable to a number of other cardiac disease contexts; it may also not apply in countries with a different health care system—where the cost of testing and treatment would have to be met by the individual or where the cost of health insurance may deny health care to the poor and to those with inherited predispositions to disease.

The particular needs of healthy but mutation-carrying (affected) children also require careful consideration. In contrast to experience from before the days of effective pharmacological therapies, the limited studies available do not suggest any major increase in psychological morbidity as a result of diagnosis and treatment through cascade testing programs, although affected children may show evidence of anger as a result of the death of their affected parent (Tonstad et al. 1996; Agård et al. 2005). It has been suggested that population screening for serum cholesterol could be applied to children between the ages of 1 and 9 years, as discrimination on the basis of cholesterol levels between those with FH and those without is best in childhood (Wald et al. 2007). There are powerful reasons for caution with this approach, however, on clinical and cost-effectiveness grounds as well as from a consideration of the psychological and social consequences of such an approach (Senior et al. 1999; Hopcroft 2007).

The "Causation" of Coronary Artery Disease

Familial predisposition to CAD is not mediated solely through FH, nor even a combination of FH and environmental factors: there are plenty of other genetic risk factors too, sufficient perhaps to justify interventions aimed at the first-degree relatives of those affected by "premature" CAD (i.e., men <55 years, women <65 years) (Chow et al. 2007). Are the other genetic risk factors identifiable? And is it clinically useful to do so? The perennial difficulty of distinguishing between association and causation, discussed ever since Hume developed his ideas during the Scottish Enlightenment, means that physicians and quacks may with equal enthusiasm promote a remedy that misses the target entirely; the standards required for proof of efficacy in this area need to be maintained most carefully. Clarity in thinking around the proof of efficacy is important and a "critical realist" position is perhaps the most straightforward perspective to adopt, acknowledging the importance of emotional, behavioral, and environmental influences on health but insisting that they are mediated through material (biological) mechanisms (Clark et al. 2007). The interaction between behaviors and genetic polymorphisms of small or modest effect are known to account for a fraction (up to one-third) of the variance of plasma cholesterol in patients affected by FH (Aalst-Cohen et al. 2005). Distinguishing between physiological and behavioral factors is not simple, with the effects of sex on CAD mortality being largely the result of gender-influenced behavioral differences (Lawlor et al. 2001). Twin studies demonstrate the high heritability of the prothrombotic state (Ariens et al. 2002) and the relevance of this finding is confirmed by the reduced mortality from CAD of female carriers of hemophilia (Sramek et al. 2003). The scope for interventions in the general population may have been systematically underestimated because of the limited duration of most studies, so that "controls" include "cases" and the endpoints used are unlikely to occur within the period of the research project (Sniderman and Furberg 2008); those at high risk may be readily identifiable at the primary care level (Marshall 2007). A number of genetic loci have been implicated in CAD—some through the recent publication of the results of large case-control, genome-wide association studies—although the pathogenetic mechanisms involved are not yet clear (Ozaki et al. 2002; Cenarro et al. 2003; Cohen et al. 2005; Kathiresan 2006; Samani et al. 2007; Wellcome Trust Case Control Consortium 2007; Rader and Daugherty 2008).

There have been periodic reassessments of whether the current state of knowledge makes it feasible to offer individualized risk assessments on the basis of single nucleotide polymorphism (SNP) typing but the consensus remains that such applications would not be warranted (Muntwyler and Lüscher 2000; Humphries et al. 2004; Janssens et al. 2008). Such information currently adds little to more conventional methods of assessing risk of cardiovascular disease (Hippisley-Cox et al. 2008), especially as measures of the apolipoproteins have now been shown to give more accurate risk assessments than any of the cholesterol ratios (McQueen et al. 2008). We know that susceptibility screening can also cause confusion and has the potential to reinforce inequities in health (Saukko et al. 2007), and that the identification of those with a "predisease" state generates feelings of uncertainty and places additional demands on the health care system (Troughton et al. 2008). Given that the interventions to be recommended would not currently be modified by such genetic data, except in the context of FH, such screening is not to be recommended (e.g., Clarke 1997a; Chaufan 2007).

In addition, there is the very real danger that individuals worried by a family history of cardiac disease may seek commercial genetic susceptibility screening for their cardiac risk in the misguided belief that this will be relevant to their family history of sudden cardiac death. Such commercially available tests usually entail testing the patients' samples with a panel of "risk profiling" SNPs but they do not usually determine the mutations present in the affected relative at the loci likely to have been responsible, such as the LDLR, the other FH-associated loci and those relevant to hypertrophic cardiomyopathy (HCM), long QT syndrome (LQTS), and so on. They may then receive false reassurance and fail to benefit from the available strategies of prevention and treatment.

Taking further the line of argument about individualized genetic risk assessment, we can see strong arguments to the effect that it is a wasteful distraction. We collectively understand well enough what to do—what health policies to implement—in order to tackle the growing problem of the complex degenerative disorders CAD, type 2 diabetes (T2D), hypertension, and obesity; in particular, there is no public health need to screen individuals to define their precise degree of predisposition to each pathology. In effect, it is not a lack of knowledge that prevents action but—as with sanitation and malnutrition in developing countries—it is a lack of political will or authority that prevents substantial progress. Further biomedical research is no substitute for implementing what we already know to be necessary (Beaglehole 2001; Færgeman 2003).

We recognize these arguments as effective against population screening for genetic susceptibility but they do not invalidate the reasons for conducting research aiming to define the genetic variation in different populations that may be relevant to the risk of developing these conditions; such research may help to elucidate the pathogenesis of these conditions whether or not it ever proves useful to screen populations to define each individual's risk. One especially important area for research that could have important implications for public health in both developed and developing countries is that of epigenetics and its relation to "fetal programming"—the contribution of transgenerational and early-life experiences to the causation of CAD and T2D (McDermott 1998; Räisänen 2006; Victora et al. 2008). The epigenetic consequences of malnutrition, especially of indigenous peoples confined to marginalized communities, may interact with income inequality and social exclusion to result in self-perpetuating cross-generational cycles of both physiological disease and demoralization from which escape is difficult for the individual, much harder still for the community.

Inherited Cardiac Disorders

We now turn to consider the less common and more clearly inherited cardiac conditions that could well have contributed to popular scepticism about the messages of health promotion noted above, through causing some of the "counter-examples" of healthy lifestyle enthusiasts dying suddenly at an early age.

Sudden Adult Death Syndrome

The large majority of sudden adult cardiac deaths are caused by CAD and in only about 4% of sudden unexplained cardiac deaths in the community is the heart structurally normal (Bowker et al. 2003; Roberts and Brugada 2003). Experience from a major referral center in the United Kingdom (Fabre and Sheppard 2006) showed that almost 60% of the 453 hearts examined postmortem of individuals aged >15 years without atherosclerosis were structurally normal but that 23% showed features of cardiomyopathy or right ventricular dysplasia and >15% showed other definite pathologies. These studies highlight both the need for and the scarcity of the specialist cardiac pathology services, including histopathology, that are required for health services to deal appropriately with the surviving family members of young adults who have died suddenly and whose relatives may be at high risk of a similar fate.

Such accounts written by pathologists make poignant reading for clinicians who meet with the families of the deceased. A typical scenario would be the grieving young woman with her two young children, both potentially at risk of serious cardiac pathology that could cause problems at any stage of life. Without a firm diagnosis in the deceased, it is difficult for the cardiologist or clinical geneticist to deal satisfactorily with the family. A normal cardiac examination and ECG give little reassurance to the clinician in these circumstances even if it temporarily satisfies the family. Unless the legal system (in England and Wales, the coroner) has exceeded its usual brief, of determining whether or not a death has occurred as a result of natural causes, the material required to conduct further investigations may well be lost to decomposition or fire. If diagnostic clarity is not achieved by pathology, it then becomes necessary to approach the immediate family of the deceased, to take a detailed family history and to assess the first-degree relatives for evidence of cardiac disease. Establishing such contact can itself be very difficult if the family is dispersed or geographically remote or if relationships between the deceased's parents and spouse are tense. Managing these circumstances requires both sensitivity and time to a degree not often readily available in (always busy) cardiology departments or (even) in clinical genetics units unless they are generously staffed with genetic counselors.

If the proband survives after presenting with cardiac symptoms, such as syncope, dyspnea, angina, or palpitations, the chance of attaining a clear diagnosis is much greater and the level of family distress is usually much less. It is then possible to approach the investigations more calmly and more efficiently. The former, more difficult circumstances, however, account for much of the work of the cardiac genetics team and it is these that set the ethos of this developing subspecialty.

The two major categories of disease encountered in the cardiac genetics clinic are (1) the inherited cardiomyopathies, especially HCM and (2) the inherited dysrhythmias, both considered below. In addition, however, there are other disorders that may be met within this setting and which must not be forgotten:

A. Congenital heart disease (Hoess et al. 2002), as an isolated phenomenon or as part of a chromosomal or syndromic disorder, will sometimes require continuing medical supervision for life. The adult cardiac phenotypes of some congenital disorders and the risk of recurrence in the children of affected individuals are both becoming clearer as survival into adult life improves. The cognitive limitations of some affected adults mean that compliance with medical advice and consent to procedures and interventions can both raise problems.
B. The inherited connective tissue disorders, especially Marfan syndrome, remain an important element in cardiac genetics. Continuing developments in drug therapy, imaging, and surgery require that all affected individuals should have access to specialist cardiac assessment; local factors will determine

whether this is best arranged through the cardiac genetics clinic or a separate, specialist cardiac service but the multiple medical, surgical, and psychological needs of those with Marfan syndrome mean that a purely cardiac clinic is not sufficient to meet their needs.

Inherited Cardiomyopathies

Recently, the European Society of Cardiology proposed a clinically oriented classification of cardiomyopathies (CMs) into specific morphological and functional phenotypes with a subclassification into familial and nonfamilial forms (Figure 37–1; Elliott et al. 2008). The most common CM in clinical practice is HCM with a prevalence of 1 in 500, a prevalence similar to familial hypercholesterolemia. DCMs are important but less frequent and also less frequently inherited. Some 25%–50% of DCM patients in Western population have evidence for familial disease with predominantly autosomal dominant inheritance (Burkett and Hershberger 2005) and the counselling issues are complex (Hanson and Hershberger 2001). The exact prevalence of restrictive cardiomyopathy (RCM) is unknown but it is probably the least common type of CM. RCM may be idiopathic, familial, or result from various systemic disorders, in particular amyloidosis, sarcoidosis, carcinoid heart disease, or scleroderma and has always been difficult to define (Elliott et al. 2008). Finally, arrhythmogenic right ventricular dysplasia (ARVD), which is rather uncommon (1:5,000) but a frequent cause of sudden cardiac death in young people.

In this paragraph we will concentrate on HCM, not only because of its frequency but also because so far it is the best studied CM from a genetic and molecular point of view and it represents the major cause of sudden death in the young and in athletes (Maron et al. 1996).

The proportion of those who develop cardiac problems (symptoms or sudden unexpected death) before 70–75 years is substantial but uncertain and lower than has been reported from highly selected clinic populations (Yu et al. 1998; ACC/ESC 2003), as is true for other inherited disorders subject to ascertainment bias (e.g., BRCA 1 and 2 mutation carriers). The prevalence of those with overt disease is of course lower still. The diagnosis and management of HCM is evolving (Semsarian and Members of the CSANZ Cardiovascular Genetics Working Group 2006) but the prognosis given to patients and families in clinic may sometimes be more pessimistic than is warranted because of this bias in publications toward the reporting of subgroups with a higher rate of sudden death and other serious complications; the extent of incomplete penetrance is still being evaluated but seems to be greater for disease-associated mutations at some loci than others.

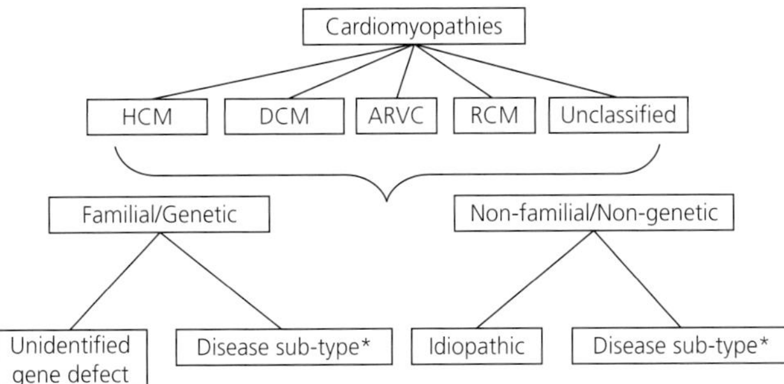

Figure 37–1 Classification of the cardiomyopathies. Reprinted from Elliott P et al. *Eur Heart J.* 2008;29(2):270–276 with permission.

As our awareness of the clinical uncertainties increases, our interpretation of molecular genetic variation of necessity also has to become more sophisticated. The mutation detection strategies employed to screen patients for disease-associated mutations are improving as high-throughput DNA sequencing methods are introduced into clinical practice (Fokstuen et al. 2008). The yield (sensitivity) of mutation screening is therefore improving but the interpretation of some identified variants can be difficult; when can a novel variant safely be assigned the blame for causing the disease in a given family? Clarifying such results can require further intensive family studies or technically challenging and time-consuming molecular functional studies. When mutation screening is offered to families, they need to be aware that the results may not be readily interpretable. Once a pathogenic mutation has been identified in a kindred, the offer of testing family members for the known variant is usually less likely to cause confusion but raises other challenges especially for asymptomatic individuals at risk.

The difficulty of giving an accurate prognosis in this clinically and genetically very heterogeneous condition, and the overestimation in published series of the risk of cardiac disease because of ascertainment bias, need to be discussed openly with those who may be at increased risk. Exaggerated risk estimates could lead some to reject genetic testing who might otherwise benefit from it either medically or psychologically. The questions posed by families seem, however, in the limited published experience, to focus more on predictive testing and reproductive risks than on the information volunteered by professionals, especially the details of diagnosis and prognosis (Charron et al. 2002).

In one study of families with a known pathogenic mutation, the uptake of predictive testing among at-risk relatives who attended for genetic counseling was very high while the proportion of at-risk first-degree relatives who attended the genetics clinic within 12 months of a mutation being identified in the family (making a predictive test available) was less than 40% (Christiaans et al. 2008). The authors concluded that efforts must be made to increase the uptake of genetic counseling. Care must be taken, however, not to achieve a higher rate of clinic attendance through offering better treatment than can be delivered. Rather than the problem being one of family ignorance, it may be that ambivalence about implantable defibrillators may contribute to this shortfall. Another reason may be that only relatives already actively seeking a predictive test attend the genetic counseling clinic and those who prefer not to know have no interest in coming. Here it would be very important that the relatives at risk are well informed about the aims of the genetic counseling clinic. They should know that it is a session of pure information that gives the basis for the decision as to whether or not to proceed with a genetic test and that there is no obligation to accept testing when they attend the clinic. It is clear that further research is required in several domains: to develop improved treatments, to describe the experiences of patients and families from their own perspectives and so to make these more accessible to professionals, and to explore with families the factors affecting the acceptability of those genetic tests and those treatments that are available.

Long QT Disorders and Brugada Syndrome

The genetic dissection of the long QT disorders, and their relationship to the epilepsies and other channelopathies, has been a fascinating story of scientific progress over the decade from 1995.

This progress and its clinical applications have been carefully set out in a consensus report from the U.S. National Heart Lung and Blood Institute, moving on from a focus on the ion channels themselves to the macromolecular signaling complex of which it is a part and whose disruption leads to a dysrrhthmogenic cardiomyopathy (Lehnart et al. 2007). The clinical application of this genetic knowledge has shown that the factors likely to trigger a dysrrhythmia (loud noise, swimming, and other exercise, sleep/rest) differ as between the different gene loci involved (Schwartz et al. 2001). It has also been shown that ethnic background can influence the frequency and severity of symptoms caused by the same disease-associated mutation within one gene—the A341V mutation in the *KCNQ1* locus (Crotti et al. 2007) and other mutations are known to cause different phenotypic effects in different members of the same family. Attempts to relate a particular gene to survival and how it interacts with gender and the duration of the QT interval have been performed (Priori et al. 2003). The authors proposed a scheme for risk stratification among patients with LQTS based on the gene mutated (*LQT1*, *LQT2*, or *LQT3*), QT measurement and sex. The risk categories were high (>50%), intermediate (30%–49%), and low (< 30%). A first cardiac arrest or SCD was highest among female patients with a mutation in the *LQT2* gene and male patients with a mutation in the *LQT3* gene. The cosegregation of two disease-associated mutations within a family can also occur, sometimes in different genes, and cause unusually severe disease in those family members who inherit both mutations (Beckmann et al. 2008).

Brugada syndrome is said to be responsible for up to 12% of all sudden deaths and approximately 20% of deaths occurring in patients with structurally normal hearts. The mean age of SCD is approximately 40 years. Clinical presentations may also include the sudden infant death syndrome (SIDS) (Priori et al. 2000) and the sudden unexpected nocturnal death syndrome, a typical presentation in young individuals from Southeast Asia (Roberts 2006). An implantable cardioverter-defibrillator (ICD) is essentially the only recommended form of therapy as most drugs are not effective.

Brugada syndrome and LQTS can both be caused by defects in the *SCN5A* gene. In general, those *SCN5A* mutations implicated in LQT3 cause gain of function of the ion channel, whereas the ones implicated in the Brugada syndrome cause a loss of channel function (Veldkamp et al. 2000). However, mutations that are associated with both diseases in the same family have been described, supporting the concept that these two disorders are part of a spectrum of "sodium channelopathies" (Grant et al. 2002).

Publications about these conditions have so far largely focused on the basic science (the molecular genetics and the electrophysiology) and on the cardiac management rather than on the genetic counseling or the social and ethical issues that arise for the families or the practitioners. That there are serious issues here, however, is not in doubt.

One issue that requires attention is how families experience and cope with being told that several of them could die at any moment. This must be greatly different from the experience of an individual being told that she has, perhaps, 4–6 months to live. And to be told that your death may be triggered by a loud noise or by swimming in cold water is likely to have immense but individually different consequences for the way such individuals and families live their lives. Very frightening is of course the fact that you could die during sleep. To be given such information about one's child results in not only immediate but also sustained distress (Hendricks et al. 2005) and you may ask the question whether one would do more harm than good discussing these topics. The crumb of comfort is that children identified as carrying such a mutation do not seem to suffer from it in the way their parents do (Smets et al. 2008), although this is a preliminary finding and it does not align well with the findings from studies of FH families (above).

An adolescent or young adult who is told that sudden loud noise or exercise or cold water or even sleep could kill them may respond in a very different fashion from their parents—or parent, if one parent has already died in just such circumstances. The stage is set for distress and conflict. We need to know more about what parents say to their at-risk children and what different patterns of coping are employed; some of the research required may be observational but some must surely entail listening to the accounts of survivors and the bereaved who are living through these difficulties.

Cardiac Genetic Clinics

The role of the cardiac genetic clinic, the required clinical approach, and the benefits for patients who attend have been well described (Chapter 36, this volume; Ingles and Semsarian 2007; Ingles et al. 2008). In addition to the advantages and disadvantages of testing from a clinical perspective, there are also issues of privacy or disclosure and coping within the family and the possible psychological consequences. In this and the following sections, we include some comments made by patients and families about their experience of the cardiac genetics service.

A 41-year-old lady who had heart transplantation at the age of 32 years because of early onset (2 years) severe familial HCM (her father died from heart failure at the age of 43 years) said:

> *My mother did her best but it was very difficult and at the time nobody offered psychological support for the family, which really should have been seen as necessary. I remember it was so hard to see my mum suffering that I forbade her to come to the hospital, which of course was a catastrophe for her but for me it was survival. This was really bad … you know how crucially important the emotional side is with the heart and the problem is different for the patient, the mother, and the healthy brothers and sisters. I think that something has to be done here.*

Preparing an individual to think through decisions about testing and perhaps facing an adverse result can be demanding on staff—on their time and their emotional energy—as can be the provision of intensive emotional support after a result (McCarthy Veach et al. 2007). Cardiologists are necessarily involved very closely in these clinics but do not usually have the time or the full set of knowledge and skills to conduct these clinics without genetics support (Langen et al. 2003).

A mother who lost her 17-year-old son from sudden cardiac death caused by ARVD said:

> *It is true that a team with a cardiologist, a geneticist, and a psychiatrist is ideal. When we asked questions of our cardiologist about genetics he could not answer. When he then had your [clinical genetics] letter he was very grateful and said that then he knew something. So it is true that a multidisciplinary approach is essential.*
>
> *I think the most important thing is to take time. You took the time. We did not have the impression of being here for only half an hour; what can you say in half an hour? You took the time to discuss with us, to listen to us, it's true that sometimes it was very long but it is really very important. It was especially important when the*

question arose of predictive testing in our son. It was not only to do the blood sampling but he had to ask himself, "What am I going to do with this, what does it mean, what will be the consequences?" and then he has the choice.

It is also possible for cardiac-trained nurses to participate in these clinics alongside and complementing the genetic counselors (Royse 2006).

Another issue that has to be considered is the potential consequences for obtaining life insurance and health insurance. The possibility of adverse consequences for obtaining insurance is likely to be at least as difficult a problem in cardiac genetics as it has become in relation to HD and familial cancers (Bombard et al. 2008; Treloar et al. 2008).

We will now consider some of these issues in more detail.

Family Communication

One of the areas that has proved most difficult in clinical genetic practice is that of difficulties with the communication of genetic information within families (Kenen et al. 2004; Keenan et al. 2005). For the full medical benefits of an early diagnosis to accrue, as for instance with FH and many other conditions, those diagnosed within a family must transmit the relevant information to their relatives. Problems with this transmission of information about the risk of disease and the health benefits of early intervention take different forms depending upon whether the information is to be passed "vertically" to a child or parent, or "horizontally" to a sibling, cousin, or other relative and also depending upon the availability of preventive and/or therapeutic strategies.

The difficulties felt by parents in transmitting such information to a child has long been clear in the context of polycystic kidney disease, where there is great potential for denial of the problem to lead subsequently both to psychological distress and to serious clinical consequences (Manjoney and McKegney 1978–1979). Similar problems have been documented in relation to other autosomal dominant disorders for which the children of an affected adult will be at risk—most notably HD (Etchegary 2006) and the Mendelian familial cancer disorders. Some difficulties have also been apparent in relation to the transmission of information about carrier status for recessive diseases and chromosomal rearrangements, especially in relation to sex-linked disorders and balanced chromosome translocations (Jolly et al. 1998; Järvinen et al. 1999). A focus group study of the impact of genetic conditions on families has shown that families (but not professionals) raised the difficulties parents have in communicating with their children as one of their major problems (McAllister et al. 2007). This field has recently been reviewed more generally by Metcalfe et al. (2008). It is clear that parents want to discuss such topics with their children but often find it very difficult; they may require active support from professionals if they are to share information in the most helpful fashion. Parents and doctors may often think to protect the child in not telling him the truth or minimizing the reasons for medical visits, but for the child's well-being and trust it seems essential to understand why she or he needs regular cardiac follow-up and what kind of investigations have to be done. As was said by the 41-year-old lady with early onset severe familial HCM (already mentioned above):

I got no explanation as to why I regularly had to go to the cardiac clinic, it was a family secret. I did not understand why I had to go and my sister did not. I just heard a few things but it was not an open discussion and that was very frightening for me. I don't recommend people to do that.

Later I heard different things like, "because of that disorder she will not have children"; but it was never an open discussion. The doctors never told me clearly what is going on and that was terrible. Finally I understood that I had the same disorder as my father and I saw how his situation got steadily worse. It got to the point where he couldn't do anything anymore, not even kneeling. I saw that it was terrible and that created a climate of fear in the family.

Passing information horizontally to other members of the family involves additional considerations. There are many reasons why the flow of information through family networks can be problematic, including the reluctance of individuals to pass on disturbing information to unaware relatives (Adelsward and Sachs 2005), the question of who counts as family (Featherstone et al. 2006), and the preexisting pattern of relationships within each family (Peterson et al. 2003). There may be specific individuals within a family system, who feel a duty of care toward specific others, to whom they would then be bound to disclose information that becomes available; furthermore, the disclosure may be the duty *of these particular individuals* so that it would be an abrogation of their role for others to perform this task (Keenan et al. 2005). There are the related but distinct issues that arise from generating such information that would then need to be passed to others; for example, some women affected by hereditary breast and ovarian cancer feel a sense of obligation to have a test performed, even if they might personally prefer not to do so, so that the family's mutation can be found—as only then does predictive testing become feasible for their female relatives (Hallowell et al. 2003; Foster et al. 2004). An interesting feature in some families is the emergence of a key family organizer who facilitates communication within the family and may organize family gatherings to ensure that all have access to the information or are able to participate (DudokdeWit et al. 1997; Featherstone et al. 2006).

We have more comments from the same mother already mentioned above, who had lost one of her two sons from sudden cardiac death due to ARVD. She developed the disorder herself after cascade screening of the family, and genetic testing in her revealed a pathogenic mutation in one of the genes associated with ARVD. She said:

There was no problem when I announced to my family that I have the same cardiac problem as (our son had) and that all my brothers and sisters need to do a cardiac evaluation, but when the mutation was identified and I informed one of my sisters about the possibility of predictive testing she said: fine, so we go and do the blood sampling. I said no, no this is not the way it should be done. It is essential to do this through a geneticist and discuss all the issues and possible consequences. So, I told them that they have to go to a geneticist, that they have to give me the address of the geneticist, and that I am going to send him or her the information. This is because you just can't simply do the blood sampling. What are you going to do afterward ? If you have the mutation what are you going to do?

Professionals can experience difficulties when important information is not passed through a family in the way they think it should be. Under what circumstances would it be permissible, or perhaps obligatory, for professionals to break their usual obligation to maintain confidentiality because of a greater duty to prevent harm to others? This raises larger questions of the obligations of a physician; do we have duties solely to the individual(s) in front of us, or also to their absent kin, or to society at large and "the general good?" The usual response of professionals in such circumstances, where there may be a conflict between the duties to protect confidentiality and at the same time to disclose personal information, is not to force disclosure but to work with the family over time to help them achieve the disclosure in an emotionally safe but effective manner (Clarke et al. 2005). There have, however, been a number of calls to define the circumstances in which professionals may or should disclose a patient's personal information to others without consent (Clarke 1997b). These have arisen largely within the anglophone world of utilitarian ethics where the difficulties of reducing incommensurable qualities to a single scalar dimension often seem not to be fully appreciated; even a sophisticated account of this view reduces essentially to the attempt to compare the problems resulting from the alternative courses of action and selecting the one assessed as leading to fewer harms (American Society of Human Genetics 1998). This effectively writes out of the account any prior Hippocratic commitment of the physician or health care professional and assumes that all manner of consequences can be reduced to a single dimension. This position is less highly regarded in continental Europe.

Efforts made by professionals to support their clients' disclosure of information to their relatives recognizes the vulnerability of those given unwelcome information and the time it can take for them to process the information and acknowledge their obligations (Forrest et al. 2008a) rather than trying to insist that they should act immediately—as if they were able instantly to weigh up these issues calmly, with objectivity and detachment. It also recognizes the complexity of relationships within a family, in which forceful medical intervention could do real harm (Gilbar 2007). This gentle approach has been shown often to be effective (Forrest et al. 2008b) and in some circumstances can be helped through a group approach (Speice et al. 2002; McKinnon et al. 2007). The need for such professionally supported communication is clear in the context of FH (Nieuwenhoff et al. 2007).

There have been a number of helpful reviews of family communication of genetic information (Wilson et al. 2004; Gaff et al. 2007; Nycum et al. 2008). Such work is useful in allowing us to anticipate some of the difficulties that may arise in families in the context of inherited cardiac disorders and sudden adult death.

Risks and Certainties

One component of genetic counseling in cardiac genetics is conveying information about risks: risks to the patient or client, risks to their relatives, and ways of modifying these risks. At one level this can entail a narrowly informational process, the impersonal transfer of cold facts; at another level, it can entail a personal contact between counselor and client when both engage with the personal meaning and significance of the information.

To focus on the narrowly delivered factual information, one can assess the effectiveness of techniques—contrasting verbal or numerical (probabilistic) or visual descriptions of risk—but this has to be just a start (e.g., Lipkus and Hollands 1999). The tendency for genetic counseling clients to convert a probability statement into the resolution of a dichotomy—converting a **maybe** into a **yes** or a **no**—has been recognized for decades (Lippman-Hand and Fraser 1979a, 1979b), so that a counselor must engage with the personal context (Julian-Reynier et al. 2003) and the significance of the possible outcome events in order to help the client appreciate the genuine uncertainties involved. This dialogical approach to risk communication has been well described in a number of nongenetic (Edwards et al. 2002) and genetic contexts (O'Doherty and Suthers 2007) although the ways in which genetic counseling clients use their understandings of risk in making decisions is yet another matter.

Decisions about genetic testing will be influenced by the professional, who has framed the choice (to have the test or not), by the client's understanding of their biological situation (Krynski and Tenenbaum 2007), and by the client's judgments about their own personal emotional responses and their assessment of the likely responses of others in their family. When the decision is not to go ahead with testing, however, or when no test is available or when the risk information simply hangs there, without one single specific decision to be made, the influence or impact of the professional will be felt in a different way. The clients have to go away and live their lives but they will take with them the way in which the information was provided; this applies especially but not only to "bad news." If these long-lasting memories of us professionals are not to be entirely negative, then we need to know our clients as individuals—as far as possible within the constraints of the health care system.

It is our personal relationship with clients, arising from empathy but without sentimentality, which gives us the opportunity to help them face these decisions. We do have to explain the facts and risks to enable them to make a realistically grounded decision but we also have to help them (those who want the help) to think through the consequences of the different possible courses of action open to them. That requires a respectful relationship that can develop over time. The centrality of the ongoing relationship between genetic services and their clients has been recognized as crucial in family-based research (Skirton 2001) and in a professional consensus of leading genetic counselors in the United States (McCarthy Veach et al. 2007).

The influence of risk perception on decision making has been studied in the context of predictive genetic testing for HD and the familial cancers. It will be important to explore the same processes in relation to familial cardiac disorders. Although this is our unsupported personal judgment, we suspect that professionals would like their clients to be making cool, rational judgments about genetic testing and practical aspects of risk management while many clients will be making decisions on quite different grounds. Whereas cardiologists, even more than genetics professionals, are likely to perceive the LQT disorders and HCMs as amenable to useful medical interventions, so that decisions about genetic testing could be made on the basis of a rational decision process, many at-risk individuals will feel differently and will perhaps stay away from both genetic and cardiac clinics. They are likely to make decisions more comparable to those made by people at risk of HD than would apply in the context of an effectively treatable cancer predisposition (such as familial polyposis coli or one of the multiple endocrine neoplasia syndromes). Substantial numbers will persist in preferring not to be tested until the family experiences of treatment confirm that the outcomes are substantially better than they have yet seen. This is particularly true for young and asymptomatic at-risk relatives. The medical benefits of predictive testing in this situation often do appear to be uncertain. This arises firstly because only limited data may so far be available about the natural history of healthy carriers (Hanson and Hershberger 2001). Secondly, the expression of the disease may be highly variable even within a family and the clinician can predict neither the age at onset of the disease nor its severity, although phenotype-genotype correlations especially for LQTS and HCM may be of some help. Thirdly, it may be that no medical treatment is effective in preventing or in lowering the occurrence of the disease. Restriction of physical activity might be recommended but its ability to counter sudden death in healthy (so far unaffected) carriers of their family's mutation remains unknown.

The only treatment that might prevent sudden death is an implantable defibrillator, which at the moment, however, is not a general recommendation for healthy mutation carriers. This option may be discussed in the context of a family with sudden death, especially in the young. For these reasons it is actually not possible to recommend systematic predictive genetic testing for inherited cardiac disorders from a medical point of view. If the test is positive, then strict medical follow-up is required that will allow the early diagnosis of symptoms and lead to improved therapeutic management. This strategy, however, can also be followed without genetic testing of the healthy at-risk relative. Interestingly, a recent study showed that only 76% of mutation carriers after predictive testing for HCM received regular cardiac follow-up which seems to indicate a need for better patient and/or physician education (Christiaans et al. 2009). If the test is negative, the individual will be reassured and the result will probably improve his or her well-being, although there might be adverse reactions as has been shown for HD (Gargiulo et al. 2009). So far the main reasons why an individual would ask for predictive cardiac genetic testing would be the psychological burden related to uncertainty and/or the wish to know the risk of transmission of the disease to their offspring (Charron et al. 2002). The psychological burden of uncertainty could, however, be replaced after an unfavorable test result by a new psychological burden of an unclear certainty of developing the disease later including eventually the risk of sudden death. Not everybody wants to know for sure about this as long as no effective preventive and/or therapeutic methods have been developed.

The knowledge of being a carrier for such a condition also has implications for reproductive decisions—it raises for discussion the eventual possibility of a prenatal diagnosis if the mutation in the family is known. Prenatal diagnosis for inherited cardiac disorders has already been performed (Charron et al. 2004) and raises complex medical, psychological, and ethical issues. From the medical point of view, the termination of an affected pregnancy may be regarded as indicated in families with malignant forms of the disease (i.e., with several cardiac deaths in the young or deaths associated with heart failure). However, the variable expression even within a given family, and the difficulty of predicting the potential phenotype, counterbalance the value of prenatal diagnosis. As for many other inherited, mainly adult onset disorders with wide clinical heterogeneity, no general rules can be given and decisions should be made after case-by-case discussion and according to a consensus between the parents and the medical team.

1. Professional Optimism, Family Scepticism

Underlying these differences in perspective there may be, on the one hand, a degree of professional optimism about the worth of one's craft and, on the other hand, the at-risk client may manifest either some measure of denial as a psychological defence, some anxiety as to what shape treatment might take or some scepticism of the professional's claims—or some combination of these. A very real issue for professionals is how to present information in a "balanced" way when what is being made available is both highly variable between centers and rapidly developing over time, so that a specialist's practice is likely to be somewhat ahead of what is justified by the published evidence. The influence of the professional on the client (the cardiologist's potential patient) will be exerted not so much by what is said but rather through the way in which the information is given; this involves both the degree of professional optimism and enthusiasm, the professional's display of professional competence and the sense of personal contact achieved between client and professional. It will be immensely important for professionals in this field to develop their self-awareness skills, to work whenever possible with a colleague from a different discipline within the same multidisciplinary team, and to seek awareness-enhancing psychological supervision. Those wishing to borrow insights from studies of HD may like to look at the findings of in-depth interviews with genetic counseling clients from HD families (such as DudokdeWit et al. 1998; Smith et al. 2002; Taylor 2004).

2. Genetic Testing of Children

Many parents of a child with serious developmental problems are initially desperate to find out why their child has these problems, and some use their knowledge of the diagnosis to exert some influence over the actions of the professionals involved with their child (Starke and Möller 2002); the "need" for a diagnosis may lessen with time as it becomes clear that no cure will be forthcoming, whatever the diagnosis. Similarly, and very understandably, many parents of a child at risk of a later-onset genetic disorder wish to find out whether their child has inherited the family's genetic disorder and is at risk of serious problems. This parental concern relates to the forgoing question of how positively professionals are to present the benefits and hazards of different approaches to cardiac management and genetic testing—what ***evaluation*** do they convey in addition to the mere facts? Testing even young children for disease manifestations, including the use of ECG and cardiac echo, will clearly be entirely appropriate as long as there is an established medical intervention available to treat, defer, or prevent complications of the condition, as is sometimes true for the HCM and LQT disorders. There will always be difficult areas of professional judgment as to the border between research and service, and how to manage a complex case that is not being included within a research study.

Predictive genetic testing of healthy children could be viewed as rather different because, in the absence of clinical, ECG, or echocardiographic evidence of current pathology, there will usually be no implications for medical management in the event of a positive genetic test result. On the other hand, not carrying out a genetic test that is available would impose continuing practical and emotional burdens on the child's family and would incur continued health care costs. Therefore, when it is available, it will usually be reasonable to discuss the offer of genetic testing with the parents of children at risk of an inherited cardiac disorder that could develop during childhood.

In practice, the focus of decision making by a child's parents will often depend upon the contextual air of optimism or caution within which the physician wraps his assessment of the medical interventions that could be offered if the child does carry the relevant mutation. This, in turn, depends upon how the physician sees the border between research and standard clinical practice. It would be possible for a clinical researcher to subject at-risk children to the potentially hazardous pharmacological provocation of electrophysiological anomalies, for example, out of both a wish to find out more about the disease (this could be termed "intellectual curiosity") and a wish to clarify the situation for this particular child; the balance between these motivations is crucial and the professional has to restrain his "curiosity" (and the legitimate wish to expand our knowledge of these diseases) when it would entail subjecting the child to additional discomfort, pain, or hazard that has not been discussed with the parents and, where appropriate, approved by an ethics review process. The cardiologist is likely to possess a greater understanding of both what is at stake and of the risks for the child than any other party involved: this is a great responsibility that calls for a very finely developed sense of professionalism. Policing this borderland is tremendously difficult and institutional attempts to prevent all misjudgment are likely to prevent all progress.

In the absence of medical interventions established as useful and applicable in childhood, or when the inherited disorder is unlikely to develop until adult life, then the case for predictive genetic testing in a child is much weaker (Clinical Genetics Society 1994; European Society of Human Genetics 2009). A special situation may arise when a child wishes to participate in competitive sports. The consequence of a positive test result would be the exclusion from this possibility that may be very difficult to accept. Thus, careful preparation and discussion of alternative options are mandatory before testing in such situations.

Adults who wished to have testing would be able to access this through a clinical genetics unit and with the support of pre- and post-test genetic counseling. The question will then arise as to whether professionals should accede to requests for testing made in their own right by adolescents of less than 18 years. In the United Kingdom, such requests are usually discussed carefully with the teenager; while it is unusual to proceed with testing for HD in such circumstances it is legally permitted if the professional assesses the teenager as possessing sufficient maturity. The legal context and professional guidance in other European jurisdictions varies, as it does internationally. A natural next question is how professionals should respond to a healthy but at-risk young adult who requests predictive genetic testing but who, upon assessment, appears to be of questionable maturity (Gaff et al. 2006; Richards 2006). If there were no medical indication for testing at that time, it would be defensible in those circumstances to defer testing while maintaining contact and encouraging further reflection. In relation to inherited cardiac disease, however, these issues are usually of little relevance as the core question is whether, or to what extent, medical surveillance and intervention will be helpful.

Conclusions

Clinical genetics and genetic counseling have been shaped by their experiences of working both with families and with colleagues from other disciplines. Clinical genetics at first emerged from pediatrics and neurology and then its pattern of working changed when its referrals increased dramatically because of developments in cancer genetics. This led to a greater focus on adult patients and to the coordination of medical management on behalf of so far unaffected family members—for example, the surveillance for tumors. The genetics professionals are not competing for work with oncologists or other specialists but work alongside these colleagues, retaining their role of working with families rather than individual patients and especially with the healthy but at-risk relatives. Genetics professionals (both medically qualified clinical geneticists and genetic counselors or genetic nurses) are currently working alongside specialists from several other medical subspecialties including cardiology. What role will they have 10–20 years into the future?

Most cardiac disease is of "complex" etiology, which may to some extent be clarified by large genetic epidemiological studies but for which individualized genetic testing or screening is unlikely to have any major role in the foreseeable future. Genetic tests may be useful in guiding treatment for those with overt disease or in population screening programs to identify those affected by FH, but those activities will not usually be carried out by genetic specialists: genetic testing for therapeutic guidance (i.e., pharmacogenetics) will be performed by generalists and population screening for FH and similar predispositions to cardiac disease will be an activity conducted within primary health care.

The central, core role of genetics professionals will remain with the uncommon, Mendelian genetic disorders and genetic counseling will continue to focus on predictive testing, especially where tests are not clearly necessary for good medical management, and on reproductive issues where individuals need to make very personal decisions that they have carefully considered. It is in the Mendelian cardiac disorders that the difficult issues will remain of (1) promoting family communication while respecting individuals' right to confidentiality and (2) making well (i.e., wisely) those difficult decisions about genetic testing and medical surveillance on behalf of young children. The disease context of sudden death ensures that these decisions are going to remain difficult and highly charged emotionally whatever scientific progress brings in terms of improved understanding, until a real cure becomes available (not just an ICD). We can offer a supportive and self-aware relationship not only to the patients seen in clinic but also to their families, which will complement the therapeutic skills of our colleagues in cardiology and will indeed help to ensure that as many at-risk family members as possible will benefit from those skills.

References

Aalst-Cohen ES van, Jansen ACM, Boekholdt SM, et al. Genetic determinants of plasma HDL-cholesterol levels in familial hypercholesterolaemia. *Eur J Hum Genet*. 2005;13:1137–1142.

ACC/ESC (American College of Cardiology/European Society of Cardiology). Clinical Expert Consensus Document on Hypertrophic Cardiomyopathy. *J Am Coll of Cardiology*. 2003;42:1687–1713.

Adelsward V, Sachs L. The meaning of 6.8: numeracy and normality in health information talks. *Soc Sci Med*. 1996;43:1179–1187.

Adelsward V, Sachs L. The messenger's dilemmas--giving and getting information in genealogical mapping for hereditary cancer. *Health Risk Soc*. 2005;5:125–138.

Agård A, Bolmsjö IA, Hermeren G, Wahlstrom J. Familial hypercholesterolaemia: ethical, practical and psychological problems from the perspective of patients. *Patient Educ Couns*. 2005;57:162–167.

American Society of Human Genetics Statement. Professional disclosure of familial genetic information. *Am J Hum Genet*. 1998;62:474–483.

Ariens RAS, Lange M de, Snieder H, Boothby M, Spector TD, Grant PJ. Activation markers of coagulation and fibrinolysis in twins: heritability of the prothrombotic state. *Lancet*. 2002;359:667–671.

Beaglehole R. Global cardiovascular disease prevention: time to get serious. *Lancet*. 2001;358:661–663.

Beckmann BM, Wilde AAM, Kääb S. Dual inheritance of sudden death from cardiovascular causes. *N Eng J Med*. 2008;358:2077–2078.

Bombard Y, Penziner E, Suchowersky O, et al. Engagement with genetic discrimination: concerns and experiences in the context of Hunrtington disease. *Eur J Hum Genet*. 2008;16:279–289.

Bowker TJ, Wood DA, Davies MJ, et al. Sudden, unexpected cardiac or unexplained death in England: a national survey. *QJM*. 2003;**96**(4):269–279.

Burkett EL, Hershberger RE. Clinical and genetic issues in familial dilated cardiomyopathy. *J Am Coll Cardiol*. 2005;45(7):969–981.

Cenarro A, Artieda M, Castillo S, et al. A common variant in the *ABCA1* gene is associated with a lower risk for premature coronary heart disease in familial hypercholesterolaemia. *J Med Genet*. 2003;40:163–168.

Charron P, Héron D, Gargiulo M, et al. Genetic testing and genetic counselling in hypertrophic cardiomyopathy: the French experience. *J Med Genet*. 2002;39:741–746.

Charron P, Héron D, Gargiulo M, et al. Prenatal molecular diagnosis in hypertrophic cardiomyopathy: report of the first case. *Prenat Diagn*. 2004;24(9):701–703.

Chaufan C. How much can a large population study on genes, environments, their interactions and common diseases contribute to the health of the American people? *Soc Sci Med*. 2007;65:1730–1741.

Chow CK, Dominiczak AF, Pell JP, Pell ACH, Walker A, O'Dowd C. Families of patients with premature coronary heart disease: an obvious but neglected target for primary prevention. *BMJ*. 2007;335:481–485.

Christiaans I, Birnie E, Bonsel GJ, Wilde AAM, Langen IM van. Uptake of genetic counselling and predictive DNA testing in hypertrophic cardiomyopathy. *Eur J Hum Genet*. 2008. advance online publication 14 May 2008; doi: 10.1038/ejhg.2008.92.

Christiaans I, Lange IM van, Birnie E, Bonsel GJ, Wilde AAM, Smets EMA. Genetic counseling and cardiac care in predictively tested hypertrophic cardiomyopathy mutation carriers: the patients' perspective. *Am J Med Genet Part A*. 149A:1444–1451.

Clark AM, MacIntyre PD, Cruickshank J. A critical realist approach to understanding and evaluating heart health programmes. *Health*. 2007;11:513–539.

Clarke A. Population screening for genetic susceptibility to disease. *BMJ*. 1995;311:35–38.

Clarke A. The genetic dissection of multifactorial disease. The implications of screening for susceptibility to disease. Chapter 7. In: Harper PS, Clarke A, (eds.). *Genetics, Society and Clinical Practice*. Oxford: Bios Scientific Publishers; 1997a:93–106.

Clarke A. Challenges to Genetic Privacy. The control of personal genetic information. Chapter 11. In: Harper PS, Clarke A. (eds.). *Genetics, Society and Clinical Practice*. Oxford: Bios Scientific Publishers; 1997b:149–164.

Clarke A. Should families own genetic information? No. *BMJ*. 2007;335:23.

Clarke A, Richards MPM, Kerzin-Storrar L, et al. Genetic professionals' reports of non-disclosure of genetic risk information within families. *Eur J Hum Genet*. 2005;13:556–562.

Clinical Genetics Society. The genetic testing of children. Report of a Working Party of the Clinical Genetics Society (UK) (chair, Clarke A). *J Med Genet*. 1994;31:785–797.

Cohen J, Pertsemlidis A, Kotowski IK, Graham R, Garcia CK, Hobbs HH. Low LDL cholesterol in individuals of African descent resulting from frequent nonsense mutations in PCSK9. *Nat Genet*. 2005;37:161–165.

Crotti L, Spazzolini C, Schwartz PJ, et al. The common long-QT syndrome mutation KCNQ1/A341V causes unusually severe clinical manifestations in patients with different ethnic backgrounds. Towards a mutation-specific risk stratification. *Circulation*. 2007;116:2366–2375.

Davison C, Frankel S, Smith GD. The limits of lifestyle: re-assessing "fatalism" in the popular culture of illness prevention. *Soc Sci Med*. 1992;34(6):675–685.

Davison C, Smith GD, Frankel S. Lay epidemiology and the prevention paradox: the implications of coronary candidacy for health education. *Social Health Illn*. 1991;13:1–19.

Dudok de Wit AC, Tibben A, Duivenvoorden HJ, et al. Distress in individuals facing predictive DNA testing for autosomal dominant late-onset disorders: comparing questionnaire results with in-depth interviews. *Am J Med Genet*. 1998;75:62–74.

Dudok de Wit AC, Tibben A, Frets PG, et al. BRCA1 in the family: a case description of the psychological implications. *Am J Med Genet*. 1997;71:63–71.

Edwards A, Elwyn G, Mulley AI. Explaining risks: turning numerical data into meaningful pictures. *BMJ*. 2002;324:827–830.

Elliott P, Andersson B, Arbustini E, et al. Classification of the cardiomyopathies: a position statement from the European Society of Cardiology Working Group on Myocardial and Pericardial Diseases. *Eur Heart J*. 2008;29(2):270–276.

Emery J, Lucassen A, Murphy M. Common hereditary cancers and implications for primary care. *Lancet*. 2001;358:56–63.

Emslie C, Hunt K, Watt G. Invisible women? The importance of gender in lay beliefs about heart problems. *Sociol Health Illn*. 2001;23:203–233.

Etchegary H. Discovering the family history of Huntington disease (HD). *J Gen Couns*. 2006;15:105–117.

European Society of Human Genetics. Genetic testing in asymptomatic minors: recommendations of the European Society of Human Genetics. *Eur J Hum Genet*. 2009;17:720–721.

Fabre A, Sheppard MN. Sudden adult death syndrome and other nonischaemic causes of sudden cardiac death. *Heart*. 2006;92:316–320.

Færgeman O. Coronary Artery Disease: genes, Drugs and the Agricultural Connection. Amsterdam: Elsevier; 2003.

Featherstone K, Bharadwaj A, Clarke A, Atkinson P. *Risky Relations. Family and Kinship in the Era of New Genetics*. Oxford: Berg Publishers; 2006.

Fokstuen S, Lyle R, Munoz A, et al. A DNA resequencing array for pathogenic mutation detection in hypertrophic cardiomyopathy. *Hum Mutat*. 2008;29(6):879–885.

Forrest LE, Burke J, Bacic S, Amor DJ. Increased genetic counselling support improves communication of genetic information in families. *Genet Med*. 2008b;10:167–172.

Forrest LE, Curnow L, Delatycki MB, Skene L, Aitken M. Health first, genetics second: exploring families' experiences of communicating genetic information. *Eur J Hum Genet*. 2008a. doi: 10.1038/ejhg.2008.104.

Foster C, Eeles R, Ardern-Jones A, Moynihan C, Watson M. Juggling roles and expectations: dilemmas faced by women talking to relatives about cancer and genetic testing. *Psychol Health*. 2004;19:439–455.

Gaff C, Clarke AJ, Atkinson PA, et al. Process and outcome in communication of genetic information within families: a systematic review. *Eur J Hum Genet*. 2007;15:999–1011.

Gaff C, Lynch E, Spencer L. Predictive testing of eighteen year olds: counseling challenges. *J Gen Couns*. 2006;15:245–251.

Gargiulo M, Lejeune S, Tanguy ML, et al. Long-term outcome of presymptomatic testing in Huntington disease. *Eur J Hum Genet*. 2009;17(2):165–171.

Gilbar R. Communicating genetic information in the family: the familial relationship as the forgotten factor. *J Med Ethics*. 2007;33:390–393.

Grant AO, Carboni MP, Neplioueva V, et al. Long QT syndrome, Brugada syndrome, and conduction system disease are linked to a single sodium channel mutation. *J Clin Invest*. 2002;110(8):1201–1209.

Hall R, Saukko PM, Evans PH, Qureshi N, Humphries SE. Assessing family history of heart disease in primary care consultations: a qualitative study. *Fam Prac*. 2007;24:435–442.

Hallowell N, Foster C, Eeles R, Ardern-Jones A, Murday V, Watson M. Balancing autonomy and responsibility: the ethics of generating and disclosing genetic information. *J Med Ethics*. 2003;29:74–79.

Hanson EL, Hershberger RE. Genetic counselling and screening issues in familial dilated cardiomyopathy. *J Gen Couns*. 2001;10:397–415.

Heath KE, Humphries SE, Middleton-Price, Boxer M. A molecular genetic service for diagnosing individuals with familial hypercholesterolaemia (FH) in the United Kingdom. *Eur J Hum Gen*. 2001:9:244–252.

Hendricks KSWH, Grosfeld FJM, Tintelen JP van, et al. Can parents adjust to the idea that their child is at risk of sudden death?: psychological impact of risk for long QT syndrome. *Am J Med Genet*. 2005;138A:107–112.

Hippisley-Cox J, Coupland C, Vinogradova Y, et al. Predicting cardiovascular risk in England and Wales: prospective derivation and validation of QRISK2. *BMJ*. 2008;336:1475–1482.

Hoess K, Goldmuntz E, Pyeritz RE. Genetic counselling for congenital heart disease: new approaches for a new decade. *Curr Cardiol Rep*. 2002;4:68–75.

Hopcroft KA. Child-parent screening may have adverse psychological effects. *BMJ*. 2007;335:683.

Horstman K, Smand C. Detecting familial hypercholesterolaemia: escaping the family history? Chapter 5. In: de Vries G, Horstman K, (eds.). *Genetics from Laboratory to Society. Societal Learning as an Alternative to Regulation*. Basingstoke: Palgrave Macmillan; 2008:90–117.

Humphries SE, Cranston T, Allen M, et al. Mutational analysis in UK patients with a clinical diagnosis of familial hypercholesterolaemia: relationship with plasma lipid traits, heart disease risk and utility in relative tracing. *J Mol Med*. 2006;84:203–214.

Humphries SE, Galton D, Nicholls P. Genetic testing for familial hypercholesterolaemia. *QJM*. 1997;90:169–181.

Humphries SE, Ridker PM, Talmud PJ. Genetic testing for cardiovascular disease susceptibility: a useful clinical management tool or possible misinformation? *Arterioscler Thromb Vasc Biol*. 2004;24:628–636.

Hunt K, Emslie C, Watt G. Lay constructions of a family history of heart disease: potential for misunderstandings in the clinical encounter? *Lancet*. 2001;357:1168–1171.

Ingles J, Lind J, Phongsavan P, Semsarian C. Psychosocial impact of specialized cardiac genetic clinics for hypertrophic cardiomyopathy... *Genet Med.* 2008;10:117–120.

Ingles J, Semsarian C. Sudden cardiac death in the young: a clinical genetic approach. *Int Med J.* 2007;37:32–37.

Janssens ACJW, Gwinn M, Bradley LA, Oostra BA, Duijn CM van, Khoury MJ. A critical appraisal of the scientific basis of commercial genomic profiles used to assess health risks and personalize health interventions. *Am J Hum Genet.* 2008;82:593–599.

Järvinen O, Aalto A-M, Lehesjoki A-E, et al. Carrier testing of children for two X linked diseases in a family based settzing: a retrospective long term psychosocial evaluation. *J Med Genet.* 1999;36:615–620.

Jolly A, Parsons E, Clarke A. Identifying carriers of balanced chromosomal translocations: interviews with family members. In: Clarke A, ed. *The genetic Testing of Children.* Oxford, Washington DC: Bios Scientific Publishers; 1998:61–90.

Julian-Reynier C, Welkenhuysen M, Hagoel L, Decruyenaere M, Hopwood P. Risk communication strategies: state of the art and effectiveness in the context of cancer genetic services. *Eur J Hum Genet.* 2003;11:725–736.

Kathiresan S for the Myocardial Infarction Genetics Consortium. A *PCSK9* missense variant associated with a reduced risk of early-onset myocardial infarction. *N Eng J Med.* 2006;358:2299–2300.

Keenan KF, Simpson SA, Wlson BJ, et al. 'It's their blood not mine': who's responsible for (not) telling relatives about genetic risk? *Health Risk Soc.* 2005;7:209–226.

Kenen R, Ardern-Jones A, Eeles R. We are talking but are they listening? Communication patterns in families with a history of breast/ovarian cancer (HBOC). *Psycho-Oncology.* 2004;13:335–345.

Krynski TR, Tenenbaum JB. The role of causality in judgement under uncertainty. *J Exp Psychol: General.* 2007;136:430–450.

Langen IM van, Birnie E, Leschot NJ, Bonsel GJ, Wilde AAM. Genetic knowledge and counselling skills of Dutch cardiologists: sufficient for the genomics era? *Eur Heart J.* 2003;24:560–566.

Lawlor DA, Ebrahim S, Davey SJ. Sex matters: secular and geographical trends in sex differences in coronary heart disease mortality. *BMJ.* 2001;323:541–545.

Lehnart SE, Ackerman MJ, Benson DW, et al. A National Heart Lung and Blood Institute and Office of Rare Diseases Workshop Consensus Report about the diagnosis, phenotyping, molecular mechanisms and therapeutic approaches for primary cardiomyopathies of gene mutations affecting ion channel function. *Circulation.* 2007;116:2325–2345.

Leren TP. Cascade genetic screening for familial hypercholesterolemia. *Clin Genet.* 2004;66:483–487.

Lipkus IM, Hollands JG. The visual communication of risk. *J Natl Can Inst Monogr.* 1999;25:149.

Lippman-Hand A, Fraser F. Genetic counselling: the post-counselling period: I. Patients' perceptions of uncertainty. *Am J Med Genet.* 1979b;4:51–71.

Lippman-Hand A, Fraser FC. Genetic counselling: provision and reception of information. *Am J Med Genet.* 1979a;3:113–127.

London IDEAS Genetics Knowledge Park. Department of Health Familial Hypercholesterolaemia Cascade Testing Audit Project. Recommendatioms to the Department of Health; 2007.

Lucassen A, Parker M, Wheeler R. Implications of data protection legislation for family history. *BMJ.* 2006;332:299–301.

Maarle MC van, Stouthard MEA, Mheen PJM van den, Klazinga NS, Bonsel GJ. How disturbing is it to be approached for a genetic cascade screening programme for familial hypercholesterolaemia? *Community Genet.* 2001;4:244–252.

Manjoney DM, McKegney FP. Individual and family coping with polycystic kidney disease: the harvest of denial. *Intl J Psychiatr Med.* 1978–1979;9:19–31.

Marks D, Wonderling D, Thorogood M, Lambert H, Humphries SE, Neil HAW. Cost effectiveness analysis of different approaches of screening for familial hypercholesterolaemia. *BMJ.* 2002;324:1303.

Maron BJ, Shirani J, Poliac LC, Mathenge R, Roberts WC, Mueller FO. Sudden death in young competitive athletes. Clinical, demographic, and pathological profiles. *JAMA.* 1996;17;276(3):199–204.

Marshall TP. Risk factors inform screening. *BMJ.* 2007;335:577.

Marteau T, Senior V, Humphries SE, et al. Psychological impact of genetic testing for familial hypercholesterolemia within a previously aware population: a randomized controlled trial. *Am J Med Genet A.* 2004;**128A**:285–293.

McAllister M, Payne K, Nicholls S, MacLeod R, Donnai D, Davies LM. Improving service evaluation in clinical genetics: identifying effects of genetic diseases on individuals and families. *J Genet Couns.* 2007;**16(1):71–83**.

McCarthy Veach P, Bartels D, LeRoy BS. Coming full circle: a reciprocal engagement model of genetic counseling practice. *J Genet Couns.* 2007;**16**(6):713–728.

McDermott R. Ethics, epidemiology and the thrifty gene: biological determinism as a health hazard. *Soc Sci Med.* 1998;47:1189–1195.

McKinnon W, Naud S, Ashikaga T, Colletti R, Wood M. Results of an intervention for individuals and families with BRCA mutations: a model for providing medical updates and psychosocial support following genetic testing. *J Genet Couns.* 2007;16:433–456.

McQueen MJ, Hawken S, Wang X, et al. Lipids, lipoproteins, and apolipoproteins as risk markers of myocardial infarction in 52 countries (the INTERHEART study): a case-control study. *Lancet.* 2008;372:224–233.

Metcalfe A, Coad J, Plumridge GM, Gill P, Farndon P. Family communication between children and their parents about inherited genetic conditions: a meta-synthesis of the research. *Eur J Hum Genet.* 2008. doi: 10.1038/ejhg.2008.84.

Muntwyler J, Lüscher TF. Assessment of cardiovascular risk: time to apply genetic risk factors? *Eur Heart J.* 2000;21:611–613.

National Screening Committee. Programme appraisal criteria Criteria for appraising the viability, effectiveness and appropriateness of a screening programme (updated June 2009). London: Department of Health; 2009.

Newson A, Humphries SE. Cascade testing in familial hypercholesterolaemia: how should family members be contacted? *Eur J Hum Genet.* 2005;13:401–408.

Nieuwenhoff HWP van den, Mesters I, Gielen C, Vries NK de. Family communication regarding inherited high cholesterol: why and how do patients disclose genetic risk? *Soc Sci Med.* 2007;65:1025–1037.

Nieuwenhoff HWP van den, Mesters I, Nellissen JJTM, Stalenhoef AF, Vries NK de. The importance of written information packages in support of case-finding within families at risk for inherited high cholesterol. *J Genet Couns.* 2006;15:29–40.

Nycum G, Avard D, Knoppers BM. Factors influencing intrafamilial communication of hereditary breast and ovarian cancer genetic information. *Eur J Hum Genet.* 2009;17(7):872 880.

O'Doherty K, Suthers GK. Risky communication: pitfalls in counselling about risk, and how to avoid them. *J Genet Couns.* 2007;16:409–417.

Ozaki K, Ohnishi Y, Iida A, et al. Functional SNPs in the lymphotoxin-α gene that are associated with susceptibility to myocardial infarction. *Nat Genet.* 2002;32:650–654.

Parsons EP, Clarke AJ, Hood K, Bradley DM, Bradley DM. Feasibility of a change in service delivery: the case of optional newborn screening for Duchenne muscular dystrophy. *Comm Genet.* 2000;3(1):17–23.

Peterson SK, Watts BG, Koehly LM, et al. How families communicate about HNPCC genetic testing: findings from a qualitative study. *Am J Med Genet.* 2003;119C:78–86.

Priori SG, Napolitano C, Giordano U, Collisani G, Memmi M. Brugada syndrome and sudden cardiac death in children. *Lancet.* 2000;355(9206):808–809.

Priori SG, Schwartz PJ, Napolitano C, et al. Risk stratification in the long-QT syndrome. *N Engl J Med.* 2003;348(19):1866–1874.

Rader DJ, Daugherty A. Translating molecular discoveries into new therapies for atherosclerosis. Nature Insight—Cardiovascular Disease. *Nature.* 2008;451:904–913.

Räisänen U, Bekkers M-J, Boddington P, Sarangi S, Clarke A. The causation of disease: the practical and ethical consequences of competing explanations. *Med Health Care Philos.* 2006;9:293–306.

Richards FH. Maturity of judgement in decision making for predictive testing for nontreatable adult-onset neurogenetic conditions: a case against predictive testing of minors. *Clin Genet.* 2006;70:396–401.

Roberts R. Genomics and cardiac arrhythmias. *J Am Coll Cardiol.* 2006;47(1):9–21.

Roberts R, Brugada R. Genetics and arrhythmia. *Annu Rev Med.* 2003:54:257–267.

Royse SD. Implications of genetic testing for sudden cardiac death syndrome. *Br J Nursing.* 2006;15:1104–1107.

Samani NJ, Erdmann J, Hall AS, et al. Genomewide association analysis of coronary artery disease. *N Eng J Med.* 2007;357:443–453.

Saukko PM, Ellard S, Richards SH, Shepherd MH, Campbell JL. Patients' understanding of genetic susceptibility testing in mainstream medicine: qualitative study on thrombophilia. *BMC Health Serv Res.* 2007;7:82.

Schwartz PJ, Priori SG, Spazzolini C, et al. Genortype-phenotype correlation in the long-QT syndrome. Gene-specific triggers for life-thereatening arrhythmias. *Circulation.* 2001;103:89–95.

Scientific Steering Committee on behalf of the Simon Broome Register Group. Mortality in treated heterozygotes for familial hypercholesterolaemia: implications for clinical management. *Atherosclerosis.* 1999;142:105–112.

Semsarian C, Members of the CSANZ Cardiovascular Genetics Working Group. Guidelines for the diagnosis and management of hypertrophic cardiomyopathy. *Heart Lung Circ.* 2007;16:16–18.

Senior V, Marteau TM. Causal attributions for raised cholesterol and perceptions of effective risk-reduction: self-regulation strategies for an increased risk of coronary heart disease. *Psychol Health.* 2007;22:699–717.

Senior V, Marteau TM, Peters TJ. Will genetic fatalism for predisposition for disease result in fatalism? A qualitative study of parents' responses to neonatal screening for familial hypercholesterolaemia. *Soc Sci Med.* 1999;48:1857–1860.

Senior V, Smith JA, Michie S, Marteau TM. Making sense of risk: an interpretive phenomenological analysis of vulnerability to heart disease. *J Health Psychol.* 2002;7:157–168.

Sever PS, Poulter NR, Dahlof B, et al. The Anglo-Scandinavian Cardiac Outcomes Trial lipid lowering arm: extended observations 2 years after trial closure. *Eur Heart J.* 2008;29(4):499–508.

Skirton H. The client's perspective of genetic counseling. A grounded theory study. *J Genet Couns.* 2001;10:311–329.

Smets EMA, Stam MMH, Meulenkamp TM, et al. Health-related quality of life of children with a positive carrier status for inherited cardiovascular diseases. *Am J Med Genet.* 2008;146A:700–707.

Smilde TJ, Wissen S van, Wollersheim H, Trip MD, Kastelein JJP, Stalenhoef AFH. Effect of aggressive versus conventional lipid lowering on atherosclerosis progression in familial hypercholesterolaemia (ASAP): a prospective randomised, double-blind trial. *Lancet.* 2001;357:577–581.

Smith JA, Michie S, Stephenson M, Quarrel O. Risk perception and decision-making processes in candidates for genetic testing for Huntington's disease: an interpretative phenomenological analysis. *J Health Psychol.* 2002;7:131–144.

Sniderman AD, Furberg CD. Age as a modifiable risk factor for cardiovascular disease. *Lancet.* 2008;371:1547–1549.

Speice J, McDaniel SH, Rowley PT, Loader S. Family issues in a psychoeducational group for women with a *BRCA* mutation. *Clin Genet.* 2002;62:121–127.

Sramek A, Kriek M, Rosendaal FR. Decreased mortality of ischaemic heart disease among carriers of haemophilia. *Lancet.* 2003;362:351–354.

Starke M, Möller A. Parents' needs for knowledge concerning the medical diagnosis of their children. *J Child Health Care.* 2002;6:245–257.

Suthers GK, Armstrong J, McCormack J, Trott D. Letting the family know: balancing ethics and effectiveness when notifying relatives about genetic testing for a familial disorder. *J Med Genet.* 2006;43:665–670.

Taylor SD. Predictive genetic test decisions for Huntington's disease: context, appraisal and new moral imperatives. *Soc Sci Med.* 2004;58:137–149.

Temple IK, Westwood G. Do once and share: clinical genetics. Department of Health—Connecting for Health; 2006.

Tod AM, Read C, Lacey A, Abbott J. Barriers to uptake of services for coronary heart disease: qualitative study. *BMJ.* 2001;323:214–217.

Tonstad S, Novik TS, Vandvik IH. Psychosocial function during treatment for familial hypercholesterolaemia. *Pediatrics.* 1996;98:249–255.

Treloar TS, Barlow-Stewart K, Stranger M, Otlowski M. Investigating genetic discrimination in Australia: a large scale survey of clinical genetics clients. *Clin Genet.* 2008;74:20–30.

Troughton J, Jarvis J, Skinner C, Robertson N, Khunti K, Davies M. Waiting for diabetes: perceptions of people with pre-diabetes: a qualitative study. *Patient Educ Couns.* 2008;72:88–93.

Umans-Eckenhausen MAW, Defesche JC, Sijbrands EJG, Scheerder RLJM, Kastelein JJP. Review of first 5 years of screening for familial hypercholesterolaemia in the Netherlands. *Lancet.* 2001;357:165–168.

Veldkamp MW, Viswanathan PC, Bezzina C, Baartscheer A, Wilde AA, Balser JR. Two distinct congenital arrhythmias evoked by a multidysfunctional Na(+) channel. *Circ Res.* 2000;86(9):E91–E97.

Victora CG, Adair L, Fall C, et al. Maternal and child undernutrition: consequences for adult health and human capital. *Lancet.* 2008;371:340–357.

Wald DS, Bestwick JP, Wald NJ. Child-parent screening for familial hypercholesterolaemia: screening strategy based on a meta-analysis. *Brit Med J.* 2007;335:599–603.

Wellcome Trust Case Control Consortium. Genome-wide association study of 14,000 cases of seven common diseases and 3,000 shared controls. *Nature.* 2007;447:661–678.

Wilcke JTR, Seersholm N, Kok-Jensen A, Dirksen A. Attitudes towards an unsolicited approach in relation to status of genetic disease: exemplified by α_1-antitrypsin deficiency. *Am J Med Genet.* 2000;94:207–213.

Wilson BJ, Forrest K, Teijlingen ER van, et al. Family communication about genetic risk: the little that is known. *Comm Gen.* 2004;7:15–24.

Yu B, French JA, Jeremy RW, et al. Counselling issues in familial hypertrophic cardiomyopathy. *J Med Genet.* 1998;35:183–188.

38

The Forensic Pathologist and Genetic Cardiovascular Disease

Stephen Leadbeatter

Introduction

In England and Wales, the coroner has a statutory duty to inquire into sudden deaths of unknown cause, violent or unnatural deaths, and deaths which occur in prison. The explanation for a sudden death of unknown cause may lie on a genetic cardiovascular disease, and that might also explain an apparently violent or unnatural death, or for a death which occurs in a prison. In the majority of inquiries into such deaths, particularly in young people, there will be a post mortem examination.

The Post-mortem Examination

So far as postmortem examination is concerned, genetic cardiovascular disease may be regarded as comprising two forms:

- Disease with features visible to the naked eye and/or under the microscope.
- Disease with morphological abnormality visible neither to the naked eye nor under the microscope.

Genetic cardiovascular disease may provide the sole explanation for death; may be the explanation for death from a cause made possible by the existence of that genetic cardiovascular disease [e.g., drowning as a consequence of arrhythmia triggered by type 1 long QT syndrome or catacholaminergic polymorphic ventricular tachycardia (Choi et al. 2004)]; or be an incidental finding that is of no relevance to how the person died (this last set of circumstances, in practice, would arise only where there was a morphological abnormality recognized by the pathologist during the investigation of cause of death—where there were no morphological abnormality, it is unlikely that the existence of such an "incidental finding" would be considered).

Whatever the role of genetic cardiovascular disease, the investigation of surviving family members may be facilitated by retention of material (e.g., a sample of spleen) from which DNA may be extracted: such investigation may be the only means of yielding the diagnosis (Tester and Ackerman 2007).

It is to be hoped that the resources, knowledge, and skills possessed by a pathologist working in any system of medicolegal investigation of death are sufficient to allow that pathologist, when faced with a death involving genetic cardiovascular disease with morphological abnormality, either to make the diagnosis alone, or to retain material—as images, and as slides for examination under the microscope—which will allow the diagnosis to be made by a more expert practitioner. There is evidence to suggest that such a hope, in England and Wales, might be in vain; that evidence suggests also that the history provided to the pathologist, regarding the antecedents of a deceased, and the circumstances of death, may be incomplete (National Confidential Enquiry into Patient Outcome and Death 2006). The Association for European Cardiovascular Pathology has "developed guidelines, which represent the minimum standard that is required in the routine autopsy practice for the adequate assessment of sudden cardiac death, including not only a protocol for heart examination and histological sampling, but also for toxicology and molecular investigation" (Basso et al. 2008).

Any pathologist involved in the medicolegal investigation of sudden death must be prepared to give guidance on what questions should be asked in relation to a death, particularly where postmortem examination yields no explanation for death. In the context of death in association with genetic cardiovascular disease, such questions would include, for example,

- in what activity was the deceased engaged when collapse occurred?
- had there been exposure to sudden noise, such as an alarm clock?
- was there a history of previous unexplained collapse, either in the individual or in family members?
- where there was such a history, what were the circumstances of the collapse?
- was there any family history of an "unusual propensity for death," for example, during swimming?

The Coroner's Inquiry

In England and Wales, where death is sudden and of unknown cause, a coroner, if of the "opinion that a post-mortem examination may prove an inquest to be unnecessary" may direct or request that a postmortem examination be made by "any legally qualified medical practitioner" [Coroners Act 1988, s.19(1)] who is "whenever practicable... a pathologist with suitable qualifications and experience and having access to laboratory facilities" (The Coroners Rules 1984, rule 6(1)(a)). If that postmortem examination yields a cause of death and there are no circumstances to suggest that an inquest is necessary (i.e., there is nothing to suggest that the death is violent, unnatural, or occurred in prison), no further investigation is required.

The human material that may be retained at a postmortem examination directed or requested by a coroner does not fall under the Human Tissue Act 2004 until the purposes of the Coroner's inquiry have been fulfilled (Human Tissue Act 2004, s.11) [i.e., when the Coroner is *functus officio* (R. v. White (1860) 3 E. & E. 137; 121 E.R.394)]. Where the "naked-eye" postmortem examination yields a morphologically obvious genetic cardiovascular disease (e.g., "classical" hypertrophic cardiomyopathy with asymmetric septal hypertrophy and endocardial fibrosis in the left ventricular outflow tract "mirroring" the anterior cusp of the mitral valve) and the circumstances of death are such that "the coroner is satisfied... that an inquest is unnecessary" [Coroners Act 1988, s.19(3)] then, given the arguments set out in recent case law [Terry v. East Sussex Coroner (2001) EWCA Civ 1094], a coroner might take the view that, whether or not he or she is *functus officio*, no further investigation—be it microscopy or DNA analysis—can be authorized without appropriate consent from the person in the "highest" qualifying relationship as set out in s.54(9) of the Human Tissue Act 2004. It is to be hoped that, in such circumstances, the possibility that the fatal disease may be inherited is raised with family members to allow them to determine whether they wish further investigations to be made (either through retention of material from the deceased, or appropriate investigations, after counseling, in surviving family members) (DH Coronary Heart Disease Team 2005).

Where the postmortem examination yields no "naked-eye" morphological explanation for death then the Coroner will not dispense with an inquest—toxicological analysis would be undertaken to exclude the role of any drug in the cause of death, and such analysis, and examination under the microscope of retained material, will take time. The possibility of genetic cardiovascular disease must be borne in mind by the pathologist who has made such a postmortem examination, and material from which DNA may be extracted to allow an attempt at diagnosis to be made must be retained and appropriately stored.

Where a pathologist retains material at postmortem examination, the Coroner must be informed of what has been retained and why; the Coroner must tell

> "(a) one of the persons referred to in rule 20(2)(a)(a parent, child, spouse, and any person representative of the deceased—The Coroners Rules 1984, rule 20(2)(a)) and
> (b) any other relative of the deceased who has notified the Coroner of his desire to attend, or be represented at the post-mortem examination"

what has been retained, for how long it will be retained, and "the options for dealing with the material" when the purposes of the Coroner's inquiry have been fulfilled [The Coroners (Amendment) Rules 2005].

It is of interest that there is no requirement to tell family members why that material is to be retained: it is possible that DNA may be extracted from that material to allow determination of cause of death by genetic analysis—the use of such DNA to determine cause of death for a coroner is an "excepted purpose," in the context of nonconsensual analysis of DNA, under schedule 4 of the Human Tissue Act 2004. Whether it is ethical to make such a diagnostic analysis without the knowledge of family members is worthy of debate. It is submitted that, where a postmortem examination yields no explanation for death, and where the possibility that death was caused by genetic cardiovascular disease exists, that possibility should be brought to the attention of family members, and appropriate counseling regarding possible further investigation made available as each family member desires: at what point this counseling and, if desired, direction into clinical investigation, should occur may differ with the views of, and resources available to, individual coroners. Within the current constraints at all stages of the coronial investigation of deaths in England and Wales, a speedy and easy resolution for family members may be difficult to achieve.

The purpose of the inquisition at inquest as stated in s.11(5) (b) of the Coroners Act 1988 is to

> "set out, so far as such particulars have been proved –
>
> (i) who the deceased was; and
> (ii) how, when and where the deceased came by his death."

It appears from current case law [Hurst, R (on the application of) v. Commissioner of Police of the Metropolis (2007) UKHL 13] that, in deaths occurring since October 2, 2000 which do not involve potential state responsibility, "how" means "by what means": whatever the meaning of "how," it will include "the cause of death."

In the absence of easily available "molecular autopsy," how coroners may formulate a cause of death where there is no morphological abnormality, no toxicological finding, and no reason to believe that a death is other than natural may differ: one coroner might regard the cause of death as "unascertained" and return an "open verdict," whereas another might regard the cause of death as from "sudden arrhythmic death syndrome" (Behr et al. 2007) and return a verdict of natural causes. The former course may cause distress to families but such families, if further information becomes available from investigation of surviving family members, may apply to the Attorney General for his *fiat* to allow application to the High Court to quash the inquisition and order another inquest (Coroners Act 1988, s.13). In the latter set of circumstances, such a *fiat* might not be forthcoming, because a new inquest would be unlikely to result in a verdict other than natural causes, the verdict at the original inquest; should the family wish to change the registered cause of death, a coroner might argue that "sudden arrhythmic death syndrome" while not so precise as (say) "Long QT syndrome, type 1" did not constitute an "error of fact or substance" capable of correction as set down in S29(4) (as amended) of the Births and Deaths Registration Act 1953 and regulation 59 of the Registration of Births and Deaths Regulations 1987.

Other Judicial Fora

The pathologist must recognize that genetic cardiovascular disease may provide an explanation for death in circumstances where there appears to be either another obvious explanation for death—such as drowning, or involvement in an inexplicable road traffic collision—or where the actions of another individual may be called in question. This latter situation is exemplified in recent case law [R. v. Carey, C and F (2006) EWCA Crim 17], although the legal points at issue in such circumstances will be determined by the facts in the individual case. In essence, however, where it is argued that the actions of an individual have set in train a chain of circumstances resulting in the death of another—say, where a person with type 1 long QT syndrome dies while swimming in an attempt to escape from an assault—then the Crown may prove unlawful act manslaughter if it is established

(a) that there was an unlawful act;
(b) that the unlawful act was such as all sober and reasonable people (having the same knowledge regarding the victim as was available to the assailant) would inevitably recognize must subject the victim to, at least, the risk of some harm resulting therefrom, albeit not serious harm; and
(c) that the unlawful act caused death.

Again, what liability might lie with the organizers of a sporting activity (or doctors involved in preparticipation screening) that results in the death of an individual with genetic cardiovascular disease would be determined only when all facts relevant to that individual case were known and judged against current clinical practice, guidelines (Mitten et al. 2005), and consensus statements (Corrado et al. 2005)—which may differ between countries—in the context of legislation in the country of action (or, in the United States of America, the individual State (Paterick et al. 2007): it appears that no legal precedent (regarding a death from genetic cardiovascular disease) has been established in the United States (Paterick et al. 2005). The role of the pathologist in such circumstances is to establish—or to provide material that will establish—the pathological condition present: questions regarding preparticipation screening and all other clinical issues are not for the pathologist to address, but are matters for those with the appropriate expertise.

Conclusions

The interaction between pathological and coroner or other judicial fora, where a genetic cardiovascular disease is a factor in an unexplained death, is complicated by the knowledge and resources available to each party, and by interpretation of current legislation. It has been said that, "....There is a lack of coherence between the regulating regime that applies during coroner's jurisdiction, and the Human Tissue Act which applies once the cause of death has been established. These problems need to be addressed by legislative changes....." (Burton et al. 2009).

References

Basso C, Burke M, Fornes P, et al. Guidelines for autopsy investigation of sudden cardiac death. *Virchows Arch.* 2008;452:11–18.

Behr ER, Casey A, Sheppard M, et al. Sudden arrhythmic death syndrome: a national survey of sudden unexplained cardiac death. *Heart.* 2007;93:601–605.

Burton H, Alberg C, Stewart A. 'Heart to Heart' Inherited Cardiovascular Conditions Services, PHG Foundation, Cambridge, 2009 (www.phgfoundation.org).

Choi G, Kopplin LJ, Tester DJ, Will ML, Haglund CM, Ackerman MJ. Spectrum and frequency of cardiac channel defects in swimming—triggered arrhythmia syndromes. *Circulation.* 2004;110:2119–2124.

Corrado D, Pelliccia A, Bjørnstad HH, et al. Cardiovascular pre-participation screening of young competitive athletes for prevention of sudden death: proposal for a coroner's European protocol. *Eur Heart J.* 2005; 26:516–524.

DH Coronary Heart Disease Team. *National Service Framework for Coronary Heart Disease*—Chapter Eight: Arrhythmias and Sudden Cardiac Death. Department of Health; 2005.

Mitten MJ, Maron BJ, Zipes DP. Legal Aspects of the 36th Bethesda Conference Recommendations. *J Am Coll Cardiol.* 2005;45:1373–1375.

National Confidential Enquiry into Patient Outcome and Death. *The Coroner's Autopsy: Do We Deserve Better?* London: NCEPOD; 2006.

Paterick TE, Paterick TJ, Fletcher GF, Maron BJ. Medical and legal issues in the cardiovascular evaluation of competitive athletes. *JAMA.* 2005;294:3011–3018.

Paterick TJ, Paterick BB, Paterick TE. Professional team physicians beware! Co-employee status may not ipso facto confer tort immunity; 2007. http://www.thesportjournal.org/2007Journal/Vol10-No3/01paterick.asp.

Tester DJ, Ackerman MJ. Postmortem long QT syndrome genetic testing for sudden unexplained death in the young. *J Am Coll Cardiol.* 2007;49:240–246.

39

Provision of Clinical Cardiovascular Genetics Services

Paul Brennan

Introduction

Within the general population there is a prevalent cohort of undetected cardiovascular disease caused by de novo or inherited genetic mutation. Affected individuals may be in a presymptomatic phase and the diagnosis may not yet be suspected. They may have symptoms or signs but the correct diagnosis may not have been made (examples being someone with a history of recurrent collapse falsely attributed to epilepsy; or someone with unrecognized physical features of Marfan syndrome). Alternatively, a diagnosis may have been made but the familial implications may not be appreciated.

Within this population there will clearly be people who are aware of their family history of inherited cardiovascular disease. Others may be completely unaware of a genuine family history, especially if relatives have been misdiagnosed or undiagnosed; or the history may be spurious and misleading (e.g., not all familial clustering of "heart attacks" equates to Mendelian disease).

The challenge for clinical teams is to respond to each of these groups and ensure that people with—or at familial risk of—inherited cardiovascular disease are identified and managed appropriately. This requires resources to be allocated to education, screening services, triage (family history assessment), and clinical service development beyond the level currently being provided in most countries.

This chapter deals with the practical issues around the provision of the genetic component of a cardiovascular genetics service. Since there is no single inherited cardiovascular disease, such services are complex, responding to a wide range of diseases affecting cardiac muscle, rhythm, connective tissue, and vessels; some diseases may have significant extracardiac pathology. All these disorders overlap in the sense that they are inherited diseases, and the genetic resources required to deal with each disease group are broadly transferable. "Cardiovascular genetics service" should therefore be seen as an umbrella term that describes a series of complex multidisciplinary services, all of which incorporate clinical and laboratory genetics services (clinical geneticists, genetic counselors, service and research laboratories) and cardiology services (cardiologists, cardiac imaging services, cardiac electrophysiology services), but will include other groups, depending on the particular clinical situation (e.g., surgeons, pathologists, clinical lipidologists, ophthalmologists, and patient support groups).

The Genetic Approach to Inherited Cardiovascular Disease

Although the genetic issues presented by an inherited cardiovascular disease service are broadly transferable from other areas of clinical genetics practice—for example, familial cancer—there are a number of specific challenges.

1. The Family History

Family history is often useful from a diagnostic point of view, since the phenotype may not be fully expressed in the proband. Assessment of an individual with a potentially inherited cardiac condition should always include a family history, although a significant proportion of cases result from de novo gene mutation. Reported diagnoses in relatives are often nonspecific; for example, the often-used term "heart attack" can mean anything from acute angina to fatal coronary artery occlusion, thoracic aortic aneurysm rupture, or sudden death caused by ventricular tachyarrhythmia. It is therefore important to supplement the family history with more detailed information (see below). In addition, the family pedigree identifies "at-risk" relatives and provides the physician with an opportunity to reduce the risk of morbidity or sudden death in relatives.

2. Age

In general terms, cardiac gene mutations predispose to earlier disease than in the general population. So, for example, a family history of myocardial infarction over the age of 60 years—especially in smokers—carries less significance than if disease presents below the age of 50 years. However, this does not hold true for all inherited cardiac conditions: presentation of hypertrophic cardiomyopathy (HCM) in older relatives is well described and may simply reflect either intrafamilial phenotypic variation, or a late onset variant (see Chapter 13).

3. Number of Affected Relatives

It is relatively unusual to encounter a family in which affected status can be confidently assigned to large numbers of relatives from the family history alone. In most families, confirmation of suspected diagnoses and clinical screening in the extended, apparently unaffected family is required. Small families create an interpretive problem in some situations; for example, the occurrence of dilated cardiomyopathy in two close relatives may have arisen by chance, since this is a common disease with multiple etiologies.

4. Relationship to the Proband

In general, if two relatives have the same cardiac phenotype, then the closer the degree of relationship, the more likely it is that those phenotypes have arisen from a shared gene mutation. Intervening "normal" relatives may be mutation carriers who do not manifest a phenotype (this is known as "variable penetrance"; see below). This also applies to intervening relatives who have died from other causes and are not available for clinical assessment.

5. Symptoms

In some circumstances, elucidation of particular symptoms may be helpful in establishing a diagnosis. For example, in a long QT syndrome (LQTS) family, particular attention should be paid to the occurrence of fainting, recurrent collapse, sudden death, congenital deafness, and "epilepsy."

6. Associated Phenotypes

A single gene mutation may manifest in different ways in different people (this is known as "variable expressivity"; see below). Marfan syndrome, for example, has a number of extracardiac disease features, which may be present to a greater or lesser degree in relatives (see Chapter 11). The person taking a family history may therefore need to specifically enquire about other phenotypes in relatives.

7. Phenocopy

A number of common phenotypes can result from a genetic disorder or secondary to a nongenetic factor. For example, left ventricular hypertrophy may represent familial HCM, the consequence of untreated hypertension, or the result of athletic training. This possibility should be borne in mind when a family history is taken.

Genetic Counseling (see also Chapter 37)

In the United Kingdom, clinical genetics services are staffed mainly by medically trained clinical geneticists and genetic counselors with a background in either nursing or science. Many definitions of "genetic counseling" exist, although many regard the definition developed by the American Society for Human Genetics to encompass the work of most genetic counselors today (Ad Hoc Committee on Genetic Counseling 1975): "A communication process which deals with human problems associated with the occurrence, or risk of occurrence, of a genetic disorder in a family."

Counseling involves an attempt by one or more appropriately trained persons to help the individual to (1) understand the medical facts, including the diagnosis, probable course of the disorder, and the available management; (2) appreciate the way heredity contributes to the disorder, and the risk of recurrence in specified relatives; (3) understand the alternatives for dealing with the risk of recurrence; (4) choose the course of action that seems to them appropriate in view of their risk, their family goals, and their ethical and religious standards, and to act in accordance with that decision; and (5) make the best possible adjustment to the disorder in an affected family member and/or the risk of recurrence of the disorder. It is clear that, in the case of inherited cardiac disease, discussion around point (1) above needs to be undertaken in close collaboration with specialist cardiology services.

Genetic Testing in a Clinical Setting

Genetic mutation analysis for many inherited cardiac diseases has become widely available in many countries in the health care setting. Genetic testing is not without its pitfalls, however (Priori et al. 1999b), and should ideally be undertaken according to consensus guidelines (e.g., Heart Rhythm U.K. Familial Sudden Death Syndromes Statement Development Group 2008). There are two broad types of genetic testing: *diagnostic* testing, in which the aim of the test is to confirm a diagnosis through the identification of a pathological sequence change (mutation) in a gene; and *predictive* testing, in which the mutation responsible for a disease has been identified elsewhere in a family, and a relative seeks to clarify his/her genetic status. In the case of inherited cardiac disease, both are complex issues that illustrate a number of potential problems.

1. Genetic Heterogeneity

A genetically heterogeneous disorder is one in which a single phenotype can result from mutations in a number of different genes (see also Chapter 3). For example, most cases of LQTS—for the purposes of this discussion a single phenotype—are caused by mutations in one of five different genes (see Chapters 17 and 18). The "mutation detection rate" in LQTS is around 80% in individuals in whom the clinical diagnosis is certain (Splawski et al. 2000), although considerably less in those in whom evidence in support of the diagnosis is weaker, limiting its use as a primary *diagnostic* test (Tester et al. 2006). It is also important to appreciate that failure to identify a gene mutation does not necessarily *exclude* the disease—in patients who do not fulfil clinical diagnostic criteria.

In those with particularly severe expression of a disease, mutation analysis should not stop when one mutation is identified, but should continue to investigate the possibility of compound mutation caused by inheritance of one mutation from each parent. Such individuals tend to have a more severe phenotype. For example, Jervell-Lange-Nielsen syndrome, the most severe (and rare) end of the LQTS spectrum, is caused by homozygosity for *KCNQ1* or *KCNE1* mutation (Schwartz et al. 2006); in addition, 5%–8% of individuals with LQTS inherit mutations in two *different* LQTS genes (termed compound heterozygosity); such patients tend to have a longer QTc, more frequent symptoms, and increased likelihood of cardiac arrest (Schwartz et al. 2003; Westenkow et al. 2004; Yamaguchi et al. 2005). Heterozygous parents and relatives of such people (who by definition only have one LQTS mutation) have much milder or even subclinical disease. Such genetic heterogeneity complicates all of the major groups of inherited cardiovascular disease.

2. Phenotypic Heterogeneity

Cardiac genetics is complicated by heterogeneity: on one level, mutation in a single cardiac gene can cause different phenotypes ("phenotypic heterogeneity" or "variable expressivity"), whereas a single phenotype may be caused by mutations in a number of different genes ("genetic heterogeneity").

For example, phenotypic heterogeneity is commonly encountered in families segregating a mutation in the *FBN1* gene: some relatives may manifest classical Marfan syndrome, whereas others may display fewer features and do not meet the Ghent diagnostic criteria (de Paepe et al. 1996). More unusually, an individual with a mutation in *MYH7* will present with dilated cardiomyopathy in a family in which the predominant phenotype is HCM (Kamisago et al. 2000); or one may encounter either LQTS or Brugada syndrome in a family segregating a *SCN5A* mutation (Bezzina et al. 1999). Variable expressivity is a potential problem in diagnosis: the proband may have an atypical or subdiagnostic phenotype, creating diagnostic uncertainty. Often, thorough family assessment will reveal the full phenotype and enable the correct diagnosis to be made, although a number of relatives may need to be seen in the process. Variable expressivity is also a potential problem when undertaking cascade genetic testing: although the term *predictive* testing is used for this activity, it can be difficult to predict the likely phenotype in an (as yet) unaffected mutation carrier (heterozygote).

In recent years, accurate and detailed phenotyping has defined a large number of overlap syndromes that share a major common feature. A simple example is LQTS: mutations in a number of different genes can cause prolongation of the QT interval (genetic heterogeneity), but when considered in detail, it is possible to define a set of closely related diseases with characteristic T-wave morphologies and arrhythmia triggers (phenotypic heterogeneity). At a clinical level it may not be possible to resolve the phenotype, in which case diagnostic genetic testing is the only option. More complex (and common) disorders include HCM, in which a variety of phenotypes are recognized, some of which appear to relate to the causative gene and may be useful in deciding which gene may be responsible. For example, severe, "classical" HCM developing in the second decade of life is typical—but not diagnostic—of mutation in the *MYH7* gene; the presence of preexcitation on the 12-lead ECG would be in keeping with the *PRKAG2* gene; X-linked inheritance in association with extracardiac disease such as renal failure, stroke, and/or cutaneous angiokeratoma would suggest Anderson-Fabry disease. Similar levels of complexity are observed with dilated cardiomyopathy and familial thoracic aneurysm syndromes, all of which may be subcategorized according to the presence of additional phenotypic features.

3. Variable Penetrance

Some mutation-carrying parents and relatives of individuals with inherited cardiovascular diseases may be symptom free and have normal cardiac investigations. In the case of LQTS it has therefore been suggested that penetrance (the proportion of heterozygotes who manifest) may be much lower than originally postulated (Priori et al. 1999a), although such nonpenetrant heterozygotes may still be at risk if they are exposed to nongenetic risk factors such as drugs that interact with the drug-binding site within the intracellular pore region of the *KCNH2* ion channel protein. Again, this phenomenon complicates cascade genetic testing, since a significant proportion of heterozygotes will never develop heart disease. This will become a greater problem in the future as effective prophylaxis (measures taken to prevent the phenotype developing), for example, pharmacological intervention or gene-based strategies become available. This is different from sudden death prophylaxis in someone with an established phenotype, such as HCM, since it may be impossible to determine which heterozygotes are truly at risk.

Interpretation of Gene Test Results

Interpretation of a sequence alteration in a gene can be difficult, particularly novel (i.e., not previously reported) missense alterations whose impact on protein function cannot easily be predicted and which have not previously been described as polymorphisms (nondisease-causing variants) in control DNA samples. A missense mutation is one that causes an amino acid substitution and does not prematurely terminate the protein by creating a "stop" codon. It is sometimes necessary to "track" a missense change through a family to confirm its segregation with the disease phenotype, although the finding of the putative mutation in a clinically unaffected relative may create further interpretive problems, and affected relatives may not be available for testing. In addition, few centers are able to study mutant protein function in vitro (e.g., using *Xenopus* oocytes in order to investigate the pathogenicity of an ion channel gene mutation).

Confirmation of a disease-causing mutation benefits the affected individual in terms of optimized management (Priori et al. 1999b; Phillips et al. 2005) and avoidance of arrhythmia trigger factors (in the case of LQTS, for example), and although genotype–phenotype correlation is not clear enough to support gene-specific therapy at present, this may be the case in the future. The main benefit lies in cascade predictive testing within the wider family. In an autosomal dominant disease, an affected individual's children have a 50% risk of having inherited the mutation; his/her siblings and parents are also potentially at risk, even in the absence of a family history of symptoms.

Predictive genetic testing in adults and children is certainly justified on medical grounds but there is very little published experience and its cost-effectiveness has not yet been established. In this context it is important to remember that a 12-lead ECG could function as a predictive test for LQTS or HCM, even though it does not examine DNA. In addition, although predictive genetic testing removes uncertainty about genetic status, it replaces it with a degree of uncertainty about disease penetrance, expressivity, and the risk of sudden death, even with prophylactic treatment. These more complex uncertainties can be particularly unsettling for patients and families. Experience from predictive testing in families affected by HCM has concluded that a supportive test protocol similar to that used by genetics services for late onset neurodegenerative diseases (e.g., Huntington's disease) and hereditary cancers should be used for LQTS families (Charron et al. 2002). Indeed, predictive testing for LQTS in children frequently causes high levels of short-term distress in their parents (Hendriks et al. 2005a); many parents of children with confirmed LQTS mutations continue to worry about the threat of arrhythmia, especially those who have experienced sudden death within the family, those with low educational levels, and those with adolescent children. Psychological support and updated information should therefore be available for families over many years through continuing contact with medical services but in general long-term distress following predictive testing is rare (Hendriks et al. 2005b, 2008).

Ethical and Legal Considerations

Information provided by a genetic test has a number of complex characteristics. Within a family, relatives share a common heredity: so, for example, the discovery of a gene mutation in an individual has immediate implications for his/her surviving relatives, and also for future generations. The information has a predictive nature, in the sense that it can predict the likelihood of future disease in someone who is currently well (although it may not be able to predict exactly how that person will be affected). Such information may therefore be of potential interest to the individual being tested, the family and third parties such as insurers and employers, and a cardiac genetics service should develop clear ethical practice around the use and disclosure of genetic information.

When dealing with genetic information within a family, the practitioner needs to balance his/her duty of confidentiality to the proband (the first person to be seen within a family) against the potential interest that a relative may have in that information (respecting the proband's "informational privacy") (Laurie 1999); and in addition, the right of a relative not to know that information (respecting their "spatial privacy"). This may seem to be an ethical minefield, yet in practice it is rarely so: patients usually understand the potential use of genetic information within the wider family and, as long as this is explicitly discussed at the time a DNA sample is taken, are usually happy for that information to be disclosed if necessary.

Refusal to disclose is rarely encountered in practice. A proband may not consent to information sharing within the wider family for reasons of family dynamics. If this happens, the practitioner needs to balance the ethical principles of patient confidentiality (proband) against the avoidance of harm (relatives); if he/she feels that to withhold genetic information from a relative would place them at significant harm, then disclosure against the will of the proband may be justified. This could certainly be argued for inherited heart diseases in which there is a risk of avoidable death. In practice, such situations can usually be avoided by careful, open discussion (Clarke et al. 2005).

In theory an insurance company may have an interest in genetic information. At present, actuarial risk calculations usually take an individual's family history into account and insurance is provided according to a "pooled risk" principle. In the United Kingdom, a voluntary moratorium currently restricts the use of genetic information by insurance companies to those individuals requesting high levels of life cover, with the exception of Huntington's disease, a chronic neurodegenerative disorder (Department of Health 2005a), so an individual undergoing genetic testing—especially predictive—is usually under no compulsion to disclose this information. The situation with respect to employers is complex. On the one hand, an employer may wish to avoid employing someone with a risk of ill-health (balanced against the limited predictive power of a genetic test), which would potentially be seen as discriminatory behavior; on the other, there may be a genuine desire to avoid placing the individual in a workplace that may precipitate or exacerbate health problems. Disclosure of genetic information to an employer may therefore be reasonable to protect the interests of employer or employee, although disclosure should certainly not be considered routine practice. In practice, this issue rarely poses a problem except in two key areas of employment: professional sport and the armed forces. Here, an individual already in employment may be unwilling to consider cascade testing for fear of losing his/her job, yet he/she may be at significant risk of harm. Conversely, either of these professions may refuse to employ someone unless he/she has had a negative predictive genetic test. Such situations need to be handled sensitively, according to core ethical principles and, where necessary, with legal advice.

It is therefore apparent that, prior to a DNA sample being taken for genetic testing (whether diagnostic or predictive), informed consent should be obtained. Consent is a process by which the practitioner and patient discuss the nature and consequences of the test. It is clearly of paramount importance that this includes a discussion around the familial nature of genetic information, and if possible prior agreement to the disclosure of that information to relatives. It is helpful to record such a discussion by asking the patient to sign a consent form, although signing such a form per se is no substitute for patient-centered discussion (Joint Committee on Medical Genetics 2006).

A cardiac genetics service needs to have a clear strategy for the dissemination of genetic information through a family ("cascade activity"). If relatives' privacy is to be respected, it may be considered inappropriate for a practitioner to approach them directly in an unsolicited manner. In most U.K. genetics centers, it is considered best practice to engage the probands, providing them with written information to pass on to their relatives. Such information includes a clear, nontechnical description of the disease and their potential risk, together with advice about how to access cardiac genetics services. Of course, cascade activity of this nature may be concerned with clinical screening (e.g., echo and ECG in the relatives of someone diagnosed with HCM) or genetic testing (e.g., the same family, once the causative gene mutation is known). A cardiac genetics nurse or a genetic counselor can facilitate this process, especially if the proband is unsure how—or reluctant to—contact his/her relatives. In many centers, unsolicited direct contact is avoided where possible, unless of course the proband steadfastly refuses to disclose. Direct contact by letter has been employed successfully in familial hypercholesterolemia families, however, and more debate is clearly needed in this area (Newson and Humphries 2005).

Service Provision in the United Kingdom

In England, the 2005 National Service Framework for Coronary Heart Disease Chapter 8: Arrhythmias and Sudden Cardiac Death (Department of Health 2005b) made two key recommendations in the context of inherited cardiac conditions: that, when a sudden cardiac death occurs, health services have systems in place to identify family members at risk and provide personally tailored, sensitive and expert support, diagnosis, treatment, information, and advice to close relatives; and that evaluation of families who may have inherited cardiac disease takes place in a dedicated clinic, with staff who are trained in diagnosis, management, and support for these families, with genetic counseling and further testing available if appropriate. The balance between genetics and cardiology depends to a large extent on local circumstances and the degree to which local services and expertise have developed. Although this recommendation was made in the context of inherited cardiac conditions associated with sudden *arrhythmic* death (essentially, ion channelopathies and HCM), they should also apply to inherited cardiovascular connective tissue disorders such as Marfan syndrome and inherited lipid disorders, the commonest of which is familial hypercholesterolemia.

For multisystem inherited cardiovascular disorders, such as Marfan syndrome, the case for collaborative clinical services extends beyond cardiology and genetics to include cardiothoracic surgery, rheumatology, orthopedics and ophthalmology, for example. In the United Kingdom, clinical genetics services for these patient groups usually function in a diagnostic capacity, sometimes part of a specific multidisciplinary clinic although more often in close collaboration with other specialties (see below).

The Public Health Genetics Foundation has conducted a comprehensive review of services for inherited cardiac conditions in the United Kingdom based on the findings of earlier unpublished surveys (PHG Foundation 2009). They have developed a series of recommendations which highlight a number of challenges for such services:

1. The need for equitable access to specialised services for inherited arrhythmia syndromes, sudden death, cardiomyopathies, arteriopathies and disorders of cholesterol metabolism associated with an increased risk of premature coronary artery disease.
2. Expertise should be concentrated in a relatively small number of centers and commissioned according to an agreed framework.
3. Services should anticipate continued growth in demand over the next 5–10 years.
4. Service development should be coordinated by a multidisciplinary Expert Advisory Group which includes health care commissioners and voluntary organisations.
5. Services should be defined by a set of agreed standards that include skill mix, clinical facilities, clinical activity, management activity, audit and research.
6. There is a need for wider education and training of clinical, laboratory, pathology and allied health care staff.
7. There is a need for systematic cascade screening protocols, enhanced by the development of IT systems that cross geographic and organizational boundaries.
8. Retention of tissue and/or DNA from victims of sudden cardiac death, and the offer of referral of surviving relatives for cardiac assessment, should become routine.
9. Genetic tests for inherited cardiac conditions should be widely available and cover the full range of disorders.
10. Services should be underpinned by a culture of collaborative audit, prospective clinical data collection and translation of emerging technologies into clinical practice.

Genetics in Mainstream Practice

Within the definition outlined in the introduction lies a key question: how do clinical genetics and "mainstream" medical specialties fit together? Specialized medical genetics services have developed in the United Kingdom as local centers of genetics expertise, often based upon health authority boundaries. Their core activities are summarized in Box 39–1. A key characteristic of such services is the development of close links between medical genetic services and other clinical specialties.

Over the past decade there has been a large, sustained increase in the number of individuals and families with a history of *cancer* referred to regional genetics services. The U.K. National Health Service Cancer Plan (Department of Health 2000) found that cancer genetics services were poorly developed in the United Kingdom at that time. Primary and secondary care teams did not always have access to the information they required to assess cancer risk. There were few expert cancer geneticists and ill-prepared laboratory services. The 2003 U.K. Government white paper "Our Inheritance, Our Future—realizing the potential of genetics in the NHS" recognized this problem and outlined a series of service development plans, focusing on a number of key areas. One major area for investment was the provision of clinical and laboratory services for people with a family history of cancer.

This activity has resulted in a range of new clinical cancer genetics services that cross the "traditional" boundary between tertiary genetics services and mainstream medical practice. These services recognize that the skills required to deal with the genetic component of a clinical situation do not necessarily reside in a highly trained professional working in a regional genetics service. In the United Kingdom, the concept of "mainstreamed" genetics skills ("competences") has now been successfully piloted in a number of noncancer genetics scenarios (e.g., renal disease, hemochromatosis, α_1-antitrypsin deficiency). A set of "core" genetics competences in mainstream patient care has been developed by the NHS National Genetics Education and Development Center (www.geneticseducation.nhs.uk) and Skills for Health (www.skillsforhealth.org.uk). These competences are summarized in Box 39–2.

A survey of Dutch cardiologists published in 2003 suggested that their genetic knowledge and skills were insufficient, creating an argument for close collaborative working relationships with their genetics colleagues (van Langen et al. 2003). Further, while most cardiologists and geneticists/genetic counselors prefer to

Box 39–1 Definition of a Genetics Service

A core genetic service is defined as an integrated clinical and laboratory service, provided for those with/concerned about a disorder with a significant genetic component and their families, offering:

Accurate clinical and genetic laboratory diagnosis
Risk estimation
Genetic counseling (including predictive genetic testing)
Accessible written and spoken information for families/other health professionals and patient support groups
Support to individuals and families (e.g., in decision making about future pregnancies)
Prevention of a disorder or complications including family follow-up (e.g., anticipatory care, prenatal care, and testing)
Expert advice to other health professionals and health care commissioners
Education and training for other health professionals including those providing genetic counseling within other specialized services and for undergraduate and postgraduate students
Participation in research and clinical audit
A family-based approach where required
Maintenance of confidential family records
Maintenance of a DNA storage service.

Source: *Specialised Services National Definitions Set* (2nd Edition). Medical Genetic Services (all ages). Definition No. 20. (http://www.dh.gov.uk/en/Managingyourorganisation/Commissioning/Commissioningspecialisedservices/Specialisedservicesdefinition/DH_4001694; accessed April 11, 2008).

Box 39–2 Core Genetics Competences for Nongenetics Health Care Staff

The nine competences:

1. Identify where genetics is relevant in your area of practice.
2. Identify individuals with or at risk of genetic conditions.
3. Gather multigenerational family history information.
4. Use multigenerational family history information to draw a pedigree.
5. Recognize a mode of inheritance wiınin a family.
6. Assess genetic risk.
7. Refer individuals to specialist sources of assistance in meeting their health care needs.
8. Order a genetic laboratory test.
9. Communicate genetic information to individuals, families, and other health care staff.

Source: http://www.geneticseducation.nhs.uk/develop/index.asp?id=44; accessed 11April 2008.

For more detailed information, including performance criteria, knowledge, and understanding requirements for each competence, download the following document from the web site above: National Genetics Education and Development Centre, November 2007. Enhancing patient care by integrating genetics in clinical practice. U.K. workforce competences for genetics in clinical practice for nongenetics health care staff.

work collaboratively in this setting, it is important to be able to separate specialist cardiology activities from core genetics activities and specialist clinical genetics activities. For example, *diagnostic* genetic testing might be a shared task in some countries, but predictive testing is widely seen as the remit of clinical genetics services (van Langen et al. 2005); whereas arrhythmia risk assessment in a LQTS gene mutation carrier—which does take family history into account—is clearly the remit of a specialist cardiologist. Very few cardiologists are accredited in genetics (and vice versa), and most services work best in collaboration. Such collaborative working can only be enhanced by the introduction of core genetics competences into the roles of associated nongenetics specialist health care staff, such as cardiology nurses.

Core Characteristics of a Cardiac Genetics Service

The identification of a proband affected by inherited heart disease in whatever setting—following sudden death, whether symptomatic or asymptomatic—should prompt referral to a cardiac genetic service in order to address the familial implications of that diagnosis. Acknowledgment that genetics competences may reside in a number of different professionals allows a flexible, integrated approach to local service provision whose key underlying principle is communication. It is important that cardiac networks identify the specialist cardiology skills required to provide high-quality, up-to-date services; or indeed outsource to other networks where those skills do not exist locally.

1. Staff/Roles

- Consultant cardiologists (adult and pediatric) with specific expertise and experience in the management of inherited heart diseases.
- Cardiology nurse specialists with training in communication, evaluation, and management of adults and children with inherited heart diseases.
- Clinical genetics staff (consultant clinical geneticist, genetic counselors) with specific expertise in inherited heart diseases to coordinate cascade clinical assessment and both diagnostic and predictive DNA testing. Regional genetics services should act as a gateway to genetic testing to ensure effective use of genetic testing budgets.
- Echocardiography technicians/cardiac physiologists with specific training in the evaluation of inherited heart diseases.
- Access to specialist cardiac pathologists with specific training in inherited heart diseases.

2. Facilities for Diagnostic Assessment (Cardiology)

- Specialist echocardiography (with access to tissue Doppler, strain rate imaging and contrast echocardiography where required).
- Cardiac magnetic resonance imaging in cardiomyopathy.
- Exercise testing.
- Ambulatory electrocardiographic monitoring.
- Signal-averaged electrocardiography.
- Facilities for noninvasive or minimally invasive electrophysiology.
- Facilities for pharmacological challenge testing (e.g., Ajmaline).

3. Facilities for Diagnostic Assessment (Genetics)

- Access to accredited, comprehensive mutation analysis for the major genes involved in HCM, LQTS, ARVC, CPVT, and Marfan syndrome and related disorders.
- Guidelines for the application of such tests in a health service setting.
- Access to research-based extended mutation analysis where appropriate.

4. Information for Service Users

- Standardized disease-specific information endorsed by service users and/or patient support groups.
- Links with patient support groups.

5. Audit

Cardiac genetics is a new and emerging specialty. Services need to engage in collaborative audit to collect their experiences and share with others. Key areas for national-level data collection will be genetic testing (to study the phenotypes associated with individual genes and mutations in a "real life" clinical setting) and the outcome of investigations into sudden cardiac death. On a more local level it is important for services to monitor referral trends, waiting times, and host of other routine measures of service delivery. It is also important to involve service users and to seek feedback from them in order to help shape local services.

Service Configuration

Although local circumstances may dictate the manner in which cardiac genetics services are provided, care should be taken to ensure that all stakeholders in the service are fully engaged and that roles and responsibilities are clearly defined by the development of care pathways and clinical management protocols. Ideally, urgent referrals (e.g., following sudden cardiac death) should be coordinated by named individuals—a cardiac genetics nurse or genetic counselor, for example—or by a national coordinating center.

1. Sudden Unexplained Death

As discussed elsewhere in this volume, a significant number of autopsies are performed in young adults who have died unexpectedly and yield potential evidence of inherited heart disease (e.g., HCM, Marfan syndrome-type aortic dissection). In addition, a proportion of *unexplained* death in young adults is the result of inherited arrhythmia (see also Chapter 33). Following such a death, the first professionals to consider the possibility of an inherited heart disease is therefore the pathologist and a legal professional (in England and Wales, one of Her Majesty's Coroners) (see also Chapter 38). It is important that the surviving relatives of the deceased individual are warned of the possibility of familial diseases, and a recommendation is made that they undergo clinical (and, if relevant, genetic) screening. Pathologists should also be encouraged to retain tissue for DNA extraction and storage, so that a retrospective genetic diagnosis may be possible. In some centers, "molecular autopsy" is now being undertaken: DNA from the deceased individual is screened for mutations in key candidate genes, such as the potassium and sodium channel genes associated with LQTS and the ryanodine receptor gene associated with catecholaminergic polymorphic ventricular tachycardia (CPVT).

In England and Wales, the publication of the Coronary Heart Disease National Service Framework chapter on arrhythmia and sudden death, has led to the establishment of a specialist cardiac pathologist network and the Department of Health is working with coroners to examine their responsibilities and relationships with medical services. It has been recommended that U.K. cardiac networks develop local care pathways that encompass the immediate care of families affected by sudden cardiac death, supported by a national coordinating center. Similar work is under way in Scotland.

2. "Independent Services" Model for Cardiac Genetics Services

Some U.K. cardiac genetics services sit most naturally in a tertiary cardiology setting. This usually develops in centers with cardiologists who have undertaken focused training in inherited heart disease and research in cardiac genetics and usually with in-house genetic counselors and/or cardiac genetics nurses. An advantage of such a model is that expertise is concentrated in a single center, although a potential disadvantage is that such services may not develop strong links with regional genetics centers.

In addition, some U.K. centers host tertiary cardiology clinics for patients with inherited heart diseases separately from genetics clinics for the same patient group. Such an approach should be reinforced by regular liaison between the specialist cardiology and genetics teams outside clinic.

3. "Parallel Service" Model

A number of U.K. cardiac genetics services are provided in a tertiary setting in which a genetics clinic is held in parallel with a cardiology clinic. This is often the case with Marfan syndrome clinics, for example. Advantages of such an approach are that the clinic provides an opportunity for shared patient care and opportunistic discussion and it avoids organizational problems associated with joint clinics (see below). On the other hand, it can be difficult to coordinate such an approach, especially if both clinics are booked to their maximum capacity.

4. "Joint Service" Model

A number of U.K. centers have been providing joint Marfan syndrome clinics in a tertiary setting for many years. In such a clinic, a variety of health care professionals assemble to provide a multidisciplinary clinic for their patients. A Marfan syndrome clinic of this type will usually consist of a cardiologist, clinical geneticist, genetic counselor, ophthalmologist, and possibly a rheumatologist. A number of centers have also established joint inherited heart disease clinics, usually with a cardiologist who has expertise in cardiac arrhythmia.

Such clinics are often challenging to organize simply because they rely on a number of busy professionals coassembling on a single day, and even more challenging for health care commissioners to commission since the input from each specialist often varies from patient to patient. Nevertheless, from the patients' point of view, such clinics provide the opportunity for a "one stop" clinic, reducing the need for multiple hospital appointments; and for the professionals involved there is a clear opportunity for professional networking and case-based discussion.

5. "Network" Model

It is becoming clearer that, as a group, inherited heart diseases are relatively common and that highly specialized tertiary clinics are unlikely to be able to coordinate clinical cascade testing across an entire health care region for reasons of workload and finance. By engaging and creating formal links with district cardiology units, establishing devolved responsibilities and agreed clinical management protocols (e.g., undertaking clinical surveillance in a HCM family in which a mutation has not yet been identified), "hub and spoke" networks can evolve in which health care is shared appropriately and there is a clear framework for communication. Within such a network it is possible to provide coordinated triage of cases and therefore demand management for tertiary "hub" clinics either using referral guidelines or by identifying key individuals at secondary care level with mainstreamed genetics skills to provide local liaison and triage (e.g., a cardiac genetics nurse). As with tertiary joint clinics, however, this approach is potentially complex from a commissioning point of view, since the patient pathway crosses a number of service provider boundaries, although it does provide a potential opportunity for equitable patient management, resource management, and comprehensive clinical networking with optimal stakeholder involvement.

6. Working with Children

Most inherited heart diseases affect children to a greater or lesser degree, and the cardiology component of a cardiac genetics service needs to take this into account, especially with respect to pediatric electrophysiology services. In the United Kingdom, the National Service Framework for Children, Young People and Maternity Services (Department of Health 2004) sets standards for clinical services designed for children, and it is clear that children should not be managed in an adult clinic setting. Thought also needs to be given to transitional arrangements for adolescents.

Genetic testing in children is potentially different to testing in adults since they may not be considered competent to give informed consent. Their rights should be protected at all times. Diagnostic genetic testing in children should only really be undertaken if the result would benefit the child being tested. If the clinical diagnosis is clear it may not be necessary to use a genetic test to confirm that diagnosis. It is unlikely that the result of a genetic test would provide *prognostic* information. Testing a child for the benefit of others within the family may be difficult to justify, unless the child is mature enough to understand the nature of the request. Predictive genetic testing in childhood also needs to be considered on a case-by-case basis. A predictive test in a child should only be considered if he/she is at risk of developing the disease during childhood and if the result will benefit the child by affecting his/her medical management. These situations demand thoughtful, comprehensive discussion with the child's parents, who are likely to be anxious and concerned about siblings, for example, and genetic testing should only be undertaken in close collaboration with specialized genetics services. An illustrative case is presented in Figure 39–1.

7. Accountability and Supervision Arrangements

In settings where clinical genetic work is undertaken in a mainstreamed fashion (e.g., a secondary care-based cardiac genetics nurse, or where cardiology units have in-house genetic counselors), it is helpful—or indeed should be considered an essential requirement—for the staff involved to have formal arrangements for clinical and counseling supervision with the regional genetics service. In this way staff work within an accountability framework, which ensures maximum support for the individual concerned and their patients. In practice this is achievable by creating links with a named member of the regional clinical genetics team and developing informal mentorship arrangements, as well as the development of regular supervision meetings at which challenging cases or situations can be discussed in a supportive setting. This work may be undertaken with an external psychology service specializing in counseling supervision.

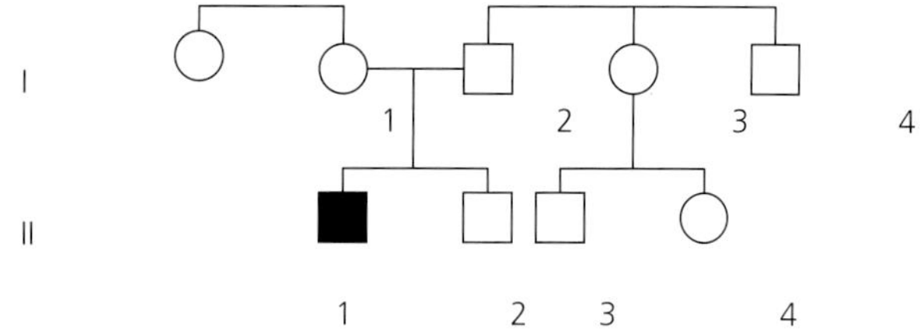

Figure 39–1 Genetic testing for inherited heart disease in children. The proband II:1 is diagnosed with LQTS following a near-drowning event in a school swimming pool at the age of 6 years. The T-wave morphology and association with swimming suggest a subdiagnosis of type 1 LQTS. He has an older male sibling aged 8 (II:2) and a paternal aunt (I:3) with a history of epilepsy. Both have normal 12-lead ECGs. She has children aged 10 and 14 years, both of whom are keen sports players.

The parents (I:1 and I:2) request genetic testing in II:1 to try and identify the causative potassium ion channel gene mutation, for use in a predictive context in the wider family, and to investigate the possibility that I:3 may in fact have LQTS. In this situation the gene test is unlikely to influence the clinical management of II:1. However, his sibling (II:2) is likely to be at 50% risk of having LQTS and is therefore at risk of cardiac arrhythmia. His paternal aunt and cousins may also be at risk. The normal 12-lead ECGs do not exclude LQTS with sufficient reassurance. After careful discussion with an experienced clinical geneticist, the parents and the pediatric cardiologist involved in his care, II:1 is able to understand the nature of the request for a blood sample and his parents give consent for genetic testing. The blood sample is taken under local anesthesia on a pediatric ward. A mutation is identified in the *KCNQ1* gene, confirming the diagnosis and allowing predictive testing. II:2 is tested for the mutation and is found not to carry it. I:3 also tests negative, and I:1 is found to be an asymptomatic heterozygote.

8. Laboratory Services

In the United Kingdom, most health service genetic testing is undertaken in accredited NHS laboratories integrated within regional genetics centers, although some occur in other laboratories; together these laboratories comprise the U.K. Genetic Testing Network (UK-GTN; www.ukgtn.nhs.uk). Genetic tests are usually funded using budgets allocated to regional genetics centers, and those funds are often restricted to tests provided by UK-GTN labs, although practice currently varies around the United Kingdom. Genetic testing undertaken in a research laboratory or in overseas laboratories may not be subject to the same quality assurance requirements as U.K. laboratories.

Laboratory services should aim to provide comprehensive services for the major clinically relevant disease genes, with a systematic strategy for service development (e.g., by adding exon dosage assays to existing sequencing-based assays; and adding new genes to existing test portfolios). Expertise should be concentrated in a small number of laboratories for reasons of quality assurance and finance (enabling low-cost testing in high-throughput settings, and regulating laboratory income). Links between service laboratories and established research groups will continue to provide translational research opportunities that should expand the number and nature of tests in coming years. Of key importance over the next decade will be the systematic collection of genotype–phenotype data, which will require close collaboration between laboratories and clinical services, and the introduction of new technologies, allowing high-throughput, more comprehensive testing. At all times, the clinical utility of such testing should be a major consideration.

Conclusions

In practice, clinical services for patients and families with inherited heart diseases need to be complex because the diseases themselves are complex from a genetic and phenotypic point of view. A host of service delivery models enable timely, expert, and coordinated care, perhaps most effectively as a multidisciplinary arrangement in which skills are recognized and used effectively. Services need to be aware of the ethical and legal framework in which they function, and develop policy around issues such as consent, genetic testing, and communication within families.

Acknowledgments

The author wishes to thank Professor John Burn for stimulating a lifelong interest in cardiac genetics and for handing over responsibility for developing a large regional cardiac genetics service.

References

Ad Hoc Committee on Genetic Counselling. American Society for Human Genetics. Genetic counseling. *Am J Hum Genet.* 1975;27:240–242.

Bezzina C, Veldkamp MW, van den Berg MP, et al. A single Na+ channel mutation causing both long-QT and Brugada syndromes. *Circ Res.* 1999;85:1206–1213.

Charron P, Heron D, Garguilo M, et al. Genetic testing and genetic counselling in hypertrophic cardiomyopathy: the French experience. *J Med Genet.* 2002;39:741–746.

Clarke A, Richards M, Kerzin-Storrar L, et al. Genetic professionals' reports of non-disclosure of genetic risk information within families. *Eur J Hum Genet.* 2005;13:556.

De Paepe A, Devereux RB, Dietz HC, et al. Revised diagnostic criteria for the Marfan syndrome. *Am J Med Genet.* 1996;62:417–426.

Department of Health. The NHS Cancer Plan: a plan for investment, a plan for reform; 2000. Available at: http://www.dh.gov.uk/en/PublicationsandstatisticsPublications/PublicationsPolicyAndGuidance/DH_4009609.

Department of Health. The National Service Framework for Children, Young People and Maternity Services; 2004. Available at: http://www.dh.gov.uk/PolicyAndGuidance/HealthAndSocialCareTopics/ChildrenServices/fs/en.

Department of Health. Concordat and moratorium on genetics and insurance; 2005a. Available at http://www.dh.gov.uk/en/Publicationsandstatistics/Publications/PublicationsPolicyAndGuidance/DH_4105905.

Department of Health. The National Service Framework for Coronary Heart Disease. Chapter 8: Arrhythmias and Sudden Cardiac Death; 2005b. Available at: http://www.dh.gov.uk/en/Healthcare/NationalServiceFrameworks/Coronaryheartdisease/DH_4117048.

Heart Rhythm UK Familial Sudden Death Syndromes Statement Development Group. Clinical indications for genetic testing in familial sudden cardiac death syndromes: an HRUK position statement. *Heart.* 2008;94:502–507.

Hendriks KS, Hendriks MM, Birnie E, et al. Familial disease with a risk of sudden death: a longitudinal study of the psychological consequences of predictive testing for long QT syndrome. *Heart Rhythm.* 2008;5:719–724.

Hendriks KWSH, Grosfeld FJM, van Tintelen JP, et al. Can parents adjust to the idea that their child is at risk for a sudden death? Psychological impact of risk for long QT syndrome. *Am J Med Genet.* 2005b;138A:107–112.

Hendriks KSWH, Grosfeld FJM, Wilde AAM, et al. High distress in parents whose children undergo predictive genetic testing for long QT syndrome. *Community Genet.* 2005a;8:103–113.

Joint Committee on Medical Genetics. *Consent and Confidentiality in Genetic Practice. Guidance on Genetic Testing and Sharing Genetic Information.* Royal College of Physicians of London;2006.

Kamisago M, Sharma SD, DePalma SR, et al. Mutations in sarcomere protein genes as a cause of dilated cardiomyopathy. *N Eng J Med.* 2000;343:1688–1696.

Laurie GT. Genetic information and the law. In: Mason JK, McCall Smith RA, eds. *Law and Medical Ethics.* London: Butterworths; 1999.

Newson AJ, Humphries SE. Cascade testing in familial hypercholesterolaemia: how should family members be contacted? *Eur J Hum Genet.* 2005;13:401–408.

Phillips KA, Ackerman MJ, Sakowski J, et al. Cost-effectiveness analysis of genetic testing for familial long QT syndrome in symptomatic index cases. *Heart Rhythm.* 2005;2:1294–1300.

Priori SG, Barhanin J, Hauer RNW, et al. Genetic and molecular basis of cardiac arrhythmias: impact on clinical management parts I and II. *Circulation.* 1999b;99:518–528.

Priori SG, Napolitano C, Schwartz PJ. Low penetrance in the long-QT syndrome. Clinical impact. *Circulation.* 1999a;99:529–533.

Public Health Genetics Foundation (2009). Heart to Heart: Inherited Cardiovascular Conditions Services. A needs assessment and service review. Available at: www.phgfoundation.org.

Schwartz PJ, Priori SG, Napolitano C. How really rare are rare diseases? The intriguing case of independent compound mutations in the long QT syndrome. *J Cardiovasc Electrophysiol.* 2003;14:1120–1121.

Schwartz PJ, Spazzolini C, Crotti L, et al. The Jervell and Lange Nielsen syndrome: natural history, molecular basis and clinical outcome. *Circulation.* 2006;113:783–790.

Splawski I, Shen J, Timothy KW, et al. Spectrum of mutations in long QT syndrome genes *KVLQT1, HERG, SCN5A, KCNE1* and *KCNE2. Circulation.* 2000;102:1178–1185.

Tester DJ, Will ML, Haglund CM, et al. Effect of clinical phenotype on yield of long QT syndrome genetic testing. *J Am Coll Cardiol.* 2006;47:764–768.

van Langen IM, Birnie E, Leschot NJ, et al. Genetic knowledge and counselling skills of Dutch cardiologists: sufficient for the genomics era? *Eur Heart J.* 2003;24:560–566.

van Langen IM, Birnie E, Schuurman E, et al. Preferences of cardiologists and clinical geneticists for future organisation of genetic health care in hypertrophic cardiomyopathy. *Clin Genet.* 2005;68:360–368.

Westenkow P, Splawski I, Timothy K, et al. Compound mutations: a common cause of severe long QT syndrome. *Circulation.* 2004;109:1834–1841.

Yamaguchi M, Shimizu M, Ino H, et al. Compound heterozygosity for mutations Asp611→Tyr in KCNQ1 and Asp609→Gly in KCNH2 associated with severe long QT syndrome. *Clin Sci.* 2005;108:143–150.

Glossary—Commonly Used Terms and Phrases in Cardiovascular Genetics

AA: antiarrhythmic.
Ablation: the removal, isolation, or destruction of cardiac tissue or conduction pathways involved in arrhythmias.
Acrocentric: a chromosome having the centromere close to one end.
Algorithm: a step-by-step method for solving a computational problem or a set of precise rules or procedures programmed into a pacemaker or defibrillator that are designed to solve a specific clinical problem.
Allele: an alternative form of a gene at the same chromosomal locus.
Allelic heterogeneity: different alleles for one gene.
Alternative splicing: a regulatory mechanism by which variations in the incorporation of coding regions (*see exon*) of the gene into messenger RNA (mRNA) lead to the production of more than one related protein or isoform.
Amino acid: a chemical subunit of a protein. Amino acids polymerize to form linear chains linked by peptide bonds called polypeptides. All proteins are made from 20 naturally occurring amino acids.
Amplification refractory mutation system (ARMS): an allele-specific PCR amplification reaction.
Annealing: the association of complementary DNA (or RNA) strands to form the double-stranded structure.
Anonymous DNA: DNA not known to have a coding function.
Annotation: the descriptive text that accompanies a sequence in a database method.
Antibody: a protein produced by the immune system in response to an antigen (*see antigen*). Antibodies bind to their target antigen to help the immune system destroy the foreign entity.
Anticipation: a phenomenon in which the age of onset of a disorder is reduced and/or severity of the phenotype is increased in successive generations.
Anticodon: the three bases of a tRNA molecule that form a complementary match to an mRNA codon and thus allow the tRNA to perform the key translation step in the process of information transfer from nucleic acid to protein.
Antigen: a molecule that is perceived by the immune system to be foreign.
Antitachycardia pacing (ATP): short, rapid, carefully controlled sequences of pacing pulses delivered by an implantable cardioverter-defibrillator (ICD) and used to terminate a tachycardia in the atria or ventricles.
Apoptosis: programmed cell death.
Arrest (Cardiac): cessation of the heart's normal rhythmic electrical and/or mechanical activity that causes immediate hemodynamic compromise.
ARVC/ARVD: arrhythmogenic right ventricular cardiomyopathy/ dysplasia; a new term of arrhythmogenic cardiomyopathy (AC) is preferred due to biventricular involvement in most cases of ARVC/ARVD.
Arrhythmia: any heart rhythm that falls outside the accepted norms with respect to rate, regularity, or sequence of depolarization. (Any abnormal or absent heart rhythm.)
Atrial fibrillation (AF): very fast, disorganized heart rhythm that starts in the atria.
Atrial flutter (AFL): fast, organized atrial rhythm.
Atrial tachycardia (AT): a rapid heart rate that starts in the atria (includes AF and AFL).
Atrioventricular (AV) node: a section of specialized neuromuscular cells that are part of the normal conduction pathway between the atria and the ventricles. (A junction that conducts electrical impulses from the atria to the ventricles of the heart.)
Atrioventricular (AV) synchrony: the normal activation sequence of the heart in which the atria contract and then, after a brief delay, the ventricles contract. The loss of AV synchrony can have significant hemodynamic effects. Dual chamber pacemakers are designed to attempt to maintain AV synchrony.
Atrium: the heart is divided into four chambers. Each of the two upper chambers is called an atrium. (Atria is the plural form of atrium.) Either of the two upper chambers of the heart, above the ventricles that receive blood from the veins and communicate with the ventricles through the tricuspid (right) or mitral (left) valve.
Autosome: any chromosome other than a sex chromosome (X or Y) and the mitochondrial chromosome.
Autozygosity: in an inbred person, homozygosity for alleles identical by descent.
Autozygosity mapping: a form of genetic mapping for autosomal recessive disorders in which affected individuals are expected to have two identical disease alleles by descent.
AVID: Antiarrhythmics Versus Implantable Defibrillators study.
Bacterial artificial chromosome (BAC): DNA vectors into which large DNA fragments can be inserted and cloned in a bacterial host.
Bioinformatics: an applied computational system that includes development and utilization of facilities to store, analyze, and interpret biological data.
Biotechnology: the industrial application of biological processes, particularly recombinant DNA technology and genetic engineering.
BLAST (Basic Local Alignment Search Tool): a fast database similarity search tool used by the NCBI that allows the world to search query sequences against the GeneBank database over the web.
Blastocyst: the mammalian embryo at the stage at which it is implanted into the wall of the uterus.
Bradycardia (Bradyarrhythmia): a heart rate that is abnormally slow; commonly defined as under 60 beats per minute or a rate that is too slow to physiologically support a person and their activities.
CABG: coronary artery bypass graft.

CAD: coronary artery disease.
CASH: Cardiac Arrest Study Hamburg.
CHD: coronary heart disease.
CHF: congestive heart failure.
CIDS: Canadian Implantable Defibrillator Study.
Candidate gene: any gene which by virtue of a known property (function, expression pattern, chromosomal location, structural motif, etc.) is considered as a possible locus for a given disease.
Cardiac arrest: failure of the heart to pump blood through the body. If left untreated, it is dangerous and life threatening.
Cardioversion: termination of an atrial or ventricular tachyarrhythmia (other than ventricular fibrillation) by a delivery of a direct low-energy electrical current, which is synchronized to a specific instant during the heart beat (during to the ventricular depolarization). Synchronization of the shock prevents shocking during periods that could cause ventricular fibrillation.
Carrier: a person who carries an allele for a recessive disease (*see heterozygote*) without the disease phenotype but can pass it on to the next generation.
Carrier testing: carried out to determine whether an individual carries one copy of an altered gene for a particular recessive disease.
Cell cycle: series of tightly regulated steps that a cell goes through from its creation to division to form two daughter cells.
"Central Dogma": a term proposed by Francis Crick in 1957—"DNA is transcribed into RNA which is translated into protein."
cDNA (complementary DNA): a piece of DNA copied in vitro from mRNA by a reverse transcription enzyme.
CentiMorgan (cM): a unit of genetic distance equivalent to 1% probability of recombination during meiosis. One centiMorgan is equivalent, on average, to a physical distance of approximately 1 megabase in the human genome.
Centromere: the constricted region near the center of a chromosome that has critical role in cell division.
Chimera: a hybrid, particularly a synthetic DNA molecule that is the result of ligation of DNA fragments that come from different organisms or an organism derived from more than one zygote.
Chromosome: subcellular structures that contain and convey the genetic material of an organism.
Chromosome painting: fluorescent labeling of whole chromosomes by a fluorescence in situ hybridization (FISH) procedure in which labeled probes each consist of complex mixture of different DNA sequences from a single chromosome.
Chronic lead: a pacemaker or ICD lead that has been implanted in the past.
Chronotropic incompetence: the inability of the heart to increase its rate appropriately in response to increased activity or metabolic need, for example, exercise, illness, and so on.
Class I antiarrhythmic drugs: drugs that act selectively to depress fast sodium channels, slowing conduction in all parts of the heart (e.g., *Quinidine, Procainamide, Flecainide, Encainide, Propafenone*).
Class II antiarrhythmic drugs: drugs that act as beta-adrenergic blocking agents (e.g., *Propanolol, Metoprolol, Atenolol*).
Class III antiarrhythmic drugs: drugs that act directly on cardiac cell membrane, prolong repolarization and refractory periods, increase VF threshold, and act on peripheral smooth muscle to decrease peripheral resistance (e.g., *Amiodarone, Sotalol*),
Clinical sensitivity: the proportion of persons with a disease phenotype who test positive.
Clinical specificity: the proportion of persons without a disease phenotype who test negative.
Clone: a line of cells derived from a single cell and therefore carrying identical genetic material.
Cloning vector: a DNA construct such as a plasmid, modified viral genome (bacteriophage or phage), or artificial chromosome that can be used to carry a gene or fragment of DNA for purposes of cloning (e.g., a bacterial, yeast, or mammalian cell).
Coagulation factors: various components of the blood coagulation system. The following factors have been identified: (Synonyms that are or have been in use are included). Factor I (fibrinogen); Factor II (prothrombin); Factor III (thromboplastin, tissue factor); Factor IV (calcium); Factor V (labile factor); Factor VII (stable factor); Factor VIII (antihemophilic globulin [AHF], antihemophilic globulin [AHG], antihemophilic factor A Factor VIII: C); Factor IX (plasma thromboplastin component [PTC], Christmas factor, antihemophilic factor B); Factor X (Stuart factor, Prower factor, Stuart-Prower factor); Factor XI (plasma thromboplastin antecedent [PTA], antihemophilic factor C); Factor XII (Hageman factor, surface factor, contact factor); Factor XIII (fibrin stabilizing factor [FSF], fibrin stabilizing enzyme, fibrinase); other factors: (prekallikrein [Fletcher factor], and high molecular weight kininogen [Fizgerald]).
Coding DNA (sequence): the portion of a gene that is transcribed into mRNA.
Codon: a three-base sequence of DNA or RNA that specifies a single amino acid.
Comparative genomics: the comparison of genome structure and function across different species in order to further the understanding of biological mechanisms and evolutionary processes.
Comparative genome hybridization (CGH): use of competitive FISH to detect chromosomal regions that are amplified or deleted, especially in tumors.
Complementary DNA (cDNA): DNA generated from an expressed messenger RNA through a process known as reverse transcription.
Complex diseases: diseases characterized by risk to relatives of an affected individual, which is greater than the incidence of the disorder in the population
Complex trait: one that is not strictly *Mendelian* (dominant, recessive, or sex linked) and may involve the interaction of two or more genes to produce a phenotype, or may involve *gene–environment* interactions.
Computational therapeutics: an emerging biomedical field concerned with the development of techniques for using software to collect, manipulate, and link biological and medical data from diverse sources. It also includes the use of such information in simulation models to make predictions or therapeutically relevant discoveries or advances.
Computer aided diagnosis [CAD]: a general term used for a variety of artificial intelligence techniques applied to medical images. CAD methods are being rapidly developed at several academic and industry sites, particularly for large-scale breast, lung, and colon cancer screening studies. X-ray imaging for breast, lung, and colon cancer screening are good physical and clinical models for the development of CAD methods, related image database resources, and for the development of common metrics and methods for evaluation. [Large-scale screening applications include (a) improving the sensitivity of cancer detection, (b) reducing observer variation in image interpretation, (c) increasing the efficiency of reading large image arrays, (d) improving efficiency of screening by identifying suspect lesions or identifying normal images, and (e) facilitating remote reading by experts (e.g., telemammography).]
Congenital: any trait, condition, or disorder that exists from birth.
Consanguinity: marriage between two individuals having common ancestral parents, commonly between first cousins; an approved practice in some communities who share social, cultural, and religious beliefs. In genetic terms two such individuals could be heterozygous by descent for an allele expressed as "*coefficient of relationship*," and any offspring could be therefore homozygous by descent for the same allele expressed as "*coefficient of inbreeding.*"
Conserved sequence: a base sequence in a DNA molecule (or an amino acid sequence in a protein) that has remained essentially unchanged throughout evolution.
Constitutional mutation: a mutation which is inherited and therefore present in all cells containing the relevant nucleic acid (same as *germline mutation*).
Contig: a consensus sequence generated from a set of overlapping sequence fragments that represent a large piece of DNA, usually a genomic region from a particular chromosome.
Copy number: the number of different copies of a particular DNA sequence in a genome.
Copy number variation (CNV): variation in copy number sequences, likely to be of pathogenic importance for certain complex disease traits.

CpG island: short stretch of DNA, often less than 1 kb, containing CpG dinucleotides that are unmethylated and present at the expected frequency. CpG islands often occur at transcriptionally active DNA.
Cytoplasm: the internal matrix of a cell. The cytoplasm is the area between the outer periphery of a cell (the cell membrane) and the nucleus (in a eukaryotic cell).
DCM: dilated cardiomyopathy.
DFT: defibrillation threshold.
Defibrillation: termination of an erratic, life-threatening arrhythmia of the ventricles by a high-energy, direct current delivered asynchronously to the cardiac tissue. The defibrillation discharge will often restore the heart's normal rhythm.
Denaturation: dissociation of complementary strands to give single-stranded DNA and/or RNA.
Demographic transition: the change in the society from extreme poverty to a stronger economy, often associated by a transition in the pattern of diseases from malnutrition and infection to the intractable conditions of middle and old age, for example, cardiovascular disease, diabetes, and cancer.
Diagnostics: data gathered by an ICD or pacemaker to evaluate patient rhythm status, verify system operation, or assure appropriate delivery of therapy options.
Diploid: a genome (the total DNA content contained in each cell) that consists of two homologous copies of each chromosome.
Disease: a fluid concept influenced by societal and cultural attitudes that change with time and in response to new scientific and medical discoveries. The human genome sequence will dramatically alter how we define, prevent, and treat disease. Similar collection of symptoms and signs (*phenotype*) may have very different underlying genetic constitution (*genotype*). As genetic capabilities increase, additional tools will become available to subdivide disease designations that are clinically identical (*see taxonomy of disease).*
Disease etiology: any factor or series of related events directly or indirectly causing a disease. For example, the genomics revolution has improved our understanding of disease determinants and provided a deeper understanding of molecular mechanisms and biological processes (see "*Systems Biology*").
Disease expression: when a pathogenic genotype is manifested in the *phenotype.*
Disease management: a continuous, coordinated health care process that seeks to manage and improve the health status of a patient over the entire course of a disease. The term may also apply to a patient population. Disease management services include disease prevention efforts as well as patient management.
Disease phenotype: includes disease related changes in tissues as judged by gross anatomical, histological, and molecular pathological changes. Gene and protein expression analysis and interpretation studies, particularly at the whole genome level, are able to distinguish apparently similar phenotypes.
Diversity, genomic: the number of base differences between two genomes divided by the genome size.
DNA (deoxyribonucleic acid): the chemical that comprises the genetic material of all cellular organisms.
DNA cloning: replication of DNA sequences ligated into a suitable vector in an appropriate host organism (see *Cloning vector*).
DNA fingerprinting: use of hypervariable minisatellite probe (usually those developed by Alec Jeffreys) on a Southern blot to produce an individual-specific series of bands for identification of individuals or relationships.
DNA library: a collection of cell clones containing different recombinant DNA clones.
DNA sequencing: technologies through which the order of base pairs in a DNA molecule can be determined.
Domain: a discrete portion of a protein with its own function. The combination of domains in a single protein determines its overall function.
Dominant: an allele (or the trait encoded by that allele) that produces its characteristic phenotype when present in the heterozygous form.
Dominant negative mutation: a mutation that results in a mutant gene product that can inhibit the function of the wild-type gene product in heterozygotes.
Dosage effect: the number of copies of a gene; variation in the number of copies can result in aberrant gene expression or associated with disease phenotype.
Drug design: development of new classes of medicines based on a reasoned approach using gene sequence and protein structure function information rather than the traditional trial and error method.
Drug interactions: refer to adverse drug interaction, drug–drug interaction, drug–laboratory interaction, drug–food interaction, and so on. It is defined as an action of a drug on the effectiveness or toxicity of another drug.
Dual-chamber pacemaker: A pacemaker with two leads (one in the atrium and one in the ventricle) to allow pacing and/or sensing in both chambers of the heart to artificially restore the natural contraction sequence of the heart. (Also called physiologic pacing.)
EF: ejection fraction.
EP: electrophysiologic.
EPS: electrophysiologic study.
ESC: European Society of Cardiology.
Electronic Health Record (EHR): a real-time patient health record with access to evidence-based decision support tools that can be used to aid clinicians in decision-making, automating, and streamlining clinician's workflow, ensuring that all clinical information is communicated. It can also support the collection of data for uses other than clinical care, such as billing, quality management, outcome reporting, and public health disease surveillance and reporting.
Ejection fraction: a measure of the output of the heart with each heartbeat (stroke volume divided by end-diastolic volume).
Electrocardiogram (ECG): a printout from an electrocardiography machine used to measure and record the electrical activity of the heart.
Electromagnetic interference (EMI): equipment and appliances that use magnets and electricity have electromagnetic fields around them. If these fields are strong, they may interfere with the operation of the ICD.
Electrophysiology (EP) study: The use of programmed stimulation protocols to assess the electrical activity of the heart in order to diagnose arrhythmias.
Embryonic stem cells (ES cells): a cell line derived from undifferentiated, pluripotent cells from the embryo.
Enhancer: a regulatory DNA sequence that increases transcription of a gene. An enhancer can function in either orientation and it may be located up to several thousand base pairs upstream or down stream from the gene it regulates.
ENTREZ: an online search and retrieval system that integrates information from databases at NCBI. These databases include nucleotide sequences, protein sequences, macromolecular structures, whole genomes, OMIM, and MEDLINE, through PubMed.
Environmental factors: may include chemical, dietary factors, infectious agents, physical and social factors.
Enzyme: a protein which acts as a biological catalyst that controls the rate of a biochemical reaction within a cell.
Epigenetic: a term describing nonmutational phenomenon, such as methylation and histone modification, that modify the expression of a gene.
Euchromatin: the fraction of the nuclear genome which contains transcriptionally active DNA and which, unlike *heterochromatin*, adopts a relatively extended conformation.
Eukaryote: an organism whose cells show internal compartmentalization in the form of membrane-bounded organelles (includes animals, plants, fungi, and algae).
Exon: the sections of a gene that code for all of its functional product. Eukaryotic genes may contain many exons interspersed with noncoding introns. An exon is represented in the mature mRNA product—the portions of an mRNA molecule that is left after all introns are spliced out, which serves as a template for protein synthesis.
Expression sequences tag (EST): partial or full complement DNA sequences that can serve as markers for regions of the genome that encode expressed products.
Family history: an essential tool in clinical genetics. Interpreting the family history can be complicated by many factors, including small families, incomplete or erroneous family histories, consanguinity, variable

penetrance, and the current lack of real understanding of the multiple genes involved in polygenic (complex) diseases.

Fibrillation: a chaotic and unsynchronized quivering of the myocardium during which no effective pumping occurs. Fibrillation may occur in the atria or the ventricles.

Fluorescence in situ hybridization (FISH): a form of chromosome in situ hybridization in which nucleic acid probe is labeled by incorporation of a *flurophore*, a chemical group that fluoresces when exposed to UV irradiation.

Founder effect: changes in allelic frequencies that occur when a small group is separated from a large population and establishes in a new location.

Founder mutation: specific mutation in a particular gene present in an ethnic migrant population that is prevalent in the indigenous population.

Frame-shift mutation: the addition or deletion of a number of DNA bases that is not a multiple of three, thus causing a shift in the reading frame of the gene. This shift leads to a change in the reading frame of all parts of a gene that are downstream from the mutation leading to a premature stop codon, and thus to a truncated protein product.

Functional genomics: the development and implementation of technologies to characterize the mechanisms through which genes and their products function and interact with each other and with the environment.

Gain-of-function mutation: a mutation that produces a protein that takes on a new or enhanced function.

Gene: the fundamental unit of heredity; in molecular terms, a gene comprises a length of DNA that encodes a functional product, which may be a polypeptide (a whole or constituent part of a protein or an enzyme) or a ribonucleic acid. It includes regions that precede and follow the coding region as well as introns and exons. The exact boundaries of a gene are often ill-defined since many promoter and enhancer regions dispersed over many kilobases may influence transcription.

Gene-based therapy: refers to all treatment regimens that employ or target genetic material. This includes (1) *transfection* (introducing cells whose genetic make-up is modified); (2) *antisense* therapy; and (3) *naked DNA* vaccination.

Gene expression: the process through which a gene is activated at a particular time and place so that its functional product is produced, that is, transcription into mRNA followed by translation into protein.

Gene expression profile: the pattern of changes in the expression of a specific set of genes that is relevant to a disease or treatment. The detection of this pattern depends on the use of specific gene expression measurement technique.

Gene family: a group of closely related genes that make similar protein products.

Gene knockouts: a commonly used technique to demonstrate the phenotypic effects and/or variation related to a particular gene in a model organism, for example, in mouse (see *Knockout*); absence of many genes may have no apparent effect upon phenotypes (though stress situations may reveal specific susceptibilities). Other single knockouts may have a catastrophic effect on the organism, or be lethal so that the organism cannot develop at all.

Gene regulatory network: a functional map of the relationships between a number of different genes and gene products (proteins), regulatory molecules, and so on that define the regulatory response of a cell with respect to a particular physiological function.

Gene therapy: a therapeutic medical procedure that involves either replacing/manipulating or supplementing nonfunctional genes with healthy genes. Gene therapy can be targeted to somatic (body) or germ (egg and sperm) cells. In *somatic gene therapy* the recipient's genome is changed, but the change is not passed along to the next generation. In *germline gene therapy*, the parent's egg or sperm cells are changed with the goal of passing on the changes to their offspring.

Genetics: refers to the study of heredity, gene, and genetic material. In contrast to genomics, the genetics is traditionally related to lower-throughput, smaller-scale emphasis on single genes, rather than on studying structure, organization, and function of many genes.

Genetic architecture: refers to the full range of genetic effects on a trait. Genetic architecture is a moving target that changes according to gene and genotype frequencies, distributions of environmental factors, and such biological properties as age and sex.

Genetic code: the relationship between the order of nucleotide bases in the coding region of a gene and the order of amino acids in the polypeptide product. It is universal, triplet, non-overlapping code such that each set of three bases (termed a codon) specifies which of the 20 amino acids is present in the polypeptide chain product of a particular position.

Genetic counseling: an important process for individuals and families who have a genetic disease or who are at risk for such a disease. Genetic counseling provides patients and other family members information about their condition and helps them make informed decisions.

Genetic determinism: the unsubstantiated theory that genetic factors determine a person's health, behavior, intelligence, or other complex attributes.

Genetic engineering: the use of molecular biology techniques such as restriction enzymes, ligation, and cloning to transfer genes among organisms (*also known as recombinant DNA cloning).*

Genetic epidemiology: a field of research in which correlations are sought between phenotypic trends and genetic variation across population groups.

Genetic map: a map showing the positions of genetic markers along the length of a chromosome relative to each other (genetic map) or in absolute distances from each other.

Genetic susceptibility: predisposition to a particular disease due to the presence of a specific allele or combination of alleles in an individual's genome.

Genome: the complete set of chromosomal and extra-chromosomal DNA/RNA of an organism, a cell, an organelle, or a virus.

Genome annotation: the process through which landmarks in a genomic sequence are characterized using computational and other means; for example, genes are identified, predictions made as to the function of their products, their regulatory regions defined, and intergenic regions characterized (see *Annotation*).

Genome project: the research and technology development effort aimed at mapping and sequencing the entire genome of human beings and other organisms.

Genomics: the study of the genome and its action. The term is commonly used to refer to large-scale, high-throughput molecular analyses of multiple genes, gene products, or regions of genetic material (DNA and RNA). The term also includes the comparative aspect of genomes of various species, their evolution, and how they relate to each other (see *comparative genomics*).

Genotype: the genetic constitution of an organism; commonly used in reference to a specific disease or trait.

Genomic instability: an increased tendency of the genome to acquire mutations when various processes involved in maintaining and replicating the genome are dysfunctional.

Genomic drugs: drugs based on molecular targets; genomic knowledge of the genes involved in diseases, disease pathways, and drug response.

Genomic profiling: complete genomic sequence of an individual including the expression profile. This would be targeted to specific requirements, for example, most common complex diseases (diabetes, hypertension, and coronary heart disease).

Genetic discrimination: unfavorable discrimination of an individual, a family, community, or an ethnic group on the basis of genetic information. Discrimination may include societal segregation, political persecution, opportunities for education and training, lack or restricted employment prospects, and adequate personal financial planning, for example, life insurance and mortgage.

Genetic screening: testing a population group to identify a subset of individuals at high risk for having or transmitting a specific genetic disorder.

Genetic test: an analysis performed on human DNA, RNA, genes, and/or chromosomes to detect heritable or acquired genotypes. A genetic test also is the analysis of human proteins and certain metabolites, which are predominantly used to detect heritable or acquired genotypes, mutations, or phenotypes.

Genetic testing: strictly refers to testing for a specific chromosomal abnormality or a DNA (nuclear or mitochondrial) mutation already known to exist in a family member. This includes diagnostic testing (postnatal or prenatal), presymptomatic or predictive genetic testing, or for establishing the carrier status. The individual concerned should have been offered full information on all aspects of the genetic test through the process of "*nonjudgmental and non-directive*" genetic counseling. Most laboratories require a formal fully informed signed consent before carrying out the test. Genetic testing commonly involves DNA/RNA-based tests for single gene variants, complex genotypes, acquired mutations, and measures of gene expression. Epidemiologic studies are needed to establish clinical validity of each method to establish sensitivity, specificity, and predictive value.

Germline cells: a cell with a haploid chromosome content (also referred to as a gamete); in animals, sperm, or egg and in plants, pollen, or ovum.

Germline mosaic (germinal mosaic, gonadal mosaic, gonosomal mosaic): an individual who has a subset of germline cells carrying a mutation that is not found in other germline cells.

Germline mutation: a gene change in the body's reproductive cells (egg or sperm) that becomes incorporated into the DNA of every cell in the body of offspring; germline mutations are passed on from parents to offspring, also called *hereditary mutation*.

HCM: hypertrophic cardiomyopathy.

Haploid: describing a cell (typically a gamete) that has only a single copy of each chromosome (i.e., 23 in man).

Haplotype: a series of closely linked loci on a particular chromosome that tend to be inherited together as a block.

Heart block: a condition in which electrical impulses are not conducted in the normal fashion from the atria to the ventricles. May be caused by damage or disease processes within the cardiac conduction system.

Hemodynamics: the forces involved in circulating blood through the cardiovascular system. The heart adapts its hemodynamic performance to the needs of the body, increasing its output of blood when muscles are working and decreasing output when the body is at rest.

Heterozygote: refers to a particular allele of a gene at a defined chromosome locus. A heterozygote has a different allelic form of the gene at each of the two homologous chromosomes.

Heterozygosity: the presence of different alleles of a gene in one individual or in a population—a measure of genetic diversity.

Holter monitoring: a technique for the continuous recording of electrocardiographic (ECG) signals, usually over 24 hours, to detect and diagnose ECG changes. (Also called ambulatory monitoring.)

Homology: similarity between two sequences due to their evolution from a common ancestor, often referred to as *homologs*.

Homozygote: refers to same allelic form of a gene on each of the two homologous chromosomes.

Human Genome Project: a program to determine the sequence of the entire 3 billion bases of the human genome.

Human Genetics Commission: established in December 1999 in order to provide strategic advice to the U.K. Government on how new developments in human genetics will impact on people and on health care. It has a particular remit to advise on the social, ethical, and legal implications of these developments. (http://www.hgc.gov.uk/)

Human gene transfer: the process of transferring genetic material (DNA or RNA) into a person; an experimental therapeutic procedure to treat certain health problems by compensating for defective genes, producing a potentially therapeutic substance, or triggering the immune system to fight disease. This may help improve genetic disorders, particularly those conditions that result from inborn errors in a single gene (e.g., sickle cell anemia, hemophilia, and cystic fibrosis), as well as with complex disorders, like cancer, heart disease, and certain infectious diseases, such as HIV/AIDS.

ICD: abbreviation for *Implantable Cardioverter-Defibrillator.* An ICD is an implanted device used to treat abnormal, fast heart rhythms. Several types of therapies are used by the ICD, including cardioversion, defibrillation, and antitachycardia pacing.

Identity by descent (IBD): alleles in an individual or in two people that are identical because they have been inherited from the same common ancestor, as opposed to *identity by state (IBS)*, which is coincidental possession of similar alleles in unrelated individuals (see *Consanguinity*).

Immunogenomics: refers to the study of organization, function, and evolution of vertebrate defense genes, particularly those encoded by the major histocompatibility complex (MHC) and the leukocyte receptor complex (LRC). Both complexes form integral parts of the immune system. The MHC is the most important genetic region in relation to infection and common disease such as autoimmunity. Driven by pathogen variability, immune genes have become the most polymorphic loci known, with some genes having over 500 alleles. The main function of these genes is to provide protection against pathogens and they achieve this through complex pathways for antigen processing and presentation.

Informatics: the study of the application of computer and statistical techniques to the management of information. In genome projects, informatics includes the development of methods to search databases quickly, to analyze DNA sequence information, and to predict protein sequence and structure from DNA sequence data.

Intron: a noncoding sequence within eukaryotic genes that separates the exons (coding regions). Introns are spliced out of the messenger RNA molecule created from a gene after transcription, prior to protein translation (protein synthesis).

Ischemia: insufficient blood flow to tissue due to blockage in the blood flow through the arteries.

Isoforms/isozymes: alternative forms of protein/enzyme.

In situ hybridization: hybridization of a labeled nucleic acid to a target nucleic acid that is typically immobilized on a microscopic slide, such as DNA of denatured metaphase chromosomes [as in fluorescent in situ hybridization (FISH)] or the RNA in a section of tissue [as in tissue in situ hybridization (TISH)].

In vitro: (Latin) literally "in glass," meaning outside of the organism in the laboratory, for example, a tissue culture.

In vivo: (Latin) literally "in life," meaning within a living organism.

Knockout: a technique used primarily in mouse genetics to inactivate a particular gene in order to define its function.

LOS: length of stay.

LQTS: long QT syndrome.

Lead: in an ICD system, the wire or catheter that conducts energy from the ICD to the heart, and from the heart to the ICD.

Left ventricular dysfunction: a heart condition in which the heart is unable to maintain normal cardiac output due to a deficiency in the left ventricle.

Library: a collection of genomic or complementary DNA sequences from a particular organism that have been cloned in a vector and grown in an appropriate host organism (e.g., bacteria or yeast).

Ligase: an enzyme that can use ATP to create phosphate bonds between the ends of two DNA fragments, effectively joining two DNA molecules into one.

Linkage: the phenomenon whereby pairs of genes that are located in close proximity on the same chromosome tend to be co-inherited.

Linkage analysis: a process of locating genes on the chromosome by measuring recombination rates between phenotypic and genetic markers (see *Lod score*).

Linkage disequilibrium: the nonrandom association in a population of alleles at nearby loci.

Locus: the specific site on a chromosome at which a particular gene or other DNA landmark is located.

Lod score: a measure of likelihood of genetic linkage between loci; a lod score greater than +3 is often taken as evidence of linkage; one that is less than –2 is often taken as evidence against linkage.

Loss-of-function mutation: a mutation that decreases the production or function (or both) of the gene product.

Loss of heterozygosity (LOH): loss of alleles on one chromosome detected by assaying for markers for which an individual is constitutionally heterozygous.

Lyonization: the process of random X chromosome inactivation in mammals.

Marker: a specific feature at an identified physical location on a chromosome, whose inheritance can be followed. The position of a gene implicated in a particular phenotypic effect can be defined through its linkage to such markers.

Meiosis: reductive cell division occurring exclusively in testis and ovary and resulting in the production of haploid cells, including sperm cells and egg cells.

Mendelian genetics: classical genetics, focuses on *monogenic* genes with high *penetrance*. The mendelian genetics is a true *paradigm* and is used in discussing the mode of inheritance (see *Monogenic disease*).

Messenger RNA (mRNA): RNA molecules that are synthesized from a DNA template in the nucleus (a gene) and transported to ribosomes in the cytoplasm where they serve as a template for the synthesis of protein (translation).

Microarrays diagnostics: a rapidly developing tool increasingly used in pharmaceutical and genomics research and has the potential for applications in high-throughput diagnostic devices. Microarrays can be made of DNA sequences with known gene mutations, polymorphisms, and selected protein molecules.

Microsatellite DNA: small array (often less than 0.1 kb) of short tandemly repeated DNA sequences.

Minisatellite DNA: an intermediate size array (often 0.1–20 kb long) of short tandemly repeated DNA sequences. *Hypervariable minisatellite* DNA is the basis of DNA fingerprinting and many VNTR markers.

Missense mutation: substitution of a single DNA base that results in a codon that specifies an alternative amino acid.

Mitochondria: cellular organelles present in eukaryotic organisms that enable aerobic respiration and generate the energy to drive cellular processes. Each mitochondria contains a small amount of circular DNA encoding a small number of genes (approximately 50).

Mitosis: cell division in somatic cells.

Model organism: an experimental organism in which a particular physiological process or disease has similar characteristics to the corresponding process in humans, permitting the investigation of the common underlying mechanisms.

Modifier gene: a gene whose expression can influence a phenotype resulting from mutation at another locus.

Molecular genetic screening: screening a section of the population known to be at a higher risk to be heterozygous for one of the mutations in the gene for a common autosomal recessive disease, for example, screening for cystic fibrosis in the North-European populations and beta-thalassemia in the Mediterranean and Middle-East population groups.

Molecular genetic testing: molecular genetic testing for use in patient diagnosis, management, and genetic counseling; this is increasingly used in presymptomatic (predictive) genetic testing of "at-risk" family members using a previously known disease-causing mutation in the family.

Mosaic: a genetic mosaic is an individual who has two or more genetically different cell lines derived from a single zygote.

Motif: a DNA-sequence pattern within a gene that, because of its similarity to sequences in other known genes, suggests a possible function of the gene, its protein products, or both.

Multifactorial disease: any disease or disorder caused by interaction of multiple genetic (polygenic) and environmental factors.

Multigene family: a set of evolutionary related loci within a genome, at least one of which can encode a functional product.

Mutation: a heritable alteration in the DNA sequence.

Myocardial infarction: death of a portion of the heart muscle tissue due to a blockage or interruption in the supply of blood to the heart muscle.

Myocardium: the middle and the thickest layer of the heart wall, composed of cardiac muscle.

Natural selection: the process whereby some of the inherited genetic variation within a population will affect the ability of individuals to survive to reproduce (*fitness*).

Neutral mutation: a change or alteration in DNA sequence that has no phenotypic effect (or has no effect on fitness).

New-born screening: performed in newborns in state public health programs to detect certain genetic diseases for which early diagnosis and treatment are available.

Noncoding sequence: a region of DNA that is not translated into protein. Some noncoding sequences are regulatory portions of genes, others may serve structural purposes (telomoeres, centromeres), while some others may not have any function.

Nonconservative mutation: a change in the DNA or RNA sequence that leads to the replacement of one amino acid with a very dissimilar one.

Nonsense mutation: substitution of a single DNA base that leads in a stop codon, thus leading to the truncation of a protein.

Northern blot hybridization: a form of molecular hybridization in which target consists of RNA molecules that have been size fractioned by gel electrophoresis and subsequently transferred to a membrane.

Nucleotide: a subunit of the DNA or RNA molecule. A nucleotide is a base molecule (adenine, cytosine, guanine, and thymine in the case of DNA), linked to a sugar molecule (deoxyribose or ribose) and phosphate groups.

Nullizygous: lacking any copy of a gene or DNA sequence normally found in chromosomal DNA, usually resulting from homozygous deletion in an autosome or from a single deletion in sex chromosomes in male.

Oncogene: an acquired mutant form of a gene that acts to transform a normal cell into a cancerous one.

OMIM: acronym for McKusick's On-line Mendelian Inheritance in Man, a regularly updated electronic catalog of inherited human disorders and phenotypic traits accessible on NCBI network. Each entry is designated by a number (*MIM number*).

Open reading frame (ORF): a significantly long sequence of DNA in which there are no termination codons. Each DNA duplex can have six reading frames, three for each single strand.

Ortholog: one set of homologous genes or proteins that perform similar functions in different species, that is, identical genes from different species, for example, *SRY* in humans and *Sry* in mice.

Paralog: similar genes (members of a gene family) or proteins (homologous) in a single species or different species that perform different functions.

Penetrance: the likelihood that a person carrying a particular mutant gene will have an altered phenotype (*see Phenotype*).

PFGE (Pulse Field Gel Eletrophoresis): a form of gel electrophoresis that permits size fractionation of large DNA molecules.

Pharmacogenomics: the identification of the genes that influence individual variation in the efficacy or toxicity of therapeutic agents and the application of this information in clinical practice.

Phenotype: the clinical and/or any other manifestation or expression, such as a biochemical immunological alteration, of a specific gene or genes, environmental factors, or both.

Physical (gene) map: a map showing the absolute distances between genes.

Point mutation: the substitution of a single DNA base in the normal DNA sequence.

Polygenic trait or character: a character or trait determined by the combined action of a number of loci, each with a small effect.

Polymerase chain reaction (PCR): a molecular biology technique developed in the mid-1980s through which specific DNA segments may be amplified selectively.

Polymorphism: the stable existence of two or more variant allelic forms of a gene within a particular population or among different populations.

Positional cloning: the technique through which candidate genes are located in the genome through their co-inheritance with linked markers. It allows genes to be identified that lack information regarding the biochemical actions of their functional product.

Posttranscriptional modification: a series of steps through which protein molecules are biochemically modified within a cell following synthesis by translation of messenger RNA. A protein may undergo a complex series of modifications in different cellular compartments before its final functional form is produced.

Predictive testing: determines the probability that a healthy individual with or without a family history of a certain disease might develop that disease.

Predisposition, genetic: increased susceptibility to a particular disease due to the presence of one or more gene mutations, and/or a combination of alleles (haplotype), not necessarily abnormal, that is associated with an increased risk for the disease, and/or a family history that indicates an increased risk for the disease.

Predisposition test: a test for a genetic predisposition (incompletely *penetrant* conditions). Not all people with a positive test result will manifest the disease during their lifetimes.

Preimplantation genetic diagnosis (PIGD): used following in vitro fertilization to diagnose a genetic disease or condition in a preimplantation embryo.

Premature atrial contraction (PAC): a contraction in the atrium that is initiated by an ectopic focus and occurs earlier than the next expected normal sinus beat.

Premature ventricular contraction (PVC or VPD): a contraction in the ventricle that is initiated by an ectopic focus and occurs earlier than the next expected normal sinus or escape rhythm beat.

Prenatal diagnosis: used to diagnose a genetic disease or condition in a developing fetus.

Presymptomatic test: predictive testing of individuals with a family history. Historically, the term has been used when testing for diseases or conditions such as Huntington's disease where the likelihood of developing the condition (known as *penetrance*) is very high in people with a positive test result.

Primer: a short nucleic acid sequence, often a synthetic oligonucleotide, which binds specifically to a single strand of a target nucleic acid sequence and initiates synthesis, using a suitable polymerase, of a complementary strand.

Probe: a DNA or RNA fragment that has been labeled in some way, and used in a *molecular hybridization* assay to identify closely related DNA or RNA sequences.

Prokaryote: an organism or cell lacking a nucleus and other membrane bounded organelles. Bacteria are prokaryotic organisms.

Promoter: a combination of short sequence elements to which RNA polymerase binds in order to initiate transcription of a gene.

Protein: a protein is the biological effector molecule encoded by sequences of a gene. A protein molecule consists of one or more polypeptide chains of amino acid subunits. The functional action of a protein depends on its three-dimensional structure, which is determined by its amino acid composition.

Proteome: all of the proteins present in a cell or organism.

Proteomics: the development and application of techniques to investigate the protein products of the genome and how they interact to determine biological functions.

Proto-oncogene: a cellular gene which when mutated is inappropriately expressed and becomes an oncogene.

Pseudoautosomal region (PAR): a region on the tips of mammalian X chromosomes that is involved in recombination during male meiosis.

Pesudogene: a DNA sequence that shows a high degree of sequence homology to a nonallelic functional gene but which is itself nonfunctional.

Recessive: an allele that has no phenotypic effect in the heterozygous state.

Recombinant DNA technology: the use of molecular biology techniques such as restriction enzymes, ligation, and cloning to transfer genes among organisms (see *genetic engineering*).

Regulatory mutation: a mutation in a region of the genome that does not encode a protein but affects the expression of a gene.

Regulatory sequence: a DNA sequence to which specific proteins bind to activate or repress the expression of a gene.

Repeat sequences: a stretch of DNA bases that occurs in the genome in multiple identical or closely related copies.

Replication: a process by which a new DNA strand is synthesized by copying an existing strand, using it as a template for the addition of complementary bases, catalyzed by a DNA polymerase enzyme.

Reproductive cloning: techniques aimed at the generation of an organism with an identical genome to an existing organism.

Restriction enzymes: a family of enzymes derived from bacteria that cut DNA at specific sequences of bases.

Restriction fragment length polymorphism (RFLP): a polymorphism due to difference in size of allelic restriction fragments as a result of restriction site polymorphism.

Ribonucleic acid (RNA): a single stranded nucleic acid molecule comprising a linear chain made up from four nucleotide subunits (A, C, G, and U). There are three types of RNA: messenger, transfer, and ribosomal.

Risk communication: an important aspect of genetic counseling that involves pedigree analysis, interpretation of the inheritance pattern, genetic risk assessment, and explanation to the family member (or the family).

RT-PCR (reverse transcriptase-PCR): a PCR reaction in which the target DNA is a cDNA copied by reverse transcriptase from an mRNA source.

Screening: carrying out of a test or tests, examination(s), or procedure(s) in order to expose undetected abnormalities, unrecognized (incipient) diseases, or defects: examples are early diagnosis of cancer using mass X-ray mammography for breast cancer and cervical smears for cancer of the cervix.

Segregation: the separation of chromosomes (and the alleles they carry) during meiosis; alleles on different chromosomes segregate randomly among the gametes (and the progeny).

Sensitivity (of a screening test): extent (usually expressed as a percentage) to which a method gives results that are free from false negatives; the fewer the false negatives, the greater the sensitivity. Quantitatively, sensitivity is the proportion of truly diseased persons in the screened population who are identified as diseased by the screening test.

Sex chromosome: the pair of chromosomes that determines the sex (gender) of an organism. In man one X and one Y chromosomes constitute a male compared to two X chromosomes in a female.

Sex selection: preferential selection of the unborn child on the basis of the gender for social and cultural purposes. However, this may be acceptable for medical reasons, for example, to prevent the birth of a male assessed to be at risk for an X-linked recessive disease. For further information visit: http://www.bioethics.gov/topics/sex_index.html

Shotgun sequencing: a cloning method in which total genomic DNA is randomly sheared and the fragments ligated into a cloning vector, also referred to as "shotgun" cloning.

Signal transduction: the molecular pathways through which a cell senses changes in its external environment and changes its gene expression patterns in response.

Silent mutation: substitution of a single DNA base that produces no change in the amino acid sequence of the encoded protein.

Single nucleotide polymorphism (SNP): a common variant in the genome sequence; the human genome contains about10 million SNPs.

Sinoatrial (SA) node: the heart's natural pacemaker located in the right atrium. Electrical impulses originate here and travel through the heart, causing it to beat.

Somatic: all of the cells in the body that are not gametes (germline).

Southern blot hybridization: a form of molecular hybridization in which the target nucleic acid consists of DNA molecules that have been size fractioned by gel electrophoresis and subsequently transferred to a nitrocellulose or nylon membrane.

Splicing: a process by which introns are removed from a messenger RNA prior to translation and the exons adjoined.

Stem cell: a cell that has the potential to differentiate into a variety of different cell types depending on the environmental stimuli it receives.

Stop codon: a codon that leads to the termination of a protein rather than to the addition of an amino acid. The three stop codons are TGA, TAA, and TAG.

Sudden cardiac death (SCD): death due to cardiac causes within 1 hour of the onset of symptoms, with no prior warning, usually caused by ventricular fibrillation.

Supraventricular tachycardia (SVT): a tachycardia originating from above the ventricles.

Syncope: fainting, loss of consciousness, or dizziness that may be due to a transient disturbance of cardiac rhythm (arrhythmia) or other causes.

Synteny: a large group of genes that appear in the same order on the chromosomes of two different species.

Systems biology: refers to simultaneous measurement of thousands of molecular components (such as transcripts, proteins, and metabolites) and integrate these disparate data sets with clinical end points, in a biologically relevant manner; this model can be applied in understanding the etiology of disease.

Tachycardia (Tachyarrhythmia): rapid beating of either or both chambers of the heart, usually defined as a rate over 100 beats per minute.

Telomere: the natural end of the chromosome.

Therapeutic cloning: the generation and manipulation of stem cells with the objective of deriving cells of a particular organ or tissue to treat a disease.

Transcription: the process through which a gene is expressed to generate a complementary RNA molecule on a DNA template using RNA polymerase.
Transcription factor: a protein that binds DNA at specific sequences and regulates the transcription of specific genes.
Transcriptome: the total messenger RNA expressed in a cell or tissue at a given point in time.
Transfection: a process by which new DNA is inserted in a eukaryotic cell allowing stable integration into the cell's genome.
Transformation: introduction of foreign DNA into a cell and expression of genes from the introduced DNA; this does not necessarily include integration into host cell genome.
Transgene: a gene from one source that has been incorporated into the genome of another organism.
Transgenic animal/plant: a fertile animal or plant that carries an introduced gene(s) in its germline.
Translation: a process through which a polypeptide chain of amino acid molecules is generated as directed by the sequence of a particular messenger RNA sequence.
Tumor suppressor gene: a gene that serves to protect cells from entering a cancerous state; according to Knudson's "two-hit" hypothesis, both alleles of a particular tumor suppressor gene must acquire a mutation before the cell will enter a transformed cancerous state.
Unequal crossing over: recombination between nonallelic sequences on nonsister chromatids of homologous chromosomes.
Ventricle: one of the two lower chambers of the heart. (See *Atrium*.)
Ventricular fibrillation (VF): very fast, chaotic, quivering heart contractions that start in the ventricles. During VF, the heart does not beat properly. This often results in fainting. If left untreated, it may result in cardiac arrest. Blood is not pumped from the heart to the rest of the body. Death will occur if defibrillation is not initiated within 6 minutes from the onset of VF.
Ventricular tachycardia (VT): a rapid heart rate that starts in the ventricles. During VT, the heart does not have time to fill with enough blood between heart beats to supply the entire body with sufficient blood. It may cause dizziness and light-headedness.
Western blotting: a process in which proteins are size-fractioned in a polyacrylamide gel prior to transfer to a nitrocellulose membrane for probing with an antibody.
X-chromosome inactivation: random inactivation of one of the two X chromosomes in mammals by a specialized form of genetic imprinting (see *Lyonization*).
Yeast artificial chromosome (YAC): an artificial chromosome produced by combining large fragments of foreign DNA with small sequence elements necessary for chromosome function in yeast cells.
Yeast two-hybrid system: a genetic method for analyzing the interactions of proteins.
Zinc finger: a polypeptide motif that is stabilized by binding a zinc atom and confers on proteins an ability to bind specifically to DNA sequences; commonly found in transcription factors.
Zoo blot: a Southern blot containing DNA samples from different species.

Index

Note: Page number in *italics* refers to figures, where as **bold** refers to tables.